This book is to be returned on or before the last date stamped below.

REFERENCE

NORD Guide to Rare Disorders

NORD Guide to Rare Disorders

*The National Organization
for Rare Disorders*

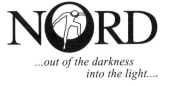

...out of the darkness
into the light....

LIPPINCOTT WILLIAMS & WILKINS
A **Wolters Kluwer** Company
Philadelphia · Baltimore · New York · London
Buenos Aires · Hong Kong · Sydney · Tokyo

Acquisitions Editor: Richard Winters
Managing Editor: Tanya Lazar
Developmental Editors: Kristen Kirchner/Karen Stoye
Supervising Editor: Mary Ann McLaughlin
Production Editor: Richard Rothschild, Print Matters, Inc.
Manufacturing Manager: Colin Warnock
Cover Designer: Karen Quigley
Compositor: Compset, Inc.
Printer: Edwards Brothers

Library of Congress Cataloging-in-Publication Data

National Organization for Rare Disorders.
    NORD guide to rare disorders / National Organization for Rare Disorders.
       p. ; cm.
    Includes bibliographical references and index.
    ISBN 0-7817-3063-5 (HC)
      1. Rare diseases—Handbooks, manuals, etc. I. Title: Guide to rare disorders. II. Title.
      [DNLM: 1. Syndrome—Handbooks. 2. Diagnostic Techniques and
Procedures—Handbooks. QZ 39 N2777n 2002]
    RC48.8 .N385 2002
    616—dc21

                                2002070232

---

10 9 8 7 6 5 4 3 2 1

We dedicate this book to the 25 million Americans who have rare disorders,
the family members who provide support and encouragement to them,
and the physicians and other medical professionals entrusted with their care.

—The National Organization for Rare Disorders

Foreword

Diagnosing rare diseases is not always an easy task for physicians. It is extremely difficult for physicians to be aware of the latest research findings and the vague and sometimes contradictory symptoms of the thousands of rare and genetic diseases. The expression of these different symptoms for the same disorder often makes a timely diagnosis difficult to obtain. The inability to obtain a prompt and correct diagnosis can be frustrating for physicians, patients, their families, and friends. With an increasing number of approved orphan products and products in investigational status, obtaining a correct diagnosis is an essential step in the treatment of rare diseases and conditions. The *NORD Guide to Rare Disorders* presents many of the signs and symptoms that can be an aid in the diagnosis and differentiation of rare diseases in addition to the possible treatment.

Stephen C. Groft, Pharm D
Director, Office of Rare Diseases
National Institutes of Health

Preface

RARE DISEASES: OUR MOST COMMON HEALTH PROBLEM

Rare diseases are, collectively, the most common and costly health problem Americans face today. According to the National Institutes of Health (NIH), there are approximately 6,000 of them affecting an estimated 25 million of us. Those numbers are expected to rise as we continue to unravel the mysteries of genetics and to study diseases at the molecular level.

In the United States, a disease is considered rare if it affects fewer than 200,000 Americans. In the European Union, "rare" indicates that no more than 5 of every 10,000 people have the disease. In Japan, the definition of rare is that fewer than 50,000 people in the nation are affected.

Regardless of the specific criteria used, rare or "orphan" diseases represent small potential markets to pharmaceutical and medical device manufacturers, and they tend to be a low priority on public health agendas. In fact, rare diseases are generally treated as if they are unimportant—except by the people who happen to have one and those who happen to love someone who has one.

In all cultures, rare diseases go undiagnosed or misdiagnosed for extensive periods of time, and there are few targeted research efforts because there is little commercial interest in developing new diagnostic tools or treatments. The families affected by rare diseases are medically disenfranchised populations that fall through the cracks of every health-care system in the world.

In 1983, the U.S. Congress enacted the Orphan Drug Act, which created incentives to entice pharmaceutical companies into developing treatments for low-incidence diseases. In the decade before the Orphan Drug Act was passed, only 10 new treatments were developed for rare diseases in the United States. Between 1983 and 2002, almost 250 orphan products were developed, approved for marketing by the U.S. Food and Drug Administration (FDA), and made available to American patients. Additionally, more than 800 orphan products are now in various stages of research. Singapore, Japan, and the European Union have enacted similar legislation, and Australia, Taiwan, and Korea have created statutes or diplomatic agreements that enable speedy importation of American orphan drugs into those countries for rare-disease patients.

Despite these major strides, there is still no universal effort to expand research on rare disorders or to find ways to reduce the time lapse between onset of symptoms and proper diagnosis. In the 1989 report to Congress from the National Commission on Orphan Diseases, the Commission found that, for 31% of rare-disease patients, it took up to 5 years to obtain an accurate diagnosis and, for 15%, it required 6 or more years. Additionally, more than half of the funding spent on rare-disease research has been devoted to approximately 200 rare forms of cancer, leaving an estimated 5,800 diseases with little or no hope for a cure.

The National Organization for Rare Disorders (NORD) is a non-profit voluntary health agency dedicated to the identification, treatment, and cure of all orphan diseases. With its many programs of education, research, advocacy, and service, NORD enhances awareness of rare diseases among the public and medical professionals to encourage prompt identification and treatment. NORD also supports clinical research on rare disorders at academic institutions throughout the world.

With this educational mission in mind, this *NORD Guide to Rare Disorders* has been created to enhance the physician's armamentarium in the battle against orphan diseases. We sought, and were blessed with, the cooperation of some of the world's leading experts on these diseases. Each disease entry in this book was written by a medical expert and reviewed by other medical experts to ensure that the information would be accurate, comprehensive, and the most current available.

This book covers about 800 of the estimated 6,000 rare diseases. To decide which diseases to include, NORD began with topics from its own rare disease database and then attempted to select diseases that, in the opinion of our medical advisors, had not been covered adequately in existing medical texts or still tended to be frequently misdiagnosed or undiagnosed. We hope to expand the number of diseases covered in future editions and would welcome suggested topics.

We are greatly indebted to Edward Gruson, NORD's medical editor, who has dedicated a full year and many sleepless nights to this project. We are also grateful to Mary Dunkle, NORD's vice president for communications, who worked with Ed to ensure the high quality of this publication. Additionally, we feel gratitude beyond what words can convey to the many physicians listed as writers and reviewers for this book. They devoted countless hours to this project without recompense, and we can never thank them enough.

The talents and expertise of many extraordinary people went into the development of this book, with the hope that it will give family physicians and other "front-line" health-care providers an additional tool to diminish pain, avert disability, and save lives. We hope you will find this book helpful, and we also invite you to visit NORD's website (*www.rarediseases.org*) for more information about rare diseases.

Abbey S. Meyers, President
National Organization for Rare Disorders

Acknowledgments

NORD is deeply indebted to the more than 600 physicians who wrote entries for this book and the 21 rare-disease experts who served as reviewers. The authors and reviewers participated in this project without compensation and as a result of their own commitment to individuals and families affected by rare diseases. Several authors wrote multiple entries. To them, we owe a special word of thanks.

The reviewers, particularly those responsible for the longer chapters, devoted many, many hours of their own time over a period of more than a year. In addition to reading each entry, they responded to our questions, provided helpful suggestions, and, without exception, remained gracious, supportive, and encouraging.

This book would never have been possible without the reviewers, who are listed below. In addition, NORD's Medical Advisory Committee provided extensive input, and several of its members served as reviewers. NORD gratefully acknowledges the assistance of our Medical Advisory Committee (see list below) in this project and many others, including our research program.

Several other physicians provided invaluable assistance in the recruitment of authors and editorial review. Bradley A. Warady, MD, professor of pediatrics at the University of Missouri—Kansas City School of Medicine and an advisor to the National Kidney Foundation, was tremendously helpful. So, too, was Mark Batshaw, MD, chief academic officer, Children's National Medical Center. Other rare-disease experts who assisted in various ways include John M. Hicks, MD, DDS, PhD, Baylor College of Medicine; John Mulliken, MD, Harvard Medical School; Joe T.R. Clarke, MD, PhD, the Hospital for Sick Children in Toronto; Nataline Kardon, MD, Mount Sinai School of Medicine; and Emily Chen, MD, PhD, Children's Hospital of Oakland.

Many voluntary health organizations played a crucial role, particularly with the recruitment of authors. NORD wishes to express its deepest gratitude to all the individuals and organizations who understood the importance of timely diagnosis and treatment, and stepped forward to help.

Finally, we thank our editorial team at Lippincott Williams & Wilkins, particularly Tanya Lazar, for patience, guidance, and unfailing good humor. We are grateful beyond measure.

The NORD Medical Advisory Committee

Sami I. Said, MD (Chair)
Professor, Pulmonary & Critical Care Medicine
State University of New York
Stony Brook Health Science Center
Associate Chief of Staff, VA Medical Center

Frederick Askari, MD, PhD
Clinical Assistant Professor of Medicine
University of Michigan Medical Center

Garrett E. Bergman, MD
Vice President, Research & Development
Octagen Corporation

Roscoe O. Brady, MD
Chief, Developmental & Metabolic Neurology Branch
National Institute of Neurological Disorders & Stroke
National Institutes of Health

Mitchell F. Brin, MD
Vice President, Botox/Neurology
The Allergan Corporation

Robert M. Campbell, Jr., MD
Associate Professor of Orthopaedics
The University of Texas
Health Science Center at San Antonio

Martha Carlson, MD, PhD
Clinical Assistant Professor
Director, Pediatric Neurology Metabolic Clinic
University of Michigan

Mervyn L. Elgart, MD
Clinical Professor of Dermatology, Medicine, and
    Pediatrics
George Washington University School of Medicine

Hugo Moser, MD
Director, Neurogenetics Research Center
Kennedy Krieger Institute
Professor of Neurology and Pediatrics
Johns Hopkins University

Mary Jean Sawey, PhD
Research Associate Professor of Radiation Oncology
Fels Institute for Cancer Research and Molecular Biology
Temple University School of Medicine

Mendel Tuchman, MD
Professor of Pediatrics, Biochemistry and Molecular
    Biology
Mary Elizabeth McGehee Joyce Chair for Genetic Research
Children's National Medical Center
The George Washington University

Susan C. Winter, MD
Chief, Metabolic Genetics Services
Valley Children's Hospital

Reviewers

Autoimmune & Connective Tissue Disorders
Robert P. Baughman, MD
Professor of Medicine
University of Cincinnati Medical Center

Cardiovascular Disorders
Leslie T. Cooper, Jr., MD
Assistant Professor of Medicine
Consultant, Cardiovascular Division
Mayo Clinic and Foundation

Chromosomal Disorders
Bruce Richard Korf, MD, PhD
Associate Professor of Neurology
Harvard-Partners Center for Genetics and Genomics
Harvard Medical School

Dermatologic Disorders
Mervyn L. Elgart, MD
Clinical Professor of Dermatology, Medicine, and
    Pediatrics
George Washington University School of Medicine

Dysmorphic Disorders
Mira B. Irons, MD
Associate Chief, Division of Genetics
Children's Hospital Medical Center, Boston
Associate Professor of Pediatrics, Harvard Medical
    School

Antonie Debra Kline, MD
Clinical Geneticist and Dysmorphologist
The Harvey Institute for Human Genetics
Greater Baltimore Medical Center

Angela E. Lin, MD
Medical Geneticist
Genetics and Teratology Unit
Massachusetts General Hospital

Emerging/Infectious Diseases
D. Peter Drotman, MD, MPH
Senior Medical Officer
National Center for Infectious Diseases
Centers for Disease Control and Prevention

Michael Schubert, MD
Formerly Executive Director
Engelhorn Foundation for Rare Diseases,
Luxembourg

Endocrine Disorders
Adda Grimberg, MD
Assistant Professor, Pediatric Endocrinology
Children's Hospital of Philadelphia
University of Pennsylvania School of Medicine

Gastroenterologic Disorders
Frederick Askari, MD, PhD
Clinical Assistant Professor of Medicine
Division of Gastroenterology
University of Michigan Medical School

Hematologic/Oncologic Disorders
Garrett E. Bergman, MD
Vice-President, Research & Development
Octagen Corporation
Bala Cynwyd, Pennsylvania

Inborn Errors of Metabolism
John H. Menkes, MD
Professor Emeritus of Neurology and Pediatrics,
UCLA School of Medicine
Director Emeritus of Pediatric Neurology
Cedars-Sinai Medical Center, Los Angeles

Neurologic Disorders
Martha Carlson, MD, PhD
Clinical Assistant Professor
Director, Pediatric Neurology Metabolic Clinic
University of Michigan

John K. Fink, MD
Associate Professor, Department of Neurology
Director, Neurogenetic Disorders Clinic
University of Michigan

Phillip Pearl, MD
Associate Professor of Neurology and Pediatrics
Children's National Medical Center
George Washington University School of Medicine

Neuromuscular Disorders
Simon Hickman, MD, MRCP
Clinical Research Fellow
NMR Research Unit
Institute of Neurology
University College, London

Phillip Pearl, MD
(See Neurologic Disorders)

Ophthalmologic Disorders
Richard A. Lewis, MD, MS
Professor, Departments of Ophthalmology,
Medicine, Pediatrics, and Molecular and Human
    Genetics
Cullen Eye Institute
Baylor College of Medicine, Houston

Pulmonary Disorders
Sami I. Said, MD
Professor, Pulmonary & Critical Care Medicine
State University of New York
Stony Brook Health Science Center
Associate Chief of Staff, VA Medical Center,
Northport, NY

Renal Disorders
Troy Dixon, MD
Chief, Renal Section, Northport VAMC
Associate Professor of Medicine
State University of New York at Stony Brook

Skeletal Disorders
Robert M. Campbell, Jr., MD
Associate Professor of Orthopaedics
University of Texas Health Science Center,
    San Antonio

Contributors

Jan Aasly, MD, PhD
Department of Neurology
University Hospital
Trondheim, Norway

Magnus Åberg, MD, PhD
Professor, Center for Craniofacial Anomalies
Department of Plastic Surgery
University Hospital MAS
Malmo, Sweden

Fatima E. Abidi, PhD
Staff Scientist
Greenwood Genetic Center
Greenwood, SC

Maria Acosta, MD
Fellow in Neurology
Children's National Medical Center
Department of Neurology
George Washington University School of Medicine
Washington, DC

Kathleen Adams, RN
President
Cyclic Vomiting Syndrome Association
Canal Winchester, OH

Ali R. Afzal, MD
Research Fellow in Medical Genetics
Department of Medical Genetics
St. George's Hospital Medical School
London, UK

Vincent Agnello, MD
Department of Laboratory Medicine
Lahey Clinic Medical Center
Burlington, MA
VA Medical Center
Bedford, MA

Amir Ahmadi, MD
Ophthalmology Section
Department of Plastic Surgery
University of Texas M.D. Anderson Cancer Center
Houston, TX

G. Eda Akbas, MD
Fellow in Reproductive Endocrinology
Department of Obstetrics & Gynecology
Yale University School of Medicine
New Haven, CT

Cem Akin, MD, PhD
Laboratory of Allergic Diseases
National Institute of Arthritis and Infectious Diseases
National Institutes of Health
Bethesda, MD

Anthony J. Aldave, MD
Francis I. Proctor Foundation
Department of Ophthalmology
University of California, School of Medicine
San Francisco, CA

Kenneth M. Algazy, MD
Clinical Associate Professor of Medicine
University of Pennsylvania
Chief, Hematology-Oncology Service
Philadelphia VA Medical Center
Philadelphia, PA

Judith E. Allanson, MB ChB
Professor of Pediatrics
University of Ottawa
Division of Clinical Genetics
Children's Hospital of East Ontario
Ottawa, ON, Canada

Uri S. Alon, MD
Professor of Pediatrics
University of Missouri—Kansas City School of Medicine
Director, Research and Education
Section of Pediatric Nephrology
Children's Mercy Hospital
Kansas City, MO

Blanche P. Alter, MD, MPH
Clinical Genetics Branch
Division of Cancer Epidemiology and Genetics
National Cancer Institute
Rockville, MD

Kingi Amin, MD, MB, MRCP
Division of Medical Genetics
Department of Genetics
University of Leicester
Leicester, UK

Charles J. Anderson, MD
Department of Ophthalmology
University of Wisconsin Medical School
Madison, WI

Karl E. Anderson, MD
Professor of Medicine
Department of Preventive Medicine and Community
    Health
University of Texas Medical Branch
Galveston, TX

Nicole J. Anderson, MD
Resident in Ophthalmology
Emory University School of Medicine
Atlanta, GA

Steven W. Anderson, PhD
Assistant Professor of Neurology
Benton Neuropsychology Laboratory
University of Iowa College of Medicine
Iowa City, IA

Gyula Ascadi, MD, PhD
Assistant Professor of Pediatrics & Neurology
Wayne State University
Detroit, MI

David Ashford, DVM, MPH, DSc
Meningitis and Special Pathogens Branch
Division of Bacterial & Mycotic Diseases
National Center for Infectious Diseases
Centers for Disease Control and Prevention
Atlanta, GA

Frederick K. Askari, MD, PhD
Clinical Assistant Professor of Medicine
Division of Gastroenterology
University of Michigan Medical School
Ann Arbor, MI

Hana Aviv, PhD
Assistant Professor
UMDNJ
New Jersey Medical School
Center for Human and Molecular Genetics
University Hospital
Newark, NJ

Felicia B. Axelrod, MD
Carl Seaman Family Professor of Dysautonomia
    Treatment and Research in Pediatrics
Professor of Neurology
Dysautonomia Treatment and Evaluation Center
New York University School of Medicine
New York, NY

Leonard L. Bailey, MD
Chair, Department of Surgery
Loma Linda University School of Medicine
Loma Linda, CA

Wendy Ballemans
PhD Candidate
Department of Medical Genetics
University of Antwerp
Antwerp, Belgium

Anne B. Ballinger, MD
Senior Lecturer
Digestive Research Center
St. Bartholomew's and the Royal London School of
    Medicine
London, UK

John Steven Bamforth, FRCP
Associate Professor of Medical Genetics
Department of Biological Sciences
University of Alberta
Medical Genetics Clinic
University of Alberta Hospital
Edmonton, AB, Canada

Michael Bamshad, MD
Department of Pediatrics and Human Genetics
Eccles Institute of Human Genetics
University of Utah
Salt Lake City, Utah

Brenda Banwell, MD, FRCPC
Assistant Professor of Pediatrics (Neurology)
Hospital for Sick Children
University of Toronto
Toronto, ON, Canada

Timothy G. Barrett, MD, MB, PhD
Hon Consultant/Clinical Senior Lecturer in Paediatric
    Endocrinology
Birmingham Children's Hospital
Birmingham, UK

Lucia Bartoloni, MD
Department of Medical & Surgical Sciences
University of Padua
Padua, Italy

Donald Basel, MB, BCh
Registrar
Department of Human Genetics
University of Connecticut Health Sciences Center
Farmington, CT

Murat Bastepe, MD, PhD
Endocrinology Unit
Department of Medicine
Massachusetts General Hospital
Instructor in Medicine
Harvard Medical School
Boston, MA

Uwe Baumert, PhD
Department of Orthodontics
University of Regensburg
Regensburg, Germany

Daniel G. Bausch, MD, MPH
Division of Viral and Rickettsial Diseases
National Center for Infectious Diseases
Centers for Disease Control and Prevention
Atlanta, GA

Kelly Becker, BA
Research Assistant
Division of Adolescent Medicine
Children's Hospital
Boston, MA

Pamela S. Becker, MD, PhD
Associate Professor of Medicine and Cell Biology
University of Massachusetts Medical School
Chief, Division of Gene Therapy
University of Massachusetts Memorial Hospital
Worcester, MA

H. Melanie Bedford, MS, MD, FRCPC
Division of Molecular Genetics
Hospital for Sick Children
Faculty of Medicine
University of Toronto
Toronto, ON, Canada

Peter Beighton, MD, PhD, FRCP
Department of Human Genetics
University of Cape Town Medical School
Cape Town, Republic of South Africa

Lenore K. Beitel, PhD
Research Scientist
Lady Davis Institute for Medical Research
Sir Mortimer B. Davis–Jewish Hospital
Montreal, PQ, Canada

Arthur L. Benton, PhD
Director Emeritus
Benton Neuropsychology Laboratory
Professor of Neurology Emeritus
University of Iowa College of Medicine
Iowa City, IA

Wilma F. Bergfeld, MD
Department of Dermatology
Cleveland Clinic Foundation
Cleveland, OH

Garrett E. Bergman, MD
Vice-President for Research & Development
OCTAGEN Corporation
Bala Cynwyd, PA

Paul D. Berk, MD
Professor of Medicine
Division of Liver Disease
Mt. Sinai Medical School
New York, NY

Ross Stuart Berkowitz, MD
William H. Baker Professor of Gynecology
Brigham & Women's Hospital
Dana Farber Cancer Institute
Harvard Medical School
Boston, MA

Gerard T. Berry, MD
Professor of Pediatrics
George Washington University School of Medicine
Chief, Division of Metabolic
Margaret Rose Children's Research Institute
Washington, DC

Ernest Beutler, MD
Professor and Chairman
Department of Molecular and Experimental Medicine
The Scripps Research Institute
La Jolla, CA

Jorge A. Bezerra, MD
Assistant Professor of Pediatrics
Division of Gastroenterology, Hepatology, and Nutrition
Children's Hospital Medical Center of Cincinnati
Cincinnati, OH

Neelakshi Bhagat, MD
Institute of Ophthalmology and Visual Science
New Jersey Medical School
University of Medicine and Dentistry of New Jersey
Newark, NJ

Martin G. Bialer, MD, PhD
Chief, Division of Medical Genetics
North Shore University Hospital
Weill-Cornell College of Medicine
Manhasset, NY

Leslie G. Biesecker, MD
Head, Human Development Section
National Human Genome Research Institute
Bethesda, MD

Valérie Biousse, MD
Third Year Resident
Neuro-Ophthalmology Unit
Emory Eye Center
Atlanta, Georgia

Mazen Bisharah, MD
Fellow in Reproductive Endocrinology and Infertility
Department of Obstetrics and Gynecology
Faculty of Medicine
McGill University
Montreal, PQ, Canada

Phyllis R. Bishop, MD
Associate Professor of Pediatric Gastroenterology
University of Mississippi Medical Center
Jackson, MS

Richard Bittar, MBBS, PhD
Department of Neurosurgery
Austin and Repatriation Medical Centre
Heidelberg, Victoria, Australia

Nenad Blau, PhD
Privatdozenten, Division of Clinical Chemistry & Biochemistry
Department of Pediatrics
University Children's Hospital
University of Zurich
Zurich, Switzerland

Oliver Bleck, MD
Department of Cell and Molecular Pathology
St. John's Institute of Dermatology
St. Thomas Hospital
London, UK

Anthony J. Bleyer, MD, MS
Associate Professor of Medicine
Section on Nephrology
Wake Forest University School of Medicine
Winston-Salem, NC

Douglas Blowey, MD
Assistant Professor of Pediatrics and Pharmacology
University of Missouri—Kansas City School of Medicine
Division of Nephrology
Children's Mercy Hospital
Kansas City, MO

Olaf Bodamer, MD, PhD
Biochemical Genetics Laboratory
University Children's Hospital
Vienna, Austria

Andreas Boeck, MD
Department of Pediatrics
University of Vienna
Vienna, Austria

A.L.M. Boehmer, MD, PhD
Department of Pediatrics
Sophia Children's Hospital/University Hospital
Rotterdam, The Netherlands

Axel Bohring, Dipl Med
Department of Paediatrics
Ostholstein Klinniken
Eutin, Germany

Herbert L. Bonkovsky, MD
Professor of Biochemistry, Molecular Pharmacology, Pediatrics & Medicine
Division of Gastroenterology
University of Massachusetts School of Medicine
Worcester, MA

Laurence M. Boon, MD
Laboratory of Human Molecular Genetics,
Université de Louvain
Brussels, Belgium

James R. Bowen, MD
Chairman, Department of Pediatric Orthopaedics
Alfred I. DuPont Hospital for Children
Wilmington, DE

Laurence A. Boxer, MD
Professor of Pediatrics
Department of Pediatrics and Communicable Diseases
Director, Pediatric Hematology/Oncology
University of Michigan Health Center and Medical School
Ann Arbor, MI

Christopher R. Braden, MD
Division of Bacterial and Myocotic Diseases
National Center for Infectious Diseases
Centers for Disease Control
Atlanta, GA

Roscoe O. Brady, MD
Chief, Developmental & Metabolic Neurology Branch
National Institute of Neurological Disorders & Stroke
National Institutes of Health
Bethesda, MD

Martin Braun, MD
Resident in Dermatology
Washington Hospital Center
Washington, DC

Nancy Braverman, MD, MS
Assistant Professor
McKusick-Nathans Institute for Genetics Medicine
Johns Hopkins Medical Center
Baltimore, MD

Mark E. Brecher, MD
Professor of Pathology and Laboratory Medicine
University of North Carolina Hospitals
Chapel Hill, NC

Carole V. Brenneise, DDS
Professor of Dentistry
Department of Oral Diagnosis
Creighton University School of Dentistry
Omaha, Nebraska

Michael Brenner, PhD
Associate Professor of Neurobiology & Rehabilitation
   Medicine
University of Alabama School of Medicine
Birmingham, AL

George J. Brewer, MD
Morton S. and Henrietta K. Sellner Professor of Human
   Genetics
Professor of Internal Medicine
University of Michigan
Ann Arbor, MI

M. Elizabeth Brickner, MD
Associate Professor of Internal Medicine
Director, Echocardiography Laboratory
Division of Cardiovascular Diseases
University of Texas Southwestern Medical Center
Dallas, TX

Scott H. Britz-Cunningham, MD, PhD
Division of Nuclear Medicine
Brigham & Women's Hospital
Department of Radiology
Harvard Medical School
Boston, MA

Margaret E. Brousseau, PhD
Assistant Research Professor of Medicine and Nutrition
Tufts University Schools of Medicine
Nutrition Science and Policy
Jean Mayer–USDA Human Nutrition Research Center on
   Aging
Boston, MA

W. Ted Brown, MD, PhD
Chairman, Department of Human Genetics
Director, George A. Jervis Clinic
Institute for Basic Research in Developmental Disabilities
Staten Island, NY

Mary Brunkow, PhD
Celltech R & D, Inc.
Bothell, WA

John C.M. Brust, MD
Professor of Clinical Neurology
Columbia University College of Physicians and Surgeons
Harlem Health Center
New York, NY

Bruce Alan Buehler, MD
Chairman of the Department of Pediatrics
Director of the Munroe-Meyer Institute for Genetics and
   Rehabilitation
University of Nebraska Medical Center
Omaha, NE

Neil R.M. Buist, MB, ChB
Professor Emeritus of Pediatrics and Molecular & Medical
　　Genetics
Oregon Health & Science University
Portland, OR

Carol Burke, MD
Center for Colon Polyps and Cancer
Cleveland Clinic Foundation
Cleveland, OH

R. Stanley Burns, MD
Professor & Head, Memory & Aging Clinic
Department of Neurology
University of Southern Illinois School of Medicine
Springfield, IL

Susan F. Burroughs, MD
Clinical Assistant Professor of Medicine
University of Connecticut Health Center
Farmington, CT

Merlin G. Butler, MD, PhD
William R. Brown/Missouri Chair of Medical Genetics
　　and Molecular Medicine
Children's Mercy Hospital
Professor of Pediatrics
University of Missouri–Kansas School of Medicine
Kansas City, MO

Jean-Claude Bystryn, MD
Professor of Dermatology
NYU School of Medicine
New York, NY

Imelda Cabalar, MD
Clinical Fellow
Connective Diseases Section
National Institute of Arthritis and Musculoskeletal and
　　Skin Diseases
Bethesda, MD

Juan F. Cabello, MD
Department of Genetics
Harvard Medical School/Children's Hospital
Boston, MA
Van Buren Hospital and
Valparaiso University Medical School
Valparaiso, Chile

Kenneth T. Calamia, MD
Division of Rheumatology
Mayo Clinic and Foundation
Jacksonville, FL

Robert M. Campbell, Jr., MD
Associate Professor of Orthopaedics
University of Texas Health Science Center
San Antonio, TX

Rebecca B. Campen, MD
Deputy Director
MGH/Harvard Cutaneous Biology Research Center
Charlestown, MA

John C. Carey, MD, MPH
Professor of Pediatrics, Obstetrics, Gynecology, and
　　Nursing
University of Utah Health Science Center
Salt Lake City, UT

Michal Carmiel, MD
Senior Fellow
Division of Liver Disease
Mt. Sinai Medical School
New York, NY

Milvia Casato, MD
Department of Clinical Medicine
University of Rome, "La Sapienza"
Rome, Italy

Suzanne B. Cassidy, MD
Professor of Pediatrics
University of California, Irvine
Director, Division of Human Genetics
University of California, Irvine, Medical Center
Orange, CA

Patrizio Caturegli, MD
Assistant Professor of Pathology
Johns Hopkins School of Medicine
Baltimore, MD

John N. Caviness, MD
Parkinson's Disease and Other Movement Disorders
　　Center
Department of Neurology
Mayo Clinic
Scottsdale, AZ

Vimal Chadha, MD
Fellow in Pediatric Nephrology
Children's Mercy Hospital
Kansas City, MO

Barbara L. Chadwick, BDS, MScD, PhD, FDSRCS
Senior Lecturer in Paediatric Dentistry
Department of Dental Health and Development
University of Wales
Cardiff, Wales, UK

Pranesh Chakraborthy, MD
Fellow in Clinical & Metabolic Genetics
Department of Paediatrics
The Hospital for Sick Children
Toronto, ON, Canada

Kenneth L. Chambliss, MD, PhD
Division of Nephrology
Department of Pediatrics
University of Texas Southwestern Medical Center
Dallas, TX

Jaideep Chandra, MS
Senior Resident in Neurosurgery
Sanjay Gandhi Post-Graduate Institute of Medicine
Lucknow, India

Taeun Chang, MD
Fellow in Neurology
Children's National Medical Center
Washington, DC

M. Shane Chapman, MD
Assistant Professor of Medicine
Department of Dermatology
Dartmouth-Hitchcock Medical Center
Lebanon, NH

Ritu Chatrath, MD
Fellow in Pediatric Cardiology
Mayo Clinic
Rochester, Minnesota

Joe T.R. Clarke, MD, PhD
Director, Genetic Metabolic Disease Program
The Hospital for Sick Children
Toronto, ON, Canada

Ray E. Clouse, MD
Professor of Medicine & Psychiatry
Washington University School of Medicine
St. Louis, MO

Bernard A. Cohen, MD
Director of Pediatric Dermatology
Johns Hopkins University Medical Center
Baltimore, MD

Kathleen M. Colleran, MD
Assistant Professor of Medicine
Program Director, Endocrinology & Metabolism
University of New Mexico Health Science Center
Albuquerque, NM

Robert W. Colman, MD
Director, The Sol Sherry Thrombosis Research Center
Chief, Hematology Division
Department of Medicine
Temple University School of Medicine
Philadelphia, PA

Anne M. Comi, MD
Instructor in Neurology
Johns Hopkins University School of Medicine
Department of Neurology
Johns Hopkins Hospital
Baltimore, MD

Brenda Conger
President
Cardio-Facio-Cutaneous Family Network
Vestal, NY

Amy M. Connell, MD
Resident in Psychiatry
University of Wisconsin
Madison, WI

Anne M. Connolly, MD
Associate Professor of Neurology & Pediatrics
Neuromuscular Disease Center
Washington University School of Medicine
St. Louis, MO

Ruth A. Cook, ANP
Foot and Ankle Service
Hospital for Special Surgery
New York, NY

Edward C. Cooper, MD, PhD
Assistant Professor of Neurology and Physiology
Department of Neurology
University of California at San Francisco School of
  Medicine
San Francisco, CA

Leslie T. Cooper, Jr., MD
Cardiovascular Medicine
Assistant Professor of Medicine
Mayo Clinic and Foundation
Rochester, MN

Michael Cornefjord, MD, PhD
Professor of Surgery
Department of Orthopedics
Sahlgrenska University Hospital
Gothenburg, Sweden

Vicki Couch, MS
Department of Medical Genetics
Mayo Clinic and Foundation
Rochester, MN

Gerald F. Cox, MD, PhD
Division of Genetics
Children's Hospital
Boston, MA
Medical Director, Clinical Research
Genzyme Corporation
Cambridge, MA

John P. Dalton, PhD
Professor of Biological Sciences
School of Biotechnology
Dublin City University
Dublin, Republic of Ireland

Christof Dame, MD
Department of Neonatology
University of Bonn
Bonn, Germany

Fernando Dangond, MD
Assistant Professor of Neurology
Harvard Medical School
Associate Neurologist
Brigham and Women's Hospital
Boston, MA

Dean J. Danner, PhD
Professor and Vice Chair
Department of Human Genetics
Emory University School of Medicine
Atlanta, GA

Mark D.P. Davis, MD
Department of Dermatology
Mayo Clinic and Foundation
Rochester, MN

Stephen J. DeArmond, MD, PhD
Division of Neuropathology
School of Medicine
University of California at San Francisco
San Francisco, CA

Elfride De Baere, MD, PhD
Molecular Laboratory
Center of Medical Genetics
University Hospital of Ghent
Ghent, Belgium

Mahlon R. DeLong, MD
Professor of Neurology
Emory University School of Medicine
Atlanta, GA

Michael A. Del Torto, MD
Fellow in Dermatology
Washington Hospital Center
Washington, DC

Pierre N.M. Demacker, PhD
Chief, Lipid Research Laboratory
Department of General Internal Medicine
University Medical Center of Nijmegen
Nijmegen, The Netherlands

David T. Dennis, MD, MPH
Chief, Bacterial Zoonoses Branch
Division of Vector-Borne Infectious Diseases
National Center for Infectious Diseases
Centers for Disease Control and Prevention
Fort Collins, CO

Natalie D. Depcik-Smith, MD
Resident in Pathology
Transfusion Medicine Service
University of North Carolina Hospitals
Chapel Hill, NC

Craig S. Derkay, MD
Professor of Otolaryngology and Pediatrics
Director of Pediatric Otolaryngology
Eastern Virginia Medical School
Norfolk, VA

Robert J. Desnick, MD, PhD
Professor and Chairman
Department of Human Genetics
Mt. Sinai School of Medicine
New York, NY

Darryl C. De Vivo, MD
Sidney Carter Professor of Neurology,
Professor of Pediatrics
Department of Neurology
College of Physicians and Surgeons
Columbia University
Director of Colleen Giblin Research Laboratories
New York Presbyterian Hospital
New York, NY

Shama Dhandha, MD
Fellow, Reproductive Genetics
Department of Obstetrics, Gynecology and Reproductive
    Sciences
Magee-Women's Hospital
Pittsburgh, PA

George A. Diaz, MD, PhD
Assistant Professor
Department of Human Genetics
Mt. Sinai School of Medicine
New York, NY

Hal Dietz, MD
Associate Investigator
Howard Hughes Medical Institute
Professor, Institute for Genetic Medicine
Johns Hopkins University School of Medicine
Baltimore, MD

Angelo M. DiGeorge, MD
Emeritus Professor of Pediatrics
Temple University Children's Medical Center
Philadelphia, PA

Mary Dinauer, MD, PhD
Nora Letzter Professor of Pediatrics, Medicine and
    Medical Genetics
Indiana University School of Medicine
Director, Herman B. Wells Center for Pediatric
    Research/Cancer Research Institute
Pediatric Hematology/Oncology
James Whitcomb Riley Hospital for Children
Indianapolis, IN

Mary Beth Dinulos, MD
Assistant Professor of Pediatrics
Division of Genetics and Child Development
Dartmouth Medical School
Lebanon, NH

Henrik J. Ditzel, MD, PhD, DMSc
Associate Professor
Department of Immunology
Scripps Research Institute
La Jolla, CA

Juan Dong, MD, PhD
Research Scientist
Department of Pediatric Dentistry
UTHSCSA Dental School
University of Texas Health Science Center at San Antonio
San Antonio, TX

Alan E. Donnenfeld, MD
Vice Chairman, Department of Obstetrics & Gynecology
Pennsylvania Hospital
Clinical Associate Professor
University of Pennsylvania School of Medicine
Philadelphia, PA

Richard M. Donner, MD
Attending Physician
Division of Pediatric Cardiology
Children's Hospital of Philadelphia
Philadelphia, PA

Mary M. Dott, MD
Epidemic Intelligence Service Officer
National Center on Birth Defects and Developmental
    Disabilities
Centers for Disease Control and Prevention
Atlanta, GA

Paul A. Dowling, BDentSc, DOrth, FDS(Orth)
Department of Public and Child Dental Health
School of Dental Science
Dublin Dental Hospital
Trinity College Dublin
Dublin, Ireland

Silvia Drechsel
Keeper, MASA Syndrome Web Site
c/o *www.masainfo.de*
Friedberg, Germany

David J. Driscoll, MD
Professor of Pediatrics
Head, Division of Pediatric Cardiology
Mayo Clinic and Foundation
Rochester, MN

F. Jane Durcan, MD
Associate Professor of Ophthalmology
John A. Moran Eye Center
University of Utah Health Sciences Center
Salt Lake City, UT

Sunil N. Dutt, MS, FRCS Ed
Associate Professor of Otolaryngology
Departments of Otolaryngology, Head and Neck Surgery,
    and Neuroradiology
Queen Elizabeth Hospital
Birmingham, UK

Rohit Dwivedi, MD
Senior Endocrinology Fellow
Division of Endocrinology & Metabolism
Indiana University School of Medicine
Indianapolis, IN

Paul Dyken, MD
Professor and Chair Emeritus
Department of Neurology
University of South Alabama College of Medicine
Mobile, AL

Simon Eaton, PhD
Institute of Child Health
Great Ormond Street Hospital for Children
London, UK

Michael J. Econs, MD
Associate Professor of Medicine
Director, Division of Endocrinology & Metabolism
Indiana University School of Medicine
Indianapolis, IN

Eli D. Ehrenpreis, MD
Assistant Professor of Clinical Medicine
Director, GI Fellowship Program
Department of Gastroenterology
University of Chicago Hospitals
Chicago, IL

Hans R.L. Eiberg, MD
Associate Professor
University Institute of Medical Biochemistry & Genetics
Copenhagen, Denmark

Daniel B. Eisen, MD
Resident in Dermatology
Washington Hospital Center
Washington, DC

Rodger Elble, MD, PhD
Professor and Chair
Department of Neurology
Southern Illinois University School of Medicine
Springfield, IL

Mervyn L. Elgart, MD
Clinical Professor of Dermatology, Medicine & Pediatrics
George Washington University School of Medicine
Washington, DC

Andrew W. Eller, MD
Associate Professor of Ophthalmology
Retina & Vitreous Service
Eye and Ear Institute
University of Pittsburgh Medical Center
Pittsburgh, PA

Alison M. Elliott, PhD
International Skeletal Dysplasia Registry
Cedars-Sinai Medical Center
Los Angeles, CA

Kathleen B. Elmer, MD
Division of Dermatology
Wilford Hall Medical Center/
Brooke Army Medical Center
San Antonio, TX

Hatem El-Shanti, MD
Department of Pediatrics
School of Medicine
Jordan University of Science and Technology
Irbid, Jordan

Beverly S. Emanuel, PhD
Professor of Pediatrics
University of Pennsylvania School of Medicine
Children's Hospital of Philadelphia
Philadelphia, PA

Charis Eng, MD, PhD
Clinical Cancer Genetics and Human Cancer Genetics
    Programs
Ohio State University
Columbus, OH

Gloria Eng, MD
Children's Hospital National Medical Center
George Washington University
Washington, DC

Kris Engelstad, BS
MELAS/MERRF Study Coordinator
Department of Neurology
College of Physicians and Surgeons
Columbia University
New York, NY

Gregory M. Enns, MD, MB, ChB
Director, Biochemical Genetics Program
Division of Medical Genetics
Stanford University School of Medicine
Stanford, CA

Tom Enta, MD
Department of Dermatology
Faculty of Medicine
University of Calgary
Calgary, AB, Canada

Nancy E. Epstein, MD
Department of Neurological Surgery
North Shore University Hospital
Manhasset, NY

Gerald Erenberg, MD
Division of Pediatric Neurology
Cleveland Clinic Foundation
Cleveland, Ohio

Niknam Eshraghi, MD
University of Washington Burn Center
Harborview Medical Center
Seattle, WA

Bita Esmaeli, MD
Assistant Professor & Chief
Ophthalmology Section
Department of Plastic Surgery
University of Texas M.D. Anderson Cancer Center
Houston, TX

Ayad A. Farjo, MD
Assistant Professor
Department of Ophthalmology
University of Iowa Hospitals & Clinics
Iowa City, IA

Simon F. Farmer, PhD, FRCP
NMR Research Unit
Department of Neurology,
National Hospital for Neurology & Neurosurgery,
University College of London
London, England, UK

Bradley K. Farris, MD
Professor of Ophthalmology
Division of Neuro-Ophthalmology
Dean A. McGee Eye Institute
Adjunct Professor of Neurology & Neurosurgery
University of Oklahoma Health Science Center
Oklahoma City, OK

Lee D. Faucher, MD
University of Washington Burn Center
Harborview Medical Center
Seattle, WA

Annette Feigenbaum, MD, ChB, FRCPC
Senior Scientist & Associate Professor of Paediatrics
Division of Clinical & Metabolic Genetics
Hospital for Sick Children
Toronto, ON, Canada

Eva L. Feldman, MD, PhD
Department of Neurology
University of Michigan Medical School
Ann Arbor, MI

Joseph L. Feldman, MD
Assistant Professor
Physical Medicine and Rehabilitation
Northwestern University Medical School
Medical Director
Evanston Northwestern Healthcare Lymphedema
    Treatment Center
Chicago, IL

J. Dominic Femino, MD
Assistant Professor of Orthopedic Surgery
USC Keck School of Medicine
Associate Medical Staff
Children's Hospital, Los Angeles
Los Angeles, CA

Ron L. Ferguson, MD
Chief of Staff
Shriners Hospital for Children
Spokane, WA

Sandra R. Fernandes, MD
Rheumatology Unit
State University of Campinas
Campinas, Sao Paulo, Brazil

Stefan Feske, MD
Center for Blood Research
Harvard Medical School
Boston, MA

Penelope P. Feuillan, MD
Developmental Endocrinology Branch
National Institute of Child Health & Human Development
    (NICHD)
Bethesda, MD

Alexandra H. Filipovich, MD
Director, Immunodeficiency and Histiocytosis Program
Division of Hematology/Oncology
Cincinnati Children's Hospital Medical Center
Cincinnati, OH

Jo-David Fine, MD, MPH
Professor of Dermatology
Clinical Professor of Epidemiology
Schools of Medicine and Public Health
University of North Carolina at Chapel Hill
Chapel Hill, NC

John K. Fink, MD
Associate Professor of Neurology
University of Michigan Medical School
Ann Arbor, MI

Richard Finnell, PhD
Professor of Cell Biology and Anatomy
College of Medicine
University of Nebraska
Omaha, NE

Brenda Finucane, MS
Elwyn Research and Training Institute
Elwyn, PA

Steven J. Fishman, MD
Assistant in Surgery
Vascular Anomalies Center
The Childrens Hospital, Boston
Assistant Professor of Surgery
Harvard Medical School
Boston, MA

Paddy Fleming, BDentSc
Senior Lecturer/Consultant
Department of Public and Child Dental Health
School of Dental Science and
Dublin Dental Hospital
Trinity College Dublin
Our Lady's Hospital for Sick Children
Dublin, Republic of Ireland

William H. Fletcher, PhD
Department of Pathology & Human Anatomy
Loma Linda University School of Medicine
Senior Research Career Scientist of the VA Medical
    Research Service
Loma Linda, CA

Mary Kay Floeter, MD, PhD
Chief, Electromyography Section
National Institute of Neurological Disorders and Stroke
    (NINDS)
National Institutes of Health
Bethesda, MD

Mona S. Foad, MD
Fellow in Dermatology
Washington Medical Center
Washington, DC

Hans Forssberg, MD, PhD
Department of Neuropediatrics
Astrid Lindgren Children's Hospital
Karolinska Hospital
Stockholm, Sweden

Robert E. Foster, MD
Cincinnati Eye Institute
Cincinnati, OH

Anne L. Foundas, MD
Associate Professor
Department of Neurology-Psychiatry
Tulane University School of Medicine
New Orleans, LA

Deborah L. French, PhD
Assistant Professor of Medicine
Division of Hematology
Mt. Sinai School of Medicine
New York, NY

Frank E. Frerman, PhD
Professor of Pediatrics and Cellular/Structural Biology
University of Colorado Health Sciences Center
Denver, CO

Jean-Pierre Fryns, MD, PhD
University Hospital, Leuven
Center for Human Genetics
Catholic University of Leuven
Leuven, Belgium

William A. Gahl, MD, PhD
Section on Human Biochemical Genetics
Heritable Disorders Branch
National Institute of Child Health and Human
    Development
National Institutes of Health
Bethesda, MD

Philippe Gailloud, MD
Assistant Professor of Radiology
Division of Neuroradiology
Johns Hopkins Medical Center
Baltimore, MD

Carlos A. Garcia, MD
Professor of Clinical Neurology
Clinical Professor of Pathology
Department of Psychiatry & Neurology
Tulane University School of Medicine
New Orleans, LA

Abhimanyu Garg, MD
Professor of Internal Medicine
Chief, Division of Nutrition and Metabolic Diseases
Endowed Chair in Human Nutrition Research
University of Texas Southwestern Medical Center
Dallas, TX

Elizabeth I.O. Garner, MD
Brigham & Women's Hospital
Dana Farber Cancer Institute
Harvard Medical School
Boston, MA

Richard A. Gatti, MD
Professor, Department of Pathology
UCLA School of Medicine
Los Angeles, California

Theresa W. Gauthier, MD
Division of Neonatal-Perinatal Medicine
Emory Children's Center
Emory University School of Medicine
Atlanta, GA

John P. Gearhart, MD, FACS
Professor & Director
Division of Pediatric Urology
Johns Hopkins Hospital
Baltimore, MD

Rita M. George, MD
Private practice in Dermatology
Goodyear, AZ

James German III, MD
Professor of Pediatrics
Cornell University Weill Medical College
New York, NY

M.J.P. Gerritsen, MD
Department of Dermatology
University Medical Centre of Nijmegen
Nijmegen, The Netherlands

Rianne Gerritsen, MD
Department of Dermatology
University Medical Centre of Nijmegen
Nijmegen, The Netherlands

Morie A. Gertz, MD
Chair, Division of Hematology
Professor of Medicine
Mayo Clinic and Foundation
Rochester, MN

C.L.M.H. Gibbons, MA, FRCS
Consultant Orthopaedic Surgeon
Nuffield Orthopaedic Centre
Headington, Oxford, UK

Nicole S. Gibran, MD
University of Washington Burn Center
Harborview Medical Center
Seattle, WA

K. Michael Gibson, PhD
Director, Biochemical Genetics Laboratory
Department of Molecular & Medical Genetics
Oregon Health & Science University
Portland, OR

Barbara Giesser, MD
Associate Professor of Clinical Neurology
Department of Neurology
Arizona Health Science Center
Tucson, AZ

Philip M. Ginsburg, MD
Department of Gastroenterology
University of Chicago Hospitals
Chicago, IL

Daniel G. Glaze, MD
Methodist Hospital
Associate Professor of Neurology
Departments of Pediatrics and Neurology
Baylor College of Medicine
Houston, TX

Joseph O. Gleeson, MD
Assistant Professor
Division of Pediatric Neurology
Department of Neurosciences
University of California at San Diego School of Medicine
La Jolla, CA

Maurice Godfrey, PhD
Associate Professor of Pediatrics and Pathology
Monroe Center for Human Genetics
University of Nebraska Medical Center
Omaha, NE

Mona Gohara, MD
Department of Dermatology
Mt. Sinai School of Medicine
New York, NY

Donna Golakovich, RN
Nurse Coordinator
Neuroradiology Toronto Hospital, Western Division
Toronto, ON, Canada

Ilan Golan, DMD
Department of Orthodontics
Center for Craniofacial Genetics
University of Regensburg
Regensburg, Germany

Barry D. Goldman, MD
Attending Physician
NYU Downtown Hospital
Clinical Instructor
Department of Dermatology
New York University School of Medicine
New York, NY

James E. Goldman, MD, PhD
Professor, Department of Pathology
Center for Neurobiology & Behavior
College of Physicians and Surgeons of Columbia
 University
New York, NY

Donald P. Goldstein, MD
Clinical Faculty
Brigham & Women's Hospital
Dana Farber Cancer Institute
Harvard Medical School
Boston, MA

Caleb González, MD
Professor of Ophthalmology
Yale Eye Center
Yale School of Medicine
New Haven, CT

Randall L. Goodman, MD
Major, USAF
Department of Ophthalmology
Wilford Hall Medical Center
Lackland Air Force Base
San Antonio, TX

Stephen I. Goodman, MD
Head, Section on Clinical Genetics
Professor of Pediatrics and Cellular/Structural Biology
University of Colorado Health Sciences Center
Denver, CO

Catherine M. Gordon, MD
Assistant Professor of Pediatrics
Harvard Medical School
Division of Endocrinology
Children's Hospital
Boston, MA

Robert J. Gorlin, DDS, MS, DSC (Athens)
Department of Oral Pathology and Genetics
University of Minnesota
Minneapolis, MN

Jerome L. Gorski, MD
Director, Division of Pediatric Genetics
Professor of Pediatrics and Human Genetics
University of Michigan Medical School
Ann Arbor, MI

Meeta Goswami, MD, MPH, PhD
Assistant Professor of Neurology
Albert Einstein College of Medicine
Montefiore Medical Center
The Bronx, NY

Bruce Gottlieb, PhD
Project Director
Lady Davis Institute for Medical Research
Sir Mortimer B. Davis–Jewish Hospital
Montreal, PQ, Canada

Gregory A. Grabowski, MD
Professor & Director
Division and Program in Human Genetics
Children's Hospital Research Foundation
Cincinnati, OH

Richard Grabowski, MD
Resident in Dermatology
Washington Hospital Center
Washington, DC

John M. Graham, Jr., MD, ScD
Director of Clinical Genetics & Dysmorphology
Cedars-Sinai Medical Center
Professor of Pediatrics
UCLA School of Medicine
Los Angeles, CA

Stephen G. Grant, PhD
Assistant Professor
Department of Environmental & Occupational Health
Graduate School of Public Health
University of Pittsburgh
Pittsburgh, PA

Sara R. Greenhill, MD
University of Pittsburgh Medical School
Pittsburgh, PA

Adda Grimberg, MD
Assistant Professor
Division of Pediatric Endocrinology
Children's Hospital of Philadelphia
University of Pennsylvania School of Medicine
Philadelphia, PA

Susan Gromacki, OD, MS
Department of Ophthalmology and Visual Science
University of Michigan Medical School
Ann Arbor, MI

John H. Growdon, MD
Department of Neurology
Massachusetts General Hospital
Professor of Neurology
Harvard Medical School
Boston, MA

Karl-Heinz Grzeschik, Prof Dr Rer Nat
Philipps-Universitaet
Marburg Zentrum-fuer Humangenetik
Marburg, Germany

Arna Gudmundsdottir, MD
Fellow in Endocrinology and Metabolism
Division of Endocrinology
Department of Internal Medicine
University of Iowa Hospitals and Clinics
Iowa City, IA

Stephen Guest, MD
Department of Clinical Ophthalmology
Moorfields Eye Hospital
Institute of Ophthalmology
London, UK

Meral Gunay-Aygun, MD, PhD
Center for Genetics & Metabolism
Children's Hospital Medical Center of Akron
Akron, OH

Nick J. Gutowski, MD
Consultant Neurologist
Royal Devon & Exeter NHS Trust Honorary Senior
    Lecturer
School of Postgraduate Medicine & Health Sciences
University of Exeter
Exeter, UK

Alan E. Guttmacher, MD
Deputy Director
National Human Genome Research Institute
National Institutes of Health
Bethesda, MD

Geetha M. Habib, MD
Department of Pathology
Baylor College of Medicine,
Houston, TX

Hoda Hachicho, MD
Resident in Neurology
Children's National Medical Center
Washington, DC

Darin H. Haivala
Dean A. McGee Eye Institute
University of Oklahoma Health Science Center
Oklahoma City, OK

Russell P. Hall III, MD
Professor and Chief, Division of Dermatology
Department of Medicine
Duke University School of Medicine
Durham, NC

Herman Hamersma, MD
Otologist
Roodepoort, Republic of South Africa

Rizwan Hamid, MD
Resident in Pediatrics
Vanderbilt University Medical Center
Nashville, TN

Heather Hampel, MS
Clinical Cancer Genetics and Human Cancer Genetics
    Programs
Ohio State University
Columbus, OH

Hideo Harigae, MD, PhD
Assistant Professor
Department of Molecular Diagnostics
Tohoku University School of Medicine
Sendai, Japan

Scott A. Harper, MD, MPH, MSc
Division of Viral and Rickettsial Diseases
National Center for Infectious Diseases
Centers for Disease Control and Prevention
Atlanta, GA

Rosanne C. Harrigan, EdD, APRN-Rx, FAAN
Dean and Professor
School of Nursing
University of Hawaii
Honolulu, HI

Malcolm Harris, MD, DSc
Emeritus Professor and Honorary Consultant in Oral and
    Maxillofacial Surgery
Eastman Dental Institute
University College
London, UK

Karen H. Harum, MD
Fellow in Neurology
Neurosciences Laboratory
Kennedy Krieger Institute
Johns Hopkins University School of Medicine
Baltimore, MD

John Moseley Hayes, DrPH, MSPH, MBA
Dengue Branch
Division of Vector-Borne Infectious Diseases
National Center for Infectious Diseases
San Juan, Puerto Rico

L. Anne Hayman, MD
Director, Herbert J. Frensley Center for Imaging Research
Professor of Radiology and Psychiatry
Baylor College of Medicine
Houston, TX

Nicole Hayre, MD
Resident in Dermatology
Washington Hospital Center
Washington, DC

Shauna Heeger, MS
Clinical Coordinator
Bone Disorders Clinic
Center for Human Genetics
University Hospitals of Cleveland
Cleveland, OH

David M. Heimbach, MD
University of Washington Burn Center
Harborview Medical Center
Seattle, WA

Wayne J. G. Hellstrom, MD
Professor of Urology
Chief, Section of Andrology and Male Sexual Dysfunction
Tulane University Health Sciences Center
New Orleans, LA

Joseph H. Hersh, MD
Professor of Pediatrics
Director, Child Evaluation Center
University of Louisville School of Medicine
Louisville, KY

Ryan P. Hester, MD
Eastern Virginia Medical School
Norfolk, VA

James E. Heubi, MD
Professor of Pediatrics
Director, Clinical Research Center
Children's Hospital Medical Center
Cincinnati, OH

Simon J. Hickman, MD, MRCP
Clinical Research Fellow
NMR Research Unit
Institute of Neurology
University College
London, UK

John M. Hicks, MD, DDS, PhD
Associate Professor and Director of Surgical and
    Ultrastructural Pathology
Texas Children's Hospital
Department of Pathology
Baylor College of Medicine
Houston, TX

Peter Higgins, MD, PhD
Fellow, Division of Gastroenterology
University of Michigan Medical School
Ann Arbor, MI

Margaret W. Hilgartner, MD
Professor of Pediatrics
Harold Weill Professor of Hematology
Weill Medical College of Cornell University
New York, NY

Anne V. Hing, MD
Assistant Professor of Pediatrics and Medical Genetics
Children's Hospital Medical Center
Seattle, WA

Kurt Hirschhorn, MD
Professor of Pediatrics, Human Genetics, and Medicine
Mt. Sinai School of Medicine
New York, NY

Anthony M.H. Ho, MSc, MD
Associate Professor
Department of Anaesthesia and Intensive Care
Chinese University of Hong Kong
Sha Tin, Hong Kong, People's Republic of China

Christeen Hodge, MD
Resident in Pediatrics
Duke University Medical Center
Durham, NC

Denice Hodgson, MD
Department of Medicine
Mayo Clinic and Foundation
Rochester, MN

Gary S. Hoffman, MD
Harold C. Schott Chair for Rheumatic and Immunologic
    Diseases
Director, Center for Vasculitis Care and Research
Cleveland Clinic Foundation
Cleveland, OH

William J. Hogan, MD, MRCPI
Division of Hematology & Internal Medicine
Mayo Clinic and Foundation
Rochester, MN

W. Allen Hogge, MD
Professor, Department of Obstetrics, Gynecology, and
    Reproductive Sciences
Medical Director, Department of Genetics
Magee-Womens Hospital
Pittsburgh, PA

Steven M. Holland, MD
Immunopathogenesis Unit
Clinical Pathophysiology Section
Laboratory of Host Defenses
National Institute of Arthritis and Infectious Diseases
Bethesda, MD

Carlin Hollar, MD
Resident in Dermatology
Wake Forest University School of Medicine
Winston-Salem, NC

Stephen Holman, MD
F. Edward Hebert School of Medicine
Uniformed Services University of the Health Sciences
Bethesda, MD

Elizabeth Holme, MD
Department of Clinical Chemistry/Transfusion Medicine
Sahlgrenska University Hospital
Gothenburg, Sweden

Timothy H. Holtz, MD, MPH
Malaria Epidemiology Branch
Division of Parasitic Diseases
National Center for Infectious Diseases
Centers for Disease Control and Prevention
Atlanta, GA

Andrew R. Hong, MD
Assistant Professor of Pediatrics & Surgery
Albert Einstein College of Medicine
Schneider Children's Hospital
New Hyde Park, NY

Robert J. Hopkin, MD
Clinical Geneticist
Children's Hospital Medical Center
Cincinnati, OH

Paul N. Hopkins, MD, MSPH
Cardiovascular Genetics Research Clinic
University of Utah Medical School
Salt Lake City, UT

Jennifer Howard, RN
Cyclic Vomiting Center
Children's Memorial Hospital
Chicago, IL

Jan C-C. Hu, BDS, PhD
Chair, Department of Pediatric Dentistry
University of Texas Health Science Center
San Antonio, TX

Glyn W. Humphreys, PhD
Professor of Cognitive Psychology, Cognitive Science,
    Cognitive Neuropsychology & Visual Cognition
University of Birmingham
Birmingham, UK

Mahmood M. Hussain, PhD, Lic Med
Professor of Anatomy and Cell Biology
Department of Anatomy & Cell Biology, and Pediatrics
SUNY Downstate Medical Center
Brooklyn, NY

Paul E. Hyman, MD
Professor, Department of Pediatrics
Chief, Pediatric Gastroenterology
University of Kansas School of Medicine
Kansas City, KS

Richard A. Insel, MD
Professor of Pediatrics
University of Rochester
Rochester, NY

Wendy J. Introne, MD
Section on Human Biochemical Genetics
Heritable Disorders Branch
National Institute of Child Health & Human Development
Bethesda, MD

Jahangir Iqbal, PhD
Postdoctoral Fellow
Department of Anatomy & Cell Biology, and Pediatrics
SUNY Downstate Medical Center
Brooklyn, NY

Alan Irvine, MD, MRCP
Senior Lecturer & Honorary Consultant
Dermatologist
Human Genetics Unit
Department of Molecular & Cellular Pathology
University of Dundee
Ninewells Hospital & Medical School
Dundee, Scotland, UK

Richard M. Irving, MD, FRCS
Consulting Neuro-otologist
Departments of Otolaryngology, Head and Neck Surgery, and Neuroradiology
Queen Elizabeth Hospital
Birmingham, UK

Elaine S. Jaffe, MD
Chief, Hematopathology Section
Center for Cancer Research
National Cancer Institute
Bethesda, MD

Peter J. Jannetta, MD
MCP Hahnemann Professor and Vice Chairman
Department of Neurosurgery
Allegheny General Hospital
Pittsburgh, PA

Thomas Jansen, MD
Department of Dermatology
Ruhr-University Bochum
Bochum, Germany

Katrien Janssens
PhD Candidate
Department of Medical Genetics
University of Antwerp
Antwerp, Belgium

J. Charles Jennette, MD
Brinkhous Distinguished Professor and Chair
Department of Pathology and Laboratory Medicine
University of North Carolina at Chapel Hill School of Medicine
Chapel Hill, NC

Robert T. Jensen, MD
Chief, Digestive Disease Branch
National Institute of Diabetes and Digestive and Kidney Diseases
Bethesda, MD

Anne B. Johnson, MD
Associate Professor of Pathology
Departments of Pathology and Neuroscience
Albert Einstein College of Medicine
The Bronx, NY

Michelle D. Johnson, MD
Pituitary Fellowship
Division of Endocrinology & Metabolism
University of Virginia Health System
Charlottesville, VA

William G. Johnson, MD
Section on Neurogenetics
Department of Neurology
Robert Wood Johnson Medical School
Piscataway, NJ

Michael V. Johnston, MD
Director, Neurosciences Laboratory
Kennedy Krieger Institute
Professor of Neurology and Pediatrics
Johns Hopkins University School of Medicine
Baltimore, MD

Gavin M. Joynt, MB BCh
Associate Professor
Department of Anaesthesia and Intensive Care
Chinese University of Hong Kong
Sha Tin, Hong Kong

Harald Jüeppner, MD
Associate Professor of Pediatrics
Harvard Medical School
Endocrine Unit
Massachusetts General Hospital
Boston, MA

James M. Jumper, MD
Major, USAF
Department of Ophthalmology
Wilford Hall Medical Center
Lackland Air Force Base
San Antonio, TX

Udaya M. C. Kabadi, MD
Professor of Medicine (Clinical)
Division of Endocrinology
Department of Internal Medicine
University of Iowa Hospitals and Clinics
Iowa City, IA

Zoltan Kaliszky, MD
Fellow in Neurology
Department of Neurology
Medical University of South Carolina
Charleston, SC

Henry J. Kaminski, MD
Associate Professor of Neurology & Neurosciences
Case Western Reserve University School of Medicine
Cleveland, OH

Bernard S. Kaplan, MD, BCh
Professor of Pediatrics and Medicine
University of Pennsylvania School of Medicine
Children's Hospital of Philadelphia
Philadelphia, PA

Frederick S. Kaplan, MD
Isaac & Rose Nassau Professor of Orthopaedic Molecular
    Medicine and Chief, Division of Metabolic Bone
    Diseases and Molecular Medicine
Department of Orthopaedic Surgery
Hospital of the University of Pennsylvania
Philadelphia, PA

Norman M. Kaplan, MD
Clinical Professor of Internal Medicine
University of Texas Southwestern Medical Center
Dallas, TX

Neil Kaplowitz, MD
Professor of Medicine and Chief Division of
    Gastrointestinal & Liver Disease
University of Southern California School of Medicine
Los Angeles, CA

Nataline B. Kardon, MD
Associate Professor of Human Genetics & Pediatrics
Director, Cytogenetics Laboratory
Mt. Sinai School of Medicine
New York, NY

Stephen C. Kaufman, MD, PhD
Director, Cornea & Refractive Surgery
Henry Ford Health System
Detroit, MI

Petra Kaufmann, MD
Assistant Professor of Neurology,
College of Physicians and Surgeons
Columbia University
Assistant Attending Neurologist
New York Presbyterian Hospital
New York, NY

Maria Inês Kavamura, MD
Dermatologist at the Center for Genetics of the Federal
    University of Sao Paulo
Sao Paulo, Brazil

Jan Kazár, MD, DSc
Head, Department of Virology
Institute of Preventive and Clinical Medicine
Bratislava, Slovak Republic

Michael J. Kelley, MD
Assistant Professor of Medicine
Department of Medicine
Duke University School of Medicine
Durham, NC

Thaddeus E. Kelly, MD, PhD
Division of Medical Genetics
University of Virginia Medical School
Director of Medical Genetics
University of Virginia Hospital
Charlottesville, VA

David P. Kelsell, BSc, MD, PhD
Center for Cutaneous Research
St. Bartholomew's & The Royal London School of
    Medicine and Dentistry
University of London
London, UK

Nigel L. Kennea, MB, BCh
Clinical Research Fellow
Imperial College School of Medicine
Hammersmith Hospital
London, UK

Ali S. Khan, MD, MPH
Division of Viral and Rickettsial Diseases
National Center for Infectious Diseases
Centers for Disease Control and Prevention
Atlanta, GA

Khalid I. Khoshhal, MD
Department of Orthopaedics
King Khalid University Hiospital
Riyadh, Saudi Arabia

William J. Kimberling, PhD
Director of the Center for the Study and Treatment of
 Usher Syndrome
Professor of Otolaryngology, Pathology, and Medical
 Sciences
Boys Town National Research Hospital
Omaha, NE

Gyula Kispal, MD
Institute of Biochemistry
University of Pecs
Pecs, Hungary

Ingrid B. Kjellin, MD
Assistant Professor of Radiology
Director, Division of Musculoskeletal Imaging
Loma Linda University Medical Center
Loma Linda, CA

Caroline M. Klein, MD, PhD
Department of Neurology
Mayo Clinic and Foundation
Rochester, MN

Jeffrey Klein, MD
Third-Year Fellow in Reproductive Endocrinology
College of Physicians and Surgeons
Columbia University
New York, NY

Antonie D. Kline, MD
Clinical Geneticist & Dysmorphologist
Harvey Institute for Human Genetics
Greater Baltimore Medical Center
Baltimore, MD

Alan P. Knutsen, MD
Division of Pediatric Immunology
St. Louis University Health Sciences Center
St. Louis, MO

Roger H. Kobayashi, MD
Clinical Professor of Pediatrics
UCLA School of Medicine
Los Angeles, CA

Dwight D. Koeberl, MD, PhD
Assistant Professor of Pediatrics
Division of Medical Genetics
Duke University Medical Center
Durham, NC

Susan Koh, MD
Assistant Clinical Professor of Pediatric Neurology
Department of Neurology
UCLA School of Medicine
Los Angeles, CA

Elena Kováčová , PhD
Department of Rickettsiology and Chlamydiology
Institute of Virology
Slovak Academy of Sciences
Bratislava, Slovak Republic

Arnold S. Kristof, MD, FRCPC
Pulmonary and Critical Care Branch
National Heart, Lung and Blood Institute
National Institutes of Health
Bethesda, MD

Thomas G. Ksiazek, DVM, PhD
Special Pathogens Branch
Division of Viral and Rickettsial Diseases
National Center for Infectious Diseases
Centers for Disease Control and Prevention
Atlanta, GA

Raj Kumar, MD
Assistant Professor
Department of Neurosurgery
Sanjay Gandhi Post-Graduate Institute of Medicine
Lucknow, India

Jeffrey S. Kutcher, MD
Department of Neurology
University of Michigan Medical School
Ann Arbor, MI

Ruben I. Kuzniecky, MD
Professor of Neurology and Neurosurgery
Director, UAB Epilepsy Center
University of Alabama
Birmingham, AL

David J. Kwiatkowski, MD, PhD
Genetics Laboratory
Division of Medical Oncology
Brigham and Women's Hospital
Boston, MA

Ave Maria Lachiewicz, MD
Assistant Clinical Professor of Pediatrics
Duke University Medical School
Medical Director
Child Development Unit
Department of Pediatrics
Duke University Medical Center
Durham, NC

Ralph S. Lachman, MD
Professor of Radiology and Pediatrics
UCLA School of Medicine
International Skeletal Dysplasia Registry
Cedars-Sinai Medical Center
Los Angeles, CA

Terry C. Lairmore, MD
Associate Professor, Endocrine & Oncologic Surgery
Washington University School of Medicine
St. Louis, MO

Stephen T.S. Lam, MBBS, FRCP
Clinical Genetic Service
Department of Health
Hong Kong, People's Republic of China

Deborah M. Lambert, MSc
Department of Human Genetics
McGill University
Montreal, PQ, Canada

Aleksandra Lange, MD, FESC
St. Andrew's Heart Institute
Brisbane, Queensland, Australia

Robert P. Langlais, DDS, MS
Professor, Division of Oral Diagnosis and Oral Medicine
Department of Dental Diagnostic Science
School of Dentistry
University of Texas Health Science Center
San Antonio, TX

James D. Lauderdale, PhD
Assistant Professor
Department of Cellular Biology
University of Georgia
Athens, GA

Renata Laxova, MD, PhD
Emeritus Professor
Department of Medical Genetics
University of Wisconsin Medical School
Madison, WI

Mark G. Lebwohl, MD
Professor and Chairman
Department of Dermatology
Mt. Sinai School of Medicine
New York, NY

Brendan Lee, MD, PhD
Associate Professor
Department of Molecular and Human Genetics
Baylor College of Medicine
Houston, TX

Kristin M. Leiferman, MD
Mayo Clinic and Foundation
Rochester, MN

Irene M. Leigh, MD, PhD
Center for Cutaneous Research
St. Bartholomew's & The Royal London School of
    Medicine and Dentistry
London, UK

Edmond G. Lemire, MD, PhD
Head, Division of Medical Genetics
Associate Professor of Pediatrics
Faculty of Medicine
University of Saskatchewan
Saskatoon, SK, Canada

Mervyn Letts, MD, FRCSC
Department of Surgery & Division of Pediatric
    Orthopaedics
Children's Hospital of Eastern Ontario
Ottawa, ON, Canada

Alexander K.C. Leung, MB, BS, FRCPC, FRCP
Clinical Associate Professor of Pediatrics
Faculty of Medicine
University of Calgary
Pediatric Consultant
Alberta Children's Hospital
Calgary, AL, Canada

Marc Levitt, MD
Department of Surgery
Children's Hospital of Buffalo
Buffalo, NY

Harvey L. Levy, MD
Associate Professor of Pediatrics
Department of Genetics
Harvard Medical School/Children's Hospital
Boston, MA

Jonathan J. Lewis, MD, PhD
Chief Medical Officer
Chairman, Medical Board
Antigenics, Inc.
New York, NY

Richard A. Lewis, MD, MS
Professor, Departments of Ophthalmology, Medicine,
    Pediatrics, and Molecular and Human Genetics
Cullen Eye Institute
Baylor College of Medicine
Houston, TX

Richard A. Lewis, MD, MS
Associate Professor
Department of Neurology
Wayne State University School of Medicine
Detroit, MI

Robert D. Lewis, MD
Resident in Nephrology
Children's Mercy Hospital
Kansas City, MO

B. U. K. Li, MD
Professor of Pediatrics
Northwestern University Medical School
Director of Gastroenterology
Director, Cyclic Vomiting Center
Children's Memorial Hospital
Chicago, IL

Joan Y. Li, MD
Attending Physician
Mills-Peninsula Hospitals
San Mateo, CA

Abraham N. Lieberman, MD
Professor of Neurology
University of Miami Medical School
Miami, FL

Michael W. Lieberman, MD
Chairman, Department of Pathology
Baylor College of Medicine
Houston, TX

Roland Lill, MD
Institut fur Zytobiologie und Zytopathologie
Philipps-Universität
Marburg, Germany

Kristy Murray Lillibridge, DVM
Meningitis and Special Pathogens Branch
Division of Bacterial & Mycotic Diseases
National Center for Infectious Diseases
Centers for Disease Control and Prevention
Atlanta, GA

Angela E. Lin, MD
Medical Geneticist
Genetics and Teratology Unit
Massachusetts General Hospital
Boston, MA

Kant Y.K. Lin, MD
Associate Professor of Plastic and Maxillofacial Surgery
Head, Division of Craniofacial Surgery
University of Virginia Medical School
University of Virginia Health System
Charlottesville, VA

Noralane M. Lindor, MD
Department of Medical Genetics
Mayo Clinics and Foundation
Rochester, MN

Irene Litvan, MD
Chief, Cognitive Neuropharmacology Unit
Henry M. Jackson Foundation
Bethesda, MD

Ivan F. M. Lo, MB, ChB, MRCP(UK)
Clinical Genetic Service
Department of Health
Hong Kong, People's Republic of China

Millie D. Long, MD
Resident in Surgery
University of Virginia Medical School
University of Virginia Health System
Charlottesville, VA

Nicola Longo, MD, PhD
Division of Medical Genetics
Department of Pediatrics
Emory University
Atlanta, GA

R. Brian Lowry, MD, DSc, FRCPC
Professor Emeritus
Department of Medical Genetics
Faculty of Medicine
University of Calgary
Calgary, AB, Canada

Mark S. Lubinsky, MD
Professor of Pediatrics
Division of Genetics
Department of Pediatrics
Medical College of Wisconsin
Milwaukee, WI

John N. Lukens, MD
Professor of Pediatrics
Division of Pediatric Hematology/Oncology
Vanderbilt University Medical Center
Nashville, TN

Henry T. Lynch, MD
Department of Hematology/Oncology
Chairman, Department of Preventive Medicine
Creighton University School of Medicine
Omaha, NE

Mary MacDougall, PhD
Professor of Dentistry
Department of Pediatric Dentistry
Associate Dean for Research
UTHSCSA Dental School
University of Texas Health Science Center at San Antonio
San Antonio, TX

William G. Mackenzie, MD
Division of Orthopaedic Surgery
Department of Orthopaedics
Alfred I. duPont Hospital for Children
Wilmington, DE

Matthias G. Maiwald, Dr Med
Privatdozent für Medizinische Mikrobiologie
University of Heidelberg
Heidelberg, Germany

Dag Malm, MD, PhD
Professor, Institute of Clinical Medicine
Senior Consultant
Tromso Mannosidosis Group
Tromso, Norway

Martha H. Manar, MD
Fellow in Neonatal-Perinatal Medicine
Emory University School of Medicine
Atlanta, GA

Grazia M. S. Mancini, MD, PhD
Department of Clinical Genetics
Erasmus University and Academic Hospital
Rotterdam, The Netherlands

Marilyn Manco-Johnson, MD
Professor of Pediatrics
Associate Professor of Pathology
University of Colorado
Health Science Center
Denver, CO

Anil K. Mandal, MD
Director, Jasti V. Ramanamma Children's Eye Care
    Centre
L.V. Prasad Eye Institute
Hyderabad, AP, India

Sylvia Mandler, MD
Fellow in Neurology
Children's National Medical Center
Washington, DC

William M. Manger, MD, PhD
Chairman, National Hypertension Association
Clinical Professor of Medicine
Division of Rehabilitation Medicine
New York University School of Medicine
New York, NY

John F. Mantovani, MD
Professor of Neurology
Washington University School of Medicine
Director of Child Neurology
St John's Mercy Medical Center
St. Louis, MO

Bala V. Manyam, MD
Professor of Neurology
Scott & White Clinic
Texas A&M University Health Science Center College of
    Medicine
Temple, TX

Jorge A. Marrero, MD
Assistant Professor of Medicine
Division of Gastroenterology
University of Michigan Medical School
Ann Arbor, MI

Jan D. Marshall, MS
Genetics Coordinator, Human Studies
Jackson Laboratory
Bar Harbor, ME

George M. Martin, MD
Professor of Pathology
Department of Pathology
University of Washington School of Medicine
Seattle, WA

Micheline M. Mathews-Roth, MD
Associate Professor of Medicine
Harvard Medical School
Physician, Brigham and Women's Hospital
Boston, MA

Gary N. McAbee, DO, JD
Chair, Department of Pediatrics
University Medical Center of New Jersey
School of Osteopathic Medicine
Stratford, NJ

Candace L. McCall, DVM, MPH
Viral and Rickettsial Zoonoses Branch
Division of Viral and Rickettsial Diseases
National Center for Infectious Diseases
Centers for Disease Control and Prevention
Atlanta, GA

Kenneth L. McClain, MD, PhD
Associate Professor of Pediatrics and Molecular
   Virology
Texas Children's Cancer Center
Baylor College of Medicine
Houston, TX

William M. McClintock, MD
Department of Neurology
George Washington University School of Medicine
Washington, DC

P. Aiden McCormick, MD, FRCP
Consultant Hepatologist, Liver Transplant Unit,
St. Vincent's University Hospital
Dublin, Ireland

Heather McDermid, PhD
Professor of Medical Genetics
Department of Biological Sciences
University of Alberta
Edmonton, AB, Canada

Jamie E. McDonald, MS
Certified Genetic Counselor
HHT Clinic
University of Utah
Salt Lake City, UT

Josh William McDonald, MD
Assistant Professor of Pathology
Department of Pathology
St. Louis University Medical Center
St. Louis, MO

Doff B. McElhinney, MD
Division of Cardiothoracic Surgery
Children's Hospital of Philadelphia & University of
   Pennsylvania School of Medicine
Philadelphia, PA

Eva M. McGhee, PhD
Assistant Professor
Department of Pediatrics
Division of Medical Genetics
University of California
San Francisco, CA

Michael McGoon, MD
Professor of Medicine
Director, Pulmonary Hypertension Clinic
Division of Cardiovascular Diseases
Mayo Clinic and Foundation
Rochester, MN

John A. McGrath, MD, MRCP
Professor of Molecular Dermatology
Department of Cell and Molecular Pathology
St. John's Institute of Dermatology
St. Thomas' Hospital
London, UK

Martina C. McGuinness, PhD
Assistant Professor of Neurology
Kennedy Krieger Institute
Johns Hopkins University School of Medicine
Baltimore, MD

Iain McIntosh, PhD
McCusick-Nathans Institute of Genetic Medicine
Johns Hopkins University School of Medicine
Baltimore, MA

Sean E. McLean, MD
Division of Pediatric Surgery
Department of Surgery
St. Louis Children's Hospital
Washington University School of Medicine
St. Louis, MO

Peter J. Meikle, PhD
Head, Metabolic, and Therapeutics
Department of Chemical Pathology
Women's and Children's Hospital
Adelaide, Australia

Shlomo Melmed, MD
Professor-in-Residence
Cedars-Sinai Research Institute
UCLA School of Medicine
Los Angeles, CA

John H. Menkes, MD
Professor Emeritus of Neurology and Pediatrics
UCLA School of Medicine
Director Emeritus of Pediatric Neurology
Cedars-Sinai Medical Center
Los Angeles, CA

Juanita L. Merchant, MD, PhD
Associate Professor of Internal Medicine and Physiology
Division of Gastroenterology
University of Michigan
Ann Arbor, MI

Ludwine Messiaen, PhD
Head, Molecular Laboratory
Center of Medical Genetics
University Hospital of Ghent
Ghent, Belgium

Albee Messing, VMD, PhD
Professor, Department of Pathobiological Sciences
Waisman Center and School of Veterinary Medicine
University of Wisconsin
Madison, WI

Dean D. Metcalfe, MD
Laboratory of Allergic Diseases
National Institute of Arthritis and Infectious Diseases
National Institutes of Health
Bethesda, MD

Kevin E. C. Meyers, MD
Pediatric Nephrologist
Children's Hospital of Philadelphia
University of Pennsylvania
Philadelphia, PA

Adam G. Mezoff, MD
Division of Gastroenterology and Nutrition
Children's Medical Center (Dayton)
Dayton, OH

Asad I. Mian, MB, BS
Research Assistant
Department of Molecular and Human Genetics
Baylor College of Medicine
Houston, TX

Virginia V. Michels, MD
Professor of Medical Genetics
Department of Medical Genetics
Mayo Clinic and Foundation
Rochester, MN

Dawn S. Milliner, MD
Division of Nephrology
Departments of Pediatrics and Internal Medicine
Mayo Clinic and Foundation
Rochester, MN

Jeffrey Ming, MD, PhD
Section on Clinical Genetics
Department of Human Genetics and Molecular Biology
Children's Hospital of Philadelphia
Philadelphia, PA

Robert K. Minkes, MD, PhD
Division of Pediatric Surgery
Department of Surgery
Washington University School of Medicine
St. Louis, MO

W. Beau Mitchell, MD
Fellow in Pediatrics
Division of Hematology/Oncology
Mt. Sinai School of Medicine
New York, NY

Alberto A. Mitrani, MD
Executive Health of Coral Gables
Department of Medicine
University of Miami Medical School
Miami, FL

Emile R. Mohler III, MD
Chief, Division of Cardiovascular Medicine
University of Pennsylvania School of Medicine
Philadelphia, PA

Mark E. Molitch, MD
Center for Endocrinology, Metabolism, and Molecular Medicine
Northwestern University School of Medicine
Chicago, IL

Charles N. Moon, MD
Resident in Orthopedic Surgery
USC Keck School of Medicine
Los Angeles, CA

Cynthia A. Moore, MD, PhD
Medical Geneticist
National Center on Birth Defects and Developmental Disabilities
Centers for Disease Control and Prevention
Atlanta, GA

Alan H. Morris, MD
Division of Pediatric & Adolescent Endocrinology/Diabetes
The Barbara Bush Children's Hospital at the Maine Medical Center
Portland, ME
Associate Clinical Professor of Medicine
University of Vermont School of Medicine
Burlington, VT

Chandra Moseley, PhD
Post-Doctoral Fellow in Pediatrics
Vanderbilt University School of Medicine
Nashville, TN

Hugo W. Moser, MD
Director, Neurogenetics Research Center
Kennedy Krieger Institute
Professor of Neurology and Pediatrics
Johns Hopkins University
Baltimore, MD

Thomas Moshang, Jr., MD
Professor of Pediatrics
University of Pennsylvania School of Medicine
Senior Endocrinologist
Children's Hospital of Philadelphia
Philadelphia, PA

Christopher A. Moskaluk, MD, PhD
Assistant Professor of Pathology, Biochemistry &
    Molecular Genetics
University of Virginia Health System
Charlottesville, VA

Joel Moss, MD, PhD
Chief, Pulmonary and Critical Care Branch
National Heart, Lung and Blood Institute
National Institutes of Health
Bethesda, MD

Kathleen J. Motil, MD, PhD
USDA/ARS Children's Nutrition Research Center
Baylor College of Medicine and Texas Children's Hospital
Houston, TX

Joseph Muenzer, MD, PhD
Division of Genetics & Metabolism
UNC Neuroscience Center
University of North Carolina at Chapel Hill
Chapel Hill, NC

Dieter Muessig, DMD
Department of Orthodontics
Center for Craniofacial Genetics
University of Regensburg
Regensburg, Germany

Andrew E. Mulberg, MD
Director, GI Fellowship Program
University of Pennsylvania Medical School
Attending Physician
Division of GI & Nutrition
Children's Hospital of Philadelphia
Philadelphia, PA

Sheila M. Muldoon, MD
Professor and Chief of Anesthesiology
F. Edward Hebert School of Medicine
Uniformed Services University of the Health Sciences
Bethesda, MD

John B. Mulliken, MD
Senior Associate in Surgery
Director, Cleft Lip and Cleft Palate Program
Department of Plastic Surgery
Children's Hospital Medical Center
Associate Professor of Surgery
Harvard Medical School
Boston, MA

Michael Mulreany, MD
Fellow in Cardiology
Children's Hospital of Philadelphia
Philadelphia, PA

William J. Murphy, PhD
Director, Basic Research Program
SAIC Frederick
National Cancer Institute
Frederick, MD

Jeffrey C. Murray, MD
Department of Pediatrics
University of Iowa Clinics & Hospitals
Iowa City, IA

Robert D. Murray, MD
Division of Endocrinology & Metabolism
Cedars-Sinai Research Institute
UCLA School of Medicine
Los Angeles, CA

Aresu A. Naderi, MD
Division of Ophthalmology
Department of Plastic Surgery
University of Texas M.D. Anderson Cancer Center
Houston, TX

Emese Nagy, MD, PhD
Post-doctoral Fellow
Center for Human Development Research
Department of Psychiatry and Behavioral Sciences
University of Texas at Houston Medical School
Houston, TX

Sumit Nanda, MD
Clinical Associate Professor
Department of Ophthalmology
Dean A. McGee Eye Institute
University of Oklahoma Health Science Center
Oklahoma City, OK

Deepak Narayan, MD
Assistant Professor of Surgery
Yale University School of Medicine
Surgeon, Section of Plastic Surgery
Yale-New Haven Medical Center
New Haven, CT

Marguerite Neerman-Arbez, PhD
Division of Medical Genetics and Division of Angiology
    and Hemostasis
Faculty of Medecine
University of Geneva
Geneva, Switzerland

Lawrence M. Nelson, MD, MBA
Senior Clinical Investigator
Head, Gynecologic Endocrinology Unit
Section on Women's Health Research
National Institute of Child Health and Human
    Development
Bethesda, MD

Richard L. Nelson, MD
Chief, Division of Colon and Rectal Surgery
University of Illinois at Chicago
College of Medicine
Chicago, IL

Giovanni Neri, MD
Professor of Medical Genetics
Universita Cattolica del Sacro Cuore
Rome, Italy

Nancy Newman, MD
Associate Professor of Neurology
Emory University School of Medicine
Neuro-Ophthalmology Unit
Emory Eye Center
Atlanta, GA

Marjan M. Nezarati, MSc, MD, FRCPC
Assistant Professor of Paediatrics
University of Toronto
Faculty of Medicine
Staff Clinical Geneticist
Hospital for Sick Children
Toronto, ON, Canada

William L. Nichols, MD
Division of Hematology & Internal Medicine
Mayo Clinic and Foundation
Rochester, MN

Inge-Merete Nielsen, MD
Consultant Pediatrician
Central Hospital
Naestved, Denmark

Geoffrey D. Nochimson, MD
Consulting Staff, Department of Emergency Medicine
Sentora-Hampton General Hospital
Hampton, VA

Michael J. Nowicki, MD
Associate Professor of Pediatric Gastroenterology
University of Mississippi Medical Center
Jackson, MS

Diane J. Nugent, MD
Division of Pediatric Hematology/Oncology
Children's Hospital of Orange County
Orange, CA

William M. Nyhan, MD, PhD
Department of Pediatrics
University of California at San Diego
San Diego, CA

Georg Oberhuber, Dr Med
Department of Clinical Pathology
Faculty of Medicine
University of Vienna
Vienna, Austria

J. Desmond O'Duffy, MD
Mayo Jacksonville
Mayo Clinic and Foundation
Jacksonville, FL

Michael S. Okun, MD
Assistant Professor of Neurology
Director, Movement Disorder Center
University of Florida College of Medicine
Gainesville, FL

Yuji Okura, MD, PhD
First Department of Internal Medicine
Niigata University School of Medicine
Niigata, Japan

Jerrold S. Olshan, MD
Director, Division of Pediatric & Adolescent
    Endocrinology/Diabetes
Barbara Bush Children's Hospital at the Maine Medical
    Center
Portland, ME
Associate Professor of Medicine
University of Vermont School of Medicine
Burlington, VT

Martin J. O'Malley, MD
Hospital for Special Surgery
Associate Professor of Orthopedic Surgery
Weill Medical College of Cornell University
New York, NY

Sandra M. O'Neill, PhD, RGN
School of Nursing
Dublin City University
Dublin, Republic of Ireland

John M. Opitz, MD
Professor of Pediatrics
Division of Medical Genetics
University of Utah Health Science Center
Salt Lake City, UT

Alfredo Orrico, MD
Center for Medical Genetics
Azienda Ospedaliera Senese
Siena, Italy

Junko Oshima, MD, PhD
Research Associate Professor
Department of Pathology
University of Washington School of Medicine
Seattle, WA

Roger J. Packer, MD
Executive Director
Center for Neuroscience and Behavioral Medicine
Children's National Medical Center
Washington, DC

Christopher D. Paddock, MD
Viral and Rickettsial Zoonoses Branch
Division of Viral and Rickettsial Diseases
National Center for Infectious Diseases
Centers for Disease Control and Prevention
Atlanta, GA

Christian E. Paletta, MD
Professor of Surgery
Division of Plastic and Reconstruction Surgery
St. Louis University School of Medicine
St. Louis, MO

Przemyslaw Palka, MD, FESC
St. Andrew's Heart Institute
Brisbane, Queensland, Australia

Anil A. Panackal, MD
Mycotic Diseases Branch
Division of Bacterial and Mycotic Diseases
National Center for Infectious Diseases
Centers for Disease Control and Prevention
Atlanta, GA

Manon Paquette, DMD
Faculty of Dentistry
University of Montreal
Montreal, PQ, Canada

Charles J. Parker, MD
Professor of Medicine
Chief, Hematology/Oncology
University of Utah School of Medicine
Salt Lake City VA Medical Center
Salt Lake City, UT

Paul H. Parker, Jr., MD
Professor of Pediatrics
Chief, Division of Pediatric Gastroenterology
University of Mississippi Medical Center
Jackson, MS

Kevin Parsons, MD
Virginia Mason Research Center
Seattle, WA

Juan Pascual, MD
Department of Physiology
College of Physicians and Surgeons
Columbia University,
New York, NY

Robert M. Pascuzzi, MD
Professor & Vice Chairman
Department of Neurology
Indiana University School of Medicine;
Chief, Wishard Health Services Section
Indianapolis, IN

Gregory M. Pastores, MD
Neurogenetics Unit
Departments of Neurology and Pediatrics
New York University School of Medicine
New York, NY

Mary Elaine Patrinos, MD
Assistant Professor
Department of Pediatrics
Division of Neonatal Medicine
John A. Burns School of Medicine
University of Hawaii
Honolulu, HI

Anirut Pattaragam, MD
Fellow in Neurology
Children's Mercy Hospital
Kansas City, MO

Marc C. Patterson, MD
Professor of Clinical Neurology and Clinical Pediatrics
Columbia University College of Physicians and Surgeons
Director of Pediatric Neurology
Neurological Institute and Children's Hospital of New
    York–Presbyterian
New York, NY

Michael A. Patton, MD
Head, Department of Medical Genetics
St. George's Hospital Medical School
London, UK

Phillip L. Pearl, MD
Associate Professor of Neurology and Pediatrics
Children's National Medical Center
George Washington University School of Medicine
Washington, DC

Alberto Peña, MD
Professor of Surgery & Pediatrics
Albert Einstein College of Medicine
Chief, Pediatric Surgery
Schneider Children's Hospital
New Hyde Park, NY

Leonardo Pereira, MD
Assistant Professor, Department of Obstetrics &
    Gynecology
Jefferson Medical College
Thomas Jefferson University
Philadelphia, PA

John A. Persing, MD
Professor of Surgery
Yale University School of Medicine
Chief, Section of Plastic Surgery
Yale–New Haven Medical Center
New Haven, CT

Lawrence D. Petz, MD
Emeritus Professor of Pathology and Laboratory Medicine
UCLA Medical Center
Los Angeles, CA

John A. Phillips III, MD
Director, Division of Medical Genetics
Vanderbilt University School of Medicine
Nashville, TN

Robert Pilarski, MS
Clinical Cancer Genetics and Human Cancer Genetics
    Programs
Ohio State University
Columbus, OH

Eniko K. Pivnick, MD
Division of Clinical Genetics
Department of Pediatrics
University of Tennessee Medical School
Memphis, TN

Gerd Plewig, MD
Department of Allergology
Ludwig-Maximilians-Universitet
Munich, Germany

Sharon E. Plon, MD, PhD
Assistant Professor
Departments of Pediatrics and Molecular and Human
    Genetics
Baylor College of Medicine
Houston, TX

Paul H. Plotz, MD
Chief, Connective Tissue Diseases Section
Chief, Arthritis and Rheumatism Branch
National Institute of Arthritis and Musculoskeletal and
    Skin Diseases
Bethesda, MD

Barbara R. Pober, MD, MPH
Associate Professor of Genetics and Pediatrics
Department of Genetics
Yale University Medical School
New Haven, CT

Ania Porazinski, MD
Department of Ophthalmology
Yale Eye Center
Yale University School of Medicine
New Haven, CT

Vijay Poreddy, MD
Hepatology Fellow—Liver Unit
University of Southern California
Downey, CA

Chandra Prakash, MD
Division of Gastroenterology
Washington University School of Medicine
St. Louis, MO

Michael R. Pranzatelli, MD
Professor of Neurology and Pediatrics
Southern Illinois University School of Medicine
Head, Section on Child Neurology
Director, National Pediatric Myoclonus Center
Springfield, IL

Richard A. Prayson, MD
Department of Anatomic Pathology
Cleveland Clinic Foundation
Cleveland, OH

Jane Pritchard, BM, BCh
Department of Neuroimmunology
Guy's, King's, and St. Thomas' School of Medicine
Guy's Hospital
London, UK

Robert Prizont, MD
Division of Gastrointestinal and Coagulation Drug
    Products
Center for Drug Evaluation and Research
U.S. Food and Drug Administration
Rockville, MD

Richard L. Proia, PhD
Chief, Genetics of Development and Disease Branch
National Institute of Diabetes & Digestive & Kidney
    Diseases
Bethesda, MD

Cynthia A. Prows, MSN, RN
Clinical Nurse Specialist, Genetics
Children's Hospital Medical Center
Cincinnati, OH

Oliver W. J. Quarrell, MD
Consultant in Clinical Genetics
Ryegate Children's Hospital
Sheffield Children's Hospital
Sheffield, UK

Niall P. Quinn, FRCP
University Department of Clinical Neurology
Movement Disorders Section
Institute of Neurology
London, UK

Ruben A. Quintero, MD
Florida Institute for Fetal Diagnosis and Therapy
University Community Hospital
Tampa, FL

Adnan I. Qureshi, MD
Department of Neurosurgery
Millard Fillmore Hospital
Toshiba Stroke Research Center
SUNY Health Science Center at Buffalo
Buffalo, NY

Irving M. Raber, MD
Wills Eye Hospital
Jefferson Medical College
Thomas Jefferson University
Philadelphia, PA

Corey Raffel, MD, PhD
Professor of Neurologic Surgery
Division of Pediatric Neurosurgery
Mayo Clinic and Foundation
Rochester, MN

Francisco A. Ramos-Caro, MD
Associate Professor of Medicine
University of Florida School of Medicine
Veterans Administration Medical Center
Gainesville, FL

A Koneti Rao, MD
Professor of Medicine
Sol Sherry Thrombosis Research Center
Temple University School of Medicine
Philadelphia, PA

Margarita J. Raygada, PhD
Laboratory for Clinical Genomics
Section on Developmental Genomics
National Institute of Child Health and Human
    Development
Bethesda, MD

Andrew P. Read, PhD
Professor of Human Genetics
University Department of Medical Genetics
St. Mary's Hospital
Manchester, UK

Kavita Reddy, MD
Cytogenics Laboratory
Quest Diagnostics
San Juan Capistrano, CA

Sashi K. Reddy, MD
Resident in Surgery
Department of Urology
Tulane University Health Sciences Center
New Orleans, LA

Westley H. Reeves, MD
Marcia Whitney Schott Professor of Medicine
Chief, Division of Rheumatology and Clinical
    Immunology
University of Florida
Gainesville, FL

Ernst Reichenberger, PhD
Harvard-Forsyth Department of Oral Biology
Harvard School of Dental Medicine
Forsyth Institute
Boston, MA

Berna K. Remzi, MD
Department of Dermatology
Cleveland Clinic Foundation
Cleveland, OH

Owen M. Rennert, MD
Scientific Director
National Institute of Child Health and Human
    Development
Bethesda, MD

Gabriela Richard, MD
Department of Dermatology & Cutaneous Biology
Jefferson Medical College
Thomas Jefferson University
Philadelphia, PA

Hanno B. Richards, MD
Assistant Professor of Medicine
Division of Rheumatology and Clinical Immunology
University of Florida
Gainesville, FL

Daniele Rigamonti, MD
Professor of Neurosurgery & Radiology
Department of Neurosurgery
Johns Hopkins University School of Medicine
Baltimore, MD

Franziska Ringpfeil, MD
Department of Dermatology & Cutaneous Biology
Jefferson Medical College
Thomas Jefferson University
Philadelphia, PA

Adelaide S. Robb, MD
Associate Professor
Department of Psychiatry & Behavioral Science
Children's National Medical Center
Washington, DC

Stephen P. Robertson, FRACP
Institute of Molecular Medicine
John Radcliffe Hospital
Oxford, UK

Brian H. Robinson, PhD
Senior Scientist and Professor of Paediatrics
Head, Metabolic Research Program
The Hospital for Sick Children
Toronto, ON, Canada

Charles R. Roe, MD
Medical Director
Institute of Metabolic Disease
Baylor University Medical Center
Dallas, TX

Jorge E. Romaguera, MD
Associate Professor of Medicine
Department of Lymphoma/Myeloma
University of Texas
M.D. Anderson Cancer Center
Houston, TX

Noel R. Rose, MD, PhD
Professor of Pathology, Molecular Microbiology &
    Immunology
Johns Hopkins University School of Hygiene and Public
    Health
Baltimore, MD

Adam Rosenblatt, MD
Clinical Director
Baltimore Huntington's Disease Center
Johns Hopkins University School of Medicine
Baltimore, MD

Tena Rosser, MD
Fellow, Department of Neurology
Children's National Medical Center
Washington, DC

Forrest S. Roth, MD
St. Louis University School of Medicine
St. Louis, MO

Alisha Rovner, BA
Division of GI and Nutrition
Children's Hospital of Philadelphia
Philadelphia, PA

Jack H. Rubinstein, MD
Cincinnati Center for Developmental Disorders
Children's Hospital Medical Center of Cincinnati
Cincinnati, OH

Bodil Rune, DDS, PhD
Former Assistant Professor at the Center for Craniofacial
    Anomalies
Department of Plastic Surgery
University Hospital MAS
Malmo, Sweden

Barry S. Russman, MD
Professor of Pediatrics and Neurology
Oregon Health Sciences University
Shriners Hospital for Children
Portland, OR

Mustafa Saad, MD
Fellow in Neurosurgery
Millard Fillmore Hospital
Toshiba Stroke Research Center
State University of New York
Buffalo, NY

Sanjiv Sahoo, MD
Resident in Neurology
Georgetown University School of Medicine
Washington, DC

Sami I. Said, MD
Professor, Pulmonary & Critical Care Medicine
State University of New York
Stony Brook Health Science Center
Associate Chief of Staff
VA Medical Center
Northport, NY

Yoriko Saito, MD
Dana-Farber/Partners Cancer Care
Harvard Medical School
Boston, MA

Rolf Salvesen, MD, PhD
Department of Neurology
University of Tromso
Nordland Sentralsykehus
Bodo, Norway

Carole A. Samango-Sprouse, EdD
Associate Professor of Pediatrics
George Washington University and Medical Center
Director, Neurodevelopment Diagnostic Center for Young
    Children
Children's National Medical Center
Washington, DC

Adil Muhib Samara, MD
Rheumatology Unit
State University of Campinas
Campinas, Sao Paulo, Brazil

Madhusudhan R. Sanaka, MD
Department of Gastroenterology
Cleveland Clinic Foundation
Cleveland, OH

Mark V. Sauer, MD
Professor and Vice Chair
Department of Obstetrics and Gynecology
College of Physicians and Surgeons
Director of Assisted Reproduction
New York–Presbyterian Hospital
New York, NY

Frank T. Saulsbury, MD
Professor of Medicine
Division of Immunology & Rheumatology
University of Virginia Health System
Charlottesville, VA

Ravi Savarirayan, MD, MB, BS, FRACP
Head, Genetics Service
Royal Children's Hospital
Fellow in Clinical Genetics
South Australia Clinical Genetic Service
Melbourne, Australia

Ernst J. Schaefer, MD
Professor of Medicine and Nutrition
Tufts University Schools of Medicine and Nutrition
    Science and Policy
Director, Lipid and Heart Disease Prevention Clinic
New England Medical Center
Chief, Lipid Metabolism Laboratory
Jean Mayer–USDA Human Nutrition Research Center on
    Aging
Boston, MA

Blake G. Scheer, MD
Division of Pediatric Immunology
St. Louis University Health Sciences Center
St. Louis, MO

Ernestina Schipani, MD, PhD
Endocrine Unit
Massachusetts General Hospital
Boston, MA

Susanne Schmandt, Dr Med
Sozialpaeditrisches Zentrum
Frankfurt, Germany

Volker Schmid, Dr Med
c/o Praxis Dr. Schuette & Dr. Schmid
Gersthofen, Germany

Robert E. Schmidt, MD, PhD
Division of Neuropathology
Department of Pathology and Immunology
Washington University School of Medicine
St. Louis, MO

Adele Schneider, MD
Clinical Assistant Professor of Pediatrics at Jefferson
    Medical College
Director, Clinical Genetics
Albert Einstein Medical Center
Philadelphia, PA

Arnold L. Schroeter, MD
Department of Dermatology
Mayo Clinic and Foundation
Rochester, MN

Christopher U. J. Schwimer, DO
Department of Anatomic Pathology
Cleveland Clinic Foundation
Cleveland, OH

Charles I. Scott, Jr., MD
Chief, Division of Medical Genetics
Department of Pediatrics
Alfred I. duPont Hospital for Children
Wilmington, DE

R. Michael Scott, MD
Director of Clinical Pediatric Neurosurgery
Children's Hospital Boston
Professor of Neurosurgery
Harvard Medical School
Boston, MA

James J. Sejvar, MD
National Center for Infectious Diseases
Centers for Disease Control and Prevention
Atlanta, GA

Elena V. Semina, PhD
Assistant Research Scientist
Department of Pediatrics
University of Iowa Clinics & Hospitals
Iowa City, IA

Raymond J. Seto, MD
Chief Resident in Ophthalmology
Eye Care Center
Vancouver Hospital
Vancouver, BC, Canada

Shama Shakir, MD
Fellow in Nephrology
Children's Mercy Hospital
Kansas City, Missouri

Robert D. Shamburek, MD
Head of Inpatient Lipid Services
Molecular Disease Branch
National Heart Lung and Blood Institute
Bethesda, MD

Stuart K. Shapira, MD, PhD
Chief, Division of Genetics and Metabolic Disorders
Department of Pediatrics
University of Texas Health Science Center
San Antonio, TX

Debbie Shears, MBBS, MRCP
Clinical Research Fellow
Institute of Child Health
London, UK

Daniel W. Sherer, MD
Department of Dermatology
Mt. Sinai School of Medicine
New York, NY

Zheng-Zheng Shi, MD
Lexicon Genetics
The Woodlands, TX

Jerry A. Shields, MD
Director, Ocular Oncology Service
Wills Eye Hospital
Professor of Ophthalmology
Jefferson Medical College of Thomas Jefferson University
Philadelphia, PA

M. Bruce Shields, MD
Yale Eye Center
Yale University School of Medicine
New Haven, CT

Raymond C. Shields, MD
Senior Associate Consultant
Division of Cardiovascular Diseases
Mayo Clinic and Foundation
Rochester, MN

Sudeep Shivakumar, BS
Research Assistant
Department of Neurology
University of California at San Francisco
School of Medicine
San Francisco, CA

John M. Shoffner, MD
Director, Molecular Medicine Laboratory
Children's Healthcare of Atlanta
Atlanta, GA

Eileen M. Shore, PhD
Research Assistant Professor
Orthopaedic Surgery and Genetics
University of Pennsylvania Health System
Philadelphia, PA

M. Priscilla Short, MD
University of Chicago Hospitals
Neurofibromatosis Clinic
Chicago, IL

Colin A. Sieff, MB, BCh
Senior Associate in Medicine
Dana-Farber Cancer Institute and Children's Hospital
Associate Professor of Pediatrics
Harvard Medical School
Boston, MA

Stavros Sifakis, MD
Departments of Pediatrics and Orthopedics
University of Connecticut Health Sciences Center
Farmington, CT

Michael H. Silber, MB, ChB
Associate Professor of Neurology
Sleep Disorders Center
Department of Neurology
Mayo Clinic and Foundation
Rochester, MN

Debra G. Silberg, MD, PhD
Assistant Professor of Medicine
Associate Director Combined Degree and Physician
    Scholar Programs
Division of Gastroenterology
University of Pennsylvania
Philadelphia, PA

Jean M. Silvestri, MD
Associate Professor of Pediatrics
Department of Pediatric Respiratory Medicine
Rush Medical College of Rush University
Rush Presbyterian–St. Luke's Medical Center
Chicago, IL

Ari M. Simckes, MD
Assistant Professor of Pediatrics
University of Missouri–Kansas City School of Medicine
Division of Nephrology
Children's Mercy Hospital
Kansas City, MO

James P. Simmer, DDS, PhD
Associate Professor
Department of Pediatric Dentistry
University of Texas Health Science Center at San Antonio
San Antonio, TX

Daniel A. Singer, MD
Epidemiological Intelligence Survey Officer
National Center for Infectious Diseases
Centers for Disease Control and Prevention
Atlanta, GA

David L. Skaggs, MD
Assistant Professor of Orthopedic Surgery
USC Keck School of Medicine
Associate Medical Staff
Children's Hospital
Los Angeles, CA

Susan Sklower-Brooks, MD
Research Scientist
Director of Genetic Testing
Biochemical Genetics
NYS Institute for Basic Research
Staten Island, NY

Ann C. M. Smith, MA, DSc(Hon)
Office of Clinical Liaison
Head, SMS Research Unit
National Human Genome Research Institute
Bethesda, MD

Kirby D. Smith, PhD
Department of Pediatrics
Johns Hopkins University School of Medicine
Baltimore, MD

Mikel D. Smith, MD
Professor of Internal Medicine/Cardiology
Director of Echocardiography
Gill Heart Institute
University of Kentucky Chandler Medical Center
Lexington, KY

Riley J. Snook, MD
Department of Neurology,
Indiana University School of Medicine
Indianapolis, IN

Edy E. Soffer, MD
Department of Gastroenterology
Cleveland Clinic Foundation
Cleveland, OH

Debbie K. Song, BS
Department of Neurology
University of Michigan
Ann Arbor, MI

Manu Sood, MD
Department of Paediatrics
University of Manchester
Manchester, UK

H. Soran, MB, BS
Department of Medicine
Royal Liverpool and Broadgreen University Hospital
Liverpool, UK

Juan Fernandez Sotos, MD
Professor of Pediatrics
Ohio State University
College of Medicine & Public Health
Section Chief, Pediatric Endocrinology & Metabolism
Children's Hospital
Columbus, OH

Andrew P. South, MD
Professor of Molecular Dermatology
Department of Cell and Molecular Pathology
St. John's Institute of Dermatology
St. Thomas Hospital
London, UK

Erik C. Spayde, MD
Department of Orthopedics
Massachusetts General Hospital
Boston, MA

Phyllis Speiser, MD
The National Adrenal Diseases Foundation
Director, Pediatric Endocrinology
North Shore–Long Island Jewish Health System
Professor of Clinical Pediatrics
NYU School of Medicine
New Hyde Park, NY

Tarak Srivastava, MD
Fellow in Nephrology
Children's Mercy Hospital
Kansas City, MO

Peter W. Stacpoole, MD, PhD
Professor of Medicine, Biochemistry and Molecular
    Biology
Director, Clinical Research Center
University of Florida
Gainesville, FL

Anton F. H. Stalenhoef, MD, PhD
Professor of Medicine and Head of Lipid Research Group
University Medical Center of Nijmegen
Nijmegen, The Netherlands

Mary Stavropoulos, MD
Assistant Professor
Department of Oral and Maxillofacial Surgery
University of Florida,
Jacksonville, FL

Barry Steinberg, MD, DDS, PhD
Chief, Department of Maxillofacial Surgery
University of Florida
Jacksonville, FL

Robin H. Steinhorn, MD
Professor of Pediatrics
Head, Division of Neonatology
Children's Memorial Hospital and Northwestern
    University
Chicago, IL

Ryan E. Stern, MD
University of Washington Burn Center
Harborview Medical Center
Seattle, WA

Cathy A. Stevens, MD
Director of Medical Genetics
Associate Professor of Pediatrics
T.C. Thompson Children's Hospital
Chattanooga, TN

David B. Stevens, MD
Chief-of-Staff Emeritus
Shriner's Hospital for Children
Lexington, KY

Roger E. Stevenson, MD
Director, Greenwood Genetic Center
Greenwood, SC

Helen Stewart, MD, MRCP
Consultant Clinical Geneticist
Churchill Hospital
Oxford, UK

James K. Stoller, MD
Vice Chairman, Division of Medicine
Head, Section on Respiratory Therapy
Department of Pulmonary and Critical Care Medicine
Cleveland Clinic Foundation
Cleveland, OH

John H. Stone, MD, MPH
Associate Professor of Medicine
Director, Vasculitis Center
Johns Hopkins University School of Medicine
Baltimore, MD

Christina Strömbeck, MD
Department of Neuropediatrics
Astrid Lindgren Children's Hospital
Karolinska Hospital
Stockholm, Sweden

Paul Sugarbaker, MD
Director, Surgical Oncology
Washington Cancer Institute
Washington Hospital Center
Washington, DC

Andrea Superti-Furga, MD
Department of Metabolic & Molecular Pediatrics
University Children's Hospital
University of Zurich
Zurich, Switzerland

Wendy S. Susser, MD
Department of Dermatology
Dartmouth-Hitchcock Medical Center
Lebanon, NH

Calum Sutherland, PhD
Lecturer & Principal Investigator
Department of Pharmacology and Neurosciences
University of Dundee
Ninewells Hospital and Medical School
Dundee, Scotland, UK

Elizabeth Sweeney, MB, ChB
Consultant Clinical Geneticist
Royal Liverpool Children's Hospital
Liverpool, UK

John W. Sweetenham, MD
Professor of Medicine
Head, Haematological Malignancies Programme
University of Colorado Medical School
Denver, CO

Virginia P. Sybert, MD
Professor of Dermatology
University of Washington School of Medicine
Seattle, WA

Yousef E. Tadros, MD
Fellow in Urology
Division of Pediatric Urology
Johns Hopkins Medical Center
Baltimore, MD

Adriaan C.I.T.L. Tan, MD, PhD
Department of Gastroenterology & Hepatology
Canisius Wilhelmina Hospital
Nijmegen, The Netherlands

Rup Tandan, MD
Associate Professor of Neurology
College of Medicine of the University of Vermont
Burlington, VT

Millicent Y. Tan-Ong, MD
Center for Vasculitis Care and Research
Cleveland Clinic Foundation
Cleveland, OH

Daniel Tarsy, MD
Chief, Movement Disorders Center
Beth Israel/Deaconess Medical Center
Associate Professor of Neurology
Harvard Medical School
Boston, MA

Shachar Tauber, MD
Department of Ophthalmology
Yale Eye Center
New Haven, CT

Bradley Taylor, OD, MPH
Department of Ophthalmology and Visual Science
University of Michigan Medical School
Ann Arbor, MI

Hugh S. Taylor, MD
Division of Reproductive Endocrinology & Infertility
Department of Obstetrics & Gynecology
Yale University School of Medicine
New Haven, CT

Ahmed S. Teebi, MD, FRCP (Edin)
Division of Molecular Genetics
Hospital for Sick Children
Professor of Paediatrics
Faculty of Medicine of the University of Toronto
Toronto, ON, Canada

Ayalew Tefferi, MD
Division of Hematology and Internal Medicine
Mayo Clinic and Foundation
Rochester, MN

I. K. Temple, MD
Department of Human Genetics
University of Southampton and Southampton University
  Hospital
Southampton, UK

Karel G. terBrugge, MD
Professor of Neuroimaging
Faculty of Medicine
Head, Division of Neuroimaging
Toronto Hospital, Western Division
Toronto, ON, Canada

Andre Terzic, MD, PhD
Department of Medicine
Mayo Clinic and Foundation
Rochester, MN

Paul Q. Thomas, PhD
Research Fellow
Murdoch Children's Research Institute
Royal Children's Hospital
Victoria, Australia

George H. Thompson, MD
Professor of Orthopedic Surgery and Pediatrics
Case Western Reserve University School of Medicine
Director, Pediatric Surgery
Rainbow Babies & Children's Hospital
Cleveland, OH

Beat Thöny, PhD
Privatdozenten, Division of Clinical Chemistry &
  Biochemistry
Department of Pediatrics
University Children's Hospital
University of Zurich
Zurich, Switzerland

Robert D. Tiegs, MD
Professor of Medicine
Division of Endocrinology, Metabolism & Nutrition
Mayo Clinic and Foundation
Rochester, MN

Cynthia J. Tifft, MD, PhD
Chair, Division of Genetics, Endocrinology, and
  Metabolism
Children's National Medical Center
Genetics of Development and Disease Branch
National Institute of Diabetes & Digestive & Kidney
  Diseases
Bethesda, MD

George E. Tiller, MD, PhD
Associate Professor of Pediatrics and Medical Genetics
Vanderbilt University Medial Center
Nashville, TN

Valdenize Tiziani, PhD
Universidade Federale de Sao Paulo
Instituto de Cirurgia Plastica Craniofacial
Campinas, Brazil
Harvard-Forsyth Department of Oral Biology
Harvard School of Dental Medicine
Forsyth Institute and Department of Cell Biology
Boston, MA

Keti P. Tokmakova, MD
Research Fellow
Department of Orthopaedics
Alfred I. duPont Hospital for Children
Wilmington, DE and Medical University
Plovdiv, Bulgaria

Helga V. Toriello, PhD
Director of Genetic Services
Spectrum Health Systems
Grand Rapids, MI

Annick Toutain, MD
Service de Genetique
Centre Hospitalo-Universitaire
Tours, France

Jeffrey A. Towbin, MD
Director of Cardiology Research
Texas Children's Hospital
Baylor College of Medicine
Houston, TX

Elias I. Traboulsi, MD
Department of Ophthalmology
Eye Center
Cleveland Clinic Foundation
Cleveland, OH

Eileen P. Treacy, MD
Division of Metabolic/Biochemical Genetics
Department of Human Genetics
McGill University
Montreal, PQ, Canada

Richard C. Trembath, MD, BSc, FRCP
Professor of Medical Genetics
Department of Genetics
University of Leicester
Leicester, UK

Jon Trent, MD, PhD
Junior Faculty Associate
University of Texas M.D. Anderson Cancer Center
Houston, TX

Mark A. Trifiro, MD
Department of Genetics
Lady Davis Institute for Medical Research
Sir Mortimer B. Davis–Jewish Hospital
Montreal, PQ, Canada

Petros Tsipouras, MD
Professor of Pediatrics
Department of Pediatrics
University of Connecticut Health Sciences Center
Farmington, CT

Togas Tulandi, MD
Professor of Obstetrics and Gynecology and Milton Leong
    Chair in Reproductive Medicine
Faculty of Medicine
McGill University
Montreal, PQ, Canada

Rossella Tupler, MD, PhD
Program in Molecular Medicine
Howard Hughes Medical Institute
University of Massachusetts Medical School
Worcester, MA

William R. Tyor, MD
Professor of Neurology
Department of Neurology
Medical University of South Carolina
Chief, V.A. Medical Center, Neurology Service
Charleston, SC

Margot I. Van Allen, MD, MSc, FRCPC
Professor, Department of Medicine
British Columbia's Children's Hospital
University of British Columbia
Vancouver, BC, Canada

Griet Van Buggenhout, MD, PhD
University Hospital, Leuven
Center for Human Genetics
Catholic University of Leuven
Leuven, Belgium

Mary Lee Vance, MD
Professor of Neurosurgery & Internal Medicine
University of Virginia Health System
Charlottesville, VA

Ignatia B. Van den Veyver, MD
Assistant Professor
Departments of Ob/Gyn and Molecular and Human
    Genetics
Baylor College of Medicine
Houston, TX

Adeline Vanderver, MD
Resident in Neurology
Children's National Medical Center
George Washington University School of Medicine
Washington, DC

Otto P. van Diggelen, PhD
Department of Clinical Genetics,
Erasmus University and Academic Hospital
Rotterdam, The Netherlands

Wim van Hul, PhD
Professor
Department of Medical Genetics
University of Antwerp
Antwerp, Belgium

Leonie van Passel-Clark, MD
Resident in Neurology
Georgetown University Medical Center
Washington, DC

Heleni Vastardis, DDS
Division of Growth & Developmental Sciences
New York University College of Dentistry
New York, NY

Angela Vincent, MB, BS, MSc
Professor, Department of Clinical Neurology
Institute of Molecular Medicine
John Radcliffe Hospital
Oxford, UK

Jerry Vockley, MD, PhD
Professor and Chair, Department of Medical Genetics
Mayo Clinic and Foundation
Rochester, MN

Axel von Herbay, Dr Med
Privatdozent für Pathologie
Pathologisches Institut
Universitätsklinikum
Heidelberg, Germany

Jens-Jörg von Lindern, MD, DMD
Department of Oral and Maxillofacial Surgery
University of Bonn
Bonn, Germany

N. Kevin Wade, MD
Eye Care Center
Vancouver Hospital
University of British Columbia
Vancouver, BC, Canada

Elisabeth Walch, MD
Department of Neonatology
Charite, Humboldt-University of Berlin
Berlin, Germany

Christopher A. Walsh, MD, PhD
Bullard Professor of Neurology
Harvard Medical School
Beth Israel–Deaconess Medical Center
Boston, MA

Bradley A. Warady, MD
Professor of Pediatrics
University of Missouri—Kansas City School of Medicine
Division of Nephrology
Children's Mercy Hospital
Kansas City, MO

Matthew L. Warman, MD
Assistant Professor of Genetics and Pediatrics
Medical School of Case Western Reserve University
Bone Disorders Clinic
Center for Human Genetics
University Hospitals of Cleveland
Cleveland, OH

Richard R. P. Warner, MD
Medical Director
Carcinoid Cancer Foundation
Clinical Associate Professor of Medicine
Mt. Sinai School of Medicine
New York, NY

David D. Weaver, MS, MD
Professor of Medical Genetics
Director of Clinical Genetics
Indiana University School of Medicine
Indianapolis, IN

Barbara Wedehase, LCSW, CGC
Executive Director
National MPS (Mucopolysaccharidoses/Mucolipidoses)
    Society, Inc
Downingtown, PA

Debra Weese-Mayer, MD
Professor of Pediatrics
Rush Medical College of Rush University
Department of Pediatric Respiratory Medicine
Rush Presbyterian–St. Luke's Medical Center
Chicago, IL

Steven R. Weiner, MD
Associate Professor of Medicine
Division of Rheumatology
UCLA School of Medicine
Los Angeles, CA

Brian Weinshenker, MD
Professor of Neurology
Mayo Clinic and Foundation
Rochester, MN

David A. Weinstein, MD, MMSc
Assistant in Medicine
Division of Endocrinology
The Children's Hospital
Boston, MA

Gil Wernovsky, MD
Director, Cardiac ICU
Children's Hospital of Philadelphia & University of
    Pennsylvania School of Medicine
Philadelphia, PA

Ursula Wesselman, MD
Associate Professor of Neurology & Biomedical
    Engineering
Johns Hopkins University School of Medicine
Baltimore, MD

Margo L. Whiteford, FRCP (Glas)
Clinical Geneticist
Duncan Guthrie Institute of Medical Genetics
Yorkhill NHS Trust
Glasgow, Scotland, UK

Donna Wicker, OD
Department of Ophthalmology and Visual Sciences
University of Michigan Medical School
Ann Arbor, MI

Peter F. Wieacker, Dr Med
Otto-von-Guericke-Universität
Institut für Humangenetik
Universitätsklinikum
Magdeburg, Germany

William R. Wilcox, MD, PhD
Associate Professor of Pediatrics
UCLA School of Medicine
Division of Medical Genetics
Cedars-Sinai Medical Center
Los Angeles, California

Steven M. Willi, MD
Associate Professor of Pediatrics
Medical University of South Carolina
Charleston, SC

Phillip L. Williford, MD, FACP
Director of Dermatological Surgery
Department of Dermatology
Wake Forest University School of Medicine
Winston-Salem, NC

Callum J. Wilson, MB, ChB, FRACP
Metabolic Unit
Great Ormond Street Hospital for Children
London, UK

Golder N. Wilson, MD, PhD
Mary McDermott Cook Distinguished Professorship of
   Pediatric Genetics
Department of Pediatrics
Director, Division of Genetics & Metabolism
University of Texas Southwestern Medical Center
Dallas, TX

Wyndham Wilson, MD, PhD
Center for Cancer Research
National Cancer Institute
Bethesda, MD

Patricia Winchester, PT, PhD
Professor and Chair, Department of Physical Therapy
University of Texas Southwest Medical Center
Dallas, TX

Susan C. Winter, MD, FAAP, FCMG
Medical Director, Metabolic Genetics
Children's Hospital, Central California
Fresno, CA

Joseph I. Wolfsdorf, MB, BCh
Associate Professor of Pediatrics
Harvard Medical School
Division of Endocrinology
Children's Hospital
Boston, MA

Fung-Ki Wong, BDS, PhD
Faculty of Dentistry
University of Hong Kong
Hong Kong, People's Republic of China

Jeffrey A. Wong, MD
Pediatric Cardiologist
Cedars Sinai Medical Center
Clinical Instructor
UCLA School of Medicine
Los Angeles, CA

Eric A. Wulfsburg, MD
Division of Pediatric Genetics
University of Maryland Medical Center
Baltimore, MD

Reuven Yakubov, BA
Student in Combined MD, PhD Program
Department of Anatomy & Cell Biology, and Pediatrics
SUNY Downstate Medical Center
Brooklyn, NY

Masayuki Yamamoto, MD, PhD
Professor, Institute of Basic Medical Sciences
Department of Clinical Genetics
University of Tsukuba School of Medicine
Tsukuba, Japan

Guy Young, MD
Division of Pediatric Hematology/Oncology
Children's Hospital of Orange County
Orange, CA

Joni C. Young, MS
TRW Systems
CISSS Project
Atlanta, GA

Neal S. Young, MD
Chief, Hematology Branch
National Heart Lung Blood Institute
National Institutes of Health
Bethesda, MD

Naveed Younis, BSc, MB, ChB
Department of Medicine
Royal Liverpool and Broadgreen University Hospital
Liverpool, UK

J. Georges Youssef, MD
Department of Pulmonary and Critical Care Medicine
SUNY Health Science Center at Stony Brook
Stony Brook, NY

Marco A. Zarbin, MD, PhD
Professor & Chair
Department of Ophthalmology
Institute of Ophthalmology and Visual Science
New Jersey Medical School
University of Medicine and Dentistry of New Jersey
Newark, NJ

Christa S. Zerbe, BSN, MS
Biologist, Genetics and Molecular Biology Branch
National Human Genome Research Institute
Bethesda, MD

John Zic, MD
Department of Dermatology
Vanderbilt University Medical Center
Nashville, TN

Leonid V. Zingman, MD
Department of Medicine
Mayo Clinic and Foundation
Rochester, MN

Contents

Dedication   v
Foreword   vii
Preface   ix
Acknowledgments   xi
Reviewers   xiii
Contributors   xv

CHAPTER 1: AUTOIMMUNE & CONNECTIVE TISSUE DISORDERS   1

1. Antiphospholipid Syndrome
2. Arachnodactyly, Congenital Contractural
3. Behçet Disease
4. Cryoglobulinemia, Mixed
5. DeBarsy Syndrome
6. Eosinophilia-Myalgia Syndrome
7. Eosinophilic Fasciitis
8. Felty Syndrome
9. Diffuse Idiopathic Skeletal Hyperostosis (Forestier Disease)
10. Graft-Versus-Host Disease
11. Hajdu-Cheney Syndrome
12. Hyper-IgE Syndrome
13. Immunodeficiency, Common Variable
14. Immunodeficiency, Severe Combined
15. Kawasaki Disease
16. Legg-Calve-Perthes Disease
17. Lymphoepithelial Lesion, Benign (Mikulicz Syndrome)
18. Marden-Walker Syndrome
19. Mediterranean Fever, Familial
20. Metatrophic Dysplasia
21. Navicular Osteochondritis (Kohler Disease)
22. Neutropenia, Cyclic
23. Neutropenia, Severe Chronic
24. Ollier Disease
25. Paget Disease of Bone
26. Peyronie Disease
27. POEMS Syndrome
28. Polyangiitis, Microscopic
29. Polyarteritis Nodosa
30. Polychondritis, Relapsing
31. Premature Ovarian Failure, Autoimmune
32. Reye Syndrome
33. Sarcoidosis
34. Scleroderma
35. Sjögren Syndrome and Cutaneous Vasculitis
36. Takayasu Arteritis
37. Thromboangiitis Obliterans
38. Vogt-Koyanagi-Harada Syndrome
39. Waldenström Macroglobulinemia
40. Wiskott-Aldrich Syndrome

CHAPTER 2: CARDIOVASCULAR DISORDERS   41

1. Atrial Septal Defects
2. Atrioventricular Septal Defects
3. Barth Syndrome
4. Brugada Syndrome
5. Cor Triatriatum
6. Eisenmenger Syndrome
7. Endomyocardial Fibrosis
8. Granulomatosis, Lymphomatoid
9. Heart Block, Congenital Complete
10. Hypoplastic Left Heart Syndrome
11. Jervell and Lange-Nielsen Syndrome
12. Myocarditis, Giant Cell
13. Myocarditis, Hypersensitivity
14. Romano-Ward Long QT Syndrome
15. Situs Inversus
16. Truncus Arteriosus, Persistent

CHAPTER 3: CHROMOSOMAL DISORDERS   57

1. Chromosome 1, Deletion of the Short Arm of
2. Chromosome 10, Distal Trisomy 10q
3. Chromosome 10, Monosomy 10p
4. Chromosome 11, Partial Monosomy 11q
5. Chromosome 11, Partial Trisomy 11q
6. Chromosome 13, Partial Monosomy 13q
7. Chromosome 14 Ring
8. Chromosome 14, Trisomy Mosaic
9. Chromosome 15, Distal Trisomy 15q
10. Chromosome 15 Ring
11. Chromosome 18, Monosomy 18p
12. Chromosome 18q- Syndrome
13. Chromosome 18 Ring
14. Chromosome 18, Tetrasomy 18p
15. Chromosome 21 Ring

16. Chromosome 22q11 Deletion Spectrum
17. Chromosome 22 Ring
18. Chromosome 22, Trisomy Mosaic
19. Chromosome 3, Monosomy 3p2
20. Chromosome 3, Trisomy 3q2
21. Chromosome 4, Monosomy 4q
22. Chromosome 4, Monosomy Distal 4q
23. Chromosome 4, Partial Trisomy Distal 4q
24. Chromosome 4 Ring
25. Chromosome 4, Trisomy 4p
26. Chromosome 5, Trisomy 5p
27. Chromosome 6, Partial Trisomy 6q
28. Chromosome 6 Ring
29. Chromosome 7, Monosomy 7p2
30. Chromosome 8, Monosomy 8p2
31. Chromosome 9, Partial Monosomy 9p
32. Chromosome 9 Ring
33. Chromosome 9, Tetrasomy 9p
34. Chromosome 9, Trisomy 9p (Multiple Variants)
35. Chromosome 9, Trisomy Mosaic
36. Pentasomy X
37. Trisomy 13 Syndrome
38. Trisomy 18 Syndrome
39. XXX Syndrome (Triple X Syndrome)
40. XXY Syndrome (Klinefelter Syndrome)
41. XYY Syndrome

CHAPTER 4: DERMATOLOGIC DISORDERS   93

1. Acrodermatitis Enteropathica
2. Alopecia Areata
3. Aplasia Cutis Congenita
4. Björnstad Syndrome
5. Bowen Disease
6. Bowenoid Papulosis
7. Cellulitis, Familial Eosinophilic (Wells Syndrome)
8. Cutis Marmorata Telangiectatica Congenita
9. Darier Disease
10. Degos Disease
11. Dermatitis Herpetiformis
12. Dermatosis, Transient Acantholytic
13. Dyskeratosis Congenita
14. Epidermal Nevus Syndrome
15. Epidermolysis Bullosa, Dystrophic
16. Epidermolysis Bullosa, Junctional
17. Epidermolysis Bullosa Simplex
18. Epidermolytic Hyperkeratosis
19. Erythema Multiforme
20. Erythrokeratodermia, Progressive Symmetric/ Erythrokeratodermia with Ataxia
21. Erythrokeratodermia Variabilis
22. Erythromelalgia
23. Fox-Fordyce Disease
24. Gianotti-Crosti Syndrome
25. Granuloma Annulare

26. Hay-Wells Syndrome
27. Hemangioma, Cavernous
28. Hidradenitis Suppurativa
29. Hypomelanosis of Ito
30. Ichthyosis
31. Incontinentia Pigmenti
32. Keratitis Ichthyosis Deafness Syndrome
33. Leiner Disease
34. LEOPARD Syndrome
35. Lichen Planus
36. Lichen Sclerosis
37. McGrath Syndrome
38. Meleda Disease
39. Mucha-Habermann Disease
40. Pachydermoperiostosis
41. Pemphigoid, Bullous
42. Pemphigoid, Cicatricial
43. Pemphigus Vulgaris and Pemphigus Foliaceus
44. Pityriasis Rubra Pilaris
45. Pseudoxanthoma Elasticum
46. Pyoderma Gangrenosum
47. Rothmund-Thomson Syndrome
48. Scleromyxedema
49. Setleis Syndrome
50. Sutton Disease
51. Sweet Syndrome
52. Toxic Epidermal Necrolysis

CHAPTER 5: DYSMORPHIC DISORDERS   141

1. Aarskog Syndrome
2. Aase Syndrome
3. Achondroplasia
4. Acrocallosal Syndrome (Schinzel Type)
5. Acrodysostosis
6. Acrogeria (Gottron Type)
7. Adams-Oliver Syndrome
8. Allan-Herndon-Dudley Syndrome
9. Amelogenesis Imperfecta
10. Amniotic Bands
11. Anencephaly
12. Angelman Syndrome
13. Anorectal Malformations
14. Apert Syndrome
15. Arthrogryposis Multiplex Congenita
16. Asphyxiating Thoracic Dystrophy
17. Atelosteogenesis Type III
18. Baller-Gerold Syndrome
19. Bardet-Biedl Syndrome
20. Bloom Syndrome
21. Blue Rubber Bleb Nevus Syndrome
22. Bowen-Conradi Syndrome
23. Branchio-Oculo-Facial Syndrome
24. C Syndrome
25. Cardiofaciocutaneous Syndrome

26. Cat Eye Syndrome
27. Catel-Manzke Syndrome
28. Caudal Regression Syndrome
29. Cerebrocostomandibular Syndrome
30. CHARGE Syndrome
31. Cherubism
32. Chondrocalcinosis, Familial Articular
33. Cockayne Syndrome
34. Coffin-Lowry Syndrome
35. Cohen Syndrome
36. Conradi-Hünermann Syndrome
37. Craniosynostosis, Primary
38. Cri-du-Chat Syndrome
39. Cystic Hygroma
40. Dentin Dysplasia
41. Dentinogenesis Imperfecta Type III
42. DiGeorge Syndrome
43. Dubowitz Syndrome
44. Dyggve-Melchior-Clausen Syndrome
45. Dyschondrosteosis
46. Dysplasia, Cleidocranial
47. Dysplasia, Craniofrontonasal
48. Dysplasia, Craniometaphyseal
49. Dysplasia, Ectodermal
50. Dysplasia Epiphysealis Hemimelica
51. Dysplasia, Maxillonasal (Binder Type Syndrome)
52. Dysplasia, Multiple Epiphyseal Type 1 (Fairbank Syndrome)
53. Dysplasia, Septooptic
54. Ear–Patella–Short Stature Syndrome
55. Esophageal Atresia
56. Exostoses, Multiple Hereditary
57. Fetal Hydantoin Syndrome
58. Fetal Valproate Syndrome
59. FG Syndrome
60. Filippi Syndrome
61. Floating Harbor Syndrome
62. Fountain Syndrome
63. Fraser Syndrome
64. Gastroschisis
65. GBBB Syndrome (Opitz Syndrome)
66. Gordon Syndrome
67. Gorlin-Chaudhry-Moss Syndrome
68. Greig Cephalopolysyndactyly Syndrome
69. Hallerman-Streiff Syndrome
70. Hanhart Syndrome
71. Heteroplasia, Progressive Osseous
72. Hyperostosis Corticalis Generalisata (van Buchem Disease)
73. Ivemark Syndrome
74. Jansen Metaphyseal Chondrodysplasia
75. Jarcho-Levin Syndrome
76. Johanson-Blizzard Syndrome
77. Kabuki Make-Up Syndrome
78. KBG Syndrome
79. Kenny-Caffey Syndrome
80. Klippel-Trenaunay Syndrome
81. Kniest Dysplasia: A Type II Collagenopathy
82. Laband Syndrome
83. Laurence-Moon Syndrome
84. Leprechaunism
85. Leri Pleonosteosis (Moore-Federman Syndrome)
86. Maffucci Syndrome
87. Marfan Syndrome
88. Marshall-Smith Syndrome
89. MASA Syndrome
90. Meckel Syndrome
91. Melnick-Needles Syndrome
92. Miller Syndrome
93. Möbius Syndrome
94. MULIBREY Nanism
95. Myhre Syndrome
96. Nager Syndrome
97. Oculocerebral Syndrome with Hypopigmentation
98. Osteogenesis Imperfecta
99. Osteopetrosis, Autosomal-Recessive
100. Oto-Palato-Digital Syndrome
101. Pallister-Hall Syndrome
102. Pallister-Killian Syndrome
103. Parkes-Weber Syndrome
104. Parry-Romberg Syndrome
105. Pentalogy of Cantrell
106. Pfeiffer Syndrome Type I
107. Pierre Robin Sequence
108. Poland Syndrome
109. Prader-Willi Syndrome
110. Progeroid Syndrome, Neonatal
111. Proteus Syndrome
112. PTEN Hamartoma Tumor Syndrome
113. Pterygium Syndrome, Multiple
114. Pterygium Syndrome, Popliteal
115. Pyknodysostosis
116. Rieger Syndrome
117. Roberts Pseudothalidomide Syndrome
118. Russell-Silver Syndrome
119. Schinzel Syndrome
120. Schinzel-Giedion Syndrome
121. Schmid Metaphyseal Chondrodysplasia
122. Sclerosteosis
123. Scott Craniodigital Syndrome
124. SHORT Syndrome
125. Simpson Dysmorphia Syndrome
126. Singleton-Merten Syndrome
127. Smith-Lemli-Opitz Syndrome
128. Smith-Magenis Syndrome
129. Sotos Syndrome
130. Split Hand/Split Foot Malformation
131. Sprengel Deformity

132. Sturge-Weber Syndrome
133. 3-M Syndrome
134. Thrombocytopenia and Absent Radius Syndrome
135. Tooth Agenesis (Anodontia)
136. Townes-Brocks Syndrome
137. Treacher-Collins Syndrome
138. Triploidy Syndrome–Partial Molar Pregnancy
139. Turner Syndrome
140. Von Hippel-Lindau Disease
141. Weaver Syndrome
142. Weill-Marchesani Syndrome
143. Weismann-Netter-Stuhl Syndrome
144. Werner Syndrome
145. Williams Syndrome
146. Winchester Syndrome
147. Wolf-Hirschhorn Syndrome
148. Wolfram Syndrome
149. XLMR-Hypotonic Facies Syndrome
150. Yunis-Varón Syndrome

CHAPTER 6: EMERGING/INFECTIOUS DISEASES   277
1. Anthrax
2. Botulism
3. Brucellosis
4. Dengue Fever
5. Ebola and Other Viral Hemorrhagic Fevers
6. Ehrlichiosis
7. Encephalitides, Selected
8. Erysipelas
9. Fascioliasis (Liver Fluke Disease)
10. Hantavirus Pulmonary Syndrome
11. Hepatitis, Idiopathic Neonatal
12. Leptospirosis
13. Listeriosis
14. Malaria
15. Plague
16. Q Fever
17. Rift Valley Fever
18. TORCH Syndrome
19. West Nile Fever
20. Whipple Disease

CHAPTER 7: ENDOCRINE DISORDERS   299
1. Achard-Thiers Syndrome
2. Acromegaly
3. ACTH Deficiency
4. Adiposis Dolorosa
5. Adrenal Hyperplasia, Congenital, Due to 21-Hydroxylase Deficiency
6. Aldosteronism, Primary
7. Alström Syndrome
8. Androgen Insensitivity Syndrome
9. Androgen Insensitivity Syndrome, Partial

10. Asherman Syndrome
11. Bartter Syndrome
12. Carcinoid Syndrome
13. Cushing Syndrome
14. Diabetes Insipidus
15. Growth Hormone Deficiency
16. HAIR-AN Syndrome
17. Hermaphroditism, True
18. Hypophosphatasia
19. Kallmann Syndrome
20. Laron Dwarfism
21. Lipodystrophy, Acquired Generalized
22. Lipodystrophy, Acquired Partial
23. Lipodystrophy, Congenital Generalized
24. Lipodystrophy, Familial Partial
25. Polycystic Ovary Syndrome
26. Precocious Puberty
27. Pseudohypoparathyroidism
28. Rickets, X-Linked Hypophosphatemic
29. Sheehan Syndrome
30. Thyroiditis, Chronic Lymphocytic
31. Zollinger-Ellison Syndrome

CHAPTER 8: GASTROENTEROLOGIC DISORDERS   331
1. Alagille Syndrome
2. Barrett Esophagus
3. Biliary Atresia
4. Byler Disease
5. Caroli Disease
6. Crigler-Najjar Syndrome
7. Cronkhite-Canada Syndrome
8. Diverticulosis, Small Bowel
9. Dubin-Johnson Syndrome
10. Gastritis, Giant Hypertrophic
11. Gastroenteritis, Eosinophilic
12. Glucose-Galactose Malabsorption
13. Hepatorenal Syndrome
14. Hirschsprung Disease
15. Intestinal Lymphangiectasia
16. Intestinal Pseudoobstruction in Adults
17. Intestinal Pseudoobstruction (Pediatric Presentation)
18. Jejunal Atresia
19. Mesenteric Panniculitis
20. Microvillus Inclusion Disease
21. Peutz-Jeghers Syndrome
22. Polyposis, Familial Adenomatous
23. Ruvalcaba-Myhre-Smith Syndrome
24. Sucrase-Isomaltase Deficiency

CHAPTER 9: HEMATOLOGIC/ONCOLOGIC DISORDERS   357
1. Abetalipoproteinemia

2. Adenoid Cystic Carcinoma
3. Afibrinogenemia, Congenital
4. Aggamaglobulinemia, X-Linked
5. Agranulocytosis, Acquired
6. Ameloblastoma
7. Anemia, Aplastic, Acquired
8. Anemia, Diamond-Blackfan
9. Anemia, Fanconi
10. Anemias, Hemolytic, Autoimmune
11. Anemia, Hemolytic, Cold Syndromes
12. Anemia, Hemolytic, Nonspherocytic Congenital
13. Anemia, Hemolytic, Spherocytic, Hereditary (Hereditary Spherocytosis)
14. Anemia, Hemolytic, Warm Antibody
15. Anemia, Sickle Cell
16. Anemia, X-Linked Sideroblastic
17. Anemia, X-Linked Sideroblastic, and Cerebellar Ataxia
18. Angioedema, Hereditary
19. Antithrombin III Deficiency, Congenital
20. Banti Syndrome
21. Bernard-Soulier Syndrome
22. Chédiak-Higashi Syndrome
23. Chylomicron Retention Disease
24. Ewing Sarcoma of Bone
25. Factor IX Deficiency
26. Factor XII Deficiency
27. Glanzmann Thrombasthenia
28. Glioblastoma Multiforme
29. Glucose-6-Phosphate Dehydrogenase Deficiency
30. Granulomatous Disease, Chronic
31. Hemochromatosis, Hereditary
32. Hemoglobinuria, Paroxysmal Cold
33. Hemoglobinuria, Paroxysmal Nocturnal
34. Hemophilias, The
35. Hermansky-Pudlak Syndrome
36. Histiocytosis, Langerhans Cell
37. Hyper-IgM Syndrome
38. Leukemia, Large Granular Lymphocyte
39. Lymphangioleiomyomatosis
40. Lymphedema, Hereditary
41. Lymphohistiocytosis, Hemophagocytic
42. Lymphoma, Angioimmunoblastic Lymphadenopathy-Type T-cell
43. Lymphoma, Mantle Cell
44. Lymphoproliferative Syndrome, X-Linked
45. Lynch Syndromes
46. Mastocytosis
47. May-Hegglin Anomaly
48. Medulloblastoma
49. Melanoma
50. Mycosis Fungoides
51. Myeloma, Multiple
52. Nezelof Syndrome
53. Pancreas, Islet Cell Tumors of the
54. Pheochromocytoma
55. Polycythemia Vera
56. Pseudomyxoma Peritonei
57. Pure Red Cell Aplasia, Acquired
58. Purpura, Henoch-Schönlein
59. Purpura, Idiopathic Thrombocytopenic
60. Purpura, Thrombotic Thrombocytopenic, and Hemolytic Uremic Syndrome of Adults
61. Shwachman-Diamond Syndrome
62. Telangiectasia, Hereditary Hemorrhagic
63. Thalassemia Major
64. Thalassemia Minor
65. Thrombocytosis, Idiopathic
66. Twin-Twin Transfusion Syndrome
67. Wegener Granulomatosis

CHAPTER 10: INBORN ERRORS OF METABOLISM   425
1. Acidemia, Glutaric Type I
2. Acidemia, Glutaric Type II
3. Acidemia, Isovaleric
4. Acidemia, Propionic
5. Acidemias, The Methylmalonic
6. Adrenoleukodystrophy, X-Linked
7. Alkaptonuria
8. Aspartylglucosaminuria
9. Carnitine Deficiency Syndromes
10. Carnitine Palmitoyl Transferase I Deficiency
11. Carnitine Palmitoyl Transferase II Deficiency
12. Carnosinemia
13. Cytochrome Oxidase Deficiency, Human
14. Dehydrogenase Deficiency, Long-Chain Acyl-CoA
15. Dehydrogenase Deficiency, Medium-Chain Acyl-CoA
16. Dehydrogenase Deficiency, Short-Chain Acyl-CoA
17. Dehydrogenase Deficiency, Very-Long-Chain Acyl-CoA
18. Dysbetalipoproteinemia, Familial
19. Erdheim-Chester Disease
20. Fabry Disease
21. Farber Disease
22. Fructose Intolerance, Hereditary
23. Fructosuria
24. Fucosidosis
25. Galactosemia
26. Gaucher Disease
27. Glut 1 Deficiency Syndrome
28. Glutathione Synthetase Deficiency
29. Glycogen Storage Disease, Type 0
30. Glycogen Storage Disease, Type I
31. Glycogen Storage Disease, Type II
32. Glycogen Storage Disease, Type III
33. Glycogen Storage Disease, Type IV

34. Glycogen Storage Disease, Type V
35. Glycogen Storage Disease, Types VI and IX
36. Glycogen Storage Disease, Type VII
37. Glycosylation, Congenital Disorders of
38. Hartnup Disease
39. Histidinemia
40. Homocystinuria
41. Hyperlipidemia, Type IV
42. Hyperoxalurias, Primary
43. Lactic Acidoses, Congenital
44. Lesch-Nyhan Syndrome
45. Lipoprotein Lipase Deficiency, Familial
46. Lowe Syndrome
47. Alpha-Mannosidosis
48. Maple Syrup Urine Disease
49. MELAS and MERRF
50. Menkes Disease
51. Methylmalonate Semialdehyde Dehydrogenase Deficiency
52. Mucolipidosis II and III
53. Mucolipidosis IV
54. Mucopolysaccharide Storage (MPS) Diseases
54a. MPS-IH (Hurler Disease)
54b. MPS-IS (Scheie Disease)
54c. MPS-II (Hunter Disease)
54d. MPS-III (Sanfilippo Disease)
54e. MPS-IV (Morquio Disease)
54f. MPS-VI (Maroteaux-Lamy Disease)
54g. MPS-VII (Sly Disease)
55. Multiple Carboxylase Deficiency (Biotinidase Deficiency)
56. Multiple Carboxylase Deficiency (Holocarboxylase Synthetase Deficiency)
57. Multiple Sulfatase Deficiency
58. Niemann-Pick Disease, Type C
59. PEPCK Deficiency
60. Peroxisomal Biogenesis Disorders
61. Phenylketonuria
62. Phenylketonuria, Maternal
63. Phosphoglycerate Kinase Deficiency
64. Porphyria, Acute Intermittent
65. Porphyria, ALA-Dehydratase–Deficient
66. Porphyria, Congenital Erythropoietic
67. Porphyria Cutanea Tarda
68. Porphyria, Variegate and Hereditary Coproporphyria
69. Protoporphyria, Erythropoietic
70. Pyruvate Kinase Deficiency
71. Sandhoff Disease
72. Sialidosis
73. Succinic Semialdehyde Dehydrogenase Deficiency
74. Tangier Disease
75. Tay-Sachs Disease
76. Tetrahydrobiopterin Deficiency
77. Trimethylaminuria
78. Tyrosinemia Type 1
79. Urea Cycle Disorders
80. Wilson Disease

CHAPTER 11: NEUROLOGIC DISORDERS   507
1. Agenesis of Corpus Callosum
2. Agnosia, Primary Visual
3. Aicardi Syndrome
4. Alexander Disease
5. Alpers Disease
6. Alternating Hemiplegia of Childhood
7. Amyotrophic Lateral Sclerosis
8. Apraxia
9. Arnold-Chiari Syndrome
10. Batten Disease
11. Beckwith-Wiedemann Syndrome
12. Binswanger Disease
13. Brown-Séquard Syndrome
14. Cerebro-Oculo-Facio-Skeletal Syndrome
15. Charcot-Marie-Tooth Polyneuropathy Syndrome
16. Chorea, Sydenham
17. Complex Regional Pain Syndrome Type 1
18. Corticobasal Degeneration
19. Cyclic Vomiting Syndrome
20. Dandy-Walker Syndrome
21. Dejerine-Sottas Syndrome
22. Diencephalic Syndrome
23. Dysautonomia, Familial
24. Empty Sella Syndrome, Primary
25. Epilepsy, Progressive Myoclonus
26. Fahr Disease
27. Frey Syndrome
28. Frontotemporal Dementia (Pick Disease)
29. Gerstmann Syndrome
30. Guillain-Barré Syndrome
31. Holoprosencephaly
32. Huntington Disease
33. Hydranencephaly
34. Hydrocephalus
35. Hyperekplexia
36. Infantile Spasms
37. Joubert Syndrome
38. Kernicterus
39. Kleine-Levin Syndrome
40. Kluver-Bucy Syndrome
41. Korsakoff Syndrome
42. Kuf Disease
43. Landau-Kleffner Syndrome
44. Lateral Sclerosis, Primary
45. Lennox-Gastaut Syndrome
46. Leukodystrophy (Canavan Disease)
47. Leukodystrophy (Krabbe Disease)
48. Leukodystrophy, Metachromatic
49. Lissencephaly, Classic

50. Locked-in Syndrome
51. Machado-Joseph Disease
52. Megalocornea and Mental Retardation
53. Melkersson-Rosenthal Syndrome
54. Ménière Disease
55. Moyamoya Syndrome
56. Multiple Sclerosis, Rare Variants of
57. Multiple System Atrophy
58. Narcolepsy
59. Neu-Laxova Syndrome
60. Neurofibromatosis Type 1
61. Neurofibromatosis Type 2
62. Neuroleptic Malignant Syndrome
63. Neuromyelitis Optica
64. Neuropathy, Congenital Hypomyelination
65. Neuropathy, Giant Axonal
66. Neuropathy, Hereditary Sensory, Type I
67. Neuropathy, Hereditary Sensory, Type II
68. Obstetric Brachial Plexus Palsy
69. Opsoclonus-Myoclonus Syndrome
70. Palsy, Progressive Supranuclear
71. Panencephalitis, Subacute Sclerosing
72. Paraplegia, Hereditary Spastic
73. Parkinson Disease
74. Parsonage-Turner Syndrome
75. Pelizaeus-Merzbacher Disease
76. Perisylvian Syndrome, Congenital Bilateral
77. Polyglucosan Body Disease, Adult
78. Polyneuropathy, Chronic Inflammatory Demyelinating
79. Pseudotumor Cerebri
80. Restless Legs Syndrome
81. Rett Syndrome
82. Rosenberg-Chutorian Syndrome
83. Santavuori Disease
84. Schwartz-Jampel Syndrome
85. Spinal Stenosis, Lumbar
86. Stiff Person Syndrome
87. Syringobulbia
88. Syringomyelia
89. Tardive Dyskinesia
90. Tarsal Tunnel Syndrome
91. Thalamic Pain Syndrome
92. Tourette Syndrome
93. Trigeminal Neuralgia
94. Tuberous Sclerosis
95. Vascular Malformation of the Brain/Brain Arteriovenous Malformation
96. Walker-Warburg Syndrome

CHAPTER 12: NEUROMUSCULAR DISORDERS   599
1. Ataxia, Baltic/Mediterranean/Unverrich-Lundborg Myoclonic Epilepsy
2. Ataxia, Episodic Type I
3. Ataxia, Episodic Type II
4. Ataxia, Friedreich
5. Ataxia, Kearns-Sayre Syndrome/Chronic Progressive External Ophthalmoplegia
6. Ataxia, Refsum Disease
7. Ataxia-Telangiectasia
8. Ataxia, with Isolated Vitamin E Deficiency
9. Central Core Disease
10. Creutzfeldt-Jakob Disease
11. Dystonia
11a. Blepharospasm
11b. Cervical Dystonia (Spasmodic Torticollis)
11c. Dopa-Responsive Dystonia
11d. Embouchure Dystonia
11e. Laryngeal Dystonia (Spasmodic Dysphonia)
11f. Myoclonic Dystonia
11g. Oromandibular Dystonia and Meige Syndrome
11h. Paroxysmal Dystonias and Dyskinesias
11i. Rapid-Onset Dystonia-Parkinsonism
11j. Writer's Cramp
11k. X-Linked Dystonia-Parkinsonism
12. Hallervorden-Spatz Disease
13. Lambert-Eaton Myasthenic Syndrome
14. Muscular Dystrophy, Becker
15. Muscular Dystrophy, Duchenne
16. Muscular Dystrophy, Emery Dreifuss
17. Muscular Dystrophy, Facioscapulohumeral
18. Muscular Dystrophy, Limb Girdle
19. Myasthenia Gravis
20. Myoclonus
21. Myopathy, Centronuclear and Myotubular
22. Myopathy, Congenital, with Fiber-Type Disproportion
23. Myopathy, Myofibrillar (Desmin and Desmin-Related)
24. Myositis, Inclusion Body
25. Myotonia Congenita
26. Neuroacanthocytosis
27. Neuroaxonal Dystrophy, Infantile
28. Neuromyotonia
29. Spinal Bulbar Muscular Atrophy
30. Spinal Muscular Atrophy
31. Wieacker-Wolff Syndrome

CHAPTER 13: OPHTHALMOLOGIC DISORDERS   639
1. Aniridia
2. Blepharophimosis-Ptosis-Epicanthus Inversus Syndrome
3. Choroideremia
4. Coats Disease
5. Cogan-Reese Syndrome
6. Duane Syndrome
7. Eales Disease

8. Epitheliopathy, Acute Posterior Multifocal Placoid Pigment
9. Horner Syndrome
10. Iridocorneal Endothelial Syndromes
11. Iris Atrophy, Essential
12. Keratoconus
13. Leber Congenital Amaurosis
14. Leber Hereditary Optic Neuropathy
15. Lenz Microphthalmia Syndrome
16. Nance-Horan Syndrome
17. Norrie Disease
18. Pars Planitis
19. Retinal Arterial Occlusion in Young Patients
20. Retinal Vein Occlusion in Young Patients
21. Retinitis Pigmentosa
22. Retinoblastoma
23. Retinoschisis, X-Linked Juvenile
24. Stargardt Disease
25. Tolosa-Hunt Syndrome
26. Usher Syndrome
27. Uveitis, Posterior
28. Wyburn-Mason Syndrome

CHAPTER 14: PULMONARY DISORDERS   669
1. Acute Respiratory Distress Syndrome
2. Alpha 1-Antitrypsin Deficiency
3. Alveolar Capillary Dysplasia
4. Central Hypoventilation Syndrome, Idiopathic Congenital
5. Churg-Strauss Syndrome
6. Ciliary Dyskinesia, Primary
7. Papillomatosis, Recurrent Respiratory
8. Pulmonary Alveolar Proteinosis
9. Pulmonary Hypertension, Primary

CHAPTER 15: RENAL DISORDERS   679
1. Alport Syndrome
2. Blue Diaper Syndrome
3. Branchio-Oto-Renal Syndrome
4. Cystinosis
5. Cystinuria
6. Cystitis, Interstitial
7. Denys-Drash Syndrome
8. Exstrophy, Bladder–Epispadias–Cloacal Exstrophy Complex
9. Galloway-Mowat Syndrome
10. Hematuria, Benign Familial
11. Hemolytic-Uremic Syndrome
12. Hemolytic-Uremic Syndrome, Inherited
13. Hepatic Fibrosis, Congenital
14. Loken-Senior Syndrome

15. Medullary Cystic Kidney Disease
16. Medullary Sponge Kidney
17. MURCS Association
18. Nephropathy, Familial Juvenile Hyperuricemic
19. Polycystic Kidney Disease, Autosomal-Recessive
20. Renal Agenesis, Bilateral
21. WAGR Syndrome

CHAPTER 16: SKELETAL DISORDERS   701
1. Acheiropodia
2. Acromesomelic Dysplasias Due to Mutations of the *CDMP-1* Gene: Grebe Syndrome and Hunter-Thompson Acromesomelic Dysplasia
3. Acromesomelic Dysplasia, Maroteaux Type
4. Antley-Bixler Syndrome
5. Borjeson-Forssman-Lehmann Syndrome
6. Campomelic Syndrome
7. Camurati-Engelmann Disease
8. Coffin-Siris Syndrome
9. Cornelia de Lange Syndrome
10. Crouzon Disease
11. Diastrophic Dysplasia
12. Femoral Hypoplasia–Unusual Facies Syndrome
13. Fibrodysplasia Ossificans Progressiva
14. Freeman-Sheldon Syndrome
15. Fryns Syndrome
16. Goldenhar Syndrome
17. Holt-Oram Syndrome
18. Hyperthermia, Malignant
19. Jackson-Weiss Syndrome
20. Klippel-Feil Syndrome
21. Marinesco-Sjögren Syndrome
22. Nail-Patella Syndrome
23. Noonan Syndrome
24. Osteolysis, Familial Expansile
25. Progeria
26. Robinow Syndrome
27. Rubinstein-Taybi Syndrome
28. Saethre-Chotzen Syndrome
29. Spondyloepiphyseal Dysplasia Congenita
30. Spondyloepiphyseal Dysplasia Tarda
31. Trichorhinophalangeal Syndrome Type I
32. Trichorhinophalangeal Syndrome Type II
33. Trichorhinophalangeal Syndrome Type III
34. Waardenburg Syndromes

List of Resource Groups   735
List of Orphan Products   769
Index   817
Figure insert falls after page 448

1

Autoimmune & Connective Tissue Disorders

1 Antiphospholipid Syndrome

William J. Hogan, MD,
and William L. Nichols, MD

DEFINITION: Primary antiphospholipid syndrome (APS) is characterized by persistently demonstrable antiphospholipid antibodies (aPL) in association with arterial or venous thromboses and/or recurrent fetal loss. The primary syndrome occurs in the absence of other autoimmune diseases such as systemic lupus erythematosus (SLE).

SYNONYMS: Antiphospholipid antibody syndrome; Hughes syndrome; Lupus anticoagulant syndrome.

DIFFERENTIAL DIAGNOSIS: SLE and related autoimmune disorders; Thrombophilic disorders.

SYMPTOMS AND SIGNS: The syndrome is a distinct entity from SLE and is generally associated with thrombosis rather than bleeding. The predominant manifestations are arterial or venous thromboses or recurrent fetal loss, particularly in the second trimester. Thrombocytopenia, autoimmune hemolytic anemia, livedo reticularis, aortic and mitral valve disease, transient cerebral ischemia, stroke, myocardial infarction, marantic endocarditis, peripheral vascular disease, transverse myelopathy or myelitis, multiple sclerosis–like syndrome, chorea, and migraine are associated manifestations. Venous thromboses occur twice as often as arterial events. Thrombosis of the placental vessels is implicated in causing obstetric complications, including spontaneous abortion, placental abruption, intrauterine growth retardation, and preeclampsia. Occasional patients with severe thrombocytopenia or associated coagulation factor deficiencies, especially prothrombin (factor II), are at risk of bleeding, particularly in the perioperative period.

ETIOLOGY/EPIDEMIOLOGY: The syndrome is an autoimmune disorder characterized by the production of aPL. The exact pathogenic mechanisms are unknown, but it is postulated that pathogenic aPLs might induce thrombosis by altering the function of vascular endothelial cells and the hemostatic system. The incidence in females may be slightly increased; the median age at presentation is 50 years. There is no known ethnic predilection.

DIAGNOSIS: Diagnosis requires the presence of the clinical manifestations described in addition to laboratory evidence of either lupus anticoagulant (LA), by coagulation based-tests, or anticardiolipin antibodies by immunologic tests, or both. Documenting persistence of aPL more than 6–12 weeks after initial detection is important, because their transient presence can accompany other conditions.

TREATMENT
Standard Therapies: Generally, patients with laboratory evidence of persistent aPL without clinical manifestations do not require specific treatment except for consideration of thrombosis prophylaxis at times of high risk. Patients with documented thrombotic manifestations may require anticoagulation or antiplatelet agents on a short-term or long-term basis; heparin or aspirin may be considered during pregnancy. Valvular heart disease may be severe and some patients may need valvular replacement surgery with appropriate perioperative monitoring. Thrombocytopenia is managed like immune thrombocytopenia and usually does not require intervention.

Investigational Therapies: Immunosuppressive drugs such as glucocorticoids and cytotoxic agents such as cyclophosphamide are under investigation. Intravenous gammaglobulin has been evaluated in the setting of pregnancy-related complications and catastrophic APS. Plasmapheresis has been tried in selected cases.

REFERENCES
Galve E, Ordi J, Barquinero J, Evangelista A, et al. Valvular heart disease in the primary antiphospholipid syndrome. *Ann Intern Med* 1992;116:293–298.

Hogan WJ, McBane RD, Santrach PJ, et al. Antiphospholipid syndrome and perioperative hemostatic management of cardiac valvular surgery. *Mayo Clin Proc* 2000;75:971–976.

Hughes GRV. The antiphospholipid syndrome: ten years on. *Lancet* 1993;342:341–344.

Italian Registry of Antiphospholipid Antibodies (IR-APA). Thrombosis and thrombocytopenia in antiphospholipid syndrome (idiopathic and secondary to SLE): first report from the Italian registry. *Haematologica* 1993;78:313–318.

Wilson WA, Gharavi AE, Koike T, et al. International consensus statement on preliminary classification criteria for definite antiphospholipid syndrome: report of an international workshop. *Arthritis Rheum* 1999;42:1309–1311.

RESOURCES
27, 250

2   Congenital Contractural Arachnodactyly

Maurice Godfrey, PhD

DEFINITION: Congenital contractural arachnodactyly (CCA) is characterized by a Marfan-like appearance with a tall, slender habitus in which arm span exceeds height. Contractures of major joints are present at birth in most patients.

SYNONYM: Beals syndrome.

DIFFERENTIAL DIAGNOSIS: Marfan syndrome; Stickler syndrome; Homocystinuria; Distal arthrogryposis.

SYMPTOMS AND SIGNS: Individuals with CCA typically have a marfanoid habitus; flexion contractures of multiple joints including elbows, knees, hips, and fingers; kyphoscoliosis (sometimes severe); muscular hypoplasia; and abnormal pinnae. Arachnodactyly is present in most patients. Most patients have "crumpled" ears that present as a folded upper helix of the external ear. Less frequent craniofacial abnormalities include mild micrognathia, high arched palate, scaphocephaly, brachycephaly, dolichocephaly, and frontal bossing. Contractures of major joints can be demonstrated at birth. Adducted thumbs and clubfoot may occur; bowed long bones and muscular hypoplasia are additional musculoskeletal findings. In most patients, contractures improve with time. Kyphosis/scoliosis is present in approximately half of patients; it begins as early as infancy and causes the greatest morbidity in CCA. Some individuals present with a more severe form of CCA known as severe/lethal CCA. In addition to the typical features of CCA, infants with severe/lethal CCA may have atrial or ventricular septal defects, interrupted aortic arch, single umbilical artery, duodenal or esophageal atresia, and intestinal malrotation.

ETIOLOGY/EPIDEMIOLOGY: CCA is inherited in an autosomal-dominant manner. It is caused by mutations in the *FBN2* gene located on chromosome 5q23-q31. There is no specific geographic or ethnic predilection. The prevalence is unknown, but appears to be less than that of Marfan syndrome.

DIAGNOSIS: The diagnosis of CCA is established by clinical findings.

TREATMENT

Standard Therapies: Management involves physical therapy—best instituted in childhood—for joint contractures to increase joint mobility and ameliorate the effects of muscle hypoplasia (usually calf muscles). As affected individuals age, spontaneous improvement in camptodactyly frequently occurs. If necessary, surgical release of contractures may be performed. Because aortic root dilatation has been observed in CCA and because of the difficulty in distinguishing CCA from Marfan syndrome, an echocardiogram should be performed. The kyphoscoliosis tends to be progressive, requiring bracing and/or surgical correction. Consultation with an orthopedist is encouraged. Because the severe/lethal form of CCA is so rare, no general recommendations exist, and defects need to be managed as they arise.

REFERENCES

Beals RK, Hecht F. Congenital contractural arachnodactyly. A heritable disorder of connective tissue. *J Bone Joint Surg [Am]* 1971;53:987–993.

Epstein CJ, Graham CB, Hodgkin WE, et al. Hereditary dysplasia of bone with kyphoscoliosis, contractures, and abnormally shaped ears. *J Pediatr* 1968;73:379–386.

Park ES, Putnam EA, Chitayat D, et al. Clustering of FBN2 mutations in patients with congenital contractural arachnodactyly indicates an important role of the domains encoded by exons 24 through 34 during human development. *Am J Med Genet* 1998;78:350–355.

Robinson PN, Godfrey M. The molecular genetics of Marfan syndrome and related microfibrillopathies. *J Med Genet* 2000;37:9–25.

Wang M, Clericuzio CL, Godfrey M. Familial occurrence of typical and severe lethal congenital contractural arachnodactyly caused by missplicing of exon 34 of fibrillin-2. *Am J Hum Genet* 1996;59:1027–1034.

RESOURCES

80, 257

3   Behçet Disease

Kenneth T. Calamia, MD

DEFINITION: Behçet disease is a chronic recurrent inflammatory condition characterized by mouth and genital ulcers, eye inflammation, and skin lesions.

SYNONYMS: Behçet syndrome; Adamantiades-Behçet syndrome; Morbus Behçet.

DIFFERENTIAL DIAGNOSIS: Crohn disease; Stevens-Johnson syndrome; Complex aphthosis; Mucous membrane pemphigoid; Lichen planus; Human immunodeficiency virus infection; Herpesvirus infection.

SYMPTOMS AND SIGNS: Oral aphthous ulcers are usually the first and most persistent feature. The buccal mucosa, tongue, or palate may be involved with single or multiple painful lesions, up to 1 cm in diameter, which heal in 1–3 weeks. Painful genital ulcers resembling oral lesions involve the scrotum, penis, labia, or vagina. Deep lesions may heal with scarring. Some patients have hypersensitivity of the skin to trauma. Small nodules or pustules may develop at sites of venipuncture. Many patients have spontaneous skin lesions, including erythema nodosum, acneform or papulopustular lesions, pyoderma, or Sweet lesions. Ocular inflammation may result in anterior uveitis, posterior uveitis, or retinal vasculitis. Recurrent eye involvement over a few years can result in partial or complete loss of vision. Joint swelling and pain, usually of knees and ankles, occurs in half of patients. Approximately one fourth of affected patients have large vessel manifestations including superficial or deep venous thrombosis, thrombosis of the vena cava or its branches, and/or aneurysms of the systemic or pulmonary circulations. Pulmonary emboli are rare, but aneurysms are apt to rupture. Single or multiple aphthous-like ulcers in the terminal ileum or colon may occur, as may aseptic meningitis or meningoencephalitis with focal infarcts of the brainstem. Symptoms of pseudotumor cerebri result from cerebral venous thrombosis.

ETIOLOGY/EPIDEMIOLOGY: The cause is unknown. Autoimmunity, perhaps triggered by exposure to certain viral or bacterial antigens, likely plays a role in the pathogenesis. Evidence exists of genetic susceptibility because of the high number of cases in certain populations. The disease is most prevalent in Turkey, other Eastern Mediterranean countries, the Middle East, and along the East Asian rim and is most commonly diagnosed in persons 25–35 years of age. Males are more severely affected. The male: female ratio is close to 1:1 in Eastern countries, but females are affected more often in the West.

DIAGNOSIS: The diagnosis is made clinically. The International Study Group has developed classification criteria that may serve as a guide. Laboratory studies may largely be normal, despite active inflammation, and biopsies of aphthous ulcers or skin lesions are nonspecific.

TREATMENT

Standard Therapies: Aphthous lesions are treated with topical or intralesional corticosteroids or dapsone. Colchicine, thalidomide, or methotrexate may be useful in treating mucocutaneous manifestations. Azathioprine may limit progression of ocular disease and improve mucosal ulcers, arthritis, and deep-vein thrombosis. Cyclosporine A is used to control uveitis. Combination treatment with cyclosporine A and azathioprine has been used when single agents fail. For uncontrolled ocular disease, central nervous system disease, and large vessel vasculitis, immunosuppression with chlorambucil or cyclophosphamide is used. Corticosteroids are useful in acute phases of the disease. Surgery is usually indicated for the treatment of systemic arterial aneurysms. Arterial vasculitis resulting in aneurysms of the systemic or pulmonary circulations should be treated with alkalating agents. If surgery is required, these agents are also necessary to minimize the high risk of anastomotic recurrences or continued disease.

Investigational Therapies: Interferon-α and anti–tumor necrosis factor agents are being investigated.

REFERENCES

Balabanova M, Calamia KT, Perniciaro C, et al. A study of the cutaneous manifestations of Behçet's disease in patients from the United States. *J Am Acad Dermatol* 1999;41:540–545.

Hamuryudan V, Özyazgan Y, Hizli N, et al. Azathioprine in Behçet's syndrome. *Arthritis Rheum* 1997;40:769–774.

International Study Group for Behçet's Disease. Criteria for diagnosis of Behçet's disease. *Lancet* 1990;335:1078–1080.

Sakane T, Takeno M, Suzuki N, et al. Behçet's disease. *N Engl J Med* 1999;341:1284–1291.

Sfakakis PP, Theodossiadis PG, Katsiari CG, et al. Effect of infliximab on sight-threatening panuveitis in Behçet's disease. *Lancet* 2001;358:295–296.

RESOURCES

28, 53

4   Mixed Cryoglobulinemia Syndrome Secondary to Hepatitis C Virus Infection

Milvia Casato, MD,
and Vincent Agnello, MD

DEFINITION: Mixed cryoglobulinemia syndrome secondary to hepatitis C virus (HCV) infection is a systemic vasculitis caused by the cold-precipitable HCV-associated immune complexes that consist of monoclonal (type II) or polyclonal (type III) IgM rheumatoid factor and polyclonal IgG.

SYNONYM: Essential mixed cryoglobulinemia.

DIFFERENTIAL DIAGNOSIS: Waldenstrom macroglobulinemia; Autoimmune diseases; Vasculitis.

SYMPTOMS AND SIGNS: Palpable purpura, usually limited to the lower extremities (Insert Fig. 1), is the hallmark of the disease, affecting more than 80% of patients. Meltzer triad (palpable purpura, arthralgias, and fatigue) occurs in approximately 50% of patients, and vasculitic symptoms and signs such as peripheral neuropathy and, less commonly, glomerulonephritis, central nervous system involvement, intestinal purpura, Raynaud phenomenon, and sicca syndrome occur variably. In virtually all patients, chronic hepatitis C that may lead to cirrhosis is present, particularly where there has been extensive immunosuppressive therapy. A minority of patients with type II cryoglobulinemia develop overt B-cell lymphoma.

ETIOLOGY/EPIDEMIOLOGY: Hepatitis C virus is the etiologic agent. Of patients with chronic HCV infection, 20%–50% have mixed cryoglobulinemia; however, only a minority of these patients, more commonly those with type II, have the clinical syndrome. The prevalence of symptomatic mixed cryoglobulinemia among HCV-infected patients is estimated to be 2%–5% in Italy and less than 1% in the United States.

DIAGNOSIS: The presence of vasculitis and the detection of mixed cryoglobulinemia and HCV infection establish the diagnosis. Cryoglobulins are assessed by placing the patient's serum, drawn and clotted at 37°C, at 4°C for 5–7 days. A white precipitate that redissolves on rewarming is diagnostic (Insert Fig. 2). Routine viral and antibody tests for HCV should be performed, because some patients can be seronegative and HCV can be sequestered in the cryoglobulins. Polymerase chain reaction assay for HCV should be performed on the cryoprecipitate when serum diagnostic test results for HCV are negative. In type II cryoglobulinemia, there is a characteristic pattern of complement activation involving the early components, particularly C4. Most patients have an elevated erythrocyte sedimentation rate and rheumatoid factor.

TREATMENT

Standard Therapies: The treatment of choice is antiviral agents, primarily interferon-α. Treatment of patients who do not meet criteria for hepatitis C therapy should be based on the severity of visceral involvement. The response of cryoglobulinemia parallels the virologic response; thus, effective protocols for treating chronic hepatitis C should be used for these patients, but the clearance of cryoglobulins as well as viremia are used for determining the end of therapy. Glucocorticoids or cyclophosphamide are contraindicated, although in patients with progressive, life-threatening, extrahepatic disease, these drugs are used despite the possibility of progression of hepatitis. Plasmapheresis can be used to treat acute disease-related events (e.g., the hyperviscosity syndrome, central nervous system vasculitis, or distal necroses).

REFERENCES

Agnello V. Mixed cryoglobulinemia and other extra hepatic manifestations of hepatitis C virus infection. In: Liang TJ, Hoofnagle JH, eds. *Hepatitis C.* New York: Academic, 2000:295.

Casato M, Agnello V, Pucillo LP, et al. Predictors of long-term response to high-dose interferon therapy in type II cryoglobulinemia associated with hepatitis C virus infection. *Blood* 1997;90:3865–3873.

Lamprecht P, Gause A, Gross WL. Cryoglobulinemic vasculitis. *Arthritis Rheum* 1999;42:2507–2516.

Meltzer M, Franklin EC, Elias K, et al. Cryoglobulinemia: a clinical and laboratory study. II. Cryoglobulins with rheumatoid factor activity. *Am J Med* 1966;40:837–856.

Monti G, Galli M, Invernizzi F, et al. Cryoglobulinemias: a multicentre study of the early clinical and laboratory manifestations of primary and secondary disease. GISC. Italian Group for the Study of Cryoglobulinemias. *Q J Med* 1995;88:115–126.

RESOURCES

27, 357

5   De Barsy Syndrome

Anthony J. Aldave, MD,
and Irving M. Raber, MD

DEFINITION: De Barsy syndrome is a progeroid syndrome associated with characteristic ocular, facial, skeletal, dermatologic, and neurologic abnormalities.

SYNONYM: De Barsy-Moens-Dierckx syndrome.

DIFFERENTIAL DIAGNOSIS: Other conditions associated with congenital corneal opacification (sclerocornea, congenital glaucoma, forceps-induced corneal trauma, corneal ulcer, mucopolysaccharidosis, Peters anomaly, and congenital hereditary endothelial dystrophy); Hutchinson-Gilford syndrome; Cockayne syndrome; Geroderma osteodysplastica; Cutis laxa; Wiedemann-Rautenstrauch syndrome.

SYMPTOMS AND SIGNS: Clinical features are generally present at birth. Ocular features include bilateral corneal opacification and cataracts. Facial signs include frontal bossing; midfacial hypoplasia; and large, dysplastic ears. Skeletal features include short stature, hyperextensibility of small joints, and multiple joint dislocations and subluxations. Dermatologic signs include cutis laxa and thin transparent skin with prominent superficial veins. Neurologic features include muscular hypotonia, brisk deep tendon reflexes, mental retardation, developmental delay, and athetoid movements.

ETIOLOGY/EPIDEMIOLOGY: The syndrome is believed to be inherited in an autosomal-recessive manner. Skin biopsy specimens demonstrate sparse, short or fragmented, irregular elastic fibers. Although many of the clinical features in this syndrome may be related to a disorder of elastogenesis, other features such as mental retardation, muscular hypotonia, and cataracts are not easily explained in this way. Abnormalities in collagen also may play a role in the phenotypic features of this disorder. Only 20 cases have been reported worldwide, and all patients described were infants or children at diagnosis. Life expectancy is unknown, although the oldest living patient in published reports was 24 years of age.

DIAGNOSIS: The unique constellation of clinical features is sufficient to establish the diagnosis. Demonstration of elastic fiber abnormalities in skin biopsy specimens may be used to confirm the diagnosis.

TREATMENT
Standard Therapies: Treatment is focused on managing the sequelae of the multisystem abnormalities. Referral to an ophthalmologist is indicated for the diagnosis and treatment of congenital cataracts or corneal opacification, to an orthopedist for evaluation and management of joint deformities, and to a neurologist for assessment of neurologic deficits. Physical therapy and special education will optimize affected patients' functional and intellectual development.

REFERENCES
Aldave AJ, Eagle RC, Streeten BW, et al. Congenital corneal opacification in De Barsy syndrome. *Arch Ophthalmol* 2001;119: 285–288.
De Barsy AM, Moens E, Dierckx L. Dwarfism, oligophrenia and degeneration of the elastic tissue in skin and cornea. A new syndrome? *Helv Paediatr Acta* 1968;3:305–313.
Karnes PS, Shamban AT, Olsen DR, et al. De Barsy syndrome: report of a case, literature review, and elastin gene expression studies of the skin. *Am J Med Genet* 1992;42:29–34.
Kunze J, Majewski F, Montgomery P, et al. De Barsy syndrome—an autosomal recessive, progeroid syndrome. *Eur J Pediatr* 1985;144:348–354.
Pontz BF, Zepp F, Stoss H. Biochemical, morphological and immunological findings in a patient with a cutis laxa–associated inborn disorder (De Barsy syndrome). *Eur J Pediatr* 1986;145:428–434.

RESOURCES
257, 351

6   Eosinophilia-Myalgia Syndrome

Joan Y. Li, MD

DEFINITION: Eosinophilia-myalgia syndrome (EMS) is a scleroderma-like multisystem disorder of undetermined etiology characterized by the acute onset of intense debilitating myalgias and eosinophilia greater than or equal to $1,000/mm^3$.

SYNONYMS: Tryptophan syndrome; L-tryptophan syndrome.

DIFFERENTIAL DIAGNOSIS: Eosinophilic fasciitis; Toxic oil syndrome; Scleroderma; Fibromyalgia.

SYMPTOMS AND SIGNS: Eosinophilia-myalgia syndrome is an inflammatory and fibrosing disorder of connective tissue. Patients present with symptoms including severe fatigue, debilitating myalgia, and often, weakness and myositis. A high eosinophil count is associated with the disorder. Scleroderma-like skin changes including morphea and rash are common, as are paraesthesias and peripheral neuropathies. Patients may present with dyspnea or cough, fever, abdominal pain, mouth ulcers, extremely painful muscle cramps, edema, hepatitis, encephalopathy, and myocarditis. Although some patients with milder disease may recover completely, others progress to chronic, lifelong illness, with permanent cutaneous abnormalities and/or neuromuscular dysfunction.

ETIOLOGY/EPIDEMIOLOGY: More than 1,500 cases, including 27 deaths, were reported to the Centers for Disease Control and Prevention (CDC) in the first year after definition of the syndrome. Of these, 83% were female, and 96% had ingested the dietary supplement L-tryptophan preceding the onset of symptoms. Patients ranged in age from 4 to 85 years (median 48 years). Epidemic EMS, first reported in the United States in 1989, has been linked to ingestion of L-tryptophan, which was contaminated with trace amounts of chemical impurities. Sporadic cases linked to lansoprazole and total parenteral nutrition containing tryptophan have also been reported. L-tryptophan–containing products were recalled by the U.S. Food and Drug Administration by early 1990, with the exception of some infant formulas, protein supplements, and intravenous and oral nutrient solutions, according to the CDC. Sporadic cases still occur, however, and EMS remains a CDC-reportable disease entity. The pathogenesis is uncertain.

DIAGNOSIS: The disorder is diagnosed clinically. Biopsies of affected organs or tissues show a microangiopathic process with diffuse inflammatory response in connective tissue. Antinuclear antibody, aldolase, and creatine kinase are elevated but nonspecific. The CDC defines EMS as severe debilitating myalgia associated with eosinophilia greater than or equal to $1,000/mm^3$.

TREATMENT
Standard Therapies: No effective treatment is known; however, corticosteroids and methotrexate may be beneficial.

REFERENCES
Centers for Disease Control and Prevention. Update: EMS associated with ingestion of L-tryptophan—United States, through August 24, 1990. *MMWR* 1990;39:587–589. Report is also accessible online at *www.cdc.gov/mmwr//preview/mmwrhtml/00001738.htm.*

De Oliveira JS, Auerbach SB, Sullivan KM, et al. Fatal EMS in a marrow transplant patient attributed to TPN with a solution containing tryptophan. *Bone Marrow Transplant* 1993;11:163–167.

Smith JD, Chang KL, Gums JG. Possible lansoprazole-induced eosinophilic syndrome. *Ann Pharmacother* 1998;32:196–200.

RESOURCES
89, 360

7   Eosinophilic Fasciitis

Joan Y. Li, MD

DEFINITION: Eosinophilic fasciitis (EF) is an inflammatory disorder involving the deep muscles, with thickening of fascia resulting in a peau d'orange appearance of overlying skin. A peripheral eosinophilia is present.

SYNONYMS: Shulman syndrome; Diffuse fasciitis with eosinophilia.

DIFFERENTIAL DIAGNOSIS: Scleroderma; Chronic carcinoid syndrome; Toxic oil syndrome; Eosinophilia-myalgia syndrome; Scleroderma-like syndromes (polyvinyl chloride exposure, bleomycin exposure).

SYMPTOMS AND SIGNS: Patients with EF report tenderness or pain, typically of the arms or legs, often following strenuous activity. The overlying skin rapidly becomes indurated and develops a puckered, woody, or peau d'orange appearance, and a groove sign or furrow can be seen on elevating the affected arm or leg, representing thickened fascia. Nailbed capillaries are normal. Carpel tunnel syndrome and flexion contractures can develop. Arthritis develops in approximately 40% of affected individuals.

ETIOLOGY/EPIDEMIOLOGY: Eosinophilic fasciitis occurs predominantly in men ages 30–60 years, with a male:female ratio of 2:1. Symptoms generally resolve on their own over several years, with recurrences being rare. The etiology of the disorder is unknown.

DIAGNOSIS: A diagnosis based on history and examination can be confirmed by a full-thickness skin biopsy, showing characteristic diffuse mononuclear inflammation and fibrosis of the deep fascia. Antinuclear antibody and RF are usually negative. Peripheral eosinophilia, hypergammaglobulinemia, and an elevated sedimentation rate are present in most patients.

TREATMENT
Standard Therapies: Prednisone is the initial treatment; resolution occurs slowly over several years. One half of all patients, however, remain permanently scarred with chronic skin changes.

REFERENCES
Giardin R, et al. T-cell ALL following Shulman's syndrome (eosinophilic fasciitis). *Hematol Cell Ther* [electronic edition]. 1996;38:1.

Graham, BS. Eosinophilic fasciitis. *www.emedicine.com/cgi-bin/foxweb.exe/showsection@d:/em/ga?book=derm&topicid=119.*

Pathology of EF. *dermatology.wustl.edu/3-98a.html.*

RESOURCES
27, 89

8   Felty Syndrome

Henrik J. Ditzel, MD, PhD

DEFINITION: Felty syndrome is an extraarticular manifestation of rheumatoid arthritis, involving neutropenia.

DIFFERENTIAL DIAGNOSIS: Neutropenia caused by other autoimmune or nonautoimmune (infections or drug induced) mechanism/diseases.

SYMPTOMS AND SIGNS: Rheumatoid arthritis–associated symptoms include joint swelling, stiffness, pain, and deformity; rheumatoid nodules; vasculitis; fatigue; general malaise; loss of appetite; weight loss (10%–15% of body weight); pallor; and a burning sensation in the eyes and/or discharge. The neutropenia-associated symptoms include recurrent bacterial or fungal infections and yellowish brown pigmentation of the skin (particularly exposed extremities). The most common infections include mucosal and cutaneous inflammations, such as gingivitis, cellulitis, furunculosis, abscesses, pneumonia, and septicemia. The neutropenia mainly occurs later in life (40–70 years) and is chronic. The type of bacterial infection depends on the severity of the neutropenia and the age of the patient. As a consequence of the lack of neutrophils, the inflammation lacks the normal clinical signs of fluctuance, induration, and exudate. Severe neutropenia may result in fulminant bacterial infections, including deep-tissue infection of the lungs, liver, or sinuses. Secondary Sjögren syndrome, lymphopenia, thrombocytopenia, anemia, leg ulcers, and pleuritis also may be associated with Felty syndrome. Felty syndrome was classically described to include splenomegaly, but it is not an essential feature of the disorder.

ETIOLOGY/EPIDEMIOLOGY: The cause of neutropenia involves several humoral and cellular immune mechanisms. Both IgG antibodies that specifically bind to the surface of neutrophils or neutrophil precursors and immune complex present in the circulation, which can bind to neutrophils through their Fc receptors, may lead to increased margination, destruction, and/or removal of neutrophils. T-cell suppression on normal bone marrow granulopoiesis may result in impaired production of neutrophils. The incidence of the disease is less than 1% of patients with rheumatoid arthritis. Women are affected 3 times as often as men. All ethnic groups are affected, but the disease is rare in blacks. A strong association with particular HLA-DRB1 class II alleles has been observed.

DIAGNOSIS: The diagnosis should be based on the findings of frequent infections combined with symptoms of rheumatoid arthritis. Laboratory analyses include hematologic cell counts to assess the neutrophil count, but also to determine whether general cytopenia or other hematologic abnormalities exist. Generally, mild neutropenia is defined as neutrophil count of 1.0 to 1.5×10^9/L, moderate neutropenia as 0.5 to 1.0×10^9/L, and severe neutropenia as less than 0.5×10^9/L. Bone marrow aspiration and biopsies are indicated to determine precursor frequency. The serum should be tested for serum-reactive protein, antinuclear antibodies, rheumatoid factor, antielongation factor 1A antibodies, antineutrophil cell surface antibodies, antineutrophil cytoplasmic antibodies, complement levels, and liver enzymes. Because neutropenia can be observed during viral infections such as hepatitis, HIV-1, parvovirus, and malaria, patients should be tested for these viruses.

TREATMENT
Standard Therapies: Therapy of autoimmune neutropenia is based on the severity of the symptoms. The overall treatment strategy aims at preventing infections rather than normalizing the neutrophil count. Granulocyte colony-stimulating factor (G-CSF) is the treatment of choice. Exogenous administration of G-CSF stimulates growth and differentiation of neutrophil precursors within the bone marrow. After an increase in neutrophil count is observed, low-dose methotrexate therapy may be added to maintain stable neutrophil levels without continuous administration of G-CSF. Splenectomy should be considered in those patients who do not respond to either G-CSF or methotrexate treatment, or in whom side effects may be too severe. In a few patients, combination of G-CSF and cyclophosphamide has resulted in normalization of neutrophil counts, where G-CSF alone had no effect. Methotrexate also may be used as the primary therapeutic approach. Therapies aimed at treating the underlying rheumatoid arthritis include D-penicillamine, gold salts, azathioprine, and cyclosporine. Appropriate antibiotic treatment of the recurrent infections also is needed.

REFERENCES
Goldberg J, Pinals RS. Felty's syndrome. *Semin Arthritis Rheum* 1980;10:52–65.
Rashba EJ, Rowe JM, Packman CH. Treatment of the neutropenia of Felty syndrome. *Blood Rev* 1996;10:177–184.
Starkebaum G. Use of colony-stimulating factors in the treatment of neutropenia associated with collagen vascular disease. *Curr Opin Hematol* 1997;4:196–199.
Starkebaum G, Singer JW, Arend WP. Humoral and cellular immune mechanism of neutropenia in patients with Felty's syndrome. *Clin Exp Immunol* 1980;39:307–314.

RESOURCES
53, 351

9 Diffuse Idiopathic Skeletal Hyperostosis (Forestier Disease)

Nancy E. Epstein, MD

DEFINITION: Diffuse idiopathic skeletal hyperostosis (DISH) is a rheumatologic disease characterized by exuberant ossification observed within ligaments throughout the body, with a predilection for the anterior longitudinal ligament of the spine. The disorder may coexist with ossification of the anterior longitudinal ligament (OALL), posterior longitudinal ligament (OPLL), and yellow ligament (OYL).

SYNONYM: Forestier disease.

DIFFERENTIAL DIAGNOSIS: Ankylosing spondylitis; Paget disease; OALL.

SYMPTOMS AND SIGNS: The disorder is prevalent in men over 60 years of age and is often characterized by dysphagia, spinal cord compression, and neural entrapment. Patients may be subject to sleep apnea. Increased pathologic motion appears to contribute to the progression of the disease. Patients often complain of a generalized stiffness, accompanied by diffuse radicular pain (root origin), or myelopathic (cord compressive) complaints. There is often a generalized decreased range of spinal motion involving the cervical, thoracic, and lumbar regions. Any type of surgical procedure may result in quadriplegia or paraplegia, and thorough knowledge of the extent of accompanying spinal disease is critical in operative planning.

ETIOLOGY/EPIDEMIOLOGY: A polygenetic mode of inheritance, perhaps autosomal dominant, appears to link DISH with the different ossification syndromes. The genetic locus of OPLL resides at site 6p, close to the HLA locus. When both HLA haplotypes appear in probands of patients with OPLL, they exhibit both radiographic and clinical evidence of the disease.

DIAGNOSIS: The disorder is radiographically typified by contiguous calcification of the anterolateral spinal vertebral bodies. This may be seen in conjunction with ossification at other spinal ligamentous sites, and can be difficult to differentiate from OALL. Alternatively, OALL is characterized by progressive hypertrophy, cartilaginous infiltration, and ossification of the anterior longitudinal ligament. Noncontrast CT, two-dimensional and three-dimensional CT reconstruction, and myelo-CT examinations directly demonstrate the calcification associated with DISH or ossification attributed to OALL, OPLL, or OYL.

TREATMENT

Standard Therapies: Prophylactic resection of DISH in asymptomatic patients may occasionally be necessary for those who are about to undergo general anesthesia for unrelated problems. Patients older than 65 years with symptomatic DISH or OALL (dysphagia), and OPLL (radiculopathy, myelopathy) in the presence of kyphosis, may be managed with anterior resection of DISH and simultaneous anterior corpectomy with fusion. Other patients presenting with DISH and severe multilevel OPLL may require anterior resection of DISH followed by multilevel anterior corpectomy with fusion and posterior wiring and fusion with halo application. If patients have asymptomatic DISH but are myelopathic from diffuse multilevel OPLL, when the cervical lordosis is well preserved, a cervical laminectomy or laminectomy with posterior wiring and fusion may provide adequate symptomatic relief.

REFERENCES

Epstein NE. Circumferential surgery for the management of cervical ossification of the posterior longitudinal ligament. *J Spinal Disord* 1998;11:200–207.

Epstein NE, Hollingsworth R. Ossification of the anterior longitudinal ligament (OALL) contributing to dysphagia: a case report. *J Neurosurg (Spine 2)* 1999;90:261–265.

Epstein NE, Hollingsworth R. Simultaneous cervical diffuse idiopathic skeletal hyperostosis and ossification of the posterior longitudinal ligament resulting in dysphagia or myelopathy in two geriatric North Americans. *Surg Neurol* 2000;53:427–431.

Mata S, Fortin PR, Fitzcharles MA, et al. A controlled study of diffuse idiopathic skeletal hyperostosis. Clinical features and functional status. *Medicine (Baltimore)* 1997;76:104–117.

McCafferty RR, Harrison MJ, Tamas LB, et al. Ossification of the anterior longitudinal ligament and Forestier's disease: an analysis of seven cases. *J Neurosurg* 1996;85:524–525.

RESOURCES

53, 351

10   Graft-Versus-Host Disease

William J. Murphy, PhD

DEFINITION: Graft-versus-host disease (GVHD) occurs when donor immunocompetent cells are placed into genetically disparate immunocompromised recipients. The disease is a major cause of morbidity after bone marrow transplantation (BMT), even with siblings matched at the human leukocyte antigen (HLA) locus. The principal mediators of GVHD are donor T cells, and multiple organs are ultimately affected including the skin, liver, and gastrointestinal tract.

SYMPTOMS AND SIGNS: The two forms of GVHD are acute and chronic. Acute GVHD manifests as early as 2–6 weeks after BMT, although a more severe form of GVHD, hyperacute GVHD, can occur within the first week after BMT. The skin is the most common organ affected; a pruritic maculopapular rash involving the neck, ears, and shoulders occurs. In severe cases, generalized erythroderma with bullous formation can occur. Liver manifestations occur as jaundice. Gastrointestinal involvement occurs in the form of diarrhea (which is often bloody), nausea, vomiting, and severe abdominal pain. Chronic GVHD is more difficult to diagnose but also involves the skin, liver, gut, and respiratory tract. The symptoms of chronic GVHD appear as "autoimmune-like" in appearance and this form is believed to have a different mode of pathogenesis than acute GVHD. Skin symptoms also include a rash and dryness of the eyes and mouth. Weight loss can occur. Pulmonary function can be affected and is compounded by immunosuppression, leaving the patient susceptible to opportunistic infections.

ETIOLOGY/EPIDEMIOLOGY: Graft-versus-host disease is affected by many variables, including the extent of genetic disparity between the donor and recipient, the type and extent of cytoreductive conditioning, the presence of T cells in the donor graft, the age of the recipient, and the use of prophylaxis. If prophylaxis is not used, the incidence of GVHD can approach 100%. Acute GVHD can occur in up to 50% of patients who receive an allogeneic HLA-matched BMT. The extent of donor/host histocompatibility is one of the biggest risk factors, with each HLA-locus mismatch increasing GVHD likelihood. The advent of using HLA-matched unrelated donors has led to an increase in GVHD (up to 70%).

TREATMENT

Standard Therapies: Prevention is the best form of treatment. Prophylaxis after BMT is widely used; despite this, acute GVHD can occur in 10%–50% of patients. Common interventions include steroids, with methylprednisolone being the first choice (2 mg/kg/day). CsA is used, as well as antithymocyte globulin.

Investigational Therapies: Removal of the donor T cells will prevent GVHD but also impairs graft-versus-tumor responses and increases the risk for marrow graft failure. Although systemic immunosuppression remains the primary treatment for GVHD, therapies are being investigated to alter the extent of donor T-cell reactivity in the recipient. Inducing anergy of donor T cells through the blockade of immune costimulatory molecules is being investigated as well. Cytokine antagonists are also being evaluated, and promoting T helper 2-type responses is being attempted to reduce acute GVHD. Gene therapy is also being assessed.

REFERENCES

Goker H, Haznedaroglu IC, Chao NJ. Acute graft-versus-host disease: pathobiology and management. *Exp Hematol* 2001;29: 259–277.

Murphy WJ, Blazar BR. New strategies for preventing graft-versus-host disease. *Curr Opin Immunol* 1999;11:509–512.

Vogelsang GB. How I treat chronic graft-versus-host disease. *Blood* 2001;97:1196–1201.

RESOURCES

81, 357

---

11   Hajdu-Cheney Syndrome

Virginia V. Michels, MD

DEFINITION: Hajdu-Cheney syndrome is a multisystem disorder characterized by acroosteolysis, skull deformities, facial anomalies, and osteoporosis. Birth defects such as cleft palate, clubfoot deformity, and congenital heart defect may also be present.

DIFFERENTIAL DIAGNOSIS: Other causes of acroosteolysis; Lysosomal storage diseases; Multiple congenital anomaly syndromes.

SYMPTOMS AND SIGNS: Common features include acroosteolysis of distal phalanges, broad stubby fingers, short stature, dolichocephaly, high or cleft palate, long philtrum, micrognathia, thick coarse hair, prominent eyebrows, basilar invaginations of the skull, hydrocephalus, wide cranial sutures, cervical spine anomalies, short neck, low-set ears, conductive hearing loss, early loss of dentition, kyphosis, scoliosis, osteoporosis, fractures, gross motor delays, joint laxity or dislocations, clubfeet, hypospadius, cryptorchidism, hernias, congenital heart defects, glomerulocystic kidneys, and normal intellect or, less frequently, mild mental subnormality. Headaches, upper airway obstruction, and vocal cord paralysis may develop. Signs and symptoms occur in variable combinations. The hallmark of the condition, acroosteolysis, may not manifest radiographically until later in life.

ETIOLOGY/EPIDEMIOLOGY: The incidence of the disease is unknown. It is transmitted in an autosomal-dominant manner, with most cases sporadic and presumed to be new mutations of an unknown gene defect. It occurs in both sexes.

DIAGNOSIS: Diagnosis is based on clinical findings, along with serial skeletal imaging.

TREATMENT
Standard Therapies: Surgical correction should be done when indicated for hydrocephalus, cord syrinx, clubfeet, congenital heart defect, and cleft palate. Hearing aids and oxygen for sleep apnea should be used as needed, as should dental care and treatment for osteoporosis.

REFERENCES
Cheney WD. Acro-osteolyses. *AJR* 1965;94:595.
Crifasi PA, Patterson MC, Bonde D, et al. Severe Hajdu-Cheney syndrome with upper airway obstruction. *Am J Med Genet* 1997;70:261–266.
Fryns JP, Stinckens C, Feenstra L. Vocal cord paralysis and cystic kidney disease in Hadju-Cheney syndrome. *Clin Genet* 1997;51:271–274.
Greenfield GB, ed. *Radiology of bone diseases*, 4th ed. Philadelphia: JB Lippincott, 1986.
Hajdu N, Kauntze R. Cranio-skeletal dysplasias. *Br J Radiol* 1948;21:42–48.

RESOURCES
257, 360

---

12   Hyper-IgE Syndrome

Christa S. Zerbe, MS, FNP,
and Steven M. Holland, MD

DEFINITION: Hyper-IgE syndrome is a primary immunodeficiency characterized by eczema, recurrent skin and lung infections, and abnormally elevated serum IgE. In addition, individuals with hyper-IgE syndrome often have a characteristic facial appearance, failure to shed baby teeth, recurrent fractures, scoliosis, and hyperextensibility.

SYNONYM: Job syndrome.

DIFFERENTIAL DIAGNOSIS: Atopic dermatitis.

SYMPTOMS AND SIGNS: Many affected individuals present in early infancy with moderate to severe eczema. Other manifestations include elevated serum IgE levels from birth and recurrent *Staphylococcus aureus* infections of the skin and lungs. Pneumonias often leave pneumatoceles; the resulting cavities predispose individuals to infection with fungi or *Pseudomonas*. Recurrent oral and vaginal thrush and fingernail involvement with yeast often start early in life. Eventually, common characteristic facial features develop in all individuals with the disease: broad nasal bridge and tip, prominent forehead, deep-set eyes, facial asymmetry, and thick facial skin. The primary teeth are not shed. Bone fractures may occur with minimal trauma; osteoporosis is typically associated. Hyperextensibility and scoliosis are also common.

ETIOLOGY/EPIDEMIOLOGY: This is a genetic disorder that occurs sporadically, in autosomal-dominant and possibly autosomal-recessive patterns. The gene(s) involved are under investigation. The frequency of the disorder is unknown.

DIAGNOSIS: The IgE level is typically greater than 2,000 IU/mL and may be greater than 50,000 IU/mL. Approximately 20% of patients have their IgE levels drop near or into the normal range in adulthood. Pneumatoceles are common and helpful in diagnosing the disorder. A scoring system has been developed and published to aid in making the diagnosis.

TREATMENT
Standard Therapies: Most experts use prophylactic antibiotics against staphylococci (e.g., dicloxacillin, trimethoprim-sulfamethoxazole), and many patients require treatment for candidiasis (e.g., fluconazole or itraconazole). Patients remain at high risk for pneumonia, and it is im-

portant to make a microbiologic diagnosis. Eczema is usually treated topically.

Investigational Therapies: Interferon gamma has been used but does not offer any clear benefits.

REFERENCES

Grimbacher B, Holland SM, Gallin JI, et al. Hyper-IgE syndrome with recurrent infections—an autosomal dominant multisystem disorder. *N Engl J Med* 1999;340:692–702.

Grimbacher B, Schaffer AA, Holland SM, et al. Genetic linkage of hyper-IgE syndrome to chromosome 4. *Am J Hum Genet* 1999;65:735–744.

O'Connell AC, Puck JM, Grimbacher B, et al. Delayed eruption of permanent teeth in hyperimmunoglobulinemia E recurrent infection syndrome. *Oral Surg Oral Med Oral Pathol Oral Radiol Endod* 2000;89:177–185.

RESOURCE

93

---

13   Common Variable Immunodeficiency

Roger H. Kobayashi, MD

DEFINITION: Common variable immunodeficiency (CVID) is a heterogeneous group of diseases characterized by recurrent bacterial infections, decreased levels of immunoglobulins, and poor antibody function.

SYNONYM: Common variable hypogammaglobulinemia.

DIFFERENTIAL DIAGNOSIS: AIDS; Hyper-IgM syndrome; Malabsorption syndrome; X-linked agammaglobulinemia.

SYMPTOMS AND SIGNS: Patients may present at any age, but most commonly in the second or third decade of life. Although recurrent sinopulmonary infections with encapsulated bacteria are characteristic, clinical manifestations may be protean. Chronic malabsorption syndrome with associated lactose intolerance, protein-losing enteropathy, villus abnormalities, or steatorrhea may confuse or delay proper diagnosis. Nodular lymphoid hyperplasia is frequent. The incidence of inflammatory bowel disease is increased, and gastrointestinal infection with a variety of organisms including giardia lamblia, cryptosporidium, and enteropathogens is common. Patients are unusually susceptible to herpes simplex infection. Autoimmune disorders include dermatomyositis-like syndrome, lupus, arthritis, immunocytopenias, pernicious anemia, and chronic active hepatitis. Malignancies are markedly increased in older patients. Reticuloendothelial and gastric cancers are common.

ETIOLOGY/EPIDEMIOLOGY: The molecular defect(s) is unknown. Impaired B-cell differentiation and function appear to be the primary abnormality in CVID, with B cells failing to mature adequately into immunoglobulin-secreting plasma cells. More than 5,000 cases have been reported in the United States.

DIAGNOSIS: Serum immunoglobulins are decreased and antibody function is absent or depressed. IgG levels rarely exceed 300 mg/dL. Most patients have normal lymphocyte subsets, but some have elevated CD8 subsets, resulting in abnormally low CD4:CD8 ratios. Up to one half of patients have depressed T-cell proliferative responses or decreased cytokine production.

TREATMENT

Standard Therapies: The mainstay of therapy includes infusion of intravenous immune globulin (IVIG) at doses ranging from 400 to 800 mg/kg every 3–4 weeks in conjunction with antibiotics when indicated. Patients with chronic bronchitis or bronchiectasis should be treated aggressively with antibiotics; those with chronic diarrhea should be examined for giardia or cryptosporidium and treated appropriately. Patients with elevated CD8 levels and splenomegaly may respond less favorably to IVIG. Older patients especially should be monitored vigilantly for autoimmune and malignant diseases.

Investigational Therapies: Natural human IL-2 and polyethylene glycol–conjugated recombinant human IL-2 have been explored as have various B-cell growth or activation factors.

REFERENCES

Buckley RH. Immunodeficiency diseases. *JAMA* 1992;268:2797–2806.

Cunningham-Rundles C, Bodian C. Common variable immunodeficiency: clinical and immunological features of 248 patients. *Clin Immunol* 1999;92:34–48.

Cunningham-Rundles C, Kazbay K, Zhou Z, et al. Immunologic effects of low-dose polyethylene-conjugated recombinant human interleukin-2 in common variable immunodeficiency. *J Interferon Cytokine Res* 1995;15:269–276.

Elenitoba-Johnson KS, Jaffe E. Lymphoproliferative disorders associated with congenital immunodeficiencies. *Semin Diagn Pathol* 1997;14:35–47.

Strober W, Eisenstein E, Jaffe E, et al. New insights into common variable immunodeficiency. *Ann Intern Med* 1993;118:720–730.

RESOURCE
218

14   Severe Combined Immunodeficiency

Stefan Feske, MD

DEFINITION: Severe combined immunodeficiencies (SCID) are a group of congenital immune disorders caused by failed or impaired development and/or function of T-lymphocytes, characterized by frequent, often opportunistic infections.

DIFFERENTIAL DIAGNOSIS: Graft-versus-host disease; Neonatal HIV infection; Reticular dysgenesis; Wiskott-Aldrich syndrome; Ataxia telangiectasia; Omenn syndrome; Di-George syndrome; Hyper-IgM syndrome; X-linked agammaglobulinemia.

SYMPTOMS AND SIGNS: The first symptoms generally occur when the affected infant is around 2–3 months of age and are predominantly due to infections that are often opportunistic. Mucocutaneous candidiasis, persistent respiratory tract infections including *Pneumocystis carinii* pneumonia (PCP), and localized or systemic bacterial infections frequently occur. Growth and weight gain typically lag behind normal development as part of a general failure to thrive, often associated with intractable diarrhea. Infections with herpes viruses as well as measles, adenovirus, and respiratory syncytial virus are common. Lethal infections after vaccination with live measles, smallpox, and bacille Calmette-Guérin vaccines have occurred. Infants with SCID are also at high risk for developing graft-versus-host disease. Untreated, infants with SCID usually die in the first years of life.

ETIOLOGY/EPIDEMIOLOGY: Severe combined immunodeficiencies occur in 1 in 50,000 to 100,000 live births with consanguinity often present in the family history. Boys are three times as likely as girls to be affected because the most common form is X linked (X-SCID). It is caused by mutations in the common g chain (cg) of the interleukin 2 (IL-2), IL-4, IL-7, IL-9, and IL-15 receptor on T and B cells. All other known forms of SCID result from au-

tosomal-recessive inheritance or occur spontaneously. Genes mutated include two enzymes of purine metabolism, adenosine desaminase and purine nucleotide phosphorylase, and the recombination-associated genes *RAG1* and *RAG2*.

DIAGNOSIS: On clinical examination, lymph nodes, tonsils, and spleen are hypoplastic or absent. The rudimentary thymus is absent on chest radiography. Total lymphocyte counts are generally low, and flow cytometric measurements show that CD3$^+$ T cells are frequently low or absent. Diagnosis requires assessment of T-cell function. *In vitro* proliferation tests of peripheral blood mononuclear cells or T cells show a decreased proliferative response to antigen-specific, antigen receptor, mitogenic, or allogeneic stimuli.

TREATMENT
Standard Therapies: Symptomatic treatment includes prevention of infections using careful hygiene, isolation of the patients and PCP prophylaxis, intravenous immunoglobulin infusions, and intravenous antibiotics in cases of bacterial infections. Bone marrow transplantation and peripheral blood stem cell transplantation are the standard therapies for all forms of SCID and should be performed as soon as possible after diagnosis. Patients with SCID who are adenosine desaminase deficient have undergone successful gene therapy in combination with regular injections of polyethylene glycol–conjugated ADA.

Investigational Therapies: Two patients with X-SCID have been successfully treated by gene therapy alone.

REFERENCES
Buckley RH. Primary immunodeficiency diseases due to defects in lymphocytes. *N Engl J Med* 2000;343:1313–1324.

Cavazzana-Calvo M, Hacein-Bey S, Basile CD, et al. Gene therapy of human severe combined immunodeficiency (SCID)-X1 disease. *Science* 2000;288:669–672.

Ochs HD, Smith CIE, Puck JM. *Primary immunodeficiency diseases.* New York: Oxford University Press, 1999.

Patel DD, Gooding ME, Parrott RE, et al. Thymic function after hematopoietic stem-cell transplantation for the treatment of severe combined immunodeficiency. *N Engl J Med* 2000;342: 1325–1332.

Rosen F, Eibl M, Roifman C, et al. Primary immunodeficiency diseases: report of an IUIS scientific committee. *Clin Exp Immunol* 1999;118(suppl 1):1–28.

RESOURCES

193, 359

15   Kawasaki Disease

Raymond C. Shields, MD

DEFINITION: Kawasaki disease (KD) is an acute febrile multisystem vasculitis disorder of unknown etiology. It predominantly affects young children and is the most common cause of acquired childhood heart disease in developed countries.

SYNONYMS: Mucocutaneous lymph node syndrome; Lymphocutaneous syndrome.

DIFFERENTIAL DIAGNOSIS: Infantile periarteritis nodosa; Nonspecific exanthema; Streptococcal staphylococcus scarlatiniform eruptions; Measles; Infectious mononucleosis; Juvenile rheumatoid arthritis; Leptospirosis; Stevens-Johnson syndrome; Toxic shock syndrome; Drug reaction; Rocky Mountain spotted fever.

SYMPTOMS AND SIGNS: The clinical course of KD typically has three phases. The acute febrile phase is characterized by fever, bilateral bulbar conjunctival injection, oropharyngeal mucosal erythema, swelling and erythema of the hands and feet, generalized erythematous polymorphous rash, and lymphadenopathy. In the subacute phase, digital desquamation of skin, polyarticular sterile arthritis, cardiovascular manifestations, and thrombocytosis are apparent. The convalescent stage is characterized by an elevated sedimentation rate. Of patients with KD, 30% have cardiovascular disease. Multisystem vasculitis with a predilection for coronary arteries accounts for most of the morbidity and mortality of KD. Other cardiovascular manifestations include pancarditis, valvular heart disease, congestive heart failure, and arrhythmia from atrioventricular conduction system inflammation.

ETIOLOGY/EPIDEMIOLOGY: Kawasaki disease is believed to be caused by an infection, but no clear etiologic agent has been identified. It has a worldwide distribution with no rural or urban proclivity. Most (80%) cases occur in children younger than 4, with a male:female ratio of 1.5:1. The average annual incidence in the United States is 1.1 cases per 100,000 children younger than 5 years.

DIAGNOSIS: Five of six clinical criteria are needed for the diagnosis, including (a) fever of at least 5 days' duration, (b) polymorphous exanthema, (c) bilateral conjunctival injection, (d) oropharyngeal changes, (e) changes in extremities and transverse fingernail grooves, and (f) cervical lymphadenopathy. KD is characterized by clinical laboratory findings of leukocytosis, thrombocytosis, elevated acute phase reactants, and pyuria. Because atypical presentations are frequent and infants have a greater risk of coronary artery aneurysms, the diagnosis should be suspected in cases that do not necessarily meet the diagnostic criteria. Echocardiography has demonstrated high sensitivity and specificity for proximal coronary artery aneurysms. Coronary angiography remains the gold standard in assessing the entire epicardial artery and the nature of complications.

TREATMENT
Standard Therapies: Therapy for KD is directed at controlling the inflammatory response and preventing thrombosis with antiplatelet therapy. Intravenous immune globulin (IVIG) in randomized trials has demonstrated reduced prevalence of coronary artery aneurysm and more rapid clinical response versus aspirin alone. Single high-dose IVIG of greater than 1 g/kg has resulted in the lowest incidence of coronary abnormalities, and this regimen along with aspirin is advocated as soon as the diagnosis is made. Indefinite aspirin therapy is recommended if coronary artery aneurysms persist on serial echocardiography. Combination of warfarin and low-dose aspirin has been advocated for persistent large (>8 mm) coronary aneurysms.

Investigational Therapies: Plasmapheresis and exchange transfusion have been reported to be effective in limited cases. Oral pentoxifylline combined with IVIG therapy had lower incidence of coronary artery lesions versus IVIG for KD patients in one small trial.

REFERENCES
Laupland KB, Davies HD. Epidemiology, etiology, and management of Kawasaki disease: state of the art. *Pediatr Cardiol* 1999;20:177–183.
Mason WH, Takahashi M. Kawasaki syndrome. *Clin Infect Dis* 1999;28:169–187.
Morens DM, Melish ME. Kawasaki disease. In: Feigin RD, Cherry JD, eds. *Textbook of pediatric infectious diseases*, 4th ed. Philadelphia: WB Saunders, 1998:995–1014.
Rowley AH, Shulman ST. Kawasaki syndrome. In: Jenson HB, Baltimore RS, eds. *Pediatric infectious diseases: principles and practice*. Norwalk, CT: Appleton & Lange, 1995:629–638.

RESOURCES
223, 359

16   Legg-Calve-Perthes Disease

Geoffrey D. Nochimson, MD

DEFINITION: Legg-Calve-Perthes disease is the name given to idiopathic osteonecrosis of the capital femoral epiphysis of the femoral head.

DIFFERENTIAL DIAGNOSIS: Sickle cell anemia; Rheumatoid arthritis; Hip fracture; Septic hip joint; Toxic synovitis.

SYMPTOMS AND SIGNS: Symptoms and signs include hip or groin pain, which may be referred to the thigh; mild or intermittent pain in the anterior thigh or knee; limp; and no history of trauma.

ETIOLOGY/EPIDEMIOLOGY: The cause is unknown. It is known that the blood supply to the capital femoral epiphysis is interrupted, which leads to bone infarction in the subchondral cortical bone. This can lead to subchondral fracture, which causes disruption to the epiphyseal growth plate. In the United States, 1 in 1,200 children younger than 15 develop the disease. Caucasians are affected more than other races, and males are affected 4–5 times more than females. It is most commonly seen in persons aged 3–12 years, with a median of 7 years. The younger the age of onset, the better the prognosis. Children who are older than 10 years in whom the disease is newly diagnosed have a high risk of developing osteoarthritis.

DIAGNOSIS: The physical examination often shows a limp, decreased range of motion especially with internal rotation and abduction, atrophy of thigh muscles secondary to disuse, muscle spasm, and short stature. Plain radiographs of the hip including frog leg views establish the diagnosis. At least four different radiographic classification systems (Waldenstrom, Catterall, Salter, and Thompson) exist, but there is no agreement on the best one.

TREATMENT

Standard Therapies: The goal of treatment is to prevent severe degenerative arthritis and permanent femoral head deformity. Once the diagnosis is suspected, the patient should be referred to an orthopedic surgeon, preferably a pediatric specialist. Medical treatment will not stop or reverse the bony changes, but analgesic medication should be given to help the pain. Nonsteroidal antiinflammatory drugs (NSAIDs) are most commonly used for the relief of mild to moderate pain. Ibuprofen remains the drug of choice, although patients may respond better to a different NSAID. The specialist may order additional tests to determine the extent of the disease, including bone scintigraphy, arthrography, and MRI. Initial orthopedic treatment involves nonsurgical containment. Various casts, braces, and crutches are used to keep the femoral head within the acetabulum so that it can act as a mold for the femoral head. Surgical procedures are done to correct gross deformities of the femoral head.

REFERENCES

Herring JA. The treatment of Legg-Calve-Perthes disease. A critical review of the literature. *J Bone Joint Surg [Am]* 1994;76:448–458.
Kaniklides C. Diagnostic radiology in Legg-Calve-Perthes disease. *Acta Radiol Suppl* 1996;406:1–28.
Molloy MK. Incidence of Legg-Perthes disease. *N Engl J Med* 1966;275:988–990.
Roy DR. Current concepts in Legg-Calve-Perthes disease. *Pediatr Ann* 1999;28:748–752.
Skaggs DL. Legg-Calve-Perthes disease. *J Am Acad Orthop Surg* 1996;4:9–16.

RESOURCES
257, 360

17   Benign Lymphoepithelial Lesion (Mikulicz Syndrome)

Alexander K.C. Leung, MB, BS, FRCPC, FRCP(UK & Ireland)

DEFINITION: Benign lymphoepithelial lesion is an autoimmune disorder characterized by diffuse and bilateral enlargement of salivary and lacrimal glands (Insert Fig. 3) with characteristic histopathologic findings, including diffuse lymphocytic infiltration of the exocrine glands and formation of epimyoepithelial islands.

SYNONYMS: Mikulicz syndrome; Mikulicz disease; Dacryosialoadenopathy.

DIFFERENTIAL DIAGNOSIS: Mumps; Uveoparotid fever; Sialoadenitis; Sialolithiasis; Amyloidosis; Hemochromatosis; Benign lymphoepithelial cysts; Tumors (pleomorphic adenoma, cylindroma, adenolymphoma, and carcinoma) of the salivary glands.

SYMPTOMS AND SIGNS: The usual clinical picture is enlargement of one or more of the salivary glands and, less frequently, the lacrimal glands. The condition is often bilateral and symptomless. Occasionally, mild local discomfort may be associated. The parotid glands are usually affected. Enlargement of the lacrimal glands may result in a bulge below the outer ends of the eyelids and narrowing of the palpebral fissures. Depending on the degree of involvement, some patients may have xerostomia and xerophthalmia. Characteristically, patients are not thirsty despite xerostomia.

ETIOLOGY/EPIDEMIOLOGY: Benign lymphoepithelial lesion may be primary (idiopathic) or caused by an underlying disease. A primary benign lymphoepithelial lesion is a clinical rarity and occurs predominately in middle-aged or older women. Secondary causes include Sjögren syndrome, which is characterized by xerostomia, keratoconjunctivitis, and a collagen vascular disease, usually rheumatoid arthritis, systemic lupus erythematosus, systemic sclerosis, or polymyositis. Rarely, benign lymphoepithelial lesion occurs in association with tuberculosis, syphilis, sarcoidosis, AIDS, leukemia, lymphomas, or thiouracil treatment.

DIAGNOSIS: The diagnosis can be confirmed by a biopsy of the involved gland. Histologically, a benign lymphoepithelial lesion is characterized by atrophy of the acinar tissue with diffuse lymphocytic infiltration and an intraductal proliferation of epithelial and myoepithelial cells with the formation of epimyoepithelial islands. A complete blood count is useful if an infection is suspected. Erythrocyte sedimentation rate, serum immunoglobulins, rheumatoid factor, antinuclear factor, and autoantibodies to nucleoprotein antigens (SSA [Ro] and SSB [La]) should be considered if Sjögren syndrome is suspected. The Mantoux test is helpful if tuberculosis is suspected.

TREATMENT

Standard Therapies: Treatment is mainly symptomatic. Xerophthalmia can be treated with artificial tears. Symptomatic xerostomia can be treated with sialogogues, provided there is some residual salivary function. Sialogogues can be mechanical, such as chewing gum; gustatory, such as citric acid–containing foods or fluids, or sweet-tasting substances; or pharmacologic, such as pilocarpine hydrochloride. For patients without functioning salivary gland parenchyma or whose salivary glands do not respond to stimulation by sialogogues, saliva substitutes can be prescribed. Effective tooth brushing with a fluoridated dentifrice and dental flossing after each meal will help prevent dental caries. Patients should be followed up regularly for further salivary or lacrimal gland involvement, autoimmune disease, and malignancy.

REFERENCES

Hochberg MC. Sjögren's syndrome. In: Goldman L, Bennett JC, eds. *Cecil textbook of medicine,* 21st ed. Philadelphia: WB Saunders, 2000:1522–1524.

Ide F, Shimoyama T, Horie N, et al. Benign lymphoepithelial lesion of the parotid gland with sebaceous differentiation. *Oral Surg Oral Med Oral Pathol* 1999;87:721–724.

Leung AK, Kao P. Xerostomia. *Singapore Paediatr J* 1999;41: 57–63.

Leung AK, Wong AL, Robson WL, Pinto A. Benign lymphoepithelial lesion (Mikulicz's syndrome) of the submandibular glands in a four-year-old boy. *Otolaryngol Head Neck Surg* 1994; 111:302–304.

RESOURCES

27, 436

18   Marden-Walker Syndrome

Alfredo Orrico, MD

DEFINITION: Marden-Walker syndrome (MWS) is a connective tissue disorder characterized by muscular hypotonia, short stature, mental retardation, failure to thrive, poorly muscled build, expressionless facies, blepharophimosis, micrognathia, high-arched or cleft palate, low-set auricles, and joint contractures.

DIFFERENTIAL DIAGNOSIS: Myotonic dystrophy; Schwartz-Jampel syndrome; Distal arthrogryposis; Marden-Walker-like syndrome without psychomotor retardation; Freeman-Sheldon syndrome.

SYMPTOMS AND SIGNS: The cardinal defects are muscular hypotonia with reduced muscle mass, growth and developmental delay, failure to thrive, immobile facies, prominent forehead, blepharophimosis, small mouth, micrognathia, narrowly high-arched or cleft palate, low-set auricles, arachnodactyly, and joint contractures. Microcephaly and scaphocephaly are frequent features, but normocephalic patients have been reported. Additional findings may be seizures, cardiomyopathy, abnormalities on MRI (Dandy-Walker malformation, hypoplasia of vermis and cerebellar hemispheres, corpus collosum hypoplasia, cerebral atrophy, and dilated ventricles), vertebral abnormalities, microcystic kidney disease, pyloric stenosis, and pancreatic insufficiency. With time, congenital muscle weakness results in scoliosis and kyphosis, mild pectus excavatum, camptodactyly, and flexion contractures in the elbows, hips, and knees. Because of the frequency of death in infancy (due to aspiration and/or cardiac failure), few surviving adult patients have been reported. Blepharophimosis, contractures, camptodactyly, growth retardation, and developmental delay persist into adulthood, whereas minor anomalies of the face may become less noticeable.

ETIOLOGY/EPIDEMIOLOGY: The condition is considered autosomal recessive because of reported cases of affected siblings and parental consanguinity. Consequently, a risk of recurrence of 0.25 seems to be appropriate. Nevertheless, most patients represent sporadic cases with a broad range of variability and potential genetic heterogeneity. Males seem to be affected more often than females, although this is not conclusive.

DIAGNOSIS: The pathogenetic mechanism for this condition, likely attributable to a single gene defect, is not yet known. Therefore, specific laboratory tests are not available. Electromyography may show mild and unspecific signs of myopathy such as low amplitude and short motor unit potentials. The electroencephalographic and muscular histologic evaluations do not show specific changes. MRI of the brain may show a broad range of nonspecific abnormalities. Diagnosis is made clinically.

TREATMENT
Standard Therapies: No specific therapies are available. Treatment involves supportive care, including use of dietary therapy and anticonvulsant drugs, when necessary. Contractures may also benefit from physical therapy.

REFERENCES
Giacoia GP, Pineda R. Expanded spectrum of findings in Marden-Walker syndrome. *Am J Med Genet* 1990;36:495–499.

King CR, Magenis E. The Marden-Walker syndrome. *J Med Genet* 1978;15:366–369.

Kotzot D, Schinzel A. Marden-Walker syndrome in an adult. *Clin Dysmorph* 1995;4:260–265.

Marden PM, Walker WA. A new generalized connective tissue syndrome: association of multiple congenital anomalies. *Am J Dis Child* 1966;112:225–228.

Orrico A, Galli L, Zappella M, et al. Additional case of Marden-Walker syndrome: confirmation of the autosomal recessive inheritance and refinement of phenotype. *J Child Neurol* 2001;16:150–152.

RESOURCES
80, 312

19   Familial Mediterranean Fever

Hatem El-Shanti, MD

DEFINITION: Familial Mediterranean fever (FMF) is a genetic multisystem disease characterized by recurrent self-limiting episodes of fever and painful polyserositis.

SYNONYMS: Benign paroxysmal peritonitis; Recurrent polyserositis; Recurrent hereditary polyserositis; Periodic disease; Periodic peritonitis.

DIFFERENTIAL DIAGNOSIS: Hyperimmunoglobulinemia D syndrome; Behçet disease; Familial hibernian fever; Muckle-Wells syndrome.

SYMPTOMS AND SIGNS: The clinical picture consists of recurrent febrile and painful attacks that are usually of acute onset, variable frequency, and without a noticeable triggering factor but often occurring with menstruation, emotional stress, or strenuous physical activity. The pain is usually severe, occurring in the abdomen, chest, and joints, owing to inflammation of the peritoneum, pleura, and synovial membrane. The attacks last from 12 to 72 hours and abort abruptly. The clinical picture, intensity of symptoms, and frequency vary from one attack to another. In between attacks, the patient has no symptoms. Abdominal pain is reported in 50% of patients as the first symptom. It can be diffuse or localized, ranging from mild bloating to real peritonitis. Chest pain is present in approximately 50% of attacks, usually in the form of unilateral pleurisy with diminished breath sounds, friction rub, and possibly effusion or collapse. Joint pain is present in approximately 50%–75% of attacks in the form of arthritis or arthralgia. The most characteristic skin lesion is the erysipelas-like erythema, occurring in 3%–45% of attacks. Uncommon manifestations include acute scrotal inflammation; myalgia that can be mild, diffuse, and of a short duration or protracted; headache, with meningeal irritation and increased cerebrospinal fluid proteins and cells; impaired female fertility; pericarditis; vasculitis; purpuric lesions; and glomerulonephritis or nephropathy. The most significant complication is amyloidosis.

ETIOLOGY/EPIDEMIOLOGY: The disorder is autosomal recessive. The gene responsible for the disorder, *MEFV*, has been cloned and mutations have been identified. The prevalence of the disease is quite high in specific ethnic groups (Jews, Turks, Armenians, and Arabs) with a carrier frequency reaching as high as 1 in 5. The male: female ratio is 1.5:1 to 2:1, probably due to reduced penetrance in females. The attacks generally start during childhood or adolescence, with approximately 80% of patients presenting before age 20 years.

DIAGNOSIS: The diagnosis is based on clinical manifestations, ethnicity, family history, and response to colchicine. The molecular test can be used as an adjunct to the clinical diagnosis. Laboratory findings during an attack include leukocytosis, elevated erythrocyte sedimentation rate, and increased acute phase reactants (C-reactive protein, serum AA, fibrinogen, haptoglobin, C3, and C4).

TREATMENT

Standard Therapies: A daily regimen of 1–2 mg of oral colchicine is the recommended treatment. It ameliorates the attacks significantly and is beneficial for the prevention of amyloidosis in all patients, in those already exhibiting proteinuria, and for the prevention of the reaccumulation of AA in a transplanted kidney. There is no role for colchicine during acute attacks.

Investigational Therapies: Interferon-α is being used as an adjuvant therapy for acute attacks in patients who still get them while taking colchicine or who are resistant to the drug.

REFERENCES

Majeed HA. Differential diagnosis of fever of unknown origin in children. *Curr Opin Rheum* 2000;12:439–444.

Majeed HA, Rawashdeh M, El-Shanti H, et al. Familial Mediterranean fever in children: the expanded clinical profile. *Q J Med* 1999;92:309–318.

Rawashdeh MO, Majeed HA. Familial Mediterranean fever in Arab children: the high prevalence and gene frequency. *Eur J Pediatr* 1996;155:540–544.

Saatci U, Ozen S, Ozdemir S, et al. Familial Mediterranean fever in children: report of a large series and discussion of the risk and prognostic factors of amyloidosis. *Eur J Pediatr* 1997;156: 619–623.

Samuels J, Aksentijevich I, Torosyan Y, et al. Familial Mediterranean fever at the millennium. Clinical spectrum, ancient mutations, and a survey of 100 American referrals to the National Institutes of Health. *Medicine (Baltimore)* 1998;77: 268–297.

RESOURCES
354, 360

20   Metatropic Dysplasia

*Charles I. Scott, Jr., MD,
and William G. Mackenzie, MD*

DEFINITION: Metatropic dysplasia is a hereditary intrinsic growth disorder of the skeleton that results in a variable pattern of disproportionately short stature, spinal deformity, and the risk of cervical spinal cord compression due to atlantoaxial instability or stenosis. Intelligence is normal. Adult height ranges from 110 to 120 cm (43.25–47.25 inches).

SYNONYMS: Metatropic dysplasia, type 2; Pseudometatropic dysplasia; Swiss-cheese cartilage dysplasia.

DIFFERENTIAL DIAGNOSIS: Achondroplasia; Morquio-type mucopolysaccharidosis; Kniest dysplasia; Spondyloepimetaphyseal dysplasia, Langer type.

SYMPTOMS AND SIGNS: Initially, affected infants show a long, narrow thorax and relatively short extremities. As kyphoscoliosis develops, these proportions reverse and the spine becomes relatively short compared with the limbs. The kyphoscoliosis may be severe, causing compressive myelopathy. Severe progressive joint contractures limit upper and lower extremity function. Osteoarthritis can result from joint surface irregularity. The stiff thorax results in restrictive lung disease. Many individuals have a small caudal appendage or skin fold ("tail") in the coccygeal region. Major radiographic findings include generalized platyspondyly, often wafer-thin, odontoid hypoplasia, and C1–2 instability or stenosis. Coronal clefts of the vertebral bodies may be seen. Kyphoscoliosis develops and is progressive. Early in life, the proximal limb long bones are dumbbell shaped. The long bones have narrow diaphyses and widely flared metaphyses. This results in the elbows, wrists, and ankles being extremely prominent and large. Ventriculomegaly/hydrocephalus may also occur.

ETIOLOGY/EPIDEMIOLOGY: Metatropic dysplasia is inherited generally as an autosomal-recessive trait, although there are reports of nonlethal autosomal-dominant inheritance in some families. There is also an exceptionally uncommon lethal autosomal-recessive form, which has been recognized prenatally. The prevalence and incidence are unknown.

DIAGNOSIS: The diagnosis is based on the family history, physical findings, and radiologic findings. The pattern of radiographic changes takes time to fully evolve.

TREATMENT
Standard Therapies: The spine must be closely monitored for cervical instability or odontoid hypoplasia, kyphoscoliosis, compressive myelopathy, respiratory compromise, and joint contractures. Complaints of arthralgias and osteoarthritis are frequent, and may be variably ameliorated by nonsteroidal antiinflammatory drugs, warm baths, massage, reassurance, and modification of physical activities. Genetic counseling is indicated, as is contact with a support group.

REFERENCES
Belik J, Anday EK, Kaplan F, et al. Respiratory complications of metatropic dwarfism. *Clin Pediatr* 1985;24:504–511.
Shohat M, Lachman R, Rimoin DL. Odontoid hypoplasia with vertebral cervical subluxation and ventriculomegaly in metatropic dysplasia. *J Pediatr* 1989;114:239–243.
Taybi H, Lachman RS. *Radiology of syndromes, metabolic disorders, and skeletal dysplasias,* 4th ed. St. Louis: CV Mosby, 1996:860–863.
Wynne-Davies R, Hall C, Apley AAG. *Atlas of skeletal dysplasias.* New York: Churchill Livingstone, 1985:274–288.

RESOURCES
188, 246

21   Navicular Osteochondritis (Kohler Disease)

Ruth A. Cook, ANP,
and Martin J. O'Malley, MD

DEFINITION: Kohler disease is an osteochondrosis that affects the tarsal navicular. It occurs in children ages 1–10 years, with most cases occurring at 3–7 years of age.

SYNONYM: Osteochondrosis of the navicular.

DIFFERENTIAL DIAGNOSIS: Tarsal scaphoiditis (Muller-Weiss disease); Navicular stress fracture.

SYMPTOMS AND SIGNS: Weight-bearing medial mid-foot pain, sometimes accompanied by swelling and erythema, is the most common symptom. The shape of the foot is not a contributing factor; however, in symptomatic patients, the foot may be held in pronation. Symptoms may be mild and patients may go months before seeking treatment.

ETIOLOGY/EPIDEMIOLOGY: The necrosis of Kohler disease may be related to trauma or mechanical overload that causes vascular compromise. The navicular does not have a physis and usually develops a single ossification center at ages 2–4 years. The center appears in girls approximately 1 year before it does in boys, but boys are 5 times more likely to develop the condition. Kohler disease is believed to result from delayed ossification. The resulting increase in the ratio of cartilage to bone causes structural weakening. A vascular ring that sends a single vessel to each ossification center surrounds the navicular. At ages 4–6 years, other vessels eventually penetrate the area. The delayed ossification, however, coupled with the increased weight gain and activity of the growing child, combine to compress the nutrient vessels and cause ischemia. The incidence in the population is approximately 2%.

DIAGNOSIS: Radiographic examination shows a flattened, sclerotic navicular with multiple areas of irregular ossification. This, combined with the common symptom of weight-bearing medial foot pain in a child aged 1–10 years, is diagnostic.

TREATMENT
Standard Therapies: Treatment may range from doing nothing to using medial support orthotics to using a weight-bearing cast. The symptoms may resolve in just a few days or may last 1–2 years. Patients treated with a cast for approximately 3 months seemed to experience more rapid resolution of symptoms. Patients treated with an orthotic had symptoms for as long as 15 months. Usually, the navicular reconstitutes to normal over 6 months to several years.

REFERENCES
Meyerson MS. *Foot and ankle disorders.* Vol. 1. Philadelphia: WB Saunders, 2000:793–796.

RESOURCE
360

22   Cyclic Neutropenia

Laurence A. Boxer, MD

DEFINITION: Cyclic neutropenia is a disorder in which blood stem cell production from the bone marrow oscillates with 21-day periodicity. Circulating neutrophils vary between almost normal numbers and zero.

SYNONYMS: Cyclic hematopoiesis; Periodic neutropenia.

DIFFERENTIAL DIAGNOSIS: Severe congenital neutropenia; Severe chronic idiopathic neutropenia; Autoimmune neutropenia.

SYMPTOMS AND SIGNS: Patients with cyclic neutropenia suffer from oropharyngeal problems (mouth ulcers and gingivitis), otitis media, respiratory infections (sinusitis, bronchitis, and pneumonia), and cellulitis and skin abscesses when their neutrophil count falls below 500 cells/mL. In addition, approximately 10% of the patients with cyclic neutropenia prior to the availability of granulocyte colony-stimulating factor (G-CSF) often developed fatal *Clostridium perfringens* infections, likely arising from dissemination of the organisms from ulcers present in the gastrointestinal tract. Most notably during periods of neutropenia, patients are prone to develop fevers.

ETIOLOGY/EPIDEMIOLOGY: This is an inherited autosomal-dominant disorder. Mutations have been identified in the neutrophil elastase (*ELA2*) gene in infected individuals. The estimated frequency of this condition is approximately one case per million population.

DIAGNOSIS: The diagnosis of cyclic neutropenia is established by obtaining blood counts 2–3 times per week for a period of 2 months, and documenting the cycle of 21 days. It can be confirmed with molecular genetic studies demonstrating mutations in the elastase gene.

TREATMENT

Standard Therapies: Recombinant human G-CSF alleviates symptoms by shortening the duration of severe neutropenia characterized by counts below 200 cells/mL from 4 to 6 days to 1 day. Infections are treated with antibiotics. Patients with inherited forms of the disease should receive genetic counseling. Other treatments depend on symptoms.

REFERENCES

Dale D, Bonilla M, Davis M, et al. A randomized controlled phase III trial of recombinant human G-CSF for treatment of severe chronic neutropenia. *Blood* 1993;81:2496–2502.

Dale D, Hammond W. Cyclic neutropenia: a clinical review. *Blood Rev* 1988;2:178–185.

Horwitz M, Benson KF, Person RE, et al. Mutations in *ELA2*, encoding neutrophil elastase, define a 21-day biological clock in cyclic haematopoiesis. *Nat Genet* 1999;23:433–436.

RESOURCES

318, 343, 431

---

23   Severe Chronic Neutropenia

Laurence A. Boxer, MD

DEFINITION: Severe chronic neutropenia (SCN) is a blood disorder in which the bone marrow does not produce adequate numbers of neutrophils, leading to susceptibility to bacterial infections. Chronic neutropenia can last for months or years, and affects both children and adults. SCN is associated with an absolute neutrophil count (ANC) below 500 cells/mL.

DIFFERENTIAL DIAGNOSIS: Severe congenital neutropenia; Kostmann syndrome; Glycogen storage disease 1b; Shwachman-Diamond syndrome; Hyperimmunoglobulin M syndrome; Cyclic neutropenia; Chronic idiopathic neutropenia.

SYMPTOMS AND SIGNS: Patients with an absolute neutrophil below 200 cells/mL have a predictable pattern of infection and inflammation; mouth ulcers, gingivitis, otitis media, respiratory infections, cellulitis, and skin abscesses. Pneumonia caused by gram-negative or anaerobic bacteria, deep tissue abscesses, and bacteremia occur infre-

quently, but are life-threatening. The most common causes of infection are *Staphylococcus aureus* and *Streptococcus*. Because most of these patients have intact monocyte and lymphocyte function at either normal or increased immunoglobulin at complement levels, infections by yeast, fungi, and parasites occur infrequently. When infections occur, they are slow in healing even with optimal antibiotic treatment. Patients with severe chronic neutropenia who maintain an absolute neutrophil count between 200 and 500 cell/mL are susceptible primarily to the oral pharyngeal problems, cellulitis, and skin abscesses.

ETIOLOGY/EPIDEMIOLOGY: Chronic neutropenia is the result of impaired production of blood cells in the bone marrow. When associated with Kostmann syndrome, over 90% of patients have had mutations in the gene for neutrophil other than cyclic neutropenia. The cause for other forms of severe chronic neutropenia remains unknown. Chronic neutropenia affects males and females equally except for the hyper-IgM syndrome, which is inherited primarily in an X-linked fashion. The estimated frequency of Kostmann syndrome is approximately 2 cases per million population.

DIAGNOSIS: Patients with Kostmann syndrome have bone marrow that shows a selective defect in neutrophil formation with an apparent arrest at the promyelocyte stage of myeloid development. Patients with severe idiopathic forms of chronic neutropenia may have an arrest at any point in myeloid cell development within the bone marrow.

TREATMENT
Standard Therapies: Infections associated with chronic neutropenia are usually managed with antibiotics. Standard treatment for severe chronic neutropenia with recurrent infection includes daily administration of recombinant human granulocyte colony-stimulating factor. Approximately 10% of patients with Kostmann syndrome have a preleukemia syndrome in which, if the patient converts to myelodysplasia/acute myelogenous leukemia, the only effective treatment is bone marrow transplantation. Genetic counseling should be considered for patients and families with Kostmann syndrome or neutropenia associated with immune deficiency.

REFERENCES
Dale D, Bonilla M, Davis M, et al. A randomized controlled phase III trial of recombinant human G-CSF for treatment of severe chronic neutropenia. *Blood* 1993;81:2496–2502.
Dale DC, Person RE, Bolyard AA, et al. Mutations in the gene encoding neutrophil elastase in congenital and cyclic neutropenia. *Blood* 2000;96:2317–2322.
Welte K, Boxer LA. Severe chronic neutropenia: pathophysiology and therapy. *Semin Hematol* 1997;34:267–278.

RESOURCES
318, 343, 431

24   Ollier Disease

C.L.M.H. Gibbons, MA, FRCS

DEFINITION: Ollier disease is a nonhereditary skeletal disorder characterized by the persistence of islands of dysplastic cartilage within several bones.

SYNONYM: Enchondromatosis.

DIFFERENTIAL DIAGNOSIS: Fibrous dysplasia; Osteochondromatosis metaphyseal chondrodysplasia.

SYMPTOMS AND SIGNS: The extent of involvement of the musculoskeletal system varies widely from limited involvement of one bone or the small tubular bones of hands and feet to extensive multifocal bony disease. In general, the more severe the skeletal involvement, the earlier in life the symptoms appear. At birth, mild shortening of the leg may be apparent without radiographic evidence of enchondromatosis. The two main clinical manifestations in children are multiple bony lumps of the fingers and toes or lower limb deformity and shortening. Because the disease predominantly affects one side, the changes are asymmetric; the limb is short with associated swelling and deformity of the affected bone. Children may also present with a pathologic fracture of an affected long bone after minor trauma. Delayed healing of the fracture may occur if intramedullary disease is extensive. In less severe cases, there is mild limb asymmetry or deformity. If one of the paired bones in the forearm or leg is affected, bowing of the radius or tibia results. A common deformity in the upper limb is shortening and bowing of the radius with overgrowth of the ulna. This leads to wrist pain and Madelung deformity. Other common findings in the lower limb are a valgus deformity of the knee if the distal femur is involved or a varus knee deformity if the proximal tibia is affected. The enchondromas generally involve the metaphysis and diaphysis of long bones. If the lesion affects the growth plate, it can cause growth arrest and foreshortening and angular deformity of the limbs. The enchondromas stop growing at puberty, and remodeling occurs with replacement of the island cartilage by matrix calcification, but foci of cartilage remain.

ETIOLOGY/EPIDEMIOLOGY: The disease is nonhereditary and has no clear sex difference. It is often unilateral.

DIAGNOSIS: The clinical and radiographic features of enchondromatosis are distinctive and often diagnostic. Skeletal radiologic surveys and isotope scans confirm the extent of the disease. There is an association between Ollier disease and chondrosarcoma. If after skeletal maturity, evidence exists of a bony swelling that is increasing in size and is painful, this should be carefully investigated to exclude malignant change. Tissue diagnosis either with trucut biopsy or open biopsy is indicated if malignant change is suspected.

TREATMENT

Standard Therapies: With lumps of the hands and feet in children, excision and curettage may be required to improve finger function and correct deformities. In the upper limb, distal radius involvement with Madelung deformity may be treated with a corrective osteotomy to improve wrist function and relieve pain. Significant angular deformity of the long bones may require a corrective osteotomy before skeletal maturity and this may be combined with limb lengthening procedures if a limb length discrepancy is associated. Limb length inequality is treated with orthotics and heel lifts, epiphysiodesis, limb lengthening, or femoral shortening. Correction of the angular deformities in a short limb can be undertaken using the Ilizarov circular frame method. This method may be combined with multiple osteotomies. In adults, pathologic fractures of the small bones of the hands and feet are common, and curettage of the bone lesion with grafting and stabilization of the fracture usually suffice if there is no suspicion of malignant change. Patients require regular clinical and radiographic surveillance, because there is a risk of secondary sarcoma transformation. With malignant change, careful clinical, radiologic, and histologic assessments are mandatory before definitive surgery that involves limb salvage reconstruction. Angular deformity of the knee and ankle occasionally requires a corrective osteotomy and bony fixation. A patient may present with coexistent degenerative joint disease, which is treated by conventional means. Asymptomatic quiescent enchondromas of long bones do not require treatment unless new symptoms develop erosion.

REFERENCES

Benson MKD, Fixen JA, MacNicol MF, eds. *Children's orthopaedics and fractures.* Edinburgh: Churchill Livingstone, 1994.

Dorfman HD, Csevnick B. *Bone tumours.* St. Louis: CV Mosby, 1998.

Kenwright J. Callus distraction in Ollier's disease. *Acta Orthop Scand* 1995;66:479–480.

Schwartz HS, et al. The malignant potential of osteochondromatosis. *J Bone Joint Surg [Am]* 1987;69:269–274.

Wynne-Davis R, Hall CM, Apley AG. Ollier's disease (enchondromatosis). In: *Atlas of skeletal dysplasia.* Edinburgh: Churchill Livingstone, 1985:533–538.

RESOURCES

360, 378

---

25 Paget Disease of Bone

Robert D. Tiegs, MD

DEFINITION: Paget disease of bone is a progressive, focal disorder of bone remodeling.

SYNONYM: Osteitis deformans.

SYMPTOMS AND SIGNS: Pain is the most common clinical presentation. Causes of pain include pagetic bone pain, fissure or complete fracture, secondary arthritis, neurologic compression syndromes, and sarcomatous transformation. Patients with skull involvement frequently have bandlike discomfort or headache. In areas such as the skull and pretibial region, increased vascularity may elevate skin temperature. Sites most commonly involved include the hip, knee, and ankle. Long bone involvement is characterized by progressive deformity. The three most common types of fracture in Paget disease are fissure fractures, complete fractures, and vertebral compression fractures. Fissure fractures commonly occur in the femur, tibia, and humerus and typically develop along the convex surface of bowed long bones. The most common site for a complete fracture is the femur, followed by the tibia and forearm.

Neurologic complications primarily develop in patients with skull and spine involvement and are among the most serious complications of the disease. Skull involvement may cause platybasia or basilar invagination and result in hydrocephalus, compression of the brainstem, entrapment of the lower cranial nerves, and vertebrobasilar insufficiency. Up to 50% of patients with skull involvement experience hearing loss. Vestibular dysfunction develops in a smaller percentage. Vertebral involvement may cause spinal stenosis, especially in the thoracic region. Compression of nerve roots may also occur. Patients with extensive skeletal involvement have increased cardiac output. In individuals with underlying cardiac disease, this may give rise to high output cardiac failure. Sarcomatous transformation is a rare but serious complication. Most of the tumors are osteosarcomas. Fibrosarcomas, chondrosarcomas, malignant fibrous histiocytomas, and giant cell tumors may also occur.

ETIOLOGY/EPIDEMIOLOGY: A viral etiology has been proposed, but the cause of the disease remains unknown. Because 15%–30% of patients have a family history of the disorder, and a first-degree relative of an individual with Paget disease has a sevenfold greater risk of developing the disease, a genetic predisposition may exist. Both men and women are affected, with a slight male predominance. The prevalence of Paget disease in the United States is estimated to be 1%–2%.

DIAGNOSIS: Radiographic findings include bony enlargement, cortical thickening, thickened trabecular markings, osteolysis, and a loss of the corticomedullary junction. In combination, these findings are diagnostic in nearly all cases. A bone scan should be considered at the time of diagnosis to define the extent of involvement.

TREATMENT
Standard Therapies: The indications for treatment are to relieve symptoms and prevent complications. The therapeutic end point should be to maintain the markers of bone turnover within the normal range, or as close to normal as possible. Treatment should be reinstituted if the symptoms recur or if there is evidence of reactivation of the disease. Therapeutic options include calcitonin and the bisphosphonates, which are the treatment of choice. Bisphosphonates approved for treatment of Paget disease in

the United States include etidronate, pamidronate, alendronate, tiludronate, and risedronate.

Investigational Therapies: Zoledronate, ibandronate, neridronate, and olpadronate are under investigation.

REFERENCES
Delmas PD, Meunier PJ. The management of Paget's disease of bone. *N Engl J Med* 1997;336:558–566.
Fleisch H. Bisphosphonates: pharmacokinetics. In: *Bisphosphonates in bone disease,* 3rd ed. Berne, Switzerland: Parthenon Publishing, 1997:58–62.
Kanis JA. Pathophysiology and histopathology. In: *Pathophysiology and treatment of Paget's disease of bone,* 2nd ed. London: Martin Dunitz, 1998:12–40.
Siris ES. Paget's disease of bone. In: Favus MJH, et al., eds. *Primer on the metabolic bone diseases and disorders of mineral metabolism,* 4th ed. Philadelphia: Lippincott Williams & Wilkins, 1999:415–425.

RESOURCES
351, 464

26 Peyronie Disease

Wayne J.G. Hellstrom, MD, and Sashi K. Reddy, MD

DEFINITION: Peyronie disease is an acquired inflammatory condition of the penis causing a plaque-like scarring of the tunica albuginea of the corpus cavernosum. This causes abnormalities of the erect penis, including pain, penile curvature, and erectile dysfunction.

SYNONYMS: Acquired curvature of the penis; Plastic induration of the penis; Penile fibromatosis.

DIFFERENTIAL DIAGNOSIS: Congenital curvature of the penis; Chordee without hypospadias; Penile malignancy.

SYMPTOMS AND SIGNS: The disease is characterized by an initial active inflammatory phase associated with scar remodeling that can last 6–18 months. Patients complain of pain with erection and significant penile curvature developing either acutely or gradually. The curvature is usually dorsal but can develop ventrally or laterally. Sometimes patients report a palpable plaque or a collection of knots

along the shaft of the penis. There also may be bottle-necking and penile shortening. As the active phase resolves, the curvature of the penis can increase, decrease, or remain stable. Some patients develop erectile dysfunction. Some also complain of softness or flaccidity of their erection distal to the plaque.

ETIOLOGY/EPIDEMIOLOGY: The etiology is not well characterized. Trauma has been proposed as the inciting event. A genetic component has been postulated with reports of chromosomal abnormalities, familial autosomal-dominant inheritance, and a possible association with the HLA-B7 antigen. The disease process affects more than 3% of the white male population (from age 40 to 70), but also occurs in African-American and Asian men with less frequency.

DIAGNOSIS: The diagnosis is usually made by history and clinical findings. Physical examination shows a palpable plaque along the midline shaft of the penis in the dorsal or ventral location depending on the direction of curvature. Because of the association with erectile dysfunction, patients may undergo penile duplex Doppler evaluation with a vasoactive agent to characterize their erectile status and measure calcification or thickening of the tunica albuginea.

TREATMENT

Standard Therapies: Treatment usually starts conservatively with either oral medications or intralesional injection therapies. Vitamin E is a common first-line oral agent. Others include colchicine, paraaminobenzoic acid, and tamoxifen. A more invasive approach involves intralesional injection of agents such as verapamil, collagenase, and interferon-α 2b. Once the plaque has stabilized, patients with erectile dysfunction or persistent curvature may become candidates for surgical correction. Most surgical procedures for patients with adequate erectile function involve incision or excision of the fibrous plaque with patching using more compliant materials, such as autografts of dermis, vein, tunica vaginalis, and temporalis fascia. Allografts are also becoming more popular and successful, including processed pericardium, dermis, and porcine small intestinal submucosa. In patients with erectile dysfunction, placement of a penile prosthetic implant is the standard of care. The plaque can be either remodeled or "cracked" to allow for penile straightening. If this modeling technique is not successful, the plaque can be incised or excised and patched with a grafting material.

Investigational Therapies: Less invasive treatment methods are being explored, including high-intensity focused ultrasonography, radiation therapy, and use of extracorporeal shock wave treatment.

REFERENCES

Devine CJ, et al. Proposal: trauma as the cause of the Peyronie's lesion. *J Urol* 1997;157:285–290.

Dunsmuir WD, et al. Francois de La Peyronie: the man and the disease he described. *Br J Urol* 1996;78:613.

Fitzuin J, Ho GT. Peyronie's disease: current management. *Am Fam Physician* 1999;60:549–554.

Hellstrom WJG, Bivalacqua TJ. Peyronie's disease: etiology, medical, and surgical therapy. *J Androl* 2000;21:347–354.

Hinman F. Etiologic factors in Peyronie's disease. *Urol Int* 1980;35:404–413.

RESOURCES

34, 372

---

27   POEMS Syndrome

Alberto A. Mitrani, MD

DEFINITION: POEMS syndrome is a plasma cell dyscrasia with systemic findings that include polyneuropathy (P), organomegaly (O), endocrinopathy (E), monoclonal protein band (M), and skin (S) changes.

SYNONYMS: Shimpo, Crow-Fukase, and Takatsukis syndrome; Osteosclerotic myeloma; PEP (polyneuropathy, endocrinopathy, plasma cell dyscrasia) syndrome.

DIFFERENTIAL DIAGNOSIS: Paraproteinemia-associated polyneuropathy syndromes; Castleman disease; Multiple myeloma and other M-protein disease.

SYMPTOMS AND SIGNS: Progressive sensorimotor polyneuropathy is an early sign that may precede the diagnosis by years. Beginning distally, segmental demyelination occurs with axonal degeneration and abnormal nerve conduction. Hepatomegaly is present in most patients; splenomegaly is detected in less than half. The endocrinopathy includes hypothyroidism and glucose intolerance, and frequently, gonadal dysfunction, symptoms of which include fatigue, erectile dysfunction or loss of libido in males, and amenorrhea in females. Adrenal insufficiency, hypoparathyroidism, and hyperprolactenemia may also be present. Monoclonal gammopathy is characteristic. Dermatologic findings include hyperpigmentation, hypertrichosis, and scleroderma-like thickening. An early cutaneous lesion may be glomeruloid hemangioma composed of anastomosing vascular channels resembling renal glomeruli. Pulmonary hypertension is seen in association with POEMS syndrome and identifies patients at higher risk for early morbidity. Additional clinical findings include lymphadenopathy, peripheral edema, flushing, bilateral optic nerve edema, Raynaud phenomenon, microangiopathic and necrotizing vasculitis, and constitutional symptoms.

ETIOLOGY/EPIDEMIOLOGY: The syndrome predominantly affects middle-aged men but has been reported in patients as young as 24 years. Men are affected more than women, with a higher incidence reported in Japan. The cause is unknown.

DIAGNOSIS: Skeletal imaging to detect the osteosclerotic lesions typical of POEMS syndrome should be done. Laboratory examinations that help support the diagnosis include fasting glucose, metabolic screening, thyroid stimulating hormone, and serum and urine immunoelectrophoresis.

TREATMENT

Standard Therapies: Irradiation or excision of the primary plasmacytoma may lead to remission. If plasma cells are not confined to a single lesion, irradiation of the primary lesion plus corticosteroids is most likely to be successful in controlling the syndrome, including the endocrinopathy and pulmonary hypertension. Plasmapheresis, interferon, chemotherapy, androgens, intravenous immunoglobulin, and all-trans-retinoic acid have been used.

REFERENCES

Belec L, et al. Human herpesvirus 8 infection in patients with POEMS syndrome associated Castleman's disease. *Blood* 1999;93:3643–3653.

Feinberg L, et al. Soluble immune mediators in POEMS syndrome with pulmonary hypertension: case report and review of the literature. *Crit Rev Oncogenesis* 1999;10:293–302.

Kishimoto S, et al. Glomeruloid hemangioma in POEMS syndrome shows two different immunophenotypic endothelial cells. *J Cutan Pathol* 2000;27:87–92.

Lesprit P, et al. Pulmonary hypertension in POEMS syndrome: a new feature mediated by cytokines. *Am J Respir Crit Care Med* 1998;157:907–911.

Modesto-Segonds A. Renal involvement in POEMS syndrome. *Clin Nephrol* 1995;43:342–345.

RESOURCES

27, 349

---

28   Microscopic Polyangiitis

J. Charles Jennette, MD

DEFINITION: Microscopic polyangiitis is a systemic necrotizing small vessel vasculitis with few or no vessel wall immune deposits. Capillaries, venules, and arterioles are most often affected.

SYNONYM: Microscopic polyarteritis.

DIFFERENTIAL DIAGNOSIS: Wegener granulomatosis; Churg-Strauss syndrome; Polyarteritis nodosa; Henoch-Schönlein purpura.

SYMPTOMS AND SIGNS: Symptoms and signs of systemic vascular inflammation are preceded by a flulike illness in most patients. Clinical presentation is extremely varied. Frequent manifestations include fever, arthritis and arthralgias, myalgias, weakness, peripheral neuropathy (especially mononeuritis multiplex), palpable purpura, hematuria and proteinuria, pulmonary infiltrates, hemoptysis, sinusitis, abdominal pain, and gastrointestinal hemorrhage. Microscopic polyangiitis is the most common cause for pulmonary renal syndrome with hemoptysis and rapidly progressive glomerulonephritis. Purpura is most frequent on the lower extremities. Cutaneous arteritis causes tender red nodules or ulcers. Evidence for vasculitic involvement of abdominal viscera includes abdominal pain, occult blood in the stools, and elevated liver or pancreatic enzymes. Approximately 90% of patients have positive serology for antineutrophil cytoplasmic autoantibodies (ANCA).

ETIOLOGY/EPIDEMIOLOGY: Microscopic polyangiitis most often occurs in older individuals. The mean age at onset is in the sixth decade of life; however, it can occur at any age. Microscopic polyangiitis has no sex predilection, and is more common in whites and Asians than blacks. The prevalence in North America and Europe is estimated at 1 in 100,000. The etiology is unknown, however, substantial evidence exists that most microscopic polyangiitis is caused by ANCA. Antineutrophil cytoplasmic autoantibodies may be capable of activating neutrophils and monocytes, which in turn cause inflammatory injury to vessels and adjacent tissues.

DIAGNOSIS: The diagnosis should be suspected in a patient, especially an older adult, who has symptoms and signs of small vessel vasculitis, especially rapidly progressive glomerulonephritis, pulmonary hemorrhage, or purpura. Positive ANCA serology or pathologic identification of necrotizing vasculitis with a paucity of immunoglobulin deposits supports the diagnosis.

TREATMENT

Standard Therapies: Microscopic polyangiitis often causes life-threatening injury to major organs, such as lungs or kidneys, if not treated promptly with substantial immunosuppression. Standard treatment is with high-dose corticosteroids, such as intravenous methylprednisolone, combined with cytotoxic drugs, such as intravenous or oral cyclophosphamide. Plasmapheresis often is used in the presence of massive pulmonary hemorrhage. After induction of remission, maintenance immunosuppression with corticosteroids or cytotoxic drugs continues for 6 months to 1 year or until adequate disease quiescence is obtained. Relapses are frequent and require reinstitution of immunosuppressive therapy.

Investigational Therapies: Mycophenolate mofetil (Cellcept) and azathioprine are being investigated, as is gamma globulin therapy in combination with other immunosuppressive agents. Experimental protocols also are evaluating the efficacy of cyclosporine, soluble tumor necrosis factor receptor antagonists, dozoxyspermaglytoline, and humanized antibodies to leukocyte antigens.

REFERENCES

Guillevin L, Durand-Gasselin B, Cevallos R, et al. Microscopic polyangiitis: clinical and laboratory findings in eighty-five patients. *Arthritis Rheum* 1999;42:421–430.

Jennette JC, Falk RJ. Small vessel vasculitis. *N Engl J Med* 1997;337:1512–1523.

Jennette JC, Falk RJ, Andrassy K, et al. Nomenclature of systemic vasculitides: the proposal of an international consensus conference. *Arthritis Rheum* 1994;37:187–192.

Jennette JC, Thomas DB, Falk RJ. Microscopic polyangiitis (microscopic polyarteritis). *Semin Diagn Pathol* 2001;18:3–13.

Lhote F, Guillevin L. Polyarteritis nodosa, microscopic polyangiitis, and Churg-Strauss syndrome. *Rheum Dis Clin North Am* 1995;21:911–947.

RESOURCES

51, 456

29   Polyarteritis Nodosa

J. Charles Jennette, MD

DEFINITION: Polyarteritis nodosa is a necrotizing vasculitis that affects arteries, especially medium-sized arteries. Polyarteritis nodosa usually is a systemic disease, although organ-limited involvement can occur.

SYNONYM: Periarteritis nodosa.

DIFFERENTIAL DIAGNOSIS: Microscopic polyangiitis (microscopic polyarteritis); Wegener granulomatosis; Churg-Strauss syndrome; Kawasaki disease.

SYMPTOMS AND SIGNS: The clinical presentation is extremely varied because different vessels in different organs can be involved in different patients. The disorder causes constitutional symptoms and signs of inflammatory disease, as well as tissue injury caused by arteritis. Constitutional symptoms include fever, malaise, arthralgias, myalgias, and anorexia. Symptoms and signs of tissue injury include peripheral neuropathy (especially mononeuritis multiplex), tender erythematous cutaneous nodules, ischemic skin ulcers, peripheral gangrene, localized muscle pain, abdominal pain, gastrointestinal hemorrhage, myocardial infarction, hypertension, hematuria, and mild proteinuria. Imaging studies may demonstrate aneurysms or obstruction of main visceral arteries, such as the mesenteric and renal arteries.

ETIOLOGY/EPIDEMIOLOGY: The disorder is most common in older adults, but can occur at any age. There is no sex predominance. The incidence is approximately 0.5 in 100,000 in Europe and North America. The etiology and pathogenesis are unknown. Limited evidence suggests that immune complex deposition in vessel walls is involved in the pathogenesis. Most patients do not have vascular deposits of immunoglobulin and complement. Infections have been proposed as the sources of antigens in immune complexes in affected patients, especially hepatitis B.

DIAGNOSIS: Arterial aneurysms, as well as narrowing and occlusion caused by arteritis, can be detected in major visceral arteries by angiography, CT, or MRI. Imaging also may demonstrate focal infarction or hemorrhage, which is indirect evidence for arteritis. Biopsy specimens may provide findings that rule out polyarteritis nodosa and confirm an alternative diagnosis. Identification of glomerulonephritis in a renal biopsy specimen indicates some form of small vessel vasculitis. Identification of necrotizing arteritis in a biopsy specimen is consistent with polyarteritis nodosa, but is not definitive, because many other types of vasculitis can cause histologically indistinguishable necrotizing arteritis, including Kawasaki disease, microscopic polyangiitis, Wegener granulomatosis, and Churg-Strauss syndrome. Serologic evaluation for antineutrophil cytoplasmic autoantibodies (ANCA) is useful in the diagnosis of systemic vasculitis. A positive ANCA result is uncommon in polyarteritis nodosa but frequent in patients with microscopic polyangiitis, Wegener granulomatosis, or Churg-Strauss syndrome.

TREATMENT

Standard Therapies: High-dose corticosteroids, often in combination with a cytotoxic drug such as cyclophosphamide, usually induce disease remission. If the disease can be managed with corticosteroids alone, a cytotoxic agent should be avoided. Surgery may be appropriate to repair a ruptured aneurysm, remove an aneurysm before rupture, or to repair occlusions. Relapses may occur but they usually respond to additional immunosuppressive therapy. Plasmapheresis should be added to the treatment regimen only if the response to conventional immunosuppression is inadequate or hepatitis B infection is present. In patients with polyarteritis nodosa caused by hepatitis B, antiviral therapy with vidarabine combined with plasmapheresis is indicated.

Investigational Therapies: Mycophenolate mofetil, rapamycin, deoxyspergualin, and azathioprine are being investigated.

REFERENCES

Guillevin L. Polyarteritis nodosa: clinical characteristics, outcome and treatment. In: Adu D, Emery P, Madaio M, eds. *Rheumatology and the kidney.* Oxford: Oxford University Press, 2001:228–245.

Jennette JC, Falk RJ. Small vessel vasculitis. *N Engl J Med* 1997;337:1512–1523.

Kirkland G, Savige J, Wilson D, et al. Classical polyarteritis nodosa and microscopic polyarteritis with medium vessel involvement—a comparison of the clinical and laboratory features. *Clin Nephrol* 1997;47:176–180.

Lhote F, Guillevin L. Polyarteritis nodosa, microscopic polyangiitis, and Churg-Strauss syndrome. *Rheum Dis Clin North Am* 1995;21:911–947.

RESOURCES

27, 359

---

30   Relapsing Polychondritis

Naveed Younis, BSc, MB, ChB, and H. Soran, MB, BS

DEFINITION: Relapsing polychondritis is a multisystem disorder characterized by episodic inflammation of cartilaginous structures resulting in tissue destruction.

SYNONYMS: Systemic chondromalacia; Panchondritis; Chronic atrophic polychondritis; Rheumatic chondritis; Diffuse perichondritis.

DIFFERENTIAL DIAGNOSIS: Connective tissue disorders; Sarcoidosis (joints); Syphilis; Wegener granulomatosis; Tuberculosis; Leprosy (nose); Infectious perichondritis (ears).

SYMPTOMS AND SIGNS: Tenderness, inflammatory swelling, and eventual destruction of cartilage, often in a cyclic fashion, are the main features. Attacks tend to vary in severity and usually last for days to weeks before resolving spontaneously. The disorder appears to affect predominantly the pinna of the ear, nasal cartilage, larynx, and trachea. Bilateral auricular chondritis with redness, swelling, tenderness, and the development of cauliflower ears in the later phase are common findings. Hearing impairment can be caused by closure of the external auditory meatus, serous otitis media, and eustachian tube obstruction. Inflammation of the middle ear and vestibular dysfunction may result in tinnitus and vertigo. Nasal cartilage involvement may result in a saddle nose deformity. Ocular inflammation often occurs manifested as episcleritis, scleritis, iritis, and keratitis. Joint involvement includes a peripheral inflammatory, nonerosive, and nondeforming polyarthritis. The involvement of the larynx and tracheobronchial tree is the most serious manifestation and is characterized by complaints of throat tenderness, hoarseness, dyspnea, wheezing, and stridor. Cardiovascular involvement includes aortic insufficiency with valvular changes as a result of aortitis and aneurysms of the aorta. Small vessel vasculitis may produce palpable purpura.

ETIOLOGY/EPIDEMIOLOGY: Relapsing polychondritis may develop at any age, with most cases diagnosed at 40–60 years of age. Sex distribution is equal; the disorder has been mainly reported in whites. The cause is unknown and no data are available on the incidence and prevalence. Tissue destruction results from release of degradative enzymes, including matrix metalloproteinases from chondrocytes and other cellular elements. The release of these enzymes is likely to be due to immune-mediated activation of the chondrocyte and other inflammatory cells. The etiology is unknown, but is probably autoimmune in nature.

DIAGNOSIS: There is no specific laboratory test, and findings are often nonspecific. Elevated erythrocyte sedimentation rate, leukocytosis, and normochromic anemia are common, and elevated titers of rheumatoid factor or antinuclear factor are occasional findings. The diagnosis is based on clinical grounds, with biopsy showing necrotizing vasculitis and cartilage destruction of affected tissue.

TREATMENT
Standard Therapies: Mild episodes of auricular/nasal chondritis and arthritis usually respond to nonsteroidal antiinflammatory drugs with or without low dosage of corticosteroids. More serious manifestations such as airway destruction respond to corticosteroids. If disease progression occurs despite these therapies, a trial of immunosuppression is warranted. Cyclophosphamide and azothio-prine have been reported to have some success, as has diaminodiphenylsulfone (dapsone). Severe respiratory tract distress requires a tracheostomy for relief. Valve replacement or valvuloplasty may be required in patients with heart failure.

REFERENCES

Eng J, Sabanathan S. Airways complications in relapsing polychondritis. *Ann Thorac Surg* 1991;51:686–692.
Fiodart JM, Abe S, Martin GR, et al. Antibodies to type II collagen in relapsing polychondritis. *N Engl J Med* 1978;229:1203–1207.
Herman J. Polychondritis. In: Kelley WN, Harris ED Jr, Ruddy S, eds. *Textbook of rheumatology,* 4th ed. Philadelphia: WB Saunders, 1993:1400–1411.
Michet CJ. Vasculitis and relapsing polychondritis. *Rheum Dis Clin* 1990;16:441–444.

RESOURCES
51, 456

31   Autoimmune Premature Ovarian Failure

Lawrence M. Nelson, MD, MBA

DEFINITION: Autoimmune premature ovarian failure is caused by a lymphocytic infiltration of the ovary. The immune attack is primarily directed at the ovarian steroid-producing cells of the theca and stroma. The resulting hypogonadism causes amenorrhea, estrogen and androgen deficiency, and infertility.

SYNONYM: Autoimmune oophoritis.

DIFFERENTIAL DIAGNOSIS: Premature ovarian failure or secondary amenorrhea due to other causes.

SYMPTOMS AND SIGNS: No characteristic menstrual pattern precedes the development of autoimmune premature ovarian failure. Patients may develop amenorrhea acutely or experience a prodrome of oligomenorrhea or dysfunctional uterine bleeding. The disorder may become apparent when menstruation fails to return after a pregnancy or after stopping oral contraceptives. The disorder may also be heralded by the onset of vasomotor symptoms. With the establishment of amenorrhea and profound estrogen deficiency, patients may develop symptoms and signs of atrophic vaginitis, including vaginal dryness and dyspareunia. In rare cases, patients may present to the emergency room with the combination of acute abdominal pain and enlarged multicystic ovaries. In about 3% of cases, autoimmune premature ovarian failure occurs concomitantly with autoimmune adrenal insufficiency. In this clinical situation, patients may also experience anorexia, nausea, weight loss, vague abdominal pain, weakness, easy fatigability, salt craving, or increased skin pigmentation. Patients who have both ovarian failure and adrenal insufficiency are profoundly deficient in circulating androgens and exhibit sparse axillary and pubic hair.

ETIOLOGY/EPIDEMIOLOGY: Most cases occur sporadically; however, the disorder is also associated with autoimmune polyglandular failure type 1, which is inherited in an autosomal-recessive manner. Approximately 1% of women develop premature ovarian failure by age 40, but it is unclear what portion of these cases is due to autoimmune oophoritis.

DIAGNOSIS: The diagnosis should be suspected in women presenting with disordered menses. It is confirmed by finding serum levels of follicle-stimulating hormone and luteinizing hormone in the menopausal range. The measurement of adrenal antibodies by commercially available assays may be helpful in the diagnosis, and is being studied.

TREATMENT

Standard Therapies: No standard treatment has been proven safe and effective. Empiric treatment with corticosteroids is to be discouraged because of the risk of osteonecrosis.

REFERENCES

Bannatyne P, Russel P, Shearman RP. Autoimmune oophoritis: a clinicopathologic assessment of 12 cases. *Int J Gynecol Pathol* 1990;9:191–207.

Kalantaridou SN, Braddock DT, Patronas NJ, et al. Treatment of autoimmune premature ovarian failure. *Hum Reprod* 1999;14:1777–1782.

Nelson LM, Anasti JN, Flack MR. Premature ovarian failure. In: Adashi EY, Rock JA, Rosenwaks Z, eds. *Reproductive endocrinology, surgery, and technology.* Philadelphia: Lippincott-Raven, 1996:1393–1410.

RESOURCES

369, 400

---

32 Reye Syndrome

James E. Heubi, MD

DEFINITION: Reye Syndrome (RS) is characterized by noninflammatory encephalopathy and fatty degeneration of the viscera. Children of all ages and, rarely, adults develop it after a prodromal illness. Liver dysfunction is transient, and morbidity and mortality relate to cerebral edema and its complications.

DIFFERENTIAL DIAGNOSIS: Urea cycle enzyme defects; Fatty acid oxidation defects; Organic acidemias; Toxins including acetaminophen and aspirin; Hepatitides caused by hepatitis A and B, Epstein Barr, varicella, cytomegalovirus, and other untypeable hepatitides; Hypoxic encephalopathy and anoxic liver injury; Central nervous system infections.

SYMPTOMS AND SIGNS: The symptoms are relatively specific but similar to the those of other metabolic or toxic conditions, or infectious processes. Typically, the child has an uncomplicated respiratory illness, varicella, or gastroenteritis. As the child is beginning to improve (usually 3–5 days from onset), repetitive vomiting begins. Low-grade fever may be present, but in most circumstances patients are afebrile. Initially, patients are well oriented but irritable and lethargic. Some patients remain lethargic to variable degrees with no progression to unconsciousness. Some patients progress to a hyperexcitable state during which they become disoriented and intermittently out of contact with their environment. Further progression to deeper coma stages may transpire over a few hours to 48 hours or longer.

ETIOLOGY/EPIDEMIOLOGY: The cause of RS remains unknown. There is strong epidemiologic association between RS and antecedent influenza and varicella infections. Similarly, a strong association has been shown between RS and exposure to aspirin. The incidence of the disease has declined substantially in recent years, attributed to reduced aspirin use and the recognition that many children suspected of RS actually have inborn errors of metabolism.

DIAGNOSIS: At presentation, most patients have had multiple episodes of emesis, and the serum SGOT (AST) and SGPT (ALT) are 3–30 times normal. Serum ammonia levels are variable. Comatose patients have elevated venous or arterial ammonia levels ranging from 2 to 20 times normal. In contrast, noncomatose patients may have normal or only mildly elevated (2–5 times normal) ammonia concentrations. Jaundice is extremely unusual and suggests an alternative diagnosis. At presentation, infants and toddlers may have hypoglycemia and marked elevation of free fatty acids. The prothrombin time may be prolonged. Results of cerebrospinal fluid examinations are normal. Additional urine and serum tests should exclude other causes.

TREATMENT

Standard Therapies: Suggested treatments include exchange transfusion, peritoneal dialysis, total body washout, and carnitine administration, but none has been demonstrated in rigorous trials to be effective. Glucose/electrolyte infusions are recommended to prevent hypoglycemia. In the noncomatose, intravenous glucose may prevent progression to deeper coma grades. All comatose patients should be managed in the intensive care setting and intracranial pressure monitored to maintain normal cerebral perfusion pressure. The use of controlled hyperventilation to reduce PCO_2, administration of mannitol, and pentobarbital all help manage cerebral edema.

REFERENCES

Belay ED, Bresee JS, Holman RC, et al. Reye's syndrome in the United States from 1991–1997. *N Engl J Med* 1999;349: 1377–1382. See also Comment in *N Engl J Med* 1999;340: 1423–1424.

Heubi JE, Partin JC, Partin JS, Schubert WK. Reye's syndrome. Current concepts. *Hepatology* 1987;7:155–164.

Hurwitz ES, Barrett MJ, Bergman D, et al. Public Health Study of Reye's syndrome and medications. Report of the main study. *JAMA* 1987;257:1905–1911. [erratum in *JAMA* 1987;257: 3366].

Rowe PC, Valle D, Brusilow SW. Inborn errors of metabolism in children referred with Reye's syndrome. *JAMA* 1988;260: 3167–3170.

RESOURCES
89, 327

33   Sarcoidosis

Leslie T. Cooper, Jr., MD

DEFINITION: Sarcoidosis is a multisystem granulomatous disorder of unknown cause, most commonly affecting the lungs and lymphatic system.

SYNONYMS: Boeck sarcoid; Löfgren syndrome.

DIFFERENTIAL DIAGNOSIS: Tuberculosis and similar microbacterial infections; Fungal infections; Lymphoma; Granulomatous lesions of unknown significance (GLUS).

SYMPTOMS AND SIGNS: The manifestations are broad, ranging from no symptoms to critical illness, and differ by ethnic group. Although sarcoidosis can present in any organ system, most patients have lung involvement. Symptoms of lung involvement include dyspnea, cough, or chest pain. Löfgren syndrome (usually self-limited and affecting those of northern European descent) is the triad of erythema nodosum, hilar lymphadenopathy, and polyarthralgia, sometimes with fever. The heart is involved clinically in 5% of patients in North America and in a higher percentage in Japan. Symptoms may include syncope from high-degree heart block or palpitations and lightheadedness from ventricular tachycardia. A minority of individuals with cardiac involvement have dyspnea and edema from congestive heart failure. Progressive cardiac sarcoidosis may require heart transplantation. Blurry vision, eye pain, and blindness can result from uveitis and glaucoma in the eye. Sarcoid skin lesions take many forms, including erythema nodosum. Large-joint polyarthralgia is relatively common as well.

ETIOLOGY/EPIDEMIOLOGY: The cause of sarcoidosis is unknown. It usually affects adults between the ages of 20 and 40. In Japan, often women over the age of 50 are affected. The incidence of ocular and cardiac involvement is higher in Japan. The incidence of sarcoidosis is estimated at 5–6 cases per 100,000 person years in the United States; it is higher in African Americans than in caucasians. Reports of temporal clustering of sarcoid cases have suggested a transmissible agent. Rarely, families have multiple affected members, suggesting a genetic component exists.

DIAGNOSIS: The diagnosis of sarcoidosis is one of exclusion, requiring a compatible clinical picture and a noncaseating granuloma on biopsy. Sites commonly subjected to biopsy include the skin, lymph nodes, and lungs. Evaluation includes a thorough history; physical examination with focus on the skin, lungs, and lymph nodes; anteroposterior chest x-ray; pulmonary function tests; complete blood count; liver and renal function studies; urinalysis; electrocardiography; tuberculosis skin test; and ophthalmologic examination.

TREATMENT
Standard Therapies: Treatment is controversial because of high rates of spontaneous improvement. Some patients have isolated lung involvement and no symptoms. Those with symptomatic lung disease may benefit from a trial of prednisone, but dose and duration of treatment are not well established. Skin and eye symptoms may respond to topical steroid treatment. Usually cardiac involvement is treated with prednisone at doses of 40–60 mg/day with a taper. Neurologic disease is often treated with steroids as well. Treatment with other immunosuppressive agents, sometimes including methotrexate or azathioprine, may be used in place of prednisone. Referral to a center with clinical expertise should be considered.

REFERENCES

Access Research Group. Design of a case control etiologic study of sarcoidosis (ACCESS). *J Clin Epidemiol* 1999;52:1173–1186.

Hunninghake GW, Costable U, Ando M, et al. ATS/ERS/WASOG statement on sarcoidosis. American Thoracic Society/European Respiratory Society/World Association of Sarcoidosis and other Granulomatous Disorders. *Sarcoidosis Vasc Diffuse Lung Dis* 1999;16:149–173.

Johns CJ, Michele TM. The clinical management of sarcoidosis. A 50-year experience at the Johns Hopkins Hospital. *Medicine* 1999;78:65–111.

Vourlekis JS, Sawyer RT, Newman LS. Sarcoidosis: developments in etiology, immunology, and therapeutics. *Adv Intern Med* 2000;45:209–257.

RESOURCES

328, 425, 426

34   Scleroderma

Westley H. Reeves, MD, and Hanno B. Richards, MD

DEFINITION: Scleroderma is a severe systemic autoimmune disorder characterized by vasculopathy and fibrosis of the skin and internal organs.

SYNONYM: Progressive systemic sclerosis.

DIFFERENTIAL DIAGNOSIS: Mixed connective tissue disease; Toxic oil syndrome; Systemic lupus erythematosus; Polymyositis; Eosinophilia-myalgia syndrome; Chronic graft-versus-host disease; Diffuse fasciitis with eosinophilia; Scleromyxedema; Paraproteinemia; POEMS syndrome.

SYMPTOMS AND SIGNS: Earliest manifestations typically include Raynaud phenomenon, fatigue, sclerodactyly, and musculoskeletal complaints. Later manifestations include progressive skin tightening in other locations and involvement of internal organs, including the gastrointestinal tract (dysphagia, diminished bowel motility), lungs (pulmonary fibrosis, pleural effusions, pulmonary hypertension), kidneys (renal failure), and heart (cardiomyopathy, conduction abnormalities). Severe Raynaud phenomenon may progress to digital ulcers and gangrene. CREST syndrome (calcinosis cutis, Raynaud phenomenon, esophageal dysmotility, sclerodactyly, telangiectasias) is a limited form generally associated with anticentromere antibodies and a mild course. Localized scleroderma includes morphea and linear scleroderma.

ETIOLOGY/EPIDEMIOLOGY: The etiology is unknown. It is 3 times more common in women and usually presents between the fourth and sixth decades of life. Genetic factors play a less important role than in other forms of systemic autoimmunity. The incidence of systemic sclerosis is 19 cases per million people per year, and the prevalence is 20–75 per 100,000. Scleroderma is associated with exposure to silica dust, and is more prevalent in masons, gold miners, and coal miners. Organic solvents (vinyl chloride, trichloroethylene) may increase the risk of scleroderma. Tainted rapeseed oil and L-tryptophan also have been associated with scleroderma-like disease.

DIAGNOSIS: The major criterion for the diagnosis is proximal scleroderma (thickening, tightening, and induration of the skin of the fingers and skin proximal to the metacarpophalangeal or metatarsophalangeal joints, including the extremities, neck, face, or trunk). Minor criteria include sclerodactyly, digital pitting scars, and bibasilar pulmonary fibrosis. Serologic tests confirm the diagnosis. Antinuclear antibodies are common, and autoantibodies against Scl-70 are associated with a poor prognosis.

TREATMENT

Standard Therapies: There is no established therapy for skin disease in systemic sclerosis, but other complications can be treated. Raynaud phenomenon is treated with calcium channel blockers (e.g., nifedipine). Topical nitrates, sympatholytic agents (e.g., prazosin), vasodilators (e.g., pentoxyphylline), or intravenous prostaglandins (prostacyclin, iloprost) may be added to calcium channel blockers. Blood pressure should be controlled aggressively (systolic ≤110), preferably with a long-acting angiotensin-converting enzyme inhibitor, such as fosinopril. Esophageal reflux may contribute to the development of scleroderma lung, and can be treated with a proton pump inhibitor.

Investigational Therapies: Cyclophosphamide is being explored for early scleroderma lung with neutrophilic alveolitis, and intravenous prostaglandins are being explored for pulmonary hypertension.

REFERENCES

Block JA, Sequeira W. Raynaud's phenomenon. *Lancet* 2001;357: 2042–2048.

Kuwana M, Kaburaki J, Okano Y, et al. Clinical and prognostic associations based on serum antinuclear antibodies in Japanese patients with systemic sclerosis. *Arthritis Rheum* 1994;37:75–83.

Steen VD. Scleroderma renal crisis. *Rheum Dis Clin North Am* 1996;22:861–878.

Steen VD, Costantino JP, Shapiro AP, et al. Outcome of renal crisis in systemic sclerosis: relation to availability of angiotensin converting enzyme (ACE) inhibitors. *Ann Intern Med* 1990; 113:352–357.

White B, Moore WC, Wigley FM, et al. Cyclophosphamide is associated with pulmonary function and survival benefit in patients with scleroderma and alveolitis. *Ann Intern Med* 2000;132:947–954.

RESOURCES

221, 428, 429

---

35 Sjögren Syndrome and Cutaneous Vasculitis

Steven R. Weiner, MD, FACP, FACR

DEFINITION: Sjögren syndrome (SS) is a chronic inflammatory/autoimmune disorder that involves infiltration of the exocrine glands by $CD4^+$ T-lymphocytes.

SYNONYMS: Sicca syndrome; Keratoconjunctivitis sicca.

DIFFERENTIAL DIAGNOSIS: Subacute cutaneous lupus erythematosus; Waldenström hypergammaglobulinemic purpura; Amyloidosis; Sarcoidosis; Idiopathic vasculitis; Leukemia.

SYMPTOMS AND SIGNS: Vasculitic skin lesions in SS most commonly manifest as palpable or nonpalpable purpura of the lower extremities. Alternatively, they may appear like urticaria, plaque, or erythema multiforme lesions, nodular or ulcerative skin lesions, or superficial poorly defined patches. Sweet syndrome with erythematous edematous plaque-like lesions containing neutrophilic infiltrates has also been described. Rarely, a larger vessel vasculitis may occur, affecting small and medium-sized arteries appearing in the skin with digital gangrene or punched-out ulcerative lesions. Vasculitic skin lesions typically burn and sting. Cutaneous vasculitis has been associated with central nervous system disease in SS.

ETIOLOGY/EPIDEMIOLOGY: The etiology of SS, as well as of the complicating vasculitis, is unknown. The disorder is more common in women (90%), with the age of onset generally older than 40. Primary and secondary SS may occur in 1%–2% of the population, depending on the criteria used for diagnosis. Vasculitis occurs in less than 20% of patients with primary SS. Dermal vasculitis accounts for approximately half of that number.

DIAGNOSIS: Diagnosis is made by a full-thickness skin biopsy, which most often shows a leukocytoclastic vasculitis.

TREATMENT

Standard Therapies: Leukocytoclastic vasculitis does not always need treatment. If treatment is necessary, antimalarials, topical steroids, or diaminodiphenylsulfones may be used. Involvement of small or medium-sized arteries may require corticosteroids and/or immunosuppressive drugs. For infectious or malignant vasculitis, the standard treatment is drug withdrawal or treatment of the infection or malignancy. In secondary SS cutaneous vasculitis, one should treat the secondary disorder.

Investigational Therapies: Plasmapheresis and interferon-α (for hepatitis C virus–associated cryoglubulinemias in SS) have been used. Other approaches being explored include tolerization to SS (Ro) proteins, gene therapy, and blocking and/or administration of various cytokines.

REFERENCES

Alexander EL, Provost TT. Cutaneous manifestations of primary Sjögren's syndrome: a reflection of vasculitis and association with anti-Ro (SSA) antibodies. *J Invest Dermatol* 1983;80: 386.

Carsons S, Harris EK, eds. *The new Sjögren's syndrome handbook.* New York: Oxford University Press, 1998.

Homma M, Sugai S, Sojo T, et al., eds. *Sjögren's syndrome: state of the art.* Amsterdam: Kugler, 1994.

Sonthumer RD, Provost TT, eds. *Cutaneous manifestations of rheumatic diseases.* Baltimore: Williams & Wilkins, 1996.

RESOURCES

53, 329, 436

36   Takayasu Arteritis

Millicent Y. Tan-Ong, MD,
and Gary S. Hoffman, MD

DEFINITION: Takayasu arteritis is an idiopathic systemic inflammatory disease that may lead to gradual segmental stenosis, occlusion, dilatation, and/or aneurysm formation of the aorta and/or the coronary or pulmonary arteries.

SYNONYMS: Pulseless disease; Young female arteritis; Middle aortic syndrome; Martorell syndrome; Occlusive thromboaortopathy; Nonspecific aortoarteritis.

DIFFERENTIAL DIAGNOSES: Vascular infections; Spondyloarthropathies with aortitis; Buerger disease; Behçet syndrome; Cogan syndrome; Kawasaki disease; Sarcoidosis; Giant cell arteritis; Ehlers-Danlos syndrome; Marfan syndrome; Fibromuscular dysplasia; Neurofibromatosis; Ergotism; Radiation fibrosis.

SYMPTOMS AND SIGNS: The disease ranges from being entirely asymptomatic to having a morbid, disabling, or fatal outcome. Vascular ischemic symptoms are the hallmark. Disease manifestations include bruits, claudication, diminished or absent pulses, asymmetric blood pressure measurements, hypertension, carotodynia, pain over inflamed arteries, Raynaud phenomenon, angina, myocardial infarction, aortic regurgitation, congestive heart failure, pericarditis, palpitations, dizziness or lightheadedness, syncope, transient ischemic attacks, cerebrovascular accidents, seizures, amaurosis fugax, diplopia, blurred vision, iritis, episcleritis, hemoptysis, dyspnea, pleural effusions, arthralgias (rarely synovitis), abdominal pain, nausea, vomiting, erythema nodosum, and, rarely, pyoderma gangrenosum and panniculitis. One or more nonspecific systemic symptoms such as fever, night sweats, malaise, fatigue, weight loss, myalgias, arthralgias, neck pain, or cervical lymphadenopathy occur in approximately half of patients at the onset of disease.

ETIOLOGY/EPIDEMIOLOGY: Although the exact etiopathogenesis of Takayasu arteritis is unknown, it is clear that vessel injury is caused by lymphocytes and macrophages. The disorder occurs most often in Asia, although cases have been recognized worldwide. Approximately 90% of patients are females of child-bearing age, but males may also be affected.

DIAGNOSIS: Diagnosis rests on a high index of suspicion, especially in the presence of ischemic manifestations in young individuals. Angiography is the procedure of choice.

TREATMENT
Standard Therapies: For control of immunoinflammatory features, glucocorticoids are given for approximately 1 month and tapered to the lowest dose required to control disease. Whenever chronic glucocorticoid therapy is employed, bone-preserving therapy should be added. If glucocorticoid therapy cannot be tapered without disease exacerbation, cytotoxic agents such as oral cyclophosphamide daily, azathioprine daily, or methotrexate weekly are added. If disease is well controlled after the addition of cytotoxic agents, corticosteroids are gradually tapered to discontinuation. Prophylactic agents for *Pneumocystis carinii* should accompany combination corticosteroid and cytotoxic therapy. Angioplasty or revascularization may be indicated in some patients. Elective surgery is generally recommended during periods of disease quiescence.

Investigational Therapies: Tacrolimus, mycophenolate mofetil, cyclosporine, and anti–tumor necrosis factor therapy (etanercept and infliximab) are being investigated.

REFERENCES
Giordano JM, Hoffman GS, Leavitt RY. Takayasu's disease: nonspecific aortoarteritis. In: Rutherford RD, ed. *Vascular surgery*. Philadelphia: WB Saunders, 1995:245–253.
Hoffman GS. Takayasu arteritis: lessons from the American National Institutes of Health experience. *Int J Cardiol* 1996; 54(suppl):99–102.
Hoffman GS. Treatment of resistant Takayasu's arteritis. *Rheum Dis Clin North Am* 1995;21:73–70.
Kerr GS, Hallahan CW, Giordano J, et al. Takayasu arteritis. *Ann Intern Med* 1994;120:919–929.
Keystone EC. Takayasu's arteritis. In: Klippel JH, Dieppe PA, eds. *Rheumatology*. Vol. 2. London: CV Mosby, 1999.

RESOURCES
27, 457, 458

37   Thromboangiitis Obliterans

Leslie T. Cooper, Jr., MD

DEFINITION: Thromboangiitis obliterans is an inflammatory vascular occlusive disease that usually affects medium to small arteries and veins in the upper and lower extremities. It is almost universally associated with the use of tobacco products.

SYNONYM: Buerger disease.

DIFFERENTIAL DIAGNOSIS: Scleroderma; Rheumatoid vasculitis; Vasculitis due to connective tissue disease; Antiphospholipid antibody syndrome; Vascular embolization.

SYMPTOMS AND SIGNS: Individuals younger than 50 years present with a history of nicotine use or exposure. In general, other risk factors for atherosclerosis, including hypertension, high cholesterol, and diabetes, are absent. Pain and pale discoloration of the hands and feet upon cold exposure may be the first sign. Pain at rest in the fingers or feet may develop after the arteries close. The decrease in blood flow may lead to dry, dark ulceration usually on the ends of the fingers and toes. These ulcers may be extremely painful; the pain is often worse with elevation and better if the limb is held in a dependent position. Superficial veins may be inflamed with symptoms of pain, redness, and local swelling.

ETIOLOGY/EPIDEMIOLOGY: Although the cause is unknown, the strong relationship between thromboangiitis obliterans and tobacco exposure suggests that a component of tobacco smoke may be essential for the disease to occur. Genetic differences are also likely because the prevalence varies significantly among ethnic groups. The disease was believed to occur almost exclusively in men, but the prevalence in women has been increasing, which may reflect an increased use of tobacco products.

DIAGNOSIS: The diagnosis is based on an appropriate clinical scenario with objective evidence of medium or small artery occlusive disease. An angiogram or noninvasive test of the arteries is usually required to confirm the diagnosis. Although a biopsy of an affected artery can be diagnostic early in the course of the disease, this is infrequently performed because of local pain and the risk of poor wound healing in the setting of decreased arterial blood supply.

TREATMENT

Standard Therapies: The primary therapy should be complete avoidance of tobacco products. The risk of ulceration and limb amputation decreases if individuals abstain from tobacco use. Conservative measures to protect affected limbs may include mittens and avoiding cold exposure. The treatment of pain in patients with thromboangiitis obliterans is frequently difficult and may require the use of medical and occasionally surgical therapies.

Investigational Therapies: Drugs that dilate the arteries and inhibit platelet function have been studied in patients, and some have been associated with modest benefits. Therapies being explored include growth factors that stimulate angiogenesis to accelerate wound healing and decrease ischemic pain, and implantable nerve stimulators to manage pain.

REFERENCES

Olin JW. Thromboangiitis obliterans (Buerger's disease). *N Engl J Med* 2000;343:864–869.

Shionoya S. Buerger's disease: diagnosis and management. *Cardiovasc Surg* 1993;1:207–214.

RESOURCE
357

38   Vogt-Koyanagi-Harada Syndrome

Robert E. Foster, MD

DEFINITION: Vogt-Koyanagi-Harada syndrome is a multisystemic, cell-mediated autoimmune disorder char-acterized by ocular, auditory, dermatologic, and meningeal involvement in middle-aged adults.

SYNONYMS: VKH; Uveomeningitic syndrome; Uveomeningoencephalitic syndrome; Alopecia-poliosis-uveitis-vitiligo-deafness-cutaneous-uveo-oto syndrome; Harada syndrome.

DIFFERENTIAL DIAGNOSIS: Sympathetic ophthalmia; Sarcoidosis.

SYMPTOMS AND SIGNS: Patients may have a brief period of inflammation and disease, or a chronic progressive course. CNS symptoms predominate initially and include headache, vertigo, stiff neck, and, less commonly, seizures, fever, coma, hemiparesis, or focal neurologic signs. Auditory and ocular symptoms tend to occur concurrently (may be presenting). Auditory symptoms, reported in >75% of patients, are central sensorineural hearing loss, dysacousis, tinnitus, and vertigo. Ocular findings tend to be bilateral and are characterized by uveitis. Anterior segment symptoms include photophobia, redness, pain, signs of conjunctival injection, microscopic cellular precipitates on the corneal endothelium, iris nodules, posterior synechiae, and a shallow anterior chamber with hypotony. Posterior symptoms include vision loss, floaters, vitritis, optic nerve head swelling, retinal edema, and exudative retinal detachment (Insert Fig. 4). Late anterior findings are cataract and secondary glaucoma. Additional late sequelae may be retinal, optic nerve head, or anterior segment neovascularization, choroidal neovascularization, and subretinal fibrosis. About 60% of patients retain good vision. The visual prognosis for the 10% with choroidal neovascularization is poor, but may be aided by extraction. About 1 in 4 patients develop cataracts, and 1 in 3 glaucoma. One third of patients develop vitiligo, alopecia, and/or poliosis, usually after the ocular and auditory symptoms.

ETIOLOGY/EPIDEMIOLOGY: The cause is unknown, but most likely autoimmune. There may be a genetic predisposition. VKH is most common in noncaucasians. Men and women seem to be affected equally.

DIAGNOSIS: Systemic findings are important in the diagnosis. No one test confirms VKH; lumbar puncture, intravenous fluorescein angiography, indocyanine green angiography, and ocular ultrasonography are useful. Early in the disease process, spinal fluid analysis reveals a nonspecific lymphocytic and monocytic pleocytosis in more than 80% of cases. Multifocal pinpoint leaks at the level of the retinal pigment epithelium on fluorescein angiography are nonspecific but helpful.

TREATMENT

Standard Therapies: Systemic corticosteroids are the mainstay of treatment for nonocular and bilateral ocular inflammatory disease. Anterior and posterior segment inflammatory ocular diseases are treated with topical steroid drops and periocular injections, respectively. With anterior segment inflammation, cycloplegic drops help prevent posterior synechiae and relieve the pain of iridocyclitis. Cyclosporine has been used, either alone or combined with steroids. Cytotoxic agents are less commonly used.

Investigational Therapies: Investigational therapies include intravenous immunoglobulin and plasmapheresis.

REFERENCES

Banares A, Jover JA, Fernandez-Gutierrez B, et al. Patterns of uveitis as a guide in making rheumatologic and immunologic diagnoses. *Arthritis Rheum* 1997;40:358–370.

Davis JL, Mittal KK, Freidlin V, et al. HLA associations and ancestry in Vogt-Koyanagi-Harada disease and sympathetic ophthalmia. *Ophthalmology* 1990;97:1137–1142.

Hayasaka S, Okabe H, Takahashi J. Systemic corticosteroids treatment in Vogt-Koyanagi-Harada disease. *Graefes Arch Clin Exp Ophthalmol* 1982;218:9–13.

Helveston WR, Gilmore R. Treatment of Vogt-Koyanagi-Harada syndrome with intravenous immunoglobulin. *Neurology* 1996;46:584–585.

Moorthy RS, Inomata H, Rao NA. Vogt-Koyanagi-Harada syndrome. *Surv Ophthalmol* 1995;39:265–292.

Nussenblatt RB, Palestine AG, Chan CC. Cyclosporin A therapy in the treatment of intraocular inflammatory disease resistant to systemic corticosteroids and cytotoxic agents. *Am J Ophthalmol* 1983;96:275–282.

Rubsamen PE, Gass JD. Vogt-Koyanagi-Harada syndrome. Clinical course, therapy, and long-term visual outcome. *Arch Ophthalmol* 1991;109:682–687.

RESOURCES

27, 355

39 Waldenström Macroglobulinemia

Morie A. Gertz, MD

DEFINITION: Waldenström macroglobulinemia is characterized by progressive bone marrow infiltration with lymphoplasmacytic or lymphoplasmacytoid cells associated with the presence of a monoclonal IgM protein in the serum.

SYNONYMS: Macroglobulinemia; Waldenström disease.

DIFFERENTIAL DIAGNOSIS: Chronic lymphatic leukemia; Low-grade non-Hodgkin lymphoma; Multiple myeloma.

SYMPTOMS AND SIGNS: Some patients with Waldenström macroglobulinemia, proven by the presence of monoclonal IgM protein and by a bone marrow biopsy, will not have symptoms and can be monitored without therapeutic intervention. IgM monoclonal gammopathies are not rare, and it is important that patients have symptoms necessitating therapeutic intervention. The clinical manifestations can occur as a result of lymphoid infiltration of the bone marrow, liver, or spleen, and most commonly produce a normochromic normocytic anemia. Some patients present with high serum levels of the IgM monoclonal protein, which lead to symptoms of increased serum viscosity, the most common of which are epistaxis, gingival bleeding, and altered mentation. Approximately 15% of patients have palpable hepatosplenomegaly, but the majority present with anemia.

ETIOLOGY/EPIDEMIOLOGY: With an incidence of approximately 4 per 1 million Americans, Waldenström macroglobulinemia represents 2% of hematologic malignancies. There is a slight male preponderance of 55% to 45%. The median age at diagnosis is 67 years. The etiology is unknown.

DIAGNOSIS: The diagnosis is verified by bone marrow infiltration with monoclonal cells that have the morphology of plasma cells, lymphocytes, or lymphoplasmacytes. Patient must have an IgM monoclonal protein to fulfill the diagnostic criteria. A CT scan of the abdomen can check the extent of hepatosplenomegaly and retroperitoneal adenopathy. One should test the level of IgM monoclonal protein by serum protein electrophoresis, urine protein electrophoresis, measurement of the β_2 microglobulin (an important prognostic factor in this disease), and the serum viscosity level.

TREATMENT
Standard Therapies: Although no consensus exists on the initial treatment, the most common classes of therapy include alkylating agents, purine nucleoside analogues, and rituximab—used singly, sequentially, and in combination. All of these treatments are designed to reduce the numbers of neoplastic cells in the bone marrow and the synthesis of the IgM monoclonal protein, thereby reducing the serum viscosity, and to improve hematopoiesis, reducing the symptoms of the associated anemia. Some patients require regular plasma exchange to manage the symptoms of hyperviscosity syndrome. Some require transfusional support with packed red blood cells for anemia not responsive to chemotherapy or supportive care with erythopoietin injections.

Investigational Therapies: These include high-dose therapy with stem cell transplantation and antiangiogenic agents.

REFERENCES
Byrd JC, White CA, Link B, et al. Rituximab therapy in Waldenström's macroglobulinemia: preliminary evidence of clinical activity. *Ann Oncol* 1999;10:1525–1527.
Dimopoulos MA, Panayiotidis P, Moulopoulos LA, et al. Waldenström's macroglobulinemia: clinical features, complications, and management. *J Clin Oncol* 2000;18:214–226.
Gertz MA, Fonseca R, Rajkumar SV. Waldenström's macroglobulinemia. *Oncologist* 2000;5:63–67.
Hellman A, Lewandowski K, Zaucha JM, et al. Effect of a 2-hour infusion of 2-cholorodeoxyadenosine in the treatment of refractory or previously untreated Waldenström's macroglobulinemia. *Eur J Haematol* 1999;63:35–41.

RESOURCES
82, 212

40   Wiskott-Aldrich Syndrome

Alexandra H. Filipovich, MD

DEFINITION: Wiskott-Aldrich syndrome (WAS) is a prematurely lethal disorder of platelets and immune cells due to deficiency of an intracellular protein, WASP, which is involved in normal structure and function of most blood cells. This deficiency leads to low platelet counts in the blood and significant risk of serious bleeding, as well as susceptibility to serious infections.

SYNONYM: X-linked thrombocytopenia.

DIFFERENTIAL DIAGNOSIS: Immune thrombocytopenic purpura (in infancy); Severe atopic eczema.

SYMPTOMS AND SIGNS: The syndrome usually presents in infancy with bloody diarrhea, mucosal bleeding, and/or petechiae. Eczema of the skin is often present. The diagnosis of recurrent middle ear infections and purulent drainage from the ears completes the classic triad of symptoms originally described. The development of *Pneumocystis carinii* pneumonia (PCP) and intracranial bleeding are possible early, life-threatening complications. In patients who survive the early years, later potential complications include hemolytic anemia, arthritis, vasculitis, and immune-mediated damage to the kidneys and liver. Patients have a high risk, increasing with age, of developing lymphomas, often in unusual locations such as the brain. These tend to occur in patients who have been exposed to Epstein-Barr virus.

ETIOLOGY/EPIDEMIOLOGY: The syndrome is inherited as an X-linked recessive disorder and is due to mutations in the *WASP* gene located on chromosome Xp11.22. Estimated incidence is 4 per million live male births; all ethnic groups are affected. Approximately one third of cases are spontaneous mutations. Female carriers of the mutation are generally healthy.

DIAGNOSIS: The diagnosis should be suspected in male infants with a history of bleeding and thrombocytopenia, especially if the findings persist for more than a few weeks and include eczema or failure to thrive. Diagnosis of PCP should lead to an investigation of primary or secondary immunodeficiency, including the possibility of WAS. On peripheral blood smear, WAS platelets are generally very small in size. Other typical laboratory findings of immune dysfunction include abnormal levels of serum immunoglobulins: low IgM, elevated IgA and IgE, decreased absolute numbers of CD8+ T cells, and decreased function of natural killer cells. Not all boys with WAS demonstrate all or many of these laboratory findings. The diagnosis can be strengthened by demonstrating lack of WASP protein in blood cells, and definitively diagnosed by molecular genetic analysis of the patient's WASP gene.

TREATMENT

Standard Therapies: The only curative treatment available is allogeneic bone marrow transplantation (BMT). Boys with WAS who receive BMT from a matched healthy sibling or closely matched unrelated donor can expect a greater than 85% probability of being cured if the procedure is performed before the fifth birthday. Preclinical studies on the use of gene therapy to treat WAS are ongoing. Supportive care after diagnosis and prior to any definitive therapy usually includes trimethoprim and sulfamethoxazole prophylaxis against PCP, topical steroid therapy for the eczema, and, often, replacement therapy with intravenous immunoglobulin every 3–4 weeks. Platelet transfusions should be administered judiciously, e.g., for significant clinical bleeding and with surgical procedures. Historically, splenectomy was widely performed to increase the platelet counts and reduce risk of fatal hemorrhage; however, removal of the spleen increases the risk of overwhelming bacterial infection and patients who have had splenectomy must take antibiotics for the rest of their lives.

REFERENCES

Derry JM, Ochs HD, Francke U. Isolation of a novel gene mutated in Wiskott-Aldrich syndrome. *Cell* 1994;78:635–644.

Filipovich AH, Stone J, Tomany, et al. Impact of donor type on outcome of bone marrow transplantation for Wiskott-Aldrich syndrome: collaborative study of the International Bone Marrow Transplant Registry and the National Marrow Donor Program. *Blood* 2001;97:1598–1603.

Ochs HD, Rosen FS. The Wiskott-Aldrich syndrome. *Cell* 1999;78:292–305.

Sullivan KE, Mullen CA, Blaese RM, et al. A multi-institutional survey of the Wiskott-Aldrich syndrome. *J Pediatr* 1994;125:876–885.

Villa A, Notarangelo L, Macchi P, et al. X-linked thrombocytopenia and Wiskott-Aldrich syndrome are allelic diseases with mutations in the *WASP* gene. *Nat Genet* 1995;9:414–417.

RESOURCES

193, 218

2

Cardiovascular Disorders

1   Atrial Septal Defects

Ritu Chatrath, MD

DEFINITION: An atrial septal defect (ASD) is an opening/deficiency in the wall between the right and the left atrium. The four types of atrial septal defects are classified according to their location in the atrial septum. An ostium secundum is the most frequent type of ASD (50%–70%) and is located in the middle part of the atrial septum in the region of the fossa ovalis. The ostium primum defect (15%–30%) lies caudal to the fossa ovalis; it is frequently associated with a cleft mitral valve and may occur in isolation or as a part of an atrioventricular septal defect. Sinus venosus defects (5%–10%) lie superior to the fossa ovalis, at the entry of the superior vena cava into the right atrium, and are commonly associated with anomalous connection of right pulmonary veins into the superior vena cava or right atrium. A coronary sinus defect is the least common type of ASD and lies anterior and inferior to the fossa ovalis, in the area where the normal coronary sinus ostium is anticipated. An "unroofed" coronary sinus results from the lack of partition between the coronary sinus and the left atrium, and is often associated with a left superior vena cava.

DIFFERENTIAL DIAGNOSIS: Lutembacher syndrome.

SYMPTOMS AND SIGNS: Infants and children with ASD are usually asymptomatic, but some may present with congestive heart failure, frequent respiratory infections, or growth failure. In adults, varying degrees of exercise intolerance, dyspnea, or fatigue may be noted. The incidence of atrial arrhythmias increases with advancing age. Paradoxic embolization through an ASD can result in cerebrovascular accidents. The risk of infective endocarditis in patients with isolated secundum ASDs is no greater than in the general population, but patients with associated cardiac anomalies and other types of ASD are at a higher risk. Spontaneous closure of a secundum ASD occurs in one third of patients. On physical examination, in patients with a large left-to-right shunt, a precordial bulge with hyperdynamic cardiac impulse is present. The auscultatory hallmark is a widely split and fixed second heart sound. The increased flow across the pulmonary valve produces an ejection systolic murmur. The increased volume of blood flowing across the tricuspid valve produces an early to mid-diastolic flow murmur. Long-term pulmonary vascular resistance may begin to gradually increase and ultimately lead to reversal of the shunt flow. These patients present with cyanosis, clubbing, erythrocytosis, and right heart failure.

ETIOLOGY/EPIDEMIOLOGY: The various types of ASD result from abnormal embryogenesis of the atrial septum. The ostium secundum defect results from either excessive resorption of the septum primum, deficient growth of the septum secundum, or an abnormal valve of the fossa ovalis. In the partial form of atrioventricular septal defect, the ostium primum defect results from a lack of closure of the ostium primum by the endocardial cushions. The morphogenesis of a sinus venosus defect is explained by an abnormal resorption of the sinus venosus close to the orifice of the superior vena cava. Coronary sinus defects occur due to the absence of a portion of wall between the left atrium and the coronary sinus. Atrial septal defects account for approximately 10% of congenital heart defects. They occur more frequently in females (2:1). Most occur sporadically. Familial occurrence of isolated ASD has been described in association with chromosome 5p.

DIAGNOSIS: Electrocardiography shows right axis deviation and an rSR' pattern in right precordial leads. Chest radiography shows enlargement of the right-sided cardiac chambers and dilatation of pulmonary arteries along with increased pulmonary vascular markings. Echocardiography allows direct visualization of the location and size of the defect. Transesophageal echocardiography is useful in demonstrating ASD if the images are not satisfactory on transthoracic imaging. A diagnostic cardiac catheterization is needed only if unanswered questions remain after an echocardiogram regarding any associated lesions or to assess pulmonary hypertension.

TREATMENT
Standard Therapies: Definite treatment is surgical closure of the defect by suture or prosthetic patch placement with the patient on cardiopulmonary bypass. Elective surgery is recommended at 3–5 years of age. It may be needed earlier if congestive heart failure is refractory to medical management with digoxin and diuretics. Except for patients with ostium secundum ASD, endocarditis prophylaxis is recommended. Device closure of secundum ASD using transcatheter techniques has had long-term use. Transesophageal or intracardiac echocardiography is used to assist placement of these devices.

Investigational Therapies: Many types of ASD closure devices are being investigated.

REFERENCES
Braunwald E, et al., eds. *Heart disease: a textbook of cardiovascular medicine*, 6th ed. Philadelphia: WB Saunders, 2001:1524–1527.

Driscoll DJ. Left-to-right shunt lesions. *Pediatr Clin North Am* 1999;46:355–368.

Formigaria R. Minimally invasive or interventional repair of atrial septal defects in children: experience in 171 cases and comparison with conventional strategies. *J Am Coll Cardiol* 2001;37:1707–1712.

Johnson MC. Echocardiographic prediction of left-to-right shunt with atrial septal defects. *J Am Soc Echocardiogr* 2000;13: 1038–1042.

RESOURCES

35, 113

2 Atrioventricular Septal Defects

Aleksandra Lange, MD, FESC, and Przemysław Palka, MD, FESC

DEFINITION: Atrioventricular septal defects can be diagnosed by the presence of several characteristic features, i.e., a common atrioventricular junction, an unwedged aorta with an often narrowed left ventricular outflow tract, and disproportion in the left ventricular aspect of the septum (inlet/outlet disproportion). The most characteristic anatomic feature is the arrangement of five atrioventricular valve leaflets that guard the common atrioventricular junction.

SYNONYMS: Atrioventricular canal defects; Atrioventricular defects; Endocardial cushion defects; Common atrioventricular orifice.

DIFFERENTIAL DIAGNOSIS: Secundum/primum atrial septal defect with or without mitral regurgitation; Anomalous pulmonary venous connection; Ventricular septal defect.

SYMPTOMS AND SIGNS: The symptoms vary greatly and depend on the severity of the malformation. Dyspnea, fatigue, and recurrent respiratory infections can occur early in life with signs of poor feeding or undergrowth. Infants with the complete form of atrioventricular septal defect develop congestive heart failure. Persistent high pulmonary vascular resistance is also common. Frequent episodes of pneumonia and bronchitis are common. Older children have an increased risk of thrombosis and subsequent arterial embolisms as well as bacterial endocarditis. Adults with untreated atrioventricular septal defects often develop Eisenmenger syndrome.

ETIOLOGY/EPIDEMIOLOGY: The exact cause is not known. This birth defect can occur alone with no apparent cause, or it can occur in association with other disorders such as Down syndrome (approximately 50%). In approximately 70% of patients, no major cardiac anomalies are associated. In approximately 10%, patent ductus arteriosus and/or tetralogy of Fallot are present. Males and females are affected in equal numbers.

DIAGNOSIS: The diagnosis of atrioventricular septal defect is often based on combined data obtained from clinical examination, electrocardiogram, and echocardiogram. Cardiac catheterization and/or MRI provide further information on the extent of malformation.

TREATMENT

Standard Therapies: Surgery is the therapy of choice and needs to be considered before the patient is 2 years of age and often before 6–12 months of age. After that age, significant pulmonary vascular obstructive disease is likely to occur. Surgical repair of complete atrioventricular septal defect in symptomatic infants is believed best done at one time even in infants younger than 6 months, because the surgical risk of banding and later complete repair is higher. Reconstruction of the left atrioventricular valve is strongly preferred over valve replacement at the time of the initial surgical procedure. Prior to surgery, congestive heart failure should be treated with the help of diuretics, angiotensin-converting enzyme inhibitors, sometimes digoxin to decrease the heart rate, and oxygen therapy. All respiratory infections should be treated early and vigorously. Because of increased risk of bacterial endocarditis, antibiotics should also be given as prophylactics before all invasive/surgical procedures (e.g., dental, urologic).

REFERENCES

Anderson RH, Becker AE, Lucchese FA, et al. *Morphology of congenital heart disease. Angiographic, echocardiographic, and surgical correlates.* City: Castle House Publications, 1983: 65–83.

Behrman RE. *Nelson textbook of pediatrics,* 14th ed. Philadelphia: WB Saunders, 1992:1169–1170.

Lange A, Mankad P, Walayat M, et al. Transthoracic three-dimensional echocardiography in the preoperative assessment of atrioventricular septal defect morphology. *Am J Cardiol* 2000;85:630–635.

Najm HK, Coles JG, Endo M, et al. Complete atrioventricular septal defects. Results of repair, risk factors, and freedom from reoperation. *Circulation* 1997;96(suppl II):311–315.

Williams WG, Rudd M. Echocardiographic features of endocardial cushion defects. *Circulation* 1974;49:418–422.

RESOURCES

35, 113

---

3   Barth Syndrome

Gerald F. Cox, MD, PhD, FACMG

DEFINITION: Barth syndrome is an X-linked genetic disorder characterized by the triad of cardiomyopathy, neutropenia, and 3-methylglutaconic aciduria in boys.

SYNONYMS: X-linked cardioskeletal myopathy and neutropenia; Endocardial fibroelastosis type 2; 3-methylglutaconic aciduria type II.

DIFFERENTIAL DIAGNOSIS: Mitochondrial myopathy, including infantile MELAS syndrome; Myocarditis; Kostmann and Shwachman-Diamond syndromes.

SYMPTOMS AND SIGNS: Barth syndrome generally occurs as heart failure in infant boys; rarely, it occurs in older children. Initially, the cardiomyopathy has a distinctive dilated and hypertrophic pattern that often includes endocardial fibroelastosis. Over time, the cardiomyopathy usually improves or resolves. Neutropenia may be cyclic or chronic and may predispose some boys to mouth ulcers and bacterial infections. Mouth ulcers may be associated with spiking fevers. Other variable symptoms include mild to moderate growth retardation, hypotonia, motor delay, and nonprogressive weakness. Affected boys often have myopathic facies and difficulty chewing.

ETIOLOGY/EPIDEMIOLOGY: The Barth syndrome gene, *G4.5*, is located on chromosome Xq28 and is predicted to encode an acyltransferase. More than 30 mutations have been described in patients with no clear phenotypic correlation. The recurrence risk to future sons is 50% if inherited from an asymptomatic carrier mother, which accounts for 80% of cases, with the rest being sporadic. The incidence may be as high as 1 in 100,000, with underdiagnosis likely. More than 50 families from North America, Europe, and Australia are known to exist.

DIAGNOSIS: The diagnosis should be suspected in any infant boy with dilated cardiomyopathy. The diagnosis is confirmed by a high level of 3-methylglutaconic acid in plasma or urine and/or a mutation in the tafazzin gene.

TREATMENT

Standard Therapies: Medical care is supportive, and physical therapy is beneficial. Standard medications, including cardiac glycosides, afterload reducers, and diuretics, are used to treat cardiomyopathy. Periodic monitoring for arrhythmias is indicated. Young boys should be observed closely for signs of infection. In the setting of fever and neutropenia, young children should be evaluated for sepsis and treated with intramuscular/intravenous broad-spectrum antibiotics until cultures are negative. Daily granulocyte colony-stimulating factor (G-CSF) given subcutaneously restores neutrophils to a normal level after a few days, but the effect is transient without regular dosing. G-CSF may be used acutely or chronically to treat recurrent infections as well as mouth ulcers and gingivitis. Some infants have received antibiotic prophylaxis. Despite lifelong neutropenia, the rate and severity of infections decrease with age. Vaccinations and normal school participation are encouraged. Although most children experience steady improvement after diagnosis during infancy, transient regression may occur during puberty.

Investigational Therapies: Pancreatic enzyme supplements for failure to thrive, vitamin supplements for mitochondrial dysfunction, and an oral formulation of cholesterol dissolved in soy oil to normalize the cholesterol level are being investigated. One critically ill patient improved after receiving intravenous pantothenic acid, but many others showed no improvement. Future clinical trials may involve dietary supplementation with specific lipids.

REFERENCES

Barth PG, Wanders RJA, Vreken P, et al. X-linked cardioskeletal myopathy and neutropenia (Barth syndrome). *J Inherit Metab Dis* 1999;22:555–567.

Bione S, D'Adamo P, Maestrini E, et al. A novel X-linked gene, G4.5, is responsible for Barth syndrome. *Nat Genet* 1996;12: 385–389.

Cox GF, Pulsipher M, Rothenberg M, et al. Correction of neutropenia in Barth syndrome by G-CSF. *Am J Hum Genet* 1995;57:177.

Johnston J, Kelley RI, Feigenbaum A, et al. Mutation characterization and genotype-phenotype correlation in Barth syndrome. *Am J Hum Genet* 1997;61:1053–1058.

Vreken P, Valianpour F, Nijtmans LG, et al. Defective remodeling of cardiolipin and phosphotidylglycerol in Barth syndrome. *Biochem Biophys Res Commun* 2000;279:378–382.

RESOURCES
66, 67

4 Brugada Syndrome

Jeffrey A. Towbin, MD

DEFINITION: Brugada syndrome is an autosomal-dominant inherited disorder characterized by ST-segment elevation in the right precordial leads (V1, V2, V3) on the surface electrocardiogram, with or without right bundle branch block and associated with ventricular fibrillation and sudden death in the absence of structural heart disease.

SYNONYMS: Idiopathic ventricular fibrillation; Syndrome of ST elevation and right bundle branch block.

DIFFERENTIAL DIAGNOSIS: Early repolarization syndrome; Idiopathic ventricular fibrillation; Arrhythmogenic right ventricular dysplasia; Long QT syndrome.

SYMPTOMS AND SIGNS: Affected individuals present with syncope, sudden death during sleep, or are asymptomatic. No obvious triggers are known, and the severity and frequency of events vary.

ETIOLOGY/EPIDEMIOLOGY: Brugada syndrome is an autosomal inherited trait caused by heterozygous mutations in the cardiac sodium channel gene *SCN5A* and probably other ion channels. It is more common in males than females and is seen worldwide. The incidence is not known.

DIAGNOSIS: The diagnosis is made on surface electrocardiography. In many cases, the electrocardiogram is nondiagnostic and electrophysiologic testing with provocation is needed. Sodium channel blocking agents such as flecainide, procainamide, and, in Europe, Ajmaline, can provoke ST-segment elevation.

TREATMENT
Standard Therapies: Implantation of an implantable cardioverter defibrillator is considered the treatment of choice because of the lack of proven pharmaceutical therapy.

Investigational Therapies: Quinidine is under investigation. Genetic testing is currently a research tool.

REFERENCES
Antzelevitch C, Brugada P, Brugada J, et al., eds. *The Brugada syndrome. Clinical approaches to tachyarrhythmias.* New York: Futura, 1999.

Brugada P, Brugada J. Right bundle-branch block persistent ST segment elevation and sudden cardiac death: a distinct clinical and electrocardiographic syndrome. A multicenter report. *J Am Coll Cardiol* 1992;20:1391–1396.

Brugada R, Brugada J, Antzelevitch C, et al. Sodium channel blockers identify risk for sudden death in patients with ST-segment elevation and right bundle branch block but structurally normal hearts. *Circulation* 2000;101:510–515.

Chen Q, Kirsch GE, Zhang D, et al. Genetic basis and molecular mechanism for idiopathic ventricular fibrillation. *Nature* 1998;392:293–296.

RESOURCES
390, 411

5 Cor Triatriatum

Mikel D. Smith, MD

DEFINITION: Cor triatriatum is a congenital heart anomaly characterized by the presence of a fibromuscular membrane, which divides the left atrium into two chambers. The membrane can obstruct inflow through the mitral valve, producing high pulmonary vein and capillary pressures.

SYNONYMS: Stenosis of the common pulmonary vein; Pulmonary sinus malformation; Left atrial membrane.

DIFFERENTIAL DIAGNOSIS: Mitral stenosis; Supravalvular mitral ring; Anomalous pulmonary venous return.

SYMPTOMS AND SIGNS: Children with severe obstructive cor triatriatum develop difficulty breathing, rapid respiratory rate, and cough, whereas infants may demonstrate irritability, difficulty feeding, and failure to thrive. If the abnormality is undetected, death may occur in the first 2 years of life. Patients with only mild obstruction may have few symptoms, even in adult life. For adults, chronic effort dyspnea, frequent bouts of pneumonia, or unexplained pulmonary edema (especially with hemoptysis) may be signs of the condition. The physical examination usually reflects evidence of chronic pulmonary hypertension, with a loud P_2 component, often without splitting, a systolic murmur of tricuspid regurgitation, and a prominent right ventricular impulse on palpation. Rarely, the left atrium–obstructing membrane itself may produce a continuous systolic/diastolic flow murmur due to a high-pressure gradient across the partition throughout the cardiac cycle. A diastolic murmur of pulmonic insufficiency due to pulmonary hypertension may also be present.

ETIOLOGY/EPIDEMIOLOGY: Cor triatriatum occurs with equal frequency in both sexes, and accounts for 0.1%–0.4% of all patients with congenital heart disease. The partitioning membrane in the left atrium embryologically represents a persistent division between the common pulmonary vein and the left atrium. A similar malformation can occur in the right atrium, where it is known as cor triatriatum dexter.

DIAGNOSIS: Cor triatriatum may be diagnosed by many imaging methods, including cardiac angiography, CT, MRI, and two-dimensional echocardiography. The presence of the abnormality is often first suspected during a standard surface (transthoracic) echo examination, seen as an echogenic ridge extending from the lateral wall of the left atrium to the interatrial septum, which produces abnormal flow patterns. Direct visualization of the left atrial membrane is best seen by transesophageal echo.

TREATMENT

Standard Therapies: Survival without surgical treatment is directly related to the size of the membrane orifice. Diagnosing obstructive cor triatriatum early is important to prevent the sequelae related to chronic pulmonary hypertension that can result from high pulmonary vein and capillary pressures. The definitive treatment is complete surgical excision of the obstructing membrane. If this operation is performed early in the course of disease, the risk for mortality is low (<1%), with excellent long-term results and no recurrence.

REFERENCES

Moss AJ, Adams FH. Stenosis of the common pulmonary vein: cor triatriatum. In: Moss AJ, Adams FH, eds. *Heart disease in infants, children and adolescents.* Baltimore: Williams & Wilkins, 1989:863–868.

Rorie M, Xie G-Y, Miles H, et al. Diagnosis and surgical correction of cor triatriatum in an adult: combined use of transaesophageal echocardiography and catheterization. *Cathet Cardiovasc Intervent* 2000;51:83–86.

Schluter M, Langstein BA, Thier W, et al. Transesophageal two-dimensional echocardiography in the diagnosis of cor triatriatum in the adult. *J Am Coll Cardiol* 1983;2:1011–1015.

Van Son J, Danielson GK, Schaff HV, et al. Cor triatriatum: diagnosis, operative approach, and late results. *Mayo Clin Proc* 1993;68:854–859.

Vuocolo LM, Stoddard MF, Longaker RA. Transesophageal two dimensional and Doppler echocardiographic diagnosis of cor triatriatum in the adult. *Am Heart J* 1992;124:791–793.

RESOURCES

35, 113, 115

6   Eisenmenger Syndrome

M. Elizabeth Brickner, MD

DEFINITION: The Eisenmenger syndrome refers to severe pulmonary vascular obstructive disease secondary to an unrepaired cardiac shunt (e.g., ventricular septal defect, patent ductus arteriosus, atrial septal defect, or other more complicated congenital defects). Patients are born with a large left-to-right shunt, then develop progressive changes in the pulmonary vascular bed leading to worsening pulmonary hypertension and ultimately resulting in reversal of the cardiac shunt (now right-to-left), causing systemic arterial desaturation.

SYNONYMS: Pulmonary vascular obstructive disease; Eisenmenger reaction or complex.

DIFFERENTIAL DIAGNOSIS: Primary pulmonary hypertension; Tetralogy of Fallot; Other unrepaired cyanotic forms of congenital heart disease.

SYMPTOMS AND SIGNS: Patients usually present in adolescence or adulthood. They often have a history of a murmur and respiratory problems (due to pulmonary congestion from a large left-to-right shunt) in infancy. Over time, spontaneous improvement occurs in symptoms as pulmonary vascular resistance increases and the size of the shunt decreases. Less commonly, adults may present with no prior history of cardiac or pulmonary problems in childhood. As the pulmonary vascular disease progresses and pulmonary hypertension worsens, patients develop increasing right-to-left shunting, resulting in cyanosis. Patients commonly present with symptoms of limited exercise tolerance, including fatigue and dyspnea. Palpitations are also common. Less common but more serious symptoms include hemoptysis and syncope. Patients have central cyanosis, most easily detected by examining the digits and the mucous membranes of the oral cavity. Clubbing of the fingers and toes is also present. The cardiac examination may be deceptive, because the murmurs resulting from the initial left-to-right shunt disappears as the patient develops severe pulmonary vascular disease. The pulmonic component of the second heart sound is increased. Lungs are clear and peripheral edema is uncommon among adolescent patients but more common among adult patients.

ETIOLOGY/EPIDEMIOLOGY: The etiology is unknown. The increased flow and pressure in the pulmonary arteries associated with the initial left-to-right shunt may cause microvascular injury, stimulating a cascade of adverse structural changes in the pulmonary vascular bed. Approximately 8% of patients with congenital heart disease develop the Eisenmenger syndrome.

DIAGNOSIS: The electrocardiogram is abnormal with right atrial enlargement and right ventricular hypertrophy. On chest radiography, heart size is usually normal with prominent central pulmonary arteries but markedly decreased peripheral vessels. Arterial blood gases or pulse oximetry will demonstrate arterial desaturation that does not resolve with the administration of supplemental oxygen. As a consequence of the arterial desaturation, a compensatory increase occurs in the hemoglobin and hematocrit (erythrocytosis). Echocardiography is the initial diagnostic tool to define the cardiac defect, confirm the right-to-left shunt, and estimate the severity of pulmonary hypertension. Echocardiography can also exclude other types of cyanotic congenital heart disease that may be amenable to repair. Cardiac catheterization is indicated to confirm the diagnosis and measure pulmonary vascular resistance.

TREATMENT

Standard Therapies: Long-term survival is possible with careful medical management. Surgical closure of the cardiac defect is contraindicated. Anesthesia must be carefully managed for noncardiac surgery. Pregnancy is absolutely contraindicated (high maternal and fetal mortality), and sterilization is recommended. Prophylaxis for bacterial endocarditis is required. Vasodilators or other medications that decrease systemic vascular resistance should be avoided, as should dehydration and anticoagulant and antiplatelet agents. Routine phlebotomy is not indicated, despite the elevated hemoglobin. Heart-lung transplantation is occasionally attempted, although outcomes are disappointing.

Investigational Therapies: Prostacyclin infusion in select patients with severe symptoms who fail to respond to medical management is being investigated.

REFERENCES

Brickner MD, Hillis LD, Lange RA. Congenital heart disease in adults: 2nd of two parts. *N Engl J Med* 2000;342:334–342.

Cantor WJ, Harrison DA, Moussadji JS, et al. Determinants of survival and length of survival in adults with Eisenmenger syndrome. *Am J Cardiol* 1999;84:677–681.

Vongpatanasin W, Brickner ME, Hillis LD, et al. The Eisenmenger syndrome in adults. *Ann Intern Med* 1998;128:748–755.

RESOURCES

97, 113, 245

7 Endomyocardial Fibrosis

Yuji Okura, MD, PhD,
and Leslie T. Cooper, Jr., MD

DEFINITION: Endomyocardial fibrosis (EMF) is characterized pathologically by fibrous endocardial thickening of the inflow portions of the right or left ventricle, or both, often with involvement of the atrioventricular valves and associated valvular regurgitation.

SYNONYMS: Davies disease; EMF of tropics and subtropics; Löffler endomyocarditis.

DIFFERENTIAL DIAGNOSIS: Other forms of primary myocardial and valvular disease, including rheumatic carditis.

SYMPTOMS AND SIGNS: The clinical picture depends on which ventricle and atrioventricular valve shows predominant involvement; left-sided involvement results in symptoms of pulmonary congestion, whereas predominant right-sided disease may present with a restrictive cardiomyopathy, with systemic venous congestion, ascites, and edema. The onset is often gradual over 1–2 years but occasionally may be rapid. The endocardial thickening may progress to obliterate the involved ventricular cavities, and extensive calcification may occur.

ETIOLOGY/EPIDEMIOLOGY: A tropical form has been observed in Sub-Saharan Africa, particularly in Uganda, and in people of low socioeconomic status in the tropical and subtropical regions of India, Brazil, Columbia, and Sri Lanka. The disorder is also seen in temperate countries as part of a hypersensitivity or hypereosinophilic syndrome. Temperate and tropical EMF may represent different disorders. The tropical form is a progressive disease of unknown cause that occurs most commonly in children and young adults residing in tropical and subtropical Africa, particularly Uganda and Nigeria. The endemic variety may be related to high levels of cerium and low levels of magnesium and has no gender predilection. Disorders associated with EMF outside of the tropics include radiation, drug reaction, helminthic infections, systemic inflammatory disorders, and storage diseases.

DIAGNOSIS: The diagnosis is based on clinical and laboratory features along with appropriate geographic location for the tropical form of EMF. A systemic drug or hypersensitivity reaction may have associated peripheral eosinophilia, rash, or hepatitis.

TREATMENT
Standard Therapies: In tropical EMF, medical treatment is often disappointing. Diuretics, angiotensin-converting enzyme inhibitors, and digoxin may be used. Surgical excision of the fibrotic endocardium and atrioventricular valve replacement have resulted in substantial symptomatic improvement. If EMF is associated with a drug or hypersensitivity reaction, withdrawal of the offending agent is essential. Corticosteroids have occasionally been associated with short-term improvement if degranulating eosinophils are present in the biopsy sample.

REFERENCES
Balakrishnan KG, Venkitachalam CG, Pillai VR, et al. Postoperative evaluation of endomyocardial fibrosis. *Cardiology* 1986;73:73–84.
Berensztein CS, Pineiro D, Marcotegui M, et al. Usefulness of echocardiography and Doppler echocardiography in endomyocardial fibrosis. *J Am Soc Echocardiography* 2000;13:385–392.
Freers J, Masembe V, Schmauz R, et al. Endomyocardial fibrosis syndrome in Uganda. *Lancet* 2000;355:1994–1995.
Goodwin JF. Cardiomyopathies and specific heart muscle diseases: definitions, terminology, classifications and new and old approaches. *Postgrad Med J* 1992;68(suppl 1):3–6.
Schneider U, Jenni R, Turina J, et al. Long-term follow-up of patients with endomyocardial fibrosis: effects of surgery. *Heart* 1998;79:362–367.

RESOURCES
35, 89, 113

8 Lymphomatoid Granulomatosis

*Elaine S. Jaffe, MD,
and Wyndham Wilson, MD, PhD*

DEFINITION: Lymphomatoid granulomatosis (LYG) is an angiocentric and angiodestructive lymphoproliferative disease involving extranodal sites, composed of Epstein-Barr virus (EBV)-positive B cells admixed with numerous reactive T cells. It has a spectrum of histologic grade and clinical aggressiveness, which is related to the proportion of large B cells. The most common mode of presentation is with pulmonary symptoms and multiple pulmonary nodules.

SYNONYM: Angiocentric immunoproliferative lesion.

DIFFERENTIAL DIAGNOSIS: Wegener granulomatosis; Churg-Strauss syndrome; Extranodal NK/T-cell lymphoma, nasal type; Pulmonary MALT lymphoma; Polyarteritis nodosa.

SYMPTOMS AND SIGNS: Patients frequently present with symptoms and signs related to the respiratory tract, such as cough (58%), dyspnea (29%), and chest pain (13%). Other constitutional symptoms are common, including fever, malaise, weight loss, neurologic symptoms, arthralgias, myalgias, and gastrointestinal symptoms. Few patients present with asymptomatic disease (<5%). Skin involvement is frequent (40%–50%), and may be manifested as papules, nodules, or, more rarely, plaque-like lesions. Larger cutaneous nodules may be ulcerated. Other frequent sites of involvement are kidneys and the central nervous system.

ETIOLOGY/EPIDEMIOLOGY: Lymphomatoid granulomatosis usually presents in adult life, but may be seen in children with immunodeficiency disorders. It affects males more often than females (at least 2:1). It is mediated by EBV, which is integrated in B cells.

DIAGNOSIS: Diagnosis is based on biopsy results of an affected organ, lung, kidney, skin, or central nervous system. A specific diagnosis is often not possible on a skin biopsy, because EBV-positive cells are frequently absent in this site. Evaluations of immune function, including flow cytometry of peripheral blood and assessment of lymphocyte function (delayed hypersensitivity tests), are helpful in the evaluation of a patient with suspected LYG.

TREATMENT
Standard Therapies: The natural history of LYG is variable. In some patients it may follow a waxing and waning clinical course, with spontaneous remissions without therapy. In most patients the disease is more aggressive, with a median survival of less than 2 years. Recent series have shown responses to aggressive combination chemotherapy for grade III lesions. Grade I and II lesions may re-spond to interferon-α 2b. Corticosteroids were frequently used in the past, but may result in further immune compromise and do not lead to long-term complete remissions. The most effective treatment for this disease is unknown. Corticosteroids and/or chemotherapy are most commonly recommended.

Investigational Therapies: Interferon-α 2b is being investigated.

REFERENCES
Beaty MW, Toro J, Sorbara L, et al. Cutaneous lymphomatoid granulomatosis: correlation of clinical and biological features. *Am J Surg Pathol* 2001;25:1111–1120.
Guinee D Jr, Jaffe E, Kingma D, et al. Pulmonary lymphomatoid granulomatosis. Evidence for a proliferation of Epstein-Barr virus infected B-lymphocytes with a prominent T-cell component and vasculitis. *Am J Surg Pathol* 1994;18:753–764.
Jaffe ES, Harris NL, Stein H, et al. Pathology and genetics of tumours of haematopoietic and lymphoid tissues. In: *World Health Organization classification of tumours.* Lyon, France: IARC Press, 2001:185–187.
Jaffe ES, Wilson WH. Lymphomatoid granulomatosis: pathogenesis, pathology and clinical implications. *Cancer Surv* 1997;30: 233–248.
Wilson WH, Kingma DW, Raffeld M, et al. Association of lymphomatoid granulomatosis with Epstein-Barr viral infection of B lymphocytes and response to interferon-alpha 2b. *Blood* 1996;87:4531–4537.

RESOURCES
27, 30, 40

---

9 Congenital Complete Heart Block

Ritu Chatrath, MD

DEFINITION: Congenital complete heart block is a conduction disorder of the heart in which the atrial impulses do not propagate to the ventricles. The atria and the ventricles beat independently, and the ventricular rate is slow and fixed because there are no conducted atrial beats.

SYNONYMS: Congenital complete atrioventricular (AV) block; Congenital third-degree AV block.

SYMPTOMS AND SIGNS: The disorder is almost uniformly irreversible. Its clinical presentation depends on the baseline heart rate and association with any structural heart disease. A fetus with the disorder may develop anasarca, lactic acidosis, and hepatomegaly due to congestive cardiac failure. This carries a high risk for morbidity and mortality, especially when associated with structural heart disease. Prenatal diagnosis of complete heart block can be made by fetal echocardiography. Children with the disorder may be asymptomatic or present with syncope, fatigue, and exercise intolerance. Patients with very slow heart rates are at risk for sudden death. In some patients, dilated cardiomyopathy may develop later in life.

ETIOLOGY/EPIDEMIOLOGY: Maternal collagen vascular diseases account for most cases; systemic lupus erythematosus being the most common. Others such as Sjö-gren syndrome, rheumatoid arthritis, and mixed connective tissue disorder have also been associated. Placental transfer of autoimmune antibodies such as anti-Ro and anti-La damages the fetal conduction system. In 25%–33% of cases, a structural cardiac abnormality such as L-transposition of great arteries or atrioventricular septal defect is present. Rare causes include familial complete heart block, fetal myocarditis, and tumors in the region of the atrioventricular node. The incidence is between 1 in 15,000 to 1 in 25,000 live births. It affects males and females equally. Familial clustering of cases has been reported.

TREATMENT

Standard Therapies: Standard treatment is pacemaker implantation. Immediate treatment of symptomatic patients includes atropine and adrenergic agonists until cardiac pacing can be initiated. Newborns with hydrops fetalis should be stabilized with inotropic agents, diuretics, and temporary pacing, and then a permanent pacemaker should be implanted.

Investigational Therapies: In pregnant women with collagen vascular diseases, steroids such as dexamethasone and prednisone have been used. Maternal plasmapheresis has been successful in some cases. Intrauterine pacing is under investigation.

REFERENCES

Boutjdir M, et al. Molecular and ionic basis of congenital complete heart block. *Trends Cardiovasc Med* 2000;10:114–122.

Brian K, et al. Congenital heart block: natural history and management. *ACC Curr J Rev* 1995;4:63–65.

Brucato A, et al. Risk of congenital complete heart block in newborns of mothers with anti-Ro/SSA antibodies detected by counterimmunoelectrophoresis: a prospective study of 100 women. *Arthritis Rheum* 2001;44:1832–1835.

Eronen M, et al. Short- and long-term outcome of children with congenital complete heart block diagnosed in utero or as a newborn. *Pediatrics* 2000;106:86–91.

Gillette PC, et al., eds. *Clinical pediatric arrhythmias,* 2nd ed. Philadelphia: WB Saunders, 1999:66–70.

RESOURCES

35, 113, 198

10   Hypoplastic Left Heart Syndrome

Michael Mulreany, MD,
and Richard M. Donner, MD

DEFINITION: Hypoplastic left heart syndrome (HLHS) is a continuum of congenital cardiac defects resulting from severe underdevelopment of the structures of the left side of the heart: mitral valve, left ventricle, aortic valve, and ascending aorta. If untreated, it is almost universally fatal (95%) within the first month of life.

SYNONYMS: Aortic atresia; Mitral atresia; Hypoplastic left ventricle syndrome.

DIFFERENTIAL DIAGNOSIS: Critical aortic stenosis and coarctation of the aorta; Interruption of the aortic arch; Cardiomyopathy (infectious, metabolic, or hypoxic); Intrauterine supraventricular tachycardia; Obstructive cardiac neoplasms; Large arteriovenous fistulae; Infant septicemia; Respiratory distress syndrome.

SYMPTOMS AND SIGNS: The clinical presentation is most often that of inadequate cardiac output and shock within the first few hours to days of life. Adequate cardiac output and oxygen delivery in affected newborns depend on continued patency of the ductus arteriosus. The right ventricle supplies both pulmonary blood flow in the usual manner and systemic blood flow across the patent ductus arteriosus to include retrograde filling of the arch vessels and coronary arteries. Pulmonary venous return to the left atrium crosses the foramen ovale and mixes with systemic venous return in the right atrium. Oxygen content of the blood ejected from the right ventricle to both the lungs and the body lies between the systemic and pulmonary venous saturations (approximately 80%–93%). Cyanosis may not be apparent clinically, but pulse oximetry in the nursery should detect the arterial desaturation. As the ductus arteriosus closes, systemic output is compromised and the infant exhibits signs of shock: tachycardia, dyspnea, rales, weak peripheral pulses, decreased blood pressure, hepatomegaly, cool extremities, and an ashen appearance. On cardiac examination, a single second heart sound, gallop rhythm, and systolic murmur are usually present. If the ductus arteriosus remains patent, heart failure from excessive pulmonary blood flow appears in days to weeks.

ETIOLOGY/EPIDEMIOLOGY: The disorder accounts for approximately 7% of all congenital heart defects with a prevalence of 1 in 100,000 live births. Most patients are males (67%), and approximately 10% have a definable genetic disorder. Inheritance appears to be multifactorial with a sibling recurrence risk of 0.5%, although some kinships express the abnormality with a frequency approaching autosomal-dominant transmission. Prenatal mechanisms that limit the blood flow from the right to the left atrium during fetal life have been postulated to result in underdevelopment of the left heart. These include premature closure of the foramen ovale and fetal cardiomyopathy.

DIAGNOSIS: Although HLHS is often suspected by routine fetal ultrasound examination and confirmed by fetal echocardiography, most patients present in the newborn nursery. Chest radiography characteristically shows pulmonary venous congestion or pulmonary edema with a varying degree of cardiomegaly. Electrocardiographic findings include right ventricular hypertrophy with minimal left-sided forces, a qR pattern in the right precordial leads, and diffuse ST segment and T wave abnormalities reflecting coronary insufficiency. Transthoracic echocardiography confirms the diagnosis.

TREATMENT
Standard Therapies: Following confirmation of the diagnosis in the newborn, prostaglandin E_1 infusion is started to maintain patency of the ductus arteriosus. At most specialized surgical centers, treatment consists of either staged surgical palliation or infant cardiac transplantation. Staged surgical palliation, usually accomplished in three operations (Norwood, hemi-Fontan, and Fontan operations) spanning the first 18–24 months of life, separates the systemic and pulmonary circulations by transforming the pulmonary artery into an aorta, creating direct connections between the vena cavae and the pulmonary arteries and ensuring an adequate pathway for pulmonary venous blood to reenter the right atrium and right ventricle. Successful infant cardiac transplantation relies on availability of donor organs, the ability to maintain ductal patency, and the proper management of heart failure for weeks to months. Excluding infants who die waiting for a donor organ, the 5-year actuarial survival for both pathways is similar, approximately 70%.

REFERENCES
Bove EL. Current status of staged reconstruction for hypoplastic left heart syndrome. *Pediatr Cardiol* 1998;19:308–315.
Johnston JK, Chinnock RE, Zuppan CW, et al. Limitations to survival for infants with hypoplastic left heart syndrome before and after transplant: the Loma Linda experience. *J Transplant Coord* 1997;7:180–184.
Williams DL, Gelijns AC, Moskowitz AJ, et al. Hypoplastic left heart syndrome: valuing the survival. *J Thorac Cardiovasc Surg* 2000;119:720–731.

RESOURCES
35, 113, 114, 356

11   Jervell and Lange-Nielsen Syndrome

Jeffrey A. Towbin, MD

DEFINITION: Jervell and Lange-Nielsen syndrome is an inherited disorder characterized by QT interval prolongation on surface electrocardiography corrected for heart rate, associated with T-wave abnormalities, relative bradycardia, ventricular tachyarrhythmias (particularly ventricular tachycardia and torsade de pointes), sudden death, and autosomal-recessive sensorineural deafness.

SYNONYMS: Cardioauditory syndrome; Autosomal-recessive long QT syndrome; Deafness, congenital and functional heart disease; Surdocardiac syndrome.

SYMPTOMS AND SIGNS: Deafness is identified early in life, followed by cardiovascular features. Affected individuals typically present with syncope or sudden death. In some instances, seizures present early. Exercise and emotion are common triggering events. Electrocardiographic features are typically severe.

ETIOLOGY/EPIDEMIOLOGY: The syndrome is characterized by autosomal-dominant long QT syndrome and autosomal-recessive sensorineural deafness caused by homozygous or compound heterozygous mutations in the potassium channel gene *KVLQT1* or *minK*. The mutations typically occur in consanguineous relationships but can occur when consanguinity is not notable. Parents usually have mild QT interval prolongation or normal electrocardiograms and no deafness. The syndrome affects an estimated 1–6 infants per 1 million live births, with males and females equally represented.

DIAGNOSIS: The diagnosis is made on serial surface electrocardiograms and by hearing tests.

TREATMENT

Standard Therapies: Beta-adrenergic blocking agents (i.e., propranolol, atenolol, nadolol) are the treatment of choice. When these are unsuccessful, left sympathectomy to remove certain apparent cardiac nerves has been used. Internal cardioverter defibrillators have been used in conjunction with β-blockers. Genetic counseling and family screening electrocardiograms should be done.

REFERENCES

Li H, Fuentes-Garcia J, Towbin JA. Current concepts in long QT syndrome. *Pediatr Cardiol* 2000;21:542–550.

Schulze-Bahr E, Wang Q, Wedekind H, et al. KCNE1 mutations cause Jervell and Lange-Nielsen syndrome. *Nat Genet* 1997;17: 267–268.

Schwartz PJ, Moss AJ, Vincent GM, et al. Diagnostic criteria for the long QT syndrome: an update. *Circulation* 1993;88:7 82–784.

RESOURCES

125, 186

12 Giant Cell Myocarditis

Leslie T. Cooper, Jr., MD

DEFINITION: Giant cell myocarditis (GCM) is characterized by widespread inflammation, giant cells with many nuclei, and evidence of heart muscle cell death (Insert Fig. 5).

DIFFERENTIAL DIAGNOSIS: Idiopathic granulomatous myocarditis; Cardiac sarcoidosis; Lymphocytic myocarditis; Hypersensitivity myocarditis.

SYMPTOMS AND SIGNS: Approximately 75% of affected individuals present with symptoms and signs of congestive heart failure. These include shortness of breath with exertion or with lying flat, and ankle swelling. A minority of patients present with sudden light-headedness or loss of consciousness from an inappropriately fast or slow heart rate. A small percentage have chest pain as their first symptom. The clinical course usually involves decreasing ejection fraction with rapidly progressive heart failure complicated by ventricular arrhythmias (usually tachycardia) and heart block (usually bradycardia). Giant cell myocarditis is usually rapidly fatal with a median time to death or cardiac transplantation of 5.5 months from the onset of symptoms. Of affected individuals, 70% die or require heart transplantation within 1 year, and the overall rate of death or cardiac transplantation is approximately 89%.

ETIOLOGY/EPIDEMIOLOGY: Approximately 200 cases have been described. The cause is not known. Up to 20% of cases occur in individuals with other autoimmune disorders, especially inflammatory bowel disease, suggesting an autoimmune link. Although genes may play a part in GCM etiology, there are no known families, regions, or ethnic groups in which this disease is particularly common. The median age of symptom onset is 42 years. Men and women are affected equally. Children younger than 15 years are rarely affected.

DIAGNOSIS: Examining a sample of heart tissue obtained from a biopsy or other specimen is the only way to diagnose GCM. Tests to rule out more common causes of heart problems should be done. These may include an echocardiogram to exclude valvular and pericardial disease, a cardiac catheterization to exclude coronary abnormalities, and sometimes serologic tests to exclude other specific causes of cardiomyopathy.

TREATMENT

Standard Therapies: No consensus exists on the best treatment. Supportive care for heart failure and standard treatments for arrhythmias are appropriate. These may include a pacemaker or implantable heart defibrillator if indicated clinically. Evaluation for heart transplantation is often initiated soon after the diagnosis is established. The GCM infiltrate recurs in approximately 25% of patients after a heart transplant; nonetheless, survival after heart transplantation may be equivalent to survival after transplantation for other causes.

Investigational Therapies: The effect of immunosuppression with muromonab-CD3, cyclosporine, and steroids in prolonging time to transplantation in patients with GCM is being investigated.

REFERENCES

Cooper LT. A review of giant cell myocarditis. *Herz* 2000; 25:291–298.

Cooper LT. Myocarditis. In: Murphy JG, ed. *Mayo Clinic cardiology review,* 2nd ed. Philadelphia: Lippincott Williams & Wilkins, 2000:483–508.

Cooper LT, Berry GJ, Shabetai R. Giant cell myocarditis: natural history and treatment. *N Engl J Med* 1997;336:1860–1866.

Desjardins V, Pelletier G, Leung TK, et al. Successful treatment of severe heart failure caused by idiopathic giant cell myocarditis. *Can J Cardiol* 1992;8:788–792.

RESOURCES
35, 113, 356

13   Hypersensitivity Myocarditis

Leslie T. Cooper, Jr., MD, and Yuji Okura, MD, PhD

DEFINITION: Hypersensitivity myocarditis (HSM) is a form of inflammatory heart disease caused by an immune reaction to a drug or exposure to a sensitizing agent. If myocyte necrosis is present, the term *acute necrotizing eosinophilic myocarditis* may be used.

DIFFERENTIAL DIAGNOSIS: Toxic myocarditis; Viral myocarditis; Giant cell myocarditis; Löffler myocarditis; Churg-Strauss syndrome.

SYMPTOMS AND SIGNS: Clinical features are relatively nonspecific, and accordingly the natural history of HSM is not well established. Most data come from autopsy series, with inherent selection bias for more severe cases. In one series, 14 patients were examined before autopsy: 64% had fever, 36% had a rash, and 50% had malaise. Eosinophilia was seen in 8 of 14 (57%) of these patients; therefore, the absence of eosinophilia does not rule out HSM. Most patients had electrocardiographic abnormalities, consisting of sinus tachycardia and nonspecific ST segment changes. Liver function studies may be elevated from concomitant hypersensitivity hepatitis or passive congestion. In acute necrotizing eosinophilic myocarditis, sudden death is often the first symptom.

ETIOLOGY/EPIDEMIOLOGY: The disorder is an idiosyncratic inflammation of the myocardium. It is caused by a delayed hypersensitivity reaction to chemically reactive metabolites of the offending drug. The precise mechanism of myocardial inflammation is not well characterized. The prevalence of clinically undetected HSM in explanted hearts ranges from 2.4% to 7%. The true incidence is unknown.

DIAGNOSIS: Early clinical suspicion and endomyocardial biopsies are essential to antemortem diagnosis. Endomyocardial biopsy should be considered for patients with peripheral eosinophilia and the new appearance of electrocardiogram changes, particularly if associated with elevations in cardiac enzymes (troponin or creatine kinase-MB), cardiomegaly, or unexplained tachycardia. Negative biopsy results do not exclude HSM. A positive biopsy result may both guide treatment and affect prognosis if necrotizing eosinophilic myocarditis or giant cell myocarditis or a granulomatous process is shown.

TREATMENT

Standard Therapies: When diagnosed early in the course, discontinuation of the offending medication, often accompanied by the addition of corticosteroids and, occasionally, intravenous immunoglobulin, has resulted in successful recovery of some patients.

REFERENCES

Beghetti M, Wilson G, Bohn D, et al. Hypersensitivity myocarditis caused by an allergic reaction to cefaclor. *J Pediatr* 1998;132:172–173.

Daniels P, Tazelaar H, Edwards W, et al. Hypersensitivity myocarditis presenting histologically with fulminant giant cell myocarditis. *Cardiovasc Pathol* 2000;9:287–291.

Fenoglio J Jr, McAllister H Jr, Mullick F. Hypersensitivity myocarditis. *Hum Pathol* 1981;12:900–907.

Garty B, Offer I, Livni E, et al. Erythema multiforme and hypersensitivity myocarditis caused by ampicillin. *Ann Pharmacother* 1994;28:730–731.

Hawkins E, Levine T, Goss S, et al. Hypersensitivity myocarditis in the explanted hearts of transplant recipients: reappraisal of pathologic criteria and their clinical implications. *Pathol Annu* 1995;30:287–305.

RESOURCES
27, 35

14   Romano-Ward Long QT Syndrome

Jeffrey A. Towbin, MD

DEFINITION: Romano-Ward long QT syndrome is characterized by QT-interval prolongation on the surface electrocardiogram corrected for heart rate, associated with T-wave abnormalities, relative bradycardia, ventricular tachyarrhythmias (particularly polymorphous ventricular tachycardia and torsade de pointes), and sudden death.

SYNONYMS: Autosomal-dominant long QT syndrome; Q-T prolongation.

DIFFERENTIAL DIAGNOSIS: Epilepsy; Acquired Q-T prolongation; Idiopathic ventricular fibrillation.

SYMPTOMS AND SIGNS: Children and adults typically present with syncope, loss of consciousness, or sudden death. In some cases, seizures are the presenting symptoms. Events are typically triggered by emotion, stress, exercise, medications, or auditory (e.g., alarm clock or phone ringing) triggers; a subset of individuals experience events during sleep. Severity and frequency of events vary among affected individuals and appear to decrease during middle age. Asthma, syndactyly, and diabetes mellitus have been noted as comorbid conditions in some individuals.

ETIOLOGY/EPIDEMIOLOGY: Romano-Ward syndrome is an autosomal-dominant trait caused by heterozygous mutations in a variety of ion channel genes (i.e., an ion channelopathy). The genes identified include *KVLQT* (*LQT1*), *HERG* (*LQT2*), *SCN5A* (*LQT3*), *minK* (*LQT5*), and *MiRP1* (*LQT6*). KvLQT1 and *HERG* encode potassium channel α-subunits, whereas *minK* and *MiRP1* encode potassium channel β-subunits. *KVLQT1* and *minK* associate to form a functional channel (I_{Ks}), and *HERG* and *MiRP1* associate to form a functional channel (I_{Kr}). *SCN5A* encodes the cardiac sodium channel. The *LQT4* gene, located on chromosome 4, is unknown. The syndrome oc-

curs in both males and females, with a male predominance. It is estimated to occur in 1 per 10,000 live births.

DIAGNOSIS: The diagnosis is made on serial surface electrocardiograms. Holter monitoring may be helpful in some patients. Electrophysiology testing is usually not necessary.

TREATMENT

Standard Therapies: Beta-adrenergic blocking agents (i.e., propranolol, atenolol, nadolol) have been well established as the treatment of choice. When unsuccessful, left sympathectomy to remove certain afferent cardiac nerves has been used. Recently, the use of internal cardioverter defibrillators (ICDs) has become popular in conjunction with β-blockers. Genetic counseling and family screening by electrocardiograms should be done.

Investigational Therapies: Sodium channel blocking agents such as mexilitine, lidocaine, and flecainide, as well as therapies to increase serum potassium such as exogenous potassium and potassium-sparing agents (e.g., spironolactone), are being investigated.

REFERENCES

Compton SJ, Lux RL, Ramsey MR, et al. Genetically defined therapy of inherited long QT syndrome: correction of abnormal repolarization by potassium. *Circulation* 1996;94:1018–1022.

Li H, Fuentes-Garcia J, Towbin JA. Current concepts in long QT syndrome. *Pediatr Cardiol* 2000;21:542–550.

Schwartz PJ, Moss AJ, Vincent GM, et al. Diagnostic criteria for the long QT syndrome: an update. *Circulation* 1993;88:782– 784.

Schwartz PJ, Priori SG, Locati ET, et al. Long QT syndrome patients with mutations of the *SCN5A* and *HERG* genes have differential responses to Na⁺ channel blockade and to increases in heart rate. *Circulation* 1995;92:3381–3386.

RESOURCES

35, 206, 451

15   Situs Inversus

George E. Tiller, MD, PhD, and Rizwan Hamid, MD

DEFINITION: Situs inversus is a condition in which the internal organs of the abdomen and thorax lie in mirror

image of their normal anatomic position. It can occur as situs inversus solitus (without any other anomalies) or as a part of a syndrome with various other defects.

SYNONYMS: Situs inversus viscerum; Situs inversus totalis; Visceral heterotaxy.

DIFFERENTIAL DIAGNOSIS: Kartagener syndrome; Ivemark syndrome; Primary ciliary dyskinesia (PCD); Asplenia with cardiovascular anomalies.

SYMPTOMS AND SIGNS: In isolated situs inversus, there is a complete mirror image transposition of the thoracic and abdominal organs with preservation of the anterior-posterior symmetry. A thorough physical examination and routine diagnostic tests can identify most cases. Dextrocardia will manifest with heart sounds and an apical impulse on the right side of the chest. Electrocardiography will show total inversion in lead I and transposition in leads II and III. The liver can be palpated on the left and the spleen on the right. When situs inversus occurs in association with syndromes such as Kartagener syndrome or primary ciliary dyskinesia, additional signs and symptoms relating to these conditions will be present. The expression of the situs inversus phenotype may be incomplete and there may be incomplete transposition of thoracic or abdominal organs, as well as additional anomalies such as congenital heart disease, polysplenia, asplenia, annular pancreas, horseshoe kidney, and diaphragmatic hernia.

ETIOLOGY/EPIDEMIOLOGY: Incidence is approximately 1 in 10,000 with a slight male predominance. Several families have been described as exhibiting autosomal-dominant, autosomal-recessive, and X-linked inheritance. Situs inversus appears to be genetically heterogeneous in humans. Mutations in the *DNAI1* gene, encoding the intermediate chain of dynein, are responsible for some cases of Kartagener syndrome and immotile cilia syndrome. Mutations in the *ZIC3* gene, a transcription factor, are responsible for X-linked visceral heterotaxy. Mutations in the *CFC1* gene have been documented in some individuals with visceral heterotaxy.

DIAGNOSIS: A thorough physical examination followed by radiographic examination of the chest and abdomen and electrocardiography will identify most cases. The main diagnostic challenge in affected individuals is the nontraditional presentation of referred pain. If a cardiac murmur is present, echocardiography may be indicated to assess for possible structural cardiac anomaly. In patients in whom symptoms of PCD predominate, the diagnostic gold standard is quantitation of abnormal structural elements, such as missing dynein arms or random orientation of cilia in nasal or bronchial biopsies or scrapings, using electron microscopy.

TREATMENT

Standard Therapies: In isolated situs inversus, no treatment may be necessary. Where situs inversus is associated with other conditions such as PCD, therapy is symptomatic. Most patients experience chronic sinusitis, otitis media, and airway disease. Appropriate antibiotic coverage for *Pneumococcus* and *Haemophilus* should be administered when indicated. Bronchodilators can also provide relief. Patients should be assessed periodically, with serial chest radiographs and pulmonary function tests when indicated.

REFERENCES

Agirbasli M, Hamid R, Jennings HS, et al. Situs inversus with cardiomyopathy in identical twins. *Am J Med Genet* 2000;91: 327–330.

Bamford RN, Roessler E, Burdine RD, et al. Loss-of-function mutations in the EGF-CFC gene *CFC1* are associated with human left-right laterality defects. *Nat Genet* 2000;26: 365–369.

Gebbia M, Ferrero GB, Pilia G, et al. X-linked situs abnormalities result from mutations in ZIC3. *Nat Genet* 1997;17:305–308.

Guichard C, Harricane M-C, Lafitte J-J, et al. Axonemal dynein intermediate-chain gene (*DNAI1*) mutations result in situs inversus and primary ciliary dyskinesia (Kartagener syndrome). *Am J Hum Genet* 2001;68:1030–1035.

Pennarun G, Escudier E, Chapelin C, et al. Loss-of-function mutations in a human gene related to chlamydomonas reinhardtii dynein IC78 result in primary ciliary dyskinesia. *Am J Hum Genet* 1999;65:1508–1519.

RESOURCES

35, 113, 357

16 Persistent Truncus Arteriosus

Doff B. McElhinney, MD, and Gil Wernovsky, MD

DEFINITION: Persistent truncus arteriosus (PTA) is a congenital cardiovascular anomaly characterized by a single arterial trunk arising from the normally formed ventricles of the heart by means of a single semilunar valve. In addition, the pulmonary arteries originate from the common arterial trunk distal to the coronary arteries and proximal to the first brachiocephalic branch of the aortic arch. The common trunk typically straddles a ventricular septal defect in the outlet portion of the interventricular septum. The pathophysiology of PTA is typified by cyanosis and systemic ventricular volume overload.

SYNONYMS: Common arterial trunk; Truncus arteriosus; Truncus arteriosus communis.

DIFFERENTIAL DIAGNOSIS: Aortopulmonary septal defect; Double-outlet right ventricle; Transposition of the great arteries; Tetralogy of Fallot; Functionally univentricular anomalies; Totally anomalous pulmonary venous return; Sepsis; Various metabolic disorders.

SYMPTOMS AND SIGNS: Symptoms are variable, and may be more or less pronounced, depending on specific anatomic features and age at presentation. The most common are cyanosis and findings related to ventricular volume overload, which typically manifest as pulmonary vascular resistance decreases and pulmonary overcirculation increases. Patients may present with symptoms and signs of high-output cardiac failure, including lethargy, metabolic acidosis, systemic hypoperfusion, hypotension, and tachypnea. Before the onset of cardiopulmonary collapse, findings may include poor feeding, diaphoresis, tachypnea, and dusky and mottled appearance. On physical examination, patients generally have a loud and harsh cardiac murmur, central cyanosis, and a decreased systemic arterial oxygen saturation. Absence of cyanosis, however, does not exclude the diagnosis.

ETIOLOGY/EPIDEMIOLOGY: The anomaly is believed to result from incomplete or failed septation of the embryonic truncus arteriosus. It may result from abnormal development of the cardiac neural crest, although the precise mechanism by which this occurs in humans has not been elucidated. Approximately 35%–40% of patients with PTA have a deletion in chromosome band 22q11.2. Persistent truncus arteriosus represents 1%–2% of congenital heart defects in live born infants, which amounts to approximately 5 to 10 per 100,000 live births. There are no known racial, ethnic, geographic, or sex predilections.

DIAGNOSIS: The definitive method of diagnosing PTA is cardiac imaging, most often echocardiography. In patients with suspected PTA or similar disease, a hyperoxia test and chest radiography will help the clinician distinguish between cardiac and noncardiac disorders.

TREATMENT
Standard Therapies: The only treatment is surgical repair. Asymptomatic or minimally symptomatic patients may be managed with anticongestive medical therapy (diuretics and digoxin) before repair, but the standard of care at most centers consists of prompt surgical repair once the patient has been stabilized. Intravenous prostaglandin therapy is generally not indicated, although it may be of benefit in patients with an associated interruption of the aortic arch. Surgical management consists of complete primary repair, with closure of the ventricular septal defect, committing the common arterial trunk to the left ventricle, and reconstruction of the right ventricular outflow tract, most often with a valved conduit.

REFERENCES
Imamura M, Drummond-Webb JJ, Sarris GE, et al. Improving early and intermediate results of truncus arteriosus repair: a new technique of truncal valve repair. *Ann Thorac Surg* 1999; 67:1142–1146.
Jahangiri M, Zurakowski D, Mayer JE, et al. Repair of the truncal valve and associated interrupted arch in neonates with truncus arteriosus. *J Thorac Cardiovasc Surg* 2000;119:508–514.
McElhinney DB, Rajasinghe HA, Mora BN, et al. Reinterventions after repair of common arterial trunk in neonates and young infants. *J Am Coll Cardiol* 2000;35:1317–1322.
Rajasinghe HA, McElhinney DB, Reddy VM, et al. Long-term follow-up of truncus arteriosus repaired in infancy: a twenty-year experience. *J Thorac Cardiovasc Surg* 1997;113:869–879.
Williams JM, de Leeuw M, Black MD, et al. Factors associated with outcomes of persistent truncus arteriosus. *J Am Coll Cardiol* 1999;34:545–553.

RESOURCES
11, 35, 113

3

Chromosomal Disorders

1   Deletion of the Short Arm of Chromosome 1

Stuart K. Shapira, MD, PhD

DEFINITION: Patients with deletion of the short arm of chromosome 1 have a multiple congenital anomaly, mental retardation syndrome that is caused by the deletion of distal chromosome 1p.

SYNONYMS: Chromosome 1p36 deletion syndrome; Monosomy 1p36.

DIFFERENTIAL DIAGNOSIS: Angelman syndrome; Prader-Willi syndrome; Alagille syndrome; Mitochondrial myopathies; Other chromosomal syndromes.

SYMPTOMS AND SIGNS: The common clinical features of the 1p36 deletion syndrome include characteristic craniofacial features, vision anomalies (particularly hyperopia), hearing deficits (particularly high-frequency sensorineural hearing loss), cleft palate and/or cleft lip, fifth finger and hand anomalies, genitourinary anomalies, minor cardiac anomalies, dilated cardiomyopathy, seizures, abusive behaviors, growth retardation, low muscle tone and developmental delay, and lack of speech. Most patients have growth retardation, although some develop obesity as a result of lack of a sense of satiety. Patients with the smallest deletion sizes may have normal speech development and only mild or borderline developmental impairment.

ETIOLOGY/EPIDEMIOLOGY: The deletion event occurs in at least 1 in 10,000 births, making it perhaps the most common terminal chromosomal deletion syndrome. Most patients have a sporadic deletion, although familial cases due to the inheritance of unbalanced chromosomal products from a parent carrying a balanced chromosomal translocation have been reported. The syndrome occurs more often in females than in males.

DIAGNOSIS: The diagnosis is usually made by cytogenetic analysis during evaluation for developmental delay or congenital anomalies. The phenotype is distinctive enough in some individuals that an experienced clinician may be able to make a diagnosis before cytogenetic analysis. Because of the subtle appearance of the deletion, it can be missed on a routine cytogenetic study. Therefore, if suspected, the deletion will need to be confirmed by fluorescence *in situ* hybridization analysis with probes for distal 1p36. Based on the clinical complications that can occur, evaluations should include an echocardiogram and electrocardiogram, a hearing evaluation by auditory brainstem evoked response testing, and an ophthalmologic examination. Hearing evaluations should occur on a yearly basis. A swallow function study should be included in the initial evaluations.

TREATMENT

Standard Therapies: If feeding difficulties and recurrent aspirations occur, early placement of a gastrostomy tube should be considered. Because functional verbal communication is unlikely to be achieved, the speech pathologists who work with these children should focus on nonverbal forms of communication, such as sign language or communication boards. The high prevalence of hypothyroidism indicates the need to obtain total thyroxine (T_4), free T_4, and thyroid-stimulating hormone levels at 6 months and 1 year of age, and then on a yearly basis. Because hypotonia and developmental delay have been observed in all patients, early referral to physical and occupational therapy is essential.

REFERENCES
Eugster EA, Berry SA, Hirsch B. Mosaicism for deletion 1p36.33 in a patient with obesity and hyperphagia. *Am J Med Genet* 1997;70:409–412.

Keppler-Noreuil KM, Carroll AJ, Finley WH, et al. Chromosome 1p terminal deletion: report of new findings and confirmation of two characteristic phenotypes. *J Med Genet* 1995;32:619–622.

Shapira SK, McCaskill C, Northrup H, et al. Chromosome 1p36 deletions: the clinical phenotype and molecular characterization of a common newly delineated syndrome. *Am J Hum Genet* 1997;61:642–650.

Slavotinek A, Shaffer LG, Shapira SK. Monosomy 1p36. *J Med Genet* 1999;36:657–663.

Wu Y-Q, Heilstedt HA, Bedell JA, et al. Molecular refinement of the 1p36 deletion syndrome reveals size diversity and a preponderance of maternally derived deletions. *Hum Mol Genet* 1999;8:313–321.

2 Chromosome 10, Distal Trisomy 10q

Nataline B. Kardon, MD

DEFINITION: Distal trisomy 10q is a chromosome disorder characterized by slow growth before and after birth; abnormal, diminished muscle tone; severe mental retardation; distinctive malformations of the head and face; characteristic hand and feet deformities; and skeletal, heart, kidney, and/or respiratory abnormalities.

SYNONYMS: Chromosome 10, partial trisomy 10q24-qter; Chromosome 10, trisomy 10q2; Distal duplication 10q; Distal trisomy 10q syndrome; Dup (10q) syndrome.

DIFFERENTIAL DIAGNOSIS: Chromosome 10; Monosomy 10p.

SYMPTOMS AND SIGNS: In most cases, abnormally slow growth occurs both before and after birth. Infants and children have severely diminished muscle tone and abnormal looseness of the joints. They may experience profound delays in the acquisition of skills that require coordination of mental and muscular activities, and have severe mental retardation. The head and facial abnormalities include a small head with a high, broad forehead, a round, slightly flattened face, prominent cheekbones, and low-set or misshapen ears. The nose is small with turned up nostrils and a broad, flat, and/or depressed nasal bridge. The mouth is bow-shaped with a prominent upper lip and an unusually small lower jaw. Some patients may have cleft palate. Other signs may be fine, highly arched eyebrows, drooping of the upper eyelids, narrowing of the eyelid folds between the upper and lower eyelids, vertical skin folds that may cover the inner corners of the eyes, and abnormally small eyes due to reduced diameter of the cornea. Abnormalities of the hands and feet consist of permanent flexion and/or overlapping of certain fingers, a large distance between the great toes and second toes, webbing between the second and third toes, and abnormal positioning of the feet. Some patients may have underdeveloped ridge patterns on the hands and feet and deep grooves in the soles of the feet. Skeletal defects include thin ribs, 11 rather than 12 pairs, an abnormally short neck, abnormal front-to-back and side-to-side scoliosis, an abnormal depression of the sternum, and delayed bone development. Approximately 50% of patients present with heart defects, respiratory abnormalities, and/or malformations of the kidneys. Approximately 50% of affected males have one or two undescended testes.

ETIOLOGY/EPIDEMIOLOGY: This syndrome is a result of the duplication of the end portion of the long arm of one chromosome 10. The duplication of bands 10q25 and 10q26 is critical for the expression of the characteristic features. More than 90% of reported cases result from a chromosomal balanced translocation in one of the parents. The disorder appears to affect males more often than females. More than 35 cases have been reported.

DIAGNOSIS: Some cases may be diagnosed before birth by amniocentesis and/or chorionic villus sampling. Ultrasonography may show characteristic findings. The laboratory testing consists of chromosome analysis performed on samples of amniotic fluid, chorionic villi, and/or peripheral blood. Specific abnormalities may be diagnosed by radiography or other imaging studies, electrocardiography, echocardiography, and/or cardiac catheterization.

TREATMENT
Standard Therapies: Treatment is symptomatic and supportive. Special education and social support services are usually needed. Genetic counseling is recommended for families.

REFERENCES
Yunis JJ, Sanchez O. A new syndrome resulting from partial trisomy for the distal third of the long arm of chromosome 10. *J Pediatr* 1974;84:567–570.

Klep-de Pater, et al. Partial trisomy 10q: a recognizable syndrome. *Hum Genet* 1979;46:29–40.

Halpern GJ, Shohat M, Merlob P. Partial trisomy 10q: further delineation of the clinical manifestations involving the segment 10q23–10q24. *Ann Genet* 1996;39:181–183.

Chen CP, Shih JC, Lee CC, et al. Prenatal diagnosis of a fetus with distal 10q trisomy. *Prenat Diagn* 1999;19:876–878.

RESOURCES
96, 120, 476

3   Chromosome 10, Monosomy 10p

Nataline B. Kardon, MD

DEFINITION: Chromosome 10, monosomy 10p is a chromosomal disorder characterized by abnormalities of the head and face, delayed development, heart defects, and abnormalities of the reproductive organs and/or urinary tract. Mental retardation often occurs.

SYNONYMS: 10p deletion syndrome (partial); Chromosome 10, 10p- partial; Chromosome 10, partial deletion (short arm).

DIFFERENTIAL DIAGNOSIS: Chromosome 22, monosomy 22q; DiGeorge syndrome.

SYMPTOMS AND SIGNS: The most common physical abnormalities are unusual features of the head and face. The head is small and the front of the head may be narrow with considerable bulging of the frontal bone. Mental retardation is variable. The facial features may include underdevelopment of the jawbone and small, underdeveloped, misshapen ears that may be associated with hearing loss. There may be abnormalities of the inner nose, unusual turned up nostrils, and extra folds of skin on the inner corners of the eyes. The eyelids may be drooping, the eye sockets may be flat, and there may be narrow openings between the margins of both the upper and lower eyelids. Developmental features consist of short stature, a short neck, widely spaced nipples, and/or underdeveloped genitalia, particularly undescended testes. Abnormalities of the heart, urinary tract, and brainstem may occur. In rare instances, a cleft lip or palate may be present.

ETIOLOGY/EPIDEMIOLOGY: This syndrome occurs as a result of a chromosomal deletion at the end of the short arm of chromosome 10. It is usually the result of a spontaneous, sporadic mutation, but it can result from a parental balanced translocation. The risk of recurrence is low, unless one of the parents carries a balanced translocation. In observed cases, males have been affected more frequently than females. Approximately 20 cases have been reported.

DIAGNOSIS: The diagnosis is made by performing chromosome analysis before or after birth.

TREATMENT
Standard Therapies: In severe cases, surgery may be necessary for the treatment of congenital defects that may obstruct feeding or breathing. Supportive therapy by a team approach consisting of special education, physical therapy, and other social, medical, or vocational services is standard. Genetic counseling is recommended for the family.

REFERENCES
Monaco G, et al. DiGeorge anomaly associated with 10p deletion. *Am J Med Genet* 1991;39:215–216.
Obregon MG, et al. Partial deletion 10p syndrome. Report of two patients. *Ann Genet* 1992;35:101–104.
Shapira M, et al. Deletion of the short arm of chromosome 10 (10p13): report of a patient and review. *Am J Med Genet* 1994; 52:34–38.
Van Esch H, et al. The phenotypic spectrum of the 10p deletion syndrome versus the classical DiGeorge syndrome. *Genet Couns* 1999;10:59–65.

RESOURCES
15, 104, 193

4   Chromosome 11, Partial Monosomy 11q

Nataline B. Kardon, MD

DEFINITION: Partial monosomy 11q is a chromosomal disorder in which a portion of the long arm of chromosome 11 is deleted or missing. It may be characterized by slow growth before and after birth, mental retardation, and psychomotor retardation. Physical abnormalities may include malformations of the head and face, abnormalities of the eyes, malformations of the hands and/or feet, and defects of the heart.

SYNONYMS: 11q syndrome, partial; Deletion 11q syndrome, partial; Jacobsen syndrome; Partial monosomy of long arm of chromosome 11.

DIFFERENTIAL DIAGNOSIS: Chromosome 11 ring; C syndrome.

SYMPTOMS AND SIGNS: Affected infants and children are characterized as moderately to severely mentally retarded. Most have severe speech impairment. The head and face abnormalities consist of premature closure of the metopic sutures, resulting in a triangular-shaped head with a prominent forehead. Other infants may present with an abnormally small head and/or the back of the head may be flat. Other signs can be an abnormally short, broad, up-turned nose, a wide, depressed nasal bridge, thin lips, downturned mouth, a small lower jaw, or low-set, mal-formed ears. The eyes may be widely spaced with drooping upper eyelids and epicanthal folds. There may be a down-ward-slanted opening between the upper and lower eye-lids, crossed eyes, and improper development of the retina. Absence of tissue from the iris has also occurred. Abnor-malities of the hands and feet consist of minor webbing of the fingers and/or toes, abnormally short bones at the ends of the fingers, a four-finger palmar crease, permanent flexion of the great toe resulting in hammer toe, clubfoot, and joint contractures. More than 50% of patients have congenital heart defects. Approximately 50% of patients have hematologic abnormalities such as low levels of platelets, and others may have low levels of all types of blood cells. Genital and urinary system abnormalities also occur and, rarely, kidney abnormalities.

ETIOLOGY/EPIDEMIOLOGY: The range and severity of symptoms depends on the exact size and location of the deletion on 11q. Most cases are sporadic, although a few have resulted from a parental balanced translocation. The region consistently missing in this disorder is band q24.1. Inheritance of a fragile site on the long arm of chromo-some 11 may play a role in causing the disorder. Females are affected more often than males. More than 40 cases have been diagnosed.

DIAGNOSIS: The diagnosis is made by performing chro-mosome analysis. Certain specific abnormalities are diag-nosed by imaging studies including radiographic studies, electrocardiography, echocardiography, and cardiac catheterization.

TREATMENT

Standard Therapies: Treatment is directed toward the specific symptoms and may require the coordinated efforts of a team of specialists, including pediatricians, surgeons, ophthalmologists, cardiologists, orthopedists, and speech-language pathologists. Complications of certain congenital heart defects may be treated with a variety of drugs to pre-vent arrhythmia and eliminate excessive fluid. Eye abnor-malities may require surgery and/or corrective lenses. Or-thopedic problems may require physical therapy and surgical procedures. Hematologic defects may be treated by transfusions of specific blood components. Supportive therapy may include special remedial education, speech therapy, and other medical, social, or vocational services. Genetic counseling is recommended for family members.

Investigational Therapies: Research is being conducted to test the theory that a larger deletion of chromosome 11q may result in more severe language difficulties.

REFERENCES
Fryns JP, et al. Distal 11q monosomy. The typical 11q monosomy syndrome is due to deletion of subband 11q24.1. *Clin Genet* 1986;30:255–260.
Histinx R, et al. Monosomy 11q: report of two familial cases and review of the literature. *Am J Med Genet* 1993;47:312–317.
Lewanda AF, et al. Two craniosynostotic patients with 11q dele-tions and review of 48 cases. *Am J Med Genet* 1995;59:193–198.

RESOURCES
1, 96, 149

---

5   Chromosome 11, Partial Trisomy 11q

Nataline B. Kardon, MD

DEFINITION: Partial trisomy 11q is caused by a duplica-tion of the end portion of the long arm of chromosome 11. It is characterized by delayed mental and physical develop-ment, retarded growth, an unusually small brain, and dis-tinctive facial features.

SYNONYMS: 11q partial trisomy; Chromosome 11, par-tial trisomy 11q13-qter; Chromosome 11, partial trisomy 11q21-qter; Chromosome 11, partial trisomy 11q23-qter; Distal trisomy 11q; Partial trisomy 11q; Trisomy 11q, partial.

DIFFERENTIAL DIAGNOSIS: Rett syndrome; Epstein anomaly; Mental retardation with dysmorphic facies.

SYMPTOMS AND SIGNS: Major symptoms include de-layed mental and physical development and an abnormally small brain. Facial abnormalities may include facial asym-metry, a short nose, low-set ears, a high–arched or incom-pletely closed palate, abnormally small jaws, and/or a very long vertical groove between the nose and upper lip. The head may be shorter and/or smaller than usual. There may be epicanthal folds, widely spaced eyes, downslanted eyes, abnormally shaped ears, and/or malformation of the collarbone. There may also be an absent or underdeveloped corpus callosum. A few individuals may have congenital heart disease, urinary tract abnormalities, malformation of the hip, loosely hanging skin, abnormal creases on the palm of the hand, a short neck, and an abnormally small penis with undescended testicles. Extra skin tags may occur in front of the ears, and umbilical hernia may be present. A small percentage of patients may have severe spinal and brain malformations.

ETIOLOGY/EPIDEMIOLOGY: The duplication of the end portion of the long arm of chromosome 11 is responsible for the symptoms, the severity and range of which may depend on the length of the duplicated portion. The cause is not known; however, it is usually the result of a spontaneous unbalanced translocation. In some cases this may result from a parental balanced translocation involving the end portion of chromosome 11 and another chromosome, most frequently chromosome 22. The disorder affects more females than males. Approximately 45 cases have been reported.

DIAGNOSIS: The diagnosis is made by chromosome analysis of amniocentesis, chorionic villus, or fetal blood samples prenatally or of peripheral blood samples postnatally.

TREATMENT
Standard Therapies: Therapy is mainly symptomatic and supportive. Special education, physical therapy, and other medical, social, or vocational services are often necessary. Genetic counseling is recommended for family members.

REFERENCES
Greig F, et al. Duplication 11(Q22-QTER) in an infant. A case report with review. *Ann Genet* 1985;28:185–188.

Pattemore PK, et al. The neonatal recognition of partial 11Q trisomy (previously "trisomy 22"). *Aust Paediatr J* 1987;23:197–199.

Pihko H, et al. Partial 11Q trisomy syndrome. *Hum Genet* 1981;58:129–134.

Wallerstein R, et al. Partial trisomy 11q in a female infant with Robin sequence and congenital heart disease. *Cleft Palate Craniofac J* 1992;29:77–79.

RESOURCES
7, 149, 462, 476

6 Chromosome 13, Partial Monosomy 13q

Nataline B. Kardon, MD

DEFINITION: Chromosome 13, partial monosomy 13q is a chromosomal disorder in which a portion of the long arm of chromosome 13 is missing.

SYNONYMS: 13q syndrome, partial; Deletion 13q syndrome, partial; Monosomy 13q, partial; Partial monosomy of the long arm of chromosome 13.

DIFFERENTIAL DIAGNOSIS: Chromosome 13 ring; C syndrome.

SYMPTOMS AND SIGNS: Infants with this disorder fail to grow at the expected rate, resulting in short stature. Severe mental retardation is present in most cases. Characteristic abnormalities consist of an unusually small head, a small jaw with a prominent maxilla, a wide flat nasal bridge, protruding front teeth, and large low-set ears. The neck may be short with webbing. Some infants may have premature closure of the metopic sutures, resulting in a triangular-shaped skull with a prominent forehead. The forebrain may develop abnormally. Rarely patients have cleft lip and/or cleft palate. Eye abnormalities include unusually small eyes, widely spaced eyes, drooping of the upper eyelids, and epicanthal folds. Cataracts or corneal opacities may be seen. Colobomas of the iris and/or choroid may be present. Some patients may also develop bilateral malignant tumors of the retina known as retinoblastomas. This presents as leukokoria, crossed eyes, diminished vision, pain and redness, and/or secondary glaucoma. Malformations of the hands or feet consist of underdeveloped or absent thumbs, fifth finger clinodactyly, fusion of certain fingers, unusually short big toes, and/or clubfoot. Additional skeletal abnormalities include rib malformations, vertebral abnormalities, and scoliosis. Genital abnormalities in males consist of hypospadias, undescended testes, and a small bifid scrotum. There may be a small penis and perineal fistulae. Anal atresia also may be present. Congenital heart defects such as atrial and ventricular septal defects may be noted. Brain abnormalities such as absence of the rhinencephalon have occurred, as have meningoceles and hydrocephaly. Hirschsprung disease and abnormalities of kidney development occur rarely.

ETIOLOGY/EPIDEMIOLOGY: The deletion of a portion of the long arm of chromosome 13 is responsible for the symptoms that characterize this disorder. There may be a correlation of specific abnormalities to various regions or breakpoints along the chromosome. Retinoblastoma is associated with deletion of band q14, but only 20% of individuals with this deletion develop the tumor. In most cases the deletion is sporadic and spontaneous. Other times a parental chromosome rearrangement such as a translocation, inversion, or insertion may produce the deletion. Chromosome 13, partial monosomy 13q appears to affect females slightly more often than males. More than 125 cases have been reported in the medical literature.

DIAGNOSIS: The diagnosis is made by performing chromosome analysis. Specialized enzyme testing for esterase D may exhibit reduced activity due to deletions involving band q14. Imaging studies, including ultrasonography, CT, and MRI, are used to diagnose retinoblastoma. Radiography, electrocardiography, and cardiac catheterization may be indicated for congenital heart defects.

TREATMENT
Standard Therapies: Treatment is symptomatic and supportive and may require the coordinated efforts of a team of specialists. Genetic counseling is recommended for family members, and chromosome analysis may be indicated for the patient's parents.

REFERENCES
Brown S, et al. Preliminary definition of a "critical region" of chromosome 13 in q32: report of 14 cases with 13 q deletions and review of the literature. *J Med Genet* 1993;26:100–104.
Tranebjaerg L, et al. Interstitial deletion 13q: further delineation of the syndrome by clinical and high-resolution chromosome analysis of five patients. *Am J Med Genet* 1988;29:739–753.

RESOURCES
326, 462

---

7 Chromosome 14 Ring

Nataline B. Kardon, MD

DEFINITION: Chromosome 14 ring is a disorder characterized by psychomotor delays, mental retardation, growth delays, and seizures, as well as distinctive abnormalities of the head and face.

SYNONYMS: r14; Ring 14; Ring chromosome 14.

DIFFERENTIAL DIAGNOSIS: Chromosome 14q terminal deletion; Chromosome 14q interstitial deletion; Chromosome abnormalities (general) with mental retardation and seizures.

SYMPTOMS AND SIGNS: Symptoms and findings vary in range and severity. They include low birth weight, slow growth, poor muscle tone, feeding difficulties in infancy, and delayed development. Recurrent seizures typically develop in infancy. The facial appearance is distinctive: a small head with a high forehead, an elongated face, and a flat nasal bridge with a prominent nasal tip and slightly upturned nostrils. The eyes may be widely spaced with downwardly slanting palpebral fissures and epicanthal folds. Patients may also have a thin upper lip, downwardly turned corners of the mouth, a high-arched palate, an unusually small jaw, and large low-set ears. Other physical features may be a short neck, abnormal skin ridge patterns, a simian crease, widely spaced nipples, and abnormalities of skin pigmentation such as vitiligo or café-au-lait spots. The retina may be characteristically pigmented. Neurologic symptoms may include ataxia and tremors, which may result in joint contractures. Congenital heart defects such as aortic stenosis and pulmonic stenosis have been described.

ETIOLOGY/EPIDEMIOLOGY: Chromosome 14 ring results from loss of genetic material from both ends of the 14th chromosome and joining of the ends to form a ring. Symptoms and features depend on the amount of genetic material lost from the chromosome and the stability of the ring during subsequent cellular divisions. The features may be a result of small deletions of genetic material from the long arm of chromosome 14, or from the occurrence of cells with extra copies of chromosome 14 due to instability of the ring chromosome during cell division. This syndrome is caused by a spontaneous or *de novo* error early during the development of the embryo. It appears to affect males slightly more often than females. More than 40 cases have been reported.

DIAGNOSIS: The diagnosis can be made prenatally by amniocentesis or chorionic villus sampling. It may be confirmed after birth by characteristic findings and chromosome analysis. Electroencephalography, CT, and MRI may be used to document neurologic findings.

TREATMENT
Standard Therapies: Anticonvulsant drugs may be necessary to reduce or control seizures. Therapeutic agents may be used to prevent or aggressively treat respiratory infections. Physical therapy may help to prevent joint contrac-

tures. Cardiac surgery may be indicated for patients with severe congenital cardiac defects. Early intervention programs, special education, and other social and/or vocational services are recommended. Genetic counseling is recommended.

Investigational Therapies: Medications for the control of certain seizure types are being studied.

REFERENCES
Fryns JP, et al. Ring chromosome 14: a distinct clinical entity. *J Genet Hum* 1983;31:367–375.
Matalon, R et al. Transmission of ring 14 chromosome from mother to two sons. *Am J Med Genet* 1990;36:381–385.
Ono J, et al. Ring chromosome 14 complicated with complex partial seizures and hypoplastic corpus callosum. *Pediatr Neurol* 1999;20:70–72.
Zelante L, et al. Ring chromosome 14 syndrome. Report of two cases, including extended evaluation of a previously reported patient and review. *Ann Genet* 1991;34:93–97.

RESOURCES
104, 145, 476

---

8   Chromosome 14, Trisomy Mosaic

Nataline B. Kardon, MD

DEFINITION: Chromosome 14, trisomy mosaic is a disorder in which some cells have three 14 chromosomes and some have the normal pair.

SYNONYMS: Trisomy 14 mosaic; Trisomy 14 mosaicism syndrome.

DIFFERENTIAL DIAGNOSIS: Incontinentia pigmenti; Hypomelanosis of Ito; UPD chromosome 14.

SYMPTOMS AND SIGNS: The prenatal course is frequently complicated by polyhydramnios and growth retardation. Infants have failure to thrive. Craniofacial malformations include a prominent forehead, wide nasal bridge, long philtrum, prominent upper jaw, and small, underdeveloped lower jaw. Many infants have deeply set, widely spaced eyes that may be covered with a translucent film. Additional abnormalities include narrow palpebral fissures, a large mouth and thick lips, small malformed low-

set ears, and a short neck. Some infants may have cleft palate. Congenital heart defect when present is usually a tetralogy of Fallot. The skin may have distinctive patches or streaks of hyperpigmentation. Some children may demonstrate facial and body asymmetry. Males may have undescended testes and an abnormally small penis.

ETIOLOGY/EPIDEMIOLOGY: An extra chromosome 14 is present in one of an individual's cell lines with at least one unaffected cell line also present. The additional chromosome is responsible for the signs and symptoms that characterize the disorder. The severity of the symptoms corresponds to the percentage of affected cells with the trisomic cell line. The disorder results from misdivision of chromosomes that occurs either in the formation of sperm or egg cells in a parent, or during cell division in the embryo. Chromosome 14, trisomy mosaic appears to affect females slightly more often than males. Approximately 20 cases have been reported.

DIAGNOSIS: Chromosome analysis is necessary to make the diagnosis. This can be done prenatally by amniocentesis and/or chorionic villus sampling or postnatally by peripheral blood sampling. Ultrasonography may show some of the features of the disorder. Cardiac evaluation may include radiography, electrocardiography, echocardiography, and cardiac catheterization.

TREATMENT

Standard Therapies: Treatment requires the coordinated efforts of pediatricians, surgeons, cardiologists, and other health-care professionals. If tetralogy of Fallot is present, hypoxic episodes may occur that require oxygen, morphine, and sodium bicarbonate. Surgical repair of the lesion may be necessary, as may other surgical corrections including craniofacial and genital repairs. Endocarditis should be averted by antibiotic prophylaxis. Other treatment is symptomatic and supportive. Early intervention and genetic counseling are recommended.

REFERENCES

Fujimoto A, et al. Natural history of mosaic trisomy 14 syndrome. *Am J Med Genet* 1992;44:189–196.

Lipson MH. Trisomy 14 mosaicism syndrome. *Am J Med Genet* 1987;26:541–544.

Ralph A, et al. Maternal uniparental isodisomy for chromosome 14 detected prenatally. *Prenat Diagn* 1999;19:681–684.

Supulveda W, et al. Twin pregnancy discordant for trisomy 14 mosaicism: prenatal sonographic findings. *Prenat Diagn* 1998;18:481–484.

RESOURCES

35, 454, 462, 476

---

9 Chromosome 15, Distal Trisomy 15q

Nataline B. Kardon, MD

DEFINITION: Distal trisomy 15q is characterized by prenatal and/or postnatal growth retardation, mental retardation, and craniofacial malformations. Other abnormalities include an unusually short neck, malformations of the fingers and/or toes, scoliosis, genital abnormalities in males, and in some cases cardiac defects.

SYNONYMS: Chromosome 15, trisomy 15q2; Distal duplication 15q; Partial duplication 15q syndrome.

DIFFERENTIAL DIAGNOSIS: Chromosome 4, partial trisomy distal 4q.

SYMPTOMS AND SIGNS: In most cases, there is prenatal and/or postnatal growth retardation, failure to thrive due to swallowing difficulties, hypotonia, and severe to profound mental retardation. Sagittal suture craniosynostosis produces an abnormally long and narrow head. There may also be microcephaly with a prominent occiput, a sloping forehead, and facial asymmetry. The palpebral fissures may be downwardly slanting, short, or narrow. Ptosis, an abnormally large, prominent, or bulbous nose, and an unusually small triangular mouth have been described. There may be a long philtrum, a crease in the midline of the lower lip, a highly arched palate, an unusually small jaw, or abnormally round, "puffy" cheeks. In some cases, the ears may be abnormally large, low-set, or dysplastic. The neck may be short and/or webbed, which may be due to cervical vertebral anomalies. Approximately one third of patients have seizures. Affected individuals may have long, thin fingers, permanently flexed fingers, or hyperextension of the thumbs. Joint contractures, scoliosis, and pectus excavatum have also been described. Male genital abnormalities may include cryptorchidism and hypogonadism, and females may have hypoplasia of the labia majora. Congenital heart defects, increased susceptibility to recurrent infections, and swallowing difficulties leading to aspiration pneumonia may also occur. Patients with trisomy 15q25-qter have tall stature, mild mental retardation, and hydrocephalus.

ETIOLOGY/EPIDEMIOLOGY: The duplication of the distal portion of chromosome 15q is the causative factor. The range and severity depend on the exact length and location of the duplicated portion. The usual breakpoints are at bands 15q21 and 15q23; however, rare cases of breaks at 15q25 have been described. In most cases, one of the parents has a balanced translocation. Males are affected approximately twice as often as females. More than 30 cases have been reported.

DIAGNOSIS: Diagnosis may be made before birth by amniocentesis and/or chorionic villus sampling. Ultrasonography may show characteristic findings that suggest a chromosome disorder. Laboratory testing consists of chromosome analysis performed on amniotic fluid, chorionic villi, and/or peripheral blood. Specific abnormalities may be diagnosed by radiographic studies, electrocardiography, electroencephalography, echocardiography, and/or cardiac catheterization.

TREATMENT
Standard Therapies: Treatment is symptomatic and supportive. It may require the coordinated efforts of a team of specialists depending on the specific presenting symptoms. Special education, early intervention, and social support services are included as part of the team. Surgical repair of certain malformations may be indicated. Physical therapy may be prescribed, as may infection surveillance. Genetic counseling is recommended for family members, and parental chromosome analysis is indicated to identify the balanced translocation.

REFERENCES
Fryns JP, et al. The fetal phenotype in 15q2 duplication. *Ann Genet* 1988;31:123–125.
Fujimoto A, et al. Inherited partial duplication of chromosome no.15. *J Med Genet* 1974;11:287–291.
Lacro RV, et al. Duplication of distal 15q: report of five new cases from two different translocation kindreds. *Am J Med Genet* 1987;26:719–728.
Orye E, et al. Mosaic and non-mosaic trisomy 15q2. *Ann Genet* 1985;28:58–60.
Schnatterly P, et al. Distal 15q trisomy: phenotypic comparison of nine cases in an extended family. *Am J Hum Genet* 1984;36:444–451.

RESOURCES
96, 113, 455

10 Chromosome 15 Ring

Nataline B. Kardon, MD

DEFINITION: Chromosome 15 ring is a chromosomal disorder characterized by delayed growth, a small head circumference, triangular-shaped face, poor muscle tone, and mental retardation.

SYNONYMS: r15; Ring 15; Ring 15, chromosome; Ring 15, chromosome (mosaic pattern).

DIFFERENTIAL DIAGNOSIS: Chromosome 15q deletion; chromosome disorders (general).

SYMPTOMS AND SIGNS: The symptoms depend on the amount of genetic material lost on the short and long arms of the chromosome, so patient presentation may vary. The most common features are mental retardation, delayed growth, a small head, poor muscle tone, a small jaw, widely spaced eyes, and underdeveloped ovaries or testes. Some patients may have congenital heart defects, short bones of the hands and feet, webbing of fingers and/or toes, curvature of the spine, seizures, abnormalities of the kidneys, and café-au-lait spots.

ETIOLOGY/EPIDEMIOLOGY: The cause of the disorder is a deletion of chromosome 15 at both ends and a joining of the ends to form a ring. The amount of lost genetic material varies from a small amount with few symptoms to a significant amount causing many symptoms. Most often, this occurs *de novo* with a low possibility of recurrence. A few cases have been the result of a parent with a balanced translocation. Some cases of mosaicism have also been reported. Females are affected more often than males. Approximately 25 cases have been reported.

DIAGNOSIS: The determination can be made only by chromosome analysis.

TREATMENT
Standard Therapies: Patients with poor muscle tone may benefit from physical therapy. Special education and early intervention are indicated. Genetic counseling is recommended.

REFERENCES
Butler MG, et al. Two patients with ring chromosome 15 syndrome. *Am J Med Genet* 1988;29:149–154.
Fryns JP, et al. Ring chromosome 15 syndrome. *Ann Genet* 1986;29:47–48.
Wilson GN, et al. Phenotypic delineation of ring chromosome 15 and Russell-Silver syndromes. *J Med Genet* 1985;22:233–236.

RESOURCES
35, 96, 188

11   Chromosome 18, Monosomy 18p

Nataline B. Kardon, MD

DEFINITION: Chromosome 18, monosomy 18p is characterized by deletion of the short arm of the 18th chromosome. Persons with the disorder have unusual facial characteristics and mild to severe mental retardation.

SYNONYM: Short arm 18 deletion syndrome.

DIFFERENTIAL DIAGNOSIS: Down syndrome (trisomy 21); Partial trisomy 14, trisomy 13 syndrome (Patau syndrome); Chromosome 18, monosomy 18q; Trisomy 18 (Edward syndrome).

SYMPTOMS AND SIGNS: Symptoms may include mild to moderate growth deficiency, hypotonia, and microencephaly with mental retardation. Affected individuals often have an IQ between 45 and 50, but some have no mental deficiency. Language is often affected; many people with the disorder do not speak simple sentences until 7 to 9 years of age. Drooping eyelids, epicanthic folds, a low nasal bridge, and unusually widely spaced eyes may be present. The patient may have a rounded face, small jaw, downturned corners of the mouth, and large protruding ears. There may also be a high frequency of dental caries, relatively small hands and feet, and depression of the breastbone. Behavioral characteristics may include restlessness, emotional instability, a fear of strangers, and inability to concentrate.

ETIOLOGY/EPIDEMIOLOGY: Monosomy 18p is characterized by deletion of the short arm of the 18th chromosome. The predominance of affected females is 60%. The average parental ages of 31.3 years for mothers and 35.7 years for fathers indicate that parental age may be related to the occurrence of this disorder in offspring.

DIAGNOSIS: Diagnosis is made by chromosome analysis of prenatal chorionic villus sampling or amniocentesis specimens or of postnatal specimens from peripheral blood.

TREATMENT
Standard Therapies: Early intervention programs in special education, physical therapy, and language development are indicated. Other treatment is symptomatic and supportive. Genetic counseling is recommended for family members.

REFERENCES
Johansson B, et al. Duplications 18p- with mild influence on the phenotype. *Am J Med Genet* 1988;4:871–874.
Liberfarb RM, et al. Multiple congenital anomalies/mental retardation (MCA/MR) syndromes due to partial 1q duplication and possible 18 p deletion: a study of four individuals in two families. *Am J Med Genet* 1979;4:27–37.

RESOURCES
96, 101, 462

12   Chromosome 18q- Syndrome

Nataline B. Kardon, MD

DEFINITION: Chromosome 18q- syndrome is caused by a deletion of a piece of the long arm (q) of chromosome 18. The most apparent and common symptoms are mental retardation, short stature, a flat midface, poor muscle tone, a small head, and unusual facial features.

SYNONYMS: 18q- syndrome; Chromosome 18 long arm deletion syndrome; Chromosome 18, monosomy 18q; Monosomy 18q syndrome.

DIFFERENTIAL DIAGNOSIS: Other chromosomal disorders involving mental retardation.

SYMPTOMS AND SIGNS: The following symptoms can be found in many patients with 18q- syndrome: mental retardation, which can vary from very mild to severe; short stature; a flat midface; poor muscle tone; and a small head. Many patients with chromosome 18q- syndrome have unusual facial features such as downturned corners of the mouth, a cleft or high palate, a broad nasal bridge, epicanthal folds, eyes spaced widely apart, and/or an outward curl of the ear. Eye abnormalities such as malformation of the optic nerve, nystagmus, and crossed eyes may occur. Long tapering fingers and toes, low-set thumbs, an abnormal crease on the palm of the hand (simian crease), fleshy tips of the fingers, abnormal placement of the second toe, and/or bowed legs may also be present. Abnormalities of the genitalia such as a small penis, undescended testicles, and a small or absent labia minor have been found in many patients. Other abnormalities include an increased number of whorl patterns on the fingertips, congenital heart disease, impaired hearing, deficient IgA, closed or narrow ear canals, widely spaced nipples, and seizures. Speech is often delayed, and behavior problems may occur.

ETIOLOGY/EPIDEMIOLOGY: Chromosome 18q- syndrome is caused by a deletion on the long arm of chromosome 18. Most chromosomal deletions occur spontaneously. The parents of the affected child typically have normal chromosomes and a very low probability of having another child with a chromosomal abnormality. In some cases, a parent may have a balanced translocation in which there is a deletion on chromosome 18 but the deleted genetic material is attached to another chromosome. Parents with such translocations are asymptomatic, but are at risk of having a child with a deletion on the long arm of chromosome 18. Some parents with chromosome 18q- syndrome have had a child with the disorder. The syndrome affects females more often than males. More than 80 cases have been reported.

DIAGNOSIS: Chromosome analysis of a peripheral blood sample will identify the disorder.

TREATMENT
Standard Therapies: Patients with chromosome 18q- syndrome and poor muscle tone may benefit from physical therapy. Special education and related services benefit pediatric patients. Genetic counseling is recommended for family members. Other treatment is symptomatic and supportive.

REFERENCES
Petty RE, et al. Chronic arthritis in two children with partial deletion of chromosome 18. *J Rheum* 1987;14:586–587.
Vogel H, et al. The brain in the 18q- syndrome. *Dev Med Child Neurol* 1990;32:732–737.

RESOURCES
101, 371, 462

13   Chromosome 18 Ring

Nataline B. Kardon, MD

DEFINITION: Chromosome 18 ring is characterized by mental retardation, unusual facial features, a small head, and poor muscle tone.

SYNONYMS: r18; Ring 18; Ring chromosome 18.

DIFFERENTIAL DIAGNOSIS: Other chromosomal disorders involving mental retardation.

SYMPTOMS AND SIGNS: The symptoms of the disorder depend on the amount of genetic material lost on the short and long arms of the chromosome; hence, patient presentation may vary. The most common features are mental retardation ranging from moderate to severe, growth retardation, a small head, poor muscle tone, unusual facial features, and repeated infections during the first year of life. More than half of patients have eye abnormalities, including a wide space between the eyes, downward-slanting lids, a small eyeball that may be displaced downward, absent or defective iris, nystagmus, and strabismus. Many patients have ear abnormalities such as unusually developed external ears, narrow ear canals, low-set ears, and deafness. Other symptoms may be a high-arched palate, small tongue, small lower jaw, protruding lower jaw, and downturned corners of the mouth. Abnormalities of the vertebrae, abnormal genitalia, small arms and legs, fingers curving inward, overlying toes, and a decrease in the antibody IgA (leading to susceptibility to respiratory infections) have also been described.

ETIOLOGY/EPIDEMIOLOGY: The disorder is caused by a deletion of chromosome 18 at both ends and a joining of the ends to form a ring. The amount of lost genetic material can vary from a small amount, causing few symptoms, to a significant amount, causing many symptoms. The condition usually occurs *de novo* with a low possibility of recurrence, but some parents with ring 18 have had a child with the disorder. Females are affected slightly more often than males. Approximately 70 cases have been reported.

DIAGNOSIS: Chromosome analysis provides the only method of definitive diagnosis.

TREATMENT
Standard Therapies: Patients with poor muscle tone may benefit from physical therapy. Special education and early intervention are indicated. Speech therapy and hearing aids may be useful. Genetic counseling is recommended for patients and their families.

REFERENCES
Donlan MA, et al. Ring chromosome 18 in a mother and child. *Am J Med Genet* 1986;24:171–174.
Petty RE, et al. Chronic arthritis in two children with partial deletion of chromosome 18. *J Rheumatol* 1987;14:586–587.

RESOURCES
101, 144, 371

14 Chromosome 18, Tetrasomy 18p

Nataline B. Kardon, MD

DEFINITION: Tetrasomy 18p is a chromosomal disorder caused by the appearance of the short arm of chromosome 18 four times in cells of the body.

SYNONYM: Tetrasomy, short arm of chromosome 18.

DIFFERENTIAL DIAGNOSIS: Trisomy 18.

SYMPTOMS AND SIGNS: Major symptoms include craniofacial abnormalities such as premature closure of the sagittal suture, producing a long and narrow head, microcephaly, and facial asymmetry. There may also be an abnormally small mouth, a highly arched palate, an unusually small jaw, malformed, low-set ears, and/or a pinched nose. Rarely, patients exhibit epicanthal folds, ocular hypotelorism, cleft palate, or gingival hypertrophy. Skeletal abnormalities are often seen such as scoliosis, kyphosis, an unusually small hipbone, or other hip deformities. The fingers or toes may be overlapped or unusually long, abnormally bent, or webbed. There may be simian creases. Affected individuals appear very thin. Neuromuscular abnormalities include hypertonia, hyperreflexia, ankle clonus, and spasticity. Older individuals exhibit an abnormal gait. Some individuals may demonstrate motor seizures. Renal abnormalities consist of double ureter, ectopic ureter, hydroureter, and hydronephrosis. Urinary reflux may occur. The kidneys may not rotate properly during development or they may fuse to produce horseshoe kidney. Other rare abnormalities include low IgA (producing a susceptibility to respiratory infections), heart murmurs, and cryptorchidism. Moderate to severe mental retardation, limited speech, and behavioral abnormalities are common.

ETIOLOGY/EPIDEMIOLOGY: An extra isochromosome consisting of the two identical short arms of 18 is usually the result of a *de novo* event and is not inherited. In a few reported cases, the isochromosome was present in the mother and therefore transmitted. Males and females appear to be affected equally. Approximately 40 cases have been reported.

DIAGNOSIS: The diagnosis is made by performing chromosome analysis either during pregnancy or after birth. Amniocentesis, chorionic villus sampling, and fetal blood sampling involve chromosomal analysis of fluid and/or tissue samples obtained prenatally.

TREATMENT
Standard Therapies: Surgical repair of malformations depends on the severity and location of the anatomic abnormalities and their associated symptoms. Other therapy is mainly symptomatic and supportive. Special education, physical therapy, and other medical, social, or vocational services are often necessary. Genetic counseling is recommended for family members.

REFERENCES
Abeliovich D, et al. Isochromosome 18p in a mother and her child. *Am J Med Genet* 1993;46:392–393.
Back E, et al. *De novo* isochromosome 18p in two patients: cytogenetic diagnosis and confirmation by chromosome painting. *Clin Genet* 1994;45:301–304.
Essmer MC, et al. Tetrasomy 18p in two cases: confirmation by *in situ* hybridization. *Ann Genet* 1994;37:156–159.
Singer TS, et al. Tetrosomy 18p in a child with trisomy 18 phenotype. *Am J Med Genet* 1990;36:144–147.

RESOURCES
96, 101, 455

15   Chromosome 21 Ring

Nataline B. Kardon, MD

DEFINITION: Chromosome 21 ring is a disorder characterized by mental retardation as well as abnormalities of the face, eyes, skeleton, and internal organs.

SYNONYMS: r21; Ring 21; Ring 21, chromosome.

DIFFERENTIAL DIAGNOSIS: Down syndrome; Chromosome 21 monosomy.

SYMPTOMS AND SIGNS: The symptoms vary depending on the amount and location of genetic material lost. Features consist of growth delays, hypotonia, and craniofacial malformations such as microcephaly or holoprosencephaly. Eye abnormalities may also be present such as dysgenesis of the anterior segment, dislocation of the lens, or hypoplasia of the optic nerve. Some individuals may have an increased predisposition to respiratory, sinus, or other infections. Some patients have had skeletal defects or visceral anomalies. Intelligence may be normal but can also include varying levels of developmental impairment. The incidence of infertility or miscarriage may also be increased.

ETIOLOGY/EPIDEMIOLOGY: The cause of the disorder is a deletion of chromosome 21 at both ends and a joining of the ends to form a ring. The amount of lost genetic material can vary from a small amount causing few symptoms to a significant amount causing many symptoms. If the ring replaces a normal 21 chromosome, the symptoms are similar to monosomy 21. If some cells contain a ring 21 in addition to the normal pair, then some features may be present that resemble Down syndrome. Most often this occurs *de novo* with a low possibility of recurrence; however, in a a few cases the ring is inherited from a parent, and in that situation the recurrence risk is 50%. Males and females are affected equally.

DIAGNOSIS: Chromosome analysis is necessary to confirm the specific abnormality.

TREATMENT
Standard Therapies: Treatment may include surgical repair of craniofacial, skeletal, visceral, or other abnormalities associated with the disorder. Treatment may also be needed to prevent or aggressively treat infections. Special education and early intervention are indicated. Genetic counseling is recommended for patients and their families.

REFERENCES
Conte RA, et al. Characterization of a ring chromosome 21 by FISH-technique. *Clin Genet* 1995;48:188–191.
Gardner RJ, et al. Ring 21 chromosome: the mild end of the phenotypic spectrum. *Clin Genet* 1986;30:466–470.
McGinniss MJ, et al. Mechanisms of ring chromosome formation in 11 cases of human ring chromosome 21. *Am J Hum Genet* 1992;50:15–28.
Melnyk AF, et al. Prenatal diagnosis of familial ring 21 chromosome. *Prenat Diagn* 1995;15:269–273.

RESOURCES
104, 476

16   Chromosome 22q11 Deletion Spectrum

Beverly S. Emanuel, PhD

DEFINITION: The 22q11.2 deletion syndrome is the most prevalent of the chromosomal microdeletion syndromes. It is a complex disorder associated with a wide variety of symptoms including conotruncal cardiac defects, cleft palate or velopharyngeal insufficiency, speech and learning disabilities, and a typical facial appearance.

SYNONYMS: DiGeorge syndrome; Velocardiofacial syndrome; Conotruncal anomaly face syndrome; CATCH22.

DIFFERENTIAL DIAGNOSIS: Autosomal-dominant "Opitz" GBBB syndrome; Cayler cardiofacial syndrome.

SYMPTOMS AND SIGNS: Congenital heart disease is the most common structural anomaly associated with the 22q11.2 deletion. The most common defect is tetralogy of Fallot, followed by interrupted aortic arch type B, conoventricular septal defect, truncus arteriosus, and a vascular ring. Children with severe cardiac defects most often present in the newborn period with cyanosis, a heart murmur, or symptoms of congestive heart failure. Palatal anomalies are frequent. Velopharyngeal incompetence is the most common, followed by submucosal cleft palate, overt cleft palate, bifid uvula, and cleft lip and/or palate. Common facial features include a prominent nasal root, bulbous nasal tip, hypoplastic alae nasae, and nasal dimple/bifid nasal tip. Other craniofacial findings include cupped, microtic, and protuberant ears, preauricular pits, preauricular tags, and overfolded and/or squared off helices. Absence or hypoplasia of the parathyroid glands can cause hypocalcemia. Hypoplasia of the thymus can cause susceptibility to infection due to a deficit of T cells. The 22q11.2 deletion has been associated with a variety of neurologic and psychologic manifestations, including hypotonia, developmental delay, and psychiatric abnormalities.

ETIOLOGY/EPIDEMIOLOGY: The 22q11 deletion occurs in approximately 1 in 4,000 live births. Males and females are equally likely to be affected, as are all ethnic groups; however, most reported patients have been caucasian, which is believed to be due to an ascertainment bias. The incidence of familial cases is estimated to be approximately 10%.

DIAGNOSIS: Clinical suspicion of the 22q11.2 deletion in a patient with one or more of the associated structural or functional findings is based on the characteristic facial appearance. The cytogenetic management should include a standard karyotype to exclude all visible structural rearrangements followed by fluorescence *in situ* hybridization with probes from within the most consistently deleted portion of 22q11.2 to detect submicroscopic deletions. The standard clinical evaluations should include cardiology,

child psychology, ear-nose-throat/audiology, immunology, plastic surgery, and speech pathology.

TREATMENT
Standard Therapies: Treatment is usually based on the systems involved. Most common surgical interventions are to repair the structural defects. Successful management for the feeding problems include G-tube placement, medication for gastrointestinal dysmotility, facilitation of bowel evacuation, treatment for gastroesophageal reflux including acid blockade and prokinetic agents, postural therapy, and spoon placement modifications. The cognitive delays, motor deficits, language delays, and speech difficulties often require early intervention services, including occupational, physical, and speech therapy.

REFERENCES
Eicher PS, McDonald-McGinn DM, Fox CA, et al. Dysphagia in children with a 22q11.2 deletion: unusual pattern found on modified barium swallow. *Pediatrics* 2000;137:158–164.
Emanuel BS, McDonald-McGinn D, Saitta SC, et al. The 22q11.2 deletion syndrome. *Adv Pediatr* 2001;48:39–73.
McDonald-McGinn DM, Kirschner R, Goldmuntz E, et al. The Philadelphia story: the 22q11.2 deletion: report on 250 patients. *Genet Couns* 1999;10:11–24.
Woodin M, Wang PP, Aleman D, et al. Neuropsychological profile of children and adolescents with the 22q11.2 microdeletion. *Genet Med* 2001;3:34–39.
Solot CB, Gerdes M, Kirschner RE, et al. Communication issues in 22q11.2 deletion syndrome: children at risk. *Genet Med* 2001;3:67–71.

RESOURCES
102, 193, 462

17 Chromosome 22 Ring

Nataline B. Kardon, MD

DEFINITION: Chromosome 22 ring is characterized by mental retardation, lack of coordination of voluntary movements, and muscle weakness. It results from breakage of the chromosome at both ends with subsequent joining of the ends to form a ring.

SYNONYMS: r22; Ring 22; Ring 22, chromosome.

DIFFERENTIAL DIAGNOSIS: Chromosome 22q deletion; DiGeorge syndrome; Opitz (BBBG) syndrome.

SYMPTOMS AND SIGNS: The symptoms depend on the amount of genetic material lost on the short and long arms

of the chromosome. The most common features are mental retardation, muscle weakness, and uncoordinated movements. Other features may be a smaller than normal nose, a large rounded nose, large ears, a high-arched palate, widely spaced eyes, epicanthal folds, and drooping eyelids. A few patients have underdeveloped toenails, syndactyly, small eyes, long eyelashes, and heart defects.

ETIOLOGY/EPIDEMIOLOGY: The cause of the disorder is a deletion of chromosome 22 at both ends and a joining of the ends to form a ring. The amount of lost genetic material varies. The condition usually occurs *de novo* with a low possibility of recurrence. The parents of the affected child typically have normal chromosomes and a low possibility of having another child with a chromosome abnormality. Males are affected more often than females. More than 40 cases have been reported.

DIAGNOSIS: The disorder is diagnosed by chromosome analysis.

TREATMENT
Standard Therapies: Patients with poor muscle tone may benefit from physical therapy. Special education and early intervention are indicated. Genetic counseling is recommended for patients and their families.

REFERENCES
Gustavson KH, et al. Deleted ring chromosome 22 in a mentally retarded boy. *Clin Genet* 1986;29:337–341.
Severien C, et al. Ring chromosome 22: a case report. *Klin Padiatr* 1991;203:467–469.

RESOURCES
102, 462

---

18   Chromosome 22, Trisomy Mosaic

Nataline B. Kardon, MD

DEFINITION: Chromosome 22, trisomy mosaic is a disorder in which some cells have three 22 chromosomes and some have the usual pair. It may be characterized by growth delays, mental retardation, unequal development of the two sides of the body, and webbing of the neck.

SYNONYMS: Trisomy 22 mosaic; Trisomy 22 mosaicism syndrome.

DIFFERENTIAL DIAGNOSIS: Trisomy 22; Turner syndrome; Noonan syndrome.

SYMPTOMS AND SIGNS: Severe growth and developmental delays and mental retardation are characteristic findings. Unilateral hearing impairment is seen in those who present with unequal development of the two sides of the body. There may be findings characteristic of Turner syndrome, such as short stature, cubitus valgus, multiple pigmented nevi, congenital heart defects involving the aorta, ptosis, webbing of the neck, a low hairline at the back of the neck, dysplastic nails, and ovarian dysgenesis. Other malformations observed include ocular hypertelorism, epicanthal folds, preauricular pits, underdeveloped digits, abnormal palmar skin creases, and renal malformations.

ETIOLOGY/EPIDEMIOLOGY: An extra chromosome 22 is present in one of an individual's cell lines with at least one unaffected cell line also present. The severity of the symptoms corresponds to the percentage of affected cells with the extra chromosome. The disorder results from an error in cell division in the formation of sperm or egg cells or in the embryo. Trisomy 22 mosaic appears to affect females slightly more often than males. About 15 cases have been reported.

DIAGNOSIS: The diagnosis is made by chromosome analysis. This can be done prenatally by amniocentesis or chorionic villus sampling or postnatally by peripheral blood sampling. Ultrasonography may show some of the features of the disorder. Cardiac evaluation may include radiography, electrocardiography, echocardiography, and cardiac catheterization. Other specialized tests may be necessary to characterize renal abnormalities, hearing impairment, or ovarian dysgenesis.

TREATMENT
Standard Therapies: Treatment requires the coordinated efforts of a team of medical professionals. Surgical repair of craniofacial and cardiovascular lesions may be necessary. Other treatment is symptomatic and supportive. Early intervention programs and genetic counseling are recommended.

REFERENCES
Crowe CA, et al. Mosaic trisomy 22: a case presentation and literature review of trisomy 22 phenotypes. *Am J Med Genet* 1997;71:406–413; comment in *Am J Med Genet* 1998;76:447.
de Pater JM, et al. Maternal uniparental disomy for chromosome 22 in a child with generalized mosaicism for trisomy 22. *Prenat Diagn* 1997;17:81–86.
Phillips OP, et al. Risk of fetal mosaicism when placental mosaicism is diagnosed by chorionic villus sampling. *Am J Obstet Gynecol* 1996;174:850–855.
Wertelecki W, et al. Trisomy 22 mosaicism syndrome and Ullrich-Turner stigmata. *Am J Med Genet* 1986;23:739–749.
Woods CG, et al. Asymmetry and skin pimentary anomalies in chromosome mosaicism. *J Med Genet* 1994;31:694–701.

RESOURCES
455, 462, 476

19   Chromosome 3, Monosomy 3p2

Nataline B. Kardon, MD

DEFINITION: Chromosome 3, monosomy 3p2 is a disorder in which the end of the short arm of chromosome 3 is missing.

SYNONYMS: Chromosome 3, deletion of distal 3p; Chromosome 3, distal 3p monosomy; Monosomy 3p2.

DIFFERENTIAL DIAGNOSIS: Other chromosomal disorders with similar features.

SYMPTOMS AND SIGNS: Symptoms are usually apparent in the first few years of life. Prenatal and postnatal growth retardation, mental retardation, microcephaly, hypertrichosis, and synophyrs are the most consistent findings. Other symptoms may include a triangular face, abnormally long head, prominent forehead, and/or unusually small jaws. Ptosis, hypertelorism, and/or epicanthal folds may also be present. Symptoms may also include low-set and malformed ears, a broad and flat nose, downturned mouth, finger abnormalities, a pectus excavatum, and/or scoliosis. Delayed sexual development has been reported in males. The following malformations have been present at birth in 1 or 2 cases: heart defects, hiatal hernia, optic atrophy, fetal lobulation of kidneys, polycystic renal dysplasia, and hypoplastic clavicles.

ETIOLOGY/EPIDEMIOLOGY: The deletion of chromosomal material from band 25 to the end of the short arm of chromosome 3 is responsible for the physical and mental abnormalities. In most reported cases, chromosome 3, monosomy 3p2 appears to have resulted from spontaneous errors during cell division. In these cases it is unlikely that subsequent offspring would have the same chromosomal abnormality. In some cases, monosomy 3p2 has appeared to result from a parental chromosome 3 inversion or a translocation involving chromosome 3p and another chromosome or chromosomes. Males and females are affected equally. Approximately 34 cases have been reported.

DIAGNOSIS: Diagnosis is possible by chromosome analysis prenatally by chorionic villus sampling or amniocentesis or postnatally based on symptoms that necessitate chromosome testing.

TREATMENT
Standard Therapies: Treatment is symptomatic and supportive. Special education, physical therapy, and other medical, social, or vocational services may be of benefit to the patient, and are often necessary for the child to reach his or her full potential. Genetic counseling may be of benefit for affected individuals and their families.

REFERENCE
Narahara J, et al. Loss of the 3p25.3 band is critical in the manifestation of del (3p) syndrome: karyotype-phenotype correlation in cases with deficiency of the distal portion of the short arm of chromosome 3. *Am J Med Genet* 1990;35: 269–273.

RESOURCES
104, 113, 462

20   Chromosome 3, Trisomy 3q2

Nataline B. Kardon, MD

DEFINITION: Trisomy 3q2 is a disorder in which a portion of chromosome 3 appears three times rather than twice in cells of the body.

SYNONYMS: Chromosome 3, distal 3q2 trisomy; Chromosome 3, distal 3q2 duplication; Partial trisomy 3q syndrome; Partial duplication 3q syndrome.

DIFFERENTIAL DIAGNOSIS: Cornelia de Lange syndrome.

SYMPTOMS AND SIGNS: The disorder is characterized by mental retardation, moderate to severe developmental delays, and hypotonia. Craniofacial abnormalities include brachycephaly, ocular hypertelorism, oblique palpebral fissures, epicanthal folds, a small nose with anteverted nares, and micrognathia. The philtrum is abnormally prominent, and the patient may have a high-arched palate, or clefting of the palate. A low hairline on the forehead and the back of the neck, an abnormally short neck with excessive skin folds, unusually long eyelashes, synophrys, and hirsutism are also characteristic. Ocular abnormalities such as glaucoma, cataracts, corneal opacities, nystagmus, strabismus, coloboma, and microphthalmia may produce varying degrees of visual impairment. Some bones within the distal phalanges may be hypoplastic, causing the hands to appear unusually short. Affected individuals may also have clinodactyly, permanent flexion of one or more digits, or syndactyly of certain toes. Cryptorchidism may be present in affected males, as may malformations of the internal genitals in females. Congenital heart defects, renal defects, and underdevelopment of certain regions of the brain may also be present.

ETIOLOGY/EPIDEMIOLOGY: The severity and range of symptoms may depend on the specific length and location of the duplicated portion of the chromosome. In addition, bands 26.3–27.3 on chromosome 3q may be a critical region in producing the syndrome. In some cases, the extra material may result from a parental chromosome rearrangement such as a balanced translocation or an inversion. In others, the duplication of the chromosome occurs *de novo* and is not likely to recur. Males and females are affected equally. At least 50 cases have been reported.

DIAGNOSIS: The diagnosis is made by chromosome analysis of prenatal or postnatal specimens.

TREATMENT
Standard Therapies: Treatment may include surgical repair of craniofacial, digital, ocular, cardiac, or other abnormalities potentially associated with the disorder. Other treatment is symptomatic and supportive. Early intervention is important. Genetic counseling is recommended for patients and their families.

REFERENCES
Aqua MS, et al. Duplication 3q syndrome: molecular delineation of the critical region. *Am J Med Genet* 1995;55:33–37.
Holder SE, et al. Partial trisomy 3q causing mild Cornelia de Lange phenotype. *J Med Genet* 1994;31:150–152.
Rosenfeld W, et al. Duplication 3q: severe manifestations in an infant with duplication of a short segment of 3q. *Am J Med Genet* 1981;10:187–192.
Tranebjaerg L, et al. Partial trisomy 3q syndrome inherited from familial t(3;9) (q26.1;p23). *Clin Genet* 1987;32:137–143.
Yunis E, et al. Partial trisomy 3q. *Hum Genet* 1979;48:315–320.

RESOURCES
455, 476

---

21   Chromosome 4, Monosomy 4q

Nataline B. Kardon, MD

DEFINITION: Chromosome 4, monosomy 4q is a chromosomal disorder caused by a partial deletion of the long arm of chromosome 4.

SYNONYMS: Chromosome 4 long arm deletion; Chromosome 4q- syndrome.

DIFFERENTIAL DIAGNOSIS: Wolf-Hirschorn syndrome (4p- syndrome); Chromosome 11, monosomy 11q; Greig cephalopolysyndactyly syndrome; Down syndrome.

SYMPTOMS AND SIGNS: Patients with monosomy 4q may have the following symptoms: abnormal skull shape, short nose with abnormal bridge, low-set malformed ears, cleft palate, small jaw, short breastbone, poor or delayed growth, moderate to severe developmental impairment, heart defects, genitourinary defects, small size, small hands and feet, unusually wide-set eyes, a pointed fifth finger and

nail which is very characteristic of this disorder, and low muscle tone. There may be agenesis of corpus callosum. In some cases, delayed growth and cognitive development may be present without obvious physical abnormalities, making it difficult to diagnose the disorder.

ETIOLOGY/EPIDEMIOLOGY: The syndrome is caused by a partial deletion of the long arm of chromosome 4. The severity and type of abnormalities depend on the size and location, whether interstitial or terminal, of the missing chromosomal piece. The disorder is present at birth, and it affects males and females in equal numbers.

DIAGNOSIS: Chromosome analysis of peripheral blood or prenatal tissue specimens confirms the diagnosis.

TREATMENT
Standard Therapies: Treatment is symptomatic and supportive. Special education, physical therapy, and vocational

services may be of benefit, as may genetic counseling for patients and their families.

REFERENCES

Caliebe A, et al. Mild phenotypic manifestations of terminal deletion of the long arm of chromosome 4: clinical description of a new patient. *Clin Genet* 1997;52:116–119.

Descartes M, et al. Terminal deletion of the long arm of chromosome 4 in a mother and two sons. *Clin Genet* 1996;50:538–540.

Robertson SP, et al. The 4q- syndrome: delineation of the minimal critical region to within band 4q31. *Clin Genet* 1998;53:70–73.

RESOURCES

104, 476

22 | Chromosome 4, Monosomy Distal 4q

Nataline B. Kardon, MD

DEFINITION: Monosomy distal 4q is a disorder in which a deletion occurs of an end piece of the long arm of chromosome 4.

SYNONYMS: Chromosome 4, deletion 4q31-qter syndrome; Chromosome 4, deletion 4q32-qter syndrome; Chromosome 4, deletion 4q33-qter syndrome; Chromosome 4, partial monosomy of distal 4q; Chromosome 4, 4q terminal deletion syndrome.

DIFFERENTIAL DIAGNOSIS: Pierre Robin sequence; Other chromosomal disorders involving mental retardation.

SYMPTOMS AND SIGNS: The major symptoms are mental retardation and unusual facial features; heart defects, developmental delays, hypotonia, and limb deformities may also be present. A small jaw, a tongue displaced downward, and cleft of the soft palate are typical. Other findings may include the absence of flexion creases on the fifth fingers and/or a pointed appearance of the fifth finger(s) and nail(s). The eyes may be widely spaced or slanted downward; the nose may be short with a broad nasal bridge; the ears may be low-set and pointed. Other findings are microcephaly, abnormalities of the kidney and skeleton, tracheoesophageal fistula, ectopic anus, seizures, and/or abnormal genitals.

ETIOLOGY/EPIDEMIOLOGY: The characteristic features of monosomy distal 4q may be a result of deletions in the region from band 31 to the end of the long arm of chromosome 4. Most chromosomal deletions occur *de novo*. The parents of the affected child typically have normal chromosomes and a low possibility of having another child with a chromosomal abnormality, although a few cases have occurred as the result of balanced translocation in the parent. When a balanced translocation occurs on the long arm of chromosome 4, the parent has a good chance of having a child with a deletion in the same area. Males and females are affected equally. Approximately 30 cases have been reported.

DIAGNOSIS: The diagnosis is made by chromosome analysis of appropriate tissues either prenatally or postnatally based on physical findings.

TREATMENT

Standard Therapies: Individuals with poor muscle tone should have physical therapy. Special education and related services are also of benefit. Infants should be observed closely for breathing difficulties. Tracheostomy may be indicated. Surgery to improve the appearance of the jaw and correct the cleft of the soft palate may also be recommended. When esophageal atresia and/or fistula are present, surgical repair may require several stages. Genetic counseling is recommended for affected individuals and their families. Other treatment is symptomatic and supportive.

REFERENCES

Fagan KA, et al. Del (4) (q33-qter): another case report of a child with mild dysmorphism. *J Med Genet* 1989;26:776–778.

Lin AE, et al. Interstitial and terminal deletions of the long arm of chromosome 4: further delineation of phenotypes. *Am J Med Genet* 1988;31:533–548.

Menko FH, et al. Robin sequence and a deficiency of the left forearm in a girl with a deletion of chromosome 4q33-qter. *Am J Med Genet* 1992;44:696–698.

Michelena DE, et al. Terminal deletion of 4q in a severely retarded boy. *Am J Med Genet* 1989;33:228–230.

RESOURCES

96, 108, 113

23   Chromosome 4, Partial Trisomy Distal 4q

Nataline B. Kardon, MD

DEFINITION: Partial trisomy distal 4q is a chromosomal disorder caused by a duplication of the end portion of the long arm of chromosome 4. The symptoms may include small head size; malformations of the arms, legs, and craniofacial area; and developmental delay.

SYNONYMS: Chromosome 4, partial trisomy 4 (q25-qter); Chromosome 4, partial trisomy 4 (q26 or q27-qter); Chromosome 4, partial trisomy 4 (q31 or 32-qter); Chromosome 4, partial trisomies 4q2 and 4q3.

DIFFERENTIAL DIAGNOSIS: Trisomy 4p; Craniofrontonasal dysplasia.

SYMPTOMS AND SIGNS: Craniofacial abnormalities may include small head, a sloping forehead, low-set and abnormally formed ears, a wide or absent nasal bridge, and epicanthal folds. Other less common abnormalities may include pursed lips, small lower jaw, a small space between the nose and the upper lip, downturned corners of the mouth, and a short neck. Affected infants may also have malformed hands, abnormalities of the thumbs, abnormally turned feet, or webbing of the toes. They may have undescended testes or renal, urinary tract, cardiac, or vascular abnormalities. A few infants may have fused eyelids, drooping eyelids, or small eyes. This disorder may also be associated with hernias, seizures, or cardiac failure. Affected individuals may experience developmental abnormalities including low birth weight, low muscle tone, and psychomotor retardation.

ETIOLOGY/EPIDEMIOLOGY: The duplication of the long arm of chromosome 4 usually results from a parental balanced translocation. This can be determined by genetic testing. Balanced translocations are usually harmless to the carrier, but are associated with a higher risk for abnormal offspring. A few cases may be *de novo*. Males and females are affected in equal numbers. Approximately 35 cases have been reported.

DIAGNOSIS: Chromosome analysis of prenatal or postnatal specimens will confirm the diagnosis. Ultrasonography and physical findings should reveal indications for performing the studies. Prenatal diagnosis can be achieved by amniocentesis or chorionic villus sampling.

TREATMENT
Standard Therapies: Surgery may correct craniofacial, cardiac, renal, or other malformations. Which procedures are performed depends on the severity of the anatomic abnormalities and the associated symptoms. A team approach may be of benefit and may include special medical, educational, and occupational services. Genetic counseling will be of benefit for affected individuals and their families. Other treatment is symptomatic and supportive.

REFERENCES
Andrle M, et al. Partial trisomy 4q in two unrelated cases. *Hum Genet* 1979;49:179–183.
Biederman B, et al. Partial trisomy 4q due to familial 2/4 translocation. *Hum Genet* 1976;33:147–153.
Cervenka J, et al. Partial trisomy 4q syndrome: case report and review. *Hum Genet* 1976;34:1–7.
Kelly TE, et al. Partial trisomy 4q resulting from a familial 4/3 translocation. *South Med J* 1979;72:1459–1461.

RESOURCES
96, 113, 462

24   Chromosome 4 Ring

Nataline B. Kardon, MD

DEFINITION: Chromosome 4 ring is a disorder in which the affected infant has a breakage of chromosome 4 at both ends, and the ends of the chromosome join together to form a ring.

SYNONYMS: Ring 4; Ring 4, chromosome; r4.

DIFFERENTIAL DIAGNOSIS: Wolf Hirschhorn syndrome; Seckle syndrome; Deletion of chromosome 4q.

SYMPTOMS AND SIGNS: The symptoms seen most often are low birth weight, slowed growth and development, and a small head. A small jaw, broad nose, and cleft palate may be present. Other signs are permanently bent fingers, ptosis, mental retardation, hypospadias, and/or abnormal ears. Speech is often delayed along with other developmental skills.

ETIOLOGY/EPIDEMIOLOGY: Most chromosomal deletions occur *de novo*. The parents of the affected child typically have normal chromosomes and a low possibility of having another child with a chromosomal abnormality. Most cases of this disorder have been a deletion of 4p16 and 4q35. Males and females are affected equally. The condition is usually detected at birth or during prenatal testing.

DIAGNOSIS: Chromosome analysis of either peripheral blood or appropriate tissue samples confirms the diagnosis.

TREATMENT
Standard Therapies: Special education as well as speech therapy are beneficial. Genetic counseling may be useful for patients and their families. Other treatment is symptomatic and supportive.

REFERENCE
Halal F, et al. Ring chromosome 4 in a child with duodenal atresia. *Am J Med Genet* 1990;37:79–82.

RESOURCES
96, 372, 476

25   Chromosome 4, Trisomy 4p

Nataline B. Kardon, MD

DEFINITION: Trisomy 4p is a disorder caused by extra short arm 4 chromosomal material. Many affected infants may have feeding and breathing difficulties, characteristic craniofacial malformations, and abnormalities of the hands and feet. Other features, such as skeletal defects, genital abnormalities in affected males, or heart defects, may be present. The disorder is also characterized by severe mental retardation.

SYNONYMS: Chromosome 4, partial trisomy 4p; Chromosome 4, trisomy 4p; Duplication 4p syndrome.

DIFFERENTIAL DIAGNOSIS: Many chromosomal disorders may have similar features.

SYMPTOMS AND SIGNS: The disorder is characterized by prenatal and postnatal growth retardation, feeding problems, and increased muscle tone in the first months of life, followed by low muscle tone. Affected infants may also have respiratory difficulties. Many infants have a small head; a relatively small, flat forehead; a flat or depressed nasal bridge with a bulbous nasal tip; and large, malformed ears. The eyes may be widely spaced with abnormal prominence of the ridges above the eyes. Additional features such as a prominent chin, a relatively large tongue, irregularities of the teeth, and a short neck may be present. Curvature of the fifth fingers, permanent flexion of one or more fingers, and "rocker-bottom" feet occur. Some affected infants may also have long fingers or underdeveloped fingernails and toenails. Other skeletal malformations may include dislocation of the hip, side to side or front to back curvature of the spine, vertebral malformations, and extra or missing ribs. Joint contractures may result in limited movements.

Affected males may have small penis, abnormal placement of the opening in the penis, or undescended testes. In some cases, inguinal hernia, congenital heart defects, renal malformations, or agenesis of the corpus callosum may be present. Some affected individuals may also have seizures. Ocular abnormalities such as small eyes or colobomata of the uvea have been described. Trisomy 4p is characterized by severe developmental impairment.

ETIOLOGY/EPIDEMIOLOGY: Trisomy of a certain region or regions of chromosome 4p is responsible for the symptoms and findings that characterize the disorder. Evidence suggests that duplication of bands 15.2 to 16.1 on chromosome 4p is a critical region. Chromosomal testing may determine whether a parent has a balanced translocation or a pericentric inversion. In some affected individuals, this occurs as a spontaneous event. Trisomy 4p appears to affect males and females in equal numbers. More than 75 cases have been reported in the medical literature.

DIAGNOSIS: The diagnosis may be suspected prenatally by ultrasonography findings and then confirmed by performing chromosome analysis on chorionic villus or amniotic fluid cell cultures. Postnatally, physical findings may lead to chromosome analysis of a peripheral blood sample. Specialized testing to characterize certain abnormalities associated with the disorder include CT or MRI and electroencephalography. Cardiac evaluation may include radiographic studies, electrocardiography, echocardiography, or cardiac catheterization.

TREATMENT
Standard Therapies: Treatment may include surgical repair of craniofacial, skeletal, genital, cardiac, or other ab-

normalities associated with the disorder. Treatment may also include measures to help prevent or aggressively treat respiratory complications. Other treatment is symptomatic and supportive. Early intervention, special education, physical therapy, and other medical, social, or vocational services are indicated. Genetic counseling will also be of benefit.

REFERENCES
de Brasi D, et al. Cloverleaf skull anomaly and *de novo* trisomy 4p. *J Med Genet* 1999;36:422–424.

Patel SV, et al. Clinical manifestations of trisomy 4p syndrome. *Eur J Pediatr* 1995;154:425–431.

Reynolds JF, et al. Trisomy 4p in four relatives: variability and lack of distinctive features in phenotypic expression. *Clin Genet* 1983;24:365–374.

Yardin C, et al. Identical chromosome imbalance in two siblings born to a mother with a double reciprocal translocation. *Ann Genet* 1997;40:232–234.

RESOURCES
113, 120, 476

26 Chromosome 5, Trisomy 5p

Nataline B. Kardon, MD

DEFINITION: Chromosome 5, trisomy 5p is a disorder in which all or a portion of the short arm of chromosome 5 (5p) appears three times in cells of the body.

SYNONYMS: Chromosome 5, trisomy 5p, complete (5p11-pter); Chromosome 5, trisomy 5p, partial (5p13 or 14-pter).

DIFFERENTIAL DIAGNOSIS: Atypical Peters anomaly; Mental retardation; Dysmorphic facial features.

SYMPTOMS AND SIGNS: Many infants with the disorder have a normal birth weight but postnatal growth retardation and hypotonia. The head may be microcephalic or, sometimes, macrocephalic. Additional craniofacial abnormalities may include ocular hypertelorism, epicanthal folds, a depressed nasal bridge, and low-set ears. Some affected infants may have a relatively large tongue and a small jaw. They may also have microphthalmia, strabismus, or iris coloboma. The child may have arachnodactyly, short first toes, or clubfeet. Some affected infants may also have congenital heart defects, such as atrial septal defects. Additional physical abnormalities may include narrowing of the larynx or seizures. Some infants may have feeding difficulties and an increased susceptibility to repeated respiratory infections. This syndrome may also be associated with psychomotor retardation and varying levels of mental retardation.

ETIOLOGY/EPIDEMIOLOGY: Evidence suggests that duplication of band 13 on chromosome 5p is a critical region in determining the severity of associated symptoms. Trisomy 5p may result from a translocation involving chromosome 5 and another chromosome. In some affected individuals, trisomy 5p may be due to unbalanced translocations that occurred *de novo*. Chromosomal testing may determine whether a parent has a balanced translocation. Trisomy 5p appears to affect females slightly more often than males. More than 30 cases have been reported.

DIAGNOSIS: The diagnosis may be suspected prenatally by ultrasonography and confirmed by chromosome analysis. Postnatal detection is based on characteristic physical findings and chromosomal analysis. In some cases, characterization of certain abnormalities such as congenital heart defects or seizure activity may be indicated.

TREATMENT
Standard Therapies: Treatment may include surgical repair of craniofacial, cardiac, or other abnormalities potentially associated with the disorder, and also measures to help prevent or aggressively treat respiratory infections. Other treatment is symptomatic and supportive. Special education and other medical, social, and vocational services may be useful. Genetic counseling is recommended for patients and their families.

REFERENCES
Avansino JR, et al. Proximal 5p trisomy resulting from a marker chromosome implicates band 5p13 in 5p trisomy syndrome. *Am J Med Genet* 1999;87:6–11.

Lorda-Sanchez I, et al. Proximal partial 5p trisomy resulting from a maternal (19; 5) insertion. *Am J Med Genet* 1997;68:476–480.

Reichenbach H, et al. *De novo* complete trisomy 5p: clinical report and FISH studies. *Am J Med Genet* 1999;85:447–451.

RESOURCES
455, 462, 476

27   Chromosome 6, Partial Trisomy 6q

Nataline B. Kardon, MD

DEFINITION: Chromosome 6, partial trisomy 6q is a disorder in which the distal portion of the long arm (q) of the 6th chromosome (6q) appears three times.

SYNONYMS: Chromosome 6, trisomy 6q2; Trisomy 6q syndrome, partial; 6q+ syndrome, partial; Trisomy 6q, partial; Distal trisomy 6q; Duplication 6q, partial; Distal duplication 6q.

DIFFERENTIAL DIAGNOSIS: Apert syndrome; Multiple pterygium syndrome.

SYMPTOMS AND SIGNS: Infants may exhibit microcephaly, a face that appears flat, ocular hypertelorism, and downwardly slanting palpebral fissures. Several abnormalities may involve the mouth, such as thin lips, a downturned mouth, and micrognathia. The soft palate may be cleft. Additional features may include arched eyebrows, a large, flat nose, and malformed ears. Often, coronal and sagittal sutures may close prematurely, causing turricephaly. As a result, the head may appear unusually long, narrow, and pointed at the top, and the forehead may be abnormally prominent. The neck may be unusually short and wide, and many affected individuals may have webbing of the anterior and/or lateral neck, which may restrict movement of the jaw and neck. In addition, the hairline on the back of the neck may be abnormally low. Flexion contractures may cause restriction of movement, and the flexor tendons may be abnormally short. Older children may have spinal abnormalities, such as scoliosis, which may result in abnormal postures and an unusual gait. Syndactyly, clubhands and/or clubfeet, and hypoplastic nails may be present. The sternum may be abnormally short, and the nipples may be widely spaced. Affected males may exhibit genital abnormalities, such as micropenis, absence of the scrotum, hypospadias, and cryptorchidism. In rare cases, various internal malformations may be present. These may include cardiac, intestinal, renal, and cerebral abnormalities. Most affected individuals also exhibit prenatal and postnatal growth retardation and/or psychomotor retardation. Mental retardation may also be present.

ETIOLOGY/EPIDEMIOLOGY: The duplicated portion of 6q may begin anywhere between bands 6q21 to q26 and then extend to the end of chromosome 6q. In most cases, this may be the result of a parental balanced chromosomal translocation. Most such translocations are of maternal origin. Rarely, this may be a sporadic *de novo* event. The disorder appears to affect males and females equally. Approximately 30 cases have been reported.

DIAGNOSIS: Partial trisomy 6q may be diagnosed prenatally by ultrasonography and amniocentesis and confirmed postnatally by a thorough clinical evaluation, characteristic physical findings, chromosomal studies, and specialized DNA tests (e.g., fluorescence *in situ* hybridization).

TREATMENT
Standard Therapies: Treatment may include surgical repair of the malformations. Physical therapy may also be prescribed for flexion contractures. Other treatment is symptomatic and supportive. Genetic counseling is recommended.

REFERENCES
Bartalena L, et al. A case of partial 6q trisomy diagnosed at birth. *Pathologica* 1990;82:549–552.

Franchino CJ, et al. Partial trisomy 6q: a case report with necropsy findings. *J Med Genet* 1987;24:300–303.

Taysi K, et al. Trisomy 6q22 leads to 6qter due to maternal 6;21 translocation. Case report review of the literature. *Ann Genet* 1983;26:243–246.

Uhrich S, et al. Duplication 6q syndrome diagnosed *in utero*. *Am J Med Genet* 1991;41:282–283.

RESOURCES
446, 462, 476

28 Chromosome 6 Ring

Nataline B. Kardon, MD

DEFINITION: Chromosome 6 ring is a disorder in which the affected infant has a breakage of chromosome 6 at both ends, and the ends of the chromosome join together to form a ring.

SYNONYMS: Ring 6; Ring 6, chromosome; r6.

DIFFERENTIAL DIAGNOSIS: Many chromosomal disorders involving mental retardation have some similar features.

SYMPTOMS AND SIGNS: The features seen most often are mild to severe mental retardation, delays in growth and psychomotor retardation, a small head circumference and jaw, low-set ears, a flat nasal bridge, and abnormalities of the eyes. Other symptoms may include widely spaced and/or downward-slanting eyes, epicanthal folds, a high-arched palate, clubfoot, hydrocephalus, webbed skin, a short neck, and widely spaced nipples.

ETIOLOGY/EPIDEMIOLOGY: Chromosome 6 ring is caused by a deletion of chromosome 6 at both ends and a joining of the ends to form a ring. The range and severity of symptoms depends on the amount of genetic material lost. No cause is apparent. Most chromosomal deletions occur spontaneously. The parents of the affected child typically have normal chromosomes and a low possibility of having another child with a chromosomal abnormality. Males are affected slightly more often than females. Approximately 17 cases have been reported.

DIAGNOSIS: The diagnosis is made by chromosome analysis of the appropriate prenatal or postnatal tissue.

TREATMENT
Standard Therapies: Patients with poor muscle tone may benefit from physical therapy. Special education and related services benefit affected children. Genetic counseling is recommended. Other treatment is symptomatic and supportive.

REFERENCES
Chitayat D, et al. Ring chromosome 6: report of a patient and literature review. *Am J Med Genet* 1987;35:145–151.
Paz-y-Mino C, et al. Ring chromosome 6: clinical and cytogenetic behavior. *Am J Med Genet* 1990;35:481–483.

RESOURCES
96, 288, 446

29 Chromosome 7, Monosomy 7p2

Nataline B. Kardon, MD

DEFINITION: Chromosome 7, monosomy 7p2 is a chromosomal disorder in which the end portion of the short arm (p) of chromosome 7 is missing.

SYNONYMS: Chromosome 7, terminal 7p deletion [del (7) (p21-p22)]; 7p2 monosomy syndrome; 7p2- syndrome; Chromosome 7, partial deletion of short arm (7p2-).

DIFFERENTIAL DIAGNOSIS: Saethre-Chotzen syndrome; Chromosomal disorders; Craniosynostosis, primary; Ventricular septal defect; Hypoplastic left heart syndrome.

SYMPTOMS AND SIGNS: The characteristic physical abnormalities involve the craniofacial region. Affected individuals often exhibit premature fusion of the skull bones. The eventual shape of the skull and the severity and complexity of the physical findings depend on how and which sutures prematurely close. Scaphocephaly may result from premature closure of the sagittal sutures and trigonocephaly or triangular shape may result from closure of the metopic sutures. Abnormalities of the hands and feet may include permanent flexion of one or more of the fingers, joint movement difficulties, and/or talipes calcaneovalgus. A variety of congenital heart defects occur, including ventricular septal defect and hypoplastic left heart syndrome. Rarely, other symptoms may include a downwardly turned or drawn back tongue; hypoplastic external genitalia; small kidneys; and/or small intestine. Affected individuals may also exhibit growth delays and developmental delays.

ETIOLOGY/EPIDEMIOLOGY: This chromosomal abnormality is caused by a deletion of the terminal segment of the short arm anywhere between bands 7p21 and 7p22-pter. The number and severity of symptoms vary depending on where the break occurs and the length of the missing portion of the chromosome. The deletion has usually occurred as the result of a spontaneous *de novo* event; future offspring would be unlikely to have the same chromosomal abnormality. Males and females are affected in equal numbers; however, in observed cases, males have been slightly more severely affected than females. Approximately 30 cases have been reported.

DIAGNOSIS: Symptoms may be discovered during prenatal testing or are evident at birth. The deletion is demonstrated on chromosome analysis of appropriate tissue specimens.

TREATMENT
Standard Therapies: Treatment may include surgery to help correct congenital heart defects and craniofacial ab-

normalities. A supportive team approach for children with this disorder may be of benefit and may include special educational services, physical and speech therapy, and other medical, social, or vocational services. Genetic counseling will be of benefit for affected individuals and their families. Other treatment is symptomatic and supportive.

REFERENCES
Aughton DJ, et al. Chromosome 7p- syndrome: craniosynostosis with preservation of region 7p2. *Am J Med Genet* 1991;40:440–443.
Chotai KA, et al. Six cases of 7p deletion: clinical, cytogenetic, and molecular studies. *Am J Med Genet* 1994;51:270–276.
Speleman F, et al. *De novo* terminal deletion 7p22.1-pter in a child without craniosynostosis. *J Med Genet* 1989;26:528–532.

RESOURCES
96, 113, 476

---

30 Chromosome 8, Monosomy 8p2

Nataline B. Kardon, MD

DEFINITION: Chromosome 8, monosomy 8p2 is a disorder in which a portion of the short arm (p) of chromosome 8 is missing.

SYNONYMS: Chromosome 8, partial deletion (short arm); Chromosome 8, partial monosomy 8p2; 8p deletion syndrome (partial); 8p- syndrome (partial); Chromosome 8, monosomy 8p21-pter.

DIFFERENTIAL DIAGNOSIS: Other chromosomal disorders.

SYMPTOMS AND SIGNS: Characteristic signs may include a head that appears abnormally long and narrow as well as unusually small; a noticeably high forehead; and/or a bulging occiput. Features may also include a flattened nose that is small and nubbed; nystagmus; epicanthal folds; a small, receding jawbone; and/or a short neck. With advancing age, some of the unusual infantile physical features may become less noticeable. Affected infants often have a ventricular septal defect. They may also have pulmonary stenosis, coronary obstructions, or more complex abnormalities. Other signs may be underdeveloped, widely spaced nipples in combination with a large rib cage that appears rounded. Symptoms may also include vertebral defects, malformed ears, an extended upper lip, mild to severe developmental delay, and/or varied degrees of speech im-

pairment. Males may have abnormalities of the genitals, including abnormal placement of the opening of the penis and/or undescended testes. Occasionally, inguinal hernia may be present. Adolescent males may sometimes have underdeveloped testes.

ETIOLOGY/EPIDEMIOLOGY: Symptoms may vary in severity and range depending on where the break in the short arm of chromosome 8 occurs. It can occur anywhere between bands 8p21 to 8pter, the terminal segment of the chromosome. In most cases, monosomy 8p2 occurred as a result of a spontaneous deletion, making it unlikely that future offspring would have the same chromosomal abnormality. Sometimes one of the parents of an affected child may have a balanced translocation, in which case the risk of recurrence in subsequent children may be increased. The disorder affects males and females in equal numbers. Approximately 20 cases have been reported.

DIAGNOSIS: Chromosome analysis of appropriate tissue by means of prenatal diagnosis or postnatal examination will confirm the diagnosis. Parental chromosomal studies are necessary to determine whether a balanced translocation is present.

TREATMENT
Standard Therapies: A supportive team approach is of benefit and may include special education, speech therapy, physical therapy, and other medical, social, or vocational

services. Other treatment is symptomatic and supportive. Genetic counseling can be of benefit for families of individuals with this disorder.

REFERENCES

Blennow E, et al. Partial monosomy 8p with minimal dysmorphic signs. *J Med Genet* 1990;27:327–329.

Hutchinson R, et al. Distal 8p deletion (8p23.1–8pter): a common deletion? *J Med Genet* 1992;29:407–411.

Pecile V, et al. Deficiency of distal 8p-: report of two cases and review of the literature. *Clin Genet* 1990;37:271–278.

RESOURCES

35, 104, 462

31   Chromosome 9, Partial Monosomy 9p

Nataline B. Kardon, MD

DEFINITION: Chromosome 9, partial monosomy 9p is a disorder in which the distal portion of the short arm (p) of chromosome 9 is deleted.

SYNONYMS: Partial deletion of short arm of chromosome 9; Deletion 9p syndrome, partial; 9p syndrome, partial; Monosomy 9p, partial; 9p partial monosomy; Distal monosomy 9p; Chromosome 9, partial monosomy 9p22; Chromosome 9, partial monosomy 9p22-pter.

DIFFERENTIAL DIAGNOSIS: Chromosome 9 ring; Down syndrome.

SYMPTOMS AND SIGNS: This disorder is usually apparent at birth and is characterized by distinctive facial features, abnormalities of the hands and feet, genital malformations, and varying degrees of mental retardation. The metopic suture between the frontal bone closes prematurely, causing the head to grow abnormally. As a result, the forehead is abnormally prominent, and the eyes are set close together; the head may also appear narrow, whereas the occiput may appear flat. Children with this finding may be at risk for abnormal development of the forebrain. Characteristic facial features include highly arched eyebrows; slightly slanted palpebral fissures; a flat, short nose; bilateral epicanthal folds; and an abnormally long philtrum. Other abnormalities of the face and head may include an unusually small jaw and mouth; a highly arched palate; and low-set, malformed ears. Additional symptoms of the disorder include a wide space between the nipples; a short, wide neck; and abnormalities of the hands and feet, including fingers and toes that appear unusually long, have a high number of ridges on the skin, a simian crease, and nails that are hyperconvex. Genital abnormalities in males may be hypospadias. In females, the labia majora may be hypoplastic, and the labia minora may be hyperplastic. Additional congenital abnormalities may be hypotonia, omphalocele, hernias, and cardiac abnormalities. In rare cases, affected infants may exhibit choanal atresia. Symptoms have also included advanced development of bone, abnormalities of the vertebrae, seizures, and precocious puberty. Developmental abnormalities may include psychomotor retardation, delayed speech, and moderate to severe mental retardation. Affected individuals tend to have an affectionate, sociable personality.

ETIOLOGY/EPIDEMIOLOGY: The deletion of the distal portion of the short arm of chromosome 9 is responsible for the symptoms. In most cases, the missing portion of chromosome 9p begins with band p22 and extends to the end of 9p. The finding is usually *de novo* and sporadic. Some cases have resulted from a familial translocation. Genetic testing can determine whether a parent has a balanced translocation. More females than males are affected. More than 100 cases have been documented.

DIAGNOSIS: Chromosome analysis of either prenatal or postnatal tissues will determine the diagnosis. Prenatal ultrasonography may detect the birth defects associated with this syndrome.

TREATMENT
Standard Therapies: Early craniofacial surgery may be performed to correct the premature closure of the frontal bone of the forehead. Surgery may also be performed to correct additional abnormalities of the face and head, cardiac lesions, genital abnormalities, omphalocele, and hernias. Choanal atresia is usually surgically corrected soon after birth. Other treatment is symptomatic and supportive. It may include special remedial education, speech therapy, physical therapy, and other medical, social, or vocational services. Genetic counseling is recommended for family members.

REFERENCES

Calzolari C, et al. A case of 9p partial monosomy caused by paternal translocation: clinical and cytogenetic aspects. *Pediatr Med Chir* 1988;10:531–534.

Huret JL, et al. Eleven new cases of del(9p) and features from 80 cases. *J Med Genet* 1988;25:741–749.

Shashi V, et al. Choanal atresia in a patient with the deletion (9p) syndrome. *Am J Med Genet* 1994;49:88–90.

RESOURCES

96, 103, 113

32   Chromosome 9 Ring

Nataline B. Kardon, MD

DEFINITION: Chromosome 9 ring is a disorder in which there is a breakage of chromosome 9 at both ends, and the ends of the chromosome join together to form a ring. Affected children may have unusual facial features, heart defects, moderate to severe mental retardation, and skeletal abnormalities.

SYNONYMS: Ring 9; Ring 9, chromosome; r9.

DIFFERENTIAL DIAGNOSIS: Many chromosomal disorders involving mental retardation have some features similar to chromosome 9 ring.

SYMPTOMS AND SIGNS: The symptoms of chromosome 9 ring depend on the amount of genetic material lost on the small and long arms of chromosome 9. The symptoms can vary greatly; they are often mild. Facial abnormalities may include a small head, a triangular-shaped forehead, downslanting eyes that protrude outward, an exaggerated arch to the eyebrows, a small chin, and/or a short neck. Heart defects, skeletal abnormalities, and cleft palate have been seen. A few affected males may have abnormal external genitalia and/or hypospadias. Mental retardation can vary from mild to severe. Some affected individuals may become agitated easily or they may be very shy and withdrawn.

ETIOLOGY/EPIDEMIOLOGY: This disorder is caused by a deletion of chromosome 9 at both ends and the joining of the ends to form a ring. Most chromosomal deletions occur spontaneously. The parents of the affected child typically have normal chromosomes and a low possibility of having another child with a chromosomal abnormality. A parent may have chromosome 9 ring with few apparent symptoms. In these cases, the affected parent has a 50% chance of having a child with this disorder. Males and females are affected equally. Approximately 12 cases have been reported, although there may be several hundred unreported cases.

DIAGNOSIS: Chromosome analysis of either prenatal or postnatal specimens will suggest the diagnosis.

TREATMENT
Standard Therapies: Special education and related services are helpful. In patients with cleft palate, surgical treatment and speech therapy may be warranted. Genetic counseling is recommended for patients and their families. Other treatment is symptomatic and supportive.

REFERENCES
Cavaliere M, et al. Phenotypic variability in the chromosome 9 ring. *Acta Biomed Ateneo Parmense* 1997;68(suppl 1):85–89.
Lanzi G, et al. Ring chromosome 9: an atypical case. *Brain Dev* 1996;18:216–219.
Manouvrier-Hanu S, et al. Ring chromosome 9: case report and review of the literature. *Ann Genet* 1988;31:250–253.
Seghezzi L, et al. Ring chromosome 9 with 9p22.3-p24.3 duplication. *Eur J Pediatr* 1999;158:791–793.

RESOURCES
35, 103, 104

33   Chromosome 9, Tetrasomy 9p

Nataline B. Kardon, MD

DEFINITION: Tetrasomy 9p is a disorder in which the short arm of chromosome 9 appears four times.

SYNONYMS: Tetrasomy 9p; Tetrasomy, short arm of chromosome 9; Chromosome 9, tetrasomy 9p mosaicism; Mosaic tetrasomy 9p.

DIFFERENTIAL DIAGNOSIS: Chromosome 9, trisomy 9p.

SYMPTOMS AND SIGNS: The symptoms can vary. Associated physical characteristics may include abnormalities of the head and facial area, such as microcephaly, abnormally wide spaces between the skull bones, widely spaced eyes, and an abnormally rounded or beaked nose. Other facial abnormalities may include epicanthal folds and/or unusually small, receding jawbones. Affected individuals may also have a short neck; low-set, misshapen ears; various malformations of the hands and fingers, such as improperly developed fingernails; fifth fingers that are abnormally bent and short; and a simian crease. Skeletal development may also be improper. Symptoms may include abnormally reduced bone mass, spina bifida occulta, kyphoscoliosis, abnormally prominent ribs, and delayed calcification of the pelvic bone or the hip bones. In some cases, cardiac malformations or abnormalities of the eyes, such as sinking in of the eyeballs or crossing of the eyes may be present. Cerebral ventricles may be dilated and result in hydrocephalus. In rare cases, affected individuals may display cleft lip and palate, renal abnormalities, or failure of one or both testes to descend. In almost all cases, individuals with tetrasomy 9p also exhibit developmental abnormalities, such as low birth weight, mild growth retardation, and moderate psychomotor retardation. Moderate to severe mental retardation may also be present.

ETIOLOGY/EPIDEMIOLOGY: In tetrasomy 9p, the short arm of chromosome 9 appears four times rather than twice in some or all of the cells of the body. When only some cells are affected, this is termed mosaicism. The disorder is sporadic, and males appear to be affected slightly more often than females. Approximately 30 cases have been reported, and mosaicism has been found in one third of those.

DIAGNOSIS: Prenatal diagnosis can be made by chromosome analysis on amniocentesis or chorionic villus sampling. Postnatal diagnosis is confirmed by clinical evaluation, characteristic physical findings, chromosome studies, and the enzymatic assay for galactose-1-phosphate uridyltransferase.

TREATMENT
Standard Therapies: Surgical repair is the standard treatment for craniofacial, cardiac, skeletal, renal, and other malformations. Other treatment is symptomatic and supportive. Genetic counseling is recommended.

REFERENCES
Andou R, et al. A case of tetrasomy 9p. *Acta Paediatr Jpn* 1994; 36:724–726.
Balestrazzi P, et al. Tetrasomy 9p confirmed by GALT. *J Med Genet* 1983;20:396–399.
Grass FS, et al. Tetrasomy 9P tissue-limited idic(9P) in a child with mild manifestations and a normal CVS report: report and review. *Am J Med Genet* 1993;47:812–816.
Jalal SM, et al. Tetrasomy 9p: an emerging syndrome. *Clin Genet* 1991;39:60–64.
Van Hove J, et al. Tetrasomy 9p: prenatal diagnosis and fetopathological findings in a second trimester male fetus. *Ann Genet* 1994;37:139–142.

RESOURCES
35, 455, 470

---

34   Chromosome 9, Trisomy 9p (Multiple Variants)

Nataline B. Kardon, MD

DEFINITION: Chromosome 9, trisomy 9p is a disorder in which part or the entire short arm of chromosome 9 is present three times rather than twice in the cells of the body.

SYNONYMS: Trisomy 9p syndrome (partial); Chromosome 9, partial trisomy 9p; Chromosome 9, complete trisomy 9p; Chromosome 9, trisomy 9 (pter-p21 to q32); Rethore syndrome.

DIFFERENTIAL DIAGNOSIS: Tetrasomy 9p; Trisomy 9 mosaic.

SYMPTOMS AND SIGNS: Most infants have hypotonia and varying degrees of mental retardation ranging from moderate to severe, growth retardation, and delayed bone maturation that typically leads to short stature. Psychomotor retardation also occurs in most children. Infants may have microcephaly and a broad and wide head; low-set, malformed, cup-shaped ears; a large, bulbous nose; downturned corners of the mouth; a short philtrum; and/or delayed closure of the sutures and fontanelles. They may also have a short, webbed neck; an abnormally small jaw; a "worried" appearance to the face; or a highly arched palate or cleft lip and palate. Eye abnormalities include widely spaced eyes, strabismus, deep-set eyes, epicanthal folds, and downwardly slanting palpebral fissures. With advancing age, kyphoscoliosis, underdevelopment of the muscles near the shoulder blade, prominent elevation or protrusion of the ischial tuberosity, dislocation of the hip, and delayed bone ossification, especially in the pubic bone, may develop. Underdevelopment of the phalanges, metacarpals, and metatarsals may occur, resulting in abnormally short fingers and toes. Other abnormalities of the hands and feet may include malformed nails, syndactyly, clinodactyly of the fifth finger, clubfoot, and a simian crease. Approximately 25% of patients have congenital heart disease, usually a ventricular septal defect. In rare cases, renal malformations, delayed onset of puberty, or umbilical hernia may occur. Cerebral ventricles may be dilated, resulting in hydrocephaly. Affected males may have genital abnormalities such as hypospadias, micropenis, or cryptorchidism.

ETIOLOGY/EPIDEMIOLOGY: The characteristics of the disorder may result from extra chromosomal material on the short arm and/or long arm of chromosome 9 or from a duplication involving the end portion of the short arm of chromosome 9. Approximately half of cases may be the result of a parental balanced chromosomal rearrangement. Other cases are sporadic. Females are affected twice as often as males. More than 100 cases have been reported.

DIAGNOSIS: The diagnosis is made by performing a chromosome analysis on amniotic fluid, tissue, or peripheral blood. Elevated levels of the galactose-1-phosphate uridyltransferase enzyme or the nucleoside triphosphate adenylatekinase enzyme may also lead one to suspect this diagnosis. Genes on the short arm of chromosome 9 regulate these enzymes.

TREATMENT
Standard Therapies: Treatment may include surgical repair of malformations. Other treatments are symptomatic and supportive. Speech therapy may help individuals who experience severe language and communication delays.

REFERENCES
Bussani Mastellone C, et al. Four cases of trisomy 9p syndrome with particular chromosome rearrangements. *Ann Genet* 1991;34:115–119.
Steinbach B, et al. Demonstration of gene dosage effects for AK3 and GALT in fibroblasts from a fetus with 9p trisomy. *Hum Genet* 1990;63:290–291.
Young RS, et al. The dermatoglyphic and clinical features of the 9p trisomy and partial 9p monosomy syndromes. *Hum Genet* 1982;62:31–39.

RESOURCES
117, 470, 476

---

35 | Chromosome 9, Trisomy Mosaic

Nataline B. Kardon, MD

DEFINITION: Chromosome 9, trisomy mosaic is a disorder in which an extra chromosome 9 is present in some cells. The severity of symptoms may depend on the percentage of cells with the extra chromosome. Characteristic features include delayed growth of the fetus, heart defects present at birth, facial abnormalities, an abnormally small head, kidney and/or genital abnormalities, skeletal abnormalities, and/or malformations of the brain.

SYNONYM: Trisomy 9 mosaic.

DIFFERENTIAL DIAGNOSIS: Goldenhar syndrome.

SYMPTOMS AND SIGNS: Major features may include delayed growth of the fetus and/or delayed development of the child after birth, structural heart defects (atrial and/or ventricular septal defects, and/or patent ductus arteriosus), malformations of the central nervous system, small head, and/or a widening of the cranial sutures. If the central nervous system is involved, the brain malformation may be similar to that which occurs in Dandy-Walker syndrome. Symptoms may also include fixed or dislocated large joints, hand abnormalities, and underdeveloped bones. Abnormalities of the genitals, kidneys, lungs, gastrointestinal tract (incomplete rotation of intestines during development), and urinary tract (e.g., hypoplastic bladder) may also occur. Facial abnormalities may include low-set and/or malformed ears, small lower jaw, deeply set eyes, a broad-based nose with a bulb-shaped tip, and an unusually small opening between the eyelids. Other characteristics of the face and head may include unusually small eyes, widely set eyes, a cleft palate, a downturned mouth, a short neck, narrow temples, and uneven development of the bones of the head. Deep furrows in the palms of the hands and soles of the feet or a single crease across the palm may occur.

ETIOLOGY/EPIDEMIOLOGY: The diagnosis is made when an extra chromosome 9 is found in one of an individual's cell populations. At least one unaffected cell population with the normal pair of ninth chromosomes is also present. The disorder appears to affect males and females in equal numbers.

DIAGNOSIS: Chromosome 9, trisomy mosaic may be detected prenatally by analysis of fetal fluid or tissue samples (such as from amniocentesis, chorionic villus sampling, and fetal blood sampling). These tests are not 100% accurate. Chromosome testing of peripheral blood or skin fibroblast cultures makes the diagnosis postnatally.

TREATMENT
Standard Therapies: Treatment is symptomatic and supportive. Special education, physical therapy, and other medical, social, and vocational services may be of benefit to the affected individual, and are often necessary for the child to reach his or her full potential. Genetic counseling may be of benefit for the families of affected individuals.

REFERENCES
Appleman Z, et al. Trisomy 9 confined to the placenta: prenatal diagnosis and neonatal follow-up. *Am J Med Genet* 1991;40: 464–466.
Diaz-Mares L, et al. Trisomy 9 mosaicism in a girl with multiple malformations. *Ann Genet* 1990;33:165–168.
Holden JA, et al. Central nervous system malformations in trisomy 9. *J Neuropathol Exp Neurol* 1993;52:71–77.

RESOURCES
113, 462, 470

---

36   Pentasomy X

Andreas Boeck, MD

DEFINITION: Pentasomy X syndrome is a sex chromosome abnormality presenting with five X chromosomes (49,XXXXX), associated with short stature, delayed psychomotor development, and other abnormalities.

SYNONYMS: Chromosome XXXXX syndrome; 49, XXXXX syndrome; Chromosome X pentasomy; Penta-X syndrome; Quintuple-X syndrome; XXXXX syndrome.

DIFFERENTIAL DIAGNOSIS: Down syndrome; 49,XX XXY syndrome.

SYMPTOMS AND SIGNS: The characteristic penta-X phenotype includes mental retardation, short stature, coarse facial features, and skeletal and limb abnormalities. Craniofacial anomalies often include microcephaly, hypertelorism, epicanthic folds, upward-slanting palpebral fissures, a depressed and/or broad nasal bridge, and a short, broad neck. Intrauterine and postnatal growth retardation are common features. Congenital heart defects usually consist of patent ductus arteriosus or a ventricular septal defect. Osseus and articular anomalies are usually present, including bilateral clinodactyly of the hands and feet, radioulnar synostosis, and generalized joint laxity with multiple dislocations. Bilateral transverse palmar creases are common. External genitalia are normally female in appearance. Several girls have been noted to have small uteri, and fertility is assumed to be reduced; no pregnancy has been reported in a 49,XXXXX woman. Patients with pentasomy X are mentally retarded, with an average IQ of 50. Speech is delayed, and communication is difficult. Most 49,XXXXX girls appear to be shy but cooperative. Immunologic abnormalities have been associated with the condition, and one patient had a coexisting primary immunodeficiency.

ETIOLOGY/EPIDEMIOLOGY: Since the first case report of pentasomy X syndrome in 1963, only some 30 additional cases have been documented. The true incidence is unknown, but may be comparable with that of 49,XXXXY, which occurs in 1 in 85,000 males. Sequential nondisjunctions in meiosis I and II in the mother were confirmed by cytogenetic and DNA analyses in 1 patient. This agrees with previous reports of X chromosome tetrasomy or pentasomy of maternal origin.

DIAGNOSIS: Cytogenetic analysis, including fluorescent *in situ* hybridization and DNA analysis, confirms the diagnosis.

TREATMENT
Standard Therapies: Somatic treatment may include heart surgery and attempts to improve the skeletal/orthopedic features. The importance of an efficient interaction between parents, school personnel, and agencies is stressed

to improve the integration and acceptance of patients with pentasomy X in daily life.

REFERENCES

Boeck A, Gfatter R, Braun F, et al. Pentasomy X and hyper IgE syndrome: co-existence of two distinct genetic disorders. *Eur J Pediatr* 1999;158:723–726.

Kassai R, Hamada I, Furuta H, et al. Penta X syndrome: a case report and review of the literature. *Am J Med Genet* 1991;40: 51–56.

Kesaree N, Wooley PV. A phenotypic female with 49 chromosomes, presumably XXXXX. *J Pediatr* 1963;63:1099–1103.

Linden MG, Bender BG, Robinson A. Sex chromosome tetrasomy and pentasomy. *Pediatrics* 1995;96:672–682.

Martini G, Carillo G, Catizione F, et al. On the parental origin of the X's in a prenatally diagnosed 49,XXXXX syndrome. *Prenatal Diagn* 1993;xx:763–766.

RESOURCES

96, 455, 476

---

37 Trisomy 13 Syndrome

John C. Carey, MD, MPH

DEFINITION: Trisomy 13 syndrome is a distinctive and recognizable pattern of malformation resulting from an extra copy of chromosome 13. The most notable features include orofacial clefts, microphthalmia/anophthalmia, and polydactyly. There is also a predisposition to infant and neonatal mortality and profound psychomotor disability.

SYNONYMS: Patau syndrome; Trisomy D syndrome.

DIFFERENTIAL DIAGNOSIS: Meckel-Gruber syndrome; Hydrolethalus syndrome; Smith-Lemli-Opitz syndrome; Pseudotrisomy 13 syndrome.

SYMPTOMS AND SIGNS: The cardinal features include orofacial clefts, microphthalmia/anophthalmia, and postaxial polydactyly. Minor anomalies that may help establish the diagnosis include glabellar hemangiomas, frontal cowlick, broad nasal tip, and ear anomalies. Congenital cardiovascular malformations occur in 80% of infants, with ventricular and atrial septal defects being the most common. Many other major congenital anomalies can occur, including omphalocele, renal malformations, and holoprosencephaly of the brain. Neonatal and infant mortality is increased compared with the general population: approximately 50% of newborns will die in the first 7 weeks of life. Approximately 90% of children die by age 1 year, most before 6 months, usually because of central apnea and/or hypoventilation. Feeding difficulties, gastroesophageal reflux, and obstructive apnea are also common in infancy.

ETIOLOGY/EPIDEMIOLOGY: The prevalence of trisomy 13 ranges from 1 in 10,000 to 1 in 20,000 births. There is no male to female predominance. The condition is caused by the presence of an extra chromosome 13. More than 80% of cases have full trisomy 13. In most of the remaining cases, the trisomy is due to an unbalanced translocation, most often a robertsonian translocation involving chromosomes 13 and 14. Partial trisomy of some of the long arm of the 18 chromosome can also account for this phenotype, but it is less common. A small minority of patients with the Patau syndrome phenotype have mosaicism of trisomy 13.

DIAGNOSIS: The diagnosis is established by performing a G-banded karyotype showing one of the above-mentioned chromosome anomalies.

TREATMENT
Standard Therapies: Because of the high mortality rate, management of children with trisomy 13 is complicated. No standard therapies exist, but symptoms can be treated medically, and surgery can be performed for many of the manifestations. Because 80% of infants have a congenital cardiovascular malformation, cardiac surgery can be considered for a child who is older than a few weeks or months, although few data exist to help in the risk/benefit decision of such intervention. Suggestions for care include neonatal echocardiography, ophthalmology consultation, referral to a feeding specialist or team, referral to early intervention, and periodic hearing tests. Older children require regular checks for scoliosis.

REFERENCES

Baty BJ, Blackburn BL, Carey JC. Natural history of trisomy 18 and trisomy 13. I. Growth, physical assessment, medical histories, survival, and recurrence risk. *Am J Med Genet* 1996; 49:175–188.

Baty BJ, Jorde LB, Blackburn BL, et al. Natural history of trisomy 18 and trisomy 13. II. Psychomotor development. *Am J Med Genet* 1994;49:189–194.

Carey JC. Trisomy 18 and trisomy 13 syndromes. In: Cassidy SB, Allanson JE, eds. *Management of genetic syndromes.* New York: Wiley-Liss, 2001:417–436.
Jones KL. *Smith's recognizable patterns of human malformation.* Philadelphia: WB Saunders, 1997:18–23.

Wyllie JP, Wright MJ, Burn J, et al. Natural history of trisomy 13. *Arch Dis Child* 1994;71:343–345.

RESOURCES
455, 462, 476

38   Trisomy 18 Syndrome

John C. Carey, MD, MPH

DEFINITION: Trisomy 18 syndrome is a distinct pattern of malformation due to the presence of an extra chromosome 18. Affected infants have a recognizable constellation of major and minor anomalies, increased neonatal and infant mortality, and a significant psychomotor disability.

SYNONYMS: Edwards syndrome; Trisomy E syndrome.

DIFFERENTIAL DIAGNOSIS: Fetal akinesia sequence; COFS syndrome; CHARGE syndrome.

SYMPTOMS AND SIGNS: The most consistent findings include prenatal growth deficiency; recognizable craniofacial features (high forehead, short palpebral fissures, small face for cranium, and external ear abnormalities), distinctive hand posturing (overriding fingers, camptodactyly, and nail hypoplasia), a short sternum, and foot deformities. Most affected infants have a congenital heart defect, most commonly a ventricular septal defect with polyvalvular dysplasia. Other major congenital anomalies include genitourinary tract malformations, omphalocele, tracheoesophageal fistula, radial aplasia, and spina bifida. Approximately 50% of affected newborns worldwide will die in the first 7 days of life. Approximately 90% of affected children die by age 1 year, most before 6 months, usually because of central apnea and/or hypoventilation. The common occurrence of congenital heart malformation also can play a role. Feeding difficulties, gastroesophageal reflux, and obstructive apnea are also common. All patients have a significant psychomotor disability. Although most affected children are not able to walk independently or speak, developmental milestones continue to progress through early and later childhood. Overall developmental skills usually are less than the 12-month level, but many individual abilities (e.g., self-feeding) are beyond the 12-month level.

ETIOLOGY/EPIDEMIOLOGY: Approximately 92% of newborns who have the phenotype have it due to a full trisomy 18. The remaining 8% of patients have the condition due either to mosaicism of trisomy 18 or a partial trisomy 18 usually involving two thirds or more of the 18 long arm and due to a translocation. The exact cause of the extra chromosome in full trisomy 18 is unknown but is presumably due to nondisjunction. The prevalence in liveborn infants ranges from 1 in 3,600 to 1 in 8,500, with the most accurate estimate being approximately 1 in 6,000. Many infants die before birth, so the actual incidence at conception is much higher.

DIAGNOSIS: Confirmation of a clinical diagnosis occurs by the performance of a standard G-banded karyotype showing the extra number 18 chromosome.

TREATMENT
Standard Therapies: No standard therapies, exist; however, surgery can be performed for the various manifestations. Because 90% of infants have a cardiovascular malformation, cardiac surgery often is considered for a child who is older than a few months, although few data exist to help assess the risk/benefit of such intervention. Suggestions for care include neonatal echocardiography, referral to a feeding specialist or team, referral to early intervention, and periodic hearing tests. Older children require regular checks for scoliosis and abdominal ultrasonography every 6 months because of the increased risk of Wilms tumor and hepatoblastoma.

REFERENCES
Baty BJ, Blackburn BL, Carey JC. Natural history of trisomy 18 and trisomy 13. I. Growth, physical assessment, medical histories, survival, and recurrence risk. *Am J Med Genet* 1996;49:175–188.
Baty BJ, Jorde LB, Blackburn BL, et al. Natural history of trisomy 18 and trisomy 13. II. Psychomotor development. *Am J Med Genet* 1994;49:189–194.
Carey JC. Trisomy 18 and trisomy 13 syndromes. In: Cassiday SB, Allanson JE. *Management of genetic syndromes.* New York: Wiley-Liss, 2001:417–436.
Embleton ND, Wyllie JP, Wright MJ, et al. Natural history of trisomy 18. *Arch Dis Child* 1996;75:38–41.
Jones KL. *Smith's recognizable patterns of human malformation.* Philadelphia: WB Saunders, 1997:14–17.

RESOURCES
75, 455, 462

39 XXX Syndrome (Triple X Syndrome)

Carole A. Samango-Sprouse, EdD

DEFINITION: Triple X syndrome (47,XXX) is a common cause of learning differences in females. It is characterized by the presence of an additional X or several X chromosomes along with the normal female complement of 46,XX. These patients have an increased incidence of learning disabilities, primarily language based, with reading disorders.

DIFFERENTIAL DIAGNOSIS: Fragile X syndrome; Marfan syndrome.

SYMPTOMS AND SIGNS: A common feature of the disorder is increased height (above the 75th percentile). Some females with 47,XXX may have reproductive and/or fertility issues, although the actual incidence is unknown. Girls with triple X syndrome are at slightly increased risk for chromosomal anomalies during pregnancy, so prenatal counseling is advisable. Intelligence is typically normal, with IQ approximately 10 to 15 points lower than siblings. Learning problems and mild developmental delay occur as early as infancy. Decreased muscle tone with motor dysfunction is evident within the first year of life. Speech delay is evident by 18 months and may be detected as early as 12 months. These children are very responsive to early intervention and treatment. If attention issues are present, they are often related to language-based learning dysfunction. Reading differences are common, with an increased incidence of dyslexia. Shyness and emotional difficulties have been described, but studies have not been well controlled. Variants include 48,XXXX or 49,XXXXX, which have similar neurodevelopmental profiles to 47,XXX but are usually more severe. Mild symptoms and fewer learning issues are consistently associated with mosaic forms (46,XX/47,XXX) of this disorder. Girls with triple X syndrome who are diag-nosed through prenatal diagnosis have fewer developmental and learning problems and higher IQ than those girls diagnosed postnatally.

ETIOLOGY/EPIDEMIOLOGY: Triple X syndrome results from nondisjunction and the presence of an additional X chromosome. Parental origin of the additional X is typically maternal. Triple X syndrome occurs in 1 in 1,000 females.

DIAGNOSIS: Triple X syndrome is usually diagnosed unexpectedly when developmental, behavioral, or learning disabilities are suspected. A growing population of children is identified through prenatal diagnosis by amniocentesis and chorionic villus sampling.

TREATMENT
Standard Therapies: Early intervention services are strongly recommended, with evaluation of muscle tone and strength done by 6 months of age. Speech and language assessment of the discrepancy between expressive and receptive domains of language should be performed by 24 months of age. Reading assessment to rule out dyslexia should be done by school age.

REFERENCES
Robinson A, Bender BG, Linden MG. Prognosis of prenatally diagnosed children with sex chromosome aneuploidy. *Am J Med Genet* 1992;44:365–368.
Rovet J, Netley C, Bailey J, et al. Intelligence and achievement in children with extra X aneuploidy: a longitudinal perspective. *Am J Med Genet* 1995;60:356–363.

RESOURCES
200, 305, 476

40 XXY Syndrome (Klinefelter Syndrome)

Carole A. Samango-Sprouse, EdD

DEFINITION: XXY syndrome (Klinefelter syndrome, 47,XXY) is the most common cause of primary hypogonadism in males. It is characterized by the presence of an additional X or several X chromosomes to the normal male complement of 46,XY. There is an increased incidence of learning disabilities, primarily language based with reading disorders (68%–80%).

SYNONYM: Klinefelter syndrome.

SYMPTOMS AND SIGNS: Affected individuals have increased height (75th percentile) with long extremities and small testes with azoospermia. Learning problems and mild developmental delay occur as early as infancy, but mental retardation is rare. Decreased muscle tonus with motor dysfunction is evident within the first year of life. Speech delay is evident by 18 months and may be detected as early as 12 months. Affected children are highly responsive to early intervention and treatment. Affected individuals usually have normal intellectual capabilities with an IQ 10 to 15 points lower than siblings. Attentional issues are present and appear related to language-based learning dysfunction. Reading differences are common, with an increased incidence of dyslexia. Variants include 48,XXXY or 49,XXXXY, which have similar neurodevelopmental profiles but are usually more severe than 47,XXY. Mosaic forms (46,XY/47,XXY) of this disorder are consistently associated with milder symptoms and fewer learning issues.

ETIOLOGY/EPIDEMIOLOGY: Klinefelter syndrome results from nondisjunction and the presence of an additional X chromosome. Paternal origin of the extra X chromosome occurs 50%–60% of the time and maternal origin approximately 40%–50%. XXY syndrome occurs 1 in 426 to 1 in 900 males.

DIAGNOSIS: The disorder is usually not diagnosed until puberty. With the development of amniocentesis and chorionic villus sampling, a growing population of children with XXY syndrome is diagnosed prenatally.

TREATMENT
Standard Therapies: Early intervention services are strongly recommended with an evaluation completed by age 6 months for muscle tonus and strength. Speech and language assessment is recommended by age 24 months to evaluate the discrepancy between expressive and receptive domains of language. Reading assessment to rule out dyslexia by school age is strongly recommended. Androgens are helpful in developing secondary sexual characteristics and promoting muscle strength and well-being. Although men with XXY syndrome are infertile, intracytoplasmic sperm injection techniques have been successful in identifying fertile sperm in men with XXY syndrome and using *in vitro* procedures for impregnation. Genetic counseling is beneficial for families.

REFERENCES
Geschwind DH, Boone KB, Miller BL, et al. Neurobehavioral phenotype of Klinefelter syndrome. *Ment Retard Dev Disabilities Res Rev* 2000;6:107–116.
Ratcliffe SG. Growth during puberty in the XXY boy. *Ann Hum Biol* 1992;19:579–587.
Robinson A, Bender BG, Linden MG. Prognosis of prenatally diagnosed children with sex chromosome aneuploidy. *Am J Med Genet* 1992;44:365–368.
Samango-Sprouse C, Law P. The neurocognitive profile of boys with XXY diagnosed through prenatal diagnosis. *Am J Hum Genet* 1999;64(suppl):161.

RESOURCES
3, 25, 362

---

41   XYY Syndrome

Carole A. Samango-Sprouse, EdD

DEFINITION: XYY syndrome (47,XYY) is a common cause of learning disabilities in males. It is characterized by the presence of an additional Y or several Y chromosomes along with the normal male complement of XY.

DIFFERENTIAL DIAGNOSIS: Klinefelter syndrome; Marfan syndrome; Sotos syndrome; Fragile X syndrome.

SYMPTOMS AND SIGNS: A common feature of this disorder is increased height, with a mean height of 187.2 cm. No significant abnormal physical features are associated with XYY syndrome. Normal intelligence is typical, with IQ approximately 10 to 15 points less than siblings. De-

creased muscle tone with learning problems and mild developmental delay occur as early as infancy. Motor dysfunction is evident within the first year of life. Speech delay is evident by 18 months and may be detected as early as 12 months. These children are very responsive to early intervention and treatment. Attention issues and increased activity level are present. Reading differences are common with an increased incidence of dyslexia. Aggression can occur in some patients, but is related to language/learning issues and impulsivity. Variants include 48,XYYY or 49,XYYYY and similar neurodevelopmental profile. Mosaic forms (46,XY/47,XYY) of this disorder are consistently associated with milder symptoms and fewer learning issues.

ETIOLOGY/EPIDEMIOLOGY: XYY syndrome results from meiotic nondisjunction and the presence of an additional Y chromosome. XXY syndrome (XYY) occurs in 1 in 894 males.

DIAGNOSIS: XYY syndrome is usually not diagnosed until learning issues are present. XYY syndrome is diagnosed in a growing population of children prenatally by amniocentesis and chorionic villus sampling.

TREATMENT

Standard Therapies: Early intervention services are strongly recommended, with an evaluation of muscle tone and strength completed by 6 months of age. Speech and language assessment should be performed by 24 months of age for the discrepancy between expressive and receptive domains of language. Reading assessment to rule out dyslexia by school age is strongly recommended.

REFERENCES

Robinson A, Bender BG, Linden MG. Prognosis of prenatally diagnosed children with sex chromosome aneuploidy. *Am J Med Genet* 1992;44:365–368.

Salbenblatt JA, Meyers DC, Bender BG, et al. Gross and fine motor development in 47,XXY and 47,XYY males. *Pediatrics* 1987;80:240–244.

RESOURCES

282, 367, 476

4

Dermatologic Disorders

1   Acrodermatitis Enteropathica

John A. McGrath, MD, MRCP, and Oliver Bleck, MD

DEFINITION: Acrodermatitis enteropathica is an inherited metabolic disorder resulting from impaired absorption of zinc from the gastrointestinal tract (Insert Fig. 6). Occasionally, the disorder may manifest in breast-fed babies whose mothers do not secrete zinc into the breast milk.

SYNONYM: Danbolt-Closs syndrome.

DIFFERENTIAL DIAGNOSIS: Acquired dietary deficiency of zinc; *Candida albicans* diaper dermatitis; Chronic mucocutaneous candidiasis; Bullous congenital ichthyosiform erythroderma; Hailey-Hailey disease; Epidermolysis bullosa.

SYMPTOMS AND SIGNS: The principal features are diarrhea, dermatitis, and failure to thrive. The skin changes include a weeping, red eczematous eruption that occurs around the mouth, genitals, anus, and distal extremities. Other signs may include softening of nail plates, paronychia, glossitis, and stomatitis. Hair is often brittle, sparse, and pale. The eyes show signs of blepharitis, keratitis, and conjunctivitis. Ataxia, depression, irritability, and lethargy also occur. Recurrent infections (e.g., with *Candida albicans* or *Staphylococcus aureus*) are frequent.

ETIOLOGY/EPIDEMIOLOGY: Acrodermatitis enteropathica is inherited in an autosomal-recessive manner. The precise underlying genetic abnormality is unknown, although there are animal models for the disease. Neither the gut type nor breast type of acrodermatitis enteropathica results from mutations in the human *ZNT4* gene on 15q21.1. Moreover, the gut type of acrodermatitis enteropathica has been mapped to 8q24.3, although no specific gene abnormalities around this locus have been identified.

DIAGNOSIS: The diagnosis should be suspected on the pattern of emerging, predominantly cutaneous, clinical signs in infants. Diagnosis can be established by measuring plasma zinc levels, which are usually (but not always) low. Blood for zinc estimation should be collected in tubes containing no additives (which may give an artificially high zinc level) but routine chemistry bottles. Other helpful diagnostic markers include reduced serum alkaline phosphatase and reduced urinary zinc excretion.

TREATMENT

Standard Therapies: Oral zinc supplementation is effective. The dose is usually 35–100 mg of elemental zinc (50–220 mg zinc sulphate heptahydrate) daily. Supplementation may need to be lifelong, although sometimes the dose can be reduced (or even stopped) around puberty. At that time, trials of stopping zinc supplementation and clinical observation may be warranted to see if maintenance therapy is still required. During pregnancy, the amount of zinc supplementation may need to be increased. For individuals with the breast type of acrodermatitis enteropathica, symptoms tend to resolve at an early age when breast-feeding is substituted with bottled milk.

REFERENCES

Bleck O, Ashton GH, Mallipeddi R, et al. Genomic localization, organization and amplification of the human zinc transporter protein gene, *ZNT4*, and exclusion as a candidate gene in different clinical variants of acrodermatitis enteropathica. *Arch Dermatol Res* 2001 (in press).

Danbolt N, Closs K. Akrodermatitis enteropathica. *Acta Derm Venerol (Stockh)* 1942;23:127–169.

Glover MT, Atherton DJ. Transient zinc deficiency in two full-term breast-fed siblings associated with low maternal breast milk zinc concentration. *Paediatr Dermatol* 1988;5:10–13.

Huang L, Gitschier J. A novel gene involved in zinc transport is deficient in the lethal milk mouse. *Nat Genet* 1997;17: 292–297.

Wang K, Pugh EW, Griffen S, et al. Homozygosity mapping places the acrodermatitis enteropathica gene on chromosomal region 8q24.3. *Am J Hum Genet* 2001;68:1055–1060.

RESOURCES

27, 351, 354

2   Alopecia Areata

Berna K. Remzi, MD,
and Wilma F. Bergfeld, MD

DEFINITION: Alopecia areata is an autoimmune disorder characterized by nonscarring hair loss. Alopecia totalis and alopecia universalis are subtypes of alopecia areata characterized by total scalp hair loss and total scalp, facial, and body hair loss, respectively (Insert Fig. 7).

DIFFERENTIAL DIAGNOSIS: Tinea capitis; Trichotillomania; Traction alopecia; Mechanical- or chemical-induced alopecia; Trichodystrophies; Telogen or anagen effluvium; Congenital alopecia; Pseudopelade; Lupus erythematosus; Lichen planopilaris; Scleroderma; Bullous pemphigoid; Syphilis; Folliculitis; Alopecia neoplastica; Granulatomatous disorders; Follicular mucinosis.

SYMPTOMS AND SIGNS: Clinical presentation varies from recurrent, small round patch of hair loss to chronic, nonscarring total hair loss of scalp, eyebrows, eyelashes, nostrils, beard, and body. Spontaneous remissions may be seen. Alopecia areata can be psychologically painful. The hair follicle changes from anagen hair to dystrophic anagen, catagen, or telogen hair due to an unknown trigger. Nail pitting may occur. Increased incidence of association with other autoimmune diseases such as Hashimoto thyroiditis and vitiligo have been reported.

ETIOLOGY/EPIDEMIOLOGY: Autoimmunity, microorganisms, genetic factors, neurogenic stimuli, emotional stress, and poor coping skills have been identified as potential causes or triggers. Various gene associations have been studied for susceptibility such as HLA-DQB1*03 and HLA-DQB1*1104. In the United States, prevalence varies from 0.2% to 2% of the population. Alopecia areata affects children and adults of both genders.

DIAGNOSIS: Careful history and physical examination are important for diagnosis. Hair pull and hair pluck tests can be done. Exclamation mark hair or telogen, catagen, or dystrophic anagen hairs may be seen. Skin biopsy of the hair loss area can confirm clinical diagnosis. Histopathology demonstrates Langerhans cell and T-cell infiltration of the perifollicular area, especially in early lesions. KOH examination and fungal culture of hairs as well as bacterial cultures can be done to exclude infectious causes of alopecia, and laboratory tests can be done to identify any associated autoimmune disorder such as Hashimoto thyroiditis.

TREATMENT

Standard Therapies: Various treatment options are available that may help healing, but they may not be curative. Intralesional and topical corticosteroids are widely used for alopecia areata, especially patchy type. Ultraviolet light therapy is effective in 19%–73% of patients, and topical anthralin is effective in 20%–75% of patients. Wig or hair addition/hairpieces are significantly helpful as a concealing method. Many patients benefit from psychosocial coping skill development and support group involvement.

Investigational Therapies: Topical sensitizers (diphenylcyclopropenone) may cause hair regrowth in 4%–75% of patients; however, the effect is limited and side effects include pruritis, moderate to severe contact dermatitis, blisters, and local lymphadenopathy. Improved delivery systems to increase penetration of topical medications to deep dermis (hair bulb) such as liposomes may be investigated.

REFERENCES

Bergfeld WF. Hair disorders. In: Moschella SL, Hurley HJ, eds. *Dermatology.* Philadelphia: WB Saunders, 1992:1545–1546.

Bertolino AP. Alopecia areata. A clinical overview. *Postgrad Med* 2000;107:81–90.

Fiedler VC. Alopecia areata. A review of therapy, efficacy, safety and mechanism. *Arch Dermatol* 1992;128:1519–1529.

Freyschmidt-Paul P, Hoffman R, Levine E, et al. Current and potential agents for the treatment of alopecia areata [review]. *Curr Pharm Des* 2001;7:213–230.

RESOURCES

283, 351

3 Aplasia Cutis Congenita

Ernst Reichenberger, PhD,
and John B. Mulliken, MD

DEFINITION: Patients with aplasia cutis congenita (ACC), are born with a localized area of skin that failed to develop normally. Typically, the lesion is on the scalp; the underlying membranous cranial bone can be absent. At birth the lesion is usually covered by a thin membrane. In rare instances, the trunk, arms, or legs can be affected. ACC can occur as part of several syndromes.

SYNONYMS: Congenital defect of cranium and scalp; Congenital scalp defect.

DIFFERENTIAL DIAGNOSIS: Epidermolysis bullosa lethalis with pyloric atresia; ACC with epibulbar dermoids; ACC with high myopia and cone-rod dysfunction; ACC with Charcot-Marie-Tooth peroneal muscular atrophy, X-linked; ACC with intestinal lymphangiectasia; ACC and coarctation of aorta; ACC of limbs, recessive; Focal facial dermal dysplasia; Adams-Oliver syndrome; Scalp-ear-nipple syndrome; Facial palsy, congenital, unilateral, or bilateral; Epidermolysis bullosa with congenital localized absence of skin and deformity of nails; Facial ectodermal dysplasia; Localized scalp infection; Small meningocele or other brain heterotopias; Sebaceous nevus of Jadassohn.

SYMPTOMS AND SIGNS: ACC of the scalp is typically in the midline. Usually there is a single defect, but two to three lesions on the vertex can occur. The defect can range from a few millimeters to more than 10 cm in diameter. In minor cases, the defect may be only a sharply marginated area of thin skin. In severe cases, the underlying calvarial bone can be absent. A newborn with extensive ACC of the scalp is at risk for thrombosis or bleeding from the sagittal sinus and meningitis. In an older patient with minor ACC, the lesion may be a hairless spot with normal cutaneous thickness. ACC can be found in association with other disorders where there is a localized hypoplastic cutaneous lesion on the trunk or extremities, or the skin can be open at birth and heal during childhood (scalp-ear-nipple syndrome).

ETIOLOGY/EPIDEMIOLOGY: Most cases are sporadic, but isolated ACC can occur as an autosomal-dominant or -recessive trait. Scalp defects are occasionally found in individuals with trisomy 13 syndrome or deletion of the short arm of chromosome 4 (Wolf-Hirschhorn syndrome). Expressivity is variable and penetrance can be incomplete.

DIAGNOSIS: If a scalp defect or other congenitally aplastic skin lesion exists, a thorough physical examination should be done to exclude a syndrome. Clinical manifestations of other syndromes include anomalies of limbs, central nervous system, cardiovascular system, alimentary system, and other cutaneous abnormalities. Ocular findings and urogenital involvement are also reported.

TREATMENT
Standard Therapies: The neonate with a large area of ACC is at high risk because of the exposed, often very thin, dura. The defect must be kept moist; intravenous antibiotics are given to prevent meningitis. Usually, the raw area will epithelialize slowly, but some defects require biologic dressings or a split-thickness skin graft. The scalp is relatively lax during infancy, so minor ACC should be considered for early excision and closure. A large area of ACC requires staged excision, and often preliminary tissue expansion, for removal and closure with normal scalp skin. A small calvarial defect usually ossifies. A large nonhealing cranial defect must be closed with a bone graft; this is usually accomplished after excision and closure of the scalp defect.

Investigational Therapies: Efforts to identify genes and mutations responsible for ACC and related disorders are ongoing.

REFERENCES
Evers ME, Steijlen PM, Hamel BC. Aplasia cutis congenita and associated disorders: an update. *Clin Genet* 1995;47:295–301.

Frieden IJ. Aplasia cutis congenita: a clinical review and proposal for classification. *J Am Acad Dermatol* 1986;14:646–660.

Kuster W, Lenz W, Kaariainen H, Majewski F. Congenital scalp defects with distal limb anomalies (Adams-Oliver syndrome): report of ten cases and review of the literature. *Am J Med Genet* 1988;31:99–115.

RESOURCE
351

4   Björnstad Syndrome

Griet Van Buggenhout, MD, PhD, and Jean-Pierre Fryns, MD, PhD

DEFINITION: Björnstad syndrome is a condition characterized by the occurrence of pili torti and sensorineural hearing loss.

SYNONYM: Pili torti and nerve deafness.

DIFFERENTIAL DIAGNOSIS: Menkes kinky hair syndrome; Monilethrix; Pseudomonilethrix; Argininosuccinic aciduria; Hyperkeratosis palmoplantaris striata-pili torti-hypodontia-sensorineural hearing loss syndrome; Acquired pili torti (trauma); Pili torti, isolated or in association with other ectodermal abnormalities.

SYMPTOMS AND SIGNS: The main clinical features are sensorineural hearing loss in association with pili torti. Patients with the most pronounced hair anomalies also tend to have the most severe hearing problems. Scalp hair, eyebrows, and eyelashes are affected. Alopecia is present. Hair structure may be coarse, dry and lusterless, and fragile.

ETIOLOGY/EPIDEMIOLOGY: Autosomal-recessive inheritance is suggested. The disease gene maps to chromosome 2q34-q36. Families were reported in which autosomal-dominant inheritance was suggested. Genetic heterogeneity may be possible.

DIAGNOSIS: The diagnosis is suspected based on the clinical findings. Scanning electron microscopy of the hairs shows flattening at irregular intervals and twisting (180 degrees).

TREATMENT
Standard Therapies: There is no specific treatment.

REFERENCES
Björnstad R. Pili torti and sensorineural loss of hearing. *Proc Fenno-Scand Assoc Derm* 1965:3.
Cremers C, Geerts S. Sensorineural hearing loss and pili torti. *Ann Otol Rhinol Laryngol* 1979;88:100–104.
Gorlin R, Toriello H, Cohen M. *Hereditary hearing loss and its syndromes.* New York: Oxford University Press, 1995:397–398.
Lubianca Neto J, Lu L, Eavey R, et al. The Björnstad syndrome (sensorineural hearing loss and pili torti) disease gene maps to chromosome 2q34–36. *Am J Hum Genet* 1998;62:1107–1112.
Petit A, Dontenwille M, Blanchet Bardon C, et al. Pili torti with congenital deafness (Björnstad's syndrome)—report of three cases in one family, suggesting autosomal dominant transmission. *Clin Exp Dermatol* 1993;18:94–95.
Reed W, Stone V, Boder E, et al. Hereditary syndromes with auditory and dermatological manifestations. *Arch Dermatol* 1967;95:456–461.
Voigtländer V. Pili torti with deafness (Björnstad syndrome). Report of a family. *Dermatologica* 1979;159:50–54.

RESOURCES
15, 75, 371

5   Bowen Disease

Daniel B. Eisen, MD, and Mervyn L. Elgart, MD

DEFINITION: Bowen disease is a form of squamous cell carcinoma *in situ* of the skin. Clinically, it is a well-demarcated, red, scaly papule, plaque, or patch. It is most commonly found on people with light colored skin in the sun-exposed regions of the body, but may occur anywhere on the skin.

DIFFERENTIAL DIAGNOSIS: Nonspecific dermatitis; Psoriasis; Lichen planus; Superficial spreading melanoma; Amelanotic melanoma; Seborrheic keratosis; Superficial basal cell carcinoma; Metastatic carcinoma; Intraepidermal epithelioma; Glomus tumors; Verruca vulgaris.

SYMPTOMS AND SIGNS: Patients typically have red, scaly, well-marginated plaques with variable degrees of pigmentation. The lesions gradually enlarge and are for the most part asymptomatic unless ulcerated. On the nail bed, it may appear as an abormal scaly papule or a crusted erosion. In the inguinal area, it may present as a nonspecific dermatitis or as an acute oozing lesion. Squamous cell carcinoma *in situ* may occur on the genital or oral mucosa. When it occurs on the glans penis as an erythematous velvety plaque, it is known as erythroplasia of Queyrat. Many consider this a distinct clinical entity from Bowen disease.

When on the oral mucosa, it appears as a red or white plaque referred to as erythroplakia and leukoplakia, respectively. These may also be separate clinical entities from Bowen disease.

ETIOLOGY/EPIDEMIOLOGY: The etiology appears to be multifactorial. A link may exist between arsenic exposure and the development of keratoses, Bowen disease, and squamous cell carcinoma. Other possible causes are ultraviolet radiation and human papilloma virus, especially type 16. Bowen disease has also been seen in congenital or acquired immunosuppression. The male:female ratio is 8:10. It can evolve into invasive squamous cell carcinoma.

DIAGNOSIS: Bowen disease is diagnosed based on clinical suspicion, with confirmation by biopsy of the lesion. The biopsy sample obtained must be deep enough to rule out invasive squamous cell carcinoma.

TREATMENT
Standard Therapies: Standard therapy includes use of topical 5. Other treatment methods include photodynamic therapy, isotretinoin, interferon-α 2a, and treatment with CO_2, Nd:YAG, or argon lasers.

REFERENCES
Campbell E, Quinn AG, Ro YS, et al. P53 mutations are common and early events that precede tumor invasion in squamous cell neoplasia of the skin. *J Invest Dermatol* 1993;100:746–748.
Cox NH, Eedy DJ, Mortaon CA. Guidelines for management of Bowen's disease. *Br J Dermatol* 1999;141;633–641.
Schwartz R, Stoll II. Epithelial precancerous lesions. In: Freedberg I, Eisen A, Wolff K, et al., eds. *Fitzpatick's dermatology in general medicine.* New York: McGraw-Hill, 1999:832– 834.
Stone MS, Noonan CA, Tschen J, et al. Bowen's disease of the feet. Presence of human papillomavirus 16 DNA in tumor tissue. *Arch Dermatol* 1987;123:1517–1520.
Thestrup-Pedersen K, Ravnborg L, Reymann F. Morbus Bowen: a description of the disease in 617 patients. *Act Derm Venereol (Stockh)* 1988;68;236–239.

RESOURCES
30, 352, 437

---

6   Bowenoid Papulosis

*Daniel B. Eisen, MD,
and Mervyn L. Elgart, MD*

DEFINITION: Bowenoid papulosis is an eruption of benign-looking, brown papules, usually seen on external genitalia. A biopsy will show intraepithelial squamous cell carcinoma–like pathology.

SYNONYMS: Pigmented penile papules with carcinoma *in situ* changes; Genital keratinocytic dysplasia; Penile carcinoma *in situ* associated with human papilloma virus infection.

DIFFERENTIAL DIAGNOSIS: Condyloma accuminata (viral warts); Melanocytic nevi; Seborrheic keratoses; Lichen planus; Zoon balanitis; Lichen simplex chronicus; Psoriasis; Squamous cell carcinoma; Melanoma; Cutaneous Hodgkin disease.

SIGNS AND SYMPTOMS: Bowenoid papulosis is usually an asymptomatic eruption of brown, warty-looking papules found most often on the penis in men and external genitalia of women. Symptoms of itching, tenderness, and pain have occasionally been reported. Bowenoid papulosis has also been reported to occur in unusual locations such as the abdomen, neck, and oral mucosa. The lesions may range in size from 0.2 to 3.3 cm in diameter. The disease almost never progresses to invasive squamous cell carcinoma and sometimes even resolves on its own. Most commonly, the papules are mistaken for warts, which when treated with cryotherapy do not resolve. A biopsy then shows squamous cell carcinoma *in situ.*

ETIOLOGY/EPIDEMIOLOGY: Bowenoid papulosis is caused by the human papilloma virus (HPV). It has been linked to HPV types 16, 18, 31, 32, 34, 39, 42, 48, and 51–54. Most affected people are young, sexually active men and women. The mean age of diagnosis is 30. The prevalence is unknown.

DIAGNOSIS: Diagnosis of bowenoid papulosis is based on clinical impression confirmed by biopsy.

TREATMENT
Standard Therapies: Standard therapies for bowenoid papulosis include electrodessication, laser, scissor excision,

cryosurgery, topical 5-fluorouracil, topical retinoic acid, low-dose interferon-α, and etretinate.

REFERENCES

Inagaki H, Nonaka M, Bimoto T. Bowenoid papulosis showing polyclonal nature. *Diagn Mol Pathol* 1998;7:122–126.

Johnson TM, Saluja A, Fader D, et al. Isolated extragenital bowenoid papulosis of the neck. *J Am Acad Dermatol* 1999; 41:867–870.

Patterson JW, et al. Bowenoid papulosis: a clinicopathologic study with ultrastructural observations. *Cancer* 1986;57:823.

Schwartz R, Janniger C. Bowenoid papulosis. *J Am Acad Dermatol* 1991;24:261–264.

Su CK, Shipley W. Bowenoid papulosis: a benign lesion of the shaft of the penis misdiagnosed as squamous carcinoma. *J Urol* 1997;157:1361–1362.

RESOURCES

89, 359, 432

---

7 Familial Eosinophilic Cellulitis (Wells Syndrome)

Mark D.P. Davis, MD,
and Kristin M. Leiferman, MD

DEFINITION: Familial eosinophilic cellulitis is an inherited chronic, recurrent skin disease with characteristic histopathologic findings and associated fluctuating peripheral blood eosinophilia.

SYNONYM: Familial Wells syndrome.

DIFFERENTIAL DIAGNOSIS: Cellulitis; Angioedema; Dermatitis; Morphea; Immunobullous disease; Any disease associated with eosinophil infiltration in the skin, including arthropod bites, infection, and drug reaction.

SYMPTOMS AND SIGNS: Signs of the disorder include annular or circinate erythematous-edematous plaques that evolve to morphea-like slate blue–colored plaques. Blistering may occur. The histologic picture is characterized by striking eosinophil infiltration and by the presence of "flame figures." Fluctuating peripheral blood eosinophilia is also characteristic. Associated features were noted in some families: in one family, short stature, dysmorphic features, and mental retardation were noted. In another family, pleural and pericardial effusions occurred.

ETIOLOGY/EPIDEMIOLOGY: Eosinophil infiltration of the skin, evidence of eosinophil degranulation in the skin, and the presence of blood and bone marrow eosinophilia suggest that the eosinophil is the cause of the clinical manifestations. An eosinophil-activating cytokine, interleukin-5, is increased in peripheral blood. The exact cause, incidence, and prevalence of the disorder are unknown. Two families have been reported with the familial form of the disease. Males and females are both affected, but the condition may be more severe in males. It occurs in both adults and children. Autosomal-dominant inheritance with variable penetrance is speculated.

DIAGNOSIS: The diagnosis is made clinically. Histology of the lesions is characterized by striking eosinophil infiltration in the dermis and subcutaneous fat, mainly around the vessels and adnexae, and the presence of flame figures.

TREATMENT

Standard Therapies: No specific treatment is known. Systemic glucocorticoids, topical glucocorticoids, colchicine, and cetirizine have been used for control of the skin manifestations. Because the toxic activities of eosinophils likely contribute to the pathogenesis, therapies directed toward minimizing or eliminating the eosinophil involvement may be helpful.

REFERENCES

Davis MD, Brown AC, Blackston RD, et al. Familial eosinophilic cellulitis, dysmorphic habitus, and mental retardation. *J Am Acad Dermatol* 1998;36:919–928.

Kamani N, Lipsitz PJ. Eosinophilic cellulitis in a family. *Pediatr Dermatol* 1987;4:220–224.

Leiferman KM. Cutaneous eosinophilic diseases. In: Fitzpatrick TB, Eisen AZ, Wolff K, et al., eds. *Dermatology in general medicine,* 5th ed. New York: McGraw-Hill, 1999:1129–1137.

Peters MS, Schroeter AL, Gleich GJ. Immunofluorescence identification of eosinophil granule major basic protein in the flame figures of Wells' syndrome. *Br J Dermatol* 1983;109: 141–148.

RESOURCES

89, 359

8   Cutis Marmorata Telangiectatica Congenita

M.J.P. Gerritsen, MD,
and Rianne Gerritsen, MD

DEFINITION: Cutis marmorata telangiectatica congenita (CMTC) is a cutaneous disease with a typical clinical presentation of a localized, segmental, or generalized persistent reticular vascular skin pattern with a bluish to deep purple appearance that is present at or shortly after birth (Insert Fig. 8).

SYNONYMS: van Lohuizen syndrome; Congenital generalized phlebectasia; Nevus vascularis reticularis; Congenital livedo reticularis.

DIFFERENTIAL DIAGNOSIS: Physiological cutis marmorata; Adams-Oliver syndrome; Other vascular syndromes.

SYMPTOMS AND SIGNS: The persistent reticular vascular pattern of the skin may be localized, segmental, or generalized. The dark lesions often show loss of dermal substance with, in some cases, superficial ulceration. The prognosis for the skin lesions is generally good. During the first years of life, the clinical improvement of the livedo markings is probably due to normal thickening and maturation of the skin and of maturation of the cutaneous vascular innervation. Approximately 50% of cases have associated abnormalities. The nature of these is variable, but the most common are body asymmetry, other vascular abnormalities, hypoplasia/aplasia, glaucoma, and psychomotor and/or mental retardation. A distinct form of CMTC is macrocephaly-CMTC, which is characterized by CMTC, macrocephaly, nevus flammeus of the philtrum and upper lip, syndactyly, a high birth weight, hypotonia, and joint laxity.

ETIOLOGY/EPIDEMIOLOGY: The exact cause is unknown. Some evidence exists for a functional malformation at the level of the terminal blood vessels. Both sexes may be affected. Most cases are sporadic. The segmental distribution with the preferred one-sided body involve-

ment may be explained by the lethal gene theory of Happle, which suggests that lethal genes survive by mosaicism. Less than 300 cases have been described.

DIAGNOSIS: The diagnosis can be made clinically. Histology does not differentiate the differential diagnoses. A full physical examination by a pediatrician and a dermatologist should always be performed. Children with associated abnormalities must be referred to an appropriate specialist. In the case of a periocular vascular lesion including CMTC, an ophthalmologic examination should be performed to exclude glaucoma or other eye abnormalities.

TREATMENT
Standard Therapies: There is no treatment for the skin lesions.

REFERENCES
Amitai DB, Fichman S, Merlob P, et al. Cutis marmorata telangiectatica congenita: clinical findings in 85 patients. *Pediatr Dermatol* 2000;17:100–104.

Bormann G, Wohlrab J, Fischer M, et al. Cutis marmorata telangiectatica congenita: laser Doppler fluxmetry evidence for a functional nervous defect. *Pediatr Dermatol* 2001;18:110–113.

Clayton-Smith J, Kerr B, Brunner H, et al. Macrocephaly with cutis marmorata, haemangioma and syndactyly—a distinctive overgrowth syndrome. *Clin Dysmorphol* 1997;6:291–302.

Gerritsen MJP, Steijlen PM, Brunner HG, et al. Cutis marmorata telangiectatica congenita: a report of 18 cases. *Br J Dermatol* 2000;142:366–369.

Moore CA, Toriello HV, Abuelo DN, et al. Macrocephaly-cutis marmorata telangiectatica congenita: a distinct disorder with developmental delay and connective tissue abnormalities. *Am J Med Genet* 1997;70:67–73.

Pehr K, Moroz B. Cutis marmorata telangiectatica congenita: long-term follow up, review of the literature, report of a case in conjunction with congenital hypothyroidism. *Pediatr Dermatol* 1993;10:6–11.

RESOURCES
344, 351, 450

9 Darier Disease

Franziska Ringpfeil, MD

DEFINITION: Darier disease is an autosomal-dominant disorder of keratinization characterized by delayed onset and highly variable progressive skin manifestations that are occasionally associated with neuropsychiatric manifestations (Insert Fig. 9).

SYNONYMS: Darier-White disease; Keratosis follicularis; Dyskeratosis follicularis; Psorospermose folliculaire vegetante.

DIFFERENTIAL DIAGNOSIS: Seborrheic dermatitis; Acrokeratosis verruciformis of Hopf; Epidermodysplasia verruciformis; Hailey-Hailey disease; Kyrle disease; Ulerythema ophryogenes; Epidermal nevus.

SYMPTOMS AND SIGNS: Darier disease is characterized by grouped, yellow or brown, rough, firm papules that are often crusted and that occur in seborrheic areas of the body, such as the chest, back, ears, nasolabial fold, forehead, scalp, or groin. Progression is marked by coalescence of papules, which in severe cases may lead to tremendously disfiguring, macerated, malodorous plaques covering the entire body. Occasionally, hemorrhagic vesicles or skin-colored, rough papules can be seen in an acral distribution. Viral, bacterial, and fungal superinfections are common, and may exacerbate the disease. Isolated segmental or linear Darier disease has been described. Skin manifestations are often accompanied by nail changes that consist of red and white longitudinal streaks, distal subungual keratoses, and V-shaped notches. The oral mucosa often shows cobblestoning and erosions and, less frequently, obstruction of salivary glands. Associated neuropsychiatric disorders encompass such disparate conditions as epilepsy, bipolar disorder, schizophrenia, and learning difficulties.

ETIOLOGY/EPIDEMIOLOGY: Darier disease is caused by mutations in *ATP2A2*, a gene on chromosome 12 that encodes a calcium pump of the endoplasmic reticulum, facilitating intracellular calcium homeostasis. With a frequency of approximately 1 in 36,000 to 1 in 100,000, Darier disease is a relatively common genodermatosis with complete penetrance that affects both genders equally. Skin manifestations occur at the end of the first or during the second decade of life and show both interfamilial and intrafamilial variability. Heat, sweating, sunlight, and stress may be exacerbating factors.

DIAGNOSIS: Skin biopsy should be performed. Histopathologic examination is characteristic for abnormal keratinization (dyskeratosis) and failure of cell-cell adhesion (acantholysis).

TREATMENT

Standard Therapies: Topical retinoids, such as tretinoin cream, adapalene gel or cream, and tazarotene gel, as well as keratolytics, such as salicylic acid in propylene glycol gel, may be used to control hyperkeratosis. More severely affected patients benefit from oral retinoids such as isotretinoin and acitretin, but long-term side effects must be carefully considered, especially in the teenage population. Avoidance of excessive heat and sun are often beneficial.

Investigational Therapies: Experimental erbium:YAG laser resurfacing is being investigated.

REFERENCES

Beier C, Kaufmann R. Efficacy of erbium:YAG laser ablation in Darier disease and Hailey-Hailey disease. *Arch Dermatol* 1999;135:423–427.

Burge S. Management of Darier's disease. *Clin Exp Dermatol* 1999;24:53–56.

Burge SM, Wilkinson JD. Darier-White disease: a review of the clinical features in 163 patients. *J Acad Dermatol* 1992; 27:40–50.

Munro CS. The phenotype of Darier's disease: penetrance and expressivity in adults and children. *Br J Dermatol* 1992; 127:126–130.

RESOURCES

162, 351

10   Degos Disease

Carlin Hollar, MD,
and Phillip L. Williford, MD, FACP

DEFINITION: Degos disease is characterized by diffuse papular skin lesions on the trunk and proximal extremities, which evolve to a classic cutaneous papule with a "porcelain white" center. The pathophysiology is believed to be primarily vasculitic, resulting in thrombosis of small vessels in the skin and other organs. The disease is often but not uniformly fatal due to complications with intestinal perforations and peritonitis.

SYNONYMS: Malignant atrophic papulosis; Külmeier-Degos disease; Degos syndrome.

DIFFERENTIAL DIAGNOSIS: Lupus erythematosus with atrophie blanche; Anetoderma.

SYMPTOMS AND SIGNS: Cutaneous manifestations often precede systemic involvement. The classic presentation is crops of asymptomatic (rarely pruritic) papules, 2–5 mm in diameter with varying shapes, located on the trunk and proximal extremities of a young caucasian male. Few lesions may be seen initially, but typically 10–40 are present at one time (can be hundreds). The palms, soles, and face are rarely involved. Oral and genital mucous membrane lesions are uncommon. Avascular patches on the bulbar conjunctiva may be present. Evolutionary stages of the papules include early flesh-colored to yellowish grey firm papules, which over a few days develop umbilicated, depressed centers with a porcelain white color and surrounding erythematous rim. These eventually result in flat, porcelain white atrophic papules without the erythematous border. Patients often have morphologically varied papules in disparate stages of evolution. Usually, involvement of the gastrointestinal system occurs years after skin manifestations. In gastrointestinal disease, white avascular patches are noted on the small intestine and peritoneum by laparoscopy or at postmortem examination. The stomach, colon, esophagus, and rectum can be involved. The most common presentation of gastrointestinal involvement is intestinal perforation and peritonitis, which is often fatal. Involvement of the central nervous system (CNS) results in varying clinical manifestations depending on the anatomic site involved.

ETIOLOGY/EPIDEMIOLOGY: The disease usually affects young adults (mean age 33 years). It rarely affects young children. Although predominantly reported in whites, a few cases have been described in black, Indian, and Japanese individuals. Case clusters in families have occurred. The etiology is unclear. Theories include primary disorder of coagulation, lymphocytic vasculitis with subsequent thrombosis and infarction, primary mucinosis, autoimmune connective tissue disorder, and infection. More than 130 cases have been reported. Some 15% of patients have had long-term survival, with disease often limited to the skin.

DIAGNOSIS: Diagnosis is made by histopathologic examination and clinical correlation.

TREATMENT
Standard Therapies: No therapy has been proven effective for treatment of this disorder. Most treatment strategies investigated are anecdotal and include immunomodulatory agents and those affecting coagulation. The combination of aspirin and dipyridamole has been reported to improve skin and ocular lesions in 2 patients with no obvious systemic involvement. Whether this could prevent progression to systemic disease is not known. Surgical treatment of patients with bowel perforation and anticoagulation of patients with CNS involvement may temporarily ameliorate symptoms, but neither has resulted in long-term survival benefits.

REFERENCES
Degos R. Malignant atrophic papulosis. *Br J Dermatol.* 1979; 100:21–35.
Harvel JD, Williford PL, White WL. Benign cutaneous Degos' disease. A case report with emphasis on histopathology as papules chronologically evolve. *Am J Dermatopathol* 2001;23: 116–123.
Margrinat G, Kerwin KS, Gabriel DA. The clinical manifestations of Degos' syndrome. *Arch Pathol Lab Med* 1989;113:354–362.
Snow JL, Muller SA. Degos syndrome: malignant atrophic papulosis. *Semin Dermatol* 1995;14:99–105.
Su WPD, Schroeter AL, Lee DA, et al. Clinical and histological findings in Degos' syndrome (malignant atrophic papulosis). *Cutis* 1985;35:131–138.

RESOURCES
135, 354

11   Dermatitis Herpetiformis

Russell P. Hall III, MD

DEFINITION: Dermatitis herpetiformis (DH) is a chronic, intensely itchy blistering disease characterized by severe itching and the occurrence of papules and vesicles that occur predominantly on extensor surfaces of the body such as the elbows, knees, buttocks, and scapula.

SYNONYM: Duhring disease.

DIFFERENTIAL DIAGNOSIS: Linear IgA dermatosis; Insect bites; Scabies; Bullous pemphigoid; Neurotic excoriations.

SYMPTOMS AND SIGNS: Patients with DH most often present with itchy, erythematous papules and vesicles over the extensor surfaces of the body. The lesions are so itchy that often the primary blister cannot be found and the patient only has multiple crusted papules and excoriated lesions. The extent of DH is variable, with some patients presenting with a few lesions and others presenting with most of their skin involved. Patients with DH have an associated gluten sensitive enteropathy (GSE). Most patients are asymptomatic and have no gastrointestinal symptoms, but approximately 10% of patients have clinical symptoms of GSE, including abdominal bloating, cramping abdominal pain, loose stools, diarrhea, or signs of malabsorption. Other diseases are often associated with the presence of DH, such as autoimmune thyroid disease, atrophic gastritis, and pernicious anemia, and an increased incidence of immune-mediated disorders such as dermatomyositis, Sjögren syndrome, and systemic lupus erythematosus.

ETIOLOGY/EPIDEMIOLOGY: The exact etiology of DH is unknown, but several factors play a critical role in the pathogenesis of the disease. Patients have an associated GSE, the presence of IgA deposits in their skin as detected by direct immunofluoresence, and an increased frequency of the HLA A-1, B8, DR3, DQ2 haplotype. The disease most often presents in the first or second decade of life, but can occur at any age. There is a slight male predominance. The prevalence of the disease is related to the genetic background of the population. In northern European and Scandinavian populations, the prevalence of the disease has been estimated to be 10 to 39 per 100,000. The disease is much less common in African-American and Asian populations, most likely due to the much lower frequency of the HLA-A1, B8, DR3, DQ2 haplotype.

DIAGNOSIS: Diagnosis is based on the presence of the typical clinical presentation and the presence of granular deposits of IgA at the dermal-epidermal junction by direct immunofluoresence examination of a perilesional or normal-appearing skin biopsy sample.

TREATMENT
Standard Therapies: Standard therapies are the use of dapsone or a diet that does not include gluten-containing grains. Although treatment with systemic corticosteroids may control symptoms, the cutaneous manifestations recur when they are discontinued. The significant long-term side effects of the high doses of corticosteroids required to control the skin lesions make this an unacceptable therapy. Treatment with dapsone controls the itching and the appearance of new skin lesions within 24 to 48 hours and is generally well tolerated. Dapsone does have significant side effects and should only be prescribed by physicians familiar with the management of those side effects. Strict adherence to a gluten-free diet can result in return of small bowel morphology to normal, cessation of the itchy skin lesions, and eventually loss of the cutaneous IgA deposits. Patients must often follow the diet for 6 to 18 months before the disease can be controlled and it may take up to a decade or longer to see the loss of IgA from the skin.

Investigational Therapies: Therapies that have been tried include the use of an elemental diet and systemic cyclosporine.

REFERENCES
Fry L. Dermatitis herpetiformis [Review]. *Baillieres Clin Gastroenterol* 1995;9:371–393.

Fry L, Leonard JN, Swain F, et al. Long-term follow-up of dermatitis herpetiformis with and without dietary withdrawal. *Br J Dermatol* 1982;107:631–640.

Garioch JJ, Lewis HM, Sargent SA, et al. 25 years' experience of a gluten-free diet in the treatment of dermatitis herpetiformis. *Br J Dermatol* 1994;131:541–545.

Hall RP III. Dermatitis herpetiformis [Review]. *J Invest Dermatol* 1992;99:873–881.

Keogh M, Hall RP III. Dermatitis herpetiformis. In: Arndt KD, Robinson JK, LeBoit PE, et al., eds. *Cutaneous medicine and surgery*. Philadelphia: WB Saunders, 1996:691–697.

RESOURCES
169, 351

12   Transient Acantholytic Dermatosis

Richard Grabowski, MD,
and Mervyn L. Elgart, MD

DEFINITION: Transient acantholytic dermatosis (TAD) is a pruritic papular eruption seen most commonly on the trunk and proximal extremities of white middle-aged males. The disease is usually self-limiting, but may be recurrent and/or persistent with initiating/exacerbating factors including sunlight, heat, and sweating.

SYNONYM: Grover disease.

DIFFERENTIAL DIAGNOSIS: Keratosis follicularis (Darier disease); Miliaria rubra; Papular urticaria; Insect bites; Scabies; Folliculitis; Acne; Dermatitis herpetiformis; Drug eruption.

SIGNS AND SYMPTOMS: Patients report variable degrees of pruritus and present with papules or papulovesicles superimposed with erosions and crusting on the trunk, neck, and proximal extremities. The palms and soles are generally not affected, and the scalp and oral mucosa are rarely involved.

ETIOLOGY/EPIDEMIOLOGY: Males are affected three times more often than females; white middle-aged males are most often affected. Older patients frequently have a more extensive and persistent eruption. Sunlight, heat, and sweating play a central role in the initiation and perturbation of this disease. Many investigators have searched for an underlying abnormality in sweating, but nothing conclusive has been found. Several underlying malignancies have been associated with TAD, but most researchers believe these links are loose at best and most likely are coincidental.

DIAGNOSIS: The diagnosis is made by histologic examination (hematoxylin and eosin stain). Results of both direct and indirect immunofluorescence are generally negative. Results for complete blood cell count, basic metabolic profile, liver function tests, antinuclear antibody, Venereal Disease Research Laboratory (LDRL) test, urinalysis, chest radiography, and viral culture are typically within normal limits.

TREATMENT
Standard Therapies: Evaluation of treatment efficacy has been difficult because TAD characteristically resolves spontaneously with or without recurrence. Patients should be counseled to avoid strenuous exercise, excessive sun exposure, and rapid changes in ambient temperature. Topical corticosteroids (classes 2–4) and soothing baths (e.g., Aveeno oatmeal baths), in conjunction with oral antihistamines (e.g., hydroxyzine, fexofenadine, loratidine, cetirizine) are helpful. Psoralen-UV-A, ultraviolet B, oral steroids (prednisone, triamcinolone), dapsone, and oral retinoids (vitamin A, isotretinoin) have been used in resistant cases.

REFERENCES
Davis MD, Dinneen AM, Landa N, et al. Grover's disease: clinicopathologic review of 72 cases. *Mayo Clin Proc* 1999;74:229–234.
Heenan PJ, Quirk CJ. Transient acantholytic dermatosis: Grover's disease. In: Freedberg IM, Eisen AZ, Wolff K, et al., eds. 5th ed. New York: McGraw-Hill, 1999:620–623.
Parsons JM. Transient acantholytic dermatosis (Grover's disease): A global perspective. *J Am Acad Dermatol* 1996;35:653–666.

RESOURCE
351

13   Dyskeratosis Congenita

Colin A. Sieff, MB, BCh

DEFINITION: Dyskeratosis congenita (DC) is an X-linked syndrome characterized by ectodermal dysplasia, progressive bone marrow failure, and an increased incidence of cancer.

SYNONYM: Zinsser-Cole-Engman syndrome.

DIFFERENTIAL DIAGNOSIS: Fanconi anemia; Acquired aplastic anemia.

SYMPTOMS AND SIGNS: The major dermal manifestations constitute a diagnostic triad: reticulate hyperpigmentation of the skin with greyish macules on an atrophic and sometimes hypopigmented background, affecting the face, neck, shoulders, and trunk; nail dystrophy, with small nail plates that develop into longitudinal ridges, hypoplasia, and eventual atrophy; and mucosal leukoplakia of oral and other mucosal surfaces. The first two signs develop in the first decade, and leukoplakia in the second. Other manifestations include eye and tooth abnormalities, developmental delay, pulmonary disease, short stature, and hyperhidrosis of palms and soles. Complications include aplastic anemia, which occurs in 50% of cases, usually during the second decade, and cancer (10%), usually of abnormal areas such as mucous membranes, gastrointestinal tract, and skin.

ETIOLOGY/EPIDEMIOLOGY: The major form is X-linked, and males constitute 86% of the patients in the dyskeratosis congenita registry. The male:female ratio is approximately 5:1. In addition, evidence exists for both autosomal-recessive and autosomal-dominant forms of the disease. Genetic linkage analysis in multiplex X-linked pedigrees narrowed the candidate region to a 1.4 Mb interval in distal Xq28, and screening of all 28 candidate genes identified a partial gene deletion in one of these genes, *DKC1,* which encoded a protein called dyskerin in a single patient and missense mutations in other patients. The autosomal-dominant form is due to mutation in the RNA component of telomerase (hTR).

DIAGNOSIS: Patients who develop aplastic anemia usually present with thrombocytopenia or anemia. Macrocytosis and elevated hemoglobin F are signs of stress erythropoiesis, and bone marrow aspirate may be hypercellular at first, but a decrease in megakaryocytes and hypocellularity develops with the aplasia. Chromosome breakage response to clastogenic agents such as mitomycin C or diepoxybutane is normal, and this distinguishes DC from Fanconi anemia.

TREATMENT
Standard Therapies: Treatment of bone marrow failure in DC is similar to that for Fanconi anemia. A study of androgens in 23 patients, usually in combination with prednisone, showed a 52% response rate. The outlook in patients who develop aplastic anemia is grim, and the interval from the onset of aplastic anemia to death is 5 years in patients who respond and 3 years in patients who fail to respond to treatment. Androgen treatment has to be continued. Supportive treatment with blood and platelet transfusions and antibiotics should be provided as indicated clinically.

Investigational Therapies: Stem cell transplantation is being investigated. Bone marrow transplantation is also being explored.

REFERENCES
Alter BP, Young NS. The bone marrow failure syndromes. In: Nathan DG, Orkin HS, eds. *Hematology of Infancy and Childhood.* Philadelphia: WB Saunders, 1998:237–335.

Dokal I. Dyskeratosis congenita in all its forms. *Br J Haematol* 2000;110:768–779.

Heiss NS, Knight SW, Vulliamy TJ, et al. I. X-linked dyskeratosis congenita is caused by mutations in a highly conserved gene with putative nucleolar functions. *Nat Genet* 1998;19:32–38.

Knight SW, Heiss NS, Vulliamy TJ, et al. Unexplained aplastic anaemia, immunodeficiency, and cerebellar hypoplasia (Hoyeraal-Hreidarsson syndrome) due to mutations in the dyskeratosis congenita gene, *DKC1. Br J Haematol* 1999;107: 335–339.

Luzzatto L, Karadimitris A. Dyskeratosis and ribosomal rebellion. *Nat Genet* 1998;19:6–7.

Vuilliamy T, Marrone A, Goldman F, et al. The RNA component of telomerase is mutated in autosomal dominant dyskeratosis congenital. *Nature* 2001:413:432–435.

RESOURCES
297, 357

---

14   Epidermal Nevus Syndrome

Richard A. Prayson, MD

DEFINITION: Epidermal nevus syndrome is a congenital neurocutaneous disorder characterized by the presence of hamartomatous epidermal nevi with involvement of the nervous, skeletal, and ophthalmologic systems.

SYNONYMS: Linear epidermal nevus syndrome; Shimmelpinning syndrome; Nevus comedonicus syndrome; Pigmented hairy epidermal nevus syndrome.

DIFFERENTIAL DIAGNOSIS: Neurocutaneous disorders including tuberous sclerosis and neurofibromatosis type I.

SYMPTOMS AND SIGNS: The disorder is marked by a variety of epidermal nevi, which may be associated with other ipsilateral malformations. Head and face nevi may be associated with malformations of the brain, eye, and craniofacial bones (hemimegaly or hypoplasia). Truncal and extremity nevi may be associated with scoliosis, hip dysplasia, and limb deformities (shortening or hypertrophy). Epidermal nevi over the scalp and face are slightly round, ovoid, or linear plaques that are devoid of hair and skin-colored in infancy. After puberty, the nevi become verrucous and orange or brown in color. Skeletal abnormalities occur in approximately 70% of patients. Approximately 50% of patients present with neurologic symptoms including mental retardation, epilepsy, or hemiparesis. Seizure onset is usually in the first year of life. A significant subset of patients with central nervous system involvement have radiographic evidence of hemimegalencephaly or cortical atrophy. Ocular involvement including the eyelids by nevi, microophthalmia, cataracts, corneal opacities, or colobomas are seen in approximately one third of cases. Other skin abnormalities, including hemangiomas, café-au-lait spots, or hypopigmentation, are less common. The extent of cutaneous disease does not necessarily correlate with the severity of disease in other organ sites.

ETIOLOGY/EPIDEMIOLOGY: The disorder may be due to an autosomal-dominant, lethal somatic mutation that occurs during early embryonic development and survives by mosaicism. There is no evidence of vertical transmission. Both sexes can be affected.

DIAGNOSIS: The diagnosis is predicated on recognition of the congenital epidermal nevi accompanied by other characteristic symptoms and signs. Nevi may be subtle, and a close inspection of the scalp or face in any patient with hemimegalencephaly or unilateral brain malformations is important. Careful ophthalmologic examination, a radiographic survey of the skeletal system, and imaging studies of the brain with electroencephalographic studies (if epilepsy is evident) may be warranted.

TREATMENT
Standard Therapies: The epidermal nevi have a potential for malignant transformation after puberty and should be removed whenever possible early in life. Correction of more severe and debilitating skeletal deformities may be warranted. Limited experience with hemispherectomy in patients with epilepsy, hemimegalencephaly, and hemiparesis has suggested some benefit for this surgical approach in selected children.

REFERENCES
Happle R. Epidermal nevus syndrome. *Semin Dermatol* 1995; 14:111–121.
Pavone L, Curatalo P, Rizzo R, et al. Epidermal nevus syndrome: a neurologic variant with hemimegalencephaly, gyral malformation, mental retardation, seizures, and facial hemihypertrophy. *Neurology* 1991;41:266–271.
Solomon LM, Esterly NB. Epidermal and other congenital organoid nevi. *Curr Probl Pediatr* 1975;6:1–56.

RESOURCES
162, 184, 345

15 Dystrophic Epidermolysis Bullosa

Jo-David Fine, MD, MPH

DEFINITION: Dystrophic epidermolysis bullosa (DEB) is one of the most severe of the three major forms of inherited epidermolysis bullosa, a group of diseases characterized by recurrent blister formation as the result of inherently mechanically fragile skin. Two major subtypes of DEB exist: dominant DEB (DDEB) and recessive DEB (RDEB) (Insert Fig. 10).

SYNONYMS: EB dystrophica; Dermolytic EB.

DIFFERENTIAL DIAGNOSIS: Herpes simplex infection; Porphyria.

SYMPTOMS AND SIGNS: Patients have widespread, painful (and/or pruritic) blisters and erosions. Skin is usually exceedingly fragile, easily shearing off as large sheets following the application of minimal lateral traction. Most wounds heal with atrophic scarring and milia formation. Nails usually become markedly dystrophic. Scarring and hair loss may occur on the scalp. In general, patients with DDEB tend to experience less severe extracutaneous disease activity than do patients with RDEB. Extracutaneous findings common to all forms of DEB include oral cavity involvement (blisters, erosions, and scarring of the tongue and other soft tissues) and esophageal strictures. Caries are common. Virtually any other epithelial-lined or -surfaced organ or structure may develop blisters, erosions, and scarring in a patient with DEB. A characteristic feature of RDEB is the development of progressive mutilating deformities (mitten deformities; pseudosyndactyly) of the hands and feet. Children with more severe RDEB tend to experience profound growth retardation and severe multifactorial anemia.

ETIOLOGY/EPIDEMIOLOGY: All forms of DEB result from mutations within the gene encoding for type VII collagen. The incidence and prevalence of DDEB in the United States in 1990 were estimated to be approximately 2.9 per million live births and 1.0 per million population, respectively, whereas the incidence and prevalence of RDEB were estimated to be approximately 2.0 per million live births and 0.9 per million population, respectively.

DIAGNOSIS: Prenatal and postnatal diagnosis of DEB is confirmed by the demonstration of sublamina densa blister formation within affected tissues, by means of either transmission electron microscopy or immunofluorescence antigenic mapping. Monoclonal antibodies (especially those for type VII collagen) also provide useful diagnostic information. Mutational analysis is now possible in selected research laboratories. Subclassification of DEB is currently based on combinations of clinical and ultrastructural findings.

TREATMENT
Standard Therapies: No specific therapies are available yet for any form of DEB. Patient management is confined to the prevention of mechanical trauma and secondary bacterial infection, the use of sterile dressings and topical antibiotics, and the treatment of any complications that arise. Chronic, aggressive nutritional support is critical in all DEB patients who have more severe disease activity. Careful, methodical surveillance for possible skin cancers should begin at about age 10 in every child with RDEB, and any clinically suspicious lesions should be immediately sampled for biopsy. Any proven squamous cell carcinomas should be widely excised. Patients should be intensively followed for the possibility of new primary cancers as well as for local recurrence or regional or distant spread from any previously treated lesions.

Investigational Therapies: Gene therapy strategies are currently being explored for both DDEB and RDEB. In RDEB, the large size of the type VII collagen gene poses many technical problems in regard to possible replacement therapy. Whether systemic isotretinoin, in RDEB, will exert a chemopreventive effect against squamous cell carcinoma is being studied.

REFERENCES
Fine J-D, Bauer EA, McGuire J, Moshell A, eds. *Epidermolysis bullosa: clinical, epidemiologic, and laboratory advances, and the findings of the National Epidermolysis Bullosa Registry.* Baltimore: Johns Hopkins University Press, 1999.

Fine J-D, Eady RAJ, Bauer EA, et al. Revised classification system for inherited epidermolysis bullosa: report of the second international consensus meeting on diagnosis and classification of epidermolysis bullosa. *J Amer Acad Dermatol* 2000; 42:1051–1066.

Fine J-D, McGrath J, Eady RA. Inherited epidermolysis bullosa comes into the new millennium: a revised classification system based on current knowledge of pathogenetic mechanisms, and the clinical, laboratory, and epidemiological findings of large, well defined patient cohorts. *J Am Acad Dermatol* 2000;43: 135–137.

RESOURCES
141, 142, 252

---

16 Junctional Epidermolysis Bullosa

Jo-David Fine, MD, MPH

DEFINITION: Junctional epidermolysis bullosa (JEB) is one of the most severe of the three major forms of inherited epidermolysis bullosa, a group of diseases characterized by recurrent blister formation as the result of the presence of inherently mechanically fragile skin. There are two major subtypes of JEB—Herlitz JEB (Insert Fig. 11) and non-Herlitz JEB—and each is typified by blister formation within the lamina lucida.

SYNONYMS: EB atrophicans; EB letalis; Generalized atrophic benign EB (GABEB).

DIFFERENTIAL DIAGNOSIS: Herpes simplex infection; Porphyria.

SYMPTOMS AND SIGNS: Patients with JEB have widespread, painful blisters and erosions. Their skin is very fragile, easily shearing off as large sheets following the application of minimal lateral traction. Wounds eventually heal with atrophic scarring. Nails either become markedly dystrophic or are shed following minimal trauma. There may be striking, permanent, pigmentary changes (either enhanced or diminished) as a result of injury to the adjacent melanocytes. In addition, a feature of the Herlitz subtype is the development of exuberant granulation tissue, usually in symmetric array around the mouth, nares, and eyelids, and along the lateral neck, axillary vaults, upper back, and proximal nail folds. Scarring alopecia may occur on the scalp. The most severe extracutaneous manifestation, seen in both major JEB subtypes, is edema and/or blister formation within the upper airway, which tends to occur within the first 2 years of life. Oral cavity involvement is common. Another feature of all forms is the presence of enamel hypoplasia. Virtually any epithelial-lined or -surfaced organ or structure may develop blisters, erosions, and scarring; a common site is the esophagus. Rarely, hand deformities may develop. Children with Herlitz JEB tend to experience profound growth retardation and severe multifactorial anemia. Rarely, patients with non-Herlitz JEB develop squamous cell carcinomas.

ETIOLOGY/EPIDEMIOLOGY: All forms of JEB are transmitted in an autosomal-recessive manner. The incidence and prevalence of JEB in the United States in 1990 were estimated to be approximately 2.0 per million live births and 0.4 per million population, respectively.

DIAGNOSIS: Prenatal and postnatal diagnosis of JEB is confirmed by the demonstration of intralamina lucida blister formation within affected tissues, either by means of transmission electron microscopy or immunofluorescence antigenic mapping. Monoclonal antibodies also provide useful diagnostic information. Mutational analysis is now possible, although it is currently available at only a few specialized laboratories worldwide. Subclassification of JEB is currently based on combinations of clinical and ultrastructural findings.

TREATMENT
Standard Therapies: No specific therapies are available yet for JEB. Patient management is confined to the prevention of mechanical trauma and secondary bacterial infection, the use of sterile dressings and topical antibiotics, and the treatment of any complications (tracheolaryngeal, esophageal, other) that arise. Nutritional support is critical in patients with more severe disease activity, because chronic malnutrition may worsen abnormal wound healing. Iron supplements are routinely prescribed in patients with severe anemia and, when necessary, transfusions are given. Aggressive preventive and restorative dental care is needed to prevent premature loss of teeth.

Investigational Therapies: The feasibility of gene therapy for at least some subtypes of JEB is being explored.

REFERENCES
Fine J-D, Bauer EA, McGuire J, Moshell A. *Epidermolysis bullosa: clinical, epidemiologic, and laboratory advances, and the findings of the National Epidermolysis Bullosa Registry.* Baltimore: Johns Hopkins University Press, 1999.
Fine J-D, Eady RAJ, Bauer EA, et al. Revised classification system for inherited epidermolysis bullosa: report of the second international consensus meeting on diagnosis and classification of epidermolysis bullosa. *J Am Acad Dermatol* 2000;42: 1051–1066.
Fine J-D, McGrath J, Eady RAJ. Inherited epidermolysis bullosa comes into the new millennium: a revised classification system based on current knowledge of pathogenetic mechanisms, and the clinical, laboratory, and epidemiological findings of large, well defined patient cohorts. *J Am Acad Dermatol* 2000;43: 135–137.

RESOURCES
141, 142, 252

17 Epidermolysis Bullosa Simplex

Jo-David Fine, MD, MPH

DEFINITION: Epidermolysis bullosa (EB) simplex is the most common of the three major forms of inherited EB, a group of diseases characterized by recurrent blister formation as the result of the presence of inherently mechanically fragile skin. There are three major subtypes of EB simplex, each typified by blister formation within the epidermis. Severity of cutaneous disease activity, as well as the frequency of extracutaneous manifestations, varies among these subtypes.

SYNONYMS: Epidermolytic EB; EB simplex superficialis; EB simplex with muscular dystrophy; EB simplex with mottled pigmentation.

DIFFERENTIAL DIAGNOSIS: Herpes simplex infection; Porphyria; Friction, thermal, or chemical burns; Contact dermatitis; Dyshidrotic eczema.

SYMPTOMS AND SIGNS: The hallmark feature of EB simplex is the presence of usually intact, tense blisters, which arise on nonerythematous skin. These blisters subsequently rupture, leaving open erosions. Not all patients may have readily demonstrable mechanical fragility on routine handling of the skin, however. As in all other forms of EB, blisters are usually associated with pain and less frequently, with itching. The distribution of lesions varies among the subtypes. In the most common subtype of EB simplex, the Weber-Cockayne variant, blisters are usually confined to the palms and soles, but may develop elsewhere if the skin is sufficiently injured (Insert Fig. 12). In more severe subtypes, particularly the Köbner and Dowling-Meara variants, blisters usually arise over virtually any skin surface site. Thickened callouses of the palms and soles eventually develop in many patients. Scarring, nail dystrophy, and/or milia may be seen in patients with more generalized subtypes of EB simplex. About one third of all patients with EB simplex experience some blisters and erosions within the oral cavity. Patients with more severe subtypes may experience repeated blistering on other epithelial-surfaced or lined surfaces, including the external surface of the eye and the esophagus. Some growth retardation and anemia may be seen in more severe subtypes of EB simplex.

ETIOLOGY/EPIDEMIOLOGY: Most forms of EB simplex are autosomal-dominantly transmitted. The incidence and prevalence of EB simplex in the United States in 1990 were estimated to be approximately 10.75 per 1 million live births and 4.60 per million population, respectively.

DIAGNOSIS: Prenatal and postnatal diagnosis of EB simplex is confirmed by demonstration of intraepidermal blister formation, by means of either transmission electron microscopy or immunofluorescence antigenic mapping. Mutational analysis is also now possible, although it is currently available through only a few specialized laboratories. Subclassification is based on combinations of clinical and ultrastructural findings.

TREATMENT
Standard Therapies: No specific therapies are available yet for EB simplex. Patient management is confined to the prevention of mechanical trauma and secondary bacterial infection, the use of sterile dressings and topical antibiotics, and the treatment of any complications that may arise.

Investigational Therapies: Preliminary *in vitro* studies are exploring the feasibility of gene therapy for at least some subtypes of EB simplex. Studies are also looking at the possible role of systemic tetracycline in the modulation of the blisters characteristic of the disease.

REFERENCES
Fine J-D, Bauer EA, McGuire J, Moshell A. *Epidermolysis bullosa: clinical, epidemiologic, and laboratory advances, and the findings of the National Epidermolysis Bullosa Registry.* Baltimore: Johns Hopkins University Press, 1999.
Fine J-D, Eady RAJ, Bauer EA, et al. Revised classification system for inherited epidermolysis bullosa: report of the second international consensus meeting on diagnosis and classification of epidermolysis bullosa. *J Am Acad Dermatol* 2000;42:1051–1066.
Fine J-D, McGrath J, Eady RAJ. Inherited epidermolysis bullosa comes into the new millennium: a revised classification system based on current knowledge of pathogenetic mechanisms, and the clinical, laboratory, and epidemiological findings of large, well defined patient cohorts. *J Am Acad Dermatol* 2000; 43:135–137.

RESOURCES
141, 142, 252

18 Epidermolytic Hyperkeratosis

*Nicole Hayre, MD,
and Mervyn L. Elgart, MD*

DEFINITION: Epidermolytic hyperkeratosis is an inherited form of ichthyosis characterized by the presentation at birth or shortly thereafter of generalized erythema, hyperkeratosis, and bullae. Crops of bullae quickly rupture, leaving denuded areas. Later, as the blistering aspect of the disease become less prominent, a characteristic gray-brown verrucous hyperkeratosis begins to predominate. This too can eventually lessen in severity, as patients with epidermolytic hyperkeratosis usually become less symptomatic as they age.

SYNONYM: Bullous congenital ichthyosiform erythroderma.

DIFFERENTIAL DIAGNOSIS: Lamellar ichthyosis; Nonbullous ichthyosiform erythroderma; X-linked ichthyosis; Epidermolysis bullosa.

SYMPTOMS AND SIGNS: Affected individuals usually present at birth or in the immediate neonatal period with generalized moist erythema and skin tenderness. Characteristic blisters are often also present at birth, or may appear within a few hours of delivery or up to a week later. These bullae appear in crops and are usually superficial, tender/painful, and contain a clear fluid. Rupture of the blisters leaves large (up to several centimeters in diameter) denuded areas that may become hyperpigmented when they heal. Within the first several months of life, blistering decreases as scales become more prominent. The scales are thick, grayish brown, verrucous, and usually found primarily in the flexure and intertriginous areas, but may be generalized. Palms, soles, and the scalp may be involved. In severe forms of the disease, an undesirable body odor is often present.

ETIOLOGY/EPIDEMIOLOGY: Epidermolytic hyperkeratosis occurs in approximately 1 in 300,000 live births. Approximately half of affected individuals inherit the disease in an autosomal-dominant fashion, whereas the rest develop the disease as a result of sporadic mutations. These mutations have been shown to cause defects in keratins K1 and K10, which leads to abnormal keratin distribution patterns, including abnormal tonofilament clumping.

DIAGNOSIS: Clinical features with supporting skin biopsy pathology will help determine the diagnosis. Prenatal diagnosis is now available through fetal skin biopsy or gene sequencing of chorionic villous samples.

TREATMENT
Standard Therapies: Both topical (retinoic acid 0.1% cream) and systemic retinoids have been shown to pro-duce clinical improvement. A 2-week course of high-dose vitamin A (750,000 units Aquasol A daily) has also been reported to be effective. Another treatment involves applying a 10% glycerin, 3% lactic acid water solution to wet skin.

REFERENCES
Hurwitz S. *Clinical pediatric dermatology: a textbook of skin disorders of childhood and adolescence,* 2nd ed. Philadelphia: WB Saunders, 1993:169–170.
Kumar S, Sehgel VN, et al. Epidermolytic hyperkeratosis. *Int J Dermatol* 1999;38:914–915.
Odom, RB, James WB, Berger TG. *Andrews' diseases of the skin: clinical dermatology,* 9th ed. Philadelphia: WB Saunders, 2000:705–706.
Otley CC, Gellis S. Epidermolytic hyperkeratosis. *Int J Dermatol* 1996;35:579–581.

RESOURCES
162, 351

19 Erythema Multiforme

Bernard A. Cohen, MD

DEFINITION: Erythema multiforme (EM) describes a group of hypersensitivity disorders manifesting with acute self-limited mucocutaneous lesions. In classic EM, skin lesions are mild, often recurrent, and involve primarily the extremities. Mucous membranes are involved only minimally or spared (Insert Fig. 13). In the unrelated Stevens-Johnson syndrome (SJS) and toxic epidermal necrolysis (TEN), skin and mucous membrane involvement is usually widespread and life threatening (Insert Fig. 14). To distinguish these disorders, some clinicians refer to classic EM as EM minor and to SJS and TEN as EM major.

DIFFERENTIAL DIAGNOSIS: Urticaria; Urticarial vasculitis; Lupus erythematosus; Viral exanthem; Staphylococcal scalded skin syndrome.

SYMPTOMS AND SIGNS: Classic EM appears abruptly in an otherwise healthy individual as multiple symmetric red papules usually less than 1.0 cm in diameter on the tops of the hands and forearms (Insert Figs. 15 and 16). Other areas of involvement may include the face, neck, palms, soles, legs, and trunk. Lesions are fixed and continue to erupt for 2–3 days. Some papules, particularly on the hands and forearms, evolve into target lesions characterized by concentric zones of color with a dusky center, surrounded by a pale ring, and finally a red border. A necrotic vesicle or crust may develop centrally. In approximately half of patients, a few mild oral vesicles or erosions appear. Most cases are preceded by an outbreak of herpes simplex virus that may still be visible at diagnosis. Classic EM tends to recur 2–3 times a year for several years before subsiding. Both SJS and TEN are usually preceded by a 2-day to 2-week prodrome of upper respiratory symptoms with fever, cough, rhinitis, sore throat, vomiting, and malaise. This is followed by abrupt onset of symmetric red macules that progress rapidly to central necrosis. Cutaneous lesions typically begin on the face, lips, neck, upper trunk, and upper arms and may become confluent and generalized. Multiple mucous membranes, including the mouth, nose, conjunctivae, genitals, and anus, become involved and this may precede the formation of skin lesions. Rarely, the esophagus and respiratory mucosa are involved. Respiratory distress has been reported, particularly in association with TEN. In SJS, cutaneous involvement is variable and may be limited, but mucous membrane lesions are usually severe. Although there is considerable overlap with SJS, cutaneous lesions in TEN are generalized from the onset. In SJS and TEN, the course is usually protracted with reepithelialization of the skin and mucous membranes occurring over 4–6 weeks. Although the risk of mortality is low in otherwise healthy individuals, it has exceeded 25% in some series. Other complications include corneal scarring and permanent visual impairment, lacrimal scarring, esophageal stricture, vaginal and urethral stenosis, and contractures when scarring occurs over joints.

ETIOLOGY/EPIDEMIOLOGY: The cause of EM is unknown; however, the association of classic EM with herpes simplex virus suggests an immunologic process initiated by the virus. In SJS and TEN, cytotoxic T-lymphocytes are believed to mediate destruction of the skin and mucous membranes in the basement membrane zone. In half the cases of EM, major drugs, particularly anticonvulsants, sulfonamides, nonsteroidal antiinflammatory drugs, and other antibiotics, have been implicated as triggering agents. Infectious organisms such as *Mycoplasma pneumoniae* and many viral agents have also been associated.

TREATMENT
Standard Therapies: Most patients with EM minor can be managed as outpatients with symptomatic therapy such as antihistamines for pruritus. In SJS and TEN, standard treatment is supportive. Patients require careful placement of fluids and electrolytes and observation for secondary infection. Transfer to a regional burn center should be considered in patients with widespread cutaneous involvement. The use of systemic steroids is controversial. The risk of complications and length of hospital stay has been longer in patients who received steroids.

Investigational Therapies: Intravenous immunoglobulin and plasmaphoresis may be useful.

REFERENCES

Garcia-Doval I, LeCeauch L, Bocquet H, et al. Toxic epidermal necrolysis and Stevens-Johnson syndrome: does early withdrawal of the causative drug reduce the risk of death? *Arch Dermatol* 2000;136:323–327.
Leaute-Labreze C, Lamireau T, Chawki D, et al. Diagnosis, classification and management of erythema multiforme and Stevens-Johnson syndrome. *Arch Dis Child* 2000;83:347–352.
Schachner LA. Erythema multiforme. *Pediatr Dermatol* 2000;16:75–83.

RESOURCES
360, 447

---

20 Progressive Symmetric Erythrokeratodermia/Erythrokeratodermia with Ataxia

Gabriela Richard, MD

DEFINITION: Progressive symmetric erythrokeratodermia (PSEK) is an inherited disorder characterized by the slowly progressive development of fixed, well-defined plaques of thickened skin with underlying redness. Erythrokeratodermia with ataxia is an autosomal-dominant disorder characterized by plaques of red, thickened, rough skin that develop during infancy and early childhood, but disappear later in life.

SYNONYMS: Erythrokeratodermia progressiva symmetrica; Gottron syndrome; Giroux-Barbeau syndrome.

DIFFERENTIAL DIAGNOSIS: Erythrokeratodermia variabilis; Keratosis palmoplantaris transgrediens et progrediens; Greither disease; Sjögren-Larsson syndrome; Chanarin-Dorfman syndrome; Refsum disease; Trichothiodystrophy.

SYMPTOMS AND SIGNS: Progressive symmetric erythrokeratodermia usually starts during early childhood with development of well-circumscribed red or red-brown plaques of thickened skin with a rough surface. They are predominantly localized at the extensor surface of the extremities, buttocks, trunk, and face (cheeks), and often involve the skin of palms and soles. These hyperkeratotic plaques are slowly progressive and increase in number and size over time. In contrast to erythrokeratodermia variabilis, there are no "migrating" red patches, and the plaques are fixed; however, there is a considerable phenotypic overlap between the skin findings in PSEK, erythrokeratodermia associated with ataxia, and erythrokeratodermia variabilis. Erythrokeratodermia with ataxia starts during infancy with the development of red plaques of thickened skin with fine, white, attached scales on the extremities. These plaques remain throughout childhood, but diminish or disappear during adulthood. During the fourth and fifth decades of life, progressive neurologic symptoms develop, including ataxia, dysarthria, nystagmus, and decreased tendon reflexes. In time, most patients become wheelchair bound.

ETIOLOGY/EPIDEMIOLOGY: The prevalence of PSEK is unknown. The disorder affects both sexes equally, has a considerable intrafamilial and interfamilial variability, and appears to be genetically heterogeneous. Most patients have sporadic cases or have affected parents and/or offspring consistent with autosomal-dominant inheritance, but autosomal-recessive transmission also occurs. The cause of PSEK is unknown. Erythrokeratodermia with ataxia has only been reported in a single family of French-Canadian origin. The disorder was transmitted over five generations in an autosomal-dominant manner, including 25 affected individuals, 14 of whom were females. It has been mapped to the locus for erythrokeratodermia variabilis on the short arm of chromosome 1, although no mutations in connexin genes clustered in this area have been identified.

DIAGNOSIS: The diagnosis of PSEK is based on clinical grounds. Psoriasis usually can be ruled out by its silvery scales and typical abnormalities seen on light microscopic examination. In the absence of a family history, erythrokeratodermia with ataxia may not be suspected until later in life, when neurologic abnormalities manifest.

TREATMENT

Standard Therapies: The treatment of PSEK and of the skin findings in erythrokeratodermia with ataxia are symptomatic and aimed at reducing thickening and cracking of the skin. Several patients with PSEK have responded well to systemic treatment with retinoids. The basic topical therapy includes emollients and keratolytics, such as urea, α-hydroxy acids, propylene glycol, salicylic acid, and topical retinoids. In erythrokeratodermia with ataxia, treatment may require the coordinated efforts of a team of specialists, including dermatologists, neurologists, and other supportive health-care professionals. Genetic counseling is helpful for affected individuals and their families.

REFERENCES

Giroux JM, Barbeau A. Erythrokeratodermia with ataxia. *Arch Dermatol* 1972;106:183–188.

MacFarlane AW, Chapman SJ, Verbov JL. Is erythrokeratoderma one disorder? A clinical and ultrastructural study of two siblings. *Br J Dermatol* 1991;124:487–491.

Ruiz-Maldonado R, Tamayo L, del Castillo V, et al. Erythrokeratodermia progressiva symmetrica: report of 10 cases. *Dermatologica* 1982;164:133–141.

21   Erythrokeratodermia Variabilis

Gabriela Richard, MD

DEFINITION: Erythrokeratodermia variabilis (EKV) is an autosomal-dominant disorder of the skin characterized by red blotches and thickened skin (Insert Fig. 17). Shortly after birth, short-lasting red patches appear. Simultaneously or over time, plaques of yellow-brown, thickened skin develop in a symmetric distribution.

SYNONYMS: Erythrokeratodermia figurata variabilis mendes de costa; Keratosis rubra figurate.

DIFFERENTIAL DIAGNOSIS: Progressive symmetric erythrokeratodermia; Erythrokeratodermia and ataxia; Giroux-Barbeau syndrome; Keratosis palmoplantaris transgrediens et progrediens; Greither disease; Ichthyosis linearis circumflexa; Erythrokeratolysis hiemalis; Psoriasis.

SYMPTOMS AND SIGNS: The hallmark of EKV is the occurrence of well-demarcated red patches, which show a remarkable variability in number, size, shape, location, and duration. This erythematous component is most prevalent during childhood, and later slowly subsides. The red spots, which are sometimes surrounded by an anemic halo, may extend to form large patches or have a targetlike appearance. The erythema usually persists for minutes to hours, although it may last for days, and may be preceded or accompanied by a burning sensation. In addition, slowly progressive, sharply outlined plaques of yellow-brown, rough, thickened skin evolve. Their surface may be ridged and verrucous, and show peeling or fine, attached scales. The plaques are almost symmetrically distributed over the limbs, buttocks, and trunk. In approximately half of patients, the thickening of the skin extends to the palms and soles. Most common are relatively fixed lesions over the knees, elbows, Achilles tendons, dorsum of the feet, and the belt area, persisting over months to years. Individual plaques may also change size and shape, and regress without residua. In some patients with severe disease, a generalized, persistent thickening of the skin occurs with prominent skin markings and fine attached scaling. After progression during infancy and childhood, EKV seems to stabilize after puberty and slowly regresses in older age.

ETIOLOGY/EPIDEMIOLOGY: The prevalence is unknown. More than 200 patients with diverse genetic backgrounds have been reported. The disorder is inherited in an autosomal-dominant fashion with nearly complete penetrance, but with considerable intrafamilial and interfamilial variability. Both sexes are affected equally. The disorder is caused by mutations in two connexin genes (*GJB3* and *GJB4*) localized on human chromosome 1p34-p35.

DIAGNOSIS: Diagnosis is usually established on clinical grounds, although microscopic examination of a skin biopsy can be helpful to rule out other disorders.

TREATMENT
Standard Therapies: The goal of therapy is to diminish thickening of the skin. Treatments of choice in extensive EKV are systemic retinoids. Isotretinoin (Accutane) or acitretin (Soriaten) can induce a dramatic improvement. The local management of EKV is symptomatic and focuses on keratolysis, lubrication, and hydration. Therapy includes emollients combined with keratolytics, such as urea, α-hydroxy acids, propylene glycol, salicylic acid, and topical retinoids. Cosmetic concerns can be limited by masking uncovered skin with makeup and camouflage. Genetic counseling is helpful for affected individuals and their families.

REFERENCES
Macari F, Landau M, Cousin P, et al. Mutation in the gene for connexin 30.3 in a family with erythrokeratodermia variabilis. *Am J Hum Genet* 2000;67:1296–1301.
Mendes da Costa S. Erythro- et keratodermia variabilis in a mother and a daughter. *Acta Derm Venerol* 1925;6:255–261.
Richard G, et al. Mutations in the human connexin gene *GJB3* cause erythrokeratodermia variabilis. *Nat Genet* 1998;20:366–369.
Sybert VP. Erythrokeratodermias. In: *Genetic skin disorders.* New York: Oxford University Press, 1997.
van de Kerkhof PC, Steijlen PM, van Dooren-Greebe RJ, et al. Acitretin in the treatment of erythrokeratodermia variabilis. *Dermatologica* 1990;181:330–333.

RESOURCES
162, 325, 351

22 Erythromelalgia

Mark D.P. Davis, MD

DEFINITION: Erythromelalgia is marked by the occurrence of red, hot, painful extremities. Classifications based on causality (primary or secondary) or age at onset (presuming that all cases of early onset are primary) have been proposed.

SYNONYMS: Erythermalgia; Erythralgia.

DIFFERENTIAL DIAGNOSIS: Peripheral neuropathy; Reflex sympathetic dystrophy; Atherosclerosis; Venous disease.

SYMPTOMS AND SIGNS: Symptoms predominantly occur in the feet and hands. Patients complain of intermittently red, painful hands or feet and an accompanying burning sensation. Affected areas are remarkably hot, both subjectively and objectively. Patients report that their symptoms are precipitated by exercise, being in a warm room, or sleeping under warm blankets. Characteristically, they seek relief by immersing the affected extremity in cold water or ice. Many report that episodes occur with increasing frequency over time; in a few patients, the interval between episodes disappears. In some patients, erythromelalgia follows a chronic or sometimes progressive and disabling course; in others, the symptoms wane and disappear.

ETIOLOGY/EPIDEMIOLOGY: The cause of symptoms in erythromelalgia is unknown. It is increasingly recognized that the syndrome is one of dysfunctional vascular dynamics. The incidence of the disorder is unknown. In Norway, the incidence is estimated to be 2.5 to 3.3 cases per million inhabitants per year. The condition is seen in both sexes but appears to be more common in females. Most reported patients were white. In one study, the mean age of the patients at presentation was 55.8 years (range, 5–91 years). The condition may be inherited in up to 5% of affected individuals. Erythromelalgia has been associated with other diseases, specifically with myeloproliferative diseases. It also has been associated with connective tissue diseases and with medications.

DIAGNOSIS: Patients with a characteristic history have erythromelalgia by definition. The diagnosis is made when the criteria given in the original description are met: intermittently or constantly red extremities (usually the feet) in combination with subjective and objective heat in the affected area. Additional specific criteria have been suggested, including burning pain in an extremity, pain aggravated by warming, relieved by cooling, redness, and increased temperature of the affected skin. A complete blood count is indicated to rule out myeloproliferative diseases. Vascular studies may confirm the increased temperature and blood flow during symptoms. In specialized centers, these have been documented with special instruments. Autonomic nerve studies and electromyography may be used to confirm the presence or absence of neuropathy.

TREATMENT
Standard Therapies: Some patients respond well to aspirin. In those who do not, erythromelalgia can be extremely difficult to treat. The various treatments used include nonsteroidal antiinflammatory drugs, β-blockers, antihistamines, biofeedback, epidural blocks, hypnosis, transcutaneous electrical nerve stimulation, vasodilators, capsaicin, anticonvulsants, antidepressants, antimigraine tablets, pentoxifylline, dipyridamole, lumbar sympathetic ganglion block, clonidine, α-blockers, calcium channel blockers, prostaglandin and epoprostenol analogues, muscle relaxants, intravenous sodium nitroprusside and prostaglandins, and intrathecal hydromorphone and clonidine.

REFERENCES
Babb RR, Alarcon-Segovia D, Fairbairn JF II. Erythermalgia: review of 51 cases. *Circulation* 1964;29:136–141.
Cohen JS. Erythromelalgia: new theories and new therapies. *J Am Acad Dermatol* 2000;43:841–847.
Davis MD, O'Fallon WM, Rogers RS III, et al. Natural history of erythromelalgia: presentation and outcome in 168 patients. *Arch Dermatol* 2000;136:330–336.
Kalgaard OM, Seem E, Kvernebo K. Erythromelalgia: a clinical study of 87 cases. *J Intern Med* 1997;242:191–197.
Sandroni P, Davis MDP, Harper CM, et al. Neurophysiologic and vascular studies in erythromelalgia: a retrospective analysis. *J Clin Neuromuscular Dis* 1999;1:57–63.

RESOURCES
146, 360

23 Fox-Fordyce Disease

Mervyn L. Elgart, MD

DEFINITION: Fox-Fordyce disease is a condition in which pruritic papules appear in the apocrine areas of the body, including the midchest, the nipples, the axillae, and sometimes the lower abdomen and pubic area.

SYNONYMS: Apocrine miliaria; Chronic itching; Papular eruption of axillae and pubes.

DIFFERENTIAL DIAGNOSIS: Molluscum contagiosum; Syringomas.

SYMPTOMS AND SIGNS: The disease usually occurs in young women, just as they begin to go through puberty. It begins with pruritic flesh-colored papules appearing in the axilla, the tissue near the breasts, and the lower abdomen. Other areas may be involved, and eccrine glands are sometimes involved. Itching may be mild or severe. Pregnancy seems to modify the severity of the symptoms, especially during the last trimester. The condition persists indefinitely, often becoming less severe after menopause.

ETIOLOGY/EPIDEMIOLOGY: The condition is caused by obstruction of the apocrine gland ducts. The reason is unknown. The blocked duct ruptures, causing an inflammatory infiltrate where the duct comes close to the follicle.

DIAGNOSIS: Diagnosis is made on the basis of the clinical picture of pruritic papules in apocrine-rich areas. A biopsy may be helpful.

TREATMENT
Standard Therapies: Pregnancy and estrogen hormones (given as estrogen-dominant oral contraceptives) have been successful, although not all patients respond. Oral retinoids have been successful for some patients, but because this disease is usually seen in women of child-bearing age, these should be used cautiously. Strong topical steroids, as well as topical solutions of clindamycin, have been helpful in some cases.

REFERENCES
Effendy I, Ossowski B, Happle R. Fox-Fordyce disease in a male patient: response to oral retinoid treatment. *Clin Exp Dermatol* 1994;19:67–69.
Feldmann R, Masouye I, Chavaz P, et al. Fox-Fordyce disease: successful treatment with topical clindamycin in alcoholic propylene glycol solution. *Dermatology* 1992;184:310–313.
Miller ML, Harford RR, Yeager JK. Fox-Fordyce disease treated with topical clindamycin solution. *Arch Dermatol* 1995;131:1112–1113.
Shelly WB, Levy E. Apocrine sweat retention in man. II: Fox Fordyce disease (apocrine miliaria). *Arch Dermatol* 1956;73:38.

RESOURCE
351

24   Gianotti-Crosti Syndrome

Richard Grabowski, MD,
and Mervyn L. Elgart, MD

DEFINITION: Gianotti-Crosti syndrome (GCS) is typically a monomorphic, papulovesicular, self-limiting childhood exanthem involving the face, extremities, and buttocks. It occurs most often in the setting of an underlying virus, classically hepatitis B virus.

SYNONYMS: Papulovesicular acrolocated syndrome; Papular acrodermatitis of childhood.

DIFFERENTIAL DIAGNOSIS: Drug eruption; Other viral exanthems.

SYMPTOMS AND SIGNS: Children present with a self-limiting (2–4 week), asymptomatic to variably pruritic, skin-toned to erythematous, papulovesicular eruption primarily on the face, extremities, and buttocks. More extensive eruptions (i.e., full body) often have more severe pruritus and accompanying systemic components (i.e., fever, lymphadenopathy, and hepatosplenomegaly). The systemic associations, when found, appear to resolve in conjunction with the skin findings.

ETIOLOGY/EPIDEMIOLOGY: Gianotti-Crosti syndrome affects children ages 6 months to 14 years. This is typically a virally induced syndrome that classically had been considered to be associated with hepatitis B virus. However, since its initial association in the early 1970s, hundreds of cases with other viral causes have surfaced. These other viral possibilities include hepatitis A and C viruses, Epstein-Barr virus, cytomegalovirus, coxsackie viruses, adenoviruses, human immunodeficiency virus, parvovirus B19, parainfluenza viruses 1 and 2, rotavirus, poliovirus, and vaccinia virus. Even immunization has been reported to induce GCS. Some children have developed GCS without a detectable viral etiology. Many now believe that this syndrome represents a reaction pattern to an underlying viral illness, such as seen in erythema multiforme and erythema nodosum, in children with a wide array of viral illnesses.

DIAGNOSIS: Diagnosis is based on history and clinical features of a self-limited, acrally located, monomorphic papulovesicular eruption in a child. Histologic examination is typically nonspecific. Given the broad range of possible inciting viral agents, checking serologic evidence may be warranted to rule out an underlying viral hepatitis or possibly HIV.

TREATMENT
Standard Therapies: Gianotti-Crosti syndrome is a self-limiting disease; thus, treatment is primarily symptomatic depending on the subjective distress of the afflicted child. Many cases require no treatment. However, frequently, antihistamines, soothing topical lotions (e.g., clioquinol lotion 1%), or mid- to low-potency topical corticosteroids are used. Infrequently, systemic steroids are used for children who are severely affected.

REFERENCES
Blauvelt A, Turner ML. Gianotti-Crosti syndrome and human immunodeficiency virus infection. *Arch Dermatol* 1994;130: 481–483.
Boeck K, Mempel M, Schmidt T, et al. Gianotti-Crosti syndrome: clinical, serologic, and therapeutic data from nine children. *Cutis* 1998;62:271–274.
Caputo R, Gelmetti C, Ermacora E, et al. Gianotti-Crosti syndrome: a retrospective analysis of 308 cases. *J Am Acad Dermatol* 1992;26:207–210.
Murphy LA, Buckley C. Gianotti-Crosti syndrome in an infant following immunization. *Pediatr Dermatol* 2000;17:225–226.

RESOURCES
89, 351

25   Granuloma Annulare

Mona S. Foad, MD,
and Mervyn L. Elgart, MD

DEFINITION: Granuloma annulare (GA) is a benign, inflammatory skin condition characterized by the development of dermal papules. It has been classified into four variants: localized GA, generalized GA, subcutaneous GA, and perforating GA.

SYNONYMS: (For subcutaneous GA): Pseudorheumatoid nodule; Subcutaneous palisading granuloma; Subcutaneous granuloma; Necrobiotic granuloma.

DIFFERENTIAL DIAGNOSIS: Tinea corporis; Lyme disease; Sarcoidosis; Annular lichen planus; Erythema annulare centrifugum; Subacute cutaneous lupus; Papular mucinosis; Secondary syphilis; Annular elastolytic giant cell granuloma; Rheumatoid nodule; Perforating collagenosis; Perforating sarcoid; Elastosis perforans serpiginosa; Molluscum contagiosum; PLEVA.

SYMPTOMS AND SIGNS: Localized GA is the most common variant, affecting primarily children and young adults. These lesions are characterized by asymptomatic, dome-shaped papules that form annular or arcuate skin-colored, erythematous, or violaceous plaques. The annular lesions tend to enlarge centrifugally, leaving behind a slightly hyperpigmented or depressed center. Solitary papules may be umbilicated. The most common location is on the dorsa of the hands and feet; 50% of lesions tend to resolve spontaneously within 2 years. Generalized GA is characterized by the development of hundreds to thousands of 1–2 mm skin-colored, tan, pink, or yellow papules. The lesions are located primarily on the trunk, or are symmetrically distributed on the neck, forearms, legs, and elbows. Annular plaques can develop, but tend to resolve unevenly, leaving behind an arcuate lesion. Lesions tend to persist for 3–4 years and respond poorly to therapy. Subcutaneous GA affects primarily children. The lesions are firm, skin-colored to pink, deep dermal or subcutaneous painless nodules, overlying or in close proximity to periosteum. They are located on the palms, lower legs, buttocks, or scalp, and may be attached to the underlying fascia or periosteum. Perforating GA is characterized by asymptomatic, grouped, 1–4 mm umbilicated papules with a central plug or crust, most commonly located on the hands, fingers, and extremities. The lesions start as erythematous papules, which evolve into yellow pustular lesions and eventually discharge a clear fluid.

ETIOLOGY/EPIDEMIOLOGY: This disorder affects primarily children and young adults, although it can occur at any age. Women are affected twice as often as men. It can appear spontaneously, but has been known to follow trauma, insect bites, tuberculin skin tests, ultraviolet light, and viral infections. The cause is unknown, but several theories exist. Genetics may also play a role.

DIAGNOSIS: Diagnosis of GA is based on clinical and histologic examination. Because laboratory results are typically within normal limits, skin biopsy is the chief diagnostic tool.

TREATMENT

Standard Therapies: Because lesions of localized GA often resolve spontaneously, they rarely require treatment. If desired, treatment options include cryotherapy, intralesional and topical steroids, radiotherapy, or intralesional interferon-γ injections. Psoralen-UV-A is the treatment of choice for generalized GA; other options include niacinamide, dapsone, antimalarials, potassium iodide, cyclosporine, and chlorambucil.

REFERENCES

Felner EL, Steinberg JB, Weinberg AG. Subcutaneous granuloma annulare: a review of 47 cases. *Pediatrics* 1997;100:965–967.

Ratnaval RC, Norris PG. Performing granuloma annulare: response to treatment with isotretinoin. *J Am Acad Dermatol* 1995;32:126–127.

Smith MD, Downie JB, DiCostanzo D. Granuloma annulare. *Int J Dermatol* 1997;36:326–333.

Toro JR, Chu P, Yen TB, et al. Granuloma annulare and human immunodeficiency virus infection. *Arch Dermatol* 1999;135: 1341–1346.

Weiss JM, Muchenburger S, et al. Treatment of granuloma annulare by local injections with low dose recombinant human interferon gamma. *J Am Acad Dermatol* 1998;39:117–119.

RESOURCE
351

---

26   Hay-Wells Syndrome

John A. McGrath, MD, MRCP, and Alan D. Irvine, MD

DEFINITION: Hay-Wells syndrome is an inherited ectodermal dysplasia resulting from impaired regulation of epidermal stem cell proliferation. Defective epidermal development leads to a spectrum of abnormalities, including skin fragility and inflammation, alopecia, eyelid malformation, cleft lip/palate, and other ectodermal anomalies.

SYNONYM: Ankyloblepharon-ectodermal dysplasia-facial clefting (AEC) syndrome.

DIFFERENTIAL DIAGNOSIS: Rapp-Hodgkin syndrome; Epidermolysis bullosa (simplex, junctional, or dystrophic);

Bullous congenital ichthyosiform erythroderma/epidermolytic hyperkeratosis; Lamellar ichthyosis/nonbullous ichthyosiform erythroderma; Popliteal pterygia syndrome; Curly hair–ankyloblepharon–nail dysplasia syndrome (CHANDS).

SYMPTOMS AND SIGNS: At birth, clefting of the palate and occasionally the lip is clinically obvious in most affected individuals. In a few patients, the clefting is limited to a small area of the palate and remains undetected until specifically examined for later in life. Skin fragility with cutaneous erosions is usually apparent at birth, although the extent and severity of the erosions varies widely. Infants with extensive skin fragility are often initially misdiagnosed with epidermolysis bullosa. Nail dystrophy is an almost universal feature in the neonate and early childhood years. Ankyloblepharon is a common but not universal sign in the neonate; ophthalmic assessment at this time may also demonstrate lacrimal duct atresia and/or punctate keratopathy. Affected infants have characteristic facies of midface hypoplasia and low-set, cup-shaped ears. In the first year of life, severe, recurrent scalp infections are often the most difficult problem to manage, and they often persist for the first few years. When infections finally abate, extensive scarring alopecia is a common sequela. Recurrent otitis media with conductive hearing loss is common; excessive skin shedding into poorly formed external auditory meati also contributes to conductive deafness. Dentition is poor with wide-spaced, conical teeth and hypoplastic enamel. Heat intolerance is often reported. Inadequate lacrimation may cause photophobia. Even after repair of cleft lip and/or palate, children may have persistent velopharyngeal insufficiency with resultant impairment of speech. Less frequent signs include supernumerary nipples, nipple hypoplasia or displacement, and hypospadias.

ETIOLOGY/EPIDEMIOLOGY: Hay-Wells syndrome is inherited in an autosomal-dominant manner, although most cases arise *de novo* with no preceding family history.

The disorder is due to heterozygous missense mutations in the p63 gene (also known as p51 or *KET*) located on chromosome 3q27. These mutations are located in the SAM (sterile-alpha-motif) domain of p63 (exons 13 and 14 of the gene).

DIAGNOSIS: The diagnosis should be suspected on the emerging pattern of clinical signs: facial clefting followed by chronic scalp erosions and alopecia, although the degree of initial skin fragility and inflammation may vary considerably. Analysis of genomic DNA for mutations in the p63 gene will help provide a diagnosis in most patients.

TREATMENT

Standard Therapies: Treatment is generally supportive. In neonates with extensive skin erosions, emollients, antiseptics, antibiotics, protective skin dressing, and attention to fluid balance and thermoregulation are important. Partial fusion of the eyelids may resolve spontaneously or require surgical correction. Scalp erosions and chronic bacterial folliculitis require treatment with oral antibiotics for several months. Surgical correction of the cleft lip and palate are carried out as for nonsyndromic cases.

REFERENCES

Fosko SW, Stenn KS, Bolognia JL. Ectodermal dysplasias associated with clefting: significance of scalp dermatitis. *J Am Acad Dermatol* 1992;27:249–256.

Hay RJ, Wells RS. The syndrome of ankyloblepharon, ectodermal defects and cleft lip and palate: an autosomal dominant condition. *Br J Dermatol* 1976;94:277–289.

McGrath JA, Duijf PHG, Doetsch V, et al. Hay-Wells syndrome is caused by heterozygous missense mutations in the Sam domain of p63. *Hum Mol Genet* 2001;10:221–229.

RESOURCES

297, 360

---

27   Cavernous Hemangioma

Martin Braun, MD,
and Mervyn L. Elgart, MD

DEFINITION: Cavernous hemangiomas are hemodynamically inactive venous malformations that are present at birth and can be found within any tissue of the body. The term *cavernous hemangioma* is now considered a misnomer, because they are vascular malformations rather than true neoplasms.

SYNONYMS: Venous malformation; Venous angioma; Cavernous angioma.

DIFFERENTIAL DIAGNOSIS: Deep hemangioma; Lymphatic malformation.

SYMPTOMS AND SIGNS: Cutaneous lesions may appear in any location, but most often appear on the head and neck, and the symptoms and signs depend on their size and location. They are most often solitary and localized, but multiple and extensive lesions also occur. Venous malformations do not tend to spontaneously regress, but persist and slowly enlarge. Clinically, cutaneous venous malformations appear as deep blue or violaceous grouped papules, plaques, or nodules that are soft and spongy on palpation. Neighboring veins may also be enlarged. Most venous malformations are asymptomatic, but as they compress adjacent structures, they may cause symptoms such as intermittent pain, hyperhidrosis over the lesions, recurrent thrombophlebitis, and swelling of the lesions when in a dependent position. Patients may present with hemorrhage when the venous malformation ruptures. Skeletal abnormalities can occur, such as bony hypertrophy or undergrowth, dental abnormalities, and facial asymmetry.

ETIOLOGY/EPIDEMIOLOGY: Most venous malformations occur sporadically as isolated lesions. When they occur as part of a syndrome, they most often are inherited autosomal dominantly. They are always present at birth, but may not become clinically apparent until later. Men and women are affected equally, and the overall incidence is estimated at 0.3%–0.5%.

DIAGNOSIS: When venous malformations are suspected, ultrasonography may assist in the diagnosis and evaluation. Accurate diagnosis and visualization of venous malformations, evaluation of their extent, and their relation to surrounding structures is accomplished by MRI.

TREATMENT
Standard Therapies: Treatment of venous malformations depends on the size of the lesion, location of the lesion, and the patient. Indications for treatment include symptoms, functional impairment, and cosmetic appearance. Compression can be accomplished with elastic bandages or tightly fitting clothing. Thrombosis can be prevented with aspirin. Sclerotherapy can reduce the size of the malformations, but the lesions tend to recur. Surgery can be curative, although it may be difficult with extensive lesions. Venous malformations tend to have significantly large and deep structures, which make laser therapy ineffective.

REFERENCES
Enjolras O, Ciabrini D, Mazoyer F, et al. Extensive pure venous malformations in the upper or lower limb: a review of 27 cases. *J Am Acad Dermatol* 1997;36:219–225.
Grevelink SV, Mulliken JB. Vascular anomalies. In: *Fitzpatrick's dermatology in general medicine*, 5th ed. New York: McGraw-Hill, 1999.
Odom RB, James WD, Berger TG. *Andrew's diseases of the skin*, 9th ed. Philadelphia: WB Saunders, 2000.
Requena L, Sangueza OP. Cutaneous vascular anomalies. Part I. Hamartomas, malformations, and dilatation of preexisting vessels. *J Am Acad Dermatol* 1997;37:523–549.

RESOURCES
172, 484

28 Hidradenitis Suppurativa

Mervyn L. Elgart, MD

DEFINITION: Hidradenitis suppurativa is a chronic scarring inflammatory disease affecting apocrine gland-bearing skin, usually the axilla or groin. Clinically, patients have draining sinuses, sinus tracts, and scarring.

SYNONYMS: Acne inversa; Verneuil disease.

DIFFERENTIAL DIAGNOSIS: Pyoderma fistulans sinifica (fox den disease); Pilonidal sinus; Perianal fistula.

SYMPTOMS AND SIGNS: The disease begins as an inflammation that closes the hair follicle in apocrine areas. This leads to inflammation in the hair follicle or in the apocrine glands, which results in apocrine gland or follicle rupture, leading to pus in the dermis, which in turn produces an inflammation with deep foci of purulent material in epithelial-lined sinuses. The final picture shows abscessing inflammation, fistulating sinus tracts, and scarring. The axillae, the groin, and the vulva have been affected. Cases have been associated with Dowling-Degos disease, presumably because of the follicular occlusion in that condition. Because of the intense inflammation, the disease is sometimes associated with arthritis, as well as pyoderma gangrenosum. Squamous cell carcinoma may eventually appear in the inflamed tissue.

ETIOLOGY/EPIDEMIOLOGY: The etiology is unknown. A follicular orifice problem probably leads to the folliculitis and deep inflammation. Men and women are affected equally. Oral lithium carbonate was associated in one case.

DIAGNOSIS: The diagnosis is made on the basis of clinical appearance. Draining pustules appear overlying long sinus tracts. These are present in the axilla and, less often, in the groin.

TREATMENT
Standard Therapies: Surgical treatment consists of either the opening and marsupialization of the sinus tracts or the excision and grafting of involved skin. Lasers (usually CO_2) have been used. Oral medications include isotretinoin or other retinoids, cyclosporine, antibiotics, and topical clindamycin.

REFERENCES
Bedlow AJ, Mortimer PS. Dowling-Degos disease associated with hidradenitis suppurativa. *Clin Exp Dermatol* 1996;21:305–306.
Boer J, Weltevreden EF. Hidradenitis suppurativa or acne inversa. A clinicopathological study of early lesions. *Br J Dermatol* 1996;135:721–725.
Brook I, Frazier EH. Aerobic and anaerobic microbiology of axillary hidradenitis suppurativa. *J Med Microbiol* 1999; 48: 103–105.
Finley EM, Ratz JL. Treatment of hidradenitis suppurativa with carbon dioxide laser excision and second-intention healing. *J Am Acad Dermatol* 1996;34:465–469.
Hamoir XL, Francois RJ, Van den Haute V, et al. Arthritis and hidradenitis suppurativa diagnosed in a 48-year-old man. *Skel Radiol* 1999;28:453–456.
Rompel R, Petres J. Long-term results of wide surgical excision in 106 patients with hidradenitis suppurativa. *Dermatol Surg* 2000;26:638–643.
Von Der Werth JM, Williams HC, Raeburn JA. The clinical genetics of hidradenitis suppurativa revisited. *Br J Dermatol* 2000; 142:947–953.

RESOURCES
182, 359, 360

---

29   Hypomelanosis of Ito

Richard A. Lewis, MD, MS

DEFINITION: Hypomelanosis of Ito is a neurocutaneous syndrome of streaky, patchy, whorl-like, or linear hypopigmentation of the skin, often associated with seizures, developmental and intellectual retardation, and other anomalies.

SYNONYMS: Ito syndrome; Incontinentia pigmenti achromians.

DIFFERENTIAL DIAGNOSIS: Naegeli-type ectodermal dysplasia syndrome (Naegeli-Franceschetti-Jadassohn syndrome); Incontinentia pigmenti (Bloch-Sulzberger syndrome); Systematized nevus depigmentosus; Leukomelanoderma; Tuberous sclerosis; Carbohydrate-deficient glycoprotein deficiency type III; Segmental vitiligo.

SYMPTOMS AND SIGNS: The disorder is characterized by asymmetric, unilateral or bilateral cutaneous patchy, whorl-like, and linear hypopigmentation, occurring on any part of the body but usually not the scalp, palms, or soles. Generally, the skin is otherwise normal (although rarely thin hair occurs in areas of scalp involvement). Associated noncutaneous features occur in approximately 90% of individuals, including infantile seizures (resistant to therapy), gross motor and psychomotor retardation, cerebellar dysfunction, neural migration defects, hypotonia, and macrocephaly. Occasionally, hypertelorism, strabismus, high or cleft palate, scoliosis or asymmetries of long bones (leg length), hip dysplasia, hemiatrophy (or hemi-growth delay), pectus excavatum, or clinodactyly may be present. Dental anomalies vary from missing teeth, pointed extra cusps on maxillary incisors, and conical anterior deciduous teeth with pitted, yellow-brown crowns. Uncommon ophthalmic features include epicanthal folds (epicanthus tarsalis), myopia, blotchy retinal pigment epithelial hypopigmentation, and ptosis.

ETIOLOGY/EPIDEMIOLOGY: Hypomelanosis of Ito is a manifestation of an etiologically heterogeneous group of disorders, some of which are associated with genetically distinct cell lines. Incidence is estimated at 1 in 8,000 to 1 in 10,000. It is usually an isolated occurrence, not inherited. The male:female ratio is 1:2.5. This condition may prove to be heterogeneous, with the streaky hypopigmentation being the only similarity among different individuals.

DIAGNOSIS: The correct dermatologic diagnosis excludes both incontinentia pigmenti and chromosomal anomalies. Diligent dermatologic history and examination should exclude identifiable antecedent inflammatory or infectious agents or evidence of vesicular or bullous eruptions. The finding of chromosomal mosaicism in epidermal keratinocytes in the hypopigmented epidermis is diagnostic. Neuroimaging for structural variants of the brain is appropriate if clinical evidence exists of neurologic involvement.

TREATMENT
Standard Therapies: No useful intervention exists for the cutaneous hypopigmentation, which is cosmetically but

not functionally altered. Ocular or dental anomalies may be managed as usual.

REFERENCES

Ito M. Incontinentia pigmenti achromians, a singular case of naevus depigmentosus systematicus bilateralis. *Tohoku J Exp Med* 1952;55(suppl):57–59.

Jelinek JE, Bart RS, Schiff GM. Hypomelanosis of Ito ('incontinentia pigmenti achromians'): report of three cases and review of the literature. *Arch Dermatol* 1973;107:596–601.

Pascual-Castroviejo I, Lopez-Rodriguez L, de la Cruz Medina M, et al. Hypomelanosis of Ito: neurological complications in 34 cases. *Can J Neurol Sci* 1988;124–129.

Ritter CL, Steele MW, Wenger SL, et al. Chromosome mosaicism in hypomelanosis of Ito. *Am J Med Genet* 1990;35:14–17.

Sybert VP. Hypomelanosis of Ito: a description, not a diagnosis. *J Invest Dermatol* 1994;103(suppl):141–143.

RESOURCES

145, 360

30 Ichthyosis

Virginia P. Sybert, MD

DEFINITION: The ichthyoses are a group of inherited disorders that share a thickened stratum corneum, which results clinically in scaling skin. These conditions are distinguished from each other by the degree and distribution of the scaling skin, the presence or absence of erythroderma, the mode of inheritance, and associated abnormalities.

DIFFERENTIAL DIAGNOSIS: Acquired ichthyoses, including nutritional deficiencies; Xerosis; Trichothiodystrophies; Gaucher disease; Erythrodermic psoriasis; Immunodeficiencies; Atopic dermatitis.

SYMPTOMS AND SIGNS: The primary skin sign is scaling. The scales may be fine and white, or thick and yellow or brown. In some of the ichthyoses, the scales are so thick that they may impede movement and respiration, as they do in harlequin fetus. The distribution of scaling may involve all skin surfaces or be restricted to certain areas. Flexures tend to be more mildly involved. Fragility of the skin, with blistering, is a feature of bullous congenital ichthyosiform erythroderma (BCIE) (epidermolytic hyperkeratosis). Underlying erythroderma or redness of the skin is a feature common to BCIE, nonbullous congenital ichthyosiform erythroderma/lamellar ichthyosis, and Netherton syndrome, and can also be seen sometimes in Conradi-Hunermann syndrome. A collodion membrane may be the first presenting sign in some of the ichthyoses. The newborn with a collodion membrane has skin that looks as if it were covered in plastic wrap. The ears can be crumpled; the digits can be held in flexion and joint movement can be restricted. The collodion membrane cracks and peels, and is usually shed by 2–3 weeks of age. Collodion membrane of the newborn, or lamellar exfoliation of the newborn, is a specific, probably autosomal-recessive, disorder in which the underlying skin is near normal, and there may be little or no evidence of ongoing problems with scaling once the membrane has shed. Secondary infection of the skin, both bacterial and fungal, is common in those conditions with thick, adherent scale and with fragility of the skin (e.g., BCIE, lamellar ichthyosis). Progressive corneal opacities, usually asymptomatic, are a feature of X-linked ichthyosis (sterol sulfatase deficiency) (Insert Fig. 18). Glistening white dots on the retina are found in Sjögren-Larsson syndrome. Macular degeneration and corneal opacities occur in a smaller percentage of individuals with this condition. Cataracts may occur in X-linked Conradi-Hunermann syndrome. Mental retardation can be found in some individuals. Progressive spastic paraparesis is part of the Sjögren-Larsson phenotype. Seizures have been reported in association with X-linked Conradi-Hunermann. Chondrodysplasia punctata and asymmetric skeletal abnormalites are found in X-linked Conradi-Hunermann syndrome. There may be an increased risk for testicular malignancy in males with X-linked sterol sulfatase deficiency. The hair in Netherton syndrome is characterized by a structural alteration referred to as trichrrhexis invaginata or bamboo hair.

ETIOLOGY/EPIDEMIOLOGY: The ichthyoses affect all racial groups. The skin changes of X-linked ichthyosis vulgaris are expressed only in males. X-linked Conradi-Hunermann is lethal in males, whereas female carriers express to varying degrees. Ichthyosis vulgaris is the most common of these disorders. X-linked sterol sulfatase deficiency occurs in approximately 1 in 6,000 male births. The other forms of ichthyosis are far less common. The underlying molecular changes responsible for some of the ichthyoses are known. X-linked ichthyosis vulgaris results from deletions of or mutations in the sterol sulfatase locus (STS) on the short arm of the X-chromosome. Mutations in keratin 1 (*KRT1*) or keratin 10 (*KRT10*) cause BCIE. Mutations in keratin 2e (*KRT2E*) are responsible for ichthyosis bullosa of Siemens. Sjögren-Larsson syndrome results from defective fatty aldehydes dehydrogenase activity (FALDH). Mutations in transglutaminase 1 (*TGM1*) cause lamellar ichthyosis/nonbullous congenital ichthyosiform erythroderma in some families. Netherton disease results from mutations in *SPINK5*, a gene that encodes a serine protease inhibitor. Refsum disease is caused by mutations in *PAHX*, which result in defective phytanoyl-CoA hydroxylase activity. X-linked chondrodysplasia punctata is caused by mutations in a gene (*EBP*) that produces an emopamil-binding protein.

DIAGNOSIS: Correct diagnosis requires a careful physical examination, a detailed family history, and knowledge about the associated features of the disorder. Microscopic examination of hair may be required. Skin biopsy for either light microscopic or electron microscopic examination or both may be required. Referral to a dermatologist is usually necessary because diagnosis can be difficult. Molecular diagnosis is clinically indicated in only a minority of conditions and instances. Fluorescent *in situ* hybridization for the STS locus is a useful and easily obtained cytogenetic examination when X-linked ichthyosis vulgaris is suspected.

TREATMENT
Standard Therapies: Treatment for the ichthyoses is varied and usually nonspecific. Topical agents that can help to reduce scale and improve hydration of the skin include standard emollients such as petroleum jelly, topical lotions and creams that contain urea, and topical agents that include α-hydroxy acids, such as lactic and glycolic acids. Scalp involvement may require the use of keratolytic agents such as salicylic acid. For more severe ichthyoses, the oral retinoids can be helpful. Monitoring for secondary infection and appropriate treatment with topical or oral antibiotics or antifungals is important. Referral to both dermatology and to medical genetics should be part of the routine evaluation and care of an individual with a suspected ichthyosis.

REFERENCES
Hernandez-Martin A, Gonzalez-Sarmiento R, De Unamuno P. X-linked ichthyosis: an update. *Br J Dermatol* 1999;141:617–627.
McGrath JA, Eady RA. Recent advances in the molecular basis of inherited skin diseases. *Adv Genet* 2001;43:1–32.
Sybert VP. *Genetic skin disorders.* New York: Oxford University Press, 1997:5–39, 105–128.
Traupe H. *The ichthyoses: a guide to clinical diagnosis, genetic counseling, and therapy.* New York: Springer-Verlag, 1989.

RESOURCES
162, 325, 351

---

31 Incontinentia Pigmenti

Jerome L. Gorski, MD

DEFINITION: Incontinentia pigmenti (IP) is a multisystemic genetic disorder affecting the skin, hair, teeth, and central nervous system (Insert Fig. 19).

SYNONYMS: Bloch-Siemens-Sulzberger syndrome; Bloch-Sulzberger syndrome; Bloch-Siemens incontinentia pigmenti melanoblastosis cutis linearis; Pigmented dermatosis, Siemens-Bloch type.

DIFFERENTIAL DIAGNOSIS: Bacterial vesicular infections; Congenital varicella; Epidermolysis bullosa; Letterer-Siwe disease; Congenital reticulohistiocytosis; Focal dermal hypoplasia; Hypomelanosis of Ito; X-linked chondrodysplasia punctata; Incontinentia pigmenti achromians; Franceschetti-Jadassohn syndrome.

SYMPTOMS AND SIGNS: The disease is characterized by progressive dermatologic abnormalities that occur in four stages, which may overlap. The first stage is present at birth or appears during early infancy and consists of redness or inflammation of the skin and blisters. In the second stage, the blisters develop a raised, wartlike appearance, and pustule-like lesions may develop scabs or thick crusts and/or areas of increased pigmentation. In the third stage, which usually occurs at 6–12 months of age, some regions of the skin appear hyperpigmented in a swirled pattern. In the fourth stage, scarring appears. Additional multisystemic abnormalities occur in at least 80% of individuals with IP. More than 65% have dental abnormalities, and approximately 35% have ocular abnormalities. Abnormal growth of blood vessels in the retina typically appears before the age of 5. Other ocular abnormalities may include strabismus, microphthalmus, and optic nerve atrophy. Severe neurologic complications and mental retardation can occur.

ETIOLOGY/EPIDEMIOLOGY: The disorder is inherited as a dominant X-linked trait. It is genetically heterogeneous with two forms: type 1 and type 2. More than 600 cases are reported in the literature. Because the presence of the gene in a male fetus usually results in a second trimester miscarriage, females are affected almost exclusively.

DIAGNOSIS: The clinical diagnosis is based on the presence of the characteristic dermatologic findings and of associated physical abnormalities. A demonstrated X-linked pattern of inheritance helps confirm the diagnosis, as does a skin biopsy.

TREATMENT

Standard Therapies: Babies born with IP must have an eye examination by an experienced pediatric ophthalmologist, and examinations should be performed every few months for the first 3 years of life. Dental abnormalities can often be treated effectively. Hair problems may require a dermatologist. Neurologic symptoms such as seizures, muscle spasms, or mild paralysis may be controlled with various drugs and/or medical devices. Any skeletal anomalies should be addressed on an individual basis. Other treatment is symptomatic and supportive. Skin abnormalities associated with IP typically do not require therapy and usually resolve spontaneously by adolescence or adulthood. Genetic counseling should be provided.

Investigational Therapies: Research is ongoing to characterize NEMO mutations that cause incontinentia pigmenti type II, and to isolate the gene responsible for incontinentia pigmenti type I.

REFERENCES
Gorski JL, Burright EN. The molecular genetics of incontinentia pigmenti. *Semin Dermatol* 1993;12:255–265.
Gorski JL, et al. Cosmids map two incontinentia pigmenti type 1 (Ip1) translocation breakpoints to a 180 Kb region within a 1.2 Mb YAC CONTIG in Xp11.21. *Genomics* 1996;35:338–345.
International Incontinentia Pigmenti (IP) Consortium. Genomic rearrangement in NEMO impairs Nf-κb activation and is a cause of incontinentia pigmenti. *Nature* 2000;405:466–472.
Makris C, et al. Female mice heterozygous for IKKΓ/MENO deficiencies develop a dermatopathy similar to the human X-linked disorder incontinentia pigmenti. *Mol Cell* 2000;5:969–979.
Schmidt-Supprian M, et al. NEMO/IKKγ-deficient mice model incontinentia pigmenti. *Mol Cell* 2000;5:981–992.

RESOURCES
194, 360

32 Keratitis-Ichthyosis-Deafness Syndrome

Michael A. Del Torto, MD, and Mervyn L. Elgart, MD

DEFINITION: Keratitis-ichthyosis-deafness (KID) syndrome is a congenital syndrome characterized by vascularizing keratitis that results in visual impairment; cutaneous ichthyosis presenting as a generalized fine scale with follicular-plugging, hyperkeratotic plaques on the cheeks and chin, and a thick, leathery hyperkeratosis of the palms and soles; and neurosensory deafness (Insert Fig. 20). Half of affected patients also get frequent, severe skin infections.

DIFFERENTIAL DIAGNOSIS: Hereditary hypohydrotic ectodermal dysplasia; Keratosis follicularis spinulosa decalvans.

SYMPTOMS AND SIGNS: Patients with KID syndrome may have skin symptoms including the following: (a) generalized, fine, dry scales and follicular hyperkeratotic spines; (b) sharply demarcated, erythematous, hyperkeratotic plaques located on the earlobes, cheeks, nose, and chin; (c) hyperkeratotic plaques over the elbows, knees, and dorsa of the hands and feet; (d) palmoplantar hyperkeratosis with a leatherlike appearance, or multiple hyperkeratotic spines with a velvety or verrucous appearance; (e) recurrent bacterial and fungal infections; and, rarely, (f) squamous cell carcinoma. Patients may also have partial or complete hair loss on the scalp, eyebrows, and eyelashes, and dystrophic nail changes including hyperkeratosis, leukonychia, dysplasia, and aplasia. Other signs include leukokeratosis, scrotal tongue, and dental abnormalities, including small malformed teeth and increased caries; neurosensory deafness, which is usually present at birth; progressive vascularizing keratitis; and corneal inflammation and progressive corneal neovascularization with pannus formation, resulting in photophobia, corneal ulcers, and opacification that may progress to blindness.

ETIOLOGY/EPIDEMIOLOGY: The etiology of KID syndrome is unknown. Approximately 30 cases have been reported, with an equal prevalence in males and females. The syndrome is present at birth. It typically occurs as an isolated case, and a sporadic new mutation is the most likely explanation, although autosomal-dominant transmission has been reported in a few cases.

DIAGNOSIS: The diagnosis is made clinically based on the presence of all three features (vascularizing keratitis, cutaneous ichthyosis, and deafness). No diagnostic laboratory test exists, and skin biopsies of involved areas are nonspecific.

TREATMENT

Standard Therapies: No known cure for KID syndrome exists; however, emollients and keratolytic agents combined with topical antibiotic and antifungal agents can provide symptomatic relief. Oral retinoids have been shown to be of some benefit in improving the skin lesions, but they have been reported to exacerbate eye lesions and to cause other adverse effects such as dryness of the skin and lips, photosensitivity, elevated serum triglycerides, and premature epiphyseal closure. The disease is best managed with a multidisciplinary approach. Patients should be referred to a dermatologist for symptomatic relief of their skin disease and for skin cancer surveillance, and referred to an ophthalmologist for lifelong eye examinations. The visual acuity of some patients has improved after superficial keratectomy. In addition, patients should be referred to an otolaryngologist to test for neurosensory deafness.

REFERENCES

Ghadially R, Chong LP. Ichthyosis and hyperkeratotic disorders. *Dermatol Clin* 1992;10:597–607.

Langer K, Konrad K, Wolf K. Keratitis, ichthyosis and deafness (KID)-syndrome: report of three cases and a review of the literature. *Br J Dermatol* 1990;122:689–697.

Nazzaro V, Blanchet-Bardon C, Lorette G, et al. Familial occurrence of KID (keratitis, ichthyosis, deafness) syndrome. *J Am Acad Dermatol* 1990;23:385–388.

Skinner BA, Greist MC, Norins AL. The keratitis, ichthyosis, and deafness (KID) syndrome. *Arch Dermatol* 1981;117:285–289.

Spitz JL. KID syndrome. In: *Genodermatoses: a full-color clinical guide to genetic skin disorders.* Baltimore: Williams & Wilkins, 1996:26–27.

RESOURCES

162, 351, 355

---

33   Leiner Disease

Martin Braun, MD, and Mervyn L. Elgart, MD

DEFINITION: Leiner disease is a congenital disease characterized by severe generalized seborrhealike dermatitis, exfoliative erythroderma, diarrhea, failure to thrive, wasting, and recurrent infections in infancy, which is believed to be the result of multiple immunologic deficiencies.

SYNONYMS: Syndrome of erythroderma; Failure to thrive; Diarrhea in infancy.

DIFFERENTIAL DIAGNOSIS: Atopic dermatitis; Seborrheic dermatitis; Multiple carboxylase deficiency; Psoriasis; SCID.

SYMPTOMS AND SIGNS: Within the first weeks to months of life, infants with Leiner disease develop severe seborrheic dermatitis of the scalp and flexural areas. These areas progressively worsen, and an affected infant may become intensely erythrodermic with profuse desquamation. Heavy crusting develops in all affected areas. The patient may have severe diarrhea or projectile vomiting. Dehydration, wasting, and failure to thrive may ensue. Gram-negative skin infections and sepsis are common. Death may occur in severe or untreated cases, usually as a result of infection.

ETIOLOGY/EPIDEMIOLOGY: Leiner disease was once believed to be a severe variant of seborrheic dermatitis, but is now believed to be a clinical phenotype that is the result of multiple immunodeficiencies. Autosomal-recessive and autosomal-dominant cases have been reported. Immunologic abnormalities may include yeast opsonification defect with C5 dysfunction, impaired deposition of C3b/C3bi, increased serum IgE with impaired neutrophil mobility, and hypogammaglobulinemia. Nutritional deficiencies may also be significant.

DIAGNOSIS: Diagnosis of Leiner disease is made on the basis of clinical manifestations and evidence of immunodeficiency. Laboratory assessment should include complement levels, immunologlobulin levels, and bacterial cultures.

TREATMENT

Standard Therapies: Management of the underlying immunodeficiency is crucial. Patients may require multiple transfusions of fresh plasma. Treatment of the skin involves topical emollients to prevent further dehydration and reduce the risk of infection. Topical corticosteroids are also beneficial. The patient should be closely monitored for signs of infection, and antibiotics should be started promptly when infection is suspected. Fluid replacement and nutritional supplements are also needed to prevent severe dehydration and wasting.

REFERENCES

Glover MT, Atherton DJ, Levinsky RJ. Syndrome of erythroderma, failure to thrive, and diarrhea in infancy: a manifestation of immunodeficiency. *Pediatrics* 1988;81:66,72.

Hurwitz S. *Clinical pediatric dermatology,* 2nd ed. Philadelphia: WB Saunders, 1993.

Spitz JT. *Genodermatoses.* New York: Williams & Wilkins; 1996.

RESOURCE

351

34   LEOPARD Syndrome

Mona S. Foad, MD,
and Mervyn L. Elgart, MD

DEFINITION: LEOPARD syndrome (LS) is an autosomal-dominant disorder characterized by many findings, reflected in the acronym: Lentigines; Electrocardiograph conduction abnormalities; Ocular hypertelorism; Pulmonary stenosis; Abnormal genitalia; Retardation of growth; Deafness, sensorineural.

SYNONYMS: Multiple lentigines syndrome; Moynahan syndrome; Cardiomyopathic lentiginosis; Lentiginosis profusa syndrome; Cardiocutaneous lentiginosis syndrome; Centrofacial lentiginosis.

DIFFERENTIAL DIAGNOSIS: Carney complex; Peutz-Jeghers syndrome; Noonan syndrome.

SYMPTOMS AND SIGNS: Lentigines are the most common manifestations of LS. They are characteristically dark brown, irregularly shaped macules, which usually develop in infancy or childhood, and are mainly found on the upper trunk and neck, but can also be found on the face, palms, soles, genitalia, and sclera. Café-au-lait macules, axillary freckling onychodystrophy, and hyperelastic skin may also be present.

Patients have conduction defects and abnormalities in cardiac structure. The most common electrocardiographic change is left axis deviation; other conduction defects include prolonged P-R intervals, ventricular conduction delay, left anterior and posterior hemiblock bundle branch block, and complete heart blocks. Hypertrophic obstructive cardiomyopathy is the most common anatomic abnormality, whereas subaortic stenosis is the most common valvular defect.

Patients may have characteristic facies, with ocular hypertelorism, low-set ears, frontal bossing, and epicanthal folds. One third of patients have short stature, and many develop skeletal abnormalities ranging from pectus excavatum or carinatum to winged scapula, scoliosis, rib abnormalities, supernumerary teeth, and retarded bone age. Mild mental retardation and sensorineural deafness are the most common neurologic abnormalities; others include abnormal electroencephalographic results, seizure disorder, nystagmus, and partial agenesis of the corpus callosum. Abnormalities in genitalia occur in 25% of patients, mostly men, and include bilateral or unilateral cryptorchidism, small penile size, and hypospadias. Female patients may have absent or hypoplastic ovaries or delayed menses. Endocrinologic abnormalities include hypothyroidism and delayed puberty.

ETIOLOGY/EPIDEMIOLOGY: LS is an autosomal-dominant disorder. It is believed that a defect in the function and development of embryonic neural crest cells leads to the cutaneous, neurologic, and cardiac defects associated with LS.

DIAGNOSIS: Most patients only have three to five of the characteristic clinical findings. A set of diagnostic criteria was proposed that divides the various abnormalities into categories: lentigines; cutaneous; cardiac; genitourinary; skeletal; endocrine; neurologic; short stature; cephalofacial dysmorphisms; and family history with autosomal inheritance. A patient is diagnosed with LS if he has lentigines and features in two separate categories, or if he does not have lentigines but has features in three separate categories and an immediate relative with LS.

TREATMENT

Standard Therapies: Therapy is directed toward screening patients for abnormalities and correcting life-threatening defects. All patients should undergo full neurologic and cardiac evaluation. Patients with hypertrophic obstructive cardiomyopathy and outlaw obstruction should be counseled to avoid strenuous exercise. In certain cases, the use of β-blockers and calcium channel blockers or surgical intervention may be warranted. Electrocardiographic abnormalities can be treated with antiarrhythmics.

REFERENCES

Arnsmeier SI, Paller AS. Pigmentary anomalies in the multiple lentigines syndrome: is it distinct from LEOPARD syndrome? *Pediatr Dermatol* 1996;13:100–104.

Bonioli E, Di Stefano A, et al. Partial agenesis of corpus callosum in LEOPARD syndrome. *Int J Dermatol* 1999;38:855–862.

Jozwiak S, Schwartz RA, Janniger CK. LEOPARD syndrome (cardiocutaneous lentiginosis syndrome). *Cutis* 1996;57:208–214.

Jozwiak S, Schwartz RA, Janniger CK, et a1. Familial occurrence of the LEOPARD syndrome. *Int J Dermatol* 1998;37:37–51.

Woywodt A, Wetzel J, et al. Cardiomyopathic lentiginosis/LEOPARD syndrome presenting as sudden cardiac arrest. *Chest* 1998;113:1415–1417.

RESOURCES

113, 188, 253

---

35   Lichen Planus

Barry D. Goldman, MD

DEFINITION: Lichen planus is an inflammatory disorder that can involve the skin, mucous membranes, and nails (Insert Fig. 21). Lichen planus is often denoted by the "five Ps": purple, polygonal, pruritic, planar, and papules.

SYNONYMS: Lichen planopilaris; Lichen nitidus.

DIFFERENTIAL DIAGNOSIS: Psoriasis; Lupus erythematosus; Prurigo nodularis; Lichen amyloidosis.

SYMPTOMS AND SIGNS: The cutaneous eruption usually consists of symmetric violaceous, flat-topped, polygonal papules. Lesions are often covered with lacy white scales called Wickham striae. Common locations include the wrists, ankles, and penis. Pruritus may range from mild to severe. Lesions often appear abruptly over a period of weeks. The skin of the face is usually spared. Oral lesions show white reticulated patches along the buccal mucosa. Occasionally, erosive lesions are seen on the tongue and genitals. Oral involvement is the sole manifestation in 15%–25% of patients. On the scalp, lichen planopilaris appears as erythematous papules with scarring of hair follicles. Lichen nitidus appears as asymptomatic monomorphic flesh-colored minute papules. Nails may show longitudinal ridging, pterygium formation, or loss of nails.

ETIOLOGY/EPIDEMIOLOGY: The cause is unknown. Infections such as hepatitis C virus have been implicated. Drugs such as β-blockers and antimalarials have been linked to a lichen planus–like eruption. Oral lichenoid drug eruptions related to dental materials such as mercury or gold have occurred. The exact incidence of lichen planus is unknown. Estimates range from 0.14% to 0.88% of the population. Most cases occur in individuals between the ages of 30 and 60. No racial predilection has been observed. Lichen nitidus is more common in blacks and children.

DIAGNOSIS: The diagnosis can be made on clinical grounds given the characteristic appearance and distribution of the lesions. Skin biopsy is useful to confirm the diagnosis, because the histology of lichen planus is distinctive. Biopsy will show liquefaction degeneration of the basal cell layer of the epidermis and a bandlike mononuclear cell dermal infiltrate. No specific laboratory abnormalities have been identified.

TREATMENT

Standard Therapies: Lichen planus is a benign disease; treatment must be tailored to the patient. Spontaneous remission can be expected in most patients after 15 months. Topical corticosteroid creams are the mainstay of treatment. Flurandrenolone tape can be applied to hypertrophic lesions. Persistent lesions can be injected with kenalog or triamcinolone solution. Oral lesions may respond to topical corticosteroids in a gel form or an oral base. Cyclosporine (500 mg/5 mL) rinses have been used for oral lesions. Topical anesthetics such as dyclonine or viscous lidocaine can reduce pain on eating. Replacement of amalgam or gold dental material has been helpful in some cases. Occasionally, squamous cell carcinoma has developed in persistent oral lesions (average 7 years). Oral prednisone over a 6-week course is effective for generalized disease. Acitretin is also effective. Other agents that have demonstrated variable efficacy include griseofulvin, antimalarials, and systemic cyclosporine.

REFERENCES
Boyd AS, Nelder KH. Lichen planus. *J Am Acad Dermatol* 1991;
    25:593–619.
Cribier B, et al. Treatment of lichen planus: an evidence-based
    medicine analysis of efficacy. *Arch Dermatol* 1998;134: 1521–
    1530.

Silverman S Jr, et al. A prospective study of findings and manage-
    ment in 214 patients with oral lichen planus. *Oral Surg Oral
    Med Oral Pathol* 1991;72:665.

RESOURCE
360

36   Lichen Sclerosis

Barry D. Goldman, MD

DEFINITION: Lichen sclerosis is a chronic inflammatory skin disorder characterized by white atrophic plaques, primarily on the genitals.

SYNONYMS: Balanitis xerotica obliterans; Lichen sclerosis et atrophicus; Kraurosis vulvae.

DIFFERENTIAL DIAGNOSIS: Lichen planus; Vitiligo; Lichen simplex chronicus; Morphea.

SYMPTOMS AND SIGNS: Shiny white atrophic plaques on the genitals are characteristic. The most common complaint is pruritus, although many patients are asymptomatic. Lesions appear as well-defined atrophic pink to depigmented plaques. Erosions, fissures, purpura, and scarring are common. The lesions in girls may be confused with signs of sexual abuse. Lesions may progress into porcelain white plaques. In women, the lesions may appear in a figure-of-eight pattern around the vulva and anus. The disease can lead to resorption of the clitoris and labia minora, leading to dyspareunia. End-stage disease can cause vaginal stenosis. Malignant degeneration occurs in up to 5% of cases. In particular, any eroded or warty vulor penile lesion should be carefully followed for evolution of a squamous cell carcinoma. Penile lesions are more commonly found in uncircumcised men and can lead to fusion of the foreskin and glans penis. Lesions are rarely found elsewhere on the body (extragenital lichen sclerosis).

ETIOLOGY/EPIDEMIOLOGY: The cause is unknown. The disease is more common in women, by a ratio of 6:1. It is found in prepubertal girls and postmenopausal women, suggesting that a hypoestrogenic state is necessary. An increased rate of autoantibodies and an increased incidence of autoimmune disease occur. A few familial cases have been found. The disease appears to be more common in caucasians. One study of adult women ages 50–59 found an incidence of 14 per 100,000 per annum.

DIAGNOSIS: The diagnosis can be made on clinical grounds. A skin biopsy is recommended. The histology of lichen sclerosis is well defined by epidermal atrophy and dermal sclerosis.

TREATMENT
Standard Therapies: Consultation with a vulor dermatology clinic is recommended. High-potency topical steroids such as clobetasol cream for several months are proven effective. Topical medication must be carefully applied to avoid steroid atrophy of adjacent normal skin. Alternatives include topical estrogen and progesterone creams. Testosterone creams are ineffective. Oral retinoids have been used but have numerous side effects. Oral antihistamines and tricyclic antidepressants have been helpful for pruritus. Circumcision in men can be curative in some cases. Surgery in women depends on the degree of scarring.

REFERENCES
Dalziel KL, Wojnarowska F. Long-term control of vulval lichen
    sclerosis after treatment with a potent topical steroid cream. *J
    Reprod Med* 1993;38:25–27.
Meffert JJ, Davis BM, Grinwood RE. Lichen sclerosis. *J Am Acad
    Dermatol* 1995;32:393–416.
Nasca MR, Innocenzi D, Micali G. Penile cancer among patients
    with genital lichen sclerosis. *J Am Acad Dermatol* 1999;
    41:911–914.
Powell JJ, Wojnarowska F. Lichen sclerosis. *Lancet* 1999;353:
    1777–1783.

RESOURCES
27, 339, 360

37   McGrath Syndrome

John A. McGrath, MD, MRCP, and Andrew P. South, MD

DEFINITION: McGrath syndrome is a genetic disorder resulting from inherited abnormalities in a structural component of desmosomes. Changes are most prominent in the skin, where loss of adhesion between keratinocytes leads to epidermal fragility that is particularly evident around the mouth and on the palms and soles.

SYNONYM: Skin fragility–ectodermal dysplasia syndrome.

DIFFERENTIAL DIAGNOSIS: Epidermolysis bullosa; Staphylococcal scalded skin syndrome; Bullous congenital ichthyosiform erythroderma.

SYMPTOMS AND SIGNS: The skin changes include erosions, scaling, and fissures, as well as alopecia, nail dystrophy, and palmoplantar hyperkeratosis. Neonates have an inflammatory desquamative rash that resembles a superficial bacterial infection. During infancy, persistent perioral fissures and inflammation occur, as do patches of scale-crust formation. The fissures on the palms and soles are painful and may impede development of motor skills and mobility. Hair at all body sites typically remains sparse or absent. Other features may include impaired sweating, dental abscesses, and astigmatism. Affected children are often small (below the 3rd percentile) but grow normally.

ETIOLOGY/EPIDEMIOLOGY: McGrath syndrome is caused by inherited mutations that result in total ablation of the protein plakophilin 1. It was first described in 1997, and only 5 cases have been reported. Plakophilin 1 is a structural component of desmosomes, and its distribution is mainly confined to the epidermis, where it has a role in stabilizing adhesion between differentiating keratinocytes. An absence of plakophilin causes the keratinocytes to separate, resulting in skin blisters or erosions. Plakophilin 1 is also expressed in the nuclei of several cells, and it may have an additional role in signal transduction and in epidermal development and morphogenesis. This may explain why patients with mutations in plakophilin 1 also have features of an ectodermal dysplasia syndrome with alopecia, nail dystrophy, and, to a variable extent, impaired sweating.

DIAGNOSIS: Clinically, the diagnosis may be suspected in neonates with congenital skin fragility in which the pattern of skin erosions seems more superficial than is typical for epidermolysis bullosa. The marked inflammation and cracking of the lips and around the mouth is also a classic feature. Primary bacterial infection should be excluded through skin swabs. Biopsy of skin adjacent to an area of scale-crust is the most useful test, particularly if the sample is examined by electron microscopy and immunofluorescence microscopy.

TREATMENT

Standard Therapies: No effective therapy for McGrath syndrome exists. Treatment is supportive. In neonates, attention should be given to fluid balance, thermoregulation, and prevention of secondary infection. In infants, protecting the hands and feet from trauma may reduce pain and help mobility. Growth and development should be monitored and regular ophthalmic and dental reviews encouraged. General skin care may include use of emollients, mild keratolytic agents, and intermittent antiseptic soaks for cracked palms and soles.

REFERENCES

McGrath JA. A novel genodermatosis caused by mutations in plakophilin 1, a structural component of desmosomes. *J Dermatol* 1999;26:764–769.

McGrath JA, Hoeger PH, Christiano AM, et al. Skin fragility and hypohidrotic ectodermal dysplasia resulting from ablation of plakophilin 1. *Br J Dermatol* 1999;140:297–307.

McGrath JA, McMillan JR, Shemanko CS, et al. Mutations in the plakophilin 1 gene result in ectodermal dysplasia/skin fragility syndrome. *Nat Genet* 1997;17:240–244.

Whittock NV, Haftek M, Angoulvant N, et al. Genomic amplification of the human plakophilin 1 gene and detection of a new mutation in ectodermal dysplasia/skin fragility syndrome. *J Invest Dermatol* 2000;115:368–374.

RESOURCES

360, 402

38   Meleda Disease

David P. Kelsell, BSc, MD, PhD,
and Irene M. Leigh, MD, PhD

DEFINITION: Meleda disease is a complex keratoderma characterized by hyperhidrosis, perioral erythema, and a diffuse "glove and stocking" keratoderma.

SYNONYMS: Keratosis palmplantaris; Transgrediens of Siemans.

DIFFERENTIAL DIAGNOSIS: Many of the other simple and complex palmoplantar keratodermas, including Papillon-Lefevre.

SYMPTOMS AND SIGNS: The disease manifests at birth or in early infancy. Symptoms and signs include the following: symmetric diffuse palmoplantar keratoderma and transgressive pachyderma of the palm and sole, often including the back of the hand and foot, giving a glove and stocking appearance; brachydactyly; nail abnormalities such as fragility and spoon-shaped nails; hyperhidrosis and susceptibility to infection, resulting in a malodorous maceration; and perioral erythema. Histologic features of affected epidermis include acanthosis, thickened stratum corneum, increased granular layer, and evidence of mild dysplasia of the basal layer. No epidermolysis is present. Sweat glands are reported to be doubled in size.

ETIOLOGY/EPIDEMIOLOGY: Meleda disease is inherited as an autosomal-recessive disorder and is due to mutations in the gene encoding *SLURP1*, which is located on chromosome 8q24.3. The protein is believed to be involved in cell signaling and adhesion. The disease was originally observed in 1826 on the island of Meleda, Yugoslavia, where the prevalence is reported to be 1 in 100,000. Elsewhere, it has been reported in a few families of Algerian and Croatian ethnicity.

DIAGNOSIS: The diagnosis depends on finding the combination of a distinctive perioral erythema with a hyperhidrotic keratoderma including transgrediens spread. The histopathologic and electron miscroscopic changes are not distinctive. Morphologic studies can exclude epidermolytic hyperkeratosis only. A molecular diagnosis would be the optimal way to define the syndrome, but biologic heterogeneity cannot be excluded.

TREATMENT
Standard Therapies: Many hyperhidrotic keratodermas become secondarily superinfected with dermatophytes and improve substantially on a course of treatment with oral terbinafine and topical antifungal agents. The hyperhidrosis may be helped by use of aluminum acetate soaks or aluminum chloride hexahydrate applications. Keratolytics are likely to aggravate the maceration of the skin, and retinoids are not of substantial benefit.

REFERENCES
Bouadjar B, Benmazouzia S, Prud'homme JF, et al. Clinical and genetic studies of 3 large, consanguineous, Algerian families with mal de Meleda. *Arch Dermatol* 2000;136:1247–1252.
Fischer J, Bouadjar B, Heilig R, et al. Mutations in the gene encoding *SLURP-1* in mal de Meleda. *Hum Mol Genet* 2001;10:875–880.
Hatsell S, Kelsell D. The diffuse palmoplantar keratodermas. *Acta Dermatovenereol APA* 2000;9:47–55.

RESOURCES
351, 371

39   Mucha-Habermann Disease

Nicole Hayre, MD,
and Mervyn L. Elgart, MD

DEFINITION: Mucha-Habermann disease is classified as a type of parapsoriasis. It consists of an abrupt eruption of papulovesicles over the trunk and extremities. The exact cause of the disease is unknown, but it is believed to be the result of a hypersensitivity reaction to an infectious agent.

SYNONYMS: Habermann disease; Pityriasis lichenoides et varioliformis acuta (PLEVA); Parapsoriasis lichenoides;

Acute guttale parapsoriasis; Parapsoriasis varioliformis acuta.

DIFFERENTIAL DIAGNOSIS: Arthropod bites; Lymphomatoid papulosis; Drug eruption; Varicella; Erythema multiforme; Gianotti-Crosti syndrome; Leukocytoclastic vasculitis; Papulonecrotic tuberculid; Psoriasis; Lichen planus; Pityriasis rosea; Secondary syphilis.

SIGNS AND SYMPTOMS: Patients typically experience abrupt onset of crops of yellowish or reddish brown, round macules, papules, and occasional vesicles, which typically evolve to include blackish brown crust, necrosis, and hemorrhage. Some lesions may be covered in a micaceous crust and have a surrounding ring of erythema. The vesicles tend to be deep seated and varicelliform. After healing, the lesions usually leave atrophic, varioliform scars, which may by hypo- or hyperpigmented. The eruption typically occurs on the anterior trunk, axillae, and flexure surfaces of the extremities, and tends to spread distally. Palms and soles may be involved. There have been rare reports of mucous membrane involvement. Patients may suffer from mild constitutional symptoms, including generalized lymphadenopathy, and occasionally may complain of pruritus. Febrile ulceronecrotic Mucha-Habermann disease (FUMHD) is a severe, febrile variant of the disease, which mainly affects children. Patients have high fever, constitutional symptoms, and large, coalescing, ulceronecrotic nodules and plaques. Lesions evolve into painful ulcers with raised red borders. There may be a prodrome of mild cutaneous disease mimicking Mucha-Habermann disease before the onset of FUMHD. This variant of the disease may be the result of a severe cutaneous allergic eruption, and patients may show mild peripheral eosinophilia.

ETIOLOGY/EPIDEMIOLOGY: Mucha-Habermann disease is more common in men than in women. The disease usually affects young adults in their second or third decade of life, but may be seen at any age. There have been case reports of infants born with lesions present.

DIAGNOSIS: The clinical presentation along with a skin biopsy will confirm the diagnosis. There are no definitive laboratory tests. Skin cultures may be positive for a variety of organisms including *Staphylococcus aureus, Streptococcus pneumoniae, and Pseudomonas aeruginosa.*

TREATMENT
Standard Therapies: Mucha-Habermann disease usually resolves in several weeks to several months. In cases of more extensive disease, systematic corticosteroids may shorten the duration of the disease. Methotrexate and dapsone may also be effective. Topical corticosteroids and systematic antihistamines may ameliorate pruritus. Erythromycin is usually recommended for treatment of children. Tetracycline may be tried in adults. Ultraviolet B is also very helpful. Febrile ulceronecrotic Mucha-Habermann disease may last from 1 month to 2 years. Occasionally, it may transform into Mucha-Habermann disease before subsiding. Several fatalities have been reported; therefore, treatment is usually aggressive. Systematic corticosteroids have been reported to reduce symptoms, but not to suppress flares of the disease. Antibiotics have been used for secondary infections. Oral 4,4-diaminodiphenyl sulfone (DDS) has been used successfully. Psoralen-UA-A and methotrexate have also been tried.

REFERENCES
Hurwitz S. Clinical pediatric dermatology. In: *A textbook of skin disorders of childhood and adolescence,* 2nd ed. Philadelphia: WB Saunders, 1993:120–121.
Odom RB, James WD, Berger TG. *Andrew's diseases of the skin: clinical dermatology,* 9th ed. Philadelphia: WB Saunders, 2000:254–255.
Puddu P, Cianchini G, et al. Febrile ulceronecrotic Mucha-Habermann's disease with fatal outcome. *Int J Dermatol* 1997;36:691–694.
Tsuji T, Kasamatsu M, et al. Mucha-Habermann disease and its febrile ulceronecrotic variant. *Cutis* 1996;58:123–131.

RESOURCES
27, 351

40 Pachydermoperiostosis

Noralane M. Lindor, MD

DEFINITION: Pachydermoperiostosis is a disorder characterized by clubbing of the fingers, thickening of the skin of the face, and hyperhidrosis. It is the complete form of idiopathic primary hypertrophic osteoarthropathy (HOA).

SYNONYMS: Rosenfeld-Kloepfer syndrome; Touraine-Solente-Gole syndrome.

DIFFERENTIAL DIAGNOSIS: Acromegaly; Secondary hypertrophic osteoarthopathy; Myxedema.

SYMPTOMS AND SIGNS: Onset of symptoms is typically around puberty and progresses for approximately 10 years. Clubbing of fingers and toes; coarse facial features with thickening, furrowing, and oiliness of the facial skin; cutis verticis gyrata (furrowing of the scalp); and excessive sweating are characteristic. Radiographs show shaggy periosteal new bone formation of the distal ends of long bones and around the insertions of tendons and ligaments, which may result in pain or synovial thickening. The manifestations are more severe in males than in females. Other skin findings include papular mucinosis, keloids, cutaneous basal and squamous cell carcinomas, seborrhea, and leg ulcerations. Nonskin findings may include acrolysis, ptosis, peptic ulcer disease, Crohn disease, compressive neuropathies, and hypertrophic gastropathy. It is unclear how many of these associations are related to the HOA.

ETIOLOGY/EPIDEMIOLOGY: The cause is unknown. Abnormality of one of several serum growth factors and/or increased sensitivity to steroid hormones is suspected. Some families clearly have an autosomal-dominant genetic trait, in which males are either more severely affected or affected more frequently than females. The disorder can also be sporadic, and autosomal-recessive pedigrees have been reported.

DIAGNOSIS: Diagnosis is made clinically. Major diagnostic criteria for HOA are digital clubbing and periostosis of the tubular bones. Three incomplete forms include clubbing alone, periostosis without clubbing, and pachydermia with any of the minor manifestations of HOA (synovial effusion, seborrheic folliculitis, hyperhydrosis, hypertrophic gastropathy, and acroosteolysis).

TREATMENT
Standard Therapies: Treatment is mostly symptomatic. Surgical resection of droopy eyelids may be indicated. Oral retinoids have been helpful for skin manifestations in some patients. Colchicine and surgical denervation have been tried for bone symptoms.

REFERENCES
Martinex-Lavin M, Matucci-Cerinic M, Jajic I, et al. Primary hypertrophic osteoarthropathy: consensus on its definition, classification, assessment and diagnostic criteria. *J Rheum* 1993;20:1386–1387.
Rimoin D. Pachydermoperiostosis (idiopathic clubbing and periostosis): genetic and physiologic considerations. *N Engl J Med* 1965;272:923–931.
Rosenthal JW, Kleopfer HW. An acromegaloid, cutis verticis gyrata, corneal leukoma syndrome. *Arch Ophthalmol* 1962:68:722–726.
Touraine A, Solente G, Gole L. Un syndrome osteodermopathique: la pachydermie plicaturee avec pachyperiostose des extremities. *Presse Med* 1935;43:1820.

RESOURCE
351

41   Bullous Pemphigoid

Jean-Claude Bystryn, MD

DEFINITION: Bullous pemphigoid is an autoimmune blistering disease of the skin. It is mediated by autoantibodies directed to antigens present at the dermal-epidermal junction.

DIFFERENTIAL DIAGNOSIS: Cicatricial pemphigoid; Herpes gestationes; Epidermolysis bullosa acquisita; Pemphigus; Urticarial drug reactions; Erythema multiforme.

SYMPTOMS AND SIGNS: Bullous pemphigoid is characterized by multiple tense bullae, which arise from large, irregular urticarial plaques. It normally begins with pruritic urticarial lesions, which differ from acute urticaria in that the lesions persist at the same location for days to weeks. Lesions occur most typically on the flexural surfaces of the extremities and then on the lower torso, but in severe cases may be generalized. The disease is chronic, but the severity fluctuates. It may occur at any age, but is most common in older individuals.

ETIOLOGY/EPIDEMIOLOGY: Bullous pemphigoid is a result of an autoimmune antibody response directed to antigens of 180 and 230 kDa, denominated BP180 and BP230. These antigens are present at the dermal-epidermal junction.

DIAGNOSIS: Diagnosis is based on the clinical appearance of the eruption, the histology, and the results of special immunologic tests. Clinically, the characteristic features are tense blisters arising from an urticarial base predominantly on the flexural surface of the extremities and on the lower torso. Characteristically, multiple blisters arise from large and irregular urticarial bases. Histologically, the blisters occur at the dermal-epidermal junction. Confirmatory immunologic tests consist of demonstrating circulating antibodies directed to the dermal-epidermal junction and the presence of abnormal linear deposits of IgG, IgM, IgA, and/or complement at the dermal-epidermal junction. By immunoblotting or immunosuppression techniques, the antibodies are directed to antigens with molecular weight of 180 to 230 kDa.

TREATMENT

Standard Therapies: Primary treatment for bullous pemphigoid is systemic steroids. The dose can range from less than 20 mg/day to more than 100 mg/day. Severe and acute disease unresponsive to high doses of systemic steroids can be treated with pulse solumedrol, plasmapheresis, or intravenous immunoglobulin. Immunosuppressive agents such as azathioprine, cyclophosphamide, methotrexate, and mycophenolic acid may reduce the need for systemic steroids. Other adjuvants include dapsone and combinations of high-dose tetracycline and niacynamide.

REFERENCES

Fitzpatrick T, Eisen A, Wolff K, et al. *Dermatology in general medicine.* Vol. II. New York: McGraw-Hill, 1971:615–619.
Rook, Wilkinson, Ebling. Bullous pemphigoid. In: *Textbook on dermatology.* Vol. 6. Oxford: Blackwell Scientific, 1998:1647–1651.

RESOURCES

27, 351, 352

---

42   Cicatricial Pemphigoid

Russell P. Hall III, MD

DEFINITION: Cicatricial pemphigoid consists of a group of symptoms that include blistering and inflammation of the mucosal surfaces of the body and occasionally the skin. The most common sites of involvement are the mouth, eyes, and nose.

SYNONYMS: Benign mucosal pemphigoid; Ocular pemphigoid.

DIFFERENTIAL DIAGNOSIS: Linear IgA dermatosis; Epidermolysis bullosa acquisita; Bullous pemphigoid; Bullous lupus erythematosus; Pemphigus vulgaris; Paraneoplastic pemphigus.

SYMPTOMS AND SIGNS: Patients most often present with involvement of the oral mucosa, and often with painful, swollen red gums that bleed easily without any obvious dental disease. Other signs in the mouth include chronic, nonhealing ulcers and erosions. These can occur on the gums, cheeks, hard and soft palate, as well as in the posterior mouth and throat. Involvement of the eyes can occur alone or along with mouth involvement. Early symptoms may include chronic redness and burning of the eyes with excessive tearing and mucus. With continued disease, patients develop scarring of the eyes that can result in a turning in of the eyelids, loss of normal tear production, and damage to the surface of the eyes. Patients with severe disease are at risk for blindness. Blisters and ulcers may develop on the skin, often localized to the head and neck. Blisters and erosions can also occur in the nasal mucosa, pharynx, larynx, and upper esophagus. Lesions may occur on the external genitalia, including the glans penis and the vaginal mucosa.

ETIOLOGY/EPIDEMIOLOGY: The estimated incidence is 1 in 12,000 to 1 in 20,000, with a slight female predominance. The disease most often occurs in patients 60 years of age and older, but can occur in childhood. Cicatricial pemphigoid is an autoimmune disease that can be caused by antibodies directed against proteins found in the basement membrane of the skin and mucous membranes. These include type VII collagen, laminan 5, β-4 integrin, and bullous pemphigoid antigens. The factors that lead to the development of these autoantibodies are not fully understood, but associations with specific HLA types have been reported.

DIAGNOSIS: The diagnosis made on the typical clinical appearance along with the findings on direct immunofluorescence of a linear band of IgG and/or C3 at the basement membrane of the mucosa. Patients often do not have evidence of circulating autoantibodies on routine indirect immunofluorescence. The use of more sensitive tests such as enzyme-linked immunosorbent assays and the use of 1 *M* NaCl split-skin substrates has resulted in increased detection of circulating autoantibodies. Routine histopathology of lesions is nonspecific.

TREATMENT

Standard Therapies: Treatment is dictated by the extent and severity of the clinical disease. Mild disease localized to the mouth can often be managed with topical therapy, including the use of potent topical corticosteroids. More significant inflammatory disease often requires the use of systemic antiinflammatory and immunosuppressive agents. Systemic corticosteroids are often required. To avoid the long-term complications associated with systemic corticosteroid therapy, other steroid-sparing antiinflammatory drugs are used. Drugs such as dapsone, azathioprine, cytoxan, and mycophenolate mofetil have been used with some success. Surgical therapy may be required to improve the structural damage that can occur, especially in the eye.

Investigational Therapies: Intravenous immune globulin may be of benefit. Monoclonal antibodies directed against cell surface receptors of T and/or B cells are also being evaluated.

REFERENCES

Fleming TE, Korman NJ. Cicatricial pemphigoid. *J Am Acad Dermatol* 2000;43:571–591.
Nguyen QD, Foster CS. Cicatricial pemphigoid: diagnosis and treatment. *Int Ophthalmol Clin* 1996;36:41–60.

RESOURCES

27, 351

---

43   Pemphigus Vulgaris and Pemphigus Foliaceus

Jean-Claude Bystryn, MD

DEFINITION: Pemphigus vulgaris and pemphigus foliaceus are autoimmune, blistering diseases of the skin, which are characterized by the presence of circulating and tissue-fixed autoantibodies directed to epidermal intercellular antigens.

DIFFERENTIAL DIAGNOSIS: Bullous impetigo; Bullous pemphigoid; Other blistering diseases.

SYMPTOMS AND SIGNS: Pemphigus vulgaris usually begins with nonhealing, painful ulcers in the oral cavity. After weeks to months, bullous lesions appear on the skin. The typical lesion is a small, flaccid bullae arising from normal skin. The blisters rapidly rupture, leaving nonhealing, painful erosions. The lesions typically appear on the scalp, face, neck, and in the "V" area of the chest and back. Lesions may be present in the esophagus and in the nasal cavity, resulting in a stuffy nose and bloody mucous discharge, and pain on swallowing. Untreated, the condition normally progresses to the eventual loss of most of the epidermis, and approximately 80% of patients die within 1.5 years. Pemphigus foliaceus is characterized by small, crusted lesions on the scalp, face, chest, and back, which gradually increase in number. Untreated, the condition will gradually progress and can resemble an exfoliative erythroderma.

ETIOLOGY/EPIDEMEOLOGY: Pemphigus vulgaris and foliaceus are both caused by autoantibodies directed to keratinocyte cell-surface antigens: desmoglein-3 in pemphigus vulgaris and desmoglein-1 in pemphigus foliaceus.

DIAGNOSIS: The diagnosis is based on the clinical appearance of the eruption, histology, and results of immunologic studies. The characteristic histology of pemphigus vulgaris is an intradermal blister occurring immediately above the basal cell layer and associated with acantholytic cells. Pemphigus foliaceus has a similar histology, but the blister occurs just below the stratum corneum. In both diseases, circulating antibodies directed to epidermal intercellular antigens are usually present in the blood and fixed in the intercellular space between keratinocytes in the epidermis.

TREATMENT

Standard Therapies: Both forms of pemphigus are treated with systemic steroids. Active disease unresponsive to high doses with steroids may be treated with pulse steroids, plasmapheresis, or therapeutic intravenous gammaglobulin. Patients in whom steroids cannot be tapered without a flare in disease activity can, in addition, be treated with immunosuppressive drugs such as azathioprine, cyclophosphamide, methotrexate, or mycophenolic acid, or with immunomodulatory drugs such as gold, dapsone, or antibiotics such as tetracycline.

REFERENCES

Fitzpatrick T, Eisen A, Wolff K, et al. *Dermatology in general medicine.* Vol. II. New York: McGraw-Hill, 1971:615–619.
Rook, Wilkinson, Ebling. Bullous pemphigoid. In: *Textbook on dermatology.* Vol. 6. Oxford: Blackwell Scientific, 1998:1647–1651.

RESOURCES

27, 323, 351

44   Pityriasis Rubra Pilaris

Mervyn L. Elgart, MD

DEFINITION: Pityriasis rubra pilaris is a disease in which there is initially erythema and keratinization of follicle openings, which then progresses to scaling of the scalp and exfoliative dermatitis. The skin is usually salmon colored, and there is hyperkeratosis of the hands and feet (Insert Fig. 22).

DIFFERENTIAL DIAGNOSIS: Psoriasis.

SYMPTOMS AND SIGNS: In the juvenile type, lesions appear before the patient is 2 years old. They rarely clear (16% in 3 years) and seem to last much longer than in the adult form. In the adult form, the signs are keratinizaton of the hair follicles, exfoliative dermatitis, thickening of the palms and soles, and an unusual salmon color. Follicular plugging and acanthosis may be present. More often, alternating orthokeratosis and parakeratosis have been reported. There is almost always an area of noninvolvement on the skin. In 80% of patients, the lesions resolve spontaneously in 3 years.

ETIOLOGY/EPIDEMIOLOGY: The etiology is unknown. Biopsy findings are often inconsistent. Psoriasis may be a factor. Some cases have been associated with AIDS, and others with underlying cancer.

TREATMENT
Standard Therapies: The best results in the adult form have been with methotrexate and/or with oral retinoids. Both isotretinoin and etretinate have been successful. Long-term treatment has occasionally resulted in keratosis of the spinal ligaments. Other treatments have included cyclosporine, azathioprine, phototherapy with either UV-B or psoralen-UV-A, extracorporeal phototherapy, and high-dose vitamin A. Topical calcipitriol (calcipitriene) may be helpful.

REFERENCES
Bonomo RA, Korman N, Nagashima-Whalen L, et al. Pityriasis rubra pilaris: an unusual cutaneous complication of AIDS. *Am J Med Sci* 1997;314:118–121.
Clayton BD, Jorizzo JL, Hitchcock MG, et al. Adult pityriasis rubra pilaris: a 10-year case series. *J Am Acad Dermatol* 1997;36:959–964.
Griffiths WAD. Pityriasis rubra pilaris: the problem of its classification. *J Am Acad Dermatol* 1992;26:140–141.
Hashimoto K, Fedoronko L. Pityriasis rubra pilaris with acantholysis and lichenoid histology. *Am J Dermatopathol* 1999; 21:491–493.
Magro CM, Crowson AN. The clinical and histomorphological features of pityriasis rubra pilaris. A comparative analysis with psoriasis. *J Cutan Pathol* 1997;24:416–424.
Sanchez-Regana M, Lopez-Gil F, Salleras M, et al. Pityriasis rubra pilaris as the initial manifestation of internal neoplasia. *Clin Exp Dermatol* 1995;20:436–438.
Van de Kerkhof PC, Steijlen PM. Topical treatment of pityriasis rubra pilaris with calcipotriol. *Br J Dermatol* 1994;130:675–678.
Vanderhooft SL, Francis JS, Holbrook KA, et al. Familial pityriasis rubra pilaris. *Arch Dermatol* 1995;131:448–453.

RESOURCES
162, 360, 394

45   Pseudoxanthoma Elasticum

Daniel W. Sherer, MD, and Mark G. Lebwohl, MD

DEFINITION: Pseudoxanthoma elasticum (PXE) is an inherited disorder of elastic tissue with many associated systemic manifestations. Fragmented and mineralized elastic fibers with resulting clinical manifestations occur mainly in the skin, ocular, gastrointestinal, and cardiovascular systems. The penetrance and expressivity of the disease is widely variable.

SYNONYM: Grönblad-Strandberg syndrome.

DIFFERENTIAL DIAGNOSIS: Eruptive xanthomas; Solar elastosis; Cutis laxa; White fibrous papulosis.

SYMPTOMS AND SIGNS: Skin signs include yellowish papules in a cobblestone appearance and plaques beginning on the lateral aspect of the neck followed by occurrence on the flexural areas of the skin, most frequently the axillae and the antecubital and popliteal fossae. In more severe cases, redundant skin folds may form. Symptoms usually begin in the second decade of life, although great variability exists, and the disease is occasionally diagnosed in childhood. Eye findings include peau d'orange, a mottled appearance of the fundus, and angioid streaks. These changes occur as a result of mineralization of the elastic lamina of Bruch membrane. These ocular findings may be the only sign of the disease for years. Disciform scarring resulting from subretinal bleeding of choroidal neovascularization can lead to vision loss, although complete blindness is rare. Mineralization of the internal elastic lamina of medium-sized arteries resulting in arterial narrowing occurs frequently. Arterial narrowing can lead to asymmetric or diminished pulses in the limbs, causing intermittent claudication of the leg and arm muscles, or angina or myocardial infarction, small strokes, intestinal angina, and renovascular hypertension. Gastrointestinal bleeding is rare, and seems to predominantly affect the stomach. The cause of bleeding is not well understood. Most women with PXE have normal pregnancies, but gastric or uterine bleeding may rarely complicate a pregnancy.

ETIOLOGY/EPIDEMIOLOGY: Prevalence has been estimated to range from 1 in 25,000 to 1 in 1 million, but the true prevalence is unknown. A mutation in the gene encoding the transporter protein ABCC6 (*MRP6*) has been found on chromosome 16. Evidence suggests that PXE is inherited in an autosomal-recessive manner; however, families with two-generation involvement have been observed. Two-generation involvement may indicate pseudodominance.

DIAGNOSIS: Until a clinically reliable molecular genetic test is available, the gold standard of diagnosis is histologic examination of a skin biopsy demonstrating a positive von Kossa stain that shows calcification of fragmented elastic fibers. Some affected individuals, however, do not have skin signs. Skin and fundus examination should be performed in all first-degree relatives of affected individuals, and flexural biopsy should be considered if there is any suggestion of disease.

TREATMENT
Standard Therapies: No treatment is known. To mitigate environmental factors, the diagnosed individual should be cautioned about engaging in contact sports, avoiding platelet inhibitors, and smoking.

REFERENCES
Bergen AA, Plomp AS, Schuurman EJ, et al. Mutations in *ABCC6* cause pseudoxanthoma elasticum. *Nat Genet* 2000;25:228–231.

Le Saux O, Urban Z, Tschuch C, et al. Mutations in a gene encoding an ABC transporter cause pseudoxanthoma elasticum. *Nat Genet* 2000;25:223–227.

Lebwohl M, Neldner K, Pope FM, et al. Classification of pseudoxanthoma elasticum: report of a consensus conference. *J Am Acad Dermatol* 1994;30:103–107.

Neldner KH. Pseudoxanthoma elasticum. *Clin Dermatol* 1988; 6:1–159.

Struk B, Neldner KH, Rao VS, et al. Mapping of both autosomal recessive and dominant variants of pseudoxanthoma elasticum to chromosome 16p13.1. *Hum Mol Genet* 1997;6:1823–1828.

RESOURCES
287, 360, 410

---

46 Pyoderma Gangrenosum

*Mark G. Lebwohl, MD,
and Mona Gohara, MD*

DEFINITION: Pyoderma gangrenosum (PG) is an ulcerative skin condition in which tender pustules/nodules erode to produce a gradually enlarging ulcer with a violaceous, overhanging, irregular, often necrotic border. It is not fatal or contagious, but can be debilitating.

DIFFERENTIAL DIAGNOSIS: Malignancy (squamous cell carcinoma, verrucous carcinoma); Infection (impetigo, herpes simplex, chancroid, syphilis, tuberculosis gumma, sporotrichosis, blastomycosis, anthrax); Collagen vascular disease; Vasculitis (Wegener granulomatosis, Churg-Strauss syndrome, hypersensitivity vasculitis); Diabetes; Trauma; Insect bites; Arterial/venous insufficiency; Other miscellaneous pathologies (Behçet syndrome, antiphospholipid antibody syndrome, aphthous stomatitis, atrophie blanche, ecthyma, Sweet syndrome).

SYMPTOMS AND SIGNS: Classic PG most commonly affects the legs and is suspected when the ulcer is deep, with a necrotic base, and confined by a violaceous, irregular border. It can occur adjacent to stoma sites, called peristomal PG. Other sites are less common. Atypical PG most often involves the face, arms, or dorsum of the hands; this variant should be considered when the ulcer is superficial, with a vesicular/pustular studded border. In both variants, patients may have concurrent fever, arthralgias, and localized tenderness associated with the ulcer. PG is associated with systemic diseases in at least 50% of patients. Pathergy is the term used for PG occurring as a result of trauma; this phenomenon occurs in 30% of affected patients.

ETIOLOGY/EPIDEMIOLOGY: The etiology of PG is ambiguous. It most likely stems from some type of alteration in the equilibrium of the immune system.

DIAGNOSIS: No specific diagnostic test exists for PG. Cultures or a skin biopsy of the lesion may facilitate the diagnostic process. Additionally, blood work and investigational techniques may be used to aid in the diagnosis of those diseases associated with PG.

TREATMENT
Standard Therapies: Treatment is intended to eradicate both the cutaneous and, if it exists, the systemic component of the disease. Topical agents, most beneficial when used in conjunction with systemic treatments, include topical corticosteroids, antiseptic solutions, cromolyn sodium 2% solution, and topical tacrolimus. Systemic agents include corticosteroids (by oral administration, pulse therapy, or intralesional injection); sulfa drugs such as dap-sone; sulfasalazine (used alone or in conjunction with corticosteroids); immunosuppressives such as cyclosporine, azathioprine, and cyclophosphamide (with or without simultaneous use of corticosteroids) in cases of PG refractory to traditional treatments; other miscellaneous agents such as tacrolimus, thalidomide, chlorambucil, clofazimine, and intravenous immune globulin. Surgery should be avoided in patients with PG because of pathergy. If, however, the patient's life is endangered, as in the case of a superimposed infection progressing toward sepsis or osteomyelitis, surgical debridement should be considered. The surgical treatment of ulcerative colitis or other associated diseases may expedite convalescence.

REFERENCES
Callen JP. Pyoderma gangrenosum. *Lancet* 1998;351:581–585.
Dyall-Smith D, Marks R. *Dermatology at the millenium.* London, UK: Parthenon Publishing, 1999:535–536.
Fitzpatrick TD, Eisen A, Wolff K, et al. *Dermatology in general medicine: textbook and atlas.* New York: McGraw-Hill, 1999: 1328–1336.
Jackson MJ. Pyoderma gangrenosum. *www.emedicine.com/derm/topic367/htm*, 2000.

RESOURCES
27, 123, 351

47 Rothmund-Thomson Syndrome

Sharon E. Plon, MD, PhD, and Stephen G. Grant, PhD

DEFINITION: Rothmund-Thomson syndrome is a genetic disorder associated with abnormal skin, including a characteristic rash (poikiloderma), photosensitivity, telangiectasias, and hyperkeratosis. Other clinical features include skeletal abnormalities, short stature, sparse hair, cataracts, and an increased risk for cancer, particularly osteosarcoma.

SYNONYM: Poikiloderma congenitale.

DIFFERENTIAL DIAGNOSIS: Fanconi anemia; Bloom syndrome; Xeroderma pigmentosum; Kindler syndrome; Werner syndrome.

SYMPTOMS AND SIGNS: The most distinctive feature is the rash. Skin is typically normal at birth. The rash begins at 3–6 months as an erythematous eruption on the cheeks. It spreads to the extremities, often sparing the trunk, and enters a chronic phase that persists throughout life with areas of hyper- and hypopigmentation. Other features include alopecia including eyebrows and eyelashes, short stature, cataracts, skeletal abnormalities including hypoplastic thumbs, dysplastic teeth and nails, hypogonadism, osteosarcoma, and acral keratoses developing into squamous cell carcinoma (which may not be restricted to sun-exposed areas).

ETIOLOGY/EPIDEMIOLOGY: More than 250 cases have been reported, almost all consistent with autosomal-recessive inheritance. Different studies have demonstrated both male and female predominance. Genetic heterogeneity is suggested clinically by the variable phenotype and at a cellular level by inconsistent photosensitivity and inconsistent reports of defects in nucleotide excision repair. Mutations in a *RecQ* helicase gene (*RECQL4*) at 8q24.3 have been found in several patients, indicating similarity with other diseases associated with loss of a *RecQ* helicase activity, Bloom syndrome, and Werner syndrome. The normal function of the *RecQ* helicases includes roles in repair, replication, senescence, and cell cycle checkpoint control.

DIAGNOSIS: The diagnosis is clinical, primarily based on the characteristic features of the skin rash, including age of onset and appearance of the chronic phase. Radiographs may show skeletal defects, and an ophthalmologic examination can identify the presence of cataracts. Photosensitivity testing may be abnormal. Karyotype may show mosaic clones with abnormalities of chromosome 8 in a minority of patients. Identification of mutations in the *RECQL4* gene by DNA sequencing is offered as part of research studies. It is unknown, however, if all patients have mutations in the *RECQL4* gene.

TREATMENT
Standard Therapies: Treatment should include constant use of sunscreen and avoidance of sun exposure, as well as annual skin examinations to monitor closely for any suspicious lesions. Pulsed dye laser has been used to treat the telangiectatic component of the rash. Lifelong annual oph-

thalmologic screening for cataracts should be performed. A complete skeletal survey by age 5 is recommended as a baseline study. Prompt evaluation of any bone changes or bone pain is warranted due to the high risk of osteosarcoma in these patients.

REFERENCES
Cumin I, et al. Rothmund-Thomson syndrome and osteosarcoma. *Med Pediatr Oncol* 1996;26:414–416.
Grant SG, et al. Analysis of genomic instability using multiple assays in a patient with Rothmund-Thomson syndrome. *Clin Genet* 2000;58:209–215.
Kitao S, et al. Mutations in *RECQL4* cause a subset of cases of Rothmund-Thomson syndrome. *Nat Genet* 1999;22:82–84.
Lindor NM, et al. Rothmund-Thomson syndrome in siblings: evidence for acquired *in vivo* mosaicism. *Clin Genet* 1996;49:124–129.
Vennos E, et al. Rothmund-Thomson syndrome: review of the world literature. *J Am Acad Dermatol* 1992;27:750–762.
Wang LL, et al. Clinical manifestations of a cohort of 41 patients with Rothmund-Thomson syndrome. *Am J Med Genet* 2001 (in press).

RESOURCES
188, 351, 355

---

48 Scleromyxedema

William J. Hogan, MD, MRCPI, and Arnold L. Schroeter, MD

DEFINITION: Scleromyxedema is a chronic fibromucinous disorder associated with a monoclonal protein.

SYNONYMS: Papular mucinosis; Generalized lichen myxedematosus.

DIFFERENTIAL DIAGNOSIS: Amyloidosis; Scleroderma; Pretibial myxedema; Follicular mucinosis; Cutaneous focal mucinosis; Colloid degeneration.

SYMPTOMS AND SIGNS: Scleromyxedema can have devastating clinical manifestations, including sclerosis of the skin with progressive pharyngeal and upper airway involvement, resulting in mortality due to respiratory complications. It is usually associated with a monoclonal protein, although overt multiple myeloma is rarely present.

ETIOLOGY/EPIDEMIOLOGY: The disease affects adults 30–70 years of age, has no gender predilection, and has a

chronic course. The etiology is uncertain; however, scleromyxedema is characterized by the accumulation of mucinous material consisting of acid glycosaminoglycan in the dermal layers of the skin.

DIAGNOSIS: Dermatologic manifestations usually include a generalized papular eruption with sclerosis. The papules may be dome shaped, firm, skin colored, or erythematous and approximately 3 mm in diameter. Extensive areas of skin may be involved; there is a predilection for the face and extensor surfaces. Histologically, focal deposition of mucin occurs in the papillary and reticular dermis, with an increased number of fibroblasts. Extracutaneous involvement can include infiltration of the pharynx and the upper airway, esophageal aperistalsis, hoarseness, inflammatory polyarthritis, proximal myopathy, neurologic dysfunction, and ophthalmic abnormalities. Laboratory abnormalities usually include a monoclonal protein (classically IgG-λ, although other monoclonal proteins also occur). The role of the associated monoclonal protein in scleromyxedema has not been elucidated. Other findings may include an increased erythrocyte sedimentation rate, leukocytosis (with or without eosinophilia), albuminuria, and monoclonal plasma cell infiltration in the bone marrow.

TREATMENT

Standard Therapies: Some patients have responded to corticosteroids and single alkylating agents, particularly melphalan. Therapeutic trials of methotrexate, cladribine, and other agents such as isotretinoin, interferon-α, dimethyl sulfoxide, mucopolysaccharidases, extracorporeal photochemotherapy, plasmapheresis, and psoralen-UV-A have had variable success.

Investigational Therapies: Autologous stem cell transplantation may be effective in selected patients with scleromyxedema, but more research is required before this approach can be widely recommended.

REFERENCES

Davis LS, Sanal S, Sangueza OP. Treatment of scleromyxedema with 2-chlorodeoxyadenosine. *J Am Acad Dermatol* 1996;35: 288–290.

Dinneen AM, Dicken CH. Scleromyxedema. *J Am Acad Dermatol* 1995;33:37–43.

Harris RB, Perry HO, Kyle RA, et al. Treatment of scleromyxedema with melphalan. *Arch Dermatol* 1979;115:295–299.

Hogan WJ, Lacy MA, Schroeter A, et al. Successful treatment of scleromyxedema with autologous peripheral blood stem cell transplantation [Abstract 5353]. *Blood* 2000;96:370b.

Rayson D, Lust JA, Duncan A, et al. Scleromyxedema: a complete response to prednisone. *Mayo Clin Proc* 1999;74:481–484.

RESOURCES

27, 360

---

49   Setleis Syndrome

Caleb González, MD

DEFINITION: Setleis syndrome is an ectodermal dysplasia syndrome characterized by leonine facies with redundant periorbital skin, wide nasal bridge, "parrot beak" nose, and thickened lips; bitemporal focal lesions resembling forceps scars; sparseness or absence of the temporal third of the eyebrows; multiple rows of lashes on the upper lids; sparse or absent lashes on the inferior lids; and hypoplastic tarsal plates with absence of meibomian glands.

SYNONYM: Forceps marks syndrome.

DIFFERENTIAL DIAGNOSIS: Focal facial dermal dysplasia syndrome (FFDD).

SYMPTOMS AND SIGNS: Signs include "dry eyes" with punctate keratopathy secondary to absent lipid layer of the tears induced by the absence of the meibomian glands, hastening evaporation of tears and amblyopia secondary to high astigmatic refractive errors.

ETIOLOGY/EPIDEMIOLOGY: The etiology is unknown. The disorder is an autosomal-recessive syndrome described in both sexes with abnormalities of the facial skin and its appendages, qualifying as an ectodermal dysplasia syndrome. The families of 10 of the 13 reported patients were traced to a small northwestern area in Puerto Rico.

DIAGNOSIS: The diagnosis is made on the basis of the autosomal-recessive inheritance, characteristic facial features (especially the bitemporal skin focal lesions), hastened evaporation of the tears, and a common Puerto Rican birthplace.

TREATMENT

Standard Therapies: Treatment is restricted to ameliorating the symptoms and signs caused by the hastened evaporation of the tears with aggressive lubrication with artificial tears. It is important to perform accurate refraction and correct the common high astigmatic refractive errors to prevent ametropic or anisometropic amblyopia.

REFERENCES

Bron AJ, Mengher LS. Congenital deficiency of meibomian glands. *Br J Ophthalmol* 1987;71:312–314.

Di Lernia V, Neri I, Patrizi A. Focal facial dermal dysplasia: two familial cases. *J Am Acad Dermatol* 1991;25:389–391.

Frederick DR, Robb RM. Ophthalmic manifestations of Setleis forceps marks syndrome. *J Pediatr Ophthalmol Strabismus* 1992;29:127–129.

Marion RW, et al. Autosomal recessive inheritance in the Setleis bitemporal "forceps marks" syndrome. *Am J Dis Child* 1987; 141:895–897.

Rudolph RI, Schwartz W, Leyden JJ. Bitemporal aplasia cutis congenita: occurrence with other cutaneous abnormalities. *Arch Dermatol* 1974a;110:615–618.

Setleis H, Kramer B, Valcárcel M, et al. Congenital ectodermal dysplasia of the face. *Pediatrics* 1963;32:540–547.

RESOURCES

96, 297, 360

50   Sutton Disease

Francisco A. Ramos-Caro, MD

DEFINITION: Sutton disease consists of mucosal, recurrent, painful, large ulcerations, usually on the mouth, which heal with scarring and deformity.

SYNONYMS: Major aphthous ulcers; Periadenitis mucosa necrotica recurrens; Major recurrent aphthous stomatitis; Stomatitis necrotica; Jacobi stomatitis neurotica chronica; Mikulicz aphthae; Loblowitz ulcus neuroticum ori.

DIFFERENTIAL DIAGNOSIS: Minor aphthous ulcers; Behçet syndrome; Syphilitic chancre; Human immunodeficiency virus oral ulcerations; Traumatic ulcers; Primary herpetic stomatitis; Wegener granulomatosis; Vincent infection; Tuberculosis; Pemphigus vulgaris.

SYMPTOMS AND SIGNS: The ulceration usually starts as a small tender nodule on the oral mucosa that gradually increases in size over the course of several days. It sloughs in the center, leaving a craterlike, painful ulceration that heals in several weeks with scarring. Lesions are usually single, but several lesions may be present at the same time. Lesions can recur for years, leaving deforming scarring on the mucous membranes. The oral mucosa, including tongue, lips, palate, and throat, are the most common areas of involvement. Occasionally, similar ulcers may occur on genitalia or ocular mucosae. Patients may experience problems ingesting nourishment during acute attacks, which can be debilitating.

ETIOLOGY/EPIDEMIOLOGY: The cause of Sutton disease is unknown. Possible autoimmune process and possible association with Behçet syndrome have been considered. It can begin at any age but is more common after puberty, and it affects females more often than males (2:1).

DIAGNOSIS: The diagnosis is mostly one of exclusion. The clinical presentation of large, recurrent, scarring ulcerations is very suggestive. Biopsies of the ulcers show dense inflammatory process and fibrosis. Minor salivary glands may be infiltrated. No organisms are usually found.

TREATMENT
Standard Therapies: Treatment is difficult. Local pain control may be necessary. Good oral hygiene is important. Topical and systemic steroids are helpful. Colchicine and azathioprine have been tried.

Investigational Therapies: Thalidomide has been used in oral aphthosis, although teratogenic potential and neuropathies caused by thalidomide are important drawbacks.

REFERENCES
Brown RS, Bottomley WK. Combination immunosuppressant and topical steroid therapy for treatment of recurrent major aphthae. *Oral Surg Oral Med Oral Pathol* 1990;69:42–44.
Chung JY, Ramos-Caro FA, Ford MJ, et al. Recurrent scarring ulcer of the oral mucosa. *Arch Dermatol* 1997;133:1161–1166.
Grispan D. Significant response of oral aphthosis to thalidomide treatment. *J Am Acad Dermatol* 1985;12:85–90.
Laccourreye O, Fadlallah JP, Pages JC, et al. Sutton's disease (periadenitis mucosa necrotica recurrens). *Ann Otol Rhinol Laryngol* 1995,104:301–304.
Stanley HR. Management of patients with persistent recurrent aphthous stomatitis and Sutton's disease. *Oral Surg Oral Med Oral Pathol* 1973;35:174–179.

RESOURCES
27, 373

51   Sweet Syndrome

Michael A. Del Torto, MD, and Mervyn L. Elgart, MD

DEFINITION: Sweet syndrome is characterized clinically by sharply marginated, rapidly expanding, tender, erythematous, or violaceous plaques that typically occur on the face, neck, upper trunk, and extremities. Four subtypes of Sweet syndrome have been described: classic (71%), associated with an inflammatory disease (16%), associated with a malignancy (11%), and associated with pregnancy (2%).

SYNONYM: Acute febrile neutrophilic dermatosis.

DIFFERENTIAL DIAGNOSIS: Erythema multiforme; Erythema nodosum; Erythema elevatum et diutinum;

Leukemia cutis; Behçet disease; Bowel bypass syndrome; Pyoderma gangrenosum.

SYMPTOMS AND SIGNS: The primary skin lesion in all four subtypes is a well-demarcated, rapidly expanding, tender, red to violaceous, elevated plaque 2–10 cm in diameter. The surface of the plaque may have a "juicy" or "mammilated" appearance due to vesiculation or pustulation. The plaques are typically located on the face, neck, upper trunk, and extremities. Fever is the most common systemic finding, occurring in 50%–80% of patients. Musculoskeletal signs include arthritis, arthralgias, or myalgias. Rarely, sterile osteomyelitis may occur. Conjunctivitis or episcleritis occurs in approximately one third of cases. Aphthae occur in approximately 10% of cases associated with a hematologic malignancy and in 2%–3% of classic cases. Pulmonary infiltrates and effusions present clinically as cough, dyspnea, and pleuritic chest pain. Rarely, cardiac, renal, intestinal, and neurologic involvement may occur.

ETIOLOGY/EPIDEMIOLOGY: No cause is known. Circulating autoantibodies, immune complexes, or cytokines may play a role.

DIAGNOSIS: The presence of both major and two of the four minor accepted criteria are needed for the diagnosis. The major criteria are (a) abrupt onset of tender or painful erythematous plaques or nodules occasionally with vesicles, pustules, or bullae; and (b) predominantly neutrophilic infiltration in the dermis without leukocytoclastic vasculitis. The minor criteria are (a) preceded by a nonspecific respiratory or gastrointestinal infection or vaccination or associated with inflammatory diseases such as chronic autoimmune disorders or infections, hemoproliferative disorders or solid malignant tumors, and pregnancy; (b) accompanied by periods of general malaise and fever; (c) laboratory values during onset of erythrocyte sedimentation rate greater than 20 mm, C-reactive protein positive, segmented neutrophils greater than 70% in the peripheral blood smear, or leukocytosis greater than 8,000 (presence of 3 of 4 of these values is necessary for diagnosis); and (d) excellent response to treatment with systemic corticosteroids or potassium iodide.

TREATMENT

Standard Therapies: The standard treatment is systemic corticosteroids in doses of 40–60 mg equivalent of oral prednisone daily. Potassium iodide is also an effective treatment. Other medications include colchicines, dapsone, doxycycline, clofazimine, indomethacin, and nonsteroidal antiinflammatory drugs. Treatment should be continued for at least 2–4 weeks.

REFERENCES
Chan HL, Lee YS, Kuo TT. Sweet's syndrome: clinicopathologic study of eleven cases. *Int J Dermatol* 1994;33:425–432.
Honigsmann H, Cohen PR, Wolf K. Acute febrile neutrophilic dermatosis (Sweet's syndrome). In: Fitzpatrick TB, Eisen AZ, Wolf K, et al., eds. *Dermatology in general medicine*, 5th ed. New York: McGraw-Hill, 1999:1117–1123.
Odom RB, James WD, Berger TG. Sweet's syndrome (acute febrile neutrophilic dermatosis). In: Odom RB, James WD, Berger TG, eds. *Andrews' diseases of the skin*, 9th ed. Philadelphia: WB Saunders, 2000:155–157.
Su WPD, Liu HNH. Diagnostic criteria for Sweet's syndrome. *Cutis* 1986;37:167–174.
von den Driesch P. Sweet's syndrome (acute febrile neutrophilic dermatosis). *J Am Acad Dermatol* 1994;31:535–556.

RESOURCE
351

52　Toxic Epidermal Necrolysis

*Niknam Eshraghi, MD,
Ryan E. Stern, MD,
Lee D. Faucher, MD,
David M. Heimbach, MD,
and Nicole S. Gibran, MD*

DEFINITION: Toxic epidermal necrolysis (TEN) is an inflammatory skin disorder marked by a severe exfoliative epidermal sloughing.

SYNONYM: Lyell syndrome.

DIFFERENTIAL DIAGNOSIS: Disseminated epidermal necrosis; Erythema multiforme major; Exudativum; Staphylococcal scalded skin syndrome.

SYMPTOMS AND SIGNS: The skin of patients who develop TEN shows multiple large flaccid bullae that become confluent and are associated with erythema and purpura. The epidermis sloughs easily, exposing a raw, red dermis. Often, areas of seemingly normal epidermis can be removed by simple wiping; this is termed Nikolsky's sign. The disorder is often associated with other manifestations including fever, conjunctivitis, and oropharyngeal and rectal mucositis.

ETIOLOGY/EPIDEMIOLOGY: What precipitates such a violent skin reaction is not known, but there appears to be a cell-mediated immune response leading to rejection of the skin and mucous membranes. Although systemic diseases and viral infections have been implicated in some cases of TEN, most involve administration of medications such as antibiotics, antiseizure medications, and nonsteroidal antiinflammatory drugs. Usually, the offending drug was introduced 7–21 days prior to the onset of the symptoms. The disease process is not drug dose dependent, and discontinuation of the medication does not alter the course of the illness. With treatment in a modern burn center, mortality has decreased from up to 75% to less than 25%.

TREATMENT

Standard Therapies: Patients have a denuded dermis that is completely viable and contains skin appendages, and if meticulously protected, the injured surfaces will reepithelialize in approximately 14 days. The wounds are first treated in the operating room with removal of all loose epidermis and blisters followed by coverage with a biologic dressing such as porcine xenograft. The patients should then be placed on an air-fluidized bed to facilitate adhesion and drying of the dressing. Daily reevaluation of all surfaces with debridement and application or reapplication of the dressing should be performed. The patient should be treated in an intensive care unit with careful pulmonary and nutritional support. An ophthalmology consultation is highly suggested because patients may also have conjunctivitis. Meticulous eye care includes daily evaluation and treatment, because blindness is possible. Occasionally, patients with milder skin conditions are treated with steroids, however, the use of steroids has not been shown to reverse the process and may even adversely influence outcomes. In contrast, administration of intravenous immune globulin in the early days of the illness and plasmapheresis have shown moderate improvement in patient outcome.

REFERENCES

Heimbach DM, Engrav LH, Marvin JA, et al. Toxic epidermal necrolysis. A step forward in treatment. *JAMA* 1987;257: 2171–2175.

Honari S, Gibran NS, Heimbach DM, et al. Toxic epidermal necrolysis in elderly patients. *J Burn Care Rehabil* 2001;22:132–135.

McGee T, Munster A. Toxic epidermal necrolysis syndrome: mortality rate reduced with early referral to regional burn center. *Plast Reconstr Surg* 1998;102:1018–1022.

Murphy JT, Purdue GF, Hunt JL. Toxic epidermal necrolysis. *J Burn Care Rehabil* 1997;18:417–420.

Smoot EC III. Treatment issues in the care of patients with toxic epidermal necrolysis. *Burns* 1999;25:439–442.

RESOURCES

141, 351

Dysmorphic Disorders

1   Aarskog Syndrome

Jerome L. Gorski, MD

DEFINITION: Aarskog syndrome is an X-linked, recessive developmental disorder that primarily affects skeletal formation.

SYNONYMS: Faciogenital dysplasia; Faciodigitogenital syndrome; Aarskog-Scott syndrome.

DIFFERENTIAL DIAGNOSIS: Noonan syndrome; Robinow syndrome; LEOPARD syndrome; Pseudohypoparathyroidism; Hydantoin embryopathy.

SYMPTOMS AND SIGNS: Males with Aarskog syndrome display a characteristic set of facial and skeletal anomalies, disproportionately short stature, and mild urogenital malformations. Facial features typically include hypertelorism, ptosis, down-slanting palpebral fissures, and anteverted nose. The philtrum is commonly long and the maxilla underdeveloped. External ear anomalies include low-set ears, posteriorly rotated auricles, and thickened overfolded helixes. Growth retardation usually occurs, and affected males rarely exceed 160 cm in height. Stature is disproportionate, and the distal extremities are most severely shortened. Hands and feet are broad and short. Interphalangeal joints are typically hypermobile. Most affected males have a pectus excavatum and inguinal hernias. The scrotum typically appears bifid, and scrotal folds commonly extend ventrally around the base of the penis. Cryptorchidism is common; penile hypospadius has also been reported. Although mild to moderate mental retardation has been described, it is not a consistent feature. Affected males have delayed eruption of teeth; some have congenitally missing teeth. Cleft lip and palate and congenital heart defects may be present. Approximately half of affected males have a cervical spine abnormality such as spina bifida occulta, odontoid hypoplasia, fused cervical vertebrae, and ligamentous laxity with subluxation. Radiographic abnormalities of the hands and feet typically consist of shortened digits, hypoplasia of the terminal phalanges, clinodactyly, fusion of the middle and distal phalanges, and delayed bone maturation. Other radiographic abnormalities include maxillary hypoplasia, additional pairs of ribs and other segmentation anomalies, and calcified intervertebral disks.

ETIOLOGY/EPIDEMIOLOGY: Genetic linkage and disease-specific familial translocations mapped the Aarskog syndrome gene to the proximal short arm of the X chromosome to region Xp11.21. Mutations in the *FGD1* gene result in Aarskog syndrome. The disease occurs with an estimated frequency of 1 per 1 million in the general population; however, since mildly affected individuals may not be detected, the actual frequency may be much higher.

DIAGNOSIS: The clinical diagnosis is based on the characteristic pattern of craniofacial abnormalities, disproportionate short stature, shortening of the distal extremities, and characteristic urogenital anomalies. Radiographic studies can identify distinctive abnormalities and distinguish patients from those with conditions that mimic Aarskog syndrome. Because this is an X-linked recessive trait, a demonstrated X-linked pattern of inheritance assists in confirming the diagnosis.

TREATMENT

Standard Therapies: Therapy is directed toward the identification and treatment of associated medical problems and congenital malformations. Patients should be referred for surgical correction of common structural malformations. Ophthalmologic and dental evaluations should be performed. Because of the associated cervical spine instability, particular care should be taken to support an affected infant's head and to avoid head and cervical spine trauma. Children with joint contractures, soft tissue syndactyly, and cervical spine anomalies should be referred to the appropriate pediatric subspecialist and to physical therapy. Endocrinologic evaluations should be performed to identify children with an isolated growth hormone deficiency. Genetic counseling should be provided to patients and carrier females.

REFERENCES

Gorski JL. Aarskog-Scott syndrome. In: Scriver CR, Beaudet AL, Sly WS, et al., eds. *The metabolic and molecular bases of inherited disease,* 8th ed. New York: McGraw-Hill, 2000 (in press).

Gorski JL, et al. Skeletal-specific expression of *Fgd1* during bone formation and skeletal defects in faciogenital dysplasia (Fgdy; Aarskog syndrome). *Dev Dynamics* 2000;218:573–586.

Pasteris NG, et al. Isolation and characterization of the faciogenital dysplasia (Aarskog-Scott syndrome) gene: a putative Rho/Rac guanine nucleotide exchange factor. *Cell* 1994;79: 669–678.

Porteous MEM, Goudie DR. Aarskog syndrome. *J Med Genet* 1991;28:44–47.

RESOURCES

6, 253

2 Aase Syndrome

Anne V. Hing, MD

DEFINITION: Aase syndrome includes the clinical findings of congenital hypoplastic anemia and triphalangeal thumbs. Some do not consider Aase syndrome a distinct entity from Diamond-Blackfan anemia, a congenital hypoplastic anemia in which as many as 34% of patients demonstrate hand anomalies, of which 18% are thumb abnormalities including triphalangeal thumb (see also Diamond-Blackfan anemia).

SYNONYMS: Aase-Smith syndrome II; Anemia and triphalangeal thumb; Diamond-Blackfan anemia.

DIFFERENTIAL DIAGNOSIS: Fanconi anemia; Thrombocytopenia with absent radius; Holt-Oram syndrome.

SYMPTOMS AND SIGNS: Individuals present with hypoplastic anemia in the first year of life. The anemia is reported to be responsive to prednisone therapy and to improve with age. Skeletal findings include bilateral triphalangeal thumbs, mild radial hypoplasia, narrow shoulders, and late closure of the fontanels. Mild growth deficiency has been reported. Some patients have additional findings, such as webbed neck and cleft lip and/or palate.

ETIOLOGY/EPIDEMIOLOGY: The incidence is unknown, because only 10–12 cases have been reported. The syndrome has been reported in both males and females, including siblings. Autosomal-recessive inheritance has been proposed because of reports of siblings with the syndrome, but there is also a report of a mother and son with congenital hypoplastic anemia with radial anomalies. Most familial forms of Diamond-Blackfan anemia are autosomal dominant, with rare exceptions of families who have normal parents and two affected siblings. Mutations in the *RBS19* gene on chromosome 19q13 have been reported in some families with dominant inheritance of Diamond-Blackfan anemia. Additional families with autosomal-dominant inheritance of Diamond-Blackfan anemia have been linked to chromosome 8p23.3.

DIAGNOSIS: The diagnosis should be considered in an infant who presents with hypoplastic anemia and normal platelet and leukocyte numbers. Evaluation by a qualified pediatric hematologist is important, and studies should include peripheral blood counts and bone marrow aspirate. Specialized chromosome studies to look for increased chromosomal breakage induced by diepoxybutane and mitomycin C can differentiate the syndrome from Fanconi anemia.

TREATMENT

Standard Therapies: Improvement in the anemia may be achieved transiently or long term with steroid (prednisone) therapy. Some children require intermittent red cell transfusions. Successful bone marrow transplantation has been reported in several individuals.

REFERENCES

Ball SE, McGuckin CP, Jenkins G, et al. Diamond-Blackfan anaemia in the U.K.: analysis of 80 cases from a 20-year birth cohort. *Br J Haematol* 1996;94:645–653.

Draptchinskaia N, Gustavsson P, Andersson B, et al. The gene encoding ribosomal protein S19 is mutated in Diamond-Blackfan anaemia. *Nat Genet* 1999;21:169–175.

Gazda H, Lipton JM, Willig T-N, et al. Evidence for linkage of familial Diamond-Blackfan anemia to chromosome 8p23.3-p22 and for non-19q non-8p disease. *Blood* 2001;97:2145–2150.

Hing AV, Dowton SB. Aase syndrome: novel radiographic features. *Am J Med Genet* 1993;45:413–415.

Hurst JA, Baraitser M, Wonke B. Autosomal dominant transmission of congenital erythroid hypoplastic anemia with radial abnormalities. *Am J Med Genet* 1991;40:482–484.

Willig T-N, Niemeyer CM, Leblanc T, et al. Identification of new prognosis factors from the clinical and epidemiologic analysis of a registry of 229 Diamond-Blackfan anemia patients. *Pediatr Res* 1999;46:553–561.

Young NS, Alter BP. Clinical features of Fanconi's anemia. In: Young NS, Alter BP, eds. *Aplastic anemia: acquired and inherited.* Philadelphia: WB Saunders, 1994:281.

RESOURCES

351, 356

3 Achondroplasia Family of Skeletal Dysplasias

John M. Hicks, MD, DDS, PhD

DEFINITION: The achondroplasia family of skeletal dysplasias includes four related but distinct entities: achondroplasia, hypochondroplasia, thanatophoric dysplasia, and SADDAN dysplasia (severe achondroplasia, developmental delay, acanthosis nigricans).

SYNONYMS: Short-stature dwarfism; Lethal dwarfism; Achondroplastic dwarfism.

DIFFERENTIAL DIAGNOSIS: Other forms of osteochondrodysplasias; Osteogenesis imperfecta; Campomelic dwarfism; Achondrogenesis; Type II collagenopathies; Craniosynostoses.

SYMPTOMS AND SIGNS: Achondroplasia proper is characterized by short stature with rhizomelic limb shortening; elbow extension limitations; genu varum; trident hands; exaggerated lumbar lordosis; frontal bossing; midface deficiency; relative macrocephaly; mild thoracolumbar kyphosis; anterior beaking of first and second lumbar vertebra; and short tubular bones. Hypochondroplasia is characterized by mild features of achondroplasia; short stature with bowed lower limbs, stubby hands, and feet; typical absence of rhizomelia, mesomelia, or acromelia; bradydactyly; mild elbow extension limitation; normal cranium and facies; increased head circumference; narrow spinal canal; lumbar lordosis; and lumbar vertebra with anteroposterior pedicle shortening. Thanatophoric dysplasia is characterized by marked shortening of limbs with micromelia; relatively normal trunk length; narrow thorax with reduced thoracic cavity and short ribs; disproportionately large head; frontal bossing; protruding eyes; low nasal bridge; cloverleaf skull; and brain malformations. SADDAN dysplasia is characterized by extremely short stature; severe tibial bowing; profound developmental delay; acanthosis nigricans; and seizures and hydrocephalus development in infancy leading to severe motor and intellectual impairment.

ETIOLOGY/EPIDEMIOLOGY: Achondroplasia proper is the most common human dwarfism and has a prevalence of 1 in 15,000 to 1 in 40,000 births. Hypochondroplasia has a prevalence of 0.2 per 10,000 births. Thanatophoric dysplasia has a prevalence of 1 in 60,000 births. The prevalence of SADDAN dysplasia is unknown. Approximately 90% of cases in the achondroplasia family of skeletal dysplasias are sporadic. All of these entities are autosomal dominant with complete penetrance. Fibroblastic growth factor receptor 3 (*FGFR3*) is mutated in achondroplasia, resulting in a gain of function. This leads to premature maturation of the skeleton and cranium. The specific mutated *FGFR3* nucleotide and its resulting amino acid substitution determine the specific phenotype of the affected individual.

DIAGNOSIS: Ultrasonography may be helpful in the prenatal diagnosis of short-limbed dwarfism for achondroplasia, thanatophoric dysplasia, and SADDAN; however, hypochondroplasia will not be detected. Specific evaluation for *FGFR3* receptor mutations by molecular means is available; however, this is only performed in cases where the parents are known to have one of the achondroplasia family skeletal dysplasias or in cases of advanced parental age with ultrasonographic results indicative of potential short-limb dwarfism features.

TREATMENT
Standard Therapies: Treatment for short stature may include recombinant growth hormone for a 1- to 2-year period; limb lengthening procedures around 10 years of age; and symptomatic treatment and surgery, as necessary, for medical complications.

REFERENCES
Baitner AC, Maurer S, Gruen MB, et al. The genetic basis of the osteochondrodysplasias. *J Pediatr Orthop* 2000;10:594–605.

Cohen MM. Achondroplasia, hypochondroplasia and thanatophoric dysplasia. *Int J Oral Maxillofac Surg* 1998;27:451–455.

Hunter A, Bankier A, Rogers J, et al. Medical complications of achondroplasia: multicentre patient review. *J Med Genet* 1998;35:705–712.

Lemyre E, Azouz E, Teebi A, et al. Achondroplasia, hypochondroplasia and thanatophoric dysplasia. *Can Assoc Radiol J* 1999;50:185–197.

Vajo Z, Francomano CA, Wilkin DJ. The molecular and genetic basis of fibroblastic growth factor 3 disorders. *Endocr Rev* 2000;1:23–39.

RESOURCES
188, 247, 351

4   Acrocallosal Syndrome (Schinzel Type)

John M. Hicks, MD, DDS, PhD

DEFINITION: Acrocallosal syndrome was initially identified in 1979 with the report of a 3-year-old boy with corpus callosum absence, macrocephaly, hypertelorism, small nose, bilateral inguinal hernias, tetramelic postaxial polydactyly, great toe duplication with syndactyly, marked growth retardation, gross motor and mental retardation, recurrent infections, cyanotic spells, and seizures. The syndrome has been further defined as an autosomal-recessively inherited syndrome with an abnormality in the short arm of chromosome 12 (12p13.3-p11.2).

SYNONYMS: Agenesis/absence of corpus callosum; Mental retardation; Polydactyly; Hallux duplication syndrome; Schinzel (type) acrocallosal syndrome.

DIFFERENTIAL DIAGNOSIS: Greig cephalopolysyndactyly syndrome; Aicardi syndrome; Cerebrooculofacioskeletal syndrome; Neu-Laxova syndrome; Orofacial digital syndrome II; Pseudotrisomy 13 syndrome; Toriello-Carey syndrome; Otopalatodigital II syndrome; Da Silva syndrome.

SYMPTOMS AND SIGNS: Characteristic findings include total or partial corpus callosum agenesis; mental retardation; hypotonia; polydactyly; craniofacial dysmorphism (prominent forehead, hypertelorism and/or broad nasal bridge, short nose with anteverted nostrils, large anterior fontanel, high-arched or cleft palate, low-set/posteriorly rotated ears, macrocephaly, and epicanthal folds); inguinal hernia; umbilical hernia; seizures; tapered fingers; hypogenitalism/hypospadias in males; congenital heart defect; cystic brain malformations; syndactyly; and great toe duplication with syndactyly. Other anomalies reported include mild conductive hearing loss; bilateral sensorineural hearing loss; narrow external ear meati; preauricular skin tags; transverse palmar crease (simian); wide gap between first and second toes; hyperextensibility of fingers; metatarsus adductus; rudimentary postaxial polydactyly of hands; frequent respiratory infections; anal atresia/stenosis; diaphragm eventration; increased birth weight; small or absent thyroid/hypothyroidism; nystagmus; bipartite clavicle; cryptorchidism; and failure to thrive.

ETIOLOGY/EPIDEMIOLOGY: At least 40 cases have been reported with a male predilection. Acrocallosal syndrome is an autosomal-recessive entity with a distinct chromosomal abnormality and is not related genetically to Greig syndrome. Sporadic cases also occur. Cytogenetic and molecular studies have defined the syndrome by an inverted tandem duplication of the short arm of chromosome 12 (12p13.3-p11.2).

DIAGNOSIS: Minimal diagnostic criteria for acrocallosal syndrome are total or partial absence of corpus callosum; minor craniofacial abnormality; moderate to severe psychomotor retardation with hypotonia; and polydactyly. Chromosome analysis is confirmatory. Prenatal cytogenetic analysis of amniotic fluid and chorionic villus samples may provide diagnostic information for genetic counseling.

TREATMENT
Standard Therapies: Symptomatic treatment depends on the phenotype of the proband.

REFERENCES
Araki T, Milbrandt J. Ninjurin2, a novel homophilic adhesion molecule, is expressed in mature sensory and enteric neurons and promotes neurite outgrowth. *J Neurosci* 2000;20:187–195.
Courtens W, Vamos E, Christophe C, et al. Acrocallosal syndrome in an Algerian boy born to consanguineous parents: review of the literature and further delineation of the syndrome. *Am J Med Genet* 1997;69:17–22.
Marafie M, Temtamy S, Rajaram U, et al. Greig cephalopolysyndactyly syndrome with dysgenesis of the corpus callosum in a Bedouin family. *Am J Med Genet* 1996;66:261–264.
Rauch A, Trautmann U, Pfeiffer R. Clinical and molecular cytogenetic observations in three cases of "trisomy 12p syndrome." *Am J Med Genet* 1996;63:243–249.
Thyan B, Asku F, Bartsch O, et al. Acrocallosal syndrome: association with cystic malformation of the brain and neurodevelopmental aspects. *Neuropediatrics* 1992;23:292–296.

RESOURCES
120, 190, 368

5   Acrodysostosis

Richard C. Trembath, MD, BSc, FRCP, and Kingi Amin, MD, MB, MRCP

DEFINITION: Acrodysostosis is a skeletal dysplasia characterized by growth retardation, nasal hypoplasia, midfacial deficiency, severe brachydactyly, and varying degrees of hearing loss and mental retardation.

SYNONYM: Peripheral dysostosis associated with nasal hypoplasia and mental retardation.

DIFFERENTIAL DIAGNOSIS: Albright hereditary osteodystrophy (AHO).

SYMPTOMS AND SIGNS: Short hands with stubby fingers reminiscent of the "trident" hand in achondroplasia are a cardinal feature. They may be apparent at birth, along with similarly affected feet and toes. The forearms are also shortened. Skeletal maturation is increased, and prenatal and subsequent growth failure are constant findings. Spinal abnormalities include decreased interpedicular distance, collapsed vertebrae, and a risk of spinal stenosis. The unusual face is due to a marked nasal bony hypoplasia, anteverted nostrils, deficient columella, and maxillary hypoplasia producing a peculiar flattening of the cheeks. By contrast, the upper alveolar process is usually prominent with an abnormally large mandible. Dental malocclusion is common. The deformities are progressive during the growth period, and the skeletal abnormalities are usually symmetric. Mild to moderate mental retardation is common. Other features include recurrent otitis media and hearing loss, hypogenitalism with menstrual irregularities in females, and pigmented nevi. Arthritic changes, which may be generalized, usually occur in hands and feet and give rise to problems with manual dexterity. The range of movement in the elbows and spine may be restricted, and children tend to walk late, probably due to difficulty balancing on their short legs.

ETIOLOGY/EPIDEMIOLOGY: Most cases are sporadic. The syndrome is believed to be the result of *de novo* dominant mutations due to advanced paternal age. Autosomal-dominant transmission has been reported. No chromosomal abnormalities have been demonstrated.

DIAGNOSIS: Diagnosis is based on the characteristic clinical findings. Metacarpophalangeal pattern profile analysis of hand roentgenograms is distinctive. Severe shortening of the metacarpals, metatarsals, and phalanges occurs with prematurely fused cone-shaped epiphyses and epiphyseal stippling. The first ray in the foot may be hyperplastic. Normal results for bone metabolic tests, absence of mutations on analysis of the *GNAS1* gene on chromosome 20, and the presence of normal bioactivity of the alpha subunit of the signal transducing protein, Gs, on erythrocyte membranes help to exclude AHO.

TREATMENT
Standard Therapies: No specific therapy exists, although patients should be monitored for complications of spinal stenosis.

REFERENCES
Butler MG, Rames LR, Wadlington WB. Acrodysostosis: report of a 13-year-old boy with review of literature and metacarpophalangeal pattern profile analysis. *Am J Med Genet* 1988;30:971–980.

Hernandez RM, Miranda M, Kofman-Alfaro. Acrodysostosis in two generations: an autosomal dominant syndrome. *Clin Genet* 1991;39:376–382.

Robinow M, Pfeiffer RA, Gorlin RJ, et al. Acrodysostosis: a syndrome of peripheral dysostosis, nasal hypoplasia, and mental retardation. *Am J Dis Child* 1971;121:195–203.

Wilson LC, Oude Luttikhuis MRM, Baraitser M, et al. Normal erythrocyte membrane Gsα bioactivity in two unrelated patients with acrodysostosis. *J Med Genet* 1997;34:133–136.

RESOURCES
246, 253, 418

6   Acrogeria (Gottron Type)

Thomas Jansen, MD,
and Gerd Plewig, MD

DEFINITION: Acrogeria is a congenital disease first described in 1941 by Heinrich Gottron, who reported two siblings with atrophy of acral skin. The changes, first noticed at age 2 years, were considered a localized variant of progeria infantum, hence the name acrogeria.

SYNONYM: Gottron syndrome.

DIFFERENTIAL DIAGNOSIS: Progeria infantum (Hutchinson-Gilford syndrome); Mandibular-acral dysplasia; Ehlers-Danlos syndrome type IV.

SYMPTOMS AND SIGNS: Acrogeria (Gottron type) is characterized by an aged appearance of the skin of the face (Insert Fig. 23) and the distal parts of the extremities (Insert Fig. 24), small stature, and skeletal abnormalities. Changes are evident at birth or noted shortly afterward. Some individuals have been born prematurely. Skin changes are prominent and may be the presenting feature. The skin of the face, hands, and feet shows loss of subcutaneous tissue with atrophy, wrinkling, dryness, and hyperpigmentation. Bruising and easy laceration after minor trauma may occur. The blood vessels on the trunk are prominent, and the facies is "pinched," with prominence of the eyes. Micrognathia is a feature in some patients. Various nail abnormalities may occur, most commonly atrophy and thickening. Elastosis perforans serpiginosa has been reported in some patients. The most striking histopathologic findings are in the dermis, which is almost always atrophic, with degeneration of both collagen and elastic fibers. The subcutaneous tissue is markedly reduced. Epidermal changes are minimal and include focal hyperkeratosis, atrophy, or patchy hypermelanosis of the basal layer. Short stature is often a feature. Spina bifida, diaphyseal thinning of long bones, talipes equinovarus, and congenital dislocation of the hips may also occur. Generally, internal organs are not involved, although cardiac murmurs of atherosclerosis have been reported in a few patients.

ETIOLOGY/EPIDEMIOLOGY: Acrogeria includes several subtypes. One is acrogeria (Gottron type) caused by type III collagen deficiency, considered to be a variant of type IV Ehlers-Danlos syndrome. The second type of acrogeria affects the acral skin but as a normal consent of type III collagen. The third group has a degree of overlap with metageria (acrometageria). Inheritance is unclear because of the small number of cases. An autosomal-recessive inheritance seems likely, but there are a few reports of mother and offspring involvement, which raises the possibility of autosomal-dominant inheritance. The disorder might be semilethal in the male fetus, because a female predominance has been noted. A mutation in the *COL3A1* gene that encodes the a(I) chain of type III collagen was identified in a patient with acrogeria (Gottron type). A variety of mutations in the *COL3A1* gene were also identified in patients with type IV Ehlers-Danlos syndrome. The prevalence of acrogeria (Gottron type) is unknown. Since its description, more than 40 cases have been reported.

DIAGNOSIS: Acrogeria (Gottron type) should be suspected with premature aging of the skin that is confined to the face and extremities and has been present from birth or shortly afterward. Skin biopsy and protein chemistry analysis (reduced type III collagen) as well as molecular analysis (mutations in the *COL3A1* gene) help confirm the clinical diagnosis.

TREATMENT
Standard Therapies: There is no specific treatment.

REFERENCES
De Groot WP, Tafelkruyer J, Woerdeman MJ. Familial acrogeria (Gottron). *Br J Dermatol* 1980;103:213–221.
Gottron H. Familiäre akrogerie. *Arch Dermatol Syphilol (Berlin)* 1941;181:571–583.
Greally JM, Boone LY, Lenkey SG, et al. Acrometageria: a spectrum of "premature aging" syndromes. *Am J Med Genet* 1992;44:334–339.
Jansen T, De Paepe A, Nuytinck L, et al. *COL3A1* mutation leading to acrogeria (Gottron type). *Br J Dermatol* 2000;142:178–180.
Venencie PY, Powell FC, Winkelmann RK. Acrogeria with perforating elastoma and bony abnormalities. *Acta Derm Venereol (Stockh)* 1984;64:348–351.

RESOURCE
209

7   Adams-Oliver Syndrome

H. Melanie Bedford, MS, MD, FRCPC, and Ahmed S. Teebi, MD, FRCP(Edin)

DEFINITION: Adams-Oliver syndrome (AOS) was first described in 1945 in an individual with severe limb reduction defects and scalp and skull abnormalities.

SYNONYMS: Congenital scalp defects with distal limb reduction anomalies; Absence defect of limbs, scalp, and skull.

DIFFERENTIAL DIAGNOSIS: Amniotic band sequence.

SYMPTOMS AND SIGNS: Distal limb deficiency is the most common manifestation. Defects are typically asymmetric, with the lower limbs more frequently and severely affected than the upper limbs. Abnormalities may include hypoplastic nails, cutaneous syndactyly, bony syndactyly, transverse reduction defects, ectrodactyly, and brachydactyly. Terminal transverse reduction defects may be highly variable in severity from shortness of any digit or nail to complete absence of the hand, foot, or limb. Rarely, constriction rings may be seen. Scalp defects are the second most common anomaly. Aplasia cutis congenita (ACC) may resemble unruptured fetal membranes or may be areas of thin atrophic skin or deeper lesions that extend from the skin through the skull to the dura. Erosion of the scalp defect through the underlying skull defect into the superior sagittal sinus has resulted in life-threatening hemorrhage. Major lesions may require skin grafting. Underlying skull defects are frequent and may include thin or deficient skull bones that may be apparent in infancy as a large anterior fontanel or widely splayed sutures. Other cutaneous manifestations include cutis marmorata telangiectatica congenita and dilated, tortuous scalp veins. Vessels may also be enlarged elsewhere on the skin. Hemangiomas and varicosities can be present. Ulceration and necrosis of the skin, including the abdomen and fingertips occur. Congenital cardiac defects are present in approximately 20% of cases. Lesions include septal defects (ventricular and atrial), tetralogy of Fallot, double-outlet right ventricle, valvular lesions (pulmonary stenosis, bicuspid aortic valve), and vascular lesion (coarctation of the aorta, portal hypertension, and pulmonary hypertension). Lymphatic abnormalities occur. Some children have been reported to have intracranial anomalies such as cortical dysplasia, pachygyria, polymicrogyria, microcephaly, and encephalocele.

ETIOLOGY/EPIDEMIOLOGY: More than 125 individuals with this condition have been reported worldwide. Inheritance is autosomal dominant with decreased penetrance and variable expressivity within and between families. Sporadic cases may reflect new mutations; however, parental nonpenetrance or gonadal mosaicism cannot be excluded. Autosomal-recessive inheritance has been postulated in some cases. The precise mechanism is unknown. Many mechanisms have been hypothesized, including trauma, intrauterine compression, intrauterine infections, amniotic band sequence, vascular disruption sequence, and placental thrombosis. AOS may be the result of abnormal small vessel structures manifesting in embryogenesis. No genes have yet been identified or linked to this condition.

DIAGNOSIS: The diagnosis is made clinically based on the presence of characteristic features or more subtle manifestations in light of a positive family history. Typically, AOS is diagnosed when terminal transverse limb defects are associated with ACC. Skeletal survey for skull and limb anomalies and echocardiogram for congenital cardiac malformations may be helpful.

REFERENCES

Al-Sanna'a N, Adatia I, Teebi AS. Transverse limb defects associated with aorto-pulmonary vascular abnormalities: vascular disruption sequence or atypical presentation of Adams-Oliver syndrome? *Am J Med Genet* 2000;94:400–404.

Amor DJ, Leventer RJ, Hayllar S, et al. Polymicrogyria associated with scalp and limb defects: variant of Adams-Oliver syndrome. *Am J Med Genet* 2000;93:328–334.

Savarirayan R, Thompson EM, Abbott KJ, et al. Cerebral cortical dysplasia and digital constriction rings in Adams-Oliver syndrome. *Am J Med Genet* 1999;86:15–19.

Swartz EN, Sanatani S, Sandor FFS, et al. Vascular abnormalities in Adams-Oliver syndrome: cause or effect. *Am Genet* 1999;82:49–52.

Zapata HH, Sletten LJ, Pierpont MEM. Congenital cardiac malformation in Adams-Oliver syndrome. *J Med Genet* 1995;47:80–84.

RESOURCES

9, 75, 351

8 Allan-Herndon-Dudley Syndrome

Martin G. Bialer, MD, PhD

DEFINITION: Allan-Herndon-Dudley syndrome is an X-linked recessive condition characterized by severe mental retardation, spastic paraplegia, muscle hypoplasia, and neck drop, with elongated facies and frequent minor ear anomalies.

SYNONYM: Allan-Herndon syndrome.

DIFFERENTIAL DIAGNOSIS: Adrenoleukodystrophy; Aqueductal stenosis/MASA; Lesch-Nyhan syndrome; Ornithine transcarbamylase deficiency; Pelizaeus-Merzbacher syndrome.

SYMPTOMS AND SIGNS: Developmental delay is typically noted in the first year of life. Speech and walking develop after 2 years of age, although a few severely affected individuals never walk or talk. Height, weight, and head circumference are normal. Muscle hypoplasia is prominent, and involvement of the trapezius muscle results in neck drop in most affected men. Patients have slowly progressive spasticity, signs of which include increased deep tendon reflexes, ankle clonus, Babinski sign, ulnar deviation of wrists, and lateral deviation of great toes. Ambulatory ability decreases with age. Scoliosis and a wide shallow pectus excavatum are often seen. Testicular volumes are normal. The face is long and thin, often with minor ear anomalies, including increased length, cupping, prominent anthelix, or flattened anthelix. Drooling and dysarthria are also typical. Patient IQs have ranged from 13 to 34. Ataxia, frontal balding, bitemporal narrowing, and midface hypoplasia are sometimes noted, and contractures may develop with age. Because of the muscle hypoplasia, affected individuals often appear tall with long hands and feet, but their measurements are in the normal range.

ETIOLOGY/EPIDEMIOLOGY: Allan-Herndon-Dudley syndrome is inherited in an X-linked recessive fashion. Carrier females are asymptomatic. The gene is reported to be linked to Xq21 markers, but it has not yet been isolated.

DIAGNOSIS: Chromosomes, fragile X DNA, and metabolic testing have been normal in all affected individuals studied. The diagnosis is based on typical clinical findings and an X-linked pattern of inheritance. Mapping to Xq21 would be supportive evidence.

TREATMENT

Standard Therapies: Treatment is supportive. Two individuals with progressive foot deformity required a triple arthrodesis.

REFERENCES
Allan W, Herndon CN, Dudley FC. Some examples of the inheritance of mental deficiency: apparently sex-linked idiocy and microcephaly. *Am J Ment Retard* 1944;48:325–334.

Bialer MG, Lawrence L, Stevenson RE, et al. Allan-Herndon-Dudley syndrome: clinical and linkage studies on a second family. *Am J Med Genet* 1992;43:491–497.

Bundey S, Comley LA, Blair A. Allan-Herndon syndrome or X-linked cerebral palsy? *Am J Hum Genet* 1991;48:1214.

Lubs H, Chiurazzi P, Arena J, et al. *XLMR* genes: update 1998. *Am J Med Genet* 1999;83:237–247.

Schwartz CE, Ulmer J, Brown A, et al. Allan-Herndon syndrome. II. Linkage to DNA markers in Xq21. *Am J Hum Genet* 1990; 47:454–458.

Stevenson RE, Goodman HO, Schwartz CE, et al. Allan-Herndon syndrome. I. Clinical studies. *Am J Hum Genet* 1990;47:446–453.

RESOURCES
371, 462, 487

9 Amelogenesis Imperfecta

Jan C-C. Hu, BDS, PhD,
and James P. Simmer, DDS, PhD

DEFINITION: Amelogenesis imperfecta (AI) is a heterogeneous group of inherited defects in dental enamel formation. The malformed enamel can be unusually thin, soft, rough, and stained.

DIFFERENTIAL DIAGNOSIS: Dental fluorosis; Enamel hypoplasia secondary to systemic disease; Tetracycline staining.

SYMPTOMS AND SIGNS: The spectrum of enamel malformations observed in patients with AI is divided into three groups based primarily on the thickness and hardness of the dental enamel. Differences in these parameters are believed to reflect differences in the timing, during amelogenesis, when the disruption occurred. Flaws in the dentino-enamel junction can result in an enamel layer that shears easily from the underlying dentin. Insufficient crystal elongation leaves the enamel layer hypoplastic. The most severe form is enamel agenesis, where there is almost no clinical or radiographic evidence of enamel. The teeth are yellowish brown, rough in texture, and widely spaced. A failure to properly remove the organic matrix and promote the hardening of the enamel layer leads to hypomaturation forms of AI. The dental crowns are of normal size and contact adjacent teeth, but the mottled, brownish yellow enamel is soft and has a radiodensity approaching dentin. X-linked forms of hypoplastic and hypomaturation AI often show a distinctive phenotype in affected females, where the enamel displays alternating vertical bands of normal and defective enamel. This phenotype is called lyonization; it results from the alternative inactivation of either the normal or the defective X chromosome in different cohorts of enamel-forming cells. In the third type, hypocalcified AI, the failure in mineralization is most extreme. The enamel layer may be of normal thickness, but is extremely soft and wears away quickly after tooth eruption. Patients with hypocalcified enamel form calculus rapidly and develop acute and chronic periodontitis.

ETIOLOGY/EPIDEMIOLOGY: Amelogenesis imperfecta, by the strict definition of inherited enamel defects in the absence of a generalized syndrome, occurs in approximately 1 of every 14,000 people. X-linked amelogenesis imperfecta, which accounts for approximately 5% of all cases, is caused by defects in the amelogenin gene (Xp22.3-p22.1). Defects in the enamelin gene (4q13-q21) also cause AI. Candidate genes for other autosomal forms include ameloblastin on chromosome 4q, tuftelin on chromosome 1q, enamelysin on 11q, and kallikrein-4 on chromosome 19q.

DIAGNOSIS: Diagnosis is made by oral examination with dental radiographs and a family history to determine mode of inheritance.

TREATMENT

Standard Therapies: Oral hygiene must be diligent with frequent professional prophylactic scalings. Extensive dental restorative and reconstructive procedures are often necessary.

REFERENCES

Bäckman B. Amelogenesis imperfecta: clinical manifestations in 51 families in a northern Swedish county. *Scand J Dent Res* 1988;96:505–516.

Seow WK. Clinical diagnosis and management strategies of amelogenesis imperfecta variants. *Pediatr Dent* 1993;15:384–393.

Witkop CJ Jr. Amelogenesis imperfecta, dentinogenesis imperfecta and dentin dysplasia revisited: problems in classification. *J Oral Pathol* 1989;17:547–553.

Witkop CJ Jr., Sauk JJ Jr. Heritable defects of enamel. In: Stewart RE, Prescott GH, eds. *Oral facial genetics.* St. Louis: CV Mosby, 1976:151–226.

RESOURCES

297, 373

---

10   Amniotic Bands

Christian E. Paletta, MD, and Forrest S. Roth, MD

DEFINITION: Amniotic bands develop subsequent to premature rupture of the fetal membranes. These mesodermic fibers disrupt embryogenesis by adhering to the fetus or embryo *in utero*. As a result, malformation of developing structures, disruption of previously formed structures, or deformation due to restricted fetal movement may occur.

SYNONYMS: Amniotic adhesion malformation syndrome; Amniotic band disruption complex/sequence; Amnion band/rupture sequence; Amniotic band syndrome; Amniotic constriction bands; Amniotic deformity-adhesion-mutilation syndrome; Congenital amputation; Congenital constricting bands; Early amnion rupture sequence; Ring constriction syndrome; Streeter anomaly/bands/dysplasia; Early amnion rupture spectrum.

DIFFERENTIAL DIAGNOSIS: Adams-Oliver syndrome; Early amnion rupture-oligohydramnios disruption; Klippel-Trenaunay syndrome; Limb-body wall defect; Oligohydramnios deformation sequence; Macrodactyly; Synbrachydactyly.

SYMPTOMS AND SIGNS: Amniotic bands are most commonly found constricting multiple limbs or digits. The head, trunk, pelvis, and umbilical cord may also be involved (Insert Fig. 25). Associated anomalies—including anencephaly, choanal atresia, cleft lip and palate, clubfeet, encephalocele, hemangioma, meningocele, microopthalmia, and scoliosis—occur in 20%–56% of affected fetuses. Although rupture of the amnion may occur at any time during pregnancy, the more severe malformations are associated with rupture during the first trimester. The distribution of involved structures is usually asymmetric; hence, no two fetuses are affected in the same manner.

ETIOLOGY/EPIDEMIOLOGY: Incidence is 1 in 1,200 to 1 in 5,000 live births, and prevalence is on the rise. Inheritance is sporadic. No genetic, gender, or ethnic preferences have been described; however, an association may exist with young mothers, first pregnancies, problem pregnancies, or premature birth.

DIAGNOSIS: Prenatal diagnosis is possible with radiography, ultrasonography, and amniocentesis. Postpartum diagnosis is made by examination of the placenta and membranes and physical evidence of an amniotic band. Radiographs of the affected limbs and digits may be helpful in evaluating bony abnormalities.

TREATMENT

Standard Therapies: Treatment depends on the location of the band and the Patterson diagnostic criteria for congenital ring constriction. Type I is a simple ring constriction that results in a soft tissue depression without neurovascular involvement. Surgical correction involves excision of the scar with multiple Z-plasties to obviate a circumferential scar. In type II, the depth of constriction is greater and results in a deformity distal to the site of involvement with or without lymphedema. This condition may require immediate surgical release or compressive garment therapy to control lymphedema. Type III is constriction with fusion of distal parts, resulting in acrosyndactyly or syndactyly. Repair should be undertaken at 1 month to 1 year of age to encourage independent finger use and unrestricted growth. Full-thickness skin grafts, web space reconstruction, and digit amputation may be required. This procedure is usually staged in two parts to prevent the possibility of vascular compromise. Finally, intrauterine amputation, or Patterson type IV, rarely requires surgical intervention because tissue healing occurs *in utero*.

Investigational Therapies: *In utero* fetoscopic correction of bands detected by ultrasonography is being explored, as is "on top" bone grafting and free tissue transfer of toes to the hand for type IV Patterson ring constrictions.

REFERENCES

Bentz ML. *Pediatric plastic surgery.* Stamford, CT: Appleton & Lange, 1998:1009–1016.

Paletta CE, Huang DB, Sabeoiro AP. An unusual presentation of constriction band syndrome. *Plast Reconstr Surg* 1999;104: 171–174.

Patterson TJ. Congenital ring constrictions. *Br J Plast Surg* 1961;14:1–31.

Walter JH, Gross LR, Laxara AT. Amniotic band syndrome. *J Foot Ankle Surg* 1998;37:325–333.

Weidrich TA. Congenital constriction band syndrome. *Hand Clin* 1998;14:29–38.

RESOURCES

75, 362

---

11   Anencephaly

*Mary M. Dott, MD,
and Cynthia A. Moore, MD, PhD*

DEFINITION: Anencephaly is a disorder of embryogenesis caused by failure of the cephalic neural tube to close, resulting in a partial or complete absence of the brain. This neural tube defect is often associated with an absence of the skull above eye level. Anencephaly with contiguous spina bifida is called craniorachischisis.

SYNONYMS: Holoanencephaly; Meroanencephaly.

DIFFERENTIAL DIAGNOSIS: Amniotic band disruption sequence; Acrania; Acalvaria.

SYMPTOMS AND SIGNS: Three quarters of mothers of affected fetuses have polyhydramnios. Elevated maternal serum or amniotic fluid α-fetoprotein may be associated with anencephaly or other neural tube defects and warrants ultrasonographic examination of the fetus.

ETIOLOGY/EPIDEMIOLOGY: From October 1995 to December 1996, anencephaly occurred in 11.6 of every 100,000 births in the United States. Affected infants are born throughout the world, and the birth prevalence is variable among countries. Rates of anencephaly at birth are highly influenced by the availability of prenatal diagnosis and elective pregnancy termination. There appears to be a female predominance among infants with anencephaly, and the prevalence of the defect is lowest in black infants. The etiology of anencephaly is believed to be multifactorial, involving both genetic and environmental factors. Possible environmental associations include maternal hyperthermia and low socioeconomic class. The evidence documenting the preventative effect of folic acid on the incidence of anencephaly is extensive, offering an opportunity for prevention.

DIAGNOSIS: Anencephaly is diagnosed after viewing the structural defect either during prenatal ultrasonography or at birth. Accompanying malformations can be craniofacial, gastrointestinal, renal, and cardiac, and can include associated single-gene or chromosomal syndromes.

TREATMENT
Standard Therapies: No treatment exists; the condition is uniformly lethal. Approximately half of affected infants are stillborn. Unless medical support is initiated, liveborn infants usually die within 48 hours of delivery. The American Academy of Pediatrics and the American Heart Association have indicated that withholding resuscitation in the delivery room is an ethical option. Primary prevention of anencephaly is the most promising medical intervention available. Increasing daily folic acid intake by women be-fore and during the first trimester of pregnancy can decrease the risk of neural tube defects, including anencephaly, by 50%. The United States Public Health Service recommends that all women capable of becoming pregnant take 400 μg (0.4 mg) of folic acid daily. Women who have had a child with a neural tube defect should take a higher daily dose (4 mg) of folic acid periconceptionally to decrease the risk in subsequent pregnancies.

REFERENCES
Botto LD, Moore CA, Khoury MJ, et al. Medical progress: neural-tube defects. *N Engl J Med* 1999;341:1509–1519.
Centers for Disease Control and Prevention. Recommendations for the use of folic acid to reduce the number of cases of spina bifida and other neural tube defects. *MMWR* 1992; 41:1–7.
Honein MA, Paulozzi LJ, Mathews TJ, et al. Impact of folic acid fortification of the US food supply on the occurrence of neural tube defects. *JAMA* 2001;285:2981–2986.
Lemire JL, Siebert JR. Anencephaly: its spectrum and relationship to neural tube defects. *J Craniofac Genet Dev Biol* 1990;10: 163–174.
Niermeyer S, Kattwinkel J, Van Reempts P, et al. International guidelines for neonatal resuscitation: an excerpt from the Guidelines 2000 for Cardiopulmonary Resuscitation and Emergency Cardiovascular Care: International Consensus on Science. Contributors and Reviewers for the Neonatal Resuscitation Guidelines. *Pediatrics* 2000;106:E29.

RESOURCES
45, 156, 368

12   Angelman Syndrome

Golder N. Wilson, MD, PhD

DEFINITION: Angelman syndrome is an inherited disorder that presents in early childhood with developmental and speech delay, jerking movements, and gelastic seizures.

DIFFERENTIAL DIAGNOSIS: Fragile X syndrome; Smith-Magenis syndrome.

SYMPTOMS AND SIGNS: The appearance of affected individuals becomes typical at age 2–3 years, with micro-brachycephaly, protrusion of the tongue and jaw, large mouth with frequent drooling, shallow midface, pale coloring, and optic pallor or atrophy. Seizures may present as unprovoked spells of laughter, grand mal, or myoclonic epilepsy. Additional neurologic abnormalities include cor-tical atrophy, strabismus, ataxic gait, hyperreflexia, truncal hypotonia with scoliosis, and tremor. Speech is severely impacted such that a vocabulary of more than 4–5 words eliminates the diagnosis. Occasional patients will have a fixation on food and obesity.

ETIOLOGY/EPIDEMIOLOGY: Angelman syndrome results from a deficient maternal imprint or a gene mutation in the chromosome 15q11-q13 region. The six causes of Angelman syndrome include (a) a microdeletion of chromosome 15, bands q11-q13; (b) chromosome rearrangements of the 15q11-q13 region; (c) paternal uniparental disomy of chromosome 15; (d) abnormal methylation of the chromosome 15q11-q13 region; (e) mutations in the *UBE3A* gene within the 15q11-q13 region; and (f) unknown. Most cases are *de novo*, but those due to inherited

UBE3A gene mutations may have a 50% recurrence risk. The incidence is estimated at 1 in 15,000 to 20,000 births with no sex predilection.

DIAGNOSIS: Fluorescent *in situ* hybridization analysis for the characteristic 15q11-q13 deletion should be obtained initially, then DNA analysis for abnormal methylation patterns (present with uniparental disomy or methylation defects), then (where available) *UBE3A* gene analysis. Electroencephalography to document epilepsy may support the clinical diagnosis.

TREATMENT
Standard Therapies: The only treatment is symptomatic for seizures and developmental disabilities.

REFERENCES
Cassidy SB, Schwartz S. Prader-Willi and Angelman syndromes. Disorders of genomic imprinting. *Medicine* 1998;77:140–151.
Laan AEM, den Boer AT, Hennekam RCM, et al. Angelman syndrome in adulthood. *Am J Med Genet* 1996;66:356–360.
Lalande M, Minassian BA, DeLorey TM, et al. Parental imprinting and Angelman syndrome. *Adv Neurol* 1999;79:421–429.
Moncla A, Malzac P, Livet MO, et al. Angelman syndrome resulting from *UBE3A* mutations in 14 patients from eight families: clinical manifestations and genetic counseling. *J Med Genet* 1999;36:554–560.
Stalker HJ, Williams CA. Genetic counseling in Angelman syndrome: the challenges of multiple causes. *Am J Med Genet* 1998;77:54–59.

RESOURCES
46, 47, 368

---

13   Anorectal Malformations

Alberto Peña, MD, Marc Levitt, MD, and Andrew R. Hong, MD

DEFINITION: Anorectal malformations (ARMs) are congenital anomalies arising from the lack of a normal rectal opening. The severity is variable, and consequently ARMs present as a wide spectrum of defects. In more than 90% of patients, the rectum has a fistulous connection with the urinary tract or the perineum. In another 5% of cases, there is no connection, and the rectum ends blindly in the pelvis. Approximately 1% of patients have a normal-looking anus with an atresia or stenosis in the rectum, located approximately 1–2 cm inside the canal.

SYNONYMS: Imperforate anus; Anal atresia; Perineal fistula.

SYMPTOMS AND SIGNS: Males have four main types of ARM: rectobulbar urethral fistulas, rectoprostatic urethral fistulas, recto-bladder neck fistulas, and perineal fistulas. More than 50% of these patients have Down syndrome, and almost all patients with Down syndrome and imperforate anus have no fistula. Females have three main types of malformations: perineal fistulas, vestibular fistulas, and complex malformations called cloacas. Typically, these patients are asymptomatic at birth, unless there is an associated problem. The diagnosis is usually made on the first newborn physical examination. If missed, patients will develop signs related to low intestinal obstruction. Abdominal distention is not present at birth, but develops within the first 24 hours of life. If the

patient remains untreated, vomiting may develop. Symptoms related to any associated defects may also be present, such as cardiovascular from a congenital cardiac anomaly, excessive salivation secondary to esophageal atresia, or vomiting from duodenal atresia. Occasionally, the patient may develop sepsis secondary to a urinary tract obstruction.

ETIOLOGY/EPIDEMIOLOGY: The etiology is unknown. The origins of these malformations are multifactorial. They occur in approximately 1 in every 4,000–5,000 newborns. There is a slight male to female predominance. Neither race nor geographic distribution plays a role.

DIAGNOSIS: The diagnosis of an ARM is easily evident. However, it is important to identify the perineal stigmata to try to determine the specific type of defect. One must suspect an ARM in a fetus that has a dilated colon, an abnormal vertebrae or sacrum, and hydronephrosis. Further work is necessary, however, before prenatal diagnosis becomes routine.

TREATMENT
Standard Therapies: Two important questions must be answered in the first 24 hours of life. The first is whether definitive repair can be performed during the newborn period without a protective colostomy. The second question is whether the patient requires urgent treatment for an associated defect that may be life threatening. Most surgeons will proceed with the definitive repair of a perineal fistula during the newborn period, without a colostomy. In al-

most all other malformations, the definitive repair is delayed, and a temporary diverting colostomy is opened shortly after birth.

REFERENCES
Levitt MA, Stein DM, Pena A. Rectovestibular fistula with absent vagina: a unique anorectal malformation. *J Pediatr Surg* 1998: 33:986–990.
Pena A, Hong AR. Anorectal malformations: the state of the art. *Colon Rectal Surg* 1999;2:1–19.
Pena A, Hong AR. Advances in the management of anorectal malformations. *Am J Surg* 2000;180:370–376.
Pena A, O'Connor-Guardino K. Colorectal problems in pediatric patients. In: Porrett T, ed. *Essential coloproctology for nurses.* London: Whurr Publishers, xxxx:332–357.
Softer SZ, Rosen NG, Hong AR, et al. Cloacal exstrophy: a unified management plan. *J Pediatr Surg* 2000;35:932–937.

RESOURCES
280, 354, 479

14   Apert Syndrome

Millie D. Long, MD,
and Kant Y.K. Lin, MD

DEFINITION: Apert syndrome is characterized by craniosynostosis, midface hypoplasia, and complex syndactyly of the hands and feet.

SYNONYM: Acrocephalosyndactyly.

DIFFERENTIAL DIAGNOSIS: Pfieffer syndrome; Carpenter syndrome; Jackson-Weiss syndrome; Crouzon syndrome; Saethre-Chotzen syndrome.

SYMPTOMS AND SIGNS: Apert syndrome is characterized by many abnormalities. Cranial findings include a prominent midline skull defect, widely patent fontanelles, and multiple fused sutures, most often coronal. Brain abnormalities of the corpus callosum and the septum pellucidum, as well as the hydrocephalus, are also seen frequently. Intelligence varies from profound mental deficiency to low-normal intellect and may be related to prolonged untreated periods of intracranial hypertension due to multiple fused cranial sutures. Facial findings include hypertelorbitism, exorbitism, and down-slanting palpebral fissures. Exotropia, strabismus, and optic atrophy are common ocular complications. Low-set ears are related to the severity of the skull deformity. The nasal bridge is often depressed and the nose is beaked with a prominent hump. Most common is a severe maxillary midface hypoplasia, which results in a malocclusion. The high frequency of cleft palate or bifid uvula can lead to substantial speech and hearing problems. If not overtly clefted, the palate can be constricted with a medial furrow and lateral palatal swellings. Pulmonary complications such as obstructive sleep apnea can be a result of the reduced nasopharyngeal dimensions. Associated limb abnormalities include complex syndactyly, often with fused spoonlike fingernails and short, broad thumbs that deviate radially. Syndactyly of the feet is similar to that of the hands, but the toenails may be at least partially segmented. Skin manifestations, particularly acne vulgaris, are common, as are hyperseborrhea and excessive sweating.

ETIOLOGY/EPIDEMIOLOGY: Apert syndrome accounts for approximately 4.5% of cases of craniosynostosis. Birth prevalence is approximately 15.5 in 1 million. Although most cases are sporadic, many instances of an autosomal-dominant inheritance pattern have been reported. Advanced paternal age has been implicated as a factor in producing fresh mutations. Gene mutations associated with Apert syndrome have been linked to the fibroblast growth factor receptor (*FGFR*) 2 gene, located on chromosome 10.

DIAGNOSIS: MRI study done early can help to define central nervous system abnormalities. DNA analysis for *FGFR* receptor mutations can often confirm the diagnosis. Prenatal diagnosis can be made on the basis of chorionic villus sampling or amniocentesis. Apert syndrome may also be suspected on ultrasonography, but usually not until the third trimester.

TREATMENT
Standard Therapies: The timing of treatment is determined by the functional problems encountered in each individual patient, and is often performed in stages throughout the early years of life. Most treatments are surgical, and early referral to a multidisciplinary craniofacial team is critical for the successful management of these patients. Generally, skull deformities are addressed in infancy, especially if evidence or suspicion exists of intracranial hypertension or hydrocephalus. Orbital and facial deformities are corrected during early childhood, as are any limb deformities, and jaw deformities are addressed during adolescence.

REFERENCES
Cohen MM, Maclean RE. *Craniosynostosis: diagnosis, evaluation and management,* 2nd ed. New York: Oxford University Press, 2000:316–353.

Gorlin RJ, Cohen MM, Levin LS, eds. *Syndromes of the head and neck,* 3rd ed. New York: Oxford University Press, 1990:520–523.

RESOURCES
48, 49, 96

15 Arthrogryposis Multiplex Congenita

Michael Bamshad, MD

DEFINITION: Arthrogryposis multiplex congenita (AMC) is a descriptive term that defines an individual with nonprogressive, congenital contractures of two or more body areas. The etiology and pathogenic mechanisms of conditions labeled as AMC are heterogeneous and inclusive of hundreds of specific diagnoses. The most common condition labeled as AMC is amyoplasia.

SYMPTOMS AND SIGNS: The primary feature of AMC is limited or fixed flexion contractures of body areas around small and large joints. Soft tissue webbing may have developed over the flexed joints, and the muscles of involved limbs may be hypoplastic, producing a tubular-shaped limb with a soft, doughy feeling. The long bones of the skeleton can be exceptionally slender, but except for some specific syndrome diagnoses, the skeletal X-rays are otherwise normal. Cleft palate and cryptorchidism may be present. Intelligence usually is average to above average. All of the symptoms and signs are dependent on the underlying etiology of the condition that is manifest as AMC.

ETIOLOGY/EPIDEMIOLOGY: The prevalence of children with a single congenital contracture is approximately 1 in 500 and of children with multiple congenital contractures is approximately 1 in 3,000. The disorder has been described in Africans, Asians, and Europeans. The number of affected males and females is approximately equal. The etiology of AMC is extremely heterogeneous. It may be caused by disorders of chromosome number or chromosome content, as well as single-gene disorders that can be transmitted in autosomal-recessive, autosomal-dominant, and X-linked patterns. Many cases of AMC are probably not heritable, however.

DIAGNOSIS: Diagnosis is generally made based on the presence of flexion contractures noted on physical examination.

TREATMENT
Standard Therapies: Standard physical therapy in the newborn period and early infancy is beneficial. Splints can be made to augment stretching exercises to increase range of motion. Removable splints for the knees and feet that permit regular muscle exercise are recommended. Surgery may be required on ankles, knees, hips, elbows, or wrists to achieve better position or greater range of motion. In some cases, tendon transfers have been performed.

REFERENCES
Staheli LT, Hall JG, Jaffe KM, et al. *Arthrogryposes.* Cambridge: Cambridge University Press, 1998.
Jones KL. *Smith's recognizable patterns of human malformation,* 4th ed. Philadelphia: WB Saunders, 1988:140–141.
Sells JM, Jaffe KM, Hall JG. Amyoplasia, the most common type of arthrogryposis: the potential for good outcome. *Pediatrics* 1996;97:225–231.

RESOURCES
54, 64, 351

16 Asphyxiating Thoracic Dystrophy

Robert M. Campbell, Jr., MD

DEFINITION: Asphyxiating thoracic dystrophy (ATD) is a genetic disorder of the thorax. Major features include a constricted rib cage, respiratory distress, shortened upper and lower extremities, and renal and hepatic dysfunction.

SYNONYMS: Asphyxiating thoracic dysplasia; Jeune syndrome; Thoracic-pelvic-phalangeal dystrophy.

DIFFERENTIAL DIAGNOSIS: Chondroectodermal dysplasia; Metatrophic dwarfism in infancy; Short rib–polydactyly syndromes.

SYMPTOMS AND SIGNS: The typical small, bell-shaped chest in patients with the disease constricts the underlying lungs, adversely affecting both lung growth and respiration. On radiography, the features of ATD are extreme narrowing of the thorax with shortened ribs, elevated "handlebar" clavicles, vertically short ilium, flattened or convex roof of the acetabulum, an inferior spur of the lateral border of the greater sciatic notch (trident pelvis), and shortening of the long bones with spurring or bulbous enlargement of the metaphysis. Early ossification of the capital femoral epiphysis is occasionally seen. Other abnormalities include short phalanges, cone-shaped epiphysis in the hands and feet, polydactyly of the hands and feet, retinitis pigmentosa, blindness, pancreatic fibrosis and cyst, and hydrocephalus. Progressive renal failure may be seen due to a combination of cystic tubular dysplasia and glomerular sclerosis.

ETIOLOGY/EPIDEMIOLOGY: Approximately 1 in 120,000 live births are affected. Males and females are affected in equal numbers.

DIAGNOSIS: Prenatal diagnosis of ATD can be made by ultrasonography as early as the 18th week of gestation.

TREATMENT
Standard Therapies: Treatment is symptomatic and supportive. Past procedures attempted to improve respiration by expanding the constrictive thorax by releasing the ribs at the costochondral junction without clear benefit. Some success has been seen by expanding the thorax through a longitudinal division of the sternum held open with bone graft, acrylic implants, metal plates, or donor bone grafts. Posterolateral expansion of the rib cages has also been accomplished with osteotomies and plate fixation. Renal dysfunction is managed with dialysis or transplantation. Liver disease is treated with phenobarbital or ursodeoxycholic acid. Genetic counseling may benefit families affected by this disorder.

Investigational Therapies: The Titanium Rib Project based at Christus Santa Rosa Children's Hospital, San Antonio, Texas, oversees the implantation of expandable prosthetic ribs in children with disorders involving malformed rib cages due to absent, fused ribs, as well as hypoplastic thorax such as seen in ATD.

REFERENCES
Borland LM. Anesthesia for children with Jeune's syndrome (asphyxiating thoracic dystrophy). *Anesthesiology* 1987;19: 86–88.
Davis JT. Lateral thoracic expansion for Jeune's asphyxiating thoracic dystrophy. *Ann Thorac Surg* 1995;60:694–696.
Jones KL. *Smith's recognizable patterns of human malformation,* 4th ed. Philadelphia: WB Saunders, 1988:292–295.
Labrune P. Jeune's syndrome and liver disease: report of three cases treated with ursodeoxycholic acid. *Am J Med Genet* 1999; 87:324–328.
Oberklaoid R, et al. Asphyxiating thoracic dysplasia: clinical, radiological, and pathological information. *Arch Dis Child* 1977; 52:756–765.
Todd DW, et al. A thoracic expansion technique for Jeune's asphyxiating thoracic dystrophy. *J Pediatr Surg* 1986;2:161–163.
Yang SS, et al. Three conditions in neonatal asphyxiating thoracic dysplasia (Jeune) and short rib–polydactyly syndrome spectrum: a clinical pathologic study. *Am J Med Genet* 1987;3 (suppl):191–207.

RESOURCES
188, 351

---

17   Atelosteogenesis Type III

Ravi Savarirayan, MD

DEFINITION: Atelosteogenesis (incomplete bone formation) type III is an inherited disorder of the skeleton of unknown cause recognizable at birth by disproportionate short stature, unusual facial appearance, and multiple large joint dislocations with specific radiographic features.

SYNONYM: Spondylo-humero-femoral hypoplasia.

DIFFERENTIAL DIAGNOSIS: Larsen syndrome (dominant form); Oto-palato-digital syndrome type II; Atelosteogenesis types I and II.

SYMPTOMS AND SIGNS: This bone dysplasia may be suspected on antenatal ultrasonography by the finding of disproportionately short limbs. At birth, these infants have disproportionately short stature with shortness of all segments, especially those closest to the trunk. In addition, they exhibit short, broad fingers and toes (which may be webbed), widely spaced eyes, depressed nasal bridge, upturned nose, midfacial hypoplasia, and a small jaw with cleft palate. Multiple large-joint dislocations are a feature of the condition, often necessitating orthopedic intervention. Infants often experience respiratory difficulties, and death may occur from this, as well as from the consequences of cervical spine instability caused by a hypoplastic odontoid process. Although many infants succumb to complications, some do survive into adulthood. The major radiographic features of this condition include large joint dislocations, unusually shaped humeri, and shortening of the small tubular bones of the hands with broad distal phalanges. The histologic appearance of the growth plate in this condition is generally unremarkable. Atelosteogenesis type III shares many clinical and radiographic features with the dominant form of Larsen syndrome, and these conditions may share a similar genetic basis.

ETIOLOGY/EPIDEMIOLOGY: Atelosteogenesis type III occurs most commonly as a sporadic condition, but dominant transmission of this trait has been documented. No gene locus or gene has been identified yet.

DIAGNOSIS: The diagnosis is based on the specific clinical and radiographic features present at birth.

No biochemical or molecular confirmatory test is available.

TREATMENT
Standard Therapies: Treatment is symptomatic. Infants who survive and have respiratory difficulties may require long-term airway management by means of tracheostomy and supplemental oxygen. Multiple orthopedic procedures may be required. Cervical spine instability may require surgical intervention. Genetic counseling is advised for families.

REFERENCES

Schultz C, Langer LO, Laxova R, et al. Atelosteogenesis type II: long-term survival, prenatal diagnosis, and evidence for dominant transmission. *Am J Med Genet* 1999;83:28–42.

Stern HJ, Graham JM, Lachman RS, et al. Atelosteogenesis type III: a distinct skeletal dysplasia with features overlapping atelosteogenesis and oto-palato-digital syndrome type II. In: Taybi H, Lachman RS, eds. *Radiology of syndromes, metabolic disorders, and skeletal dysplasias,* 4th ed. New York: CV Mosby, 1996.

RESOURCES
96, 351

---

18   Baller-Gerold Syndrome

I. K. Temple, MD

DEFINITION: The major features of the Baller-Gerold syndrome are craniosynostosis, usually involving the coronal suture, and radial aplasia, which can be asymmetric and include absence of the thumb and bowing of the ulna.

DIFFERENTIAL DIAGNOSIS: Fanconi pancytopenia; VACTERL association; Roberts syndrome; Rothmund-Thomson syndrome; KID syndrome; Saethre-Chotzen syndrome/TWIST mutation syndrome.

SYMPTOMS AND SIGNS: Affected children have craniosynostosis associated with radial defects. The many associated features include vertebral and other skeletal anomalies, renal defects, and anal atresia or stenosis. Short stature is common. Structural brain anomalies, hearing loss, dysplastic external ears, and congenital cardiac anomalies have been reported. Some children have developmental delay.

ETIOLOGY/EPIDEMIOLOGY: Baller-Gerold syndrome is likely inherited in an autosomal-recessive manner. The supposition is based on the observation of affected siblings of both sexes and three families with consanguinity; however, many of the early patients have not been tested for other conditions such as Fanconi pancytopenia, and an autosomal-recessive gene has not yet been identified. In 1999, researchers identified a mutation in the TWIST gene in a patient with craniosynostosis and radial aplasia, which is inherited as an autosomal-dominant gene.

DIAGNOSIS: The diagnosis is one of exclusion, but rests on the presence of craniosynostosis and radial defects. The described associated features are common. All patients meeting the diagnostic criteria should have hematologic investigations. It is important to actively exclude Fanconi pancytopenia by looking for excessive chromosome damage using DEB (diepoxybutane) as the clastogenic agent. Karyotyping should also include looking for premature centromere separation, thereby excluding Roberts syndrome. The skin abnormalities noted in Rothmund-Thomson syndrome do not appear until age 6 months.

TREATMENT
Standard Therapies: Surgery for craniosynostosis may be required. Screening for deafness, cardiac anomalies, and congenital renal anomalies is important.

REFERENCES
Cohen MM Jr, Toriello HV. Editorial comment: is there a Baller-Gerold syndrome? *Am J Med Genet* 1996;61:63–64.

Galea P, Tolmie JL. Normal growth and development in a child with Baller-Gerold syndrome (craniosynostosis and radial aplasia). *J Med Genet* 1990;27:784–787.

Gripp KW, Stolle CA, Celle L, et al. TWIST gene mutation in a patient with radial aplasia and craniosynostosis: further evidence for heterogeneity of Baller-Gerold syndrome. *Am J Med Genet* 1999;82:170–176.

Huson SM, Rodgers CS, Hall CM, et al. The Baller-Gerold syndrome: phenotypic and cytogenetic overlap with Roberts syndrome. *J Med Genet* 1990;27:371–375.

RESOURCES
96, 149, 351

---

19   Bardet-Biedl Syndrome

Richard A. Lewis, MD, MS

DEFINITION: Bardet-Biedl syndrome (BBS) is an autosomal-recessive disorder characterized by postnatal obesity, postaxial polydactyly, progressive retinal dystrophy, hypogenitalism, learning difficulties, and malformations of the kidney.

SYNONYMS: Laurence-Moon-Bardet-Biedl syndrome; Laurence-Moon-Biedl syndrome.

DIFFERENTIAL DIAGNOSIS: Acrocephalopolysyndactylia; Alstrom syndrome; Biemond syndrome Type II; Carpenter syndrome; Cohen syndrome; Laurence-Moon syndrome; McKusick-Kaufman syndrome; Meckel-Gruber syndrome; Prader-Willi syndrome.

SYMPTOMS AND SIGNS: The primary defining features are (a) a retinal dystrophy combining both rod and cone deterioration, beginning with night blindness but including myopia, strabismus, loss of side vision, eventual loss of central vision, occasional nystagmus, and a retinal appearance by the teenage years similar to retinitis pigmentosa; (b) postaxial polydactyly, brachydactyly, short, wide, flat feet with no arch, and syndactyly; (c) obesity; (d) learning disabilities (developmental delay and poor gross and fine motor skills) and distinctive speech pathology (breathiness, high pitch, difficulty phonating certain labial and dental sounds); (e) hypogenitalism (most obvious in males with small penis, reduced testicular volume, or frank cryptorchidism; females occasionally have vaginal atresia, persistent urogenital sinus, hydrometrocolpos, septate vagina, and uterine hypoplasia); and (f) renal anomalies (including structural and functional anomalies, fetal lobulation, communication cysts of the collecting system, and nephrogenic diabetes insipidus with inability to concentrate urine, leading to renal failure, dialysis, and rarely, transplantation). Secondary features include recurrent otitis media and conductive hearing loss from "glue ear," labile personality, short stature compared with siblings and parents, asthma and reactive airway disease, congenital heart disease, acquired left ventricular hypertrophy, diabetes mellitus, and fibrosis of the liver.

ETIOLOGY/EPIDEMIOLOGY: This syndrome is an autosomal-recessive mendelian trait that is genetically highly heterogeneous, including mapped loci at chromosomes 11q13 (*BBS1*), 16q21 (*BBS2*), 3p12–13 (*BBS3*), 15q23 (*BBS4*), 2q31 (*BBS5*), and 20p12 (*BBS6*). Approximately 20%–25% of families cannot be assigned to any known locus, suggesting that at least one more locus remains to be identified. Some families are triallelic, however; that is, they require two homologous mutations in one gene and a third mutation in another *BBS* gene to cause an abnormal phenotype. Population frequency is estimated at approximately 1 in 150,000, except in Newfoundland and Kuwait, where it is approximately 1 in 13,500.

DIAGNOSIS: The diagnosis of BBS requires four primary features (including retinal disease) or three primary and two secondary features. The *BBS2, BBS4,* and *MKKS/BBS6* genes are available for mutational analysis.

TREATMENT
Standard Therapies: No proven therapies are available for the retinal dystrophy. Standard ophthalmic care is recommended for refractive errors and low vision assistance. For polydactyly, rudimentary skin tags can be tied off after birth, but larger accessory digits may require orthopedic reconstruction. Obesity may be managed with age-appropriate diet regimens, behavioral modifications, and exercise pro-

grams. Intervention for kidney disease depends on the structural and/or functional natures of the problem. Hormonal supplementation in males for hypogonadism requires confirmation of low testosterone levels.

REFERENCES

Beales PL, Elcioglu N, Woolf AS, et al. New criteria for improved diagnosis of Bardet-Biedl syndrome: results of a population survey. *J Med Genet* 1999;36:437–446.

Katsanis N, Ansley SJ, Badano JL, et al. Triallelic inheritance in Bardet-Biedl syndrome, a Mendelian recessive disorder. *Science* 2001;294:2256–2259.

Katsanis N, Beales PL, Woods MO, et al. Mutations in *MKKS* cause obesity, retinal dystrophy and renal malformations associated with Bardet-Biedl syndrome. *Nat Genet* 2000;26:67–70.

Katsanis N, Eichers ER, Ansley SJ, et al. *BBS4* is a minor contributor to Bardet-Biedl syndrome and may also participate in tri-allelic inheritance. *Am J Hum Genet* 2002 (in press).

Leppert M, Baird L, Anderson KL, et al. Bardet-Biedl syndrome is linked to DNA markers on chromosome 11q and is genetically heterogeneous. *Nat Genet* 1994;7:108–112.

RESOURCES

31, 232, 286

---

20   Bloom Syndrome

James German III, MD

DEFINITION: Bloom syndrome (BS) is a genetically determined form of dwarfism characterized clinically by proportional smallness at all ages and, at maturity, infertility. It usually is accompanied by sun-sensitive facial erythema and immunodeficiency, with or without additional less constant features. The genetic material in BS somatic cells is abnormally unstable; a wide variety of neoplasms arise unusually frequently and at exceptionally early ages.

DIFFERENTIAL DIAGNOSIS: Russell-Silver dwarfism.

SYMPTOMS AND SIGNS: The predominating and constant clinical feature of BS is small body size, both pre- and postnatally, proportioning being fairly normal except for a slightly disproportionately small brain/head and dolichocephaly. Subcutaneous fat is conspicuously scanty. The facies is characteristic, somewhat keel shaped because of malar and mandibular hypoplasia, and a prominent nose. The ears are often unusually prominent. Facial erythema, characteristically limited to the butterfly area of the face, usually appears in infancy following sun exposure. This lesion sometimes extends to other areas of the face, ears, and neck and may affect the dorsa of the hands and forearms. It is variable in severity and sometimes is absent, especially in dark-complexioned individuals. The skin in other areas is not hypersensitive to sunlight. Another dermal feature is an excessive number of circumscribed areas of hyper- and hypopigmentation. The voice is characteristically high pitched, and of somewhat coarse timbre. During infancy, vomiting and diarrhea are increased in many patients; severe gastroesophageal reflux has been diagnosed in some. Typically, affected infants and young children show relatively little interest in eating; in a few cases, surgically placed tubes into the stomach for supplementary feeding have permitted weight gain due to an increase in fat depo-

sition. Immunodeficiency is demonstrable in most affected individuals, and most are prone to respiratory infections complicated by otitis media and pneumonia. Several adults have had bronchiectasis and fatal chronic lung disease. Intelligence usually is average to low average, although several persons with BS have been mentally defective. Generally, affected individuals are infertile, although some women have had normal children. Diabetes mellitus develops in more than 10% of adults with BS. Both benign and malignant neoplasms arise unusually frequently. During infancy and childhood, acute leukemia and lymphoma predominate; carcinomata predominate in adulthood.

ETIOLOGY/EPIDEMIOLOGY: BS is transmitted as an autosomal-recessive trait. More than 60 mutations causing BS have been identified, but all at a single locus, *BLM*, in chromosome band 15q26.1.

DIAGNOSIS: The appearance of persons with BS is striking, which facilitates their recognition. The clinical diagnosis can be confirmed cytogenetically: dividing BS cells have excessive numbers of gaps, breaks, and rearrangements in their chromosomes. A uniquely increased tendency for exchange to take place between DNA strands is demonstrable as an increase in sister-chromatid exchanges (SCEs); an SCE analysis is the standard way to confirm the diagnosis, including prenatally. Molecular methods are applicable when the BS-causing mutation segregating in a given family has been identified.

TREATMENT

Standard Therapies: Measures to increase height in BS, including administration of growth hormone, have not been found effective. The skin lesion requires protection of the face from the sun. Increased surveillance for carcinoma is advisable in adults. Cancer chemotherapy in BS is unusually challenging because of hypersensitivity to many DNA-damaging agents; reduced dosage is often required to avoid fatal ablation of enteric tract mucosae and bone marrow. Potential HLA-matched bone marrow donors (usually unaffected siblings) can be identified.

REFERENCES

German J. Bloom syndrome: a Mendelian prototype of somatic mutational disease. *Medicine* 1993;72:393–406.

German J. Bloom's syndrome. XX. The first 100 cancers. *Cancer Genet Cytogenetics* 1997;93:101–107.

German J, Ellis NA. Bloom syndrome. In: Schriver CR, Beaudet AL, Sly WS, et al., eds. *The metabolic and molecular bases of inherited disease,* 8th ed. New York: McGraw-Hill, 2000: 733–752.

21   Blue Rubber Bleb Nevus Syndrome

Steven J. Fishman, MD,
and John B. Mulliken, MD

DEFINITION: Blue rubber bleb nevus syndrome (BRBNS) is a subcategory of familial venous malformations. It presents as multiple, small, domelike cutaneous venous lesions in association with multifocal lesions of the gastrointestinal (GI) tract. Venous lesions can also occur in solid organs and occasionally in muscle and bone.

SYNONYM: Bean syndrome.

DIFFERENTIAL DIAGNOSIS: Venous malformation, multiple cutaneous and mucosal.

SYMPTOMS AND SIGNS: The cutaneous lesions appear during infancy and childhood; they are soft, blue, and generally compressible but sometimes nodular. They occur anywhere on the body, but with a predilection for the trunk, palms, and soles of the feet. The lesions increase in size and become more obvious with age. Lesions on the palms and plantar areas become hyperkeratotic. BRBNS is the most common vascular anomaly that causes severe, chronic GI bleeding. The lesions are distributed throughout the gut, most commonly in the small bowel. In addition to bleeding, the GI mucosal lesions can cause intussusception and other types of obstruction. Venous malformations are usually asymptomatic in the liver, gallbladder, mesentery, retroperitoneum, lungs, and brain.

ETIOLOGY/EPIDEMIOLOGY: Most cases are sporadic, but there are well-documented pedigrees showing autosomal-dominant inheritance.

DIAGNOSIS: Cutaneous lesions vary from the size of a pinhead to 1.5 cm in diameter. Often the dome-shaped lesions can be emptied easily by compression. Large intramuscular venous malformations also occur, as well as lesions in skeletal venous malformations. Gastrointestinal lesions are easily diagnosed by endoscopy or by technetium-tagged red blood cell study. The lesions have a typical purplish, berry-like, polypoid appearance.

TREATMENT
Standard Therapies: The cutaneous lesions can be injected (sclerotherapy), treated with laser (Nd:YAG), or surgically excised. Multiple GI lesions should be addressed if repeated transfusions become necessary because of anemia caused by bleeding. Endoscopic therapy using band ligation, injection sclerosis, or snare electrocautery is useful for lesions in the esophagus, stomach, duodenum, and colorectum. Lesions may be mucosal, intramural, or transmural. Thus, endoscopic therapy has a high risk of penetration. Surgical resection is required for multiple lesions in the small intestine.

Investigational Therapies: Clinical studies are ongoing. The genetic cause of BRBNS is being investigated.

REFERENCES

Bean WB. Blue rubber bleb naevi of the skin and gastrointestinal tract. In: *Vascular spiders and related lesions of the skin.* Springfield, IL: Charles C Thomas, 1958:178–185.

Fishman SJ, Burrows PE, Leichtner AM, et al. Gastrointestinal manifestations of vascular anomalies in childhood: varied etiologies require multiple therapeutic modalities. *J Pediatr Surg* 1998;33:1163–1167.

Hales K, Connally LP, Drubach LA, et al. Tc-99m RBC imaging of blue rubber bleb nevus syndrome. *Clin Nucl Med* 2000;25: 835–837.

22 Bowen-Conradi Syndrome

*Edmond G. Lemire, MD, PhD,
and R. Brian Lowry, MD, DSc, FRCPC*

DEFINITION: Bowen-Conradi syndrome is a lethal autosomal-recessive condition characterized by intrauterine growth retardation, failure to thrive, microcephaly, rocker-bottom feet, and joint deformities. Most cases have occurred in the Hutterite religious isolate.

SYNONYMS: Bowen-Hutterite syndrome; Bowen-Conradi-Hutterite syndrome.

DIFFERENTIAL DIAGNOSIS: Bowen syndrome; Cerebro-oculo-facial-skeletal syndrome; Trisomy 18.

SYMPTOMS AND SIGNS: Antenatally, fetuses with Bowen-Conradi syndrome present with intrauterine growth retardation, microcephaly, rocker-bottom feet, and abnormal finger posture. The symptoms are often mistaken for trisomy 18 until cytogenetic studies are available. At delivery, presentation is often breech. Features noted at birth include low birth weight, microcephaly, prominent nose, micrognathia, joint limitation including camptodactyly and abnormal finger posture, and rocker-bottom feet. Inguinal hernias and cryptorchidism in males are common. Feeding difficulties with failure to thrive are apparent from birth. The prognosis is very poor. Many infants have a history of pneumonia and often succumb within the first year of life. Some infants have been known to survive for several years with severe failure to thrive and profound psychomotor retardation.

ETIOLOGY/EPIDEMIOLOGY: Bowen-Conradi syndrome is inherited in an autosomal-recessive fashion. Most cases have occurred in members of the Hutterite religious isolate, but occasionally infants with Bowen-Conradi syndrome have been born to parents of non-Hutterite descent.

DIAGNOSIS: The diagnosis should be suspected in microcephalic infants with low birth weight thought to have trisomy 18 (Edwards syndrome), but who have normal chromosomes. Ethnicity (especially Hutterite) and consanguinity are important elements in the family history. Imaging studies may identify evidence of congenital heart disease, central nervous system malformations, renal anomalies, and vertebral defects. The diagnosis is usually made clinically.

TREATMENT
Standard Therapies: Treatment is supportive. Gastrostomy feeding has been considered in some cases because of the severe failure to thrive.

REFERENCES
Bowen P, Conradi GJ. Syndrome of skeletal and genitourinary anomalies with unusual facies and failure to thrive in Hutterite sibs. *Birth Defects Orig Art Series* 1976;6:1–108.
Gupta A, Phadke SR. Bowen-Conradi syndrome in an Indian infant: first non-Hutterite case. *Clin Dysmorphol* 2001;10:155–156.
Hunter AGW, Woerner SJ, Montalvo-Hicks LDC, et al. The Bowen-Conradi syndrome—a highly lethal autosomal recessive syndrome of microcephaly, micrognathia, low birth weight and joint deformities. *Am J Med Genet* 1979;3:269–279.
LeMarec B, Paty E, Roussey M, et al. La phénocopie de la trisomie 18: une maladie autosomique récessive. *Arch Fr Pediatr* 1981;38:253–259.

RESOURCES
149, 360, 362

23 Branchio-Oculo-Facial Syndrome

Angela E. Lin, MD

DEFINITION: Branchio-oculo-facial (BOF) syndrome is a distinctive multiple malformation syndrome with variable severity. Craniofacial anomalies are characteristic, with frequent renal malformations and rare skeletal, cardiac, and brain malformations.

DIFFERENTIAL DIAGNOSIS: Branchio-oto-renal syndrome; Oculo-cerebro-cutaneous syndrome.

SYMPTOMS AND SIGNS: Patients present as newborns with unusual skin defects and multiple craniofacial anomalies. The branchial skin defects are usually linear ellipses, with erythematous wrinkled skin. Draining fistulae may be present. Rarely, they occur in the superior or posterior auricular region. Ocular abnormalities include nasolacrimal duct stenosis or atresia, true microphthalmia, small palpebral fissures, up-slanted palpebral fissures, and coloboma. Facial abnormalities include dolichocephaly, high forehead, malformed nose, cleft lip with or without cleft palate, incomplete cleft lip, and low-set and posteriorly rotated ears with cupped pinnae and upturned lobules. Frequent ectodermal anomalies are sparse hair, prematurely gray hair, absent or small teeth, and small fingernails. Renal anomalies are the most common noncraniofacial abnormality. Major brain, skeletal, and cardiac malformations are uncommon. Postnatal growth retardation, as well as developmental delays, low normal function, and mild mental retardation occur in approximately one third of affected individuals.

ETIOLOGY/EPIDEMIOLOGY: Although a causative mutant gene has not yet been detected, autosomal-dominant inheritance is well supported by vertical transmission and male-to-male transmission. Prevalence has not been estimated. No ethnic preference has been observed.

DIAGNOSIS: The diagnosis usually can be made from the physical examination without supportive tests. The presence of unusual cervical skin defects with aplastic and/or erythematous skin is sufficient to suspect BOF syndrome. When malformed ears, cleft lip, and microphthalmia are

also present, the diagnosis is certain. Although no chromosome abnormality has been found in any patients with BOF syndrome, a chromosome analysis is worthwhile. Renal ultrasonography, eye examination, and hearing test should be performed.

TREATMENT
Standard Therapies: Treatment is directed at repairing the skin defects, which should not be merely cauterized. Additional reconstructive surgery can repair the oral lips, improve malformed nose and upturned lobules, enlarge small orbits, and repair stenotic or atretic nasolacrimal ducts. Although this is not a syndrome with mental retardation, vision and hearing losses may present special learning challenges that should be addressed.

REFERENCES
Lin AE, Gorlin RJ, Lurie IW, et al. Further delineation of the branchio-oculo-facial syndrome. *Am J Med Genet* 1995;56: 42–59.
Lin AE, Semina EV, Daack-Hirsch S, et al. Exclusion of the branchio-oto-renal syndrome locus (EYA1) from patients with branchio-oculo-facial syndrome. *Am J Med Genet* 2000;91: 327–390.

RESOURCES
240, 298

---

24   C Syndrome

Axel Bohring, Dipl Med

DEFINITION: C syndrome is a disorder in which affected individuals have a characteristic appearance with a triangular-shaped skull with metopic suture prominence, fleshy epicanthal folds, strabismus, multiple folds of mucosa that attach the inside of the lips to the gums, abnormal palate that is deeply furrowed, low nasal bridge with a short nose, short neck, short stature with short hands and feet, loose body skin, and joint dislocation, with hyperextensibility and crepitation. Developmental and learning disabilities are common.

SYNONYMS: Opitz trigonocephaly syndrome; C trigonocephaly syndrome.

DIFFERENTIAL DIAGNOSIS: Autosomal-dominant trigonocephaly; Bohring-Opitz syndrome; Kabuki make-up syndrome.

SYMPTOMS AND SIGNS: Signs of C syndrome include trigonocephaly/ridged metopic suture with hypotelorism, anterior hair whorl, glabellar hemangioma, low and broad nasal bridge, up-slanting palpebral fissures, epicanthic folds, strabismus, highly arched palate, thick/wide alveolar ridges, buccolabial frenula, abnormally modeled/low-set ears, sternum anomalies, widely spaced nipples, diastasis recti, cryptorchidism, short stature/limbs/hands, hexadactyly, syndactyly, joint dislocation/hyperextensibility/crepitation, sacral dimple, skin laxity, muscular weakness, heart failure, feeding problems, agenesis of the corpus callosum, seizures, mental retardation, and developmental delay. Neurologic manifestations often improve. An affected child's receptive skills may be better than his or her expressive responses.

ETIOLOGY/EPIDEMIOLOGY: C syndrome affects males and females in equal numbers. Approximately 70 cases are known to exist. A gene causing C syndrome has not been identified. A mostly sporadic occurrence with a few familial cases and apparently normal parents suggests the disorder is the result of new mutation/autosomal-dominant inheritance, with occasional parental germ cell mosaicism explaining the rare familial occurrence.

DIAGNOSIS: High-resolution chromosome studies are necessary to rule out similar disorders with chromosome abnormalities (deletion of part of chromosomes 1, 2, 3, 6, 7, 9, 11, 15, or 16 or partial duplication of chromosome 3, 4, 5, or 13).

TREATMENT

Standard Therapies: There is no causal therapy. Symptomatic and supportive therapies include the placement of a gastric tube in cases of sucking/swallowing problems. In cases of frequent vomiting and true gastroesophageal reflux, a Nissen fundoplication may be indicated. No evidence exists that craniotomy improves psychomotor development and neurologic deficits; however, when trigonocephaly is severe, surgery may relieve pressure on optic nerves (and brain) and "improve" facial appearance. Some children have had repeat craniotomies because of rapid reclosure of the metopic suture after surgery. Treatment with growth hormones is frequently considered for short stature, but this should be restricted to children with C syndrome who have true growth hormone deficiency. A pediatric endocrinologist should be consulted.

Investigational Therapies: Research on birth defects and their causes is ongoing, including research aimed at mapping the gene(s) of C syndrome.

REFERENCES

Antley RM, Hwang DS, Theopold W, et al. Further delineation of the C (trigonocephaly) syndrome. *Am J Med Genet* 1981;9: 147–163.

Bohring A, Silengo M, Lerone M, et al. Severe end of Opitz trigonocephaly (C) syndrome or new syndrome? *Am J Med Genet* 1999;85:438–446.

Opitz JM, Johnson RC, McCreadie SR, et al. The C syndrome of multiple congenital anomalies. *Birth Defects Orig Art Series* 1969;2:161–166.

Sargent C, Burn J, Baraitser M, et al. Trigonocephaly and the Opitz C syndrome. *J Med Genet* 1985;22:39–45.

RESOURCE

149

---

25 Cardiofaciocutaneous Syndrome

Maria Inês Kavamura, MD,
Giovanni Neri, MD, John M. Opitz, MD,
and Brenda Conger

DEFINITION: Cardiofaciocutaneous (CFC) syndrome is a genetic disorder first described in 1986 based on the observation of eight unrelated patients with similar facial appearance characterized by unusually sparse, brittle, curly hair, macrocephaly, a prominent forehead, and bitemporal constriction; mental retardation; failure to thrive; congenital heart defect; short stature; and ectodermal abnormalities.

DIFFERENTIAL DIAGNOSIS: Noonan syndrome; Costello syndrome.

SYMPTOMS AND SIGNS: Most patients are initially referred because of feeding difficulties (poor suck) and failure to thrive; later, because of psychomotor developmental delay and other clinical manifestations. Affected individuals may have macrocephaly and high forehead and abnormal narrowing of the sides of the forehead. The ears are posteriorly angulated. The nose is short and bulbous, and has anteverted nostrils. There is also hypoplasia of the ridges of the bone above the eyes, ocular hypertelorism, downward slant of eyelid openings, and ptosis. All patients have some kind of ectodermal abnormality of skin, hair, or nails. Patients usually have sparse, slowly growing, curly scalp hair that is friable. They also have absent or sparse eyebrows and eyelashes. Skin involvement ranges from dry skin to hyperkeratosis, including keratosis pilaris, ichthyosis, eczema, hemangiomas, hyperelastic skin, hyperkeratosis of palms and soles, café-au-lait spots, generalized hyperpigmentation, and cutis marmorata. Congenital heart defect is present in 77.8% of reported patients, particularly valpulmonary stenosis or atrial septal defects. Hypertrophic cardiomyopathy is present in 11% of patients with cardiac involvement. Some 90% of patients have mild to severe mental retardation, most having moderate retardation. Motor delays are reported in 81.5% of patients and speech delay in 46.3%. Short stature; webbed neck; abnormal shape of the thorax; joint hyperextension; hypotonia, especially during the first years of life; seizures; apparent hydrocephalus; hepatomegaly; or splenomegaly may be present. Undescended testes are present in approximately half of male patients.

ETIOLOGY/EPIDEMIOLOGY: Males and females are affected equally, and patients are reported from all continents. The number of published cases is close to 100, but many more unpublished cases are known. All patients represent sporadic cases born to nonconsanguineous parents with no history of genetic disease. They also have apparently normal chromosomes. Statistical evidence exists of increased paternal age, which suggests a new mutation of an autosomal-dominant gene as the cause of the syndrome. Chromosomal rearrangements have been described in two CFC patients, inherited in both from phenotypically normal mothers.

DIAGNOSIS: The diagnosis is clinical, based on the aforementioned traits. None of them are pathognomonic or obligatory and it is their general pattern that makes the diagnosis.

TREATMENT
Standard Therapies: Treatment is symptomatic. Gastrostomy has been helpful for patients with severe feeding problems. Cryptorchidism must be corrected surgically in the first years of life to avoid malignant transformation of the testes. Seizures, if present, must also be well controlled,

and the heart condition must be followed regularly and carefully. The skin condition, in general, responds well to moisturizers and ointments applied regularly.

REFERENCES
Grebe TA, Clericuzio C. Neurologic and gastrointestinal dysfunction in cardio-facio-cutaneous syndrome: identification of a severe phenotype. *Am J Med Genet* 2000;95:135–143.

Krajewska-Walasek M, Chrzanowska K, Jastrzbska M. The cardio-facio-cutaneous (CFC) syndrome: two possible new cases and review of the literature. *Clin Dysmorph* 1996;5: 65–72.

Legius E, Schollen E, Matthijs G, et al. Fine mapping of Noonan/cardio-facio-cutaneous syndrome in a large family. *Eur J Hum Genet* 1998;6:32–37.

McDaniel CH, Fujimoto A. Intestinal malrotation in a child with cardio-facio-cutaneous syndrome. *Am J Med Genet* 1997;70: 284–286.

Rauen KA, Cotter PD, Bitts SM, et al. Cardio-facio-cutaneous syndrome phenotype in an individual with an interstitial deletion of 12q: identification of a candidate region for CFC syndrome. *Am J Med Genet* 2000;93:219–222.

26   Cat Eye Syndrome

Heather McDermid, PhD,
and John Steven Bamforth, FRCPC (Can)

DEFINITION: Cat eye syndrome (CES) is a chromosomal disorder characterized by abnormalities of the eyes, heart, anus, kidneys, genitourinary tract, skeleton, and face, as well as by mild mental retardation. The features present and their severity are highly variable.

SYNONYMS: Schmid-Fraccaro syndrome; Chromosome 22, partial tetrasomy (22pter-22q11); Chromosome 22, partial trisomy (22pter-22q11); Chromosome 22, inverted duplication (22pter-22q11).

DIFFERENTIAL DIAGNOSIS: Townes-Brocks syndrome.

SYMPTOMS AND SIGNS: The name *cat eye syndrome* originates from the presence of unilateral or bilateral colobomata, although this feature is present in only half of patients. The variability of this syndrome is extensive. Features may include the following: preauricular pits or skin tags, ear anomalies (reduced auricles, atresia of the external auditory canal), ocular coloboma, hypertelorism, downslanting palpebral fissures, epicanthal folds, other ocular

abnormalities (microphthalmia, Duane anomaly), broad flat nasal bridge, micrognathia, congenital heart defects, anal anomalies (anal atresia or stenosis), renal anomalies (hypoplasia, unilateral agenesis), genital anomalies (hypospadias, cryptorchidism), skeletal anomalies (scoliosis), and mild mental retardation. Total anomalous pulmonary venous drainage/return represents approximately half of the heart defects detected, but also seen are tetralogy of Fallot, septal defects, interrupted aortic arch, patent ductus arteriosus, and coarctation of the aorta.

ETIOLOGY/EPIDEMIOLOGY: CES is usually caused by the presence of an extra chromosome of chromosome 22 origin. Rare cases have been caused by three copies of the region of chromosome 22. The incidence in northeastern Switzerland has been estimated to be 1 in 50,000 to 1 in 150,000. A person with CES has an approximately 50% chance of passing the chromosome to each child (autosomal-dominant inheritance).

DIAGNOSIS: Because the clinical features of this syndrome are highly variable, a suspected diagnosis must be confirmed cytogenetically, showing the presence of a chromosome 22 abnormality. Abnormalities on ultrasonography (especially congenital cardiac defects involving abnormal pulmonary vein connections) may prompt prenatal cytogenetic studies.

TREATMENT

Standard Therapies: Treatment is symptomatic. Surgical intervention is usually required to correct the heart and anal problems. Education may require special resources, and assessment of needs should begin at least 1 year before school entry to allow placement planning, if indicated. Growth hormone therapy may be indicated for patients with a deficiency.

Investigational Therapies: Research is being done on the genes involved and the structure of the CES chromosome.

REFERENCES

Liehr T, Pfeiffer RA, Trautmann U. Typical and partial cat eye syndrome: identification of the marker chromosome by FISH. *Clin Genet* 1992;42:91–96.

McKusick VA, ed. Online Mendelian Inheritance in Man (OMIM) [database online]. Bethesda, MD: National Center for Biotechnology Information, National Library of Medicine; 2000. Entry No: 115470; Last Update: July 13, 2000.

McTaggart KE, Budarf ML, Driscoll DA, et al. Cat eye syndrome chromosome breakpoint clustering: identification of two intervals also associated with 22q11 deletion syndrome breakpoints. *Cytogenet Cell Genet* 1998;81:222–228.

Mears AJ, Duncan AMV, Biegel JA, et al. Molecular characterization of the marker chromosome associated with cat eye syndrome. *Am J Hum Genet* 1994;55:134–142.

Schinzel A, Schmid W, Fraccaro M, et al. The "cat eye syndrome": decentric small marker chromosome probably derived from a 22 (tetrasomy 22pter;q11) associated with a characteristic phenotype. Report of 11 patients and delineation of the clinical picture. *Hum Genet* 1981;57:148–158.

RESOURCES

102, 253, 292

---

27 Catel-Manzke Syndrome

Golder N. Wilson, MD, PhD

DEFINITION: Catel-Manzke syndrome is a pediatric syndrome characterized by Pierre Robin sequence and hyperphalangism of the index finger.

SYNONYM: Pierre Robin sequence with hyperphalangism.

DIFFERENTIAL DIAGNOSIS: Otopalatodigital syndromes; Desbuquois skeletal dysplasia syndrome.

SYMPTOMS AND SIGNS: The Robin anomaly with cleft soft palate, small jaw, and glossoptosis is found in 90% of cases; extra phalanges and clinodactyly of the index fingers in 100%. Low birth weight, postnatal growth retardation, and mild developmental disability are common. Cardiac anomalies include septal and aortic defects, and skeletal changes other than the hyperphalangy include fifth finger clinodactyly, short fingers and toes, clubfeet, vertebral or rib anomalies, pectus excavatum, and joint laxity with dislocations.

ETIOLOGY/EPIDEMIOLOGY: Occurrence is usually sporadic, but three families with two or more cases have been reported. The presence of 4 females among 18 reported cases, male-to-male transmission, and affected siblings suggest genetic heterogeneity.

DIAGNOSIS: Examination to document Robin anomaly and a skeletal radiographic survey to document index finger hyperphalangy are sufficient for diagnosis. The full skeletal survey and an echocardiogram are mandated by the frequency of cardiac and skeletal anomalies.

TREATMENT

Standard Therapies: Neonates with Pierre Robin sequence should be placed prone to sleep to facilitate jaw extension and airway patency. Surgery to correct palatal defects is indicated to reduce otitis media and improve speech, but catch-up jaw growth will normally obviate the need for mandibular surgery.

REFERENCES

Brude E. Pierre Robin sequence and hyperphalangy—a genetic entity (Catel-Manzke syndrome). *Eur J Pediatr* 1984;142: 222–223.

Kant SG, Oudshoorn A, Gi CV, Zonderland et al. The Catel-Manzke syndrome in a female infant. *Genet Couns* 1998; 9:187–190.

Shohat M, Lachman R, Gruber HE, et al. Desbuquois syndrome: clinical, radiographic, and morphologic characterization. *Am J Med Genet* 1994;52:9–19.

Wilson GN, King TE, Brookshire GS. Index finger hyperphalangy and multiple anomalies: Catel-Manzke syndrome? *Am J Med Genet* 1993;46:176–179.

RESOURCES

360, 392, 492

28   Caudal Regression Syndrome

Axel Bohring, Dipl Med

DEFINITION: The term *caudal regression* describes a group of well-known, serious, complex malformations affecting the lower part of the body, including anomalies of lumbar and sacral vertebrae and pelvis, contractures of the hip and knees, clubfeet, and renal and genital anomalies. Additional anomalies of the gastrointestinal tract, heart, upper limbs, and thoracic and cervical spine are common.

SYNONYMS: Caudal dysgenesis; Caudal dysplasia.

DIFFERENTIAL DIAGNOSIS: VATER; VACTERL; Sirenomelia; Potter sequence; OEIS complex; Mayer-Rokitansky-Küster-Hauser syndrome.

SYMPTOMS AND SIGNS: Common findings are lumbar and sacral spine anomalies, sacral dimple, distal spinal cord anomalies which may lead to neurologic impairments such as defective bladder and bowel control, flexion contractures of lower limbs, popliteal pterygia, and clubfeet. Occasional findings include imperforate anus, meningomyelocele, anomalies of the upper vertebral spine, and facial anomalies. Renal agenesis or multicystic kidneys may cause oligohydramnios and the Potter sequence.

ETIOLOGY/EPIDEMIOLOGY: This condition represents a polytopic developmental field defect due to disturbed blastogenesis either by environmental or genetic causes that may interrupt the pattern forming signaling cascades necessary for normal early development. The incidence is 1 to 5 in 100,000 live births. Mostly sporadic occurrence suggests new mutation or environmental/teratogenic effects. Maternal diabetes mellitus is reported in 16%–28% of patients. Alcohol and retinoic acid have been reported as causes. Occasional familial occurrence suggests a genetic cause in some cases. The human homeobox gene *HLXB9* has been identified as the major locus for dominantly inherited sacral agenesis.

DIAGNOSIS: The diagnosis can be made easily on the basis of clinical findings, but no correlation is known between clinical appearance and cause. Careful examination is necessary to rule out additional anomalies. High-resolution chromosome studies are suggested in all cases.

TREATMENT
Standard Therapies: There is no causal therapy. Maternal diabetes mellitus should be well controlled before conception and during pregnancy, and all women trying to conceive should take at least 400 μg of folic acid daily beginning 1 month before conception. Alcohol and isotretinoin should be avoided. Very high doses of vitamin A may be teratogenic. Symptomatic and supportive therapy depends on the special needs of the patient and includes orthopedic, urologic, surgical, and physical therapy; however, severe malformations including bilateral renal agenesis and severe congenital heart defects may be fatal.

REFERENCES
Bohring A, Lewin SO, Reynolds JF, et al. Polytopic anomalies with agenesis of the lower vertebral column. *Am J Med Genet* 1999;87:99–114.
Duhamel B. From the mermaid to anal imperforation. The syndrome of caudal regression. *Arch Dis Child* 1961;36:152–155.
Passarge E, Lenz W. Syndrome of caudal regression in infants of diabetic mothers: observation of further cases. *Pediatrics* 1966;37:672–675.
Ross AJ, Ruiz-Perez V, Wang Y, et al. A homeobox gene, *HLXB9*, is the major locus for dominantly inherited sacral agenesis. *Nat Genet* 1998;20:358–361.

RESOURCES
360, 418

29   Cerebrocostomandibular Syndrome

Matthew L. Warman, MD, and Shauna Heeger, MS

DEFINITION: Cerebrocostomandibular syndrome (CCMS) describes a constellation of congenital malformations including rib gap defects, resulting thorax deformity, and micrognathia. The oral findings often include the complete Robin anomaly of micrognathia, glossoptosis, and cleft palate.

SYNONYM: Rib gap defects with micrognathia.

DIFFERENTIAL DIAGNOSIS: Robin anomaly, either isolated or syndromic; Other short rib skeletal dysplasias.

SYMPTOMS AND SIGNS: Infants born with CCMS are immediately noted to have micrognathia. Coupled with cleft palate (67%) and glossoptosis (73%), this often leads to neonatal respiratory distress. Half of the infants have prenatal growth retardation, half are microcephalic. Radiographic studies reveal gaps in the posterior portion of the ribs. These gaps are present at birth, usually asymmetric, and can create a flail chest appearance. Lower ribs can be underdeveloped or absent. A wide range of additional anomalies is reported in approximately 50% of affected individuals. These most often include tracheal malformations, vertebral anomalies, and hearing loss. Neonatal death, postnatal growth retardation, and developmental delay (50%) are also reported.

ETIOLOGY/EPIDEMIOLOGY: CCMS was first described in 1966; approximately 100 affected individuals have been reported worldwide. This may be an underrepresentation, as half of affected children die in the neonatal period due to respiratory insufficiency. The disorder has been seen in both genders, with all ethnic groups represented. The genetics of CCMS are poorly defined, with most instances representing a single occurrence in a family. Sibling pairs and consanguineous parents (suggesting autosomal-recessive inheritance) as well as parent-to-child transmission (suggesting autosomal-dominant inheritance) have also been reported.

DIAGNOSIS: The diagnosis is made radiographically on the basis of posterior rib gap deformities in conjunction with micrognathia.

TREATMENT
Standard Therapies: Respiratory insufficiency, cleft palate repair, dental difficulties, and hearing loss are treated with traditional therapies as needed. Approximately half of affected children will require special education services.

Investigational Therapies: Investigation centers on localizing and identifying the gene for this condition.

REFERENCES
Hennekam RC, Beemer FA, Huijbers WA, et al. The cerebro-costo-mandibular syndrome: third report of familial occurrence. *Clin Genet* 1985;28:118–121.
Plotz FB, van Essen AJ, Bosschaart AN, et al. Cerebro-costo-mandibular syndrome. *Am J Med Genet* 1996;62:286–292.
Van den Ende JJ, Schrander-Stumpel C, Rupprecht E, et al. The cerebro-costo-mandibular syndrome: seven patients and review of the literature. *Clin Dysmorphol* 1998;7:87–94.

RESOURCES
88, 108, 462

30 CHARGE Syndrome

John M. Graham, Jr., MD, ScD

DEFINITION: CHARGE association was initially delineated as a nonrandom pattern of congenital anomalies that occurred together more frequently than one would expect on the basis of chance. Within the group of children diagnosed with CHARGE association, a subgroup clearly exists with such distinctive clinical characteristics that they appear to manifest a recognizable syndrome. Major diagnostic criteria include those findings that occur commonly in CHARGE association, but are relatively rare in other conditions: coloboma, choanal atresia, cranial nerve involvement, and characteristic ear abnormalities.

SYNONYMS: CHARGE association; Hall-Hittner syndrome; Choanal atresia multiple anomalies syndrome.

DIFFERENTIAL DIAGNOSIS: DiGeorge sequence; Velocardiofacial syndrome (VCFS); Retinoic acid embryopathy; PAX2 abnormalities; Coloboma; Choanal atresia; Heart defects.

SYMPTOMS AND SIGNS: Major diagnostic criteria include those findings that occur commonly in CHARGE association, but are relatively rare in other conditions: coloboma, choanal atresia, cranial nerve involvement (particularly asymmetric facial palsy and neurogenic swallowing problems), and characteristic ear abnormalities including both the distinctive asymmetric auricular defects and the temporal bone anomalies. The ears have a triangular concha, small lobule, and extension of the antihelix toward the helical rim, where the lower helical fold is often thin or absent. Minor diagnostic criteria that occur less frequently (or are less specific to CHARGE syndrome) include heart defects, genital hypoplasia, orofacial clefting, tracheoesophageal fistula, short stature, and developmental delay. Other occasional less specific findings include renal anomalies, thymic/parathyroid hypoplasia, hand and spine anomalies, webbed neck, sloping shoulders, nipple anomalies, characteristic facial features, and abdominal defects. When orofacial clefting is present, the choanae are usually patent, so this finding can substitute for choanal atresia, particularly if the remaining findings are characteristic for CHARGE syndrome.

ETIOLOGY/EPIDEMIOLOGY: Most cases of CHARGE association have been sporadic occurrences in an otherwise normal family. In some families there is a clear genetic component, with parent-to-child transmission suggesting autosomal-dominant inheritance, and recurrences among siblings born to normal parents suggesting possible germ cell line mosaicism. No well-documented cases of CHARGE syndrome have had a detectable chromosome anomaly or a submicroscopic fluorescent *in situ* hybridization (FISH) deletion of 22q11 (VCFS), 7q36 (holoprosencephaly), or 10q25 (PAX2). These findings support the strong possibility that most patients with CHARGE association have a fresh dominant mutation or submicroscopic chromosomal deletion involving an unknown gene. The syndrome occurs with an estimated rate of 1 in 10,000–15,000 live births, and in both sexes.

DIAGNOSIS: The diagnosis is made on the basis of clinical features. High-resolution chromosome analysis should be performed in new and old cases of CHARGE association to identify any associated chromosome abnormality, and FISH for 22q11 deletion should also be done when DiGeorge sequence is associated, to rule out VCFS.

TREATMENT
Standard Therapies: Choanal atresia requires surgical repair with nasal stents. Gastrostomy feeding tubes are often used to manage feeding difficulties. Although gastrostomy tubes may improve growth and reduce the risk of aspiration pneumonia, problems with oral hypersensitivity may develop. In the preschool years, some catch-up growth occurs in children with CHARGE syndrome, but it is usually inadequate. Hormone therapy with ethinyl estradiol may be helpful, and pelvic ultrasonography to assess internal genitalia may be necessary. When full pubertal progression or breakthrough bleeding occurs, a change to low-dose oral contraceptive pills or adult hormone replacement therapy becomes necessary. Boys usually require testosterone replacement for adequate masculinization and normalization of penile size.

REFERENCES
Blake K, Davenport SH, Hall BD, et al. CHARGE association: an update and review for the primary pediatrician. *Clin Pediatr* 1998;37:159–174.
Hall BD. Choanal atresia and associated multiple anomalies. *J Pediatr* 1979;95:395–398.
Hittner HM, Hirsch NJ, Kreh GM, et al. Colobomatous microphthalmia, heart disease, hearing loss and mental retardation: a syndrome. *J Pediatr Ophthalmol Strabismus* 1979;16:122–128.
Tellier AL, Cormier-Daire V, Abadie V, et al. CHARGE syndrome: report of 47 cases and review. *Am J Med Genet* 1998;76:402–409.

RESOURCES
75, 91, 113

---

31   Cherubism

Ernst Reichenberger, PhD,
and Valdenize Tiziani, MD

DEFINITION: Cherubism is a genetic disorder restricted to the maxilla and mandible that manifests as excessive localized bony degradation and results in the formation of cystlike cavities that fill with fibrous tissue. The process is benign and self-limiting.

DIFFERENTIAL DIAGNOSIS: Caffey disease; Ramon syndrome; Gingival fibromatosis; Noonan-like multiple giant cell lesion syndrome; McCune-Albright syndrome; Giant cell granuloma; Giant cell tumor.

SYMPTOMS AND SIGNS: The onset is typically between the ages of 18 months and 14 years, although most patients present at the age of 3–4 years. The first symptom is painless, usually symmetric, swelling of the jaws. Radiographs show cystlike, multilocular degradation in the maxilla and mandible. The localized bone destruction can cause dental abnormalities such as hypodontia, displacement of teeth, noneruption, and root resorption. Fibrous tissue fills the intraosseous cystic spaces, and the process rapidly expands over the next few years, leading to the typical facial appearance. Mandibular swelling is more obvious and frequently occurs before maxillary enlargement. The severity of the phenotype is widely variable even within the same family. In more severe cases, the tumor-like tissue pushes the orbital floors upward, and the sclera are exposed above the lower eyelids, hence the cherub-like facial expression. Mastication, swallowing, and speech can be affected by the swelling. Enlarged submandibular lymph nodes can be a result of prolonged inflammatory processes caused by the disease. The symptoms and signs usually regress after puberty, often without the need for intervention. After the swelling disappears in adulthood, the bony lesions remain and are eventually filled with compact bone.

ETIOLOGY/EPIDEMIOLOGY: The disorder is autosomal dominant and has been mapped to chromosome 4p16.3. Cherubism occurs in equal frequency in both sexes and there is no sex difference in expressivity or penetrance.

DIAGNOSIS: Radiographs of the skull and ribs are used to assess the status of bony degradation and dentition. Patients with cherubism present with normal levels of blood calcium, phosphorus, and parathyroid hormone. Histology of the soft fibrous tissue shows dense fibroblastoid stroma with well-developed vasculature and clusters of multinucleated cells.

TREATMENT
Standard Therapies: Usually, the only treatment necessary is monitoring the progression of symptoms and signs. Early dental intervention may be appropriate. Surgical removal of abnormal tissue may be necessary in severe cases to prevent orbital compression and impact on speech or mastication.

Investigational Therapies: The locus of the gene and mutations for the autosomal-dominant form of cherubism are being investigated. The possibility that there are other mutations and genes causing cherubism has not been excluded.

REFERENCES
Katz JO, Underhill TE. Multilocular radiolucencies [Review]. *Dent Clin North Am* 1994;38:63–81.
Southgate J, Sarma U, Townend JV, et al. Study of the cell biology and biochemistry of cherubism. *J Clin Pathol* 1998;51:831–837.
Tiziani V, Reichenberger E, Buzzo CL, et al. The gene for cherubism maps to chromosome 4p16. *Am J Hum Genet* 1999;65:158–166.

RESOURCES
96, 351

32 Familial Articular Chondrocalcinosis

J. Desmond O'Duffy, MD

DEFINITION: Familial articular chondrocalcinosis is an inborn error of metabolism in which crystalline deposits of calcium pyrophosphate infiltrate joint cartilages, resulting in eventual damage to the joints.

SYNONYMS: Calcium pyrophosphate dihydrate (CPPD) deposition disease; Pseudogout; Chondrocalcinosis articularis.

DIFFERENTIAL DIAGNOSIS: Gout; Osteoarthritis; Rheumatoid arthritis; Other metabolic diseases such as hemochromatosis, hyperparathyroidism, and hypomagnesemia.

SYMPTOMS AND SIGNS: Few or no symptoms may be apparent in the first several decades of life. In presymptomatic individuals, radiography of the joints, especially the knees and wrists, may detect the calcifications. As the disease develops, symptoms can be acute, with sudden attacks of inflammation, called pseudogout, with pain and swelling in one or more joints. Attacks of pseudogout are caused by the release of calcium pyrophosphate crystals into the joint. Most patients present at age 60 or older. They often have pain and stiffness with little or no inflammation. The knees, hips, wrists, and shoulders are most often clinically involved. CPPD deposits in the spinal intervertebral discs often lead to their premature degeneration.

ETIOLOGY/EPIDEMIOLOGY: In most patients the cause of the disease is uncertain. Overproduction of CPPD deposits in joints is believed to result from excessive activity of an enzyme nucleoside triphosphate pyrophosphohydrolase (NTPPPH), but no broad agreement exists on the cause. All ethnic groups can be affected. Inheritance in an individual may be difficult to prove, but in some families it may be a dominant trait and in others a recessive trait.

DIAGNOSIS: The microscopic demonstration of CPPD crystals in the acute joints of pseudogout attacks combined with characteristically linear calcifications in radiographed joints confirm the diagnosis. The family history may be negative or positive.

TREATMENT

Standard Therapies: Pseudogout attacks can be treated with intraarticular corticosteroid injection or by nonsteroidal antiinflammatory drugs (NSAIDs). Attacks that recur frequently can be prevented by very low doses of oral colchicine. Joints that are damaged beyond repair are often replaced by joint arthroplasty. Most patients require little treatment, aside from NSAIDs or common analgesics. In the future, enzymatic replacement therapy may be offered.

REFERENCES

McCarty DJ, Kohn NN, Faires JS. The significance of calcium phosphate crystals in the synovial fluid of arthritic patients. *Ann Intern Med* 1962;56:711–737.

Ryan LM, McCarty DJ. Calcium pyrophosphate crystal deposition disease, pseudogout, and articular chondrocalcinosis. In: Koopman, ed. *Arthritis and allied conditions: a textbook of rheumatology,* 13th ed. Baltimore: Williams & Wilkins, 1997: 2103–2125.

Smyth CJ, Holers VM, eds. *Gout, hyperucemia and other crystal-associated arthropathies.* New York: Marcel Dekker, 1999.

RESOURCE
360

---

33   Cockayne Syndrome

Susanne Schmandt, Dr Med, and Phillip L. Pearl, MD

DEFINITION: Cockayne syndrome (CS) is a multisystem disorder characterized by severe brain and somatic growth failure, progressive cachexia, photosensitivity, and retinal, cochlear, and neurologic degeneration related at least in part to defective DNA repair.

DIFFERENTIAL DIAGNOSIS: XP-CS complex; COFS syndrome; CAHMR syndrome; CAMFAK syndrome; DeSanctis-Cacchione syndrome; Rothmund-Thomson syndrome; Aminoacidopathies; Mitochondrial disease; Pelizaeus-Merzbacher disease; Congenital infections; Skeletal dysplasias; Genetic syndromes with dwarfism.

SYMPTOMS AND SIGNS: Three types are differentiated by their severity: type I CS or classic CS, the most common subtype with survival into adolescence/young adulthood; type II CS, with early onset and death; and a mild type. Predictors for severe disease are prenatal growth failure, severe neurologic dysfunction from birth, congenital structural eye anomalies, and cataracts within the first 3 years of life. In classic CS, growth failure including of the brain starts postnatally, although with onset in the first year of life. It is accompanied by progressive loss of adipose tissue, resulting in a cachectic, microencephalic dwarfism with a senile appearance. The facies are characteristic, with sunken orbits, a relatively large, beaklike nose, and a narrow mouth and chin. Other features include cognitive decline in the presence of a rather well-preserved sociability; progressive spasticity with contractures of hips, knees, and ankles, resulting in a characteristic stooped gait or nonambulatory

status; variable reflexes due to a concurrent clinically mild demyelinating neuropathy; cerebellar involvement with tremor and ataxia; optic atrophy; pigmentatory retinopathy; nystagmus; miotic pupils; decreased lacrimation; sensorineural deafness; dental caries; photosensitivity; renal hypertension; underdeveloped sexual characteristics; and skeletal changes with variable bone age. Mean age of death is approximately 12 years, although some affected individuals live into their late twenties.

ETIOLOGY/EPIDEMIOLOGY: No more than 200 cases have been reported. In 90% of cases, CS arises due to mutations in the *CSA* or *CSB* gene, which result in type I and II CS, respectively. Patients with certain mutations in the genes *XPB, XPD,* and *XPG* overwhelmingly present with a CS phenotype of variable severity, whereas the xeroderma pigmentosum phenotype is mild (XP-CS complex). Mutations in these five genes are responsible for UV sensitivity and deficient post-UV DNA repair. In CS specifically, transcription coupled repair of UV-induced damage is deficient. Transcription coupled repair may be a prerequisite for nucleotide excision repair as well as base excision repair and allows continuation of blocked transcription.

DIAGNOSIS: Clinical observation, assays of UV light sensitivity and DNA repair, cell fusion studies to assign complementation groups, and DNA sequencing for mutation analysis are used in the diagnosis. Imaging studies are among the most valuable screening tools, showing calcifications of the basal ganglia and dentate nucleus, ventriculomegaly, and leukodystrophy. Elevated cerebrospinal fluid protein and abnormal audiometry, funduscopy, electroretinogram, nerve conduction, nerve biopsy, and evoked potentials support the diagnosis.

TREATMENT

Standard Therapies: Symptomatic treatment and avoidance of sun exposure are the mainstays of therapy. The role of antioxidants or free radical scavengers is not yet established. Treatment with 5-hydroxytryptophan is also being explored.

REFERENCES

Cockayne EA. Dwarfism with retinal atrophy and deafness. *Arch Dis Child* 1936;21:52–54.

Ellaway CJ, Duggins A, Fung VS, et al. Cockayne associated with low CSF 5-hydroxyindole acetic acid levels. *J Med Genet* 2000;37:553–557.

Hanawalt PC. The bases for Cockayne syndrome. *Nature* 2000;405:415–416.

Rapin I, Lindenbaum Y, Dickson DW, et al. Cockayne syndrome and xeroderma pigmentosum. *Neurology* 2000;55:1442–1449.

RESOURCES

188, 253, 433

---

34   Coffin-Lowry Syndrome

Karen H. Harum, MD,
and Michael V. Johnston, MD

DEFINITION: Coffin-Lowry syndrome is an X-linked mental retardation disorder characterized by the constellation of specific hand and facial features, short stature, and skeletal malformations. The disorder is due to mutations of the *RSK2* gene, located on the short arm of the X chromosome (Xp22.2).

DIFFERENTIAL DIAGNOSIS: Alpha-thalassemia mental retardation; Williams syndrome; Mucopolysaccharidoses or other "storage disorders"; 10q deletion syndrome.

SYMPTOMS AND SIGNS: Infants present with hypotonia and global developmental delays. The severely affected child may have no speech development and may be significantly cognitively impaired. The affected individual's temperament is usually gentle and affectionate. Although the child may be shy, there is typically no autistic overlay. Characteristic facial features are coarse and include prominence of the forehead due to a thickened cranium, hypertelorism, thick lips, thickened nasal septum, prominent chin and ears, delays in dental eruption, premature dental exfoliation, and tooth malformations. Additional physical features include forearm and hand fullness due to increased fat accumulation, hypothenar crease, brachydactyly, "champagne cork" appearance to the distal phalanges on radiography, scoliosis, vertebral malformations, and short stature. Drop attacks (cataplexy) are described as atypical, exaggerated startle episodes during which all muscle tone is lost following an unexpected noise or emotional event. Full consciousness is maintained during the episodes, which are approximately 1 second in duration followed immediately by recovery of muscle tone. The episodes can result in significant injury due to unexpected falls. Epileptic seizures can also develop. Occasionally, congenital heart defects are present. Sensorineural hearing loss develops over time and may be difficult to ascertain in a nonverbal individual.

ETIOLOGY/EPIDEMIOLOGY: RSK2 is a protein kinase important in intracellular molecular signaling and is a member of the RAS/MAPK signaling cascade, which is known to be important in cognitive function. Various mutations have been identified at the *RSK2* gene, each with variable functional impact on the RSK2 protein product. If the protein product is truncated or unstable, CLS is usually fully manifested. Minor missense mutations that result in less impairment of the RSK2 protein result in nonsyndromic, X-linked mental retardation or learning disabilities. The prevalence of this disorder is unknown; it is most certainly underdiagnosed in those with nonsyndromic mental retardation. There appears to be no ethnic predilection. This X-linked semidominant disorder is most likely to manifest in its classic form in males; however, females with unfavorable X chromosome inactivation can also present with the classic clinical picture, although with less cognitive impairment.

DIAGNOSIS: The clinical diagnosis can be confirmed by mutation analysis of the *RSK2* gene. No abnormalities of the mutated X chromosome are visible by high-resolution banded karyotype.

TREATMENT

Standard Therapies: No specific therapies exist for the associated cognitive impairment, apart from that which may be offered to persons with nonsyndromic mental retardation. Early diagnosis and treatment of scoliosis and sensorineural hearing loss, both of which may be progressive, significantly improve quality of life. Anticipation of difficult airway management and hemodynamic instability related to cardiac defects may require special anesthetic techniques. The best theoretical treatment for cataplexy includes the selective serotonin reuptake inhibitors and clomipramine. Benzodiazapenes have demonstrated moderate efficacy. Surgical correction of the scoliosis may also resolve the cataplectic spells.

REFERENCES

Delaunoy JP, Abidi F, Zeniou M, et al. Mutations in the X-linked *RSK2* gene (*RPS6KA3*) in patients with Coffin-Lowry syndrome. *Hum Mutat* 2001;17:103–116.

Gilgenkrantz S, Mujica P, Gruet P, et al. Coffin-Lowry syndrome: a multicenter study. *Clin Genet* 1988;34:230–245.

Stevenson RE, Schwartz CE, Schroer RJ. *X-linked mental retardation.* New York: Oxford University Press, 2000.

RESOURCES

111, 351, 368

---

35   Cohen Syndrome

Meral Gunay-Aygun, MD, PhD

DEFINITION: Cohen syndrome is an autosomal-recessive disorder characterized by mental retardation, obesity, and typical facial features. Chorioretinal degeneration and granulocytopenia are seen in a subset of patients.

SYNONYMS: Pepper syndrome; CHS1; COH1.

DIFFERENTIAL DIAGNOSIS: Prader-Willi syndrome; Bardet-Biedl syndrome.

SYMPTOMS AND SIGNS: Clinical features are highly variable. Characteristic physical findings include typical facial appearance consisting of down-slanting palpebral fissures, high nasal bridge, short philtrum, high narrow palate, prominent central incisors and open mouth, and narrow hands and feet with long, tapering fingers. The space between toes 1 and 2 is usually increased. All affected individuals have mental retardation, and approximately half of patients have mild to moderate microcephaly. Infantile hypotonia is frequent. Developmental delay becomes obvious at 6–12 months of age. Most children walk between 2 and 5 years of age. Approximately two thirds of patients have delayed puberty, and more than half have short stature. Newborns have low-normal weights; the onset of obesity is generally in midchildhood. Severe obesity is rare and some patients may not develop obesity at all. Granulocytopenia associated with gingival and skin infections and chorioretinal degeneration are described in all Finish patients with Cohen syndrome. The earliest retinal changes are pale fundus and disc with or without pigment granularity, followed by narrowed vessels, pigment clumps, and bone spicule-like pigment accumulations by 10–20 years of age. Cataracts, progressive high-grade myopia, and astigmatism are also common. Granulocytopenia may be associated with recurrent gingivitis. No endocrine or significant cardiac abnormalities were found except for a decreased left ventricular function with advancing age. Kyphosis and scoliosis are other common features. Patients with chorioretinal involvement are also reported from other countries.

ETIOLOGY/EPIDEMIOLOGY: The inheritance pattern of the disorder is autosomal recessive, and is seen in both sexes. More than 100 cases have been reported. Although it is diagnosed in various populations, most cases are reported from Finland and Israel. Pathogenesis is unknown. Increase in neutrophil adhesive capability and a generalized neutrophil activation are shown. Some patients have high levels of urinary hyaluronic acid, suggesting a metabolic abnormality in the extracellular matrix. Cohen syndrome is mapped to chromosome 8q22-q23.

DIAGNOSIS: Diagnosis should be suspected based on clinical findings. Tests that can support the diagnosis include ophthalmologic examination and/or electroretinography to look for retinal degeneration; a white blood cell count for granulocytopenia; and MRI of the brain showing a relatively enlarged corpus callosum in a microcephalic head and normal gray and white matter.

TREATMENT

Standard Therapies: There is no specific treatment. Granulocytopenia is generally responsive to granulocyte colony-stimulating factor.

REFERENCES

Cohen MM Jr, Hall BD, Smith DW, et al. A new syndrome with hypotonia, obesity, mental deficiency, and facial, oral ocular and limb anomalies. *J Pediatr* 1973;83:280–284.

Kivitie-Kallio S, Eronen M, Lipsanen-Nyman M, et al. Cohen syndrome: evaluation of its cardiac, endocrine and radiological features. *Clin Genet* 1999;56:41–50.

Kivitie-Kallio S, Summanen P, Raitta C, et al. Ophthalmologic findings in Cohen syndrome. A long-term follow-up. *Ophthalmology* 2000;107:1737–1745.

Kolehmainen J, Norio R, Kivitie-Kallio S, et al. Refined mapping of the Cohen syndrome gene by linkage disequilibrium. *Eur J Hum Genet* 1997;5:206–213.

Okamoto N, Hatsukawa Y, Arai H, et al. Cohen syndrome with high urinary excretion of hyaluronic acid. *Am J Med Genet* 1998;76:387–388.

RESOURCES

112, 368

36   Conradi-Hünermann Syndrome

Nancy Braverman, MS, MD

DEFINITION: Conradi-Hünermann syndrome is an X-linked dominant genetic disorder caused by a defect in the *EBP* gene, located on Xp11.22–23. Affected females have chondrodysplasia punctata, asymmetric limb shortening, short stature, skin changes, and cataracts. The disorder is presumed to be lethal in males in the early embryonic period.

SYNONYMS: Chondrodysplasia punctata, X-linked dominant; CDPX2.

DIFFERENTIAL DIAGNOSIS: Rhizomelic chondrodysplasia punctata, types 1, 2, and 3 (RCDP1, 2, and 3); CHILD syndrome; Congenital hemidysplasia with ichthyosiform nevus and limb defects; CDPX1; Chondrodysplasia punctata X-linked recessive; *In utero* exposure to warfarin; Maternal lupus; Maternal vitamin K deficiency.

SYMPTOMS AND SIGNS: The classic abnormalities involve bone, skin, and lens. Radiologic studies in infancy show punctate epiphyseal calcifications along the vertebral column, ribs, sternum, clavicle, scapulae, pelvis, and long bones. Coronal clefts can be present. Although the calcifications resolve during childhood, epiphyseal irregularity may result. In addition, Asymmetric shortening of the long bones frequently involves the humerus and/or femur. Joint contractures, hip dysplasia, vertebral anomalies, kyphoscoliosis, and postaxial polydactyly may occur. Adult stature is reduced. Newborns have an ichthyosiform erthyroderma with thick adherent scales arrayed in a linear and swirled pattern. This hyperkeratotic eruption clears spontaneously by 6 months and is replaced by follicular atrophoderma and patchy areas of alopecia on the scalp. A linear and whorled pattern of hyperpigmentation has been observed. Hair may be sparse, coarse, and lusterless. Cataracts may be present at birth or develop in infancy. They are often asymmetric and sectorial. Rarely, other eye abnormalities occur such as microphthalmia and optic atrophy. Characteristic facial features include frontal bossing, depressed nasal bridge, flat facies, and anteverted nostrils. Facial asymmetry occurs.

ETIOLOGY/EPIDEMIOLOGY: The incidence is approximately 1 in 100,000. The phenotypic severity in females ranges from stillborn to mildly affected individuals identified in adulthood. Although many cases are isolated in families and represent *de novo* mutations in the *EBP* gene, familial cases are reported. Both the range of severity and the asymmetry of skeletal and eye findings, along with the linear and whorled pattern of skin involvement, result from random X-inactivation in heterozygous females. Affected males are rarely observed and are either 47,XXY individuals or, presumably, have the disorder as a consequence of a postzygotic mutation. The recurrence risk for each pregnancy for an affected female is 50% for female offspring. The pathogenesis is unknown. It has been suggested that relative cholesterol deficiency or the accumulation of a teratogenic sterol precursor may be a pathogenic factor.

DIAGNOSIS: The disorder is suspected on clinical examination and confirmed by plasma sterol analysis. This test employs gas chromatography/mass spectroscopy analysis of plasma.

TREATMENT

Standard Therapies: Treatment is supportive and involves the team care of a geneticist, orthopedist, ophthalmologist, and dermatologist. Orthopedic interventions may be required. Cataracts are extracted when they interfere with vision. Emollients may help to decrease the irritation associated with the hyperkeratosis.

REFERENCES

Braverman N, Lin P, Moebius FF, et al. Mutations in the gene encoding 3β-hydroxysteroid-Δ8,Δ7-isomerase cause X-linked dominant Conradi-Hünermann syndrome. *Nat Genet* 1999; 22:291–294.

Happle R. X-linked dominant chondrodysplasia punctata. Review of literature and report of a case. *Hum Genet* 1979;53:65–73.

Has C, Bruckner-Tuderman L, Muller D, et al. The Conradi-Hunermann-Happle syndrome (CDPX2) and emopamil binding protein: novel mutations, and somatic and gonadal mosaicism. *Hum Mol Genet* 2000;12:1951–1955.

Herman GE. X-Linked dominant disorders of cholesterol biosynthesis in man and mouse. *Biochim Biophys Acta* 2000;1529: 357–373.

Kelley R, Wilcox W, Smith M, et al. Abnormal sterol metabolism in patients with Conradi-Hunermann-Happle syndrome and sporadic lethal chondrodysplasia punctata. *Am J Med Genet* 1999;83:213–219.

RESOURCES

162, 351, 418

37   Primary Craniosynostosis

Kant Y. K. Lin, MD,
and Millie D. Long, MD

DEFINITION: Primary craniosynostosis occurs in the absence of an associated syndrome or known cause and is defined as the premature fusion of cranial vault suture(s) resulting in craniostenosis.

DIFFERENTIAL DIAGNOSIS: Positional skull molding; Crouzon syndrome; Apert syndrome; Pfieffer syndrome; Jackson-Weiss syndrome; Saethre-Chotzen syndrome; Secondary craniosynostosis.

SYMPTOMS AND SIGNS: With primary craniosynostosis, growth of the cranial vault cannot occur at right angles to the fused suture. The skull is forced to expand in compensation at other sutures that have remained patent. The location of the affected suture(s) and the timing during development of when the fusion occurs directly determines the resulting skull shape. When the sagittal suture is involved, the resulting head shape is long and narrow, described as scaphocephaly. Metopic suture synostosis results in a triangular-shaped skull, described as trigonocephaly. Unilateral coronal suture synostosis results in an oblique head shape with a flattened forehead and brow, described as an anterior plagiocephaly. Bilateral coronal suture involvement leads to a shortened and/or a towerlike skull described respectively as brachycephaly or turricephaly. Lambdoidal suture synostosis results in an oblique-shaped skull posteriorly, described as a posterior plagiocephaly. Mental development likely depends on the presence or absence of intracranial hypertension.

ETIOLOGY/EPIDEMIOLOGY: Primary craniosynostosis is an isolated finding and occurs irrespective of race. It is not associated with other facial, limb, or organ anomalies as is seen with the approximately 70 known craniosynostosis syndromes. Primary craniosynostosis occurs sporadically with a frequency of 0.6 in 1,000 newborns. Rare familial instances of craniosynostosis have been reported in an autosomal-dominant inheritance pattern. There is a male preponderance with sagittal synostosis and a female preponderance with coronal synostosis.

DIAGNOSIS: The diagnosis is made on physical examination through a careful assessment of cranial shape, seeking the presence of sutural ridging as well as the presence of other skull compensations. Additional confirmatory tests include CT and plain film skull radiography. A thorough birth and family history along with a full body physical examination is necessary to exclude the possibility of syndromal involvement.

TREATMENT

Standard Therapies: The treatment is surgical release of the fused suture and cranial vault remodeling and reconstruction to correct both the deficient areas as well as the areas of compensatory growth on the skull. Early referral to a multidisciplinary craniofacial team is recommended.

REFERENCES

Cohen MM, Maclean RE, eds. *Craniosynostosis: diagnosis, evaluation and management,* 2nd ed. New York: Oxford University Press, 2000:51, 119–120.

Gorlin RJ, Cohen MM, Levin LS, eds. *Syndromes of the head and neck,* 3rd ed. New York: Oxford University Press, 1990:519–520.

Kapp-Simon KA, Figueroa A, Jocher CA, et al. Longitudinal assessment of mental development in infants with nonsyndromic craniosynostosis with and without cranial release and reconstruction. *Plast Reconstr Surg* 1993;92:831–839.

RESOURCES

96, 149, 303

38 Cri-du-Chat Syndrome

Adam G. Mezoff, MD

DEFINITION: A rare chromosomal disorder characterized by a catlike cry at birth, failure to thrive, microcephaly, moderate to severe developmental delay, and facial abnormalities.

SYNONYMS: 5p-syndrome; Cat cry syndrome; Deletion 5p syndrome.

SYMPTOMS AND SIGNS: At birth, almost all patients have a high-pitched, weak, catlike cry. Failure to thrive and mental impairment (IQ rarely above 35) are virtually always present. Most (85%) patients have short stature. Up to half of patients older than 10 can communicate verbally. Other findings include infantile hypotonia, constipation, low birth weight (<2,500 g), congenital heart disease (patent ductus arteriosis is most common), inguinal hernia, and gastroesophageal reflux. Phenotypical abnormalities include microcephaly, broad based nose, micrognathia, low-set or poorly formed ears, abnormal palate (high-arched or broad or flat), hypertelorism, epicanthal folds, down-slanting palpebral fissures, simian crease, and distal axial triradius.

ETIOLOGY/EPIDEMIOLOGY: Cri-du-chat syndrome occurs as a result of a partial deletion (variable length) on the short arm, or p region, of chromosome 5. Approximately 85% of cases arise from *de novo* deletions; the other 15% are due to chromosomal translocation. The incidence is approximately 1 in 20,000. Females are affected more often than males. Small deletions in 5p15.3 and/or 5p15.2 can lead to cat-cry phenotype without associated mental impairment.

DIAGNOSIS: Diagnosis is suspected on a clinical basis and verified by karyotyping, which shows simple deletion of the short arm of chromosome 5. Occasionally, mosaicism or ring formation can result in 5p deletion.

TREATMENT
Standard Therapies: There is no treatment for the underlying disorder. With early aggressive supportive therapy, some children can function at the level of a 5- to 6-year-old. Patients often require a multidisciplinary approach including genetic counseling, a developmental specialist, a pediatric gastroenterologist, an orthopedist, a speech therapist, and occupational and physical therapy.

REFERENCES
Gersh M, et al. Evidence for a distinct region causing a cat-like cry in patients with 5p deletion. *Am J Hum Genet* xxxx;56: 1404.
Jones KL, ed. *Smith's recognizable patterns of human malformation,* 5th ed. Philadelphia: WB Saunders, 1997:44–45.
Mezoff AG, et al. Cri-du-chat: gastrointestinal manifestations and feeding practices [Abstract]. *J Pediatr Gastroenterol Nutr* 1995;3:338.
Wilkins LE, et al. Psychomotor development in 65 home reared children with Cri-du-chat syndrome. *J Pediatr* 1980;97:401.

RESOURCES
5, 104, 462

39 Cystic Hygroma

Hana Aviv, PhD

DEFINITION: Cystic hygroma is a congenital malformation of the lymphatic system characterized by single or multiple fluid-filled lesions that occur at sites where the lymphatic system connects to the venous system, most commonly in the back of the neck.

SYNONYMS: Lymphangioma; Cervical lymphocele; Jugular lymphatic obstruction.

DIFFERENTIAL DIAGNOSIS: Posterior encephalocele; Cervical meningocele or meningomyelocele; Benign cystic teratoma; Neck edema.

SYMPTOMS AND SIGNS: Cystic hygromas arise during fetal development due to failure of the jugular lymph sacs to connect and drain into the jugular veins. This leads to a series of events termed the jugular-lymphatic obstruction sequence. This is manifested in overgrowth of overlying skin, alterations in hair growth and patterning, protrusion of the lower ear, prominence of pads on the fingers, and narrow, hypoconvex nails. The lack of lymphatic drainage also leads to increased flow to the venous system, resulting in large veins and flow-related cardiac defects. In the prenatal period, cystic hygromas can be seen on ultrasonography as a mass with multiple echolucent cysts of varying size in the posterior and lateral aspect of the neck. Postnatally, the clinical manifestations are painless soft or semi-firm cystic masses in the neck and lower portion of the face. In children, cystic hygromas can also be found in the oral cavity. In adults, they are more commonly seen in the sublingual, submandibular, and parotid spaces.

ETIOLOGY/EPIDEMIOLOGY: The etiology of cystic hygroma is diverse. More than 60% of affected persons have an associated chromosomal abnormality. The most common cause is Turner syndrome (45,X or variants) and other chromosomal trisomies, such as trisomy 13, 18, and 21, and partial trisomies or monosomies. Cystic hygromas have also been associated with many inherited disorders and syndromes with normal karyotypes. Among autosomal-dominant syndromes are Noonan syndrome and achondroplasia. Autosomal-recessive syndromes include isolated cystic hygroma, lethal multiple pterygium syndromes, Roberts syndrome, Cumming syndrome, Cowchock syndrome, and achondrogenesis type II. Teratogenic causes of cystic hygroma include prenatal exposure to alcohol, amethopterin, or trimethadione. At 9–15 weeks of gestation, the prevalence may be as high as 1 in 200 fetuses. Males and females are equally affected. In children, the diagnosis is usually made before the second year of life.

DIAGNOSIS: Cystic hygroma is detected prenatally by ultrasonography. Chorionic villus sampling or amniocentesis can detect associated chromosome defects. In children or adults, detection of a painless soft cervical mass on clinical examination is followed by ultrasonographic examination to delineate its size, extent, and relationship to surrounding structures. CT can be used to evaluate soft tissue planes adjacent to larger masses and detect calcifications and vascularity of lesions. MRI may be important for preoperative planning.

TREATMENT
Standard Therapies: Complete excision of the lesion is the treatment of choice. This can be accomplished without difficulty in superficial lesions. If the lesion involves adjacent vital structures, such as cranial nerves, major vascular structures, or soft tissues such as the hypopharynx, parotid gland, and trachea, complete removal may involve multiple operations or may not be possible.

Investigational Therapies: Bleomycin, a sclerosing agent, and OK-432, a lyophilized mixture of low virulence *Su* strain of *Streptococcus pyogenes* of human origin, are being investigated.

REFERENCES
Edwards MJ, Graham JM. Posterior nuchal cystic hygroma. *Clin Perinatol* 1990;17:611–640.
Gallagher PG, Mahoney MJ, Gosche JR. Cystic hygroma in the fetus and newborn. *Semin Perinatol* 1999;23:341–356.
Koeller KK, Alamo L, Adir CF, et al. Congenital cystic masses of the neck: radiologic-pathologic correlation. *Arch AFIP* 1999;19:121–146.

RESOURCES
93, 128, 310

---

40   Dentin Dysplasia

Carole V. Brenneise, DDS, MS

DEFINITION: Dentin dysplasia (DD) is an inherited, autosomal-dominant, developmental defect that results in disorganization of the dentin tubules, producing abnormalities of the teeth that are evident in both primary and permanent dentitions. DD is divided into type I (radicular DD), which causes root abnormalities, and type II (coronal DD), which produces abnormalities of the coronal pulp chambers.

SYNONYMS: Rootless teeth; Opalescent dentin; Pulpless teeth; "Thistle tube" teeth.

SYMPTOMS AND SIGNS: The radiographic findings in DD type I include abnormal root formation (usually short and conical); pulpal obliteration with residual crescent-shaped pulp chambers; and periapical radiolucencies. These changes are seen most often in the permanent dentition but have also been documented in the primary dentitions. The abbreviated root formation and periapical changes result in early exfoliation of the primary teeth and unexpected mobility and early loss of permanent teeth. The shape and coloration of the crowns of permanent teeth are normal, however, giving no hint of the abnormal root formation. The alteration seen in DD type II includes brownish opalescent coloration of the primary teeth with progressive obliteration of the pulp chambers by the formation of abnormal dentin. The permanent teeth exhibit "thistle tube"–shaped, abnormally large pulp chambers, which the progressive formation of pulp calcifications eventually fills. Because the mantle dentin is normal, both the crown and the roots of these teeth are externally normal.

DIAGNOSIS: The diagnosis of DD type I is usually made on the radiographic appearance or early exfoliation of permanent teeth. DD type II may be diagnosed in children by the unusual coloration of the teeth and in the permanent dentition by the radiographically evident abnormal coronal pulp formation.

TREATMENT
Standard Therapies: When the alteration in root morphology in DD type I produces a root so short that retention of the teeth in the jaw is impossible, extraction and construction of full dentures is the treatment of choice. If the roots are adequate for retention, general dental care can

be performed. These teeth are extremely brittle, however, and the crown often fractures off with minimal force. DD type II requires no unusual treatment of permanent teeth.

REFERENCES
Brenneise CV, Conway KR. Dentin dysplasia, type II: report of 2 new families and review of the literature. *Oral Surg* 1999;87: 752–755.
Brenneise CV, Dwornik RM, Brenneise EE. Clinical radiographic and histological manifestations of dentition dysplasia, type I: report of case. *J Am Dent Assoc* 1989;119:721–723.
Shields ED, Bixler D, El-Kafrawy AM. A proposed classification for heritable human dentine defects with a description of a new entity. *Arch Oral Biol* 1973;18:543–553.
Witkop CJ Jr. Hereditary defects of dentition. *Dent Clin North Am* 1975;19:31–32.
Witkop CJ Jr. Amelogenesis imperfecta, dentinogenesis imperfecta and dentition dysplasia revisited: problems in classification. *J Oral Pathol* 1988;17:547–553.

RESOURCES
297, 320

41   Dentinogenesis Imperfecta Type III

*Mary MacDougall, PhD,
and Juan Dong, MD, PhD*

DEFINITION: Dentinogenesis imperfecta type III (DGI-III) is an autosomal-dominant disease affecting both deciduous and permanent teeth. It is the most common dental disease affecting an isolated population in southern Maryland, known as the Brandywine isolate. The disease in one kindred is caused by a compound mutation (insertion and deletion) within the dentin phosphoprotein (DPP) domain of the dentin sialophosphoprotein (DSPP) gene. The teeth are bluish brown with an amber opalescent appearance. They wear easily due to abnormal dentin mineralization and chipping of the overlying enamel layer.

SYNONYMS: Shields type III; Brandywine type dentinogenesis imperfecta.

DIFFERENTIAL DIAGNOSIS: Dentinogenesis imperfecta type I (with osteogenesis imperfecta); Dentinogenesis imperfecta type II; Dentin dysplasia type I; Dentin dysplasia type II.

SYMPTOMS AND SIGNS: Teeth are discolored, appearing brown to bluish gray, sometimes referred to as an amber opalescent appearance. The deciduous and permanent teeth wear rapidly after eruption, and multiple pulp exposures may occur. The enamel is often pitted, and can chip from the underlying dentin surface. Radiographs show large pulp chambers and root canals during early tooth development and radiolucencies at the apices of teeth without pulp exposures. The teeth are often referred to as "shell teeth." Anterior open bites are reported in most patients.

ETIOLOGY/EPIDEMIOLOGY: The disorder is inherited in an autosomal-dominant manner. Within the Brandywine isolate, the prevalence is estimated at 1 in 15. The disease in one large kindred is due to a mutation in the DPP domain of DSPP located on chromosome 4q21 within a 6.6 cM region defined by markers D4S2691 and D4S2692. The DGI-III locus overlaps with the critical loci for DGI type II and dentin dysplasia type II. The Brandywine isolate is an inbred triracial population consisting of caucasians, African Americans, and Native American Indians.

DIAGNOSIS: The diagnosis should be suspected based on the findings of the discoloration of the teeth first evident in the deciduous teeth and a positive family history. Dental radiographs should confirm the diagnosis.

TREATMENT

Standard Therapies: Children are fitted with dental crowns as early as possible for cosmetic benefit and to minimize tooth surface wear. Adults may undergo tooth extraction and replacement with dentures or implants. Early and correct diagnosis is imperative to allow early intervention preventing tooth loss and to allow optimal treatment. Affected family members may benefit from genetic counseling.

Investigational Therapies: Genetic studies are being performed to determine the possibility of other DSPP mutations being present within Brandywine isolate families, and are being designed to screen potential DGI-III patients before tooth eruption, allowing earlier dental intervention.

REFERENCES

Hursey RJ, Witkop CJ Jr, Miklashek D, et al. Dentinogenesis imperfecta in a racial isolate with multiple hereditary defects. *Oral Surg* 1956;9:641–658.

Levin LS, Leaf SH, Jelmini RJ, et al. Dentinogenesis imperfecta in the Brandywine isolate (DI type III): clinical, radiologic, and scanning electron microscopic studies of the dentition. *Oral Surg Oral Med Oral Pathol* 1983;56:267–274.

MacDougall M. Refined mapping of the human dentin sialophosphoprotein (DSPP) gene within the critical dentinogenesis imperfecta type II and dentin dysplasia type II loci. *Eur J Oral Sci* 1998;106(suppl 1):227–233.

MacDougall M, Jeffords LG, Gu TT, et al. Genetic linkage of the dentinogenesis imperfecta type III locus to chromosome 4q. *J Dent Res* 1999;78:1277–1282.

Witkop CJ Jr, MacLean CJ, Schmidt PJ, et al. Medical and dental findings in the Brandywine isolate. *Ala J Med Sci* 1966;3:382–403.

RESOURCES
297, 320

---

42   DiGeorge Syndrome

Angelo M. DiGeorge, MD

DEFINITION: DiGeorge syndrome originally encompassed congenital defects of the heart, thymus, and parathyroid glands and has been expanded to include ear, nose, and throat; facial; genitourinary; developmental; and psychiatric disorders.

SYNONYMS: Chromosome 22q11 deletion syndrome; Shprintzen velo-cardio-facial (VCF) syndrome; DiGeorge/VCF syndrome; Conotruncal anomaly face syndrome; Cayler syndrome; Opitz GBBB syndrome (some patients).

DIFFERENTIAL DIAGNOSIS: Deletion of chromosome 10p; Retinoic acid embryopathy; CHARGE association.

SYMPTOMS AND SIGNS: Most patients (75%) have cardiac defects, particularly tetralogy of Fallot, interrupted aortic arch, truncus arteriosis, and other conotruncal defects. Neonatal hypocalcemia due to aplasia or hypoplasia of the parathyroid glands occurs in approximately 60% of patients and usually presents as seizures. In many of these patients, the hypocalcemia is transient. Late onset hypocalcemia during childhood and later occurs less often. Aplasia of the thymus, which occurs in about 1% of patients, results in severe immune deficiency. Ectopia of the thymus occurs more often and may cause mild and transient immune deficiency; these patients are usually clinically asymptomatic. Patients with the predominantly velo-cardio-facial phenotype manifest velopharyngeal insufficiency, which causes nasal regurgitation and difficulty swallowing in infancy and a marked nasal quality to the voice later. Cleft lip, cleft palate, choanal atresia, and facial dysmorphism may be present. Behavioral problems and learning difficulties are common. In adults, psychiatric disorders are increased. Other findings include renal disorders, growth hormone deficiency, and autoimmune disorders. These manifestations may vary widely from patient to patient.

ETIOLOGY/EPIDEMIOLOGY: Affected patients have a deletion of chromosome 22q11. The incidence is 1 in 400 live births, and the disorder affects males and females equally. Prenatal diagnosis is possible. Most often the condition occurs sporadically, but in 5%–10% of patients the deletion was inherited from one parent.

DIAGNOSIS: The deletion is readily detected using the fluorescence *in situ* hybridization test.

TREATMENT
Standard Therapies: Infantile seizures and other symptoms caused by hypocalcemia are readily treated by administration of calcium and vitamin D. Most of the cardiac de-

fects are surgically correctible. Infants with complete aplasia of the thymus have been successfully treated by transplantation of thymus tissue. Early recognition of developmental delay is important. Testing of both parents of affected children and genetic counseling are indicated.

REFERENCES

Lindsay EA, Citelli F, Su H, et al. Tbxl, haploinsufficiency in the DiGeorge syndrome region causes aortic arch defects in the mouse. *Nature* 2001;410:97–101.

Ryan AK, Goodship JA, Wilson DJ, et al. Spectrum of clinical features associated with interstitial chromosome 22q11 deletions: a European collaboration study. *J Med Genet* 1997;34:795–804.

Scambler PJ. The 22q11 deletion syndromes. *Hum Mol Genet* 2000;9:2421–2426.

Schinke M, Izumo S. Deconstructing DiGeorge syndrome. *Nat Genet* 2001;27:238–240.

Thomas JA, Graham GM Jr. Chromosome 22q11 deletion syndrome: an update and review for the primary pediatrician. *Clin Pediatr* 1997;253–266.

RESOURCES

102, 362

---

43   Dubowitz Syndrome

John M. Opitz, MD

DEFINITION: Dubowitz syndrome is a genetic multiple congenital anomalies syndrome with characteristic facial appearance and minor anomalies, predisposition to developmental delay, eczema, cervical vertebral and other skeletal anomalies, agenesis of the corpus callosum, and possible hematologic/oncologic complications.

DIFFERENTIAL DIAGNOSIS: Fanconi syndrome; Nijmegen (chromosome) breakage syndrome.

SIGNS AND SYMPTOMS: Signs of Dubowitz syndrome include intrauterine growth retardation; postnatal growth failure (primordial shortness of stature); small head (true microcephaly, i.e., disproportionately small head for height); craniosynostosis in a few cases (at times requiring craniosynostectomy); hypotelorism; asymmetric ptosis; small palpebral fissures; upward slant of palpebral fissures; persistence of epicanthic folds, flat eyebrow (supraorbital) ridges; prominent, somewhat rounded tip of nose; relatively short upper lip with thin lip vermilion; relatively sparse hair and lateral eyebrows; predisposition to eczema; diarrhea and/or constipation; submucous (rarely complete) cleft palate; and occasional velopharyngeal incompetence with somewhat hypernasal, high pitched, hoarse voice. Developmental signs include speech delay; however, borderline to normal intelligence is often present. Most patients also show attention deficit/hyperactivity disorder; fascination with sound vibrations (touching music speakers); hypospadias; rare vascular anomalies (abnormal carotid or subclavian arteries); headaches; rare anorectal anomalies; agenesis (or other corpus callosum abnormalities); recurrent respiratory tract infections; and transient or aplastic anemia. Rarely, patients develop bone marrow failure or solid tumors or sarcomas.

ETIOLOGY/EPIDEMIOLOGY: Although 200 cases are recognized worldwide, the condition is probably more common because the diagnosis in mildly affected patients is difficult. About a dozen familial cases exist; hence, it was initially thought to be an autosomal-recessive trait with 25% recurrence risk. Most are sporadic cases representing new mutations, however, and evidence is mounting of rare manifestations (e.g., small head) in a parent. Thus, autosomal-dominant inheritance is postulated.

DIAGNOSIS: Diagnosis is made purely on a clinical basis: characteristic appearance, small size, eczema, diarrhea/constipation, rare skeletal anomalies (duplicated/malformed thumbs, cervical vertebral anomalies, spina bifida occulta); rare mild heart defects (as seen on echocardiography); rare agenesis of corpus callosum (on MRI).

TREATMENT

Standard Therapies: Treatment is symptomatic and empiric for attention deficit/hyperactivity disorder, eczema, diarrhea and constipation; possible surgery to correct (submucous) cleft palate; PE tubes for chronic middle ear infection; special pedagogic and speech therapy support for developmental and speech delay; and always, psychological/emotional support.

REFERENCES

Al-Nemri AR, Kilani RA, Salih MAM, et al. Embryonal rhabdomyosarcoma and chromosomal breakage in a newborn infant with possible Dubowitz syndrome. *Am J Med Genet* 2000;92:107–110.

Berthold F, Fuhrmann W, Lampert F. Fatal aplastic anaemia in a child with features of Dubowitz syndrome. *Eur J Pediatr* 1987;146:605–607.

Dubowitz V. Familial low birthweight dwarfism with an unusual facies and a skin eruption. *J Med Genet* 1965;2:12–17.

Hansen KE, Kirkpatrick SJ, Laxova R. Dubowitz syndrome: long-term follow-up of an original patient. *Am J Med Genet* 1995;55:161–164.

Kuster W, Majewski F. The Dubowitz syndrome. *Eur J Pediatr* 1986;144:574–578.

OMIM * 223370 Dubowitz syndrome (probably *not* an autosomal recessive trait, asterisk and 223370 number notwithstanding). *www.nchi.nlm.nih.gov/htbin-post/omim/dispmim?223370.*

Tsukahara M, Opitz JM. Dubowitz syndrome: review of 141 cases including 36 previously unreported patients. *Am J Med Genet* 1996;63:277–289.

RESOURCES
361, 462

44   Dyggve-Melchior-Clausen Syndrome

David D. Weaver, MS, MD

DEFINITION: Dyggve-Melchior-Clausen (DMC) syndrome is a bone dysplasia caused by a rough endoplasmic reticulum storage disorder. Microcephaly, mental retardation, short stature, and skeletal abnormalities characterize the condition.

SYNONYMS: Dyggve-Melchior-Clausen disease, dysplasia, or dwarfism; Smith-McCort syndrome or dwarfism; X-linked Dyggve-Melchior-Clausen syndrome.

DIFFERENTIAL DIAGNOSIS: Hurler syndrome; Morquio syndrome; Spondyloepiphyseal dysplasia, congenita; Spondyloepiphyseal dysplasia, tarda.

SYMPTOMS AND SIGNS: The newborn with DMC syndrome is normal in appearance but may be small. During infancy there may be delayed development, feeding problems, and onset of short stature and other dysmorphic features. Subsequently, other features may develop, including microcephaly, coarse facies, mandibular prognathism, barrel-shaped chest with protruding sternum, thoracic kyphosis, excessive lumbar lordosis, mild clawing of the fingers, joint contractures, waddling gait, disproportional short stature with a short trunk, and mental retardation. Adult height may reach only 82 cm. Some radiographic features are present by age 4. Vertebral changes include hypoplasia of the odontoid process with atlantoaxial instability; platyspondyly; and deep central notching, irregular superior and inferior surfaces, and anterior beaking of the vertebral bodies. In the pelvis, the ilia are small and broad with a lacelike appearance to the iliac crests. The sacrum is broad with small sacrosciatic notches, the pubic symphysis is wide, and the acetabulae are irregular and flat. The long bones are short and have both epiphyseal and metaphyseal changes. The proximal femoral epiphyses are flat and irregular, and often laterally displaced. The femoral necks are short. The carpal bones are small and irregular. The metacarpals, metatarsals, and phalanges are short, resulting in brachydactyly. The odontoid process defect can lead to excessive laxity, spinal cord compression, and paralysis. Mental retardation occurs in approximately two thirds of patients and may be severe. Dislocated hips and restricted joint mobility can develop with time.

ETIOLOGY/EPIDEMIOLOGY: The syndrome generally is inherited in an autosomal-recessive fashion; however, an X-linked recessive form has been reported. The maximum recurrence risk for parents with an affected child of either form would be 25%. Smith-McCort syndrome is the same syndrome but without mental retardation. The disorder has been reported in several different ethnic groups.

DIAGNOSIS: The combination of disproportional short stature with a short, barrel-shaped chest and shortened limbs suggests the diagnosis. Diagnosis is established from the radiographic abnormalities. Particularly useful are the notching of the vertebral bodies, the lacelike appearance of the iliac crests, and the small and irregular carpal bones.

TREATMENT
Standard Therapies: The C1 and C2 vertebrae should be fused if there is odontoid hypoplasia and excessive instability. Appropriate orthopedic management is indicated. Otherwise, treatment is symptomatic, such as analgesics for joint pain.

REFERENCES
Nakamura K, Kurokawa T, Nagano A, et al. Dyggve-Melchior-Clausen syndrome without mental retardation (Smith-

McCort dysplasia): morphological findings in the growth plate of the iliac crest. *Am J Med Genet* 1997;72:11–17.

Spranger J. X-linked Dyggve-Melchior-Clausen syndrome. *Clin Genet* 1981;19:304.

Spranger J, Bierbaum B, Herrmann J. Heterogeneity of Dyggve-Melchior-Clausen dwarfism. *Hum Genet* 1976;33:279–287.

Taybi H, Lachman RS. Dyggve-Melchior-Clausen (DMC). In: Taybi H, Lachman RS, eds. *Radiology of syndromes, metabolic disorders, and skeletal dysplasias,* 4th ed. St. Louis: CV Mosby, 1996:805–807.

Yunis E, Fontalvo J, Quintero L. X-linked Dyggve-Melchior-Clausen syndrome. *Clin Genet* 1980;18:284–290.

RESOURCES

188, 253

---

45   Dyschondrosteosis

Debbie Shears, MBBS, MRCP

DEFINITION: Dyschondrosteosis is a skeletal dysplasia characterized by disproportionate short stature with shortening of the forearms and lower legs. A Madelung deformity is often present.

SYNONYMS: Leri-Weill dyschondrosteosis; Mesomelic dwarfism-Madelung deformity.

DIFFERENTIAL DIAGNOSIS: Madelung deformity due to trauma or infection; Madelung deformity associated with Turner syndrome; Hypochondroplasia; Acrodysostosis; Langer mesomelic dysplasia syndrome; Nievergelt syndrome; Reinhardt-Pfeiffer syndrome; Robinow syndrome.

SYMPTOMS AND SIGNS: In early childhood, disproportionate short stature may be present with mesomelic limb shortening. The Madelung deformity, which is due to shortening and bowing of the radius with dorsal subluxation of the distal ulna, may not be clinically apparent at this stage, although radiographs may show subtle abnormalities. During the pubertal growth spurt, the Madelung deformity becomes more obvious, leading to symptoms such as wrist and elbow pain, reduced supination and pronation of the forearm, limitation of wrist extension, and poor grip. Mild bowing of the tibia as well as knee or ankle pain can occur. Wide variation in the clinical spectrum exists even within families, ranging from mild short stature with little disproportion to marked short stature with obvious disproportion and severe Madelung deformity. In the longer term, osteoarthritis may occur, particularly of the knee, elbow, and wrist. Langer mesomelic dysplasia is characterized by severe short stature and both proximal and mesomelic limb shortening, with mandibular hypoplasia. Hypoplasia of the ulnae and fibulae is marked, with very short, thick, curved radii and tibiae.

ETIOLOGY/EPIDEMIOLOGY: The disorder is caused by deletion or mutation of the short-stature homeobox gene (*SHOX*), located at the tip of the short arm of the X and Y chromosomes. Despite its location on the sex chromosomes, dyschondrosteosis shows an autosomal-dominant pattern of inheritance. The condition occurs in both males and females, although females are generally more severely affected. Prevalence is generally given as 3–7 per million, but this is likely an underestimate.

DIAGNOSIS: The diagnosis is made on the basis of the clinical features supported by the typical radiologic findings. It is confirmed by fluorescent *in situ* hybridization studies of the chromosomes to detect the deletion of *SHOX*, or by DNA sequencing to detect a *SHOX* point mutation. Chromosome analysis (karyotype) should be performed, because occasional cases are associated with XY translocation, Turner syndrome (45,X), or with a larger Xp or Yp deletion.

TREATMENT

Standard Therapies: In many cases no specific treatment is required, apart from monitoring growth. If the Madelung deformity causes pain, functional impairment, or cosmetic problems, it can be surgically corrected by procedures such as wedge subtraction osteotomy of the radius and shortening osteotomy of the ulna. This may improve grip strength and range of movement of the wrist and forearm. Genetic counseling may be beneficial.

Investigational Therapies: Recombinant human growth hormone treatment to increase final height is being studied. Leg-lengthening procedures have been used to increase final height or to correct asymmetry.

REFERENCES

Binder G, Schwarz CP, Ranke MB. Identification of short stature caused by SHOX defects and therapeutic effect of recombinant human growth hormone. *J Clin Endocrinol Metab* 2000; 85:245–249.

Blaschke RJ, Rappold GA. SHOX: growth, Leri-Weill and Turner syndromes. *Trends Endocrinol Metab* 2000;11:227–230.

Carter PR, Ezaki M. Madelung's deformity. Surgical correction through the anterior approach. *Hand Clin* 2000;16:713–721.

Shears DJ, Vassal HJ, Goodman FR, et al. Mutation and deletion in the pseudoautosomal gene *SHOX* cause Leri-Weill dyschondrosteosis. *Nat Genet* 1998;19:70–73.

Thuestad IJ, Ivarsson SA, Nilsson KO, et al. Growth hormone treatment in Leri-Weill syndrome. *J Paediatr Endocrinol Metab* 1996;9:201–204.

RESOURCES
188, 253

---

46   Cleidocranial Dysplasia

Ilan Golan, DMD, Uwe Baumert, PhD, and Dieter Muessig, DMD

DEFINITION: Cleidocranial dysplasia (CCD) is an autosomal-dominant skeletal dysplasia with variable expressivity, characterized by short stature, abnormal clavicles, typical facies, delayed closure of sutures and fontanelles, supernumerary teeth, and delayed tooth eruption.

SYNONYMS: Cleidocranial dysostosis; Scheuthauer-Marie-(Sainton) syndrome; Osteodental dysplasia.

DIFFERENTIAL DIAGNOSIS: Osteogenesis imperfecta; Pycnodysotosis; Hajdu-Cheney syndrome; Mandibuloacral dysplasia.

SYMPTOMS AND SIGNS: The phenotype shows short stature, a typical facial appearance, and narrow sloping shoulders caused by defective or aplastic clavicles. The skeletal system shows a wide range of developmental, structural, and morphologic anomalies. Major findings include hypoplasia or aplasia of clavicular bones, narrow and abnormally shaped pelvic and pubic bones, and deformations in the thoracic region. The most prominent findings are osseous malformations in the cranial base and skull. Due to disturbed bone formation and delayed maturation, the skull is formed by a large number of Wormian bones, which develop from multiple supernumerary centers of ossification. Closure of sutures and the anterior fontanel is delayed, at times remaining patent through adulthood. Bossing of the frontal bones, prominent chin, and maxillary hypoplasia typify the characteristic facial appearance. Although the deciduous teeth develop relatively normally, permanent dentition shows unique disturbances, including persistence of the milk teeth, retention of regular permanent teeth, and the development of a large number of supernumerary permanent tooth germs. The development of follicular cysts as a result of these dental anomalies is common. Clefting of the palate occurs with the same frequency as in the general population.

ETIOLOGY/EPIDEMIOLOGY: The disorder is inherited in an autosomal-dominant fashion with complete penetrance and variable expressivity. Since it was first described in 1898, approximately 1,000 cases, including the rare autosomal-recessive Yunis-Varon form, have been reported. Male and females are affected equally. The incidence is 1 in 1 million.

DIAGNOSIS: Although dental findings are constant, skeletal involvement may be variable. The disease gene has been mapped to chromosome 6p21 containing the core binding factor ∀1 gene (*CBFA1/RUNX2*; OMIM 600211), and mutations in this gene have been identified in affected individuals.

TREATMENT
Standard Therapies: The symptoms and signs may appear distinct, but are entirely benign. Treatment of the overall medical condition is not obligatory. According to most patients, the disturbances of the dentition are the main cause for reduction in life quality. Treatment requires an interdisciplinary approach involving orthodontics, maxillofacial surgery, and prostodontics. Protective head gear should be worn until the skull bones close or maturity is reached. Genetic consultation is advised for family planning.

REFERENCES
Becker A, Lustmann J, Shteyer A. Cleidocranial dysplasia: part 1—general principles of the orthodontic and surgical treatment modality. *Am J Orthod Dentofac Orthop* 1997;111:28–33.

Fleischer-Peters A, Schuch P. Befindlichkeit und Lebensschicksal von Patienten mit Dysostosis cleidocranialis. *Kinderarzt* 1983; 14:1059–1067.

Golan I, Preising M, Wagener H, et al. A novel missense mutation of the *CBFA1* gene in a family with cleidocranial dysplasia (CCD) and variable expressivity. *J Craniofac Genet Dev Biol* 2000;20:113–120.

Marie P, Sainton P. Sur la dysostose cleido-crânienne héréditaire. *Rev Neurol* 1898;6:835–838.

Mundlos S. Cleidocranial dysplasia: clinical and molecular genetics. *J Med Genet* 1999;36:177–182.

RESOURCES
96, 149, 351

47 Craniofrontonasal Syndrome

Ernst Reichenberger, PhD, and John B. Mulliken, MD

DEFINITION: Craniofrontonasal syndrome (CFNS) is a rare, X-linked skeletal disorder. The most prominent features are hypertelorism, coronal synostosis, bifidity of the nasal tip, and shoulder and limb anomalies.

SYNONYMS: Craniofrontonasal dysplasia (CFND); Craniofrontonasal dysostosis.

DIFFERENTIAL DIAGNOSIS: Frontonasal dysplasia; Greig cephalopolysyndactyly syndrome; Frontofacionasal dysostosis; Teebi hypertelorism syndrome.

SYMPTOMS AND SIGNS: Females are usually more severely affected than are males. Characteristic craniofacial features include coronal synostosis (unilateral more often than bilateral), frontal bossing, low-set posteriorly angled ears, hypertelorism, down-slanting palpebral fissures, broad nasal bridge, bifidity of the nasal tip, broad face (euryprosopia), and pterygium colli. Also in females, unusual thick, wiry, and curly hair often appears, usually at 2–3 months of age. Synostotic phenotypes can appear as dolicho-, brachy-, plagio-, or acrocephaly. Extracranial skeletal anomalies include short clavicles, narrow/sloping shoulder girdles, and unilateral short limbs. Unilateral glandular breast hypoplasia (postpubertal) is observed in 11% of females, and three reports link CFNS with Poland syndrome. Pronounced longitudinal ridging of nails (grooves) is frequently observed. Digits can be broad or long, and minor soft tissue webbing, syndactyly, fifth finger clinodactyly, and hyperextensive joints have also been reported. In males, a wide nasal bridge (hypertelorism) may be the only sign of the disorder. Potentially, a male may be clinically unaffected but can be a carrier of the mutation.

ETIOLOGY/EPIDEMIOLOGY: The syndrome is rare; most cases are sporadic and usually occur in females. There are reported pedigrees showing vertical transmission. This disorder maps to Xp22. The more severe expression in females is unusual for an X-linked disorder. The reasons for this are not understood.

DIAGNOSIS: Radiologic findings include unilateral or bilateral coronal synostosis, hypertelorism, and midfacial hypoplasia. A wide variety of findings can accompany these features. For the diagnosis of an apparent sporadic case, it may be appropriate to have the patient's parents undergo a detailed medical diagnosis, because the father may be an obligate carrier of the disease gene and therefore without stigmata.

TREATMENT
Standard Therapies: Most patients have coronal synostosis and have frontoorbital advancement (unilateral/bilateral) in infancy. The bifid nose can be surgically narrowed. Midfacial advancement and correction of hypertelorism and pterygium colli may be considered in childhood.

Investigational Therapies: Efforts to find the genetic cause for CFNS are underway in several laboratories.

REFERENCES
Cohen MM, MacLean RE, eds. *Craniosynostosis: diagnosis, evaluation, and management,* 2nd ed. New York: Oxford University Press, 2000:380–384.
Feldman GJ, Ward DE, Lajeunie-Renier E, et al. A novel phenotypic pattern in X-linked inheritance: craniofrontonasal syndrome maps to Xp22. *Hum Mol Genet* 1997;6:1937–1941.
Pulleyn LJ, Winter RM, Reardon W, et al. Further evidence from two families that craniofrontonasal dysplasia maps to Xp22. *Clin Genet* 1999;55:473–477.
Saavedra D, Richieri-Costa A, Guion-Almeida ML, et al. Craniofrontonasal syndrome: study of 41 patients. *Am J Med Genet* 1996;61:147–151.

RESOURCES
96, 149

48   Craniometaphyseal Dysplasia

*Ernst Reichenberger, PhD,
and John B. Mulliken, MD*

DEFINITION: Craniometaphyseal dysplasia (CMD) is a craniotubular bone disorder; the characteristic features are sclerosis of the skull and metaphyseal widening of long bones. The flared metaphyses exhibit decreased bone density, while the diaphyses appear normal.

SYNONYMS: Craniometaphyseal dysplasia Jackson type (CMDJ), autosomal dominant; Craniometaphyseal dysplasia, recessive type.

DIFFERENTIAL DIAGNOSIS: Pyle disease; Craniodiaphyseal dysplasia; Frontometaphyseal dysplasia; Osteopathia striata with cranial sclerosis; Sclerosteosis; Osteitis fibrosa cystica.

SYMPTOMS AND SIGNS: CMD is often diagnosed within the first weeks of life because of breathing or feeding problems due to choanal stenosis. Cranial radiographs show beginning sclerosis of the cranial base; in time there is progressive diffuse hyperostosis of the cranial base, cranial vault, facial bones, and mandible. Facial features include a wide nasal bridge, paranasal bossing, increased bizygomatic width, and hypertelorism. Dolichocephaly has been reported in a number of patients due to frontooccipital hyperostosis. In severe cases, progressive sclerosis can result in narrowing of the cranial foramina, including the foramen magnum, causing symptoms of Chiari I anomaly, such as headaches and vomiting. Pressure on cranial nerves can result in facial palsy, blindness, or deafness. The long bone phenotype develops within the first years of life and is restricted to metaphyseal widening (Erlenmeyer flask shape) with decreased bony density in the metaphyses. The flaring is most prominently seen in the femur and tibia. Ribs and the medial (endochondral) portion of clavicles can be sclerotic in younger children but show normal bone density by the time they are 5 years old.

ETIOLOGY/EPIDEMIOLOGY: Craniometaphyseal dysplasia has been reported in approximately 160 cases. It occurs as an autosomal-dominant or autosomal-recessive disorder or sporadically. Penetrance seems to be complete, but expressivity can vary considerably even within one family. Both sexes are affected equally.

DIAGNOSIS: Radiologic findings in infants are increased bony density at the cranial base. Audiologic, ophthalmologic, neurologic, and otolaryngologic examination is appropriate. Blood calcium and phosphate levels have been shown to be within normal limits, but serum alkaline phosphatase and parathyroid hormone levels can be elevated.

TREATMENT
Standard Therapies: The first reported surgical procedure for CMD was osteotomy of the femoral condyles to correct genu valgum. Craniofacial techniques can be used for contour reduction of the facial bones through an incision under the upper lip. Bony overgrowth of the nasal, forehead, and cranial regions can be contoured through a coronal scalp incision. Orbital decompression should be considered to save vision. Surgical decompression of the facial nerve canal or narrowed foramen magnum (Chiari I anomaly) is also technically possible.

Investigational Therapies: Gene mutations for autosomal-dominant CMD have been found in ANK, a multipass transmembrane protein. Studies on the function of ANK are being conducted at the Forsyth Institute/Harvard School of Dental Medicine, Boston.

REFERENCES
Beighton P. Craniometaphyseal dysplasia (CMD), autosomal dominant form. *J Med Genet* 1995;32:370–374.

Millard DR Jr, Maisels DO, Batstone JHF, et al. Craniofacial surgery in craniometaphyseal dysplasia. *Am J Surg* 1967;113:615–621.

Reichenberger E, Tiziani V, Watanabe S, et al. Autosomal dominant craniometaphyseal dysplasia (CMD) is caused by mutations in the transmembrane protein ANK. *Am J Hum Genet* 2001;68:1321–1326.

Vanhoenacker FM, De Beuckeleer LH, Van Hul W, et al. Sclerosing bone dysplasias: genetic and radioclinical features. *Eur Radiol* 2000;10:1423–1433.

RESOURCES
96, 149

49 Ectodermal Dysplasia

Kathleen J. Motil, MD, PhD

DEFINITION: The ectodermal dysplasia (ED) syndromes are a group of inherited disorders that affect the ectodermal-derived tissues of the body, including skin, hair, and nails; sebaceous, sweat, and mammary glands; teeth; eyes (lens, conjunctiva); ears; nipples; and respiratory and gastrointestinal tract. The ED syndromes are divided into two major groups, hypohidrotic and hidrotic, based on whether affected persons can sweat normally.

SYNONYMS: Hypohidrotic (anhidrotic) ectodermal dysplasia; Christ-Siemens-Touraine syndrome; Hidrotic ectodermal dysplasia (Clouston type); Ectrodactyly-ectodermal dysplasia-clefting; Rapp-Hodgkin ectodermal dysplasia; Robinson-type ectodermal dysplasia.

DIFFERENTIAL DIAGNOSIS: Fever of unknown origin (FUO).

SYMPTOMS AND SIGNS: Features of the ED syndromes include sparse, fine hair; varying degrees of conical-shaped and missing teeth; decreased number of sweat and mucous glands; thin, hypoplastic skin; and hyperthermia with increased ambient temperature. Some of the individual syndromes may have overlapping features, and not all features may be present in an affected individual or within members of a family. The hypohidrotic form (HED) is characterized by a triad of clinical features including hypohidrosis, anomalous dentition (missing or malformed), and hypotrichosis.

ETIOLOGY/EPIDEMIOLOGY: More than 100 clinical patterns can be classified as ED syndromes. The hypohidrotic form is the most common, occurring in 1 to 7 per 10,000 births, and is found in all racial groups and in all areas of the world.

DIAGNOSIS: The diagnosis of ED syndromes should be suspected on the basis of clinical and dental examination. The diagnosis of HED can be established by clinical examination. Oral radiographs may show hypo- or anodontia. A palmer skin biopsy shows absent or reduced sweat glands and ducts, but is rarely required for diagnosis. The technique of sweat pore counts can be misleading, especially in carrier detection. Diagnosis in females at risk to be carriers may be problematic; molecular studies may be helpful.

TREATMENT

Standard Therapies: Children with HED are at risk for heat-related illness and must be protected from exposure to increased ambient temperatures. Avoiding warm clothing, overexertion, and exposure to hot weather are important preventative measures, and cooling with water, drinking cool fluids, or wearing wet T-shirts is imperative in an overheated individual. Early treatment of respiratory infections is mandatory. Early dental evaluation is necessary; properly fitted dentures and possibly dental implants can improve the child's speech, facial appearance, and nutrition. Difficulty chewing and swallowing can be offset with the increased consumption of fluids or by the use of artificial saliva preparations. In other ED syndromes, cleft deformities may require surgery. Hearing aids may alleviate hearing difficulties and assist in speech and language development.

REFERENCES

Celli J, Duijf P, Hamel BC, et al. Heterozygous germline mutations in the p53 homolog p63 are the cause of EEC syndrome. *Cell* 1999;99:143–153.

Guckes AD, Roberts MW, McCarthy GR. Pattern of permanent teeth present in individuals with ectodermal dysplasia and severe hypodontia suggests treatment with dental implants. *Pediatr Dent* 1998;20:278–280.

Lamartine J, Pitaval A, Soularue P, et al. A 1.5-Mb physical map of the hidrotic ectodermal dysplasia (Clouston syndrome) gene region on human chromosome 13q11. *Genomics* 2000;67:232–236.

Munoz F, Lestringant G, Sybert V, et al. Definitive evidence for an autosomal recessive form of hypohidrotic ectodermal dysplasia clinically indistinguishable from the more common X-linked disorder. *Am J Hum Genet* 1997;61:94–100.

Pinheiro M, Freire-Maia N. Ectodermal dysplasias: a clinical classification and causal review. *Am J Med Genet* 1994;53:153–162.

RESOURCES

297, 373

50   Dysplasia Epiphysealis Hemimelica

Charles N. Moon, MD,
J. Dominic Femino, MD,
and David L. Skaggs, MD

DEFINITION: Dysplasia epiphysealis hemimelica is an intraarticular dysplasia of bone and cartilage. It is a developmental lesion histologically identical to an osteochondroma, arising from an epiphysis and consisting of cortical and cancellous bone that is continuous with the underlying normal bone, ending in a cartilage cap.

SYNONYMS: Trevors disease; Tarsomegalie; Tarsoepiphyseal aclasis.

DIFFERENTIAL DIAGNOSIS: Chondroblastoma; Osteochondroma; Osteochondritis dissecans; Synovial chondromatosis; Loose body.

SYMPTOMS AND SIGNS: Typically, the lesion is found in the epiphysis or the tarsal or flat bones of a single extremity. The ankle is most commonly affected, although assorted other joints throughout the body have been involved. Approximately two thirds of patients have multiple lesions. Patients may report pain, deformity, limitation of motion, or subluxation or dislocation of the involved joint. The lesion is often not visible on plain radiographs, because it may not have begun ossification. Once mineralization has begun, it appears as a secondary ossification center. Once mature, there is cortical and medullary continuity between the lesion and the normal bone with a cartilage cap.

ETIOLOGY/EPIDEMIOLOGY: The etiology is unknown. There is one report of a family with a hereditary pattern of cartilage tumors including dysplasia epiphysealis hemimelica, but the disease does not appear to be hereditary in general.

DIAGNOSIS: Plain radiographs are most commonly used to make the diagnosis; however, before the ossification of the lesion, radiographs often appear normal. When the secondary ossification center of the lesion appears, the diagnosis can be made readily. MRI is useful to image cartilaginous lesions and possibly in delineating the location and morphology of the immature lesion.

TREATMENT
Standard Therapies: Treatment is somewhat controversial. Some clinicians advocate surgical excision of symptomatic lesions because these are typically symptomatic and cause functional problems with joint motion. Others believe that because articular lesion excision is technically difficult and may further compromise the joint, these lesions should simply be observed.

REFERENCES
Azouz EM, Slomic AM, Marton D, et al. The variable manifestations of dysplasia epiphysealis hemimelica. *Pediatr Radiol* 1985;15:44–49.
Fairbank TJ. Dysplasia epiphysealis hemimelica (tarso-epiphyseal aclasis). *J Bone Joint Surg [Br]* 1956;38:237–257.
Kuo RS, Bellemore MC, Monsell FP, et al. Dysplasia epiphysealis hemimelica: clinical features and management. *J Pediatr Orthop* 1998;18:543–548.
Silverman FN. Dysplasia epiphysealis hemimelica. *Semin Roentgenol* 1989;24:246–258.
Skaggs DL, Moon CN, Kay RM, et al. Dysplasia epiphysealis hemimelica of the acetabulum. *J Bone Joint Surg [Am]* 2000; 82:409–414.
Wynne-Davies R. Dysplasia epiphysealis hemimelica. In: *Atlas of skeletal dysplasias.* 1985:539–543.

RESOURCES
351, 418

51   Maxillonasal Dysplasia (Binder Type Syndrome)

Bodil Rune, DDS, PhD,
and Magnus Åberg, MD, PhD

DEFINITION: Maxillonasal dysplasia is a congenital anomaly with phenotypic expression and undefined inheritance pattern. It is characterized by retrusion of the midface with aplasia or hypoplasia of the anterior nasal spine and has been associated with other congenital defects including cervical spine anomalies (in approximately 50% of cases), influencing head posture. The pattern of abnormalities does not represent a causally defined entity, so the word *syndrome* might be inappropriate.

SYNONYMS: Binder syndrome; Dishface, scaphoid face, and nasomaxillary hypoplasia.

DIFFERENTIAL DIAGNOSIS: Maxillary retrusion/mandibular protrusion; Chondrodysplasia punctanta, rhizomelic type; Fetal warfarin syndrome.

SYMPTOMS AND SIGNS: The typical facial appearance is a frontonasal angle of almost 180 degrees, a short columella, a convex upper lip, underdevelopment of the anterior facies of the maxilla, dysplasia of the anterior part of the hard palate, and flattening of the anterior maxillary dental arch. An anterior dental cross-bite is common (seen in approximately 50% of cases), whereas the occlusal relationship of the lateral segments may be normal. The frontal sinuses may be absent or underdeveloped. A slope instead of a fossa in the anterior nasal floor is found in approximately 6% of cases. The nostrils are crescent shaped, often described as *oreilles de chat*. In many cases the nasal septum is atrophic, with resulting airway obstruction. The sense of smell is unaffected. The symptoms do not change with growth, i.e., the appearance at birth coincides with that in adulthood.

ETIOLOGY/EPIDEMIOLOGY: The anomaly appears to occur randomly, but a few cases of familial occurrence have been reported. The etiology is unclear. The anomaly either may be caused by an autosomal-recessive allele or is of a quantitative genetically multifactorial character with a threshold. It might be a mild form of arhinocephaly. The anomaly is seen in approximately equal numbers in males and females; the incidence has not been established.

DIAGNOSIS: Maxillonasal dysplasia should be suspected based on the clinical facial appearance of the patient with a lack of familial resemblance. A lateral roentgenogram showing absence/hypoplasia of the anterior nasal spine and underdevelopment of the anterior maxilla confirms the diagnosis.

TREATMENT
Standard Therapies: Early heavy extraoral traction on an orthodontic mask has been advocated, possibly combined with orthodontic correction of an anterior cross-bite. Surgery is best delayed until facial growth has stopped. Psychosocial considerations may prompt earlier intervention with iliac bone reconstruction of the ridge and tip of the nose and the columella together with onlay bone to the perialar region. The patient and family must be aware, however, that additional treatment may be necessary, e.g., orthognatic surgery to the maxilla and the mandible. Bone grafts to the nose may be displaced or resorbed, but no correlation has been found with the clinical outcome of surgery. The characteristic appearance of individuals with maxillonasal dysplasia seems to be predetermined by biologic boundaries. As long as the predisposing biologic mechanisms remain unclear, long-term treatment outcomes are unpredictable.

REFERENCES
Greenberg SA. Binder's syndrome (nasomaxillary dysplasia): an uncommonly common disorder. *J La State Med Soc* 1991;143:27–38.
Holmström H. Clinical and pathologic features of maxillonasal dysplasia (Binder's syndrome): significance of the prenasal fossa on etiology. *Plast Reconstr Surg* 1986;78:559–582.
Olow-Nordenram M. Maxillonasal dysplasia (Binder's syndrome). A study of cranofacial morphology, associated malformations and familial relations. *Swed Dent J Suppl* 1987; 47:1–38.
Rune B, Åberg M. Bone grafts to the nose in Binder's syndrome (maxillonasal dysplasia): a follow-up of eleven patients with the use of profile roentgenograms. *Plast Reconstr Surg* 1998; 101:297–304.
Tessier P, Tulasne JF, Delaire J, et al. Aspects thérapeutiques de la dysostose maxillo-nasale de Binder. *Rev Stomatol Chir Maxillofac* 1979;80:363–372.

RESOURCES
298, 360

52 Multiple Epiphyseal Dysplasia Type 1 (Fairbank Syndrome)

Erik C. Spayde, MD

DEFINITION: Fairbank syndrome is a subtype of multiple epiphyseal dysplasia (MED) characterized by moderately short limbs, waddling gait, and painful joints.

SYNONYM: Multiple epiphyseal dysplasia, Fairbank type.

DIFFERENTIAL DIAGNOSIS: Ribbing type of MED; Metaphyseal chondrodysplasia; Spondyloepiphyseal dysplasia; Achondroplasia.

SYMPTOMS AND SIGNS: The Fairbank type of MED is usually evident in childhood, characterized by moderately shortened upper and lower extremities, waddling gait, and painful joints. Radiographs demonstrate generalized epiphyseal involvement. Typically, affected individuals are 145–170 cm in height. The knees and hips are usually involved; however, the shoulder, elbow, ankle, wrist, hand, foot, and spine may also be affected. Early-onset severe osteoarthritis of weight-bearing joints is common in the 3rd and 4th decades of life. This is unlike the milder ribbing form of MED, which may not be detected until adolescence and typically affects only the hips.

ETIOLOGY/EPIDEMIOLOGY: Fairbank syndrome is usually inherited in an autosomal-dominant manner. The disease results from mutations in several genes and may be variable in severity. Mutations have been discovered in three genes: cartilage oligomeric matrix protein gene (*COMP*), *COL9A2*, and *COL9A*. These genes encode molecules that are believed to play a significant role in maintaining the integrity of articular cartilage, thus explaining the premature breakdown of articular surfaces and premature degenerative arthritis observed in the disorder.

DIAGNOSIS: Diagnosis is achieved by both clinical and genetic correlation through familial linkage analysis.

TREATMENT
Standard Therapies: Treatment consists primarily of symptomatic relief of the early-onset arthritis. Severe osteoarthrosis may require surgical intervention, including osteotomy or total joint replacement.

REFERENCES
Klippel JH, Weyand CM, Wortmann RL, eds. *Primer on rheumatic diseases,* 11th ed. Atlanta: Arthritis Foundation, 1997:375–376.
Spayde EC, Joshi AP, Wilcox WR, et al. Exon skipping mutation in the *COL9A2* gene in a family with multiple epiphyseal dysplasia. *Matrix Biol* 2000;19:121–128.

RESOURCES
362, 418

53   Septooptic Dysplasia

Paul Q. Thomas, PhD

DEFINITION: Septooptic dysplasia (SOD) is a congenital disorder that results from incomplete development of the embryonic forebrain and pituitary gland. The three defining features are optic nerve hypoplasia, abnormalities of midline brain structures such as the corpus callosum and septum pellucidum, and hypopituitarism.

SYNONYM: De Morsier syndrome.

DIFFERENTIAL DIAGNOSIS: Other causes of congenital hypopituitarism; Holoprosencephaly.

SYMPTOMS AND SIGNS: Infants with SOD may develop neonatal hypoglycemia and jaundice due to combined growth hormone (GH) and corticotropin deficiencies. Boys may have micropenis due to GH deficiency with or without gonadotrophin deficiency. Their testes may be undescended. They commonly have ocular nystagmus, strabismus, and blindness caused by optic nerve hypoplasia. Diabetes insipidus in infancy is manifested as polyuria, failure to thrive, and hypernatremic dehydration.

Some patients have developmental delay and disturbed motor function due to disordered neuronal migration. Growth is retarded from early childhood due to GH deficiency, yet some patients may show early pubertal development, indicating that gonadotrophin secretion can be retained independent of GH status.

ETIOLOGY/EPIDEMIOLOGY: The prevalence is estimated at 1 in 50,000, and the disorder affects equal numbers of males and females. This disorder is mainly sporadic in occurrence, although there are reports of familial SOD with an autosomal-recessive mode of inheritance. Direct evidence for environmental causes is lacking. At least some forms of familial SOD are known to result from mutation of the *HESX1* gene, which is the only one known to be associated with SOD; however, the existence of SOD pedigrees in which no *HESX1* mutation has been detected indicates that mutations in other developmental genes are also associated with this disorder.

DIAGNOSIS: Diagnosis is made by complete ophthalmologic examination. Cranial ultrasonography and CT (to examine septum pellucidum and optic nerves) should be performed. Assessment of serum cortisol and GH at a time of hypoglycemia or, in the absence of spontaneous hypoglycemia, GH and cortisol responses to glucagon stimulation help confirm the diagnosis, as does *HESX1* gene mutational analysis.

TREATMENT

Standard Therapies: Hormone replacement therapy is indicated as appropriate (human growth hormone, hydrocortisone, thyroxine, induction of puberty using either testosterone or estradiol, desmopressin).

REFERENCES

Dattani MT, Martinez-Barbera J-P, Thomas PQ, et al. Mutations in the homeobox gene *HESX1/Hesx1* associated with septo-optic dysplasia in human and mouse. *Nat Genet* 1998;19: 125–133.

de Morsier G. Etudes sur les dysraphies cranio-encephaliques. III. Agenesie du septum lucidum avec malformation du tractus optique: la dysplaie septo-optique. *Schweiz Arch Neurol Psychiatr* 1956;77:267–292.

Hoyt WF, Kaplan SL, Grumbach MM, et al. Septo-optic dysplasia and pituitary dwarfism. *Lancet* 1970;1:893–894.

Thomas PQ, Dattani MT, Brickman JM, et al. Heterozygous *HESX1* mutations associated with isolated congenital pituitary hypoplasia and septo-optic dysplasia. *Hum Mol Genet* 2001;10:39–45.

RESOURCES

79, 188, 430

---

54 Ear–Patella–Short Stature Syndrome

Marjan M. Nezarati, MSc, MD, FRCPC, and Ahmed S. Teebi, MD, FRCP(Edin)

DEFINITION: Ear–patella–short stature syndrome is a disorder characterized by short stature, microtia, delayed skeletal development, and absence of the patellae.

SYNONYM: Meier-Gorlin syndrome.

DIFFERENTIAL DIAGNOSIS: Coxoauricular syndrome; 3M syndrome; Russell-Silver syndrome; Gloomy face syndrome.

SYMPTOMS AND SIGNS: Individuals with this condition have severe proportionate short stature of prenatal onset. The craniofacial features include microcephaly, microtia, micrognathia, small mouth, and short palpebral fissures. Some individuals have ptosis; some have hypogonadism. Characteristic radiologic findings are absent patellae, generalized joint laxity, and delayed bone age. Other findings include slender long bones, early closure of the sutures or craniosynostosis, increased convolutional markings on skull radiographs, hooked clavicles, flat glenoid fossae, and abnormal epiphyses. Psychomotor development is generally normal to borderline normal, although some patients have had mild to moderate developmental delay.

ETIOLOGY/EPIDEMIOLOGY: Fewer than 15 patients have been reported. Several affected sibling pairs and one case of parental consanguinity suggest autosomal-recessive inheritance.

DIAGNOSIS: The diagnosis is made on clinical grounds, and is based on the presence of the characteristic findings previously described. A skeletal survey would be helpful in delineating some of the characteristic radiographic features.

TREATMENT

Standard Therapies: There is no specific treatment for this condition.

REFERENCES

Boles RG, Teebi AS, Schwartz D, et al. Further delineation of the ear-patella-short stature syndrome (Meier-Gorlin syndrome). *Clin Dysmorphol* 1994;3:207–214.

Buebel MS, Salinas CF, Pai S, et al. A new Seckel-like syndrome of primordial dwarfism. *Am J Med Genet* 1996;64:447–452.

Cohen B, Temple IK, Symons JC, et al. Microtia and short stature: a new syndrome. *J Med Genet* 1991;28:786–790.

Fryns JP. Meier-Gorlin syndrome: the adult phenotype. *Clin Dysmorphol* 1998;7:231–232.

Gorlin RJ. Microtia, absent patellae, short stature, micrognathia syndrome. *J Med Genet* 1992;29:516–517.

Hurst JA, Winter RM, Baraitser M. Distinctive syndrome of short stature, craniosynostosis, skeletal changes, and malformed ears. *Am J Med Genet* 1988;29:107–115.

Teebi AS, Gorlin RJ. Not a new Seckel-like syndrome but ear-patella-short stature syndrome. *Am J Med Genet* 1997;70:454.

RESOURCES

144, 360, 371

55 Esophageal Atresia

Alberto Peña, MD,
and Andrew R. Hong, MD

DEFINITION: Esophageal atresia refers to a congenital condition in which a portion of the esophagus is maldeveloped and lacks a normal lumen. Tracheoesophageal fistula refers to an abnormal connection between the trachea and esophagus. Esophageal atresia and tracheoesophageal fistula commonly occur together. In 85% of cases, the upper esophagus ends blindly, and the distal esophagus connects to the trachea. This is called proximal esophageal atresia with distal fistula. In the second most common type (10% of cases), known as pure or long-gap esophageal atresia, both the lower and the upper esophagus end blindly, and there is no tracheal fistula. Other types of esophageal atresia include proximal tracheoesophageal fistula and distal esophageal atresia, double fistula, and the H-type fistula, in which there is no real atresia.

SYNONYM: Congenital esophageal obstruction.

SYMPTOMS AND SIGNS: An antenatal history of polyhydramnios is almost always present. After birth, the child is unable to swallow his or her own saliva, and excessive, foamy secretions develop in the mouth. In addition, respiratory symptoms may be present if the patient has pneumonia secondary to aspiration or reflux of gastric contents into the trachea. Tracheomalacia is frequently present, and intermittent episodes of cyanosis may occur. The most common associated anomalies are cardiovascular.

ETIOLOGY/EPIDEMIOLOGY: The abnormality occurs as a result of abnormal development of the laryngeotracheal bud, but the exact cause is unknown. This group of malformations occurs in approximately 1 in 4,000 newborn babies.

DIAGNOSIS: The diagnosis of esophageal atresia should be suspected in any newborn infant with an antenatal history of polyhydramnios and excessive salivation or secretions. An attempt should be made to pass a catheter through the mouth or nose into the esophagus. Resistance when the tip is at approximately 9–10 cm is significant. A plain chest film will confirm the diagnosis if it shows the curled catheter in the dilated upper pouch of the esophagus. If the film shows gas in the stomach, a communication between the lower esophagus and the trachea is evi-

dent. Lack of gas in the gastrointestinal tract with a blind upper esophageal pouch establishes the diagnosis of a long-gap esophageal atresia with no fistula.

TREATMENT
Standard Therapies: Without surgery, esophageal atresia is a lethal condition. With surgery, most patients can expect to lead a normal life. Most repairs are undertaken shortly after birth. The esophagus is approached through the right chest, except in cases with a right aortic arch. The chest is opened, the lower esophagus is separated from the trachea, and the tracheal opening is repaired. An end-to-end anastomosis between the upper and lower esophagus is performed. In a full-term infant with esophageal atresia with tracheoesophageal fistula, one should expect 100% survival if no cardiovascular abnormalities are associated. The survival rate decreases when patients are born prematurely or if they have significant associated cardiac defects. In a patient with pure esophageal atresia, achieving an end-to-end esophageal connection primarily is often difficult. Several treatment options are available. Some surgeons use intermittent suction in the upper pouch to handle the secretions, and perform stretching maneuvers over a period of weeks or months to decrease the size of the gap and allow a repair without the use of bowel. Other surgeons will bring the end of the upper esophagus out to the neck as a cervical esophagostomy to allow the secretions to drain and to avoid aspiration. In either case, a gastrostomy is placed for feeding purposes. Later, an attempt can be made to bring both ends of the esophagus together, or a piece of intestine can be placed in the chest as a conduit, or the stomach can be pulled up into the chest and anastomosed to the proximal esophagus. There is still controversy regarding the best way to treat this specific type of defect.

REFERENCES
Engum SA, Grosfeld JL, West KW, et al. Analysis of morbidity and mortality in 227 cases of esophageal atresia and/or tracheoesophageal fistula over two decades. *Arch Surg* 1995;130: 502–508.
Holder TM, Cloud DT, Lewis JE Jr, et al. Esophageal atresia and tracheoesophageal fistula: a survey of its members by the Surgical Section of the American Academy of Pediatrics. *Pediatrics* 1964;34:542–549.
Spitz L. Esophageal atresia: past, present, and future. *J Pediatr Surg* 1996;31:19–25.

RESOURCES
143, 354, 461

56   Multiple Hereditary Exostoses

George H. Thompson, MD

DEFINITION: Multiple hereditary exostoses is a common skeletal disorder consisting of multiple cartilage-capped exostoses.

SYNONYMS: Multiple hereditary osteochondromatosis; Multiple cartilaginous exostoses; Hereditary multiple exostoses; Osteochondromatosis; Diaphyseal aclasia.

DIFFERENTIAL DIAGNOSIS: Skeletal dysplasia; Solitary osteochrondromas.

SYMPTOMS AND SIGNS: Mild short stature and palpable masses, particularly around joints with the greatest growth potential, are the most common features. Angular deformities involving the wrist (Madelung-type deformity), knee (genu valgum), and ankle (ankle valgus) occur frequently. Limb length discrepancies and symptoms related to pressure on contiguous structures also occur. Upper extremity involvement usually involves the shoulders and wrist. Scapular involvement may cause pain and crepitation with scapulothoracic motion. The elbow is usually minimally involved, although radial head dislocation can occur when there is wrist and forearm involvement. Shortening and bowing of the forearm are common. The ulna is more involved than is the radius, leading to radial bowing and ulnar tilt to the distal radial epiphysis and wrist joint (Insert Fig. 26). Spinal involvement is uncommon, but intraspinal exostoses have been reported, usually in the cervical spine (Insert Fig. 27). Neurologic signs and symptoms, such as pain, muscle weakness, and deep tendon hyperreflexia may be indicative of an intraspinal lesion. Lower extremity involvement is very common, particularly of the distal femur and proximal tibia and fibula (Insert Fig. 28). The fibula is disproportionately short, resulting in tibia valga or genu valgum (Insert Fig. 29) and an oblique orientation of the distal tibial epiphysis and the ankle joint (Insert Fig. 30). Shortening of the lower extremity is common but usually symmetric. Involvement of the proximal femur and femoral neck can result in subluxation of the femoral head. A lesion between the distal tibia and fibula can produce ankle diastasis and pain.

ETIOLOGY/EPIDEMIOLOGY: The etiology of multiple hereditary exostosis is unknown. It is an autosomal-dominant trait with mutation occurring in three distinct genes: 8q24, 11p11–12, and 19p. This disorder is considered a familial neoplastic trait.

DIAGNOSIS: Diagnosis is suspected by physical examination and confirmed radiographically. Solitary osteochrondromas or exostoses are extremely common. The presence of multiple lesions on a skeletal survey confirms the diagnosis.

TREATMENT

Standard Therapies: Surgical intervention is the major treatment for multiple hereditary exostoses. These lesions are excised when they are large, disfiguring, cause pain, have a potential for producing deformity, or when they occur in close proximity to neurovascular structures that may cause a problem at a later time. Deformity correction, when present, is also an indication for treatment. This can include osteotomies, as well as procedures to alter growth, such as epiphyseal stapling or closure, to correct angular deformities or limb length inequality.

Investigational Therapies: Gene therapy to correct the cause is the ultimate goal but is not available at this time.

REFERENCES

Arms DM, Strecker WB, Manske PR, et al. Management of forearm deformity in multiple hereditary osteochondromatosis. *J Pediatr Orthop* 1997;17:450–454.

Carroll KL, Yandow SM, Ward K, et al. Clinical correlation to genetic variations of hereditary multiple exostosis. *J Pediatr Orthop* 1999;19:785–791.

Kivioja A, Ervasti H, Kinnunen J, et al. Chondrosarcoma in a family with multiple hereditary exostoses. *J Bone Joint Surg [Br]* 2000;82:261–266.

Oga M, Nakatani F, Ikuta K, et al. Treatment of cervical cord compression, caused by hereditary multiple exostosis, with laminoplasty: a case report. *Spine* 2000;25:1290–1292.

Porter DE, Emerton ME, Villanueva-Lopez F, et al. Clinical and radiographic analysis of osteochondromas and growth disturbance in hereditary multiple exostoses. *J Pediatr Orthop* 2000; 20:246–250.

RESOURCES

263, 264, 351

57   Fetal Hydantoin Syndrome

*Bruce Alan Buehler, MD,
and Richard Finnell, PhD*

DEFINITION: Fetal hydantoin syndrome results when a susceptible fetus is exposed to the anticonvulsant drug Dilantin.

SYNONYMS: Dilantin embryopathy; Phenytoin embryopathy.

DIFFERENTIAL DIAGNOSIS: Fetal alcohol syndrome; Maternal phenylketonuria fetal embryopathy; Carbamazepine embryopathy.

SYMPTOMS AND SIGNS: Pregnant women taking Dilantin (phenytoin) for seizure control or other medical reasons have a 7%–10% risk of having their fetus exhibit some or all of the following features. Affected children have mild developmental delays, hypotonia, hirsutism, elongated upper lip with poorly developed philtrum, nail hypoplasia, and intrauterine growth retardation. Approximately 90% of affected children have no signs at birth of any teratogenic effect. As these children age, the developmental delays improve, but studies suggest that children remain slightly behind unexposed siblings. The growth delays remain throughout life, as does the hirsutism. Approximately 3% of exposed infants have brain malformations, cleft lip and palate, and severe developmental delays.

ETIOLOGY/EPIDEMIOLOGY: Exposed infants with decreased epoxide hydroxylase activity have shown symptoms of fetal hydantoin syndrome. Those with normal activity did not exhibit any symptoms at birth. Other additive factors that may increase teratogenicity include decreased folic acid levels due to Dilantin binding and the genetic implications of epilepsy. Approximately 2 million women worldwide are exposed to Dilantin during pregnancy.

DIAGNOSIS: The diagnosis is made clinically on the basis of the findings of the features described along with a history of Dilantin exposure.

TREATMENT
Standard Therapies: To lower the potential risk of Dilantin teratogenicity, women should be treated with a single anticonvulsant before conception and throughout pregnancy. Changing medications in pregnancy should be avoided, and lowest dose therapy is recommended. Additionally, women should take 0.4–4 mg of folic acid and a multivitamin daily before conception. Smoking and alcohol are potential additive teratogens and should be avoided.

REFERENCES
Buehler BA, Delimont D, van Waes M, et al. Prenatal prediction of the fetal hydantoin syndrome. *N Engl J Med* 1990;322: 1567–1571.
McKusick VA, ed. Online Mendelian Inheritance in Man (OMIM) [database online]. Bethesda, MD: National Center for Biotechnology Information, National Library of Medicine; 1999. Entry no. 132810; last update 9/16/99.

RESOURCES
257, 462

58   Fetal Valproate Syndrome

Joseph H. Hersh, MD

DEFINITION: Fetal valproate syndrome (FVS) results from maternal valproic acid (VPA) use *in utero* and is characterized by minor facial anomalies, occasional major organ structural abnormalities, and a developmental disorder.

SYNONYM: Valproic acid embryopathy.

DIFFERENTIAL DIAGNOSIS: Teratogenic effects from other anticonvulsants taken during pregnancy.

SYMPTOMS AND SIGNS: Common craniofacial abnormalities include metopic suture ridging or trigonocephaly; macrocephaly with a high, broad forehead and bifrontal narrowing; epicanthal folds connecting with an infraorbital groove; hypertelorism; flat nasal bridge; broad nasal root; small, broad nose; anteverted nares; abnormal ear position or size; long, flat philtrum; long upper lip with thin vermilion border; small mouth with downturned corners; and micrognathia or retrognathia. Low spina bifida lesions occur in about 2% of infants exposed to VPA *in utero*. Other possible congenital anomalies include cardiovascular defects; oral clefting; respiratory tract/thoracic cage abnormalities, including tracheomalacia, subglottic stenosis, abnormal lung lobulation, and pulmonary hypoplasia; genital anomalies, such as hypospadias, hypoplastic scrotum, undescended testes, and rarely, incomplete fusion of müllerian duct structures in affected females; limb anomalies, including arachnodactyly, camptodactyly, nail hypoplasia, radial ray defects, and talipes equinovarus; abdominal wall defects; inguinal hernia; and minor anomalies of the skin and, occasionally, brain and renal abnormalities. Postnatal growth deficiency and microcephaly have occurred in affected individuals who were exposed to VPA when used in combination with other anticonvulsants. The risk for a developmental disorder is significant, and an association with autism and FVS also exists.

ETIOLOGY/EPIDEMIOLOGY: Some of the manifestations may result from VPA disturbing the balance of retinoids in the developing embryo, leading to impaired regulation of *HOX* gene expression in the neuronal organization of the developing rhombomeres of the hindbrain. Clinical manifestations are the result of first-trimester exposure, with a greater risk for major malformations possibly related to higher daily doses. Although the exact risk for structural and developmental abnormalities from maternal VPA exposure during pregnancy is not known, the risk is believed to be significant. The syndrome has been reported in at least seven sibling pairs, indicating that risk for recurrence in a subsequent pregnancy exposed to VPA may be high. Males and females are equally affected.

DIAGNOSIS: The diagnosis is made clinically based on the presence of a characteristic facial phenotype following maternal VPA use during pregnancy.

TREATMENT
Standard Therapies: Early identification is important to implement appropriate management strategies to address potential complications secondary to major organ malformations and a developmental disorder. The typical lower location of the spinal defect usually is associated with fewer neurologic sequelae than is a higher lesion. Treatment of a cardiac defect depends on the nature of the lesion. Oral clefting requires surgical repair in infancy. Management of other structural abnormalities depends on the type of defect. Given the increased risk for a developmental disorder including autism, close monitoring of the affected child is warranted, including screening for social, communication, and play skills at about 18 months of age.

REFERENCES
Ardinger H, Atkin J, Blackston RP, et al. Verification of the fetal valproate syndrome phenotype. *Am J Med Genet* 1988;29:171–185.

Clayton-Smith J, Donnai D. Fetal valproate syndrome. *J Med Genet* 1995;32:1724–1727.

Kozma C. Valproic acid embryopathy: report of two siblings with further expansion of the phenotypic abnormalities and a review of the literature. *Am J Med Genet* 2001;98:168–175.

Thisted E, Ebbeson F. Malformations, withdrawal manifestations and hypoglycaemia after exposure to valproate in utero. *Arch Dis Child* 1993;69:288–291.

Williams G, King J, Cunningham M, et al. Fetal valproate syndrome and autism: additional evidence of an association. *Dev Med Child Neurol* 2001 (in press).

RESOURCES
351, 445

---

59   FG Syndrome

John M. Graham, Jr., MD, ScD

DEFINITION: FG syndrome is an X-linked recessive form of mental retardation associated with complete or partial agenesis of the corpus callosum, mild facial dysmorphism, relative macrocephaly, congenital hypotonia, chronic constipation with or without anal anomalies, broad thumbs and halluces, prominent fetal fingerpads, failure to thrive, and characteristic friendly, loquacious, hyperactive behavior with occasional aggressive outbursts.

SYNONYMS: Opitz-Kaveggia syndrome; Keller syndrome.

DIFFERENTIAL DIAGNOSIS: Fragile X syndrome; Other types of X-linked mental retardation.

SYMPTOMS AND SIGNS: Partial agenesis of the corpus has been seen in many cases, and neuropathologic findings include megalencephaly, midline fusion of mammillary bodies, and neuroglial heterotopias. The associated congenital hypotonia with joint hyperlaxity usually progresses to contractures with spasticity and unsteady gait in later life. Lethality during infancy has been reported in as many as one third of patients, as a consequence of bronchopulmonary problems and/or heart defects, but once patients have survived infancy, death is rare. The presence of subtle dysmorphic facial features (macrocephaly, broad forehead with frontal upsweep), with broad thumbs and toes with persistent fetal pads, and characteristic behaviors (hyperactive behavior, affability, excessive talkativeness) facilitates diagnosis in midchildhood. Constipation, with or without anal anomalies, is a distinctive major finding. Mental retardation is a universal finding, and sensorineural hearing loss or seizures have sometimes occurred. Other nonspecific occasional features have included abnormal pinnae, hypertelorism, pyloric stenosis, cryptorchidism, hypospadius, hernia, single transverse palmar creases, syndactyly, and camptodactyly. Congenital hypotonia secondary to central nervous system involvement is also frequent. Maternal carriers may manifest constipation, broad forehead with or without frontal cowlick, macrocephaly, ocular hypertelorism, and/or congenital hypotonia.

ETIOLOGY/EPIDEMIOLOGY: More than 50 cases have been reported. Linkage analysis in some families with FG syndrome has resulted in a broad localization of the gene from Xq12 to Xq22, but other families do not link to this locus, suggesting genetic heterogeneity.

DIAGNOSIS: The diagnosis should be considered in boys with congenital hypotonia and anorectal anomalies and in older males with mental retardation, congenital hypotonia, joint contractures, chronic constipation, and characteristic facial appearance and personality. The presence of complete or partial agenesis of the corpus callosum helps make the diagnosis.

TREATMENT
Standard Therapies: Early intervention with physical, occupational, and speech therapy should be initiated at the time of diagnosis. Because initial hypotonia may progress to spasticity, long-term physical therapy should be undertaken throughout childhood. Additional referral to pediatric gastroenterology for constipation may be necessary. Occasional seizures and hearing loss may require additional treatment.

REFERENCES
Graham JM Jr, Superneau D, Rogers RC, et al. Clinical and behavioral characteristics in FG syndrome. *Am J Med Genet* 1999;85: 470–475.

Graham JM Jr, Tackels D, Dibbern K, et al. FG syndrome: report of three new families with linkage to Xq12-q21.1. *Am J Med Genet* 1998;80:145–156.

Kato R, Niikawa N, Nagai T, et al. Japanese kindred with FG syndrome [Letter]. *Am J Med Genet* 1994;52:242–243.

Opitz JM, Richieri-da Costa A, Aase JM, et al. FG syndrome update 1988: note of 5 new patients and bibliography. *Am J Med Genet* 1988;30:309–328.

Ozonoff S, Williams BJ, Rauch AM, et al. Behavioral phenotype of FG syndrome: cognition, personality, and behavior in eleven affected boys. *Am J Med Genet* 2000;97:112–118.

RESOURCE
155

---

60   Filippi Syndrome

Susanne Schmandt, Dr Med, and Phillip L. Pearl, MD

DEFINITION: Filippi syndrome is a multiple congenital anomalies/mental retardation syndrome characterized by syndactyly, clinodactyly, variable phalangeal abnormalities, unusual facial features, microcephaly, and mental and growth retardation.

SYNONYM: Syndactyly type I with microcephaly and mental retardation.

DIFFERENTIAL DIAGNOSIS: Scott craniodigital syndrome with mental retardation; Chitayat syndrome; Zerres syndrome; Kelly syndrome; Woods syndrome.

SYMPTOMS AND SIGNS: At birth, affected children typically present with short stature, low birth weight, microcephaly, clinodactyly of the fifth finger, and variable soft-tissue syndactyly of toes and fingers. Finger syndactyly is not a consistent finding, but when present, involvement of fingers 3–4 appears to be a distinctive finding. Other abnormalities of the hands include brachydactyly/brachymesophalangy, tapered fingers, small hands, and a single palmar crease. Syndactyly of the toes often involves toes 2–4. Almost complete syndactyly of toes 2–3 is characteristic. Cryptorchidism is noted in some males. Later, mild facial dysmorphism becomes evident, including a broad and high nasal bridge, abnormalities of the alae nasi (e.g., thin alae nasi), and a broad nasal tip. Usually short stature persists. Just a few patients have gained normal height over the years. Bone age may be delayed. Additional features including skeletal abnormalities are reported, but confirmation in more patients is needed before these can be considered characteristic. Developmental delay becomes obvious within the first year, often resulting in severe mental retardation. Speech and language acquisition is especially affected. Many children speak only single words or simple sentences.

ETIOLOGY/EPIDEMIOLOGY: The etiology is unknown. Chromosomal analysis is normal. Mutations of genes expressed in the developing brain and limb, such as sonic hedgehog, may be causative. An autosomal-recessive trait is assumed, because males and females are affected equally and pedigrees show only affected siblings except in one family in which the mother had mild bilateral cutaneous syndactyly of toes 2–3. Including patients who are difficult to classify, no more than 16 cases are known. Consanguinity existed in 1 of 11 families.

DIAGNOSIS: Diagnosis is based on clinical observation. X-rays should be performed if skeletal abnormalities are suspected.

TREATMENT
Standard Therapies: Treatment is symptomatic.

REFERENCES
Fryer A. Filippi syndrome with mild learning difficulties. *Clin Dysmorphol* 1996;5:35–39.
Heron D, Billette de Villemeur T, Munnich A, et al. Filippi syndrome: a new case with skeletal abnormalities. *J Med Genet* 1995;32:659–661.
Orrico A, Hayek G. An additional case of craniodigital syndrome: variable expression of the Filippi syndrome? *Clin Genet* 1997; 52:177–179.
Toriello HV, Higgins JV. Craniodigital syndromes: report of a child with Filippi syndrome and discussion of differential diagnosis. *Am J Med Genet* 1995;55:200–204.
Walpole IR, Parry T, Goldblatt J. Expanding the phenotype of Filippi syndrome: a report of three cases. *Clin Dysmorphol* 1999;8:235–240.
Williams MS, Williams JL, Wargowski DS, et al. Filippi syndrome: report of three additional cases. *Am J Med Genet* 1999;87: 128–133.

RESOURCES
296, 351

---

61 Floating Harbor Syndrome

Mark S. Lubinsky, MD

DEFINITION: Floating harbor syndrome is a disorder in which affected individuals have characteristic triangular facies with a large, bulbous nose; deep-set eyes; short philtrum and thin lips; and a wide, downturned mouth. Infants have low birth weight and short length.

SYNONYM: Pelletier-Leisti syndrome.

DIFFERENTIAL DIAGNOSIS: Velo-cardio-facial syndrome.

SYMPTOMS AND SIGNS: Affected individuals have characteristic triangular facies with the aforementioned features. Low birth weight and short length develop into short stature significantly below the 5th percentile. Bone age is typically delayed. Boys may have an underdeveloped penis. Major early speech delays tend to improve, and there may be mild mental retardation. There seem to be a variety of cognitive issues that are not yet well defined. Trigonocephaly may occur in infancy but become less prominent with age. Some children have a high-pitched voice, and occasional heart findings, supernumerary upper incisor, and clavicular pseudoarthroses. Celiac disease also seems to be common.

ETIOLOGY/EPIDEMIOLOGY: The disorder is likely autosomal dominant. Both sexes are affected.

DIAGNOSIS: The main diagnostic test is radiography for delayed bone age.

TREATMENT
Standard Therapies: Speech therapy with an emphasis on communication may be important for early difficulties. Careful assessment of specific cognitive impairments may help older patients.

REFERENCES
Hersh JH, et al. Changing phenotype in floating harbor syndrome. *Am J Med Genet* 1998;76:58–61.
Midro AT, et al. Floating harbor syndrome: case report and further delineation of the syndrome. *Ann Genet* 1997;40:133–138.
Rosen AC, et al. A further report of a case of floating harbor syndrome in a mother and daughter. *J Clin Exp Neuropsychol* 1998;20:483–495.

RESOURCES
157, 188, 351

62   Fountain Syndrome

Griet Van Buggenhout, MD, PhD, and Jean-Pierre Fryns, MD, PhD

DEFINITION: Fountain syndrome is an autosomal-recessive condition with cardinal features of mental retardation, sensorineural deafness, skeletal abnormalities, and coarse face with full lips.

DIFFERENTIAL DIAGNOSIS: Coffin-Lowry syndrome; Alpha-thalassemia syndrome; Melkersson-Rosenthal syndrome.

SYMPTOMS AND SIGNS: Fountain described a family with four members (three brothers and a sister) with mental retardation, deafness, and skeletal abnormalities. Two of them developed progressive swelling of the lips, and in one of them an eroded granulomatous mass appeared in the lower lip. Spina bifida was present in one of the siblings. Other patients have presented with congenital deafness due to an inner ear anomaly, facial plethorism, and skeletal anomalies (thickening of the calvaria and short stubby hands with broad terminal phalanges). Accessory features of the syndrome may include epilepsy, short stature, large head circumference, broad and plump hands, and friendly behavior.

ETIOLOGY/EPIDEMIOLOGY: Occurrence in siblings with normal parents suggests an autosomal-recessive inheritance.

DIAGNOSIS: The diagnosis is suspected based on the clinical findings.

TREATMENT
Standard Therapies: There is no specific treatment.

REFERENCES
Fountain RB. Familial bone abnormalities, deaf mutism, mental retardation and skin granuloma. *Proc R Soc Med* 1974;67: 878–879.

Fryns JP. Fountain's syndrome: mental retardation, sensorineural deafness, skeletal abnormalities, and coarse face with full lips. *J Med Genet* 1989;26:722–724.

Fryns JP, Dereymaeker A, Hoefnagels M, et al. Mental retardation, deafness, skeletal abnormalities and coarse face with full lips: confirmation of the Fountain syndrome. *Am J Med Genet* 1987;26:551–555.

Van Buggenhout GJCM, van Ravenswaaij-Arts CMA, Renier WO, et al. Fountain syndrome: further delineation of the clinical syndrome and follow-up data. *Genet Couns* 1996;7:177–186.

RESOURCES
145, 351

63   Fraser Syndrome

Cathy A. Stevens, MD

DEFINITION: Fraser syndrome is an autosomal-recessive condition characterized by cryptophthalmos, syndactyly, abnormal genitalia, and other features, including malformations of the nose and ears, cleft lip and palate, laryngeal abnormalities, and renal agenesis.

SYNONYMS: Fraser cryptophthalmos syndrome; Cryptophthalmos syndrome; Cryptophthalmos-syndactyly syndrome.

DIFFERENTIAL DIAGNOSIS: Isolated cryptophthalmos; Fraser-like syndrome.

SYMPTOMS AND SIGNS: The major features of Fraser syndrome include unilateral or bilateral cryptophthalmos, cutaneous syndactyly of the fingers and/or toes, and abnormalities of the internal and external genitalia. Cryptorchidism and hypospadias are common in males, whereas females may have enlarged clitoris and labia majora, vaginal atresia, and uterine malformations. Bilateral or unilateral renal agenesis is also common. Laryngeal atresia or stenosis may occur, leading to pulmonary hyperplasia in some cases. Other craniofacial features include broad nose with depressed bridge, coloboma of the alae nasi, midline groove of the nasal tip, malformed and/or low-set ears, and clefts of the lip and/or palate. Although cryptophthalmos is not an obligate feature of Fraser syndrome, those who have it often lack eyebrows and eyelashes and sometimes have a tongue of hair over the temple, forehead, or eye area. Mental retardation is present in most affected individuals.

ETIOLOGY/EPIDEMIOLOGY: Fraser syndrome is inherited in an autosomal-recessive fashion. The gene locus has not been identified. More than 100 cases have been reported; the sex distribution is equal.

DIAGNOSIS: Clinical features establish the diagnosis. Renal and pelvic ultrasonography may detect renal agenesis and other internal urogenital malformations. Imaging studies of the brain may show structural anomalies. Prenatal diagnosis has been made using ultrasonography and fetoscopy.

TREATMENT

Standard Therapies: No treatment is available if bilateral renal agenesis is present. Surgical correction of cryptophthalmos is possible; however, associated eye malformations often result in poor visual function. Many of the other anomalies involving the urogenital system, craniofacies, and extremities can be surgically corrected.

REFERENCES

Boyd PA, Keeling JW, Lindenbaum RH. Fraser syndrome (cryptophthalmos-syndactyly syndrome): a review of 11 cases with postmortem findings. *Am J Med Genet* 1988;31:159–168.

Gattuso J, Patton MA, Baraitser M. The clinical spectrum of the Fraser syndrome: report of 3 new cases and review. *J Med Genet* 1987;24:549–555.

Gorlin RJ, Cohen MM, Hennekam RCM, eds. *Syndromes of the head and neck,* 4th ed. New York: Oxford University Press, 2001:1016–1019.

Stevens CA, McClanahan C, Steck A, et al. Pulmonary hyperplasia in the Fraser cryptophthalmos syndrome. *Am J Med Genet* 1994;52:427–431.

Thomas IT, Frias JL, Felix V, et al. Isolated and syndromic cryptophthalmos. *Am J Med Genet* 1986;25:85–98.

RESOURCES

96, 308

64 Gastroschisis

Sean E. McLean, MD, and Robert K. Minkes, MD, PhD

DEFINITION: Gastroschisis is a congenital defect of the anterior abdominal wall with associated herniation of abdominal viscera.

DIFFERENTIAL DIAGNOSIS: Omphalocele; Congenital hernia of the umbilical cord.

SYMPTOMS AND SIGNS: Gastroschisis is characterized by a 2–5 cm opening in the anterior abdominal wall lateral to a normal umbilical cord, most commonly on the right side. Abdominal viscera protrude through the defect without a covering sac. Stomach, small intestine, and large intestine are the most common organs to herniate in gastroschisis. Liver herniation is rare, but evisceration of the gallbladder, uterus, fallopian tubes, ovaries, urinary bladder, and testes may be apparent. The bowel develops serositis and may be edematous, thickened, shortened, and covered with a thick fibrous peel. Malrotation is invariably present, and the exposed bowel is at risk for strangulation and vascular compromise due to the small size of the abdominal wall defect. Bowel function is delayed in most infants due to malabsorption and hypomotility. Intestinal atresia and other gastrointestinal tract abnormalities occur in as many as 10% of infants with gastroschisis, and affected infants are often small for their gestational age.

ETIOLOGY/EPIDEMIOLOGY: The etiology and embryogenesis of gastroschisis is unknown. Theories include defects in differentiation of the lateral folds of the abdominal wall and gestational vascular accidents involving the omphalomesenteric artery. Consistent chromosomal or genetic abnormalities have not been defined. The incidence of gastroschisis ranges from 1 in 1,500 to 1 in 13,000 and it is more common in women of low gravidity younger than age 30 years. There is no sex predilection.

DIAGNOSIS: The diagnosis can be made by prenatal ultrasonography and is differentiated from omphalocele by the presence of freely floating viscera in the amniotic cavity. Other anomalies should be noted and the degree of bowel dilatation should be followed with serial examinations. Dilated or thickened bowel suggests intestinal atresia or ischemia. The finding of eviscerated bowel after delivery confirms the diagnosis.

TREATMENT

Standard Therapies: Women with pregnancies complicated by gastroschisis should undergo delivery at a tertiary care center where neonatal and pediatric surgical expertise is available. Prenatal consultation is advisable. Outcomes after cesarean section and vaginal delivery are similar. Planned induction at 37–40 weeks' gestation may prevent bowel ischemia. Initial management of infants born with gastroschisis includes intravenous fluid, electrolyte and antibiotic therapy, monitoring of urine output, and placement of a nasogastric tube. The exposed bowel should be covered in moist sterile guaze and placed in a bowel bag or wrapped in cellophane to prevent heat loss. The infant should be placed in a lateral position to prevent kinking of the bowel and vascular compromise. Surgery is needed to close the abdominal wall defect. Postoperatively, ventilatory support is needed because of the increase in intra-abdominal pressure. Total parenteral nutrition is needed until the bowel regains function, usually in 2–4 weeks. Techniques that allow gentle reduction of the herniated bowel followed by closure of the defect on an elective basis are being advocated by many centers. One such technique uses a spring-loaded silo that is placed at the bedside without anesthesia or suturing and is associated with fewer complications and a shorter hospital stay.

REFERENCES

Cooney DR. Defects of the abdominal wall. In: O'Neill JA, Rowe MI, Grosfeld JL, et al., eds. *Pediatric surgery,* 5th ed. St. Louis: CV Mosby, 1998:1045–1069.

Dykes EH. Prenatal diagnosis and management of abdominal wall defects. *Semin Pediatr Surg* 1996;5:90–94.

Fonkalsrud EW, Smith MD, Shaw KS, et al. Selective management of gastroschisis according to the degree of visceroabdominal disproportion. *Ann Surg* 1993;218:742–747.

Langer JC. Gastroschisis and omphalocele. *Semin Pediatr Surg* 1996;5:124–128.

Minkes RK, Langer JC, Mazziotti MV, et al. Routine insertion of a silastic spring-loaded silo for infants with gastroschisis. *J Pediatr Surg* 2000;35:843–846.

RESOURCES

135, 354

---

65   GBBB Syndrome (Opitz Syndrome)

John M. Opitz, MD

DEFINITION: Opitz or GBBB syndrome refers to a highly variable condition affecting mostly derivatives of the midline, including monozygotic twinning and development of brain, facial midline, lip, palate, heart, tracheobronchial tree, esophagus, and genitalia (in males). There are two forms: X-linked and autosomal dominant.

SYNONYMS: For the X-linked form: Opitz G/BBB syndrome, X-linked; Opitz syndrome, X-linked, OSX; Opitz-G syndrome, type I, OGS1; Opitz BBBG syndrome, type I, BBBG1; Opitz G/BBB syndrome type I; Midline 1, *MID1*; Midline 1 ring finger gene; Midin. For the autosomal dominant form: G syndrome; Hypospadias dysphagia syndrome; Opitz-Frías syndrome; Opitz-G syndrome, type II, OGS2; Telecanthus with associated anomalies; BBB syndrome; Hypertelorism, hypospadias syndrome; Telecanthus hypospadias syndrome; Opitz BBBG syndrome; Opitz oculogenito laryngeal syndrome, type II.

SYMPTOMS AND SIGNS: Intrauterine growth usually is normal; however, there may be polyhydramnios with hypertelorism, agenesis of corpus callosum, cleft lip and/or palate, congenital heart defect, or abnormal genitalia in a male. Neonatally, the condition should be suspected in any infant with wide-set eyes, cleft scrotum, hypospadias, congenital hypotonia, stridor, and repeated choking and spluttering on initial feedings. A laryngeal cleft may be found with dysphagia and/or gastroesophageal reflux, causing aspiration into the lungs. Congenital heart defects may be present, as may imperforate anus, frequent constipation, and intestinal malrotation. The trachea may be short with high carina and bifurcation into main-stem bronchi; therefore, extreme caution should be used during bronchoscopy. Rarely, there may be congenital pulmonary hypoplasia, malformed sinuses with frequent sinus, middle ear and tonsil infections, and small ear canals. Most patients have borderline or normal psychomotor development; mental retardation is rare. Some affected individuals have seizures, behavior abnormalities, sensory integration dysfunction, oral defensiveness, or scoliosis.

ETIOLOGY/EPIDEMIOLOGY: The X-linked form is caused by mutations of the *MID1* gene at Xp22.3. An apparent gene duplication is present on the long arm of the X chromosome and is referred to as *MID2*. Its role in the X-linked GBBB syndrome is yet to be established. The autosomal-dominant form maps to 22q11, in the close vicinity of the DiGeorge region. The actual gene involved is unknown.

DIAGNOSIS: All pregnant women, especially those with polyhydramnios, should have an ultrasonographic evaluation. All children with bilateral cleft lip/palate have some degree of hypertelorism, but usually not a widow's peak, minor ear anomalies, micrognathia, stridor, or dysphagia with aspiration. Such infants should have laryngoscopy/

bronchoscopy to rule out tracheobronchial cleft or tracheoesophageal fistula. If dysphagia with aspiration is diagnosed, studies of gastroesophageal reflux are indicated. Echocardiography should be performed. Renal ultrasonography should also be done, as should MRI and electroencephalography if the patient has seizures.

TREATMENT

Standard Therapies: Treatment should include repair of cleft lip/palate, as well as prevention and treatment of middle ear infections. Emergent treatment of pulmonary aspiration with placement of gastrostomy tube, in some cases even jejunostomy tube, with Nissen fundoplication may be necessary. Other treatment should include treatment/repair of heart defects, intestinal malrotation, hypospadias, cleft scrotum, cryptorchidism, and imperforate anus. Patients with gastroesophogeal reflux without aspiration should be treated with the usual medications. Special pedagogic support may be needed for patients who have developmental delays.

REFERENCES

Fryburg JS, Lin KY, Golden WL. Chromosome 22q11.2 deletion in a boy with Opitz (G/BBB) syndrome. *Am J Med Genet* 1996;62:274–275.

Cainarca S, Messali S, Ballabio A, et al. Functional characterization of the Opitz syndrome gene product (midin): evidence for homodimerization and association with microtubles throughout the cell cycle. *Hum Mol Genet* 1999;8:1387–1396.

Quaderi NA, Schweiger S, Gaudenz K, et al. Opitz G/BBB syndrome, a defect of midline development, is due to mutations in a new RING finger gene on Xp22. *Nat Genet* 1997;17:285–291.

Robin NH, Feldman GJ, Aronson AL, et al. Opitz syndrome is genetically heterogeneous, with one locus on Xp22, and a second locus on 22qll.2. *Nat Genet* 1995;11:459–461.

Robin NH, Opitz JM, Muenke M. Opitz G/BBB syndrome: clinical comparisons of families linked to Xp22 and 22q, and a review of the literature. *Am J Med Genet* 1996;62:305–317.

RESOURCES

2, 351, 380

---

66 Gordon Syndrome

Angela Vincent, MB, BS, FRCPath, and Helen Stewart, MD, MRCP

DEFINITION: Gordon syndrome is a congenital condition characterized by talipes, camptodactyly, and cleft palate.

SYNONYM: Arthrogryposis multiplex congenita, dominant distal, type IIA.

DIFFERENTIAL DIAGNOSIS: Distal arthrogryposis type I; Aase-Smith syndrome; Oro-facial-digital syndrome type I; Freeman-Sheldon syndrome.

SYMPTOMS AND SIGNS: The limbs may show talipes and fixed camptodactyly of the proximal interphalangeal joints, sparing the thumbs. Some patients have mild syndactyly of the fingers. These features are congenital and bilateral, but may be asymmetric. The spectrum of palatal abnormalities includes cleft palate, multiple palatal defects, or bifid uvula. Cleft palate is the least frequently manifested trait, occurring in 20% of cases. Additional features of the syndrome include ptosis, epicanthic folds, nevus flammeus of the face, pterygium colli, omphalocele, short stature in 50% of patients, cryptorchidism, hip dislocation, and congenital vertebral anomalies in 33% of patients (lumbar lordosis, kyphoscoliosis). The more severe contractures are seen in individuals with shortness of stature and cleft palate. Cognitive development is normal.

ETIOLOGY/EPIDEMIOLOGY: Gordon syndrome is inherited in an autosomal-dominant manner, with variable expressivity and incomplete penetrance. Females are less severely affected than males. Fertility is normal in affected individuals.

DIAGNOSIS: The diagnosis is not difficult if the patient has the full syndrome or a family history. If the patient has an isolated case, the diagnosis may be made clinically by the presence of two or more of the cardinal features: talipes, camptodactyly, and cleft palate. Routine laboratory investigations and chromosome analysis are normal. Radiographs confirm the presence of skeletal abnormalities.

TREATMENT

Standard Therapies: Surgical correction of palatal abnormalities and orthopedic treatment of the limb defects may be required. All patients with Gordon syndrome walk but have short feet with residual clubbing.

REFERENCES

Gordon H, Davies D, Berman MM. Camptodacty, cleft palate, and club foot: syndrome showing the autosomal-dominant pattern of inheritance. *J Med Genet* 1969;6:266–274.

Halal F, Fraser FC. Camptodactyly, cleft palate and club foot (the Gordon syndrome): a report of a large pedigree. *J Med Genet* 1979;16:149–150.

Hall JG, Reed SD, Greene G. The distal arthrogryposes: delineation of new entities—review and nosologic discussion. *Am J Med Genet* 1982;11:185–239.

Ioan DM, Belengeanu V, Maximillian C, et al. Distal arthrogryposis with autosomal dominant inheritance and reduced penetrance in females: the Gordon syndrome. *Clin Genet* 1993;43:300–302.

Robinow M, Johnson GF. The Gordon syndrome: autosomal dominant cleft palate, camptodactyly, and club feet. *Am J Med Genet* 1981;9:139–146.

Say B, Barber DH, Thompson RC, et al. The Gordon syndrome. *J Med Genet* 1980;17:405.

RESOURCES

64, 351

---

67   Gorlin-Chaudhry-Moss Syndrome

Deepak Narayan, MD, and John A. Persing, MD

DEFINITION: Gorlin-Chaudhry-Moss (GCM) syndrome is characterized by short stature, hypertrichosis, low frontal hairline, brachycephaly secondary to craniosynostosis, midface hypoplasia, abnormally shaped teeth, and genital hypoplasia.

DIFFERENTIAL DIAGNOSIS: Saethre-Chotzen syndrome; Lopez Hernandez syndrome; Crouzon syndrome; Cornelia de Lange syndrome.

SYMPTOMS AND SIGNS: Children with this syndrome have characteristic coarse facial features; a flattened midface and nose; a short, wide head (brachycephaly secondary to premature coronal suture fusion); a low frontal hairline; and down-slanting palpebral fissures. Orbital/ocular anomalies may include orbital hypoplasia, microophthalmia, synophrys, colobomas of the upper eyelid, hyperopia, astigmatism, and lacrimal duct stenosis. Oral anomalies include a high arched palate, microdontia, and class III malocclusion. Characteristic dental defects include bell-shaped dental crowns, spindle-shaped roots, and small or missing pulp chambers. Audiologic investigation shows bilateral conductive hearing loss. Hypertrichosis involving the arms, legs, and back is consistent in all patients. Hypoplastic labia majora are the most common sign of genital hypoplasia. Acral defects are characterized by hypoplastic distal phalanges and toes. Intelligence is normal.

ETIOLOGY/EPIDEMIOLOGY: No chromosomal abnormalities have been reported with this syndrome. All affected patients described have been female. The finding of two affected siblings with unaffected parents and relatives suggests an autosomal-recessive inheritance.

DIAGNOSIS: Diagnosis is made clinically based on the presence of the features described. CT can confirm craniosynostosis in early cases; radiography of the hands and feet show the characteristic shortened distal phalanges. Chromosomal studies are required to rule out an abnormal karyotype.

TREATMENT

Standard Therapies: Treatment of all anomalies is surgical, directed toward a specific deformity. Such procedures may include release of syndactyly, augmentation of hypoplastic areas such as the nasal dorsum and the maxilla, and cranial vault reshaping for craniosynostosis.

REFERENCES

Ippel PF, Gorlin RJ, Lenz W, et al. Craniofacial dysostosis, hypertrichosis, genital hypoplasia, ocular dental and digital defects. *Am J Med Genet* 1992;44:518–522.

McKusick VA, ed. Online Mendelian Inheritance in Man (OMIM) [database online]. Bethesda, MD: National Center for Biotechnology Information, National Library of Medicine; 2000. Entry no. 233500.

Pries S, Kawel EV, Majewski F. Gorlin-Chaudhry-Moss or Saethre-Chotzen syndrome. *Clin Genet* 1995;47:267–269.

RESOURCES

96, 149, 363

68 Greig Cephalopolysyndactyly Syndrome

Karl-Heinz Grzeschik, Prof Dr Rer Nat

DEFINITION: Greig cephalopolysyndactyly syndrome (GCPS) is an autosomal-dominant developmental disorder caused by defects in the zinc finger transcription factor GLI3. The phenotype is characterized by preaxial and postaxial polydactyly, syndactyly of fingers and toes, and macrocephaly resulting in apparent hypertelorism.

SYNONYM: Polysyndactyly with peculiar skull shape.

DIFFERENTIAL DIAGNOSIS: Acrocallosal syndrome; Oral-facial-digital syndrome IV or VI.

SYMPTOMS AND SIGNS: In GCPS, limb and craniofacial development are affected. Hand and foot malformations are mostly bilateral. Postaxial polydactyly is common in the hands and preaxial polydactyly in the feet. The thumbs are frequently broad due to a malformed distal phalanx, sometimes with a bifid tip. Radiography can show preaxial polydactyly of the hands not noted on physical examination. Postaxial polydactyly is the presence of a well-formed digit on the ulnar or fibular side of the limb (type A, PAP-A), or a rudimentary digit (pedunculated postminimus, nubbin, type B, PAP-B). Syndactyly is mostly cutaneous in the feet, varying from mild webbing between the first two or three toes to complete cutaneous fusion, sometimes also with nail fusion.

In the hands, bony fusion can involve the distal phalanges fingers 3–4 or 3–5. The craniofacial manifestations consist of macrocephaly, in some cases with a broad prominent forehead, a broad nasal root, and brachycephaly. In individuals with large crania, the interpupillary distance is increased, giving the impression of hypertelorism.

ETIOLOGY/EPIDEMIOLOGY: The disorder is inherited in an autosomal-dominant manner. It is caused by a mutation affecting one copy of the GLI3 gene, which is located on chromosome 7p13. Point mutations within the gene, deletions involving GLI3, or chromosomal rearrangements affecting GLI3 expression have been described. The phenotype shows full penetrance, but marked interfamilial and intrafamilial variability. It is seen in both sexes, and all ethnic groups are affected. Mutations in GLI3 have also been associated with Pallister-Hall syndrome, postaxial polydactyly type A (PAP-A), and preaxial polydactyly type IV. These phenotypes and GCPS are grouped under the term GLI3 morphopathies.

DIAGNOSIS: The diagnosis should be considered if preaxial or postaxial polydactyly, syndactyly of fingers 3–4 and toes 1–3, macrocephaly, and hypertelorism are present. Molecular genetic testing of GLI3 on a research basis employing SSCP, DHPLC, and genomic sequencing detects point mutations in approximately 60% of patients, loss of heterozygosity analysis finds large deletions of all or part of GLI3, and Giemsa-banding cytogenetics uncovers chromosomal rearrangements involving chromosome 7p13.

TREATMENT
Standard Therapies: Surgical repair of polydactyly and syndactyly of the hand may be undertaken, where appropriate. Surgical correction of the feet for cosmetic benefits should be balanced against possible orthopedic complications.

REFERENCES
Gorlin RJ, Cohen MM Jr, Levin LS. Greig cephalopolysyndactyly syndrome. In: *Syndromes of the head and neck.* New York: Oxford University Press, 1990:799–800.
Kalff-Suske M, Wild A, Topp J, et al. Point mutations throughout the GLI3 gene cause Greig cephalopolysyndactyly syndrome. *Hum Mol Genet* 1999;8:1769–1777.
Kang S, Graham JM, Olney AH, Biesecker LG. GLI3 frameshift mutations cause autosomal dominant Pallister-Hall syndrome. *Nat Genet* 1997;15:266–268.
Radhakrishna U, Bornholdt D, Scott HS, et al. The phenotypic spectrum of GLI3 morphopathies includes autosomal dominant preaxial polydactyly type-IV and postaxial polydactyly type-A/B; no phenotype prediction from the position of GLI3 mutations. *Am J Hum Genet* 1999;65:645–655.
Radhakrishna U, Wild A, Grzeschik KH, et al. Mutation in GLI3 in postaxial polydactyly type A. *Nat Genet* 1997;17:269–271.

RESOURCES
96, 160, 351

69   Hallermann-Streiff Syndrome

John M. Graham, Jr., MD, ScD

DEFINITION: Hallermann-Streiff syndrome (HSS) is a congenital syndrome characterized by distinctive craniofacial abnormalities, including dyscephaly; a small, underdeveloped lower jaw; an unusually small mouth; and a characteristic beak-shaped nose.

SYNONYMS: François syndrome; Oculomandibulodyscephaly.

DIFFERENTIAL DIAGNOSIS: Progeria; Wiedemann-Rautenstrauch syndrome; Mandibulofacial dysostosis; Autosomal-recessive pseudoprogeria/Hallermann-Streiff syndrome.

SYMPTOMS AND SIGNS: Constant features include dyscephaly, small eyes and congenital cataracts, and short stature. Most infants with HSS have a small head that is unusually broad with a prominent forehead and a small face with a birdlike appearance. Ossification of the cranial sutures and closure of the anterior fontanel may be delayed. Scalp hair is often sparse or absent. Additional craniofacial abnormalities may include an abnormally small jaw, underdeveloped cheekbones, small nostrils, and underdeveloped cartilage in the nose. There may also be an abnormally small mouth, an unusually high palate, and glossoptosis. Recurrent respiratory infections or tracheomalacia may occur. Microphthalmia, strabismus, nystagmus, and/or blue sclera also may occur, as well as decreased visual acuity, iris atrophy, and short palpebral fissures. Approximately 36% of infants with HSS are born prematurely and/or have a low birth weight. Intelligence is usually normal, but mental retardation may be present. Infants with HSS may have neonatal or natal teeth, and many affected children have malformed and/or abnormally crowded teeth, resulting in malocclusion. Severe tooth decay, enamel dysplasia, and/or extra or missing teeth may occur. Most infants with HSS also have abnormalities affecting the skin and hair, including atrophy of skin on the scalp and over the middle of the face. Some may have underdeveloped clavicles and/or ribs, scoliosis or lordosis, winged scapula, or pectus excavatum. Males may have hypogonadism or cryptorchidism. Approximately 5% of patients have cardiac defects, and some patients develop cor pulmonale.

ETIOLOGY/EPIDEMIOLOGY: More than 180 cases have been reported. The cause is unknown. Most cases appear to occur randomly. The disorder is likely autosomal dominant, with almost all cases being the result of fresh mutation.

DIAGNOSIS: The diagnosis is usually made shortly after birth based on the identification of characteristic physical findings and symptoms. The diagnosis may be confirmed by a thorough clinical evaluation and a detailed patient history.

TREATMENT

Standard Therapies: Treatment is aimed at specific symptoms and may require the coordinated efforts of a team of specialists. Surgical correction may be done for micrognathia, an underdeveloped mandible, and glossoptosis. Tracheostomy may be required for severe breathing difficulties. Affected individuals may experience complications during surgical procedures requiring anesthesia because of their narrowed air passages, which make intubation difficult. Snoring or daytime hypersomnolence are indications for sleep studies. Affected individuals should receive frequent eye and dental examinations. Surgery may be performed to remove congenital cataracts.

REFERENCES

Christian CL, Lachman RS, Aylsworth AS, et al. Radiological findings in Hallermann-Streiff syndrome: report of five cases and a review of the literature. *Am J Med Genet* 1991;41:508–514.

Cohen MM Jr. Hallermann-Streiff syndrome: a review. *Am J Med Genet* 1991;41:488–499.

David LR, Finlon M, Genecov D, et al. Hallermann-Streiff syndrome: experience with 15 patients and review of the literature. *J Craniofac Surg* 1999;10:160–168.

Robinow M. Respiratory obstruction and cor pulmonale in the Hallermann-Streiff syndrome. *Am J Med Genet* 1991;41:515–516.

Salbert BA, Stevens CA, Spence JE. Tracheomalacia in Hallermann-Streiff syndrome. *Am J Med Genet* 1991;41:521–523.

RESOURCES

96, 246, 355

70   Hanhart Syndrome

Stephen P. Robertson, FRACP

DEFINITION: Hanhart syndrome is characterized by hypoplasia/aplasia of the tongue and mandible in addition to defects of the limbs.

SYNONYMS: Aglossia adactylia; Oromandibular-limb hypoplasia complex; Peromelia with micrognathism.

DIFFERENTIAL DIAGNOSIS: Splenogonadal fusion complex; Acheiropodia.

SYMPTOMS AND SIGNS: The primary abnormalities are hypoplasia/agenesis of the tongue and limb defects affecting the upper and/or lower limbs in an asymmetric fashion. An anomalous attachment of the tongue is a commonly associated finding. The mandible is hypoplastic with resultant oligodontia or hypodontia; the oral aperture can be very small, complicating feeding. Disordered or anomalous vasculature, demonstrable on arteriography, can complicate surgery. In addition to the characteristic transverse limb defects, combinations of ectrodactyly, syndactyly, and hypodactyly also occur. Stature and intelligence generally appear unaffected. Other defects include abnormalities of the temporal bone and auditory apparatus, leading to deafness; cleft palate; bowel atresia; cranial nerve palsies; colobomatous microphthalmia; and brain defects.

ETIOLOGY/EPIDEMIOLOGY: No established prevalence figures are available for the condition; milder phenotypes may go undiagnosed. Both sexes are affected. The etiology is in dispute. The evidence seems to point to a nongenetic cause with a low risk of recurrence.

DIAGNOSIS: The diagnosis is a clinical one. A prerequisite is hypoplasia/agenesis of the tongue with resultant limitation of movement.

TREATMENT
Standard Therapies: Feeding may be severely compromised and tube feeding or gastrostomy may be required. Surgical intervention to aid ambulation and improve hand function may be indicated. Dental surgery may also improve oral function and cosmesis. Supportive therapy is the keystone to management. Occupational therapy and speech and language therapy may be required. Attainment of intelligible speech and full oral feeding is possible.

REFERENCES
Kaplan P, Cummings C, Fraser FC. A "community" of face-limb malformation syndromes. *J Pediatr* 1976;89:241.
Lipson AH, Webster WS. Transverse limb deficiency, oromandibular limb hypogenesis sequences, and chorionic villus biopsy. Human and animal experimental evidence for a uterine vascular pathogenesis. *Am J Med Genet* 1993;47:1141.

RESOURCES
60, 96, 160

71   Progressive Osseous Heteroplasia

Eileen M. Shore, PhD, and Frederick S. Kaplan, MD

DEFINITION: Progressive osseous heteroplasia (POH) is a disabling autosomal-dominant disorder characterized by dermal ossification during infancy and progressive heterotopic ossification of subcutaneous fat, skeletal muscle, and deep connective tissue.

DIFFERENTIAL DIAGNOSIS: Fibrodysplasia ossificans progressiva (FOP); Albright hereditary osteodystrophy (AHO).

SYMPTOMS AND SIGNS: The first sign occurs during infancy with the appearance of islands of heterotopic bone in the dermis. Over time, the islands of heterotopic bone coalesce into plaques with subsequent involvement of subcutaneous fat, skeletal muscle, and deep connective tissue. Extensive ossification of the deep connective tissues results in ankylosis of affected joints and focal growth retardation of involved limbs. Spicules of dermal bone may protrude through the epidermis, although bone formation does not originate in the epidermis.

ETIOLOGY/EPIDEMIOLOGY: The disorder may be sporadic or familial. Offspring of affected individuals inherit the disease in an autosomal-dominant manner with widely variable expression. Males and females are affected equally. Occasional reports of mild heterotopic ossification in AHO, and a report of two AHO patients with atypically extensive heterotopic ossification, suggest a common genetic basis for POH and AHO. AHO, a complex disorder characterized by developmental dysmorphologies and commonly associated with multiple hormone resistance, is caused by heterozygous inactivating mutations in the *GNAS1* gene, resulting in decreased expression or function of the a subunit of the stimulatory G protein ($G_s\alpha$) of adenylyl cyclase. Paternally inherited heterozygous inactivating mutations of the *GNAS1* gene have been reported as a cause of POH. These observations suggest that POH may lie at one end of a clinical spectrum of ossification disorders mediated by abnormalities in *GNAS1* expression and impaired activation of adenylyl cyclase.

DIAGNOSIS: POH can be distinguished from FOP by the presence of cutaneous ossification, the absence of congenital malformations of the skeleton, the absence of inflammatory tumorlike swellings, the asymmetric mosaic distribution of lesions, the absence of predictable regional patterns of heterotopic ossification, and the predominance of intramembranous rather than endochondral ossification. It can be distinguished from AHO by the progression of heterotopic ossification from skin and subcutaneous tissue into skeletal muscle, the presence of normal endocrine function, and the absence of a distinctive habitus associated with AHO. The results of routine laboratory studies in POH are usually normal, although elevated levels of serum alkaline phosphatase have been observed. Typically, serum levels of calcium, inorganic phosphate, parathyroid hormone, and vitamin D metabolites are normal. Elevated serum levels of lactate dehydrogenase and creatine phosphokinase have been observed and may reflect bone deposition in skin and skeletal muscle.

TREATMENT

Standard Therapies: No effective treatments or preventions exist for POH. Areas of well-circumscribed heterotopic ossification may rarely be removed successfully; surgical removal of POH tissue has led to recurrence in most patients.

REFERENCES
Kaplan FS, Craver R, MacEwen GD, et al. Progressive osseous heteroplasia: a distinct developmental disorder of heterotopic ossification. *J Bone Joint Surg [Am]* 1994;76:425–436.

Kaplan FS, Shore EM. Progressive osseous heteroplasia. *J Bone Miner Res* 2000;15:2084–2094.

Rosenfeld SR, Kaplan FS. Progressive osseous heteroplasia in male patients. *Clin Orthop Rel Res* 1995;317:243–245.

Shore EM, Ahn J, Jan de Beur S, et al. Paternally inherited inactivating mutations of the *GNAS1* gene in progressive osseous heteroplasia. *N Engl J Med* 2002;346:99–106.

Urtizberea JA, Testart H, Cartault F, et al. Progressive osseous heteroplasia. *J Bone Joint Surg [Br]* 1998;80:768–771.

RESOURCES
351, 405

---

72 Hyperostosis Corticalis Generalisata (van Buchem Disease)

John M. Hicks, MD, DDS, PhD, and Wendy Ballemans

DEFINITION: Hyperostosis corticalis generalisata is an osteosclerotic disease involving the skull, mandible, clavicles, ribs, and diaphyses of long bones.

SYNONYMS: van Buchem disease; Hyperphosphatemia tarda; Endosteal hyperostosis; Bone dystrophy; Generalized leontiasis ossea.

DIFFERENTIAL DIAGNOSIS: Hyperostosis corticalis generalista, benign form of Worth, with torus palatinus; Osteopetrosis, recessive form; Hyperostosis interna; Osteosclerosis, autosomal dominant; Hyperostosis cranialis interna; Craniodiaphyseal dysplasia; Sclerosteosis.

SYMPTOMS AND SIGNS: The characteristic findings are cranial hyperostosis; optic atrophy from cranial nerve compression; hearing loss; headaches; cranial nerve palsy; and osteosclerosis of long bones, cranium, mandible, clavicles, and ribs on radiographic examination. The signs and symptoms usually begin during adolescence, with striking hyperostosis of the cranium and mandible. In most affected individuals, this results in facial paralysis, optic atrophy, and hearing loss due to compression of the cranial nerves. This disease may have an onset in early childhood.

Microscopic examination of bone shows preservation of the lamellar structures with bone hypertrophy. The bone is qualitatively normal and does not have features of metabolic bone disease or bone dysplasia.

ETIOLOGY/EPIDEMIOLOGY: This disease has an autosomal-recessive inheritance pattern. Molecular studies have identified a region on the long arm of chromosome 17—the van Buchem disease gene region (chromosome 17q11.2). This region is the locus for the thyroid hormone receptor alpha-1 gene. Because thyroid hormones stimulate bone resorption, this gene may be altered in van Buchem disease and result in failure to induce appropriate bone resorption. This gene may be intimately involved in the etiology, pathogenesis, and progression of the disease.

DIAGNOSIS: Clinical and radiologic findings provide support for the diagnosis. Laboratory studies show serum hyperphosphatemia. Molecular studies for alterations in the chromosome 17q11.2 region may help to confirm the diagnosis.

TREATMENT
Standard Therapies: Surgery is necessary to relieve intracranial pressure, to decompress cranial nerves, to correct bone deformities, and for aesthetic considerations.

REFERENCES
Balemans W, van den Ende J, Paes-Alves A, et al. Localization of the gene for osteosclerosis to the van Buchem disease-gene region on chromosome 17q12-q21. *Am J Hum Genet* 1999; 64:1661–1669.
Cook J, Phelps P, Chandy J. van Buchem's disease with classical radiological features and appearances on cranial computed tomography. *Br J Radiol* 1989;62:74–77.
Schendel SA. van Buchem disease: surgical treatment of the mandible. *Ann Plast Surg* 1988;20:462–467.
Scopelliti D, Orsini R, Ventucci E, et al. van Buchem disease. Maxillofacial changes, diagnostic classification and general principles of treatment. *Minerva Stomatol* 1999;48:227–234.
Van Buchem F, Hadders J, Hansen J, et al. Hyperostosis corticalis generalisata: report of seven cases. *Am J Med* 1962;33:387–397.
Van Hul W, Balemans W, Van Hul E, et al. van Buchem disease (hyperostosis corticalis generalisata) maps to chromosome 17q12.-21. *Am J Hum Genet* 1998;62:391–399.

RESOURCES
351, 355, 371

73 Ivemark Syndrome

*Scott H. Britz-Cunningham, MD, PhD,
Leonard L. Bailey, MD,
and William H. Fletcher, PhD*

DEFINITION: Ivemark syndrome is a severe subtype of visceroatrial heterotaxia (VAH) in which splenic agenesis is combined with complex, life-threatening heart malformations and laterality defects (situs ambiguous) of most organs. It is best described as a generalized failure to establish normal left/right asymmetry.

SYNONYMS: Asplenia syndrome; Right isomerism sequence.

DIFFERENTIAL DIAGNOSIS: Polysplenia syndrome; Kartagener syndrome; Primary splenic agenesis; Often, but incorrectly, lumped with less severe forms of VAH.

SYMPTOMS AND SIGNS: Cyanosis is moderate to marked at birth. The echocardiogram is usually normal but may show aberrant conduction pathways. Cardiovascular defects may include right atrial isomerism, bilateral sinoatrial nodes, univentricular heart, common atrium, absent coronary sinus, common atrioventricular valve, pulmonic stenosis or atresia, bilateral superior vena cavae, total anomalous pulmonary venous return, transposition of the great arteries, and/or double-outlet right ventricle. Pulmonary defects include right bronchopulmonary isomerism (both lungs trilobed and short epiarterial bronchii). By Ivemark's definition, the spleen must be absent, the liver transverse (midline), the gallbladder is on the left, and the bowel is malrotated with a left-sided cecum. Lacking a spleen, patients may be prone to sepsis.

ETIOLOGY/EPIDEMIOLOGY: Ivemark syndrome is clearly multigenetic in origin, but maternal or environmental factors may also contribute. Many genes have been described that are involved in left/right axis formation. Somatic mutations of the *connexin43* gap junction gene have been found in heart tissue from 17 children: 11 with Ivemark, 5 with polysplenia, and 1 with no defined syndrome. Family members have no *connexin43* defects.

DIAGNOSIS: Fetal ultrasonography may provide the earliest detection of heart defects, asplenia, and other abnormalities of laterality. Fetal echocardiography can provide a definitive diagnosis as early as 20–24 weeks of gestation. The child's appearance at birth, along with echocardiography, clarify cardiovascular problems. Howell-Jolly bodies in blood specimens are common due to absence of the spleen.

TREATMENT

Standard Therapies: Surgical intervention is palliative. The distressed newborn whose pulmonary circulation is ductus dependent is temporarily maintained by an infusion of prostaglandin E1 until a modified Blalock-Taussig shunt is completed. When anomalous pulmonary venous connection is present, repair is accomplished in early infancy. The second intervention involves takedown of the modified Blalock-Taussig shunt, which is replaced with bilateral, bidirectional superior cavopulmonary shunts. The final intervention is a lateral tunnel Fontan procedure (inferior vena cava and hepatic veins diverted directly to the pulmonary artery). This effectively separates the pulmonary and systemic circulations and abolishes the infant's cyanosis. If the infant's cardiovascular pathophysiology and/or anatomy preclude conventional surgical palliation, cardiac transplantation provides the only other means for survival and would be the primary procedure of choice if donor hearts were readily available.

REFERENCES

Britz-Cunningham SH, Shah M, Zuppan CW, et al. Mutations of the *connexin43* gap junction gene in patients with heart malformations and defects of laterality. *N Engl J Med* 1995;332: 1323–1329.

Ivemark BI. Implications of agenesis of the spleen on the pathogenesis of cono truncus anomalies in childhood: an analysis of the heart malformations in the splenic agenesis syndrome, with fourteen new cases. *Acta Paediatr (Uppsala)* 1955;44 (suppl 104):1–110.

Levin M, Johnson RL, Stern CD, et al. A molecular pathway determining left-right asymmetry in chick embryogenesis. *Cell* 1995;82:803–814.

Oh SP, Li E. The signaling pathway mediated by the type IIB activin receptor controls axial patterning and lateral asymmetry in the mouse. *Genes Dev* 1997;11:1812–1826.

RESOURCE

217

---

74   Jansen Metaphyseal Chondrodysplasia

Ernestina Schipani, MD, PhD

DEFINITION: Jansen metaphyseal chondrodysplasia is an autosomal-dominant disorder characterized by short limb dwarfism secondary to severe abnormalities of the growth plate, and hypercalcemia, despite normal blood concentrations of parathyroid hormone (PTH) and PTH-related peptide (PTHrP).

SYNONYMS: Jansen disease; Jansen dysostosis.

DIFFERENTIAL DIAGNOSIS: Rickets; Achondroplasia.

SYMPTOMS AND SIGNS: Clinical, radiologic, and biochemical abnormalities may be present at birth, but often the disease becomes manifest only within the first 2 years of life. Clinical findings include severe short stature, disproportionately short limbs, and micrognathia. The radiologic features during infancy are partially suggestive of rickets: the metaphyseal ends are wide, cupped, and ragged. However, metacarpals and metatarsals are also involved; thickness of the calvarial bones is increased and the base of the skull is sclerotic, which may lead to cranial nerve compression. During childhood the radiologic findings in almost all long bones show irregular patches of partially calcified cartilage that protrudes into the diaphyses. These abnormalities resolve later in life, resulting in extreme short stature. The increase in trabecular bone, the loss of cortical thickness, and subperiosteal bone resorption appear to be similar to the findings in hyperparathyroidism. The bone and growth plate abnormalities are associated with severe and asymptomatic hypercalcemia, hypophosphatemia, decreased tubular reabsorption of phosphate, increased urinary excretion of cAMP, and elevated circulating levels of $1,25\text{-}(OH)_2$ vitamin D, and normal or undetectable concentrations of PTH and PTHrP. Bone remodeling is increased in affected patients.

ETIOLOGY/EPIDEMIOLOGY: Jansen metaphyseal chondrodysplasia is an autosomal-dominant disorder caused by activating mutations in the PTH/PTHrP receptor gene, located on chromosome 3p21.1. Most cases are sporadic; the disease affects various ethnic groups.

DIAGNOSIS: The diagnosis should be suspected based on short-limbed dwarfism, PTH-independent hypercalcemia, characteristic radiologic changes, and often, nephrocalcinosis.

TREATMENT
Standard Therapies: No therapy is available.

Investigational Therapies: Treatment with bisphosphonates is being explored.

REFERENCES
Charrow J, Poznanski AK. The Jansen type of metaphyseal chondrodysplasia: conformation of dominant inheritance and review of radiographic manifestations in the newborn and adult. *J Med Genet* 1984;18:321–327.

Frame B, Poznanski AK. Conditions that may be confused with rickets. In: DeLuca HF, Anast CS, eds. *Pediatric diseases related to calcium.* New York: Elsevier, 1980:269–289.

Parfitt AM, Schipani E, Rao DS, et al. Hypercalcemia due to constitutive activity of the PTH/PTHrP receptor. *J Clin Endocrinol Metab* 1996;81:3584–3588.

Schipani E, Langman CB, Parfitt AM, et al. Constitutively activated receptors for parathyroid hormone and parathyroid hormone–related peptide in Jansen's metaphyseal chondrodysplasia. *N Engl J Med* 1996;335:708–714.

Silverthorn KGHC, Duncan BP. Murk Jansen's metaphyseal chondrodysplasia with long-term follow-up. *Pediatr Radiol* 1983; 17:119–123.

RESOURCES
188, 246, 351

---

75   Jarcho-Levin Syndrome

Robert M. Campbell, Jr., MD

DEFINITION: Jarcho-Levin syndrome is characterized by severe foreshortening of the chest due to congenital thoracic vertebral and rib malformations with associated deformities of the face, head, and extremities.

SYNONYMS: For classic Jarcho-Levin syndrome: Spondylothoracic dysostosis. For Jarcho-Levin syndrome type II: Spondylocostal dysostosis; Spondylothoracic dysostosis; Spondylocostal dysplasia; Spondylothoracic dysplasia; Occipital-facial-cervical-thoracic-abdominal-digital dysplasia.

DIFFERENTIAL DIAGNOSIS: Thanatophoric dysplasia.

SYMPTOMS AND SIGNS: Classic Jarcho-Levin syndrome is characterized by cranial facial abnormalities, including prominent occiput, low hairline, wide nasal bridge, anteverted nares, and upward-slanted eyelids. Syndactyly and camptodactyly are commonly seen, as is a protuberant abdomen. Caudal dysgenesis occurs in 90% of patients, and central nervous system abnormalities in 50%. The thorax is extremely shortened but barrel shaped and stiff, and has a fan- or crab-shaped configuration on radiography without intrinsic rib abnormalities. The spine is lordotic in many patients, with infrequent scoliosis. Spina bifida is present in 25% of patients; congenital diaphragmatic hernia is seen in 30%. Congenital heart disease is infrequent. Approximately 81% of patients die in infancy from respiratory insufficiency. Jarcho-Levin syndrome type II is characterized by less marked thoracic deformation and hemivertebra of the thoracic spine. Congenital heart disease, renal abnormalities, urogenital abnormalities, polydactyly, and tracheal and esophageal fistulas can be seen. Radiographic studies show intrinsic changes in the ribs such as broadening and fusion, and combinations of rib absence and fused chest wall. Central nervous system abnormalities are seen in 19% of patients, and 56% have caudal dysgenesis. Some patients have died in infancy, but most survive long-term.

ETIOLOGY/EPIDEMIOLOGY: The inheritance of classic Jarcho-Levin syndrome is autosomal recessive. The gene responsible is found on chromosome 19q13. Type II is seen mostly with autosomal-dominant inheritance, but with some mild recessive inheritance. Males and females are affected equally. Most cases have occurred in children of Puerto Rican descent.

TREATMENT
Standard Therapies: There is no standard treatment.

Investigational Therapies: One patient with classic Jarcho-Levin syndrome was treated with rib osteotomies for clustered ribs with a polypropylene mesh/methylmethacrylate chest wall prosthesis for associated rib defect. There was improvement in respiratory insufficiency, but rib refusion and scoliosis due to a fixed dimension chest wall prosthesis required reoperation.

The implantation of expandable prosthetic ribs in children with disorders involving malformed rib cages due to absent or fused ribs, as well as hypoplastic thorax, is being explored.

REFERENCES

Ayme S, Treus M. Spondylocostal/spondylothoracic dysostosis: the clinical basis for prognosticating and genetic counseling. *Am J Med Genet* 1986;24:599–606.

Martinez-Frias M-L, et al. Severe spondylocostal dysostosis associated with other congenital anomalies: a clinical/epidemio-logical analysis and description of ten cases from the Spanish Registry. *Am J Med Genet* 1994;51:203–212.

McCall CP, et al. Jarcho-Levin syndrome: unusual survival in a classical case. *Am J Med Genet* 1994;49:328–332.

Roberts AP, et al. Spondylothoracic and spondylocostal dysostosis, hereditary forms of spinal deformity. *J Bone Joint Surg [Br]* 1988;70:123–126.

Turnpenny PD. A gene for autosomal recessive spondylocostal dysostosis maps to 19 Q 13.1-Q 13.3. *Am J Hum Genet* 1999; 65:175–182.

RESOURCES

351, 418

---

76   Johanson-Blizzard Syndrome

*Chandra Prakash, MD,
and Ray E. Clouse, MD*

DEFINITION: Johanson-Blizzard syndrome is an autosomal-recessive disorder characterized by pancreatic hypoplasia, orofacial malformations, and other associated congenital defects. The most distinctive features of the syndrome are a small, beaklike nose with aplasia or hypoplasia of the alae nasae, dental abnormalities, sensorineural deafness, and pancreatic insufficiency with severe malabsorption and growth retardation.

DIFFERENTIAL DIAGNOSIS: Cystic fibrosis; Schwachman syndrome; Pancreatic agenesis; Down syndrome; Klinefelter syndrome.

SYMPTOMS AND SIGNS: The disorder usually is diagnosed in infancy from the characteristic facial appearance and growth retardation. A small, beaklike nose with aplastic or hypoplastic alae nasi is the hallmark orofacial anomaly. Other features include a mouth with downturned corners, a long and narrow upper lip, an everted lower lip, a small and pointed chin, and sparse hair with an abnormal frontal upsweep. The deciduous teeth are small and often carious, and permanent teeth are absent. Profound sensorineural deafness is characteristic. Growth retardation typically starts in the intrauterine period and continues throughout childhood. Pancreatic hypoplasia with resultant exocrine insufficiency, malabsorption, and profound steatorrhea is largely responsible. Diabetes mellitus is a later outcome. Associated but less consistent features include hypothyroidism, congenital heart disease, imperforate anus with dilated distal colon, genitourinary anom-alies (including clitoromegaly, bicornuate uterus, septate vagina, micropenis, and cryptorchidism), and abnormal nipples. Intelligence varies considerably. Mental retardation is common, although high intelligence has been reported.

ETIOLOGY/EPIDEMIOLOGY: More than 30 cases have been reported. The disorder is inherited as an autosomal-recessive trait without gender predilection. A singular inherited defect responsible for the manifestations has not been described. Loss of pancreatic acinar tissue is evident and, along with a primary acinar cell defect, appears responsible for exocrine insufficiency; fatty replacement of the gland and ultimate loss of endocrine function occur in patients surviving childhood.

DIAGNOSIS: Prenatal ultrasonographic features include severe intrauterine growth retardation, beaklike nose, and dilated sigmoid colon from anal atresia. After birth, profound steatorrhea and growth retardation in conjunction with the typical facial features allow a clinical diagnosis. Subjective hearing tests and auditory evoked brainstem potentials confirm associated hearing loss. CT of the abdomen can demonstrate fatty replacement of the pancreas.

TREATMENT

Standard Therapies: The mainstay of treatment is pancreatic enzyme replacement and management of pancreatic exocrine insufficiency. Correcting malabsorption can arrest or reverse growth retardation and prevent early death. Diabetes mellitus requires insulin management. Hypothyroidism should be treated with thyroid hormone supplementation. Anal atresia requires early surgical intervention. The more severe facial anomalies have been corrected surgically, using a freely vascularized iliac bone graft and osteotomy to adjust the shape of the orbit and elongate the hypoplastic maxilla.

REFERENCES

Auslander R, Nevo O, Diukman R, et al. Johanson-Blizzard syndrome: a prenatal ultrasonographic diagnosis. *Ultrasound Obstet Gynecol* 1999;13:450–452.

Gershoni-Baruch R, Lerner A, Braun J, et al. Johanson-Blizzard syndrome: clinical spectrum and further delineation of the syndrome. *Am J Med Genet* 1990;35:546–551.

Jones NL, Hofley PM, Durie PR. Pathophysiology of the pancreatic defect in Johanson-Blizzard syndrome: a disorder of acinar development. *J Pediatr* 1994;125:406–408.

Steinbach WJ, Hintz RL. Diabetes mellitus and profound insulin resistance in Johanson-Blizzard syndrome. *J Pediatr Endocrinol Metab* 2000;13:1633–1636.

Trellis DR, Clouse RE. Johanson-Blizzard syndrome. Progression of pancreatic involvement to adulthood. *Dig Dis Sci* 1991;36: 365–369.

RESOURCES

253, 354, 363

77 Kabuki Make-Up Syndrome

Ivan F.M. Lo, MB, ChB, MRCP(UK), FHKAM, and Stephen T.S. Lam, MBBS, FRCP, FHKAM

DEFINITION: Kabuki make-up syndrome (KMS) is a multiple congenital anomalies/mental retardation syndrome defined by five cardinal manifestations: characteristic craniofacial dysmorphic features, short stature, mental retardation, skeletal abnormalities, and dermatoglyphic abnormalities.

SYNONYMS: Kabuki syndrome; Niikawa-Kuroki syndrome.

DIFFERENTIAL DIAGNOSIS: Turner syndrome; Robinow syndrome.

SYMPTOMS AND SIGNS: Patients typically do not present until they are found to have stunted growth and global delay in development. Some patients may present earlier in infancy with congenital heart defects. The most telltale signs are the craniofacial dysmorphic features, which are often not notable until the child is several years of age, including high arching eyebrows with lateral flaring, long palpebral fissures with eversion of the lateral third of the lower eyelids, short nasal septum, and prominent ears. These facial features are reminiscent of the actor's make-up in the Kabuki opera of Japan, hence the name of the syndrome. Other features often present are highly arched or cleft palate, brachydactyly, bilateral clinodactyly of fifth fingers, and persistent fetal finger pads. Most but not all patients have variable degrees of proportionate short stature.

Mental retardation is usually of mild to moderate grade. Dermatoglyphic abnormalities are nonspecific and include excessive ulnar loops, absent digital triradius c or d, and hypothenar loops. Skeletal abnormalities include mainly minor vertebral defects and a short middle phalanx of the little fingers. Scoliosis is present in nearly half of all patients. Urinary tract malformations are present in 12% of patients.

ETIOLOGY/EPIDEMIOLOGY: The disorder has an estimated prevalence of 1 in 30,000 to 1 in 60,000 in school-aged children. Although the name of the syndrome implies a Japanese origin, the disease has been widely reported in different ethnic groups. There is no predilection for either sex. Most cases are sporadic; however, familial cases have also been described, and all suggested autosomal-dominant inheritance. The cause is unknown. Chromosomal abnormalities involving chromosomes 1p, 4p, 6q, 12q, 13, 15q, 17q, X, and Y have been reported in patients with KMS, but the gene locus is unknown.

DIAGNOSIS: Diagnosis is made primarily on clinical grounds, but no generally agreed-on diagnostic criteria exist. Although all five cardinal manifestations are not needed to make the diagnosis, it is not convincing if the Kabuki face is not present. Chromosome analysis is essential, because some patients with Turner syndrome, those with a ring X or ring Y chromosome in particular, share features of Kabuki face, short stature, and mental retardation. Getting a readable handprint for dermatoglyphic examination can be difficult, especially when the patient cannot cooperate. One can examine the palms carefully with a magnifying glass under bright light. The minor skeletal abnormalities can be seen only on a radiographic survey of the whole skeleton. Echocardiography and ultrasonography of the kidneys should be offered routinely.

TREATMENT

Standard Therapies: Treatment is supportive. Congenital heart defects should be managed with drugs and/or surgery if necessary. Developmental problems should be addressed early on with appropriate physical, occupational, and language therapy. Physicians should be mindful of the common complications of otitis media, congenital hip dislocation, scoliosis, and precocious puberty in female patients.

REFERENCES

Lo IFM, Cheung LYK, Ng AYY. Interstitial dup(1p) with findings of Kabuki make-up syndrome. *Am J Med Genet* 1998;78: 55–57.

McGinniss MJ, Brown DH, Burke LW. Ring chromosome X in a child with manifestations of Kabuki syndrome. *Am J Med Genet* 1997;70:37–42.

Niikawa N, Kuroki Y, Kajii T. Kabuki make-up (Niikawa-Kuroki) syndrome: a study of 62 patients. *Am J Med Genet* 1988;31: 565–589.

RESOURCE

222

---

78   KBG Syndrome

Paul A. Dowling, BDentSc, DOrth, MDentSc, MOrth, FDS(Orth), P. Fleming, BDentSc, FDS, FFD, MSc, and Robert J. Gorlin, DDS, MS, DSc(Athens)

DEFINITION: The KBG syndrome is an autosomal-dominant condition characterized by short stature, mild developmental delay, craniofacial dysmorphism, and characteristic dental and skeletal features.

DIFFERENTIAL DIAGNOSIS: Aarskog syndrome; Noonan syndrome.

SYMPTOMS AND SIGNS: The cardinal features are mild developmental delay, short stature, characteristic facies, and characteristic dental anomalies. The face is round with prominent arched and broad eyebrows, telecanthus, flat philtrum, and a bow-shaped upper lip. The skeletal anomalies may include cervical ribs, short femoral vertebrae, and delayed bone age. The dental anomalies include macrodontia of the permanent incisors and hypodontia. Macrodontia is one of the most consistent features of the syndrome. The association of developmental delay and macrodontia of the maxillary central incisors has not been documented in any other syndrome. Dermatoglyphic findings consist of a single palmar crease and distal axial triradius.

ETIOLOGY/EPIDEMIOLOGY: Both familial cases and sporadic occurrences have been reported. The pattern of inheritance is believed to be autosomal dominant with variable expressivity, particularly with regard to developmental delay. In the reported cases, there is a male-to-female predominance.

DIAGNOSIS: Once the maxillary permanent central incisors erupt, the characteristic appearance of the macrodont teeth in association with short stature and developmental delay facilitates the diagnosis. Accurate diagnosis is important for genetic counseling.

TREATMENT

Standard Therapies: Standard therapies include investigation for developmental delay and appropriate supportive therapy. Orthodontic opinion and management should be sought on eruption of macrodont teeth.

REFERENCES

Devriendt K, Holvoet M, Fryns JP. Further delineation of the KBG syndrome. *Genet Couns* 1998;9:191–194.

Dowling PA, Fleming P, Gorlin RJ, et al. The KBG syndrome, characteristic dental findings: a case report. *Int J Paediatr Dent* 2001;11:131–134.

Fryns JP, Haspeslagh M. Mental retardation, short stature, minor skeletal anomalies, craniofacial dysmorphism and macrodontia in two sisters and their mother. Another variant example of the KBG syndrome? *Clin Genet* 1984;26:69–72.

Herrmann J, Pallister PD, Tiddy W, et al. The KBG syndrome: a syndrome of short stature, characteristic facies, mental retardation, macrodontia and skeletal anomalies. *Birth Defects* 1975;11:7–18.

Parloir C, Fryns JP, Deroover J, et al. Short stature, craniofacial dysmorphism and dento-skeletal abnormalities in a large kindred. A variant of K.B.G. syndrome or a new mental retardation syndrome. *Clin Genet* 1977;12:263–266.

RESOURCES

351, 363, 377

79 Kenny-Caffey Syndrome

George A. Diaz, MD, PhD

DEFINITION: Kenny-Caffey syndrome (KCS) causes short stature and hypoparathyroidism. Additional features include cortical thickening of the long bones, patent anterior fontanel, hypermetropia, and microorchidism. An autosomal-recessive variant has been described in which patients have mental retardation and may have immune deficits.

SYNONYMS: Kenny syndrome. For the recessive form: Sanjad-Sakati syndrome; HRD (hypoparathyroidism, retardation, dysmorphism).

DIFFERENTIAL DIAGNOSIS: Albright hereditary osteodystrophy.

SYMPTOMS AND SIGNS: The triad of hypoparathyroidism, short stature, and medullary stenosis of the long bones is characteristic. Growth retardation may be intrauterine or postnatal; thus, evaluation for skeletal dysplasia may be delayed until growth failure becomes apparent. As a result, patients may come to attention secondary to manifestations of hypocalcemia in the neonatal period. Hypocalcemia may be transient or may not manifest until periods of metabolic stress (i.e., postoperative period, infection). In addition, patients generally have ocular malformations, typically microphthalmos, and males may have microorchidism or cryptorchidism. Patients with the typical sporadic or dominantly inherited form are generally of normal intelligence, whereas those with the recessive form usually have significant developmental delay. Three patients are reported to have developed diabetes mellitus in adulthood or adolescence, suggesting that this may be a later-onset feature.

ETIOLOGY/EPIDEMIOLOGY: Incidence is unknown. The condition can occur sporadically or can be inherited in a dominant or recessive fashion. Males and females are affected, but male-to-male transmission has not been documented. Sporadic and dominant cases have been reported in multiple ethnic groups. The recessive form has been described mostly in Arab populations and has been linkage mapped to chromosome 1q43. The genetic basis for both forms is unknown.

DIAGNOSIS: Key diagnostic features include growth retardation of prenatal or postnatal onset, hypoparathyroidism, cortical thickening of the long bones and/or hyperostosis of the calvarium, and ocular abnormalities. Ophthalmologic evaluation should be performed to document these.

TREATMENT

Standard Therapies: No specific therapies exist. Hypocalcemia is treated with vitamin D and calcium supplementation. Ocular abnormalities generally require corrective lenses. Patients with the recessive form may be susceptible to recurrent bacterial infections and should be monitored with heightened vigilance.

REFERENCES

Caffey J. Congenital stenosis of medullary spaces in tubular bones and calvaria in two proportionate dwarfs—mother and son; coupled with transitory hypocalcemia. *AJR* 1967;100:1–11.

Diaz GA, Khan KTS, Gelb BD. The autosomal recessive Kenny-Caffey syndrome maps to 1q42-q43. *Genomics* 1998;54:13–18.

Kenny FM, Linarelli L. Dwarfism and cortical thickening of tubular bones. *Am J Dis Child* 1966;111:201–207.

Khan KTS, Uma R, Usha R, et al. Kenny-Caffey syndrome in six Bedouin sibships: autosomal recessive inheritance is confirmed. *Am J Med Genet* 1997;69:126–132.

Majewski F, Rosendahl W, Ranke M, et al. The Kenny syndrome, a rare type of growth deficiency with tubular stenosis, transient hypoparathyroidism and anomalies of refraction. *Eur J Pediatr* 1981;136:21–30.

RESOURCES

188, 191

80   Klippel-Trenaunay Syndrome

David J. Driscoll, MD

DEFINITION: Klippel-Trenaunay syndrome (KTS) consists of the triad of cutaneous capillary vascular malformations, bone and soft tissue hypertrophy, and venous varicosities.

SYNONYM: Klippel-Trenaunay-Weber syndrome.

DIFFERENTIAL DIAGNOSIS: Parkes-Weber syndrome; Proteus syndrome; Lymphedema; Servelle-Martorell syndrome; Sturge-Weber syndrome.

SYMPTOMS AND SIGNS: The venous involvement in KTS can range from subtle abnormalities to massive varicosities and absence of important deep venous structures. The venous abnormalities usually involve the affected extremity and are apparent as superficial varicose veins. Dilatation of superficial varicose veins may not be apparent in infancy but becomes so with increasing age. Not all patients have superficial venous varicosities. In at least 20% of patients, abnormal venous malformations can involve pelvic or abdominal organs. Many patients have abnormalities of the lymphatic system. A broad spectrum of cutaneous manifestations of KTS exists, most commonly a port-wine stain, which can be light in color to deep maroon, and can be flat or elevated. Other cutaneous manifestations include phlebectasias, hyperhidrosis, lymphangioma circumscripta, angiokeratoma circumscripta, hyperthermia, and hypertrichosis. Patients are prone to cellulitis. In one series, 95 of 144 patients had one extremity longer than the other, and 100 of 144 patients had a swollen or circumferentially enlarged extremity. Most commonly a lower extremity is affected, but in 25% of patients an upper extremity is involved. In addition to bony hypertrophy, many patients have soft tissue hypertrophy, which is usually fatty and contains variable amounts of venous structures. Other limb findings include syndactyly, clinodactyly, polydactyly, split-hand deformity, metatarsal and phalangeal agenesis, osteolysis, congenital dislocation of the hip, and peripheral neuropathy.

ETIOLOGY/EPIDEMIOLOGY: The disorder occurs in 1 of 20,000 to 40,000 live births. It affects males and females equally. The cause is unknown.

DIAGNOSIS: The diagnosis is made by clinical examination. Because expression of the condition is variable and covers a broad spectrum, the appropriate tests must be individualized.

TREATMENT

Standard Therapies: Appropriate treatment must be individualized. Most patients with lower extremity involvement experience some degree of lower extremity edema. Compression therapy is helpful in controlling swelling and may slow the progression of lower extremity varicose veins. Unsightly or painful superficial varicose veins can be removed in selected patients. Epiphysiodeses are done to assure relatively equal leg lengths at full maturation. This procedure is necessary only if the projected limb length discrepancy exceeds 2.0 cm. Amputation of digits and portions of an extremity should only be undertaken to improve function of the extremity and to manage otherwise uncontrollable infection or bleeding. The potential complications of such debulking procedures should be considered carefully. Laser therapy can be used to reduce the discoloration of capillary hemangiomas and to treat superficial venular blebs.

REFERENCES

Gloviczki P, Stanson A, Stickler G, et al. Klippel Trenaunay syndrome: the risks and benefits of vascular interventions. *Surgery* 1991;110:469–479.

Jacob A, Driscoll D, Shaugnessy W, et al. Klippel Trenaunay syndrome: its spectrum and management. *Mayo Clinic Proc* 1998;73:28–36.

McGrory, Amadio PC. Klippel Trenaunay syndrome: orthopedic considerations. *Orthop Rev* 1993;22:41–50.

Samuel M, Spitz L. Klippel-Trenaunay syndrome: clinical features, complications and management in children. *Br J Surg* 1995;82:757–761.

Stickler G. Klippel Trenaunay syndrome. In: Gomez M, ed. *Neurocutaneous diseases: a practical approach.* Boston: Butterworths, 1987.

RESOURCES

226, 368, 450

81 | Kniest Dysplasia: A Type II Collagenopathy

John M. Hicks, MD, DDS, PhD

DEFINITION: Kniest dysplasia is an autosomal-dominant chondrodysplasia with characteristic clinical and radiographic features and a defining mutation in the type II collagen gene.

SYNONYMS: Metatropic dwarfism type II; Metatropic dysplasia type II; Type II collagenopathy.

DIFFERENTIAL DIAGNOSIS: Achondrogenesis type II; Hypochondrogenesis; Spondylepimetaphyseal dysplasia congenital; Late-onset spondylepimetaphyseal dysplasia; Stickler dysplasia; Goldblatt syndrome; Campomelic dwarfism; Achondroplasia; Hypochondroplasia; Classic metatropic dwarfism (autosomal recessive); SADDAN dysplasia.

SYMPTOMS AND SIGNS: Kniest dysplasia is characterized phenotypically by disproportionate dwarfism with short trunk, small pelvis, and short limbs; prominent joints with decreased mobility; kyphoscoliosis; premature osteoarthritis; inability to form a fist; violaceous hue to skin of palms; midface hypoplasia; cleft palate; downturned mouth; skull asymmetry; sensorineural hearing loss; retinal detachment with early-onset myopia and glaucoma leading to blindness; shallow supraorbital ridges; prominent eyes; flat face; and respiratory distress and feeding difficulties due to tracheomalacia. Radiographic features include dumbbell-shaped femora; platyspondylia with anterior wedging of vertebral bodies; thoracic vertebra with coronal clefts; low broad ilia; osteoarthritis; and short tubular bones with broad metaphyses and deformed large epiphyses.

ETIOLOGY/EPIDEMIOLOGY: Kniest dysplasia is an autosomal-dominant osteochondrodysplasia with a mutation in the type II collagen gene located on the long arm of chromosome 12.

DIAGNOSIS: Clinical phenotype and radiologic features help define Kniest dysplasia in the affected neonate and infant. Prenatal diagnosis may be made on ultrasonographic findings of disproportionate dwarfism with short trunk, small pelvis, and short limbs. Molecular analysis of amniotic fluid and/or chorionic villus samples for mutations in the *COL2A1* gene confirms the clinical and radiographic impression.

TREATMENT
Standard Therapies: Treatment is medical and surgical intervention for symptomatic relief of complications associated with the effects of defective type II collagen incorporation into cartilage, the inner ear, eye, trachea, and intervertebral discs. During the neonatal period or infancy, tracheotomy may be necessary to relieve respiratory distress and to avoid feeding difficulties associated with tracheomalacia and/or cleft palate.

REFERENCES
Biatner A, Maurer S, Greun MB, DiCesare P. The genetic basis of the osteochondrodysplasias. *J Pediatr Orthop* 2000;20:594–605.

Freisinger P, Bonaventure J, Stoess H, et al. Type II collagenopathies: are there additional family members? *Am J Med Genet* 1996;63:137–143.

Gilbert-Barness E, Langer L Jr, Opitz J, et al. Kniest dysplasia: radiologic, histopathological and scanning electronmicroscopic findings. *Am J Med Genet* 1996;63:34–45.

Hicks J, DeJong A, Barrish J, et al. Tracheomalacia in a neonate with Kniest dysplasia: histopathologic and ultrastructural features. *Ultrastruct Pathol* 2001;25:79–83.

Wilkins D, Artz A, South S, et al. Small deletions in the type II collagen triple helix produce Kniest dysplasia. *Am J Med Genet* 1999;85:105–112.

RESOURCES
188, 227

82   Laband Syndrome

Barbara L. Chadwick, BDS, MScD, PhD, FDSRCS

DEFINITION: Laband syndrome is an inherited disorder characterized by gingival fibromatosis, abnormalities of the nose and/or ears, and absence or hypoplasia of the nails or terminal phalanges of the hands and feet. Other more variable features include hyperextensibility of joints, hepatosplenomegaly, mild hirsutism, mental retardation, and anterior open bite.

SYNONYM: Zimmermann-Laband syndrome.

DIFFERENTIAL DIAGNOSIS: Gingival fibromatosis with hypertichosis; Epilepsy and mental retardation; Murray-Puretic-Drescher syndrome; Rutherford syndrome; Cowden syndrome; Cross syndrome.

SYMPTOMS AND SIGNS: Gingival fibromatosis involves the upper arch in almost all cases, with both papillary and rugose enlargement present. Hypertrophy may result in delayed eruption of teeth. As the patient ages, the enlargement may become unsightly and cover the surfaces of the teeth, making oral hygiene difficult. An anterior open bite has been noted in more than half of reported cases. There are also abnormalities of the face, typically thickened or bulbous nose and/or ears with the lips also affected, although less frequently. As the patient ages, these features become coarser. The terminal phalanges of some or all of the fingers and toes may be hypoplastic or absent, whereas the nails may be normal, hypoplastic, or missing. Hyperextensible joints are another common finding, with spinal abnormalities in some cases. Hepatomegaly is reported in one third of cases, with splenomegaly less common. These changes may be present in the first few months of life, and biopsies have shown fibrous changes within the organs. Hirsutism is less common and may be present from birth but is usually mild and may only affect the eyelashes and eyebrows. Patients may be of normal intelligence or present with mild or profound retardation.

ETIOLOGY/EPIDEMIOLOGY: There are 31 reported cases, 11 of which from two families show clear evidence of autosomal-dominant transmission. However, 2 cases from marriages of first cousins strongly suggest autosomal-recessive inheritance in some families.

DIAGNOSIS: Gingival fibromatosis must be present to make the diagnosis, and all reported cases include bulbous facial features, and toe and/or finger abnormalities, all of which are usually present within the first few months of life. Hepatosplenomegaly, hirsutism, and joint hyperextensibility are more variable features. Although some of these findings are suggestive of a storage disorder, no biochemical defect has been described.

TREATMENT

Standard Therapies: There is no specific treatment. Surgical correction of the gingival fibromatosis is recommended to improve appearance, but no data exist on the long-term results of this therapy. Genetic counseling for sporadic cases has been recommended.

REFERENCES

Chadwick BL, Hunter B, Hunter L, et al. Laband syndrome. Report of two cases, review of the literature, and identification of additional manifestations. *Oral Surg Oral Med Oral Pathol* 1994;78:57–63.

Laband PF, Habib G, Humphreys GS. Hereditary gingival fibromatosis. *Oral Surg Oral Med Oral Pathol* 1964;17:339–351.

Pina Neto JM, Soares LRM, Souza AHO. A new case of Zimmermann-Laband syndrome with mild mental retardation, asymmetry of limbs and hypertrichosis. *Am J Med Genet* 1988;31:691–695.

Zimmermann. Uber Anomalien der Ektoderms. *Vjschr Zahnheilkd* 1928;44:419–434.

RESOURCES

360, 363

83   Laurence-Moon Syndrome

Richard A. Lewis, MD, MS

DEFINITION: Laurence-Moon syndrome is an autosomal-recessive disorder characterized by developmental retardation, obesity, pigmentary retinal dystrophy, and spastic paraplegia, but not polydactylia.

SYNONYM: Laurence-Moon-Bardet-Biedl syndrome.

DIFFERENTIAL DIAGNOSIS: Acrocephalopolysyndactylia; Alstrom syndrome; Bardet-Biedl syndrome; Carpenter syndrome; Cohen syndrome; McKusick-Kaufman syndrome; Prader-Willi syndrome.

SYMPTOMS AND SIGNS: Laurence-Moon syndrome consists of mental retardation, pigmentary retinopathy with severe visual impairment, hypogenitalism, and spastic paraplegia. It was first reported in 1866 in a family with four affected siblings. No reports mention polydactylia in any affected individual, thus distinguishing the disorder nosologically from Bardet-Biedl syndrome. Although hypogenitalism, especially in males, should be notable at birth, slow development, delayed motor milestones and ataxic gait, and night blindness may not be noticed until childhood. The ataxia progresses to paraplegia in adolescence, and affected individuals become bedridden in adulthood.

ETIOLOGY/EPIDEMIOLOGY: Laurence-Moon syndrome is consistent with an autosomal-recessive mode of inheritance and is often confused with the more prevalent Bardet-Biedl syndrome. Population estimates are unknown but are likely less than 1 in 250,000.

DIAGNOSIS: The clinical diagnosis requires the simultaneous concurrence of progressive pigmentary retinopathy, developmental retardation, hypogenitalism, and spastic paraparesis. In some instances, overlap between Laurence-Moon syndrome and Bardet-Biedl syndrome may occur from lack of expressed features.

TREATMENT
Standard Therapies: Visual disabilities should be treated by conventional ophthalmologic assessment of errors of refraction and low vision assistance. Appropriate dietary modification and exercise programs may be helpful in obesity. Learning and speech difficulties should be assessed and managed early. The spastic paraparesis progresses and requires physical therapy and mechanical assistance.

REFERENCES
Bowen P, Ferguson-Smith M, Mosier D, et al. The Laurence-Moon syndrome. Association with hypogonadotrophic hypogonadism and sex-chromosome aneuploidy. *Arch Intern Med* 1965;116:598–604.

Farag TI, Teebi AS. Bardet-Biedl and Laurence-Moon syndromes in a mixed Arab population. *Clin Genet* 1988;33: 78–82.

Laurence JZ, Moon RC. Four cases of retinitis pigmentosa occurring in the same family and accompanied by general imperfection in development. *Ophthalmol Rev* 1866;2:32–41.

McKusick VA, ed. Online Mendelian Inheritance in Man (OMIM) [database online]. Bethesda, MD: National Center for Biotechnology Information, National Library of Medicine; 1994. Entry no. 245800; last update 6/3/94.

Schachat AP, Maumenee IH. The Bardet-Biedl syndromes and related disorders. *Arch Ophthalmol* 1982;100:285–288.

RESOURCES
232, 288, 462

84   Leprechaunism

Nicola Longo, MD, PhD

DEFINITION: Leprechaunism is an inborn error of metabolism caused by a defect in the insulin receptor, which is essential for the stimulation of metabolism and growth.

Milder alterations of the same receptor cause Rabson-Mendenhall syndrome (pineal hyperplasia, insulin-resistant diabetes mellitus, and somatic abnormalities).

SYNONYM: Donohue syndrome.

DIFFERENTIAL DIAGNOSIS: Congenital absence of the pancreas; Costello syndrome; Chromosomal anomalies; Berardinelli lipodystrophy syndrome.

SYMPTOMS AND SIGNS: The intrauterine growth of affected fetuses stops at approximately 7 months of gestation. At birth, newborns are small for gestational age and have peculiar dysmorphic features, including prominent eyes, thick lips, gingival hyperplasia giving the appearance of an inverted V-shaped palate, upturned nostrils, low-set, posteriorly rotated ears, hirsutism, acanthosis nigricans, thick skin with lack of subcutaneous fat, distended abdomen, breast hyperplasia, enlarged genitalia in the male, and cystic ovaries in the female with enlargement of the clitoris. Patients have an increased incidence of congenital heart disease and cardiac hypertrophy or cardiomyopathy. Shortly after birth, affected infants have abnormal glucose levels, with both hypoglycemia before meals and hyperglycemia after feeding. Insulin levels are grossly increased above the normal range. Children not identified at birth have severe failure to thrive and most fail to attain normal milestones. They tend to have frequent infections and most affected children die before age 1 year during one of these episodes. Rabson-Mendenhall syndrome is a milder variant of leprechaunism. Affected children have additional dysmorphic features, including premature or dysplastic teeth and enlargement of the pineal gland. They survive to age 5–20 years and have progressive worsening of metabolic imbalance, leading first to constant hyperglycemia, then to diabetic ketoacidosis and death.

ETIOLOGY/EPIDEMIOLOGY: Leprechaunism and Rabson-Mendenhall syndrome are inherited as autosomal-recessive traits. They are due to mutations in the insulin receptor gene located on chromosome 19p13. The prevalence of these disorders is unknown, but believed to be approximately 1 in 1 million. All ethnic groups are affected.

DIAGNOSIS: The diagnosis should be suspected on clinical grounds based on the characteristic dysmorphic features. Chromosome testing should exclude other causes of dysmorphism. A screening test is provided by the measurement of blood glucose and simultaneous insulin levels, which are usually approximately 100 times above normal. The diagnosis is confirmed by the demonstration of defective insulin binding in skin fibroblasts. Sequencing of the insulin receptor gene is available on a research basis. Prenatal diagnosis is available once causative mutations in the insulin receptor gene have been identified.

TREATMENT

Standard Therapies: Treatment is generally supportive. The goal is to maintain blood glucose levels as constantly as possible with the use of frequent or continuous feeds and complex carbohydrates. Insulin is not effective at normal doses. Minimal effects on glucose levels can be seen with extra large doses of insulin (up to 9 U/kg per hour).

Investigational Therapies: The use of insulin sensitizers (thazolidinediones and metformin) to improve residual insulin action is under investigation. Insulinlike growth factor 1 at high doses in divided doses or as continuous subcutaneous infusion has been effective in a few patients.

REFERENCES

Longo N, Langley SD, Griffin LD, et al. Two mutations in the insulin receptor gene of a patient with leprechaunism: application to prenatal diagnosis. *J Clin Endocrinol Metab* 1995; 80:1496–1501.

Longo N, Wang Y, Pasquali M. Progressive decline in insulin levels in Rabson-Mendenhall syndrome. *J Clin Endocrinol Metab* 1999;84:2623–2629.

Nakae J, Kato M, Murashita M, et al. Long-term effect of recombinant human IGF-I on metabolic and growth control in a patient with leprechaunism. *J Clin Endocrinol Metab* 1998;83:542–549.

Taylor SI, Kadowaki T, Kadowaki H, et al. Mutations in insulin-receptor gene in insulin-resistant patients. *Diabetes Care* 1990;13:257–279.

RESOURCES
96, 188, 362

85 Leri Pleonosteosis

John M. Hicks, MD, DDS, PhD

DEFINITION: Leri pleonosteosis is an autosomal-dominant syndrome characterized by short stature, limb abnormalities, decreased joint mobility, and laryngeal stenosis. It shares similar phenotypic features with syndromes in the differential diagnosis.

SYNONYMS: Dwarfism with joint stiffness.

DIFFERENTIAL DIAGNOSIS: Moore-Federman syndrome; Acromicric dysplasia; Weill-Marchesani syndrome; GEMSS (glaucoma-lens ectopia-microspherophakia-stiffness-shortness) syndrome; Gelophysic dysplasia; Laryngotracheal stenosis, progressive, with short stature and arthropathy.

SYMPTOMS AND SIGNS: The characteristic findings of Leri pleonosteosis are short stature, brachydactyly, genu recurvatum, short, spadelike hands, broad thumbs in valgus position, decreased joint mobility, thick planar and forearm fasciae, shuffling gait, Mongoloid facies, enlarged posterior neural arches of cervical vertebrae, and laryngeal stenosis.

ETIOLOGY/EPIDEMIOLOGY: The various conditions that share the underlying phenotype of dwarfism with joint stiffness have few affected families, case series, and individual cases available for cytogenetic and molecular genetic studies. The similarity in the underlying phenotype may imply that a specific gene, with alterations in various regions, is responsible for the variety of phenotypes in these apparently related syndromes.

DIAGNOSIS: Clinical and radiologic findings support the diagnosis of dwarfism with joint stiffness. The specific clinical phenotype and radiologic findings are helpful in classifying the affected proband into the appropriate syndrome. No cytogenetic or molecular genetic marker is available for prenatal or postnatal diagnosis.

TREATMENT
Standard Therapies: Symptomatic treatment depends on the phenotype of the affected individual. No therapy is available.

REFERENCES
Hennekam R, van Bever Y, Oorthuys J. Acomicric dysplasia and gelophysic dysplasia: similarities and differences. *Eur J Pediatr* 1996;155:311–314.
Hilton R, Wentzel J. Leri's pleonosteosis. *Q J Med* 1980;49:419–429.
Hopkin R, Cotton R, Langer L, Saal H. Progressive laryngotracheal stenosis with short stature and arthropathy. *Am J Med Genet* 1998;80:241–246.
Pontz B, Stoss H, Henschke F, et al. Clinical and ultrastructural findings in three patients with geleophysic dysplasia. *Am J Med Genet* 1996;63:50–54.
Verloes A, Hermia J, Galand A, et al. Glaucoma-lens ectopia-microspherophakia-stiffness-shortness (GEMSS) syndrome: a dominant disease with manifestations of Weill-Marchesani syndrome. *Am J Med Genet* 1992;44:48–51.

RESOURCES
188, 360

---

86   Maffucci Syndrome

Laurence M. Boon, MD, and John B. Mulliken, MD

DEFINITION: Maffucci syndrome is characterized by cutaneous venous-like anomalies, typically occurring in the distal extremities and in association with multiple enchondromas.

SYNONYMS: Enchondromatosis; Hemangiomatosis osteolytica; Spindle-cell hemangioendothelioma.

DIFFERENTIAL DIAGNOSIS: Ollier disease; Blue rubber bleb nevus syndrome; Familial cutaneous-mucosal venous malformation; Familial glomuvenous malformations.

SYMPTOMS AND SIGNS: Although Maffucci syndrome is a congenital disorder, the features usually do not manifest until early to mid-childhood. Enchondromas develop first in the long bones, typically near the epiphysis and in the hands and feet. Pathologic fractures are common, as are deformities and shortening of the extremities. The cutaneous lesions begin typically around age 4–5 years as firm, domelike, bluish spots on a finger or toe. Later, they can become knotty, verrucose vascular masses that contain phleboliths. The lesions are either unilateral or bilateral and do not necessarily overlie enchondromas. Patients tend to be of short stature, and may develop scoliosis. The disorder seems to stabilize with completion of skeletal growth. As many as 40% of patients develop malignancy, especially chondrosarcoma.

ETIOLOGY/EPIDEMIOLOGY: The syndrome affects males and females equally. No pedigrees of multiple affected family members have been reported. Karyotyping is usually normal.

DIAGNOSIS: Endochondral involvement results in severe distortion and deviation of the hands and feet. Plain radiology or computed tomography demonstrate the typical radiolucent enchondromas. The cutaneous venous anomalies are compressible early in the course of the disorder; later they become firm. Rarely, venous lesions occur on mucosal surfaces of the oral cavity and gastrointestinal tract. Phleboliths are typical of mature vascular lesions.

TREATMENT

Standard Therapies: The cutaneous venous lesions can be injected with sclerosing agents and/or surgically excised. A specialist in hand surgery should be involved if skeletal distortion causes loss of function or recurrent fracture. The enchondromal lesions can be resected; bone grafting may be needed. Orthopedic consultation is needed for correction of leg length discrepancy, scoliosis, and other bony deformities.

REFERENCES

Fanburg JC, Meis-Kindblom JM, Rosenberg AE. Multiple endochondromas associated with spindle-cell hemangioendotheliomas. An overlooked variant of Maffucci's syndrome. *Am J Surg Pathol* 1995;19:1029–1030.

Kaplan RP, Wang JT, Amron DM, et al. Maffucci's syndrome: two case reports with a literature review. *J Am Acad Dermatol* 1993;29:894–899.

Lewis RJ, Ketcham AS. Maffucci's syndrome: functional and neoplastic significance. Case report and review of the literature. *J Bone Joint Surg [Am]* 1973;55:1465–1479.

Sun T-C, Swee RG, Shives TD, et al. Chondrosarcoma in Maffucci's syndrome. *J Bone Joint Surg [Am]* 1985;67:1214–1219.

RESOURCES

351, 356, 378

---

87   Marfan Syndrome

Hal Dietz, MD

DEFINITION: Marfan syndrome is a systemic disorder of connective tissue caused by defective or deficient fibrillin-1.

DIFFERENTIAL DIAGNOSIS: Familial ectopia lentis; Familial thoracic aortic aneurysm; Isolated skeletal features; Mitral valve prolapse syndrome; MASS phenotype; Homocystinuria.

SYMPTOMS AND SIGNS: Marfan syndrome shows extreme clinical variability. Cardinal manifestations involve the ocular, skeletal, and cardiovascular systems. An elongated globe, iris hypoplasia, early and severe myopia, and a predisposition for displacement of the ocular lens characterize the eye. Less common features include retinal detachment, glaucoma, and early cataract formation. The skeleton shows joint laxity and overgrowth of the long bones. Most patients show dolichostenomelia. Common manifestations include anterior chest deformity, scoliosis, and medial rotation of the medial malleolus. Craniofacial features include down-slanting of palpebral fissures, a long and narrow face, dolichocephaly, high-arched palate, enophthalmos, malar hypoplasia, micrognathia, and retrognathia. Affected individuals show progressive enlargement of the aortic root at the level of the sinuses of Valsalva. Many individuals have redundancy and thickening of the mitral valve leaflets and mitral valve prolapse. Other cardiovascular manifestations include tricuspid valve prolapse, dilatation of the main pulmonary artery, and aneurysm in descending thoracic or abdominal aortic segments. Patients often develop widening of the dural sac in the lumbosacral region (dural ectasia) that can lead to bone erosion and nerve impingement. Other features in the skin and integument include recurrent or incisional hernias and skin stretch marks. Patients can show a lack of muscularity and a paucity of subcutaneous fat.

ETIOLOGY/EPIDEMIOLOGY: Marfan syndrome is inherited in an autosomal-dominant manner. Approximately 25% of cases are sporadic due to spontaneous mutations. Penetrance is complete, but with marked clinical variability. The disease is caused by mutations in the gene (*FBN1*) encoding fibrillin-1 on chromosome 15q21.1. The prevalence is estimated at 1–2 in 10,000, without any ethnic or sex preference.

DIAGNOSIS: Many features of the disease have diagnostic significance only when they are seen in combination. Although both DNA and protein-based molecular studies are available, they lack complete sensitivity and specificity for Marfan syndrome and only serve as adjuncts in the clinical diagnosis. In the absence of a family history for the disease, one must observe major involvement of two body systems with minor involvement of a third. Once the diagnosis has been established in a proband, the requirements for diagnosis of a first-degree family member include major involvement of one organ system with minor involvement of a second. These criteria also apply if an individual is shown to carry an *FBN1* mutation that has previously been associated with Marfan syndrome or an *FBN1* haplotype inherited by descent.

TREATMENT

Standard Therapies: The cardiovascular features require close follow-up and aggressive management. Echocardiograms should be performed at regular intervals. Many centers prescribe β-blockers to reduce hemodynamic stress and reduce the rate of aortic growth. Prophylactic surgical repair of the aorta is recommended when the maximal dimension exceeds 5.0–5.5 cm in adults. Patients with valve regurgitation should receive SBE prophylaxis for dental work or other procedures expected to contaminate the bloodstream with bacteria. MRI or CT scans should be used to assess the status of aortic segments beyond the ascending aorta. Ocular abnormalities can generally be managed with eyeglasses. A freely mobile lens or a displaced lens that disrupts vision may need to be surgically removed. Eye examinations should be performed yearly by an ophthalmologist who has specific expertise with the disorder. Selected skeletal manifestations require management by an orthopedist. Progressive scoliosis may require surgical stabilization.

REFERENCES

DePaepe A, Devereux RB, Dietz HC, et al. Revised diagnostic criteria for the Marfan syndrome. *Am J Med Genet* 1996;62:417–426.

Dietz HC. Molecular etiology, pathogenesis and diagnosis of Marfan syndrome. *Prog Pediatr Cardiol* 1996;5:159–166.

Dietz HC, Pyeritz RE. In: Scriver CR, Beaudet AL, Sly WS, et al, eds. *The metabolic and molecular bases of inherited disease,* 8th ed. New York: McGraw-Hill, 2001:5287–5312.

Robinson PN, Godfrey M. The molecular genetics of Marfan syndrome and related microfibrillopathies. *J Med Genet* 2000; 37:9–25.

RESOURCES

313, 351

---

88 Marshall-Smith Syndrome

Merlin G. Butler, MD, PhD

DEFINITION: Marshall-Smith syndrome is a congenital condition characterized by advanced bone age, chronic pulmonary disease, a small face with a prominent forehead and eyes, micrognathia, anteverted nares, choanal atresia, hypertrichosis, and failure to thrive (Insert Figs. 31 and 32).

DIFFERENTIAL DIAGNOSIS: Weaver syndrome; Elejalde syndrome; Simpson-Golabi-Behmel syndrome.

SYMPTOMS AND SIGNS: Although it is described as an overgrowth syndrome, this disorder probably involves unknown defects of the cartilage, bone, and connective tissue rather than a generalized or localized cellular hyperplasia. It is characterized by advanced skeletal maturation of prenatal onset with the bone age at birth often exceeding that of a 2-year-old. Patients have increased skeletal radiodensity, craniofacial disproportion, slender tubular bones, and broad middle phalanges. Structural brain anomalies can include macrogyria, cerebral atrophy, optic atrophy, absence of corpus callosum, and cerebellar hypoplasia. Craniofacial features include a flattened nasal bridge, prominent forehead, shallow orbits with prominent eyes, bluish sclera, anteverted nares, micrognathia, and a small face. Choanal atresia/stenosis, hypertrichosis, umbilical hernia, instability of the cranial cervical junction with spinal stenosis, abnormal larynx, and dysplastic teeth are other possible findings. Patients have persistent respiratory difficulties manifested by stridor, hyperextension of the neck, and an obstructive airway. Recurrent aspiration, atelectosis, hemorrhagic pneumonia, and pulmonary hypertension with serious pulmonary compromise are frequent complications. Hydronephrosis has been reported, as well as polyhydramnios and preterm delivery. Overall intellectual performance is usually in the lower range of normal, but patients generally lack speech and may have conductive hearing loss. Most patients die by 20 months of age; the oldest reported patient is 15 years. Cause of death is generally related to pulmonary and central nervous system problems.

ETIOLOGY/EPIDEMIOLOGY: The cause of this syndrome is unknown, although it appears to be sporadic in the families reported. The male:female ratio is 1:1.

DIAGNOSIS: The diagnosis is suspected in babies with markedly accelerated skeletal maturation, particular facial anomalies, and failure to thrive. The estimated bone age in the wrist, elbow, and femoral epiphysis may be 3–6 years in relationship to a chronologic age of under 6 months. Radiographic studies are important for diagnosis.

TREATMENT

Standard Therapies: Careful attention to airway anatomy should be given. Infants with this condition may have repeated episodes of low oxygen saturation due to choanal atresia and upper airway obstruction requiring supplemental oxygen. Respiratory complication is a major component of this syndrome, as are anatomic abnormalities of the respiratory tract, including choanal atresia/stenosis, laryngeal malacia, unusual laryngeal positioning, and defects of the vocal cords. Intubation may be difficult because of laryngeal positioning. Tracheostomy is frequently required to maintain the airway.

REFERENCES

Eich GF, Silver MM, Weksberg R, et al. Marshall-Smith syndrome: new radiographic, clinical and pathologic observations. *Radiology* 1991;181:183–188.

Hoyme HE, Byers PH, Guttmacher AE. Marshall-Smith syndrome: further evidence of an osteochondrodysplasia in long-term survivors. *Proc Greenwood Genet Ctr* 1993;12:70.

Johnson JP, Carey JC, Glassy FJ, et al. Marshall-Smith syndrome: two case reports and a review of pulmonary manifestations. *Pediatrics* 1983;71:219–224.

Seidahmed MZ, Rooney DE, Salih MA, et al. Case of partial trisomy 2q3 with clinical manifestations of Marshall-Smith syndrome. *Am J Med Genet* 1999;85:185–188.

Summers D, Cooper HA, Butler MG. Marshall-Smith syndrome: case report of a newborn male and review of the literature. *Clin Dysmorphol* 1999;8:207–210.

RESOURCES

188, 253, 351

---

89   MASA Syndrome

Volker Schmid, Dr Med, and Silvia Drechsel

DEFINITION: MASA syndrome is an inborn disease caused by defects in the development of the nervous system during embryonic development. The acronym *MASA* stands for mental retardation, aphasia, shuffling gait, and adducted thumbs.

SYNONYMS: Adducted thumbs syndrome; Congenital clasped thumbs with mental retardation; CRASH syndrome.

DIFFERENTIAL DIAGNOSIS: X-related and other forms of hydrocephalus; Isolated adduction of thumbs; Complicated X-linked spastic paraplegia; Uncomplicated X-related spastic paraplegia; X-linked mental retardation renpenning type; Bickers-Adams syndrome.

SYMPTOMS AND SIGNS: Infants may have hypotonia, low muscle tone, spacticities, adducted thumbs (usually symmetric), and an excessive Moro reflex or other reflex abnormalities. Symptoms such as squinting or psychomotor retardation may occur in later infancy or early childhood. Grasping can be affected as well as gait and speech. The ventricles of the brain may be enlarged and an aqueductal stenosis or agenesis of the corpus callosum may be diagnosed. Other physical findings may include abnormalities of the spine (lordosis, kyphosis, scoliosis), the feet (flat feet, clubfeet), or the hips (anteversion). The knees can be bowed. Hydrocephalus or microcephaly may be present. Affected individuals may express mild to severe learning difficulties. Patients may have sleeping problems, problems with sensoric integration, vomiting (weak stomach muscles), or caries. An unusually small body size or mild short stature also may be found.

ETIOLOGY/EPIDEMIOLOGY: MASA syndrome is inherited in a gonosomal-recessive manner. Therefore, it usually affects males only. It is the result of a mutation in the cell adhesion molecule gene *L1CAM* located on chromosome Xq28, which plays an important role in the development of the nervous system. The prevalence is estimated at 50 cases (13 families).

DIAGNOSIS: A reliable prenatal diagnosis is possible by chorionic villus biopsy or amniocentesis followed by molecular analysis of the *L1CAM* gene. Sometimes it is possible to exclude MASA syndrome by creating an ultrasonographic image of the fetus's unflexed thumbs. The presence of hydrocephalus, agenesis of the corpus callosum, and/or aqueductal stenosis can be confirmed by CT or MRI and by ultrasonography of the fontanelles during infancy. The clinical evaluation must include a detailed patient history, identification of characteristic findings, and advanced imaging techniques. A molecular analysis shows whether an asymptomatic female is a carrier.

TREATMENT

Standard Therapies: Treatment is directed toward the symptoms (e.g., physiotherapy can improve muscle tone). Adequate treatment requires comprehensive therapy planning and coordinated efforts of all specialists.

RESOURCES

303, 368

90   Meckel Syndrome

*Leonardo Pereira, MD,
and Alan E. Donnenfeld, MD*

DEFINITION: Meckel syndrome is an autosomal-recessive disorder classically defined by the triad of polycystic kidneys, occipital encephalocele, and polydactyly.

SYNONYMS: Meckel-Gruber syndrome; Dysencephalia splanchnocystica.

DIFFERENTIAL DIAGNOSIS: Smith-Lemli-Opitz syndrome; Potter syndrome; Trisomy 13; Ellis–van Creveld syndrome; Joubert syndrome; Short rib–polydactyly syndromes; Infantile polycystic kidneys; Cystic dysplasia of the kidneys.

SYMPTOMS AND SIGNS: The classic triad of Meckel syndrome consists of enlarged polycystic kidneys, polydactyly, and occipital encephalocele. Oligohydramnios, the sequelae of Potter syndrome, and a decreased head-to-body ratio in the fetus are also seen. Other cranial findings include occipital encephalocele, microcephaly, and enlarged lateral ventricles. Findings such as eye anomalies, cleft lip, cleft palate, anencephaly, Dandy-Walker malformation, Arnold-Chiari malformation, and cerebellar dysplasia have been seen sporadically. Ultrasonographic findings often include an increased abdominal circumference secondary to bilaterally enlarged kidneys and hepatomegaly. The liver may appear cystic as well as enlarged. Renal anomalies associated with the disorder include urethral malformations and absence or hypoplasia of the bladder. Genital tract malformations may be identified postnatally. Polydactyly when present typically involves the hand.

ETIOLOGY/EPIDEMIOLOGY: The Meckel syndrome is inherited in an autosomal-recessive manner. The risk of recurrence is 25% in subsequent pregnancies. The disorder accounts for up to 5% of all neural tube defects. It has been reported in males and females with equal frequency. It is typically lethal in the perinatal period.

DIAGNOSIS: Multicystic dysplasia of the kidney is the most commonly reported abnormality, and the most crucial for diagnosis. In its absence, a diagnosis of Meckel syndrome may not be valid. Some have advocated that fibrosis of the liver also be included as a necessary element. At least two of the typical features must be present for the diagnosis to be made. The diagnosis can be suggested prenatally by an elevated maternal serum α-fetoprotein or elevated amniotic fluid α-fetoprotein level. Typical findings on ultrasonography include oligohydramnios and postaxial polydactyly, as well as cranial and abdominal abnormalities. Postnatal ultrasonography can show cerebral atrophy with enlarged lateral ventricles, and can easily confirm the presence of bilaterally enlarged echogenic kidneys. Autopsy can confirm the prenatal findings.

TREATMENT

Standard Therapies: No therapeutic intervention exists for this syndrome. The rare infant that survives the perinatal period is developmentally delayed, and generally dies from hepatorenal failure within the first 3 years of life.

REFERENCES

Fraser FC. Spectrum of anomalies in the Meckel syndrome. *Am J Med Genet* 1981;9:67–73.

Lowry RB. Survival and spectrum of anomalies in the Meckel syndrome. *Am J Med Genet* 1983;14:417–421.

Salonen R. The Meckel syndrome. *Am J Med Genet* 1984;18: 671–689.

Summers M, Donnenfeld A. Dandy-Walker malformation in the Meckel syndrome. *Am J Med Genet* 1995;55:57–61.

RESOURCE
362

91   Melnick-Needles Syndrome

Jeffrey A. Wong, MD

DEFINITION: Melnick-Needles syndrome is a disorder composed of abnormal bone modeling, characteristic facial anomalies, and occasional other multiple anomalies.

SYNONYM: Melnick-Needles osteodysplasty.

DIFFERENTIAL DIAGNOSIS: Cleidocranial dysplasia; Multiple epiphyseal dysplasia.

SYMPTOMS AND SIGNS: Affected individuals are usually identified by an abnormal gait and bowing of the extremities. More common findings include a narrow thorax, delayed closure of the anterior fontanel, exophthalmos, full and protruding cheeks, a high and narrow forehead, micrognathia, malaligned teeth, and large ears. Other clinical findings include dislocation of the hips, scoliosis, pectus excavatum, incurved distal thumb segments, short upper arms, and distal phalanges. In females, a contracted pelvis may result in a difficult vaginal delivery. Eventually, osteoarthritis of the back and/or hips may develop. Cardiopulmonary defects have also been noted, including ventricular septal defect, double-outlet right ventricle, complete atrioventricular canal defect with tetralogy of Fallot or pulmonary atresia, mitral or tricuspid valve prolapse, noncompaction of the ventricular myocardium, and primary pulmonary hypertension. Renal and abdominal wall anomalies have also been reported, including ureteral stenosis or ureterovesicle obstruction, leading to hydronephrosis. Psychomotor development and adult stature are usually normal.

ETIOLOGY/EPIDEMIOLOGY: Melnick-Needles syndrome is postulated to be a primary disorder of early fetal development, possibly from a defect in collagen synthesis. It is an X-linked dominant trait either severely affecting or lethal in males. Surviving affected males are believed to represent new mutations. An autosomal-recessive form has been reported.

DIAGNOSIS: The diagnosis is first suspected because of the characteristic clinical features, which can be seen at varying ages. Radiographic evaluation may confirm the diagnosis by revealing characteristic skeletal anomalies, which include a small thoracic cage with irregular ribbon-like ribs, irregular and uneven thickening of the cortices of the long bones; lateral bowing of the radius and tibia; flaring of the distal humeral, tibial, and fibular metaphyses; tall vertebrae with anterior concavity of the vertebral bodies; supraacetabular iliac wing narrowing with iliac wing flaring; a small mandible; and sclerosis of the skull base (Insert Figs. 33 and 34). Cardiac and renal evaluation is also warranted as clinically indicated.

TREATMENT

Standard Therapies: Treatment is symptomatic and supportive. Correction of skeletal, cardiac, and renal anomalies should be undertaken as needed. No specific therapy is available. Genetic counseling may be helpful.

REFERENCES

Coste F, Maroteaux P, Chouraki L. Osteoplasy (Melnick-Needles syndrome). *Ann Rheum Dis* 1968;27:360.

Donnenfeld AE, Connard KA, Roberts NS, et al. Melnick-Needles syndrome in males: a lethal multiple congenital anomalies syndrome. *Am J Med Genet* 1987;27: 159–173.

Melnick JC, Needles CF. An undiagnosed bone dysplasia. *AJA* 1966;97:39.

Haar B, Hamel B, Hendriks J, et al. Melnick-Needles syndrome: indication for an autosomal recessive form. *Am J Med Genet* 1982;13:469–477.

RESOURCE

260

---

92   Miller Syndrome

Eric A. Wulfsberg, MD

DEFINITION: Miller syndrome is a genetic acrofacial (hand-face) dysostosis with malar hypoplasia, down-slanting palpebral fissures, ear anomalies, and absence or abnormalities of the fifth (postaxial) fingers and/or toes.

SYNONYMS: Postaxial acrofacial dysostosis; Genee-Wiedemann syndrome.

DIFFERENTIAL DIAGNOSIS: Treacher-Collins syndrome; Nager syndrome; Other acrofacial dysostoses.

SYMPTOMS AND SIGNS: Miller syndrome is recognizable in the newborn period. The facial features are similar to those of Treacher-Collins syndrome and include malar hypoplasia with hypoplasia of the zygoma and maxilla, down-slanting palpebral fissures, and lower eyelid colobomas with partial to complete absence of the lower eyelashes. The external ears are typically small and cup shaped, and many patients have conductive deafness or hearing impairment. Mandibular hypoplasia may be severe and may be associated with cleft lip or cleft palate, feeding difficulties, and airway obstruction. Limb anomalies include absence or hypoplasia of the hands and feet, especially of the fifth digits, with variable syndactyly of the remaining digits. The thumbs may also be affected. The forearms and lower legs may be mildly shortened, with radial, ulnar, tibial, and fibular hypoplasia. Intelligence is generally normal.

ETIOLOGY/EPIDEMIOLOGY: The syndrome is a suspected autosomal-recessive genetic condition, based on a limited number of cases with recurrence in siblings. The gene has not been identified. The incidence is unknown.

DIAGNOSIS: The diagnosis is generally made by observing the typical features on careful craniofacial examination. Although Miller syndrome is not a chromosomal syndrome, karyotype is recommended to rule out similar-appearing phenocopies. Consultation with a clinical geneticist to confirm the diagnosis and provide recurrence risk counseling is recommended.

TREATMENT

Standard Therapies: Surgical treatment is best accomplished at a craniofacial center with expertise including plastic surgery, otolaryngology, orthodontics, and dentistry. Radiography and three-dimensional CT are indicated in the presurgical evaluation of patients. Hearing augmentation requires consultation with an experienced otolaryngologist.

Investigational Therapies: New surgical procedures and hearing aid technologies are constantly being developed.

REFERENCES

Ogilvy-Stuart AL, Parsons AC. Miller syndrome (postaxial acrofacial dysostosis): further evidence for autosomal recessive inheritance and expansion of the phenotype. *J Med Genet* 1991;28:695–700.

Opitz JM, Mollica F, Sorge G, et al. Acrofacial dysostoses: review and report of a previously undescribed condition: the autosomal or X-linked dominant Catania form of acrofacial dysostosis. *Am J Med Genet* 1993;47:660–678.

RESOURCES

149, 163

---

93 Möbius Syndrome

John B. Mulliken, MD

DEFINITION: The cardinal features of Möbius syndrome are congenital sixth and seventh nerve palsy, often in association with limb and truncal defects. Möbius syndrome may not be a distinct entity; there are overlapping features with other oromandibular-limb hypogenesis syndromes.

SYMPTOMS: Congenital facial paralysis; Congenital facial diplegia syndrome; Congenital oculofacial paralysis.

DIFFERENTIAL DIAGNOSIS: Isolated seventh nerve palsy secondary to birth trauma; Hemifacial microsomia with expanded spectrum; Hypoglossia-hypodactylia syndrome; Hanhart syndrome; Glossopalatine ankylosis syndrome; Limb deficiency–splenogonadal fusion syndrome; Charlie M. syndrome.

SYMPTOMS AND SIGNS: From birth, affected children exhibit a mask-like expression that is particularly obvious when crying or laughing. The eyelid(s) remain open during sleep; this can cause corneal ulceration. In addition to the unilateral or bilateral VIIth nerve paresis or palsy, the VIth nerve is affected in most patients; cranial nerves IX, X, XI, and XII may also be involved. Feeding during infancy may be difficult. Auricular anomalies occur in a spectrum from protrusion to microtia to anotia. Microphthalmia is a rare associated abnormality. The tongue can be affected as hypo- to aglossia. Defects in the upper extremity manifest from hypoplasia to absence of the humerus, radius, ulna, or digits; defects in the lower extremity include syndactyly, clubfoot, and axial hypoplasia. Truncal abnormalities include pectoral and breast hypoplasia, as well as scoliosis and scapular hypoplasia. Other anomalies may be secondary, such as micrognathia and temporomandibular joint dysfunction, caused by neural involvement, muscular weakness or diminished intrauterine movement, and cleft palate as a result of micrognathia.

ETIOLOGY/EPIDEMIOLOGY: Almost all known cases are sporadic; rare instances occur of familial seventh and sixth nerve paralysis. Pathogenesis may involve disruption of the developing vascular system, resulting in ischemic or hypoxic insult to the fetus. Other proposed causes include gestational hyperthermia and first trimester exposure to a prostaglandin E1 analogue. Postmortem studies have shown agenesis and necrosis of brainstem nuclei, prenatal encephalomalacic lesions, and hypoplasia of cranial nerve trunks and facial musculature.

DIAGNOSIS: In addition to facial diplegia and abducens palsies, diagnosis is made on the clinical appearance of abnormalities of the extremities and trunk.

TREATMENT

Standard Therapies: Surgical procedures utilize the muscles of mastication innervated by the uninvolved Vth cranial nerve. Traditional operations are transfer of temporalis muscle for eyelid closure and transfer of masseter muscle to the corner of the mouth. A new procedure is microvascular transplantation of the gracilis muscle to the face, innervated by the trigeminal motor branch. This gives an average of 1.37 cm excursion of the corner of the mouth and also helps speech and control of drooling. Specialized surgical procedures are used to correct extremity defects, auricular deformities, and pectoral/mammary hypoplasia.

REFERENCES

Abramson DL, Cohen MM Jr, Mulliken JB. Möbius syndrome: classification and grading system. *Plast Reconstr Surg* 1998; 102:961–967.

Gorlin JJ, Cohen MM Jr, Levin LS. *Syndromes of the head and neck,* 3rd ed. New York: Oxford University Press, 1990: 666–674.

Pastuszak AL, Schuler L, Speck-Martins CE, et al. Use of misoprostol during pregnancy and Möbius syndrome in infants. *N Engl J Med* 1998;338:1881–1885.

Zuker RM, Goldberg CS, Manktelow RT. Facial animation in children with Möbius syndrome after segmental gracilis muscle transplant. *Plast Reconstr Surg* 2000;106:1–8.

RESOURCES

96, 267, 268

---

94 MULIBREY Nanism

Adda Grimberg, MD

DEFINITION: Muscle-liver-brain-eyes (MULIBREY) nanism is an autosomal-recessive syndrome involving growth failure and anomalies of mesodermal tissues. Constrictive pericarditis is a characteristic feature not included in the original acronym.

SYNONYMS: Pericardial constriction with growth failure; Perheentupa syndrome.

DIFFERENTIAL DIAGNOSIS: Russell-Silver syndrome; Robinow syndrome; Primary empty sella syndrome (dwarfism with abnormal sella turcica); Late purulent or tuberculous pericarditis; Pericarditis due to chest radiation or tumor invasion into the pericardium; Restrictive cardiomyopathy (constrictive pericarditis).

SYMPTOMS AND SIGNS: Progressive growth failure of prenatal onset is a constant finding. More than 90% of patients have a J-shaped sella turcica. Triangular facies and features suggest persistence of infantile craniofacial structural relationships. Voice is characteristically high pitched. Yellow dots on the fundi and other ocular abnormalities are frequently seen, but visual acuity is normal. Pericardial constriction with occasional calcification manifests as prominent jugular veins, hepatomegaly, and congestive heart failure. Muscle hypotonia is frequently seen, as is fibrous dysplasia of the tibia. The abnormally large cerebral ventricles and cysternae, included in the acronym, are uncommon findings, as is retarded motor development; most affected individuals have normal intelligence.

ETIOLOGY/EPIDEMIOLOGY: MULIBREY nanism is an autosomal-recessive condition arising from mutations in MUL on chromosome 17q22-q23. Most reported patients are from Finland, although others have been seen in North America, South America, Central America, Spain, France, and Egypt. Their families show increased risk for abortions and infant death, likely due to early heart failure and susceptibility to pneumonia.

DIAGNOSIS: The major diagnostic criteria are short stature, growth failure, abnormally shaped sella turcica, yellow dots in ocular fundi, pericardial constriction, and a peculiar face.

TREATMENT

Standard Therapies: Constrictive pericarditis is treated with pericardiectomy; some patients require diuretics and digoxin for progressive congestive heart failure. Hormonal replacement should be offered to children with deficiencies (growth hormone deficiency, delayed puberty, oligomenorrhea, hypothyroidism, hypoadrenocorticism, and abnormal gonads). Patients should be monitored closely for ovarian tumors and Wilms tumor.

REFERENCES

Avela K, Lipsanen-Nyman M, Idanheimo N, et al. Gene encoding a new RING-B-box-coiled-coil protein is mutated in mulibrey nanism. *Nat Genet* 2000;25:298–301.

Lapunzina P, Rodriguez JI, de Matteo E, et al. MULIBREY nanism: three additional patients and a review of 39 patients. *Am J Med Genet* 1995;55:349–355.

Perheentupa J, Autio S, Leisti S, et al. MULIBREY nanism, an autosomal recessive syndrome with pericardial constriction. *Lancet* 1973;2:351–355.

Tarkkanen A, Raitta C, Perheentupa J. MULIBREY nanism, an autosomal recessive syndrome with ocular involvement. *Acta Ophthalmol* 1982;60:628–633.

Zapata JM, Pawlowski K, Haas E, et al. TEFs: a diverse family of proteins containing TRAF domains. *J Biol Chem* 2001; Feb 21 (in press).

RESOURCES

188, 190, 355

95 | Myhre Syndrome

Margo L. Whiteford, FRCP(Glas)

DEFINITION: Myhre syndrome is associated with mental retardation, short stature, generalized muscle hypertrophy, and a distinctive facial appearance.

DIFFERENTIAL DIAGNOSIS: GOMBO (growth retardation, ocular abnormalities, microcephaly, brachydactyly, oligophrenia) syndrome.

SYMPTOMS AND SIGNS: The main presenting features are short stature, muscular build, mental retardation, deafness, limited joint movement, and dysmorphic facial features. These consist of maxillary hypoplasia, prominent jaw, short palpebral fissures, short philtrum, and a small mouth. The intellectual deficit is usually within the moderate range. The radiologic abnormalities include thickened calvarium, broad ribs, hypoplastic iliac wings, short tubular bones, and platyspondyly. The facial features tend to become coarser with age, and the muscle hypertrophy becomes more evident. Nonspecific changes have been detected on electromyography and muscle ultrasonography, but only in 1 of the 3 patients in whom a muscle biopsy was performed was an abnormality detected (hypertrophic muscle fibers). Three of the adult patients developed hypertension. Other reported features include blepharophimosis, cardiac anomalies, cleft lip and palate, facial nerve paralysis, genital anomalies, inguinal hernia, seizures, cataract, velopharyngeal incompetence, and gallstones.

ETIOLOGY/EPIDEMIOLOGY: Only 6 cases of Myhre syndrome have been reported, and all affected individuals were males. Chromosome analysis is normal. The condition may occur as a result of an underlying metabolic defect. The average age of the fathers of affected individuals was advanced, indicating that Myhre syndrome is likely to occur as a result of a new dominant gene mutation.

DIAGNOSIS: The diagnosis is based on the identification of the clinical features and the detection of the radiologic abnormalities on skeletal survey. In suspected cases, assessment of hearing, electromyography/muscle ultrasonography/muscle biopsy, and echocardiography may give additional helpful information. Chromosome abnormality should be excluded.

TREATMENT

Standard Therapies: There is no specific treatment other than the provision of hearing aids and support from a learning disability team. Complications should be treated as they arise. Regular blood pressure measurements are advisable.

REFERENCES

Garcia Cruz D, Figuera LE, Feria-Velazco A, et al. The Myhre syndrome: report of two cases. *Clin Genet* 1993;44:203–207.

Myhre SA, Ruvalcaba RHA, Graham CB. A new growth deficiency syndrome. *Clin Genet* 1981;20:1–5.

Soljak MA, Aftimos S, Gluckman PD. A new syndrome of short stature, joint limitation and muscle hypertrophy. *Clin Genet* 1983;23:441–446.

Whiteford ML, Doig WB, Raine PAM, et al. A new case of Myhre syndrome. *Clin Dysmorphol* 2001;10:135–140.

RESOURCES

188, 246

96   Nager Syndrome

Eric A. Wulfsberg, MD

DEFINITION: Nager syndrome is an acrofacial (hand-face) dysostosis with malar hypoplasia, ear anomalies, and structural abnormalities or absence of the thumb and/or radius.

SYNONYMS: Nager acrofacial dysostosis; Preaxial acrofacial dysostosis.

DIFFERENTIAL DIAGNOSIS: Treacher-Collins syndrome; Miller syndrome; Other acrofacial dysostoses.

SYMPTOMS AND SIGNS: Nager syndrome is recognizable in the newborn period. The facial features are similar to those of Treacher-Collins syndrome and include malar hypoplasia with hypoplasia of the zygoma and maxilla, down-slanting palpebral fissures, and lower eyelid colobomas with partial to complete absence of the lower eyelashes. The external and internal ears are small and dysplastic, and many patients have conductive deafness or hearing impairment. Mandibular hypoplasia may be severe and may be associated with cleft palate, feeding difficulties, and airway obstruction. Limb anomalies include absence or hypoplasia of the thumb and/or radius with shortening of the forearm and radioulnar synostosis. Intelligence is generally normal.

ETIOLOGY/EPIDEMIOLOGY: Nager syndrome appears to be genetically heterogeneous. Most cases have been sporadic, but families showing both autosomal-dominant and autosomal-recessive inheritance have been described. The incidence is unknown.

DIAGNOSIS: The diagnosis is generally made by finding typical features on careful craniofacial examination. Although Nager syndrome is not a chromosomal syndrome, karyotype is recommended to rule out similar-appearing phenocopies. Consultation with a clinical geneticist to confirm the diagnosis and provide recurrence risk counseling is recommended.

TREATMENT
Standard Therapies: Surgical treatment is best accomplished at a craniofacial center with expertise in plastic surgery, otolaryngology, orthodontics, and dentistry. Radiography and three-dimensional CT are indicated in the presurgical evaluation of patients. Hearing augmentation requires consultation with an experienced otolaryngologist.

Investigational Therapies: New surgical procedures and hearing aid technologies are constantly being developed.

REFERENCES
Danziger I, Brodsky L, Perry R, et al. Nager's acrofacial dysostosis. *Int J Pediatr Otorhinolaryngol* 1990;20:225–240.
Opitz C, Stoll C, Ring P. Nager syndrome. Problems and possibilities of therapy. *J Orofacial Orthop* 2000;61:226–236.
Opitz JM, Mollica F, Sorge G, et al. Acrofacial dysostoses: review and report of a previously undescribed condition: the autosomal or X-linked dominant Catania form of acrofacial dysostosis. *Am J Med Genet* 1993;47:660–678.

RESOURCES
96, 163

97   Oculocerebral Syndrome with Hypopigmentation

Elias I. Traboulsi, MD

DEFINITION: This syndrome combines gingival fibromatosis, ocular abnormalities, skin and hair hypopigmentation, and cerebral defects manifested by developmental delay, spasticity, and athetoid movements.

SYNONYMS: Cross syndrome; Kramer syndrome.

DIFFERENTIAL DIAGNOSIS: Oculocutaneous albinism; Syndromes with microphthalmia and multiple malformations such as Lenz syndrome; Lowe syndrome; Cystinosis.

SYMPTOMS AND SIGNS: Generalized pigment dilution is noted at birth. Athetoid movements, suckling sounds, and a high-pitched cry are present by age 3 months. Patients are usually unable to hold the head up, sit, or walk. Flexion contractures of the limbs, shoulders, and hips develop in late infancy. Deep tendon reflexes are exaggerated. Hyperemia of the skin is noted on exposure to sunlight. Growth and weight are below normal for age. Underdeveloped sexual characteristics are usually present. The ocular findings are microphthalmia, uveal depigmentation, nystagmus, and diffuse corneal opacities that become vascularized.

ETIOLOGY/EPIDEMIOLOGY: This is an autosomal-recessive disorder. Slightly more than 10 cases, including two sets of siblings, have been reported since the original description in 1967. The exact cause is unknown.

DIAGNOSIS: The diagnosis is established when most clinical signs and symptoms are present. The diagnostic workup should include a neuroimaging study to identify possible associated brain malformations.

TREATMENT
Standard Therapies: Treatment is supportive. Protection from excessive UV exposure is advisable, although skin cancer and actinic skin damage have not been reported or emphasized in this disorder.

REFERENCES
Courtens W, Broeckx W, Ledoux M, et al. Oculocerebral hypopigmentation syndrome (Cross syndrome) in a Gipsy child. *Acta Paediat Scand* 1989;78:806–810.
Fryns JP, Dereymaeker AM, Heremans G, et al. Oculocerebral syndrome with hypopigmentation (Cross syndrome): report of two siblings born to consanguineous parents. *Clin Genet* 1988;34:81–84.
Lerone M, Pessagno A, Taccone A, et al. Oculocerebral syndrome with hypopigmentation (Cross syndrome): report of a new case. *Clin Genet* 1992;41:87–89.
Passarge E, Fuchs-Recke S. Oculocerebral syndrome with hypopigmentation. *Birth Defects Orig Art Series* 1975;21:466–467.
Tezcan I, Demir E, Asan E, et al. A new case of oculocerebral hypopigmentation syndrome (Cross syndrome) with additional findings. *Clin Genet* 1997;51:118–121.
White CP, Waldron, M, Jan JE, et al. Oculocerebral hypopigmentation syndrome associated with Bartter syndrome. *Am J Med Genet* 1993;46:592–596.

RESOURCES
351, 355

---

98 Osteogenesis Imperfecta

Alison M. Elliott, PhD,
and Ralph S. Lachman, MD

DEFINITION: Osteogenesis imperfecta (OI) is a group of hereditary skeletal disorders leading to a susceptibility to fracture and severe skeletal deformity. Osteopenia is the hallmark feature. This clinically heterogeneous group of disorders is divided into four major types (OI I–IV). Within each group, clinical severity and radiographic findings are extremely variable. Considerable overlap exists among the four groups.

SYNONYMS: "Brittle bone" disease/fragilitas ossium; Osteopsathyrosis; Ekman-Lobstein disease; Vrolik disease.

DIFFERENTIAL DIAGNOSIS: Trauma X (child abuse); Juvenile idiopathic osteoporosis (types I, IV); Blue sclera and keratoconus (type I); Blue sclera, familial nephrosis, thin skin, and hydrocephalus (type I); Cole-Carpenter (type III).

SYMPTOMS AND SIGNS: Type OI I is characterized by osteopenia leading to a susceptibility to fractures, blue sclera, presenile conductive hearing loss, easy bruising, some dentinogenesis imperfecta, joint hypermobility, and minimal deformity. There is usually spontaneous improvement in adolescence and exaggerated postmenopausal bone loss. Type OI II is the most severe form, with beaded ribs/crumpled bones *in utero* leading to pulmonary insufficiency and perinatal death. Type OI III occurs in newborns or infants and is characterized by severe bone fragility and multiple fractures leading to progressive deformity of the skeleton, sclera that are normal or light blue, triangular facies, poor longitudinal growth, and progressive kyphoscoliosis. Type OI IV is characterized by osteopenia without the typical features of OI type I (blue sclera, deafness); however, sclera may be blue at birth (which eventually resolves).

ETIOLOGY/EPIDEMIOLOGY: Type OI I affects approximately 1 in 30,000 individuals and is seen in both sexes. Most affected patients have either a reduction in the production of normal type I collagen or synthesize abnormal collagen as a result of mutations in the type I collagen genes (chromosome 17q21). Most cases are autosomal dominant. An affected individual has a 50% chance of having an affected child. Many cases are the result of sporadic mutations with no family history in which case the recurrence risk is approximately 7% for the unaffected parents to have another affected child.

DIAGNOSIS: The diagnosis can be made radiographically in most patients by the presence of generalized osteopenia. A full genetic skeletal survey should be performed. Other radiographic findings include fractures, healed fractures, wormian bones, and deformities of the bone. Diagnosis can sometimes be confirmed with analysis of type I collagen, either biochemically (skin biopsy) or by molecular analysis of a blood sample. Prenatal diagnosis by these means may be available for certain at-risk families (with previous identification of the mutation in the proband). Second-trimester prenatal ultrasonography may show signs of limb shortening, widening (femurs), or fractures, or rib fractures or shortening in the fetus.

TREATMENT
Standard Therapies: Treatment includes physical therapy to improve mobility and muscle strength; orthopedic care with appropriate management of fractures to minimize deformity and maximize mobilization; and intramedullary rodding (mainly for type III) to improve mobility, prevent fractures, and correct deformity.

Investigational Therapies: Bisphosphonates are being studied.

REFERENCES
Glorieux FH, Bishop NJ, Plotkin H, et al. Cyclic administration of pamidronate in children with severe osteogenesis imperfecta. *N Engl J Med* 1998;339:947–952.
Pepin M, Atkinson M, Starman BJ, et al. Strategies and outcomes of prenatal diagnosis for osteogenesis imperfecta: a review of biochemical and molecular studies completed in 129 pregnancies. *Prenat Diagn* 1997;17:559–570.
Sillence DO. Disorders of bone density, volume and mineralization. In: Rimoin DL, Connor JM, Pyeritz RE, eds. *Emery and Rimoin's principles and practice of medical genetics,* 3rd ed. New York: Churchill Livingston, 1996:2817–2835.
Taybi H, Lachman RS. *Radiology of syndromes, metabolic disorders and skeletal dysplasias,* 4th ed. St. Louis: Mosby–Year Book, 1996:876–882.
Thompson EM, Young ID, Hall CM, et al. Recurrence risks and prognosis in severe sporadic osteogenesis imperfecta. *J Med Genet* 1987;24:201–206.

RESOURCES
95, 360, 384

---

99   Autosomal-Recessive Osteopetrosis

Callum J. Wilson, MB, ChB, FRACP

DEFINITION: Autosomal-recessive osteopetrosis is a congenital disorder of bone resorption. This impaired bone remodeling results in bone marrow obliteration, brittle bones, and bony encroachment of the nerves.

SYNONYMS: Infantile "malignant" osteopetrosis; Brittle bone disease.

DIFFERENTIAL DIAGNOSIS: Autosomal-dominant adult disease; Carbonic anhydrase II deficiency syndrome.

SYMPTOMS AND SIGNS: Affected children usually present within the first year of life, frequently within the first 3 months. Parental concern regarding the child's vision is frequently the presenting complaint. Other presentations include failure to thrive, recurrent infection, anemia, seizures, and/or fractures. Failure of the bone to remodel results in obliteration of the bone marrow, which leads to anemia. The liver and spleen take over the marrow's function in producing blood and are thus greatly enlarged. This abnormal bone also impinges on nerves, most importantly the optic nerve. Children therefore have increasing visual impairment as the disease progresses. Hearing is less commonly involved. Children often have problems with sufficient nutrition and hydration and may require nasogastric tube feeding. Recurrent infections are also a problem, secondary to the bone marrow involvement, bony involvement of the ears and nose, and poor overall nutrition. The bones become brittle and fracture easily. The fractures can be difficult to treat.

ETIOLOGY/EPIDEMIOLOGY: The disease occurs equally in both sexes. It is inherited in an autosomal-recessive manner. Incidence is unknown but is less than 1 in 200,000. There appear to be several different genetic causes for the disease. All these genetic defects involve the osteoclasts.

DIAGNOSIS: Infants with visual impairment and bone marrow failure should undergo skeletal radiography. Very dense bones are highly suggestive of osteopetrosis. A bone biopsy confirms the diagnosis. A genetic diagnosis may be possible and, although not necessary for treatment purposes, is likely to be the best way to diagnose the disease prenatally.

TREATMENT
Standard Therapies: Initial management should focus on treating the anemia, biochemical abnormalities, and infection as indicated. Adequate nutrition is also important. Bone marrow transplantation (BMT), by replacing the faulty osteoclasts, will halt the progression of the disease. Tissue typing should be arranged, and based on the availability of a suitable donor, BMT should be performed as soon as is practical to save the patient's vision. A 5-year survival rate of at least 80% would be expected after BMT with a well-matched donor.

Investigational Therapies: Corticosteroids, high-dose calcitriol, and interferon-γ have all been reported to be helpful in the treatment of osteopetrosis.

REFERENCES
Gerritsen EJA, Vossen JM, Fasth A, et al. Bone marrow transplantation for osteopetrosis. A report from the working party on inborn errors of the European bone marrow transplantation group. *J Pediatr* 1994;125:896–902.

Gerritsen EJA, Vossen JM, van Loo IHG, et al. Autosomal recessive osteopetrosis: variability of findings at diagnosis and during the natural course. *Paediatrics* 1994;93:247–253.

Key LL, Rodriguiz RM, Willi SM, et al. Long-term treatment of osteopetrosis with recombinant human interferon. *N Engl J Med* 1995;332:1594–1599.

Wilson CJ, Vellodi A. Autosomal recessive osteopetrosis: diagnosis, treatment and management. *Arch Dis Child* 2000;83:449–452.

RESOURCES
348, 351, 464

100   Oto-Palato-Digital Syndrome

Ravi Savarirayan, MD, FRACP

DEFINITION: Oto-palato-digital syndrome is an X-linked, multiple congenital anomaly syndrome characterized by specific clinical and radiographic features.

SYNONYM: Oto-palato-digital syndrome, types I and II.

DIFFERENTIAL DIAGNOSIS: Atelosteogenesis type 3; Melnick-Needles syndrome.

SYMPTOMS AND SIGNS: Males with this condition have a characteristic facial appearance, with down-slanting eyes, small chin, cleft palate, overlapping flexed fingers (tree frog–like), and bowed limbs. The condition may be severe and detected at antenatal ultrasonography with the finding of bowed lower limbs and abnormal hands and feet. Many other extraskeletal abnormalities have been described in the condition, including defects of the anterior abdominal wall. The condition has several radiographic hallmarks, including bowing of the long bones, absent fibula, and irregular ossification of the small bones of the hands and feet. Histologic examination of bone and cartilage suggests defects in both membranous ossification and bone remodeling. Female carriers of the condition may have subtle suggestive facial, hand, and feet findings.

ETIOLOGY/EPIDEMIOLOGY: The disorder is inherited as an X-linked recessive trait. The gene for the condition has been linked to Xq28 and oto-palato-digital syndrome types I and II are most likely due to mutations in the same gene.

DIAGNOSIS: The diagnosis is based on the specific clinical and radiographic features and inheritance pattern. No biochemical or molecular confirmatory test is available.

TREATMENT
Standard Therapies: Treatment is symptomatic. Infants may have respiratory difficulties and require long-term airway management. Orthopedic and other surgical procedures to correct deformity may be required. Genetic counseling of families is advised.

REFERENCES
Fitch N, Jequier S, Papageorgiou A. A familial syndrome of cranial, facial, oral and limb abnormalities. *Clin Genet* 1976;10: 226–231.

Robertson SP, Walsh S, Oldridge M, et al. Linkage of otopalatodigital syndrome type 2 (OPD2) to distal Xq28: evidence for allelism with OPD1. *Am J Hum Genet* 2001;69:223–227.

Savarirayan R, Cormier-Daire V, Unger S, et al. Oto-palato-digital syndrome, type II: report of three cases with further delineation of the chondro-osseous morphology. *Am J Med Genet* 2000;95:193–200.

Taybi H, Lachman RS. *Radiology of syndromes, metabolic disorders, and skeletal dysplasias*, 4th ed. St. Louis: Mosby–Year Book, 1996.

RESOURCES

96, 149, 298

---

101 Pallister-Hall Syndrome

Penelope P. Feuillan, MD, and Leslie G. Biesecker, MD

DEFINITION: Pallister-Hall syndrome (PHS) is characterized by hypothalamic hamartoma (HH), bifid epiglottis, polydactyly, malformations of the kidneys, and imperforate anus.

SYNONYMS: Congenital hypothalamic hamartoblastoma syndrome; CAVE (cerebro-acro-visceral early lethality) complex; Hall-Pallister syndrome.

DIFFERENTIAL DIAGNOSIS: Oral-facial-digital syndromes; McKusick-Kaufman syndrome; Greig cephalopolysyndactyly syndrome; Short rib–polydactyly (Beemer-Langer) syndrome; Familial holoprosencephaly; Bardet-Biedl syndrome.

SYMPTOMS AND SIGNS: Diagnosis is usually made at birth, when polydactyly and imperforate anus are observed. Other skeletal abnormalities may include osseous syndactyly and short limbs. More severely affected infants may have impaired pituitary function, causing micropenis, hypothyroidism, growth hormone deficiency and, rarely, hypocortisolemia and diabetes insipidus. Laryngoscopy may show a bifid epiglottis. The diagnosis is often confirmed when MRI shows HH. Some patients may develop precocious puberty. Growth hormone deficiency may also be diagnosed in later childhood. Some patients have seizures. Intelligence and school and job performance are usually normal, although some patients have behavioral problems and some adults have complained of anxiety or depression. Headaches appear to be common. Fertility appears to be unaffected in patients with intact pituitary function.

ETIOLOGY/EPIDEMIOLOGY: PHS is associated with heterozygous mutations in the *GLI3* gene, which regulates other genes in early development of the fetus. Many cases are isolated; others have an autosomal-dominant inheritance, and multiple generations may be affected. Males and females are affected equally. The disorder has an estimated prevalence of less than 1,000 patients in the developed world.

DIAGNOSIS: In addition to a careful physical examination, evaluation should include a thorough family history, including the occurrence of polydactyly or endocrine dysfunction. Radiographic studies include a full skeletal survey to exclude skeletal dysplasia and MRI of the cerebrum to identify and estimate the dimensions of a hamartoma. Additional studies include renal ultrasonography to evaluate the kidneys and collecting system, and indirect or fiberoptic laryngoscopy to evaluate the epiglottis. The endocrine evaluation should include measurement of pituitary factors. If morning cortisol is low, adrenal function should be tested with a corticotropin stimulation test. A Giemsa-banded karyotype may help to distinguish patients with PHS from those with related disorders.

TREATMENT

Standard Therapies: Extra digits are customarily removed in infancy for social or biomechanical reasons. If the endocrine evaluation shows hormonal deficiencies, replacement with appropriate doses of hydrocortisone, thyroid hormone, or injections of human growth hormone is initiated. Precocious puberty is treated with one of the long-acting GnRH agonist-analogues, such as Lupron. Because HH is almost always a benign lesion that can be identified radiographically, neither biopsy nor surgery is recommended, except in unusual circumstances. Seizures may be treated with an anticonvulsant such as carbamazepine.

REFERENCES

Biesecker LG, Abbott M, Allen J, et al. Report from the workshop on Pallister-Hall syndrome and related phenotypes. *Am J Med Genet* 1996;65:76–81.

Feuillan P, Peters KF, Cutler Jr GB, et al. Evidence for decreased growth hormone in patients with hypothalamic hamartoma and the Pallister-Hall syndrome. *J Pediatr Endocrinol Metab* 2001;14:141–149.

Kang S, Graham JM, Olney AH, et al. *GLI3* frameshift mutations cause the Pallister-Hall syndrome. *Nat Genet* 1997;15:266–268.

Topf KF, Kletter G, Kelch RP, et al. Autosomal dominant transmission of the Pallister-Hall syndrome. *J Pediatr* 1993;123:943–946.

RESOURCES
29, 190, 386

102 Pallister-Killian Syndrome

*Shama Dhandha, MD,
and W. Allen Hogge, MD*

DEFINITION: Pallister-Killian syndrome (PKS) is characterized by multiple congenital anomalies, characteristic facial features, and mental retardation.

SYNONYMS: Tetrasomy 12p; Isochromosome 12p mosaicism.

DIFFERENTIAL DIAGNOSIS: Fryns syndrome; Wolf-Hirschhorn syndrome.

SYMPTOMS AND SIGNS: Patients with PKS have characteristic facies that are present at birth, but become more pronounced with age. Facial features are coarse, often with frontal bossing, temporofrontal balding, localized alopecia, absence of lateral or medial eyebrows and eyelashes, low-set or dysplastic ears, hypertelorism, exophthalmos, shallow upper orbital ridges, upward-slanting palpebral fissures, inner epicanthic folds, small nose, upturned nares, full cheeks, long and simple philtrum, and prominent upper lip. Affected individuals may also have a large mouth with downturned corners, high-arched palate, and short, often webbed, neck with excess nuchal skin. Hypopigmentation or hyperpigmentation of the skin may be present. From infancy, patchy depigmentation may be seen on Woods light examination. Other findings on physical examination include disproportionate shortness of upper and lower extremities, supernumerary nipples, anal atresia/stenosis, or anteriorly placed anus. Males may have a small scrotum or cryptorchidism. One fourth of patients have congenital heart defects. Ventricular septal defect is most frequent, but coarctation of the aorta, patent ductus arteriosus, atrial septal defect, and aortic stenosis may also occur. Congenital diaphragmatic hernia is also commonly seen. Other congenital anomalies may include cystic or dysplastic kidneys, neural tube defects, and abdominal wall defects. Patients usually have onset of seizures in early infancy. There is severe to profound mental and motor retar-dation. Most affected patients die prenatally, perinatally, or in the early postnatal period. Long-term survival has been reported, however, with 5 of 42 reported patients surviving to adulthood. With age, frontotemporal alopecia diminishes or disappears, the facies becomes increasingly coarse, lips thicken, the tongue increases in size and protrudes, and the mandible becomes large and protruding. Patients may develop kyphoscoliosis and joint contractures. Adult patients are nonverbal and generally lack all self-help skills. Most never learn to walk.

ETIOLOGY/EPIDEMIOLOGY: Pallister-Killian syndrome is due to mosaic tetrasomy for the short arm of chromosome 12. The proposed mechanisms involve centromeric misdivision and nondisjunction during maternal meiosis. This results in three copies of the short arm of chromosome 12 and one copy of the long arm of chromosome 12 in the oocyte. When fertilized with a normal sperm, the end result is four copies of the short arm of chromosome 12. It is associated with advanced maternal age and occurs sporadically.

DIAGNOSIS: The diagnosis is made by chromosome analysis. The aberrant chromosome is not found in lymphocytes, but can be identified in fibroblasts. Therefore, both blood and skin samples should be sent for karyotype. Prenatal diagnosis is possible with amniocentesis. Interphase fluorescence *in situ* hybridization on uncultured amniocytes may improve detection, because the isochromosome is often lost in culture.

TREATMENT
Standard Therapies: No treatment is available.

REFERENCES
Horneff G, Majewski F, Hildebrand B, et al. Pallister-Killian syndrome in older children and adolescents. *Pediatr Neurol* 1993;9:312–315.

Mowery-Rushton PA, Stadler M, Kochmar S, et al. The use of interphase FISH for prenatal diagnosis of Pallister-Killian syndrome. *Prenat Diagn* 1997;17:255–265.

Schinzel A. Tetrasomy 12p (Pallister-Killian syndrome). *J Med Genet* 1991;28:122–125.

Smulian J, Guzman E, Mohan C, et al. Genetics casebook. Pallister-Killian syndrome. *J Perinatol* 1996;16:406–412.

Struthers JL, Cuthbert CD, Khalifa MM. Parental origin of the isochromosome 12p in Pallister-Killian syndrome: molecular analysis of one patient and review of reported cases. *Am J Med Genet* 1999;84:111–115.

RESOURCES
387, 462

103   Parkes-Weber Syndrome

John B. Mulliken, MD

DEFINITION: Parkes-Weber syndrome denotes diffuse, microscopic arteriovenous fistulae, involving all tissues of the upper or lower limb.

SYNONYM: Giant limb of Robertson.

DIFFERENTIAL DIAGNOSIS: Klippel-Trenaunay syndrome; Diffuse, macular hemangioma of the limb and perineum with arteriovenous (AV) shunting.

SYMPTOMS AND SIGNS: This combined fast-flow vascular anomaly is obvious at birth. The lower limb is more commonly affected than the upper limb. The involved extremity is warm to the touch and covered by a geographic, pink, macular stain. In the lower limb, the capillary stain often extends into the buttock and lower abdomen. The limb is enlarged symmetrically, often with disparity in length. High-output congestive heart failure may be present at birth or appear later. Later complications include ischemic ulceration and pain.

DIAGNOSIS: Cutaneous warmth is increased in the limb in the areas of capillary blush. A bruit usually can be appreciated by auscultation and AV shunting is confirmed by Doppler study. MRI demonstrates muscular and skeletal overgrowth that exhibits an abnormal signal and enhancement. Magnetic resonance (MR) angiography and MR venography show generalized arterial and venous dilatation. Catheter angiography delineates discrete arteriovenous shunts, particularly at the joints. Lymphatic anomalies, including lymphedema and chylous reflux into the limb, have been reported.

TREATMENT
Standard Therapies: Emergent embolization is required for the rare congenital congestive heart failure. Embolization and sclerotherapy are useful for control of pain and to assist healing of cutaneous ulceration. Epiphyseal arrest is indicated if there is significant axial overgrowth.

REFERENCE
Mulliken JB, Young AE. *Vascular birthmarks: hemangiomas and malformations.* Philadelphia: WB Saunders, 1988:246–247, 264–265.

RESOURCES
357, 483

104   Parry-Romberg Syndrome

Wendy S. Susser, MD, and M. Shane Chapman, MD

DEFINITION: Parry-Romberg syndrome is an acquired progressive hemifacial atrophy involving the dermis, subcutaneous fat, muscle, and, sometimes, underlying bone. This hemiatrophy may rarely involve the ipsilateral or contralateral side of the body.

SYNONYMS: Progressive facial hemiatrophy; Progressive hemifacial atrophy; Romberg syndrome.

DIFFERENTIAL DIAGNOSIS: Linear scleroderma (en coup de sabre); Hemifacial microsomia; Goldenhar syndrome; Partial lipodystrophy; Posttraumatic atrophy.

SYMPTOMS AND SIGNS: Onset is usually in the first or second decade of life, although the diagnosis has been made in both neonates and older patients. The initial sign may be hyperpigmentation or hypopigmentation followed by atrophy of the deeper layers of skin and underlying structures. In contrast to linear scleroderma, where the skin appears to be sclerotic and bound down, there is only minimal cutaneous sclerosis. Typically, these changes are first noted superior to the eyebrow or just below the lower eyelid with slow progressive involvement of the ipsilateral face. Rarely, the trunk and extremities, either ipsilateral or contralateral to the facial atrophy, may also be affected. Ocular symptoms are reported in 10%–40% of cases. Enophthalmos secondary to orbital fatty tissue atrophy is the most common orbital finding, and seizures are the most common neurologic manifestation. Other neurologic abnormalities include hemiparesis, cranial nerve palsies, trigeminal neuralgia, hemiplegic migraines, ipsilateral cerebral calcification, intracranial aneurysms, vascular malformations, and cognitive abnormalities. Patients may also develop multiple benign tumors, hamartomas, muscle malformations, and dental anomalies. The course of this disorder is variable, because progression may cease at any time, resulting in a wide spectrum of clinical manifestations. The pathologic changes usually reach maximum severity 2–10 years after onset.

ETIOLOGY/EPIDEMIOLOGY: The etiology is unknown. Theories include sympathetic nerve dysfunction (abnormal sympathetic nerve development or inflammation of the sympathetic nervous system), meningoencephalitis, slow viral infection, trauma, cortical dysgenesis, autoimmunity, and disturbance of angiogenesis during growth and development.

DIAGNOSIS: The diagnosis is based primarily on clinical features. Central nervous system imaging may be indicated. A skin biopsy can be used to rule out localized sclerosis (en coup de sabre), but histology of skin samples of Parry-Romberg syndrome is nondiagnostic.

TREATMENT
Standard Therapies: Treatment is palliative. Atrophic areas may be augmented with filler substances such as silicone, collagen, inorganic implants, and fat transfer for cosmetic improvement. In addition, more complex reconstructive surgical procedures may be appropriate to restore facial contour defects; however, surgery should be deferred until the disease process has stabilized. Physical therapy referral may be indicated to prevent contractures. Associated neurologic disorders should be treated on a case-by-case basis.

REFERENCES
Chapman MS, Peraza JE, Spencer SK. Parry-Romberg syndrome with contralateral and ipsilateral extremity involvement. *J Cutan Med Surg* 1999;3:260–262.
Mazzeo N, Fisher JG, Mayer MH, et al. Progressive hemifacial atrophy (Parry-Romberg syndrome). Case report. *Oral Surg Oral Med Oral Pathol* 1995;79:30–35.
Miller MT, Spencer MT. Progressive hemifacial atrophy. A natural history study. *Trans Am Ophthalmol Soc* 1995;93:203–215.
Rodgers BO. *Progressive facial hemiatrophy: Romberg's disease: a review of 772 cases.* Washington, DC: Excerpta Medica Foundation, 1963:682–689. International congress series 66.
Woolfenden AR, Tong DC, Norbash AM, et al. Progressive facial hemiatrophy: abnormality of intracranial vasculature. *Neurology* 1998;50:1915–1917.

RESOURCES
368, 421

105 Pentalogy of Cantrell

Ingrid B. Kjellin, MD

DEFINITION: Pentalogy of Cantrell is a congenital syndrome characterized by defects of the lower sternum, anterior diaphragm, diaphragmatic pericardium, midline supraumbilical abdominal wall, and cardiac anomalies. The syndrome occurs in various degrees of severity.

SYNONYMS: Cantrell pentalogy; Cantrell syndrome; Cantrell deformity.

DIFFERENTIAL DIAGNOSIS: Isolated thoracic cardiac ectopy; Ectopia cordis associated with amniotic band syndrome; Body stalk anomaly syndrome.

SYMPTOMS AND SIGNS: In its most extreme manifestation, pentalogy of Cantrell presents at birth with both ectopia cordis and omphalocele. The abdominal wall defect may be limited to an umbilical hernia or diastasis of the rectus abdominis muscles. Varying degrees of sternal defects are seen, from a sternal cleft to absence of the xyphoid. Depending on the associated intracardiac anomalies, the degree of cardiovascular insufficiency varies. Prolonged cardiorespiratory support is often required. Other midline anomalies such as cleft lip, with or without cleft palate, and neural tube defects have been described.

ETIOLOGY/EPIDEMIOLOGY: The syndrome may result from a defect in the developmental field with failure of a segment of the lateral mesoderm at approximately 14 to 18 days of embryonic life. As a consequence, the transverse septum of the diaphragm does not develop. The intrinsic causes are probably heterogeneous and may include major gene mutation, teratogens, and mechanical teratogenesis by means of amniotic bands. Most cases are sporadic, and both sexes can be affected. The pentalogy of Cantrell has been reported to occur with trisomy 18. The prevalence of pentalogy of Cantrell is estimated to be 5.5 in 1 million live births.

DIAGNOSIS: Prenatal diagnosis is possible using ultrasonography, and is made on the basis of ectopia cordis and omphalocele. Chromosome analysis should be considered in every fetus and infant with suspected pentalogy of Cantrell. Echocardiography should be performed for evaluation of congenital heart disease. Anterior diaphragmatic and pericardial defects can be difficult to diagnose accurately with conventional radiography or sonography, and may have to be evaluated further with MRI. Other associated midline defects, such as neural tube defects, can also be studied further with MRI.

TREATMENT

Standard Therapies: In patients with severe congenital heart disease, emergency palliation procedures, such as balloon atrial septostomy, balloon pulmonary valvuloplasty, and Blalock-Taussig shunt placement may be necessary immediately after birth. A staged repair has been advocated in the most severe cases of pentalogy of Cantrell. The first operation immediately after birth provides separation of the peritoneal and pericardial cavities, coverage of the midline skin defect, and repair of the omphalocele. After appropriate growth of the thoracic cavity and lungs, the second stage procedure consists of intracardiac repair and return of the heart to the chest. Bilateral pectoralis muscle flaps can be created to support the underlying bifid sternum. At the age of 2 or 3 years, reconstruction of the lower sternum and epigastrium may be needed to give solid protection to the heart.

REFERENCES

Abdallah HI, Marks LA, Balsara RK, et al. Staged repair of pentalogy of Cantrell with tetrology of Fallot. *Ann Thorac Surg* 1993;56:979–980.

Cantrell JR, Haller JA, Ravitch MM. A syndrome of congenital defects involving the abdominal wall, sternum, diaphragm, pericardium and heart. *Surg Gynecol Obstet* 1958;107:602–614.

Carmi R, Boughman JA. Pentalogy of Cantrell and associated midline anomalies: a possible ventral midline developmental field. *Am J Med Genet* 1992;42:90–95.

Song A, McLeary MS. MR imaging of pentalogy of Cantrell variant with an intact diaphragm and pericardium. *Pediatr Radiol* 2000;30:638–639.

Toyama WM. Combined congenital defects of the anterior abdominal wall, sternum, diaphragm, pericardium, and heart: a case report and review of the syndrome. *Pediatrics* 1972;50:778–792.

RESOURCE

92

---

106   Pfeiffer Syndrome Type I

Millie D. Long, BA, and Kant Y.K. Lin, MD

DEFINITION: Pfeiffer syndrome consists of craniosynostosis, broad great toes and thumbs, and soft tissue syndactyly of the hands. Other common associated features include hypertelorism, down-slanting palpebral fissures, and midface hypoplasia.

DIFFERENTIAL DIAGNOSIS: Apert syndrome; Crouzon syndrome; Jackson-Weiss syndrome; Saethre-Chotzen syndrome.

SYMPTOMS AND SIGNS: Cranial vault features include craniosynostosis involving the coronal sutures, leading to a turribrachycephaly. Facial deformities include maxillary hypoplasia and mandibular prognathism. The nose can be beaked and the nasal bridge depressed. Pfeiffer syndrome shares many of the same features as Apert syndrome, but in a milder form. Eye anomalies include hypertelorbitism, down-slanting palpebral fissures, ocular proptosis, and strabismus. Infants with Pfeiffer syndrome type I usually are of normal intelligence, although mental deficiency has been noted. Common central nervous system anomalies include progressive hydrocephalus, calvarial midline defects, and cerebellar herniation. The extremities have a characteristic appearance with broad great toes and thumbs, usually varus in nature, along with brachydactyly and clinodactyly of the terminal phalanges.

ETIOLOGY/EPIDEMIOLOGY: Pfieffer syndrome is often familial. Inheritance is autosomal dominant with complete penetrance and variable expressivity. Genetic mutations have been found in the fibroblast growth factor receptor (*FGFR1*) gene located on chromosome 8, and the *FGFR2* gene on chromosome 10.

DIAGNOSIS: A familial history with a specific known mutation can allow for prenatal diagnosis of Pfeiffer syndrome type I. Diagnosis can be made by chorionic villus sampling or amniocentesis. After birth, a thorough physical examination usually suggests the diagnosis. CT and plain skull films can delineate the craniosynostosis and define the craniofacial skeletal deformities. DNA analysis can con-firm the diagnosis when the known mutations at *FGFR1* and *FGFR2* are identified.

TREATMENT
Standard Therapies: The timing and nature of the treatment are dictated by the functional disturbances in each individual patient. Most treatments are surgical, and early referral to a multidisciplinary craniofacial team can optimize the prognosis.

REFERENCES
Cohen MM, Maclean RE, eds. *Craniosynostosis: diagnosis, evaluation and management,* 2nd ed. New York: Oxford University Press, 2000:284–285, 354–360.
Gorlin RJ, Cohen MM, Levin LS, eds. *Syndromes of the head and neck,* 3rd ed. New York: Oxford University Press, 1990: 526–527.

RESOURCES
96, 121, 371

107 Pierre Robin Sequence

Cynthia A. Prows, MSN, RN, and Robert J. Hopkin, MD

DEFINITION: Pierre Robin sequence (PRS) is a syndrome characterized by micrognathia, glossoptosis, and cleft palate.

DIFFERENTIAL DIAGNOSIS: Stickler syndrome; Velo-cardio-facial syndrome; Fetal alcohol syndrome.

SYMPTOMS AND SIGNS: Newborns present with micrognathia and/or retrognathia, glossoptosis, and cleft palate. The glossoptosis can be severe enough to cause obstructive apnea.

ETIOLOGY/EPIDEMIOLOGY: PRS is seen equally in both males and females and has an incidence of approximately 1 in 3,000 to 1 in 30,000 live births. In PRS, micrognathia is the primary congenital anomaly, which results in secondary defects: glossoptosis and cleft palate. The abnormal mandible displaces the tongue back and up into the nasopharynx, preventing the palatal shelves from fusing at the midline during the 7–11 weeks postconception. The result can range from a bifid uvula or a submucous cleft palate to a complete cleft of the secondary palate.

The four broad etiologic categories for abnormal mandibular development in PRS are mechanical, terato-genic, genetic, and multifactorial. Mechanical factors that result in uterine constraint—such as intrauterine fibroids, bicornate uterus, and transverse positioning of the fetus—can inhibit normal development of the fetal mandible. Teratogenic agents include Accutane, alcohol, and tobacco. Genetic factors are the most common cause of PRS. These include chromosome abnormalities or single gene mutations that result in a syndrome or disorder that have specific patterns of congenital anomalies, which include micrognathia. Micrognathia can also be caused by a combination of genetic and environmental factors (multifactorial etiology).

DIAGNOSIS: Clinical identification of the classic triad of micrognathia, glossoptosis, and cleft palate is the first step in a diagnostic workup. Once PRS has been identified in a newborn, assessment by a clinical geneticist, together with evaluations of prenatal, perinatal, medical, and comprehensive family histories, determine which laboratory tests, imaging studies, and procedures are necessary.

TREATMENT
Standard Therapies: Treatment involves prevention or management of complications and surgical intervention for structural abnormalities. Obstructive apnea is a life-threatening complication and may not be clinically apparent at birth. Objective measurement with polysomnog-

raphy is strongly recommended. Keeping the resting neonate in a prone position can sometimes prevent obstructive apnea; however, newborns who experience intermittent or partial airway obstruction despite positioning require additional interventions. These may include the following: placement of a nasopharyngeal airway with or without continuous positive airway pressure; glossopexy; hyomandibulopexy; subperiosteal release of the floor of the mouth musculature on the mandible; or tracheotomy. Failure to thrive, a possible serious complication, can be prevented or reversed by using specialized cleft palate nursers and upright positioning during oral feedings or by using some form of gavage feeding to assure adequate caloric intake. Conductive hearing loss due to Eustachian tube dysfunction is another complication that can be prevented with aggressive management at the first signs of otitis media and myringotomy and insertion of percutaneous Eustachian tubes before or at the time of surgical palate repair. Surgical interventions include closure of the cleft palate (usually by 1 year) and, if the mandibular in-

volvement is severe enough, mandibular bone expansion (distraction osteogenesis).

REFERENCES

Caouette-Laberge L, Bayet B, Larocque Y. The Pierre Robin sequence: review of 125 cases and evolution of treatment modalities. *Plast Reconstr Surg* 1994;93:934–942.

Cohen SR, Simms C, Burstein FD, et al. Alternatives to tracheostomy in infants and children with obstructive sleep apnea. *J Pediatr Surg* 1999;34:182–187.

Holder-Espinasse M, et al. Pierre Robin sequence: a series of 117 consecutive cases. *J Pediatr* 2001;139:588–590.

Singer L, Sidoti EJ. Pediatric management of Robin sequence. *Cleft Palate Craniofac J* 1992;29:220–223.

Wilson A, Moore D, Moore M, et al. Late presentation of upper airway obstruction in Pierre Robin sequence. *Arch Dis Child* 2000;83:435–438.

RESOURCES

149, 392

108 Poland Syndrome

David B. Stevens, MD

DEFINITION: Poland syndrome is a sporadic, infrequent congenital deformity of the upper extremity manifested by a constant absence of the sternocostal head of the pectoralis muscle with inconstant retardation of breast development and deficiencies in the distal ipsilateral extremity, usually symbrachydactyly.

DIFFERENTIAL DIAGNOSIS: Isolated deficiencies of the upper extremity; Absence of ribs; Other congenital muscle defects of the thoracic wall; Klippel-Feil anomaly; Sprengel deformity.

SYMPTOMS AND SIGNS: The condition is recognizable at birth with the absence of the pectoralis major and the hand deformity, if present. Retardation of breast development is apparent in affected females at puberty. Dextrocardia may occur rarely.

ETIOLOGY/EPIDEMIOLOGY: The incidence has been reported at 1 in 32,000 births without familial occurrence. The etiology is uncertain. It may be genetic (with incomplete expression) or caused by some interruption of normal embryonic development. Isolated cases of familial involvement are rare, but have been reported. The leading theory of etiology is the subclavian artery supply disruption sequence. For some undefined reason, in the fifth to

sixth week of gestation, a disruption of the artery occurs, interrupting the internal thoracic artery, which supplies the chest wall origin of the pectoralis major and the breast. Such a blockage can also interfere with hand or distal extremity development. At a slightly different site in the artery and at a slightly different time, the same disruption is postulated to result in Moebius syndrome, Klippel-Feil anomaly, Sprengel anomaly, and possibly distal transverse limb deficiencies. Proponents of this theory attribute the disruption to some abnormality of embryonic development. None of the theories has been confirmed with laboratory or clinical evidence.

DIAGNOSIS: The diagnosis is established by an adequate physical examination of the entire person. As with any congenital deformity, a careful and thorough family history is indicated with examination of any family members with known defects. Careful questioning may reveal a defect of the chest wall previously ignored or forgotten. Genetic investigation with appropriate DNA analysis would be helpful in defining the natural history of the condition. A chest radiograph may discover a previously unknown dextrocardia.

TREATMENT
Standard Therapies: No treatment exists to change the individual's development. Little, if any, functional deficit results from the absent pectoralis major. Some have advo-

cated transfer of other chest wall muscles to replace the absent muscle. With such a minimal functional problem, however, major procedures would result in little gain. Breast augmentation or prosthetic replacement to achieve symmetry and relieve the cosmetic defect seem rational and worthwhile. For certain of the hand deformities, invasive procedures can be helpful, such as syndactyly release or thumb reconstruction. With one normal upper extremity and one helping hand, the low likelihood of further functional benefit should limit the extent of ongoing surgical procedures.

REFERENCES

Bouwes Bavinck JN, Weaver DD. Subclavian artery supply disruption sequence hypothesis of a vascular etiology for Poland, Klippel-Feil, and Moebius anomalies. *Am J Med Genet* 1986; 23:903–918.

McGillivray BC, Lowry RB. Poland syndrome in British Columbia: incidence and reproductive experience of affected persons. *Am J Med Genet* 1977;1:65–74.

Poland A. Deficiency of the pectoral muscles. *Guy's Hospital Rep* 1841;6:191–193.

Stevens DB, Fink BA, Prevel C. Poland's syndrome in one identical twin. *J Pediatr Orthop* 2000;20:392–395.

Weaver DD. Vascular etiology of limb defects: the subclavian artery supply disruption sequence. In: Herring JA, Birch JG, eds. *The child with a limb deficiency*. Chicago: American Academy of Orthopaedic Surgeons, 1998:25–37.

RESOURCES

75, 351

109 Prader-Willi Syndrome

Suzanne B. Cassidy, MD

DEFINITION: Prader-Willi syndrome (PWS) is a complex multisystem abnormality caused by a deficiency of paternal chromosome 15(q11-q13) that includes infantile hypotonia, early childhood–onset obesity, hypogonadism, developmental disability, behavioral abnormalities, mild short stature, and a characteristic facial appearance.

SYNONYM: Paternal chromosome 15(q11-q13) deficiency; HHHO syndrome.

DIFFERENTIAL DIAGNOSIS: Congenital myotonic dystrophy; Myopathies; Neuropathies; Spinal muscular atrophy; Albright hereditary osteodystrophy; Bardet-Biedl syndrome; Cohen syndrome; Borjeson-Forssman-Lehmann syndrome; Fragile X syndrome with obesity; 6q deletion; 1p36 deletion; Acquired hypothalmic insufficiency (Froehlich syndrome).

SYMPTOMS AND SIGNS: Severe hypotonia with poor suck and failure to thrive in early infancy are followed by excessive eating starting at 1–6 years of age, with resultant obesity unless externally controlled. Hypogonadotrophic hypogonadism is present in both males and females and is manifested by genital hypoplasia (small penis, hypoplastic scrotum, and cryptorchidism in males; hypoplasia of labia minora and clitoris in females) and pubertal insufficiency (lack of normal beard growth, voice change, male body habitus, and body hair in males; amenorrhea or oligomenorrhea in females). Mild short stature is associated with growth hormone deficiency. Characteristic facial appearance includes narrow bifrontal diameter, almond-shaped palpebral fissures, and a downturned mouth with a thin upper lip. All patients have some degree of cognitive impairment, usually mild mental retardation. The distinctive behavioral phenotype includes temper tantrums and obsessive-compulsive behavior. Sleep disturbance (excessive sleeping), scoliosis, high pain threshold, skin picking, and decreased saliva flow are common.

ETIOLOGY/EPIDEMIOLOGY: Prader-Willi syndrome is due to deficiency of the paternal contribution to chromosome 15(q11-q13) from interstitial deletion 15(q11-q13), maternal uniparental disomy 15, or imprinting defect. Frequency is 1 in 10,000 to 1 in 15,000, and it occurs in both sexes and all ethnic groups.

DIAGNOSIS: All cases are detected by abnormality on DNA methylation analysis using the methylation-sensitive *SNRPN* probe. Deletion cases are detected by fluorescence *in situ* hybridization (FISH) for *SNRPN*. Uniparental disomy cases are identified by microsatellite analysis of parental and child DNA. Imprinting defects are diagnosed by abnormal (maternal only) methylation analysis with negative FISH and uniparental disomy results.

TREATMENT

Standard Therapies: Therapy includes assurance of adequate caloric intake in early infancy, often requiring gavage but not gastrostomy feeding, as it is transient. Supportive treatment for excessive eating and obesity consists of an approximately 1,000 kcal/day diet due to decreased caloric requirement, exercise, and restricted access to food. Other treatments include growth hormone replacement therapy, sex hormone replacement, special education, behavioral therapy, and sometimes use of psychoactive medication such as specific serotonin reuptake inhibitors. No surgical therapies are effective for obesity. Scoliosis is managed as in the general population.

Investigational Therapies: Growth hormone replacement in adults is being explored.

REFERENCES

Cassidy SB. Prader-Willi syndrome [Syndrome of the Month]. *J Med Genet* 1997;34:917–923.

Greenswag LR, Alexander RA, eds. *Management of Prader-Willi syndrome*, 2nd ed. New York: Springer-Verlag, 1995.

Holm VA, Cassidy SB, Butler MG, et al. Prader-Willi syndrome: consensus diagnostic criteria. *Pediatrics* 1993;91:398–402.

Report of the ASHG/ACMG Test and Technology Transfer Committee. Diagnostic testing for Prader-Willi and Angelman syndromes. *Am J Hum Genet* 1996;58:1085–1088.

Ritzen EM, Lindgren AC, Hagenas L, et al. Growth hormone treatment of patients with Prader-Willi syndrome. Swedish Growth Hormone Advisory Group. *J Pediatr Endocrinol Metab* 1999;12(suppl 1):345–349.

RESOURCES

362, 399

---

110   Neonatal Progeroid Syndrome

Eniko K. Pivnick, MD

DEFINITION: Neonatal progeroid syndrome (NPS) is an autosomal-recessive disorder composed of generalized lipoatrophy except for fat pads in the suprabuttock areas; hypotrichosis of the scalp hair, eyebrows, and eyelashes; relative macrocephaly; triangular face; natal teeth; and micrognathia.

SYNONYM: Wiedemann-Rautenstrauch syndrome.

DIFFERENTIAL DIAGNOSIS: Hallerman-Streiff syndrome; De Barsy syndrome; Hutchinson-Gilford syndrome; Cockayne syndrome; Berardinelli-Seip syndrome; Leprechaunism syndrome; Carbohydrate deficient glycoprotein syndrome type 1.

SYMPTOMS AND SIGNS: Infants with NPS have a peculiar appearance at birth, including a head that is disproportionately large for the face; prominent scalp veins; triangular, aged face; wrinkled skin; and decreased subcutaneous fat. Natal teeth are variably present. Paradoxic caudal fat accumulation is present in approximately half of patients. Severe intrauterine growth retardation, later growth retardation, and failure to thrive are typical. The disease is usually lethal by 7 months; however, on rare occasions, patients have survived into infancy or the teens. Radiologic abnormalities are common in NPS, including a large neurocranium, wide cranial sutures, trident configuration of the acetabula, and irregular metaphyses of the long bones. Endocrine abnormalities including hypothyroidism, hypertriglyceridemia, and hyperprolactinemia have been reported. Genital anomalies, particularly cryptorchidism, are common. Neuropathologic findings in NPS include generalized demyelination of the white matter in the central nervous system with or without an accumulation of neutral fats in macrophages. Other central nervous system abnormalities include ventricular dilatation with cortical atrophy and Dandy-Walker malformation. Psychomotor retardation is another variable manifestation. Most patients show significant developmental delay at an early age and die in early childhood.

ETIOLOGY/EPIDEMIOLOGY: NPS is inherited in an autosomal-recessive manner. Pathogenesis is not clear. Fewer than 30 cases have been reported. No racial predilection exists, and males and females are affected equally.

DIAGNOSIS: Diagnosis is based on clinical presentation. Patients should be tested for insulin resistance, abnormalities of lipid metabolism, and dysfunction of the hypothalamic–pituitary axis at birth and at periodic follow-up evaluations.

TREATMENT
Standard Therapies: There is no effective treatment.

REFERENCES

Hou JW, Wang TR. Clinical variability in neonatal progeroid syndrome. *Am J Med Genet* 1995;58:195–196.

Martin JJ, Ceuterick CM, Leroy JG, et al. The Wiedemann-Rautenstrauch or neonatal progeroid syndrome: neuropathological study of a case. *Neuropediatrics* 1984;15:43–48.

Obregon MG, Bergami GL, Gianotti A, et al. Radiographic findings in Wiedemann-Rautenstrauch syndrome. *Pediatr Radiol* 1992;22:474–475.

Pivnick EK, Angle B, Kaufman RA, et al. The neonatal progeroid (Wiedemann-Ratenstrauch) syndrome. Report of five new cases and review of the literature. *Am J Med Genet* 2000; 90:131–140.

Rautenstrauch T, Snigula F, Wiedemann HR. Neonatales progeroides syndrome (Wiedemann-Rautenstrauch): Eine follow-up-Studie. *Klin Pediatr* 1994;206:440–443.

Wiedemann HR. An unidentified neonatal progeroid syndrome: follow-up report. *Eur J Pediatr* 1979;130:65–70.

RESOURCES
209, 368

---

111 Proteus Syndrome

Leslie G. Biesecker, MD

DEFINITION: Proteus syndrome is an overgrowth condition that affects the body in a patchy or mosaic manner. It causes overgrowth of bones, fatty tissues, and skin.

SYNONYM: Encephalocraniocutaneous lipomatosis.

DIFFERENTIAL DIAGNOSIS: Hemihyperplasia with multiple lipomatosis; Mafucci syndrome; Enchondromatosis; Klippel-Trenaunay syndrome.

SYMPTOMS AND SIGNS: Patients are commonly born without noticeable abnormalities, although occasional patients are born with large, complex mixed vascular malformations. Congenital capillary vascular malformations are common. In infancy, parents generally note overgrowth, usually digital. This often begins as enlargement of phalanges near the epiphysis with overlying thickening and hardening of the soft tissues. This also commonly occurs at the knees but can occur in any part of the body in an irregular pattern. The spine is commonly affected with resulting scoliosis. In childhood, patients also develop linear epidermal nevi. A characteristic lesion is the connective tissue nevus, also called the moccasin sole or cerebriform lesion. The progressive nature of the bony overgrowth limits the range of motion of the affected joints, with the end result that the joint is massively overgrown and fixed. Other affected organs include the spleen, thymus, uterus, and colon. Patients may develop progressive pulmonary cystic dysplasia. Infiltrative lipomas may involve large portions of the limbs and trunk, and can invade the spinal canal. Another serious complication is deep venous thrombosis and pulmonary embolism. Some patients have mental retardation, often associated with central nervous system malformations or hemimegencephaly. Seizures have been reported. A predisposition to tumors exists, especially cystadenomas of the ovary and tunica albuginea in young children and mesothelioma.

ETIOLOGY/EPIDEMIOLOGY: The disorder is hypothesized to be caused by a mutation in a growth regulatory gene that occurs after fertilization of the embryo. Affected persons are mosaics and the mutation is lethal in the non-mosaic state. Proteus syndrome affects several hundred persons in the developed world.

DIAGNOSIS: Diagnosis is made using published clinical diagnostic criteria. Useful diagnostic modalities include plain radiography, CT for skull lesions, high-resolution CT of the lungs for pulmonary cysts, and MRI of the brain, abdomen, pelvis, and limbs, as indicated. Ultrasonography is used for scrotal or ovarian masses. Encephalocraniocutaneous lipomatosis is considered to be a form of Proteus syndrome that is limited to the head and neck.

TREATMENT
Standard Therapies: Surgical therapy is indicated for symptoms such as the bony overgrowth that interferes with joint function, scoliosis, and angular deformities (most commonly of the knees and ankles). Splenectomy is indicated in patients with thrombocytopenia or red cell sequestration. Similarly, reduction surgery or resection for overgrown tissues such as thymus, uterus, and ovaries is indicated. All surgical patients must be closely monitored for deep venous thrombosis and pulmonary embolism. The same is true for patients who may be immobilized for long periods of time. At this time, chronic anticoagulation is not indicated.

REFERENCES
Biesecker LG. Multifaceted challenges of Proteus syndrome: NIH Clinical Center Grand Rounds. *JAMA* (in press).
Biesecker LG, Happle R, Mulliken JB, et al. Proteus syndrome: diagnostic criteria, differential diagnosis, and patient evaluation. *Am J Med Genet* 1999;84:389–395.
Biesecker LG, Peters KF, Darling TN, et al. Clinical differentiation between Proteus syndrome and hemihyperplasia: description of a distinct form of hemihyperplasia. *Am J Med Genet* 1998; 79:311–318.
Gordon PL, Wilroy RS, Lasater OE, et al. Neoplasms in Proteus syndrome. *Am J Med Genet* 1995;57:74–78.
Slavotinek AM, Vacha SJ, Peters KF, et al. Sudden death caused by pulmonary thromboembolism in Proteus syndrome. *Clin Genet* 2000;58:386–389.

RESOURCES
184, 351, 406

112 PTEN Hamartoma Tumor Syndrome

Robert Pilarski, MS,
Heather Hampel, MS,
and Charis Eng, MD, PhD

DEFINITION: The PTEN hamartoma tumor syndrome (PHTS) includes hamartomas and cancer characterized by germline PTEN mutations. Clinically, PHTS includes Cowden syndrome (CS) and Bannayan-Riley-Ruvalcaba syndrome (BRR). CS is a multiple hamartoma syndrome with a high risk of benign and malignant tumors of the thyroid, breast, and endometrium (Insert Fig. 35). BRR is characterized by macrocephaly, intestinal polyposis, lipomas, and pigmented macules of the glans penis.

SYNONYMS: For CS: Multiple hamartoma syndrome. For BRR: Bannayan-Zonana syndrome; Riley-Smith syndrome; Ruvalcaba-Myhre-Smith syndrome (see entry in Gastrointestinal Disorders).

DIFFERENTIAL DIAGNOSIS: Proteus syndrome; Peutz-Jeghers syndrome; Sotos syndrome; Juvenile polyposis; Darier-White disease.

SYMPTOMS AND SIGNS: The pathognomonic signs for CS are mucocutaneous—at least 99% of affected individuals have these findings, which include trichilemmomas and papillomatous papules. Acral and plantar keratoses are also common. Individuals with CS usually have macrocephaly and dolicocephaly, as well as a high risk for breast, thyroid, and endometrial cancers. Skin cancers, renal cell carcinomas, and brain tumors are occasionally seen. Common features of BRR, in addition to those mentioned, include large birth weight, developmental delay and mental deficiency, a myopathic process in proximal muscles and joint hyperextensibility, pectus excavatum, and scoliosis. Patients with BRR with *PTEN* gene mutations are believed to have the cancer risks associated with CS. The gastrointestinal hamartomatous polyps in BRR may occasionally be associated with intussusception, but rectal bleeding and oozing of "serum" are more common.

ETIOLOGY/EPIDEMIOLOGY: PHTS is an autosomal-dominant condition caused by mutations in the *PTEN* gene, located on chromosome arm 10q. Approximately 80% of individuals diagnosed with CS and 50% of individuals diagnosed with BRR have a detectable *PTEN* gene mutation. CS is estimated to affect 1 in 300,000 individuals worldwide, but is underdiagnosed. The incidence of BRR is unknown. Germline *PTEN* mutations have been found to be responsible for a proportion of patients with Proteus syndrome (see Proteus Syndrome entry) and a Proteus-like syndrome.

DIAGNOSIS: Consensus diagnostic criteria for CS have been developed; pathognomonic criteria consist of facial trichilemmomas, acral keratoses, papillomatous lesions, and mucosal lesions. Major criteria for diagnosis are breast and thyroid cancers; macrocephaly; Lhermitte-Duclos disease; and endometrial carcinoma. Minor criteria are other thyroid lesions; mental retardation; gastrointestinal hamartomas; fibrocystic disease of the breast; lipomas; fibromas; and genitourinary tumors or malformation. Diagnostic criteria for BRR are based heavily on the presence of the aforementioned cardinal features.

TREATMENT

Standard Therapies: Women with CS should undergo increased breast cancer screening. Men should also perform monthly breast self-examinations. Women should receive endometrial cancer screening. Both men and women with CS should receive a comprehensive annual physical examination starting at age 18 (or 5 years before the youngest component cancer diagnosis in the family). Individuals with CS should undergo a baseline colonoscopy at age 50 (unless symptoms arise earlier). They should also undergo annual urinalysis to help detect renal carcinoma. Screening recommendations have not been established for BRR; however, patients with BRR and a germline *PTEN* mutation should undergo the same surveillance as CS patients. Patients with BRR should be monitored for complications related to gastrointestinal hamartomatous polyposis, which can be more severe than in CS. Myopathy in BRR has been treated successfully with carnitine in some patients.

REFERENCES

Eng C. Will the real Cowden syndrome please stand up?: revised diagnostic criteria. *J Med Genet* 2000;37:828–830.

Eng C, Parsons R. Cowden syndrome. In: Vogelstein B, Kinzler K, eds. *The genetic basis of human cancer.* New York: McGraw-Hill, 1998.

Gorlin RJ, Cohen MM, Condon LM, et al. Bannayan-Riley-Ruvalcaba syndrome. *Am J Med Genet* 1992;44:307–314.

Marsh DJ, Kum JB, Lunetta KL, et al. *PTEN* mutation spectrum and genotype-phenotype correlations in Bannayan-Riley-Ruvalcaba syndrome suggest a single entity with Cowden syndrome. *Hum Mol Genet* 1999;8:1461–1472.

Zhou XP, Hampel H, Thiele H, et al. Association of germline mutation in the *PTEN* tumor suppressor gene and Proteus and Proteus-like syndromes. *Lancet* 2001;358:210–211.

RESOURCES

351, 462

113 Multiple Pterygium Syndrome

Gregory M. Enns, MB, ChB

DEFINITION: Multiple pterygium syndrome is an autosomal-recessive condition that features minor facial anomalies, short stature, vertebral defects, joint contractures, and pterygia of the neck, axillae, antecubital and popliteal fossae, intercrural area, and digits.

SYNONYMS: Escobar syndrome; Multiple pterygium syndrome of Escobar type.

DIFFERENTIAL DIAGNOSIS: Popliteal pterygium syndrome; Lethal multiple pterygium syndrome; Fetal akinesia sequence; Femoral hypoplasia–unusual facies syndrome; Neck pterygia are common in Turner, Noonan, and LEOPARD syndromes.

SYMPTOMS AND SIGNS: Down-slanting palpebral fissures, epicanthic folds, long philtrum, low-set ears, and a pointed, receding chin are common facial features. Ptosis and cleft palate may be present. Patients typically have short stature. Pterygia occur in the cervical area in nearly all patients, but involvement of the axillae, popliteal and antecubital fossae, and digits is also common. Intercrural webs are seen in 40% of patients. Cryptorchidism and absent labia majora occur in more than 50% of patients. Popliteal pterygia may cause an unusual stance and interfere with walking. The pterygia tend to become more severe with time and may cause traction deformities. Camptodactyly, syndactyly, and rocker-bottom feet are relatively frequent findings. Kyphoscoliosis and vertebral segmentation anomalies, especially fusion defects, affect approximately two thirds of patients. Abnormal ossicles may lead to conductive hearing loss. Other skeletal anomalies include rib fusions, radial head and hip dislocations, talipes calcaneovalgus or equinovarus, and absent or dysplastic patellae.

ETIOLOGY/EPIDEMIOLOGY: Multiple pterygium syndrome is an autosomal-recessive condition of unknown cause. The population frequency is unknown.

DIAGNOSIS: Multiple pterygium syndrome is diagnosed based on clinical features and should be considered in patients with webs across different body joints. The subtle facial features described above may also assist in making a diagnosis. Skeletal anomalies, especially vertebral defects, are relatively common; radiographs of the complete skeleton should be obtained. Diagnostic abnormalities are not apparent on histologic examination of muscle or nerve. Multiple pterygium syndrome has overlapping features with popliteal pterygium syndrome, but lower lip pits and autosomal-dominant inheritance in the latter condition may assist in distinguishing these disorders. A detailed family history is essential to obtain. The lethal multiple pterygium syndrome is a separate entity that is characterized by stillbirth or early neonatal death and autosomal-recessive inheritance. These patients typically have lung hypoplasia and other anomalies, including diaphragmatic hernia, and heart, renal, and brain defects.

TREATMENT

Standard Therapies: Therapy is supportive and depends on the severity of the pterygia and kyphoscoliosis. Scoliosis develops before age 5 in most patients, and orthopedics should be involved with patient care from the start. A small thoracic cage, secondary to kyphoscoliosis, increases the risk of developing pneumonia. Respiratory problems cause significant morbidity and even mortality in infancy, and any infection must be treated promptly. Contracture releases have been performed with variable outcome. Physical therapy is important to help minimize contractures. Ptosis may interfere with vision, so early ophthalmology referral is prudent. The risk of conductive hearing loss is significant; patients should have a formal audiology evaluation.

REFERENCES

Chen H, Chang C-H, Misra RP, et al. Multiple pterygium syndrome. *Am J Med Genet* 1980;7:91–102.

Escobar V, Bixler D, Gleiser S, et al. Multiple pterygium syndrome. *Am J Dis Child* 1978;132:609–611.

Gorlin RJ, Cohen MM, Levin LS. Multiple pterygium syndrome. In: *Syndromes of the head and neck*, 3rd ed. New York: Oxford University Press, 1990:626–629.

Hall JG. Arthrogryposis multiplex congenita: etiology, genetics, classification, diagnostic approach, and general aspects. *J Pediatr Orthop* 1997;6:159–166.

Ramer JC, Ladda RL, Demuth WW. Multiple pterygium syndrome: an overview. *ADJC* 1988;142:794–798.

RESOURCE

351

114   Popliteal Pterygium Syndrome

Fung-Ki Wong, BDS, PhD

DEFINITION: Popliteal pterygium syndrome (PPS) is a congenital condition with multiple malformations and high clinical variability. Major features include cleft lip with or without cleft palate, paramedial pits or mucous cysts on the lower lip, popliteal pterygium, and digital and genital anomalies.

SYNONYM: Facial-genito-popliteal syndrome.

DIFFERENTIAL DIAGNOSIS: Bartsocas-Papas syndrome; Escobar syndrome; Hay-Wells syndrome.

SYMPTOMS AND SIGNS: Oral-facial findings include cleft lip with or without cleft palate, paramedial pits or mucous cysts on the lower lip, syngnathia (intraoral tissue bands), and ankyloblepharon. Cutaneous and musculoskeletal findings include popliteal pterygium, hypoplasia or absence of digits, variable syndactyly of the second to fifth toes, pyramidal skin over the hallux, hypoplastic toenails, spina bifida, scoliosis, or lordosis. Genitourinary findings include cryptorchidism; absent, cleft, or ectopic scrotum; small penis; and inguinal hernia in males and absence or displacement of the labia majora, enlarged clitoris, and hypoplastic uterus in females.

ETIOLOGY/EPIDEMIOLOGY: The etiology of PPS is unknown, but genetic linkage to the van der Woude syndrome locus at chromosome 1q32 has been suggested. The incidence of PPS is 1 in 300,000 births. Most cases are sporadic, but familial cases appear as autosomal dominant with reduced penetrance and variable expressivity.

DIAGNOSIS: Popliteal pterygium, the hallmark of PPS, may not appear in every case. Toe syndactyly is a useful diagnostic sign. However, cleft lip with or without cleft palate together with the pyramidal skin over the hallux is sufficient for the diagnosis.

TREATMENT

Standard Therapies: Treatment of PPS involves surgical correction of ankyloblepharon and syngnathia to facilitate eye and mouth opening and surgical repair of cleft lip, palate, and lower lip pits. Surgery on the popliteal pterygium must be performed with caution because of the superficial location of the sciatic nerve, popliteal artery, and abnormal muscle connections.

REFERENCES
Gorlin RJ, Cohen MM Jr, Levin LS. Popliteal pterygium syndrome (facio-genito-popliteal syndrome). In: *Syndromes of the head and neck.* Oxford: Oxford University Press, 1990: 629–631.
Hunter A. The popliteal pterygium syndrome: report of a new family and review of the literature. *Am J Med Genet* 1990;36: 196–208.
Lees MM, Winter RM, Malcolm S, et al. Popliteal pterygium syndrome: a clinical study of three families and report of linkage to the Van der Woude syndrome locus on 1q32. *J Med Genet* 1999;36:888–892.
Wong FK, Gustafsson B. Popliteal pterygium syndrome in a Swedish family—clinical findings and genetic analysis with the van der Woude syndrome locus at 1q32-q41. *Acta Odontol Scand* 2000;58:85–88.

RESOURCES
96, 351

115   Pyknodysostosis

Malcolm Harris, DSc, MD, FDSRCS, FRCS(Edin)

DEFINITION: Pyknodysostosis is a sclerosing osteochondrodysplasia.

DIFFERENTIAL DIAGNOSIS: Osteopetrosis; Cleidocranial dysostosis.

SYMPTOMS AND SIGNS: Dwarfism, osteopetrosis, abbreviated terminal phalanges (acroosteolysis), clavicular dysplasia, and hypoplasia of the mandibular angles and cranial anomalies (including frontal and occipital bossing) occur. The dwarfism is due to short limbs rather than a short trunk. Affected individuals also may have narrow shoulders, partial or complete aplasia of the clavicles, exophthalmos, and fractures in response to minimal trauma. Orofacial features include underdeveloped facial bones and relative mandibular prognathism, persistent deciduous teeth, and enamel hypoplasia and a grooved palate. The hypoplastic mandible may predispose patients to obstructive sleep apnea. Radiologic features include hypoplastic paranasal sinuses, wormian bones in the lamboidal area, persistence of fontanelles, and failure of suture closure.

ETIOLOGY/EPIDEMIOLOGY: The disorder is an idiopathic condition with autosomal-recessive inheritance. Only 133 cases were reported in the 1998 literature.

DIAGNOSIS: Diagnosis is suggested by characteristic short stature and facies, with increased thickness of bones due to increased density of the trabecular bone, but with a tendency for fractures. Histologically, the osteoclasts appear to be normal in both appearance and their attachment to the bone surface, with ruffled borders and adjacent clear zone. Large, intracellular vacuoles containing collagen fibrils may be present, indicating a defect in intracellular lysosomal degradation of the organic matrix. The osteoclast has a cathepsin K deficiency (a major matrix resorbing protease-cysteine protease), which is responsible for impaired type 1 collagenolytic, elastinolytic, and gelatinolytic activity. There is slow but satisfactory bone healing.

TREATMENT
Standard Therapies: No specific therapy exists, apart from advancing the mandible and/or the hyoid bone to relieve the obstructive sleep dyspnea.

REFERENCES
Gorlin RJ, Cohen MM, Levin LS. *Syndromes of the head and neck,* 3rd ed. Oxford: Oxford University Press, 1990:285–287.
Hunt NP, Cunningham SJ, Adnan N, et al. The dental, craniofacial, and biochemical features of pyknodysostosis: a report of three cases. *J Oral Maxillofac Surg* 1998;56:497–504.
Maroteaux P, Lamy M. The malady of Toulouse-Lautrec. *JAMA* 1965;191:715.

RESOURCES
7, 96, 351

116 Rieger Syndrome

Jeffrey C. Murray, MD, and Elena V. Semina, PhD

DEFINITION: Rieger syndrome is a hereditary developmental disorder characterized by anomalies of the anterior segment of the eye, face, dentition, and umbilicus caused by mutations in the transcription factors *PITX2, FOXC1,* or other yet unknown genes.

SYNONYMS: Axenfeld-Rieger syndrome; Iridogoniodysgenesis syndrome.

DIFFERENTIAL DIAGNOSIS: Axenfeld-Rieger anomaly; Iris hypoplasia; Peter plus syndrome; Aarskog syndrome; Robinow syndrome; SHORT syndrome; Cataract-dental syndrome.

SYMPTOMS AND SIGNS: Rieger syndrome is an association of specific ocular features with some systemic abnormalities, mostly of the craniofacial, dental, and umbilical regions. Ocular features affect the anterior segment of the eye and include posterior embryotoxon (a white ring in the peripheral cornea that is believed to be an anteriorly displaced Schwalbe line of trabecular meshwork), irido-corneal adhesions, iris hypoplasia, and glaucoma, which is the most debilitating feature and affects approximately 50% of patients. Dental anomalies may include missing incisors, microdontia, oligodontia, and misshapen teeth. Umbilical anomalies include failure of the periumbilical skin to involute, umbilical hernia, and omphalocele in severe cases. The most frequent other associated features include flattened midface, hearing loss, growth hormone deficiency and pituitary anomalies, cardiac defects, and hypospadius in males.

ETIOLOGY/EPIDEMIOLOGY: The prevalence is estimated to be 1 in 200,000. Rieger syndrome is transmitted by autosomal-dominant inheritance in most families. Within any single pedigree there is complete penetrance, but variable expressivity of the symptoms may be due to influence of modifying genes and/or environmental factors. Variation of the phenotype between families can also be attributed to significant genetic heterogeneity of the disorder: four different linkage loci with two causative genes, *PITX2* and *FOXC1,* have been identified.

DIAGNOSIS: The diagnosis should be suspected based on clinical findings: identification of characteristic ocular, dental, or umbilical features. Presence of the other classic features and other affected family members confirms the diagnosis.

TREATMENT

Standard Therapies: The glaucoma associated with Rieger syndrome is difficult to control with medication, and surgery is often unsuccessful. The iridocorneal adhesions are often surgically removed. The dental defects require orthodontic and prosthodontic treatment because of malocclusion associated with multiple missing teeth. The umbilical features are cosmetic in most patients, but umbilical hernias and omphalocele require surgical intervention in severe cases.

REFERENCES

Alward WLM. Axenfeld-Rieger syndrome in the age of molecular genetics. *Am J Ophthalmol* 2000;130:107–115.

Amendt BA, Semina EV, Alward WL. Rieger syndrome: a clinical, molecular, and biochemical analysis. *Cell Mol Life Sci* 2000; 57:1652–1666.

Mirzayans F, Gould DB, Heon E, et al. Axenfeld-Rieger syndrome resulting from mutation of the *FKHL7* gene on chromosome 6p25. *Eur J Hum Genet* 2000;8:71–74.

Nishimura DY, Searby CC, Borges AS, et al. Identification of a fourth Rieger syndrome locus at 16q24. *Am J Hum Genet* 2000;67:2146.

Phillips JC, del Bono EA, Haines JL, et al. A second locus for Rieger syndrome maps to chromosome 13q14. *Am J Hum Genet* 1996;59:613–619.

Semina EV, Reiter R, Leysens NJ, et al. Cloning and characterization of a novel bicoid-related homeobox transcription factor gene, *RIEG*, involved in Rieger syndrome. *Nat Genet* 1996;14: 392–399.

RESOURCES

297, 355

---

117   Roberts Pseudothalidomide Syndrome

Anil K. Mandal, MD

DEFINITION: Roberts syndrome (RS) is a recessively inherited condition characterized by symmetric limb defects, craniofacial abnormalities, and prenatal and postnatal growth retardation, with or without mental retardation.

SYNONYMS: Pseudothalidomide syndrome; SC-phocomelia syndrome.

DIFFERENTIAL DIAGNOSIS: Baller-Gerold syndrome.

SYMPTOMS AND SIGNS: The most severely affected infants have phocomelia involving all four extremities, clefting of the lip and palate, and striking prenatal growth retardation. The limb abnormalities range from mild reduction in the number and length of bones of the arms and legs to complete absence of all extremities except for rudimentary digits (Insert Fig. 36). The upper limbs tend to be more severely affected than the lower limbs. Flexion contractures of joints are common. Craniofacial abnormalities also show variable severity. Microcephaly is common, although hydrocephaly has been noted. Some patients have craniosynostosis, causing confusion with Baller-Gerold syndrome. Ophthalmologic abnormalities may include shallow orbits with resulting proptosis, hypertelorism, telecanthus, cloudy corneas (Insert Fig. 37) cataracts, and glaucoma. The nasal alae tend to be hypoplastic. Capillary hemangiomas of the face are frequently present. Radiologic investigation may show dysplastic shoulder joints and ab-

sence of both ulnae and radii. In the lower extremities, there may be hypoplastic hip joints, shortened and deformed tibiae, and absence of both fibulae. Among the less frequent abnormalities are encephalocele, exencephaly, and congenital heart disease. Both prenatal and postnatal growth retardation occur. The length of survival correlates directly with the severity of craniofacial and limb involvement. Severely affected children rarely survive past 1 month of age. Mental retardation is characteristic of most children who survive the neonatal period.

ETIOLOGY/EPIDEMIOLOGY: The pattern of tissues affected in RS suggests that the mutated gene or genes may be involved in basic cell metabolism, with those organs that are most sensitive to a reduction in growth rate being affected to the greatest degree. RS has been identified in individuals of variable ethnic backgrounds. The small number of reported cases and the high incidence of consanguinity imply that RS is a rare genetic disorder.

DIAGNOSIS: The clinical diagnosis may be confirmed by chromosomal analysis demonstrating a characteristic premature centromere separation in mitotic cells. This separation is often referred to as puffing, and the chromosome may have a "railroad track" appearance because of the absence of the constriction at the centromere. The characteristic centromere puffing has allowed prenatal diagnosis using samples obtained by chorionic villus sampling and amniocentesis. Fetal ultrasonographic examinations may also be valuable, although abnormalities in the limbs may not be apparent until 16 weeks' gestation.

TREATMENT

Standard Therapies: The primary treatment is prevention. Prenatal ultrasonographic examinations combined with amniocyte chromosome analysis are powerful tools for prenatal diagnosis. Families at risk can monitor subsequent pregnancies and make informed decisions. Patients with phenotypically mild abnormalities may require surgery to repair craniofacial or limb anomalies and minimal to full-time care depending on their degree of mental retardation.

REFERENCES

Holden KR, Jabs EW, Sponseller PD. Roberts pseudothalidomide syndrome and normal intelligence: approaches to diagnosis and management. *Dev Med Child Neurol* 1992;34:534–538.

Huson SM, Rodgers CS, Hall CM, et al. The Baller-Gerold syndrome: phenotypic and cytogenetic overlap with Roberts syndrome. *J Med Genet* 1990;27:371–375.

Mandal AK, Singh AP, Rao L, et al. Roberts Pseudothalidomide syndrome. *Arch Ophthalmol* 2000;118:1462–1463.

Otano L, Matayoshi T, Gadow EC. Roberts syndrome: first-trimester prenatal diagnosis. *Prenat Diagn* 1996;16:770–771.

Robins DB, Ladda RL, Thieme GA, et al. Prenatal detection of Roberts-SC phocomelia syndrome: report of 2 sibs with characteristic manifestations. *Am J Med Genet* 1989;32:390–394.

Van Den Berg DJ, Francke U. Roberts syndrome: a review of 100 cases and a new rating system for severity. *Am J Med Genet* 1993;47:1104–1123.

RESOURCES

7, 60, 96

---

118 Russell-Silver Syndrome

Margot I. Van Allen, MD, MSc, FRCPC(Med Gen), DABMG, DABP, DCCMG

DEFINITION: Russell-Silver syndrome is characterized by prenatal and postnatal growth deficiency, proportionate short stature, relative macrocephaly, a typical facial gestalt, brachyclinodactyly of the fifth finger, hemihypertrophy, and other associated anomalies.

SYNONYM: Silver-Russell syndrome.

DIFFERENTIAL DIAGNOSIS: Hypopituitarism and growth hormone deficiency; In utero exposures (e.g., cigarettes, alcohol); Mild skeletal disorders; Psychosocial short stature; Wilms tumor aniridia syndrome; 11p deletions; SHORT syndrome; MULIBREY nanism; X-linked short stature with skin pigmentation abnormalities; 3M syndrome; Chromosome 15 ring; Partial 15q deletion; Partial 1q duplication; Diploid-triploid mixoploidy.

SYMPTOMS AND SIGNS: Prenatally, the disease is characterized by a normal-appearing fetus, with *in utero* growth retardation and sparing of head size usually seen in the last trimester. At birth, the infant appears otherwise normal or mildly dysmorphic and is small for gestational age. The face is triangular shaped, and the facial features are delicate, giving the typical gestalt of this disorder. There is a broad, high frontal area, retrused hair line, and late closure of the anterior fontanelle, with a fine small nose, short philtrum, and thin upper lip. The chin is pointed and the jaw is small relative to the frontal area. Oral findings include microdontia, congenital absence of teeth, primary double molars, and blunted condyles. Body asymmetry is evident at birth, and becomes more apparent with time. Brachyclinodactyly of the fifth finger is a usual feature. Associated structural anomalies include a variety of cardiac anomalies. Genitourinary anomalies are common, including hypospadius, cryptorchidism, and ureteral and renal anomalies. Café-au-lait spots are common. Hyperhydrosis is reported. Postnatal growth is slow. Delayed bone age and late closure of the anterior fontanelle occur even in those with normal growth hormone study results. Developmental delays and learning problems may occur. Limb length discrepancy can result in scoliosis and pelvic tilt. Endocrine abnormalities including growth hormone deficiency, nocturnal hypoglycemia, abnormal growth hormone pulsatility, absence of catch-down growth after growth hormone therapy, and inappropriate advancement of bone age during the middle childhood years may occur.

ETIOLOGY/EPIDEMIOLOGY: The incidence is unknown, but the condition appears to be relatively common. The syndrome is etiologically heterogeneous. Identified causes include placental insufficiency, selective deficiencies of placental growth factors, placental chromosomal mosaicism, and uniparental disomy for chromosome 7.

DIAGNOSIS: Diagnostic criteria are clinical, without confirmatory laboratory or diagnostic investigations. Placental pathology and chromosome analysis looking for mosaicism are indicated. Patient chromosomal studies are recommended. If there is abnormal upper-to-lower segment ratio and/or arm span–to-height ratio, skeletal surveys are recommended to exclude an underlying skeletal disorder. Uniparental disomy studies are available at a limited number of centers, and *GRB10* mutation analysis is available in research laboratories.

TREATMENT

Standard Therapies: No treatment interventions are available, other than those for associated endocrine disorders. Symptomatic treatment of leg length discrepancy may include shoe inserts, orthotics, and ultimately epiphyseal ablation at puberty.

Investigational Therapies: Treatment with growth hormone is being investigated.

REFERENCES

Azcona C, Albanese A, Bareille P, et al. Growth hormone treatment in growth hormone-sufficient and -insufficient children with intrauterine growth retardation/Russell-Silver syndrome. *Horm Res* 1998;50:22–27.

Baily W, Popovich B, Jones KL. Monozygotic twins discordant for Russell-Silver syndrome. *Am J Med Genet* 1995;58:101–105.

Bernard LE, Penaherrara MS, Van Allen MI, et al. Clinical and molecular findings in two patients with Russell-Silver syndrome and UPD7: comparison with non-UPD7 cases. *Am J Med Genet* 1999;87:230–236.

Stanhope R, Albanese A, Azcone C. Growth hormone treatment of Russell-Silver syndrome. *Horm Res* 1998;49(suppl):47.

Yoshihashi H, Maeyama K, Kosaki R, et al. Imprinting of human GRB10 and its mutations in two patients with Russell-Silver syndrome. *Am J Hum Genet* 2000;67:476–482.

RESOURCES
188, 360, 452

119   Schinzel Syndrome

Michael Bamshad, MD

DEFINITION: Schinzel syndrome is an autosomal-dominant disorder characterized by defects of the posterior skeletal elements of the upper limb, teeth, genitourinary system, and apocrine glands, including the breast.

SYNONYMS: Ulnar-mammary syndrome; Pallister-ulnar-mammary syndrome.

DIFFERENTIAL DIAGNOSIS: Poland syndrome; Limb-mammary syndrome; Scalp-ear-nipple syndrome.

SYMPTOMS AND SIGNS: Individuals with Schinzel syndrome typically have duplication or deletions of the posterior skeletal elements of the upper limb. Deletions range from hypoplasia of the terminal phalanx of digit 5 to phocomelia; however, anterior elements of the upper limb are affected only if the more posterior elements are affected first. Virtually unique to Schinzel syndrome is that the ventral surface of digit 5 is sometimes dorsalized, including the presence of a duplicated nail bed that can replace the finger pad. Upper limb defects are commonly bilateral and asymmetric. Mammary defects range from polythelia to nipple hypoplasia to complete absence of a breast. Unilateral or bilateral reduction or absence of axillary hair and sweating are common. Dental defects include extra or ectopic canine teeth. Genitourinary defects include micropenis, cryptorchidism, and hypospadias in males and structural defects of the uterus in females. Males with Schinzel syndrome commonly have delayed puberty.

ETIOLOGY/EPIDEMIOLOGY: No accurate estimates of prevalence exist; approximately 25 families have been described. Schinzel syndrome is inherited as an autosomal-dominant trait. It has been described in Africans, Asians, and Europeans. Males and females are affected equally. The syndrome is caused by mutations in *TBX3*, a T-box gene, located on chromosome 12q24.

DIAGNOSIS: Usually, the diagnosis of Schinzel syndrome is based solely on clinical findings. Ancillary studies that may facilitate the diagnosis include radiographs of the upper limbs and ultrasonographic examination of the genitourinary system.

TREATMENT

Standard Therapies: Treatment of individuals with Schinzel syndrome is dependent on the severity of limb involvement, and typically includes surgical removal of an extra digit or reconstruction of a limb with a reduction defect to improve its functional capabilities. Surgical reconstruction of the breast and uterus is sometimes indicated. Responses to the use of exogenous testosterone in males with delayed puberty have been inconsistent. Services that benefit the physically disabled may be helpful. Genetic counseling is recommended for patients and their families.

REFERENCES

Bamshad M, Le T, Watkins WS, et al. The spectrum of mutations in *TBX3*: genotype-phenotype relationship in ulnar-mammary syndrome. *Am J Hum Genet* 1999;64:1550–1562.

Bamshad M, Root S, Carey JC. Clinical analysis of a large kindred with the Pallister-ulnar-mammary syndrome. *Am J Med Genet* 1996;65:325–331.

Schinzel A. Ulnar-mammary syndrome. *J Med Genet* 1987;12:778–781.

RESOURCES

60, 360, 452

120   Schinzel Giedion Syndrome

Oliver W.J. Quarrell, MD

DEFINITION: Schinzel Giedion syndrome causes multiple congenital anomalies. It is recognized from a combination of facial features, problems with the renal and genital tract, skeletal dysplasia, severe developmental delay, and seizures.

DIFFERENTIAL DIAGNOSIS: Storage disorders; Rudiger syndrome.

SYMPTOMS AND SIGNS: The characteristic facial features have been described as being "like a figure 8." The forehead is tall, the temples narrow, and the cheeks chubby. The midface is retracted and there is often a groove under the eyes. The fontanelles are wide open. Various radiographic changes have been noted, but among the most consistent are increased density of the bones at the base of the skull and wide occipital synchondrosis that is seen as a gap on the radiograph. Developmental delay is severe, and seizures are common. Abnormalities of the renal tract occur, frequently with hydronephrosis. Abnormalities of the genital tract also have been noted in many affected children. Other problems include cardiac anomalies, choanal stenosis, polydactyly and syndactyly, and sacrococcygeal tumors.

ETIOLOGY/EPIDEMIOLOGY: Fewer than 30 cases have been reported. The disorder is presumed to be autosomal recessive because the condition has been seen in a brother and sister twice. The underlying cause of the syndrome has not been established.

DIAGNOSIS: The diagnosis is suspected from the unusual pattern of features and because the standard chromosome and metabolic investigations are normal. No specific blood test positively confirms the diagnosis.

TREATMENT

Standard Therapies: Standard supportive and symptomatic treatments are given for the variety of features seen in affected children.

REFERENCES

Al-Gazali LI, Farndon P, Burn J, et al. The Schinzel-Giedion syndrome. *J Med Genet* 1990;27:42–47.

Laburne P, Lyonnet S, Zupan V, et al. Three new cases of the Schinzel-Giedion syndrome and review of the literature. *Am J Med Genet* 1994;50:90–93.

McPherson E, Clemens M, Hoffner L, et al. Sacral tumors in Schinzel Giedion syndrome. *Am J Med Genet* 1998;79:62–63.

Schinzel A, Giedion A. A syndrome of severe midface retraction, multiple skull anomalies, clubfeet and cardiac and renal malformations in sibs. *Am J Med Genet* 1978;1:361–375.

Verloes A, Moës D, Palumbo L, et al. Schinzel Giedion syndrome. *Eur J Pediatr* 1993;152:421–423.

RESOURCES

96, 462

121   Schmid Metaphyseal Chondrodysplasia

Ravi Savarirayan, MD, MB, BS, FRACP

DEFINITION: Schmid metaphyseal chondrodysplasia is an autosomal-dominant disorder of the skeleton, predominantly affecting the long bone metaphyses.

SYNONYM: "Japanese" type spondylo-metaphyseal dysplasia.

DIFFERENTIAL DIAGNOSIS: Rickets; Other metaphyseal bone dysplasias; Metaphyseal anadysplasias.

SYMPTOMS AND SIGNS: This bone dysplasia is not detectable clinically or radiographically at birth and usually manifests in early childhood with bowed legs and a "waddling" gait. There is also mild to moderate limb shortening with disproportionate short stature in most cases. The facial appearance is normal. Radiographically there are diffuse metaphyseal changes (flaring, irregularity, and widening) that are typically most severe at the knees with coxa vara. The spine can also be variably affected in approximately 10% of cases, and the short tubular bones of the hands and feet can exhibit metaphyseal changes. Secondary degenerative arthritic changes may occur in the affected joints and the spine in later life. The condition is limited to the skeleton. Intelligence is normal. The histologic appearance of the growth plate in this condition is nonspecific.

ETIOLOGY/EPIDEMIOLOGY: The disorder is inherited as an autosomal-dominant trait and is caused by heterozygous mutations in the gene coding for collagen type X (*COL XA1*). The mutations in this gene appear to cluster predominantly in the carboxyl (NC1) terminal. Considerable inter- and intrafamilial variability exists in the severity of the disorder.

DIAGNOSIS: The diagnosis is based on the characteristic clinical and radiographic features present in childhood and is confirmed by the finding of a type X collagen mutation on DNA analysis. Prenatal diagnosis can be offered if a mutation is known within a family.

TREATMENT
Standard Therapies: Treatment is symptomatic. Rotational osteotomies of the hips are sometimes required. Growth hormone treatment is not effective to increase final adult height. Genetic counseling of families is advised.

REFERENCES
Lachman RS, Rimoin DL, Spranger J. Metaphyseal chondrodysplasia, Schmid type, clinical and radiographic delineation with review of the literature. *Pediatr Radiol* 1988;18:93–102.
Savarirayan R, Cormier-Daire V, Lachman RS, et al. Schmid type metaphyseal chondrodysplasia: a spondylometaphyseal dysplasia identical to the "Japanese" type. *Pediatr Radiol* 2000;30: 460–463.
Schmid F. Beitrag zur dysostosis enchondralis metaphysaria. *Monatsschr Kinderheilk* 1949;97:393.

RESOURCES
96, 188, 362

122   Sclerosteosis

*Peter Beighton, MD, PhD, FRCP,
Herman Hamersma, MD,
and Mary Brunkow, PhD*

DEFINITION: Sclerosteosis is an autosomal-recessive disorder characterized by progressive skeletal overgrowth, gigantism, distortion of the facies, elevation of intracranial pressure, and entrapment of the 7th and 9th cranial nerves. Syndactyly of the second and third fingers is an important diagnostic discriminant.

SYNONYM: Endosteal hyperostosis.

DIFFERENTIAL DIAGNOSIS: van Buchem disease; Osteopetrosis.

SYMPTOMS AND SIGNS: The manifestations of sclerosteosis arise from skeletal overgrowth. The onset of the condition usually occurs in early childhood with episodes of facial palsy resulting from pressure on the 7th cranial nerve in the bony foramina of the skull. By midchildhood, deafness may develop owing to compression of the 8th cranial nerve. At this stage, tall stature and overgrowth of the mandible may be apparent. Variable syndactyly ranging from minor skin webbing to complete bony fusion of the second and third fingers is a frequent syndromic component. Radiographs show widening and increased bone density of the calvarium after the age of 5 years, and thereafter hyperostosis of the skull and the cortices of the long bones become increasingly apparent. By adulthood, affected persons have excessive height and weight. The bones are resistant to fracture. Facial distortion is compounded by facial palsy, and deafness may be an additional problem. Increasing width of the vault of the skull leads to progressive elevation of intracranial pressure, which manifests as intractable headaches. There is a high risk for sudden death due to impaction of the medulla oblongata in the foramen magnum. Intellect is unimpaired, although psychosocial problems are frequent.

ETIOLOGY/EPIDEMIOLOGY: Sclerosteosis is inherited as an autosomal-recessive trait. The underlying molecular fault is a mutation in the *SOST* gene at the chromosomal locus 17q12-q21. Most affected persons are members of the Afrikaner community of South Africa, where more than 60 affected persons have been documented since the 1970s. Sclerosteosis has also been documented in individuals or families in the United States, Germany, Japan, Brazil, Spain, and Senegal.

DIAGNOSIS: The diagnosis is suspected clinically in the Afrikaner community in any child with a combination of facial palsy and partial or complete syndactyly of the second and third fingers. In other populations, diagnosis may be delayed until increased bone density and overgrowth become radiologically evident.

TREATMENT
Standard Therapies: Surgical decompression of cranial foramina may alleviate facial palsy and deafness. The results of these procedures are variable. In adulthood, progressive elevation of intracranial pressure frequently necessitates extensive craniectomy. Surgical correction of the syndactyly may improve the cosmetic appearance and function of the digits. The skull and skeleton are extremely resistant to trauma, and surgical instruments may be blunted during operation. Provision of a hearing aid and orthodontic measures may be indicated and psychosocial support may be necessary. No medicinal therapy is available. Genetic counseling is provided on the basis of autosomal-recessive inheritance. Carrier detection by molecular techniques is possible but not widely available.

REFERENCES
Beighton P. Sclerosteosis. *J Med Genet* 1988;25:200–203.
Beighton P, Davidson J, Durr L, et al. Sclerosteosis—an autosomal recessive disorder. *Clin Genet* 1977;11:1–7.
Beighton P, Hamersma H. The clinical features of sclerosteosis. *Ann Intern Med* 1976;84:393–397.
Brunkow ME, Gardner J, Van Ness J, et al. Sclerosteosis results from disruption of a novel secreted factor with potential activity as a BMP antagonist. *Am J Hum Genet* 2001;68: 577–589.

RESOURCES
360, 362

---

123 Scott Craniodigital Syndrome

Helga V. Toriello, PhD

DEFINITION: Scott craniodigital syndrome is a condition that has only been found in two families. The manifestations of this X-linked condition include unusual head shape, growth and developmental delay, and mild webbing between the fingers and toes.

SYNONYM: Craniodigital syndrome of Scott.

DIFFERENTIAL DIAGNOSIS: Fillipi syndrome; Chitayat syndrome; Zerres syndrome; Kelly syndrome; Woods syndrome.

SYMPTOMS AND SIGNS: Individuals with Scott craniodigital syndrome have a combination of mental and growth retardation, minor craniofacial anomalies, and syndactyly. Birth weight and length are typically within normal limits, but subsequent growth retardation occurs. The head shape is brachycephalic. In addition, affected individuals have long eyelashes, a small chin, a small and pointed nose, and a thin upper lip. Partial soft tissue webbing occurs between fingers 2 and 4 and between toes 2 and 3. Spina bifida occulta may also be seen. There is moderate developmental delay, with patients generally walking after age 2 years. Speech occurs, but is also delayed.

ETIOLOGY/EPIDEMIOLOGY: This is presumably an X-linked recessive trait, based on the presence of the condition in males only. Carrier females have very mild manifestations. Only two families have been described with the condition, so the true gene frequency is unknown.

DIAGNOSIS: The diagnosis is made on clinical findings. No laboratory tests are helpful, and bone age may or may not be delayed.

TREATMENT

Standard Therapies: These individuals do not have any particular health problems, so no treatment is necessary.

REFERENCES

Lorenz P, Hinkel GK, Hoffmann C, et al. The craniodigital syndrome of Scott: report of a second family. *Am J Med Genet* 1990;37:224–226.

Scott CR, Bryant JI, Graham CB. A new craniodigital syndrome with mental retardation. *J Pediatr* 1971;78:658–663.

RESOURCES
96, 362

---

124   SHORT Syndrome

Margarita J. Raygada, PhD,
and Owen M. Rennert, MD

DEFINITION: SHORT syndrome is characterized by short stature, hyperextensibility of joints and/or inguinal hernia, ocular depression, Rieger anomaly, and tooth eruption delay. Other characteristic features include intrauterine growth retardation, slow weight gain, frequent illnesses, triangular face, anteverted ears, telecanthus, deeply set eyes, chin dimple, micrognathia, partial lipodystrophy, hearing loss, delayed bone age, delayed speech, glucose intolerance, and insulopenic diabetes.

DIFFERENTIAL DIAGNOSIS: Rieger syndrome; Russell-Silver syndrome; Seckel syndrome; Leprechaunism.

SYMPTOMS AND SIGNS: Intrauterine growth retardation is usually present. Infants with this disorder have difficulty gaining weight and may exhibit frequent illnesses. Hyperextensibility of the joints is also noted early in life. The typical facial characteristics include triangular face, telecanthus, deeply set eyes, Rieger anomaly, wide nasal bridge, hypoplastic alae, micrognathia, anteverted ears, short philtrum, and chin dimple. Patients with SHORT syndrome have been described as having partial lipodystrophy, especially involving the face and upper body. Other physical characteristics are clinodactyly, inguinal hernia, and short stature. Tooth eruption is frequently delayed. Intellectual function is usually normal, but some patients have delayed speech development and developmental delay. Hearing loss has also been noted. Radiologic findings include delayed bone age, large epiphyses, gracile diaphyses, and coned epiphyses. Congenital glaucoma was seen in 1 reported case. During the second decade of life, diabetes is common, usually preceded by hyperglycemia.

ETIOLOGY/EPIDEMIOLOGY: Evidence regarding the pattern of inheritance is conflicting. A specific mutation has not been identified. Few cases of SHORT syndrome have been reported, and data are inadequate to establish its incidence.

DIAGNOSIS: The diagnosis is made based on the association of the physical characteristics, including short stature, Rieger anomaly, hyperextensibility of the joints, ocular depression, inguinal hernia, tooth eruption, low birth weight, partial lipodystrophy, and hearing loss.

TREATMENT

Standard Therapies: No specific therapy exists. Symptoms should be treated as they arise.

REFERENCES

Aarsk D, Ose L, Pande H, et al. Autosomal dominant partial lipodystrophy associated with Rieger anomaly, short stature, and insulinopenic diabetes. *Am J Med Genet* 1983;15:29–38.

Brodsky MC, Whiteside-Michel J, Merin LM. Rieger anomaly and congenital glaucoma in the SHORT syndrome. *Arch Ophthalmol* 1996;114:1146–1147.

Gorlin RJ. A selected miscellany. *Birth Defects Orig Art Ser* 1975:11:46–48.

Joo S, Raygada M, Rennert OM. Case report on SHORT syndrome. *Clin Dysmorphol* 1999;8:219–221.

Sensenbrenner JA, Hussels IE, Levin LS. A low birth weight syndrome, Rieger syndrome. *Birth Defects Orig Art Ser* 1975; 11:423–426.

Toriello HV, Wakefield S, Komar K, et al. Report of a case and further delineation of the SHORT syndrome. *Am J Med Genet* 1985;22:311–314.

RESOURCES
188, 351, 355

125 Simpson Dysmorphia Syndrome

Gregory M. Enns, MB, ChB

DEFINITION: Simpson dysmorphia syndrome (SDS) is an X-linked recessive disorder in which patients have prenatal and postnatal overgrowth, a coarse face, visceral and skeletal defects, and a predisposition to develop certain embryonal tumors.

SYNONYMS: Simpson-Golabi-Behmel syndrome; Golabi-Rosen syndrome.

DIFFERENTIAL DIAGNOSIS: Beckwith-Wiedemann syndrome; Weaver syndrome; Perlman syndrome; Pallister-Killian syndrome.

SYMPTOMS AND SIGNS: The spectrum of clinical features is variable both within and between families, ranging from a lethal neonatal form with hydrops fetalis to mild disease in carrier females. Most patients are not severely mentally retarded, although impaired intelligence may be present in some cases. Relatively frequent abnormalities include overgrowth of prenatal onset, hypotonia, supernumerary nipples, cardiac conduction defects, organomegaly, umbilical and/or inguinal hernias, vertebral segmentation defects, broad thumbs and great toes, postaxial polydactyly of the hands, and syndactyly of the second and third fingers and toes. Characteristic craniofacial features include macrocephaly, a coarse facial appearance, hypertelorism, down-slanting palpebral fissures, broad nasal bridge, short nose, dental malocclusion, macroglossia, and a midline groove of the lower lip. Less frequent manifestations include cleft lip with or without cleft palate, ear pits/tags, cardiac defects, diaphragmatic hernia, gastrointestinal anomalies (intestinal malrotation, polysplenia, Meckel diverticulum), genitourinary anomalies (large kidneys, renal cysts, hydronephrosis, hypospadias), and brain abnormalities (hydrocephalus, agenesis of the corpus callosum, cerebellar hypoplasia). Patients have an increased risk of developing embryonal tumors, especially Wilms tumor and neuroblastoma. Approximately 50% of patients die before age 6 months from unknown causes, although complications secondary to underlying anomalies undoubtedly play a role.

ETIOLOGY/EPIDEMIOLOGY: The syndrome is an X-linked recessive condition of unknown incidence. Mild expression in heterozygous females may occur. The gene for SDS has been cloned and localized to Xq26. The syndrome is caused by point mutations, deletions, or translocations involving the glypican-3 gene, *GPC3*, a heparan sulfate proteoglycan that may function as a cell surface receptor. The glypican-3 protein plays a central role in mesodermal tissue embryonic development, but its mechanism of action is not yet understood. An additional locus for a severe form of SDS has been mapped to Xp22, but a candidate gene has not yet been found.

DIAGNOSIS: DNA mutation analysis is only available on a limited basis; therefore, diagnosis is primarily clinical. The syndrome should be considered in patients with overgrowth and multiple anomalies, especially involving the skeletal, cardiovascular, and genitourinary systems. A detailed family history is essential. A skin biopsy for chromosome analysis on cultured fibroblasts may be necessary to exclude tetrasomy 12p (Pallister-Killian syndrome). Screening studies include a complete skeletal radiographic survey, echocardiography, electrocardiography, and abdominal ultrasonography. Selected patients may also require neuroimaging studies.

TREATMENT

Standard Therapies: Treatment is supportive and depends on the severity of the condition in the individual patient. A multidisciplinary approach to care is needed, involving specialists in genetics, orthodontics, plastic surgery, cardiology, orthopedics, gastroenterology, and urology. Appropriate psychological and social support is crucial for patients to achieve their life goals.

REFERENCES

Chen E, Johnson JP, Cox VA, et al. Simpson-Golabi-Behmel syndrome: congenital diaphragmatic hernia and radiologic findings in two patients and follow-up of a previously reported case. *Am J Med Genet* 1993;46:574–578.

Jones KL. Simpson-Golabi-Behmel syndrome. In: *Smith's recognizable patterns of human malformation,* 5th ed. Philadelphia: WB Saunders, 1997:168–169.

Neri G, Gurrieri F, Zanni G, et al. Clinical and molecular aspects of the Simpson-Golabi-Behmel syndrome. *Am J Med Genet* 1998;79:279–283.

Pilia G, Hugh-Benzie RM, MacKenzie A, et al. Mutations in *GPC3,* a glypican gene, cause the Simpson-Golabi-Behmel overgrowth syndrome. *Nat Genet* 1996;12:241–247.

Veugelers M, De Cat B, Muyidermans SY, et al. Mutational analysis of the *GPC3.GPC4* glypican gene cluster on Xq26 in patients with Simpson-Golabi-Behmel syndrome: identification of loss-of-function mutations in the *GPC3* gene. *Hum Mol Genet* 2000;9:1321–1328.

RESOURCES
69, 96, 355

126 Singleton-Merten Syndrome

Emile R. Mohler III, MD

DEFINITION: Singleton-Merten syndrome is characterized by progressive calcification of the thoracic aorta, calcific aortic stenosis, osteoporosis, dental dysplasia, and expansion of the marrow cavities in hand bones.

DIFFERENTIAL DIAGNOSIS: Atherosclerotic aortic disease; Syphilitic aortitis; Gaucher disease; Hypoparathyroidism; Vitamin D intoxication; Progeria.

SYMPTOMS AND SIGNS: Patients usually present at a young age with a history of difficulty walking due to a gradual onset of lower extremity weakness. By age 12 years, patients may lose permanent teeth. A generalized psoriaform skin eruption may occur. Ambulation may be inhibited by bilateral flexion contractures of the knees. Abnormal physical findings may include generalized dry and scaly skin lesions and a loud grade systolic ejection murmur heard in the aortic region with conduction to the carotid vessels and possible radiation to the apex. The fingernails and toenails may have a spadelike appearance with onycholysis. Generalized hypotonia and hyperreflexia may be present. If the aortic valve disease progresses to the point of hemodynamic compromise, dizziness and fainting episodes may occur.

ETIOLOGY/EPIDEMIOLOGY: Although the exact genetic abnormality is unclear given the small number of cases, this is likely an autosomal-dominant condition with variable expressivity. As of 2001, only 6 cases of Singleton-Merten syndrome had been reported.

DIAGNOSIS: The diagnosis should be suspected if the following constellation of symptoms and signs are present: calcification of the aorta and aortic valve, unique radiographic changes (especially of the hands), abnormal dentition, and lower extremity weakness, possibly in conjunction with the psoriaform skin eruption.

TREATMENT
Standard Therapies: Treatment is generally palliative. The presence of bilateral pes cavus deformity can be treated with Dwyer osteotomies. Fainting spells should be investigated for possible development of complete heart block, which can be treated with insertion of a cardiac pacemaker. The patient should be carefully monitored for the development of pulmonary infections as well as endocarditis. Antibiotic prophylaxis before dental work or other procedures that may involve bacteremia is recommended. The cause of death is typically due to congestive heart failure secondary to progressive calcific aortic stenosis. It is unknown whether aortic valve replacement will prolong survival in these patients.

REFERENCES
Feigenbaum A, Kumar A, Weksberg R. Singleton-Merten (S-M) syndrome: autosomal dominant transmission with variable expression [Abstract]. *Am J Hum Genet* 1988;43:48.
Galvin KM, Donovan MJ, Lynch CA, et al. A role for smad6 in development and homeostasis of the cardiovascular system. *Nat Genet* 2000;24:171–174.
Gay B Jr, Kuhn JP. A syndrome of widened medullary cavities of bone, aortic calcification, abnormal dentition, and muscular weakness (the Singleton-Merten syndrome). *Radiology* 1976; 118:389–395.
Singleton EB, Merten DF. An unusual syndrome of widened medullary cavities of the metacarpals and phalanges, aortic calcification and abnormal dentition. *Pediatr Radiol* 1973;1:2–7.

RESOURCES
348, 357, 360

127 Smith-Lemli-Opitz Syndrome

John M. Opitz, MD

DEFINITION: Smith-Lemli-Opitz syndrome (SLOS) is a common, autosomal-recessive, at times lethal malformation/mental retardation syndrome due to a defect in the pre- and postnatal synthesis of cholesterol, due to mutations in the 7-dehydrocholesterol reductase (*DHCR7*) gene.

SYNONYMS: RSH syndrome; *DHCR7* abnormality.

DIFFERENTIAL DIAGNOSIS: The biochemical and genetic diagnostic data are definitive.

SIGNS AND SYMPTOMS: Smith-Lemli-Opitz syndrome may be suspected prenatally if the values determined on the maternal serum triple screen test are abnormally low. Ultrasonography may demonstrate a range of anomalies, including holoprosencephaly/cyclopia, cleft palate and/or lip, small mandible (micrognathia), lymphedema, extra fingers or toes, gross heart defects, abnormal external genitalia in a male, and renal cysts or malformations. After birth, symptoms include growth failure, microcephaly, cleft palate, congenital heart defect, postaxial polydactyly and other digit malformations, syndactyly hypospadias and other degrees of incomplete genital development in males, severe congenital hypotonia with obtunded/semi-comatose sensorium and risk of seizures, and, occasionally, cataracts. Children with SLOS have a characteristic appearance, with a small head, ptosis (usually asymmetric), a "heavy-lidded" appearance, and many fine wrinkles of the skin of the upper and lower eyelids. Other signs of SLOS include anteversion of the nostrils; long upper lip; inverted V shape of the upper lip; micrognathia; boad or thick alveolar ridges, excessively "rugose" anteriorly; invariant ear anomalies of mostly large auricles with molding anomalies and soft cartilages; and occasional branchial arch fistulae in the neck. Other signs are congenital hypotonia, frequently with increased deep tendon reflexes, delayed motor development, and, occasionally, mild spasticity of the lower limbs, as well as unusual sensitivity to light, photophobia, a tendency to sunburn quickly, and immune deficiency.

ETIOLOGY/EPIDEMIOLOGY: SLOS is caused by biparental mutations in the *DHCR7* gene located at 11q13. Thus, SLOS is an autosomal-recessive condition with 25% recurrence risk. Carriers can easily be identified with appropriate gene tests. A 2% gene frequency predicts a 4% carrier frequency, and birth prevalence of 1 in 2,500. Newborn screening detects 1 in 20,000 to 1 in 22,000; thus, 5 of 6 of all tested babies may be stillborn. This suggests that SLOS be suspected in all idiopathic stillbirths.

DIAGNOSIS: Diagnosis is made by determining the ratio of total cholesterol to 7-dehydrocholesterol (C:7DHC) in an infant's blood. Total cholesterol determination by ordinary means will not yield the C:7DHC ratio accurately, but with mass spectrometry the test can be performed reliably in a university hospital or an appropriate commercial laboratory. Prenatal diagnosis is accurate and reliable on the basis of the C:7DHC ratio in amniotic fluid and detection and measurement of unusual steroid hormones excreted in the mother's urine. If *DHCR7* mutations are known, molecular analysis may be performed on chorionic villus cells or amniocytes.

TREATMENT
Standard Therapies: Standard therapies are used for nonspecific individual manifestations, such as cleft palate, cataracts, ptosis, strabismus, congenital heart defects, polydactyly, and seizures. One of the apparently most effective ways of increasing plasma cholesterol and of lowering plasma 7DHC levels is to supplement the infant's diet with egg yolk. In the short term, this increases plasma cholesterol levels from an average of 53 to 82 mg/dL; in the long term, studies show mean plasma 7DHC decreased from 11.3 to 3.5 mg/dL, and cholesterol increased from 53 to 114 mg/dL.

REFERENCES
Fitzky BU, Glossmann H, Utermann G, et al. Molecular genetics of the Smith-Lemli-Opitz syndrome and post-squalene sterol metabolism. *Curr Opin Lipidol* 1999;10:123–131.
Kelley RI. Inborn error of cholesterol biosynthesis. *Adv Pediatr* 2000;47:1–53.
Kelly RI, Hennekam RCM. The Smith-Lemli-Opitz Syndrome. *J Med Genet* 2000;37:321–335.
Linck LM, Lin DS, Flavell D, et al. Cholesterol supplementation with egg yolk increases plasma cholesterol and decreases plasma 7-dehydrocholesterol in Smith-Lemli-Opitz syndrome. *Am J Med Genet* 2000;93:360–365.
Opitz JM. RSH (so-called Smith-Lemli-Opitz) syndrome. *Curr Opin Pediatr* 1999;11:363–362.
Shackleton CHL, Roitman E, Kratz L. Dehydro-oestriol and dehydro-pregnanetriol are candidate analytes for prenatal diagnosis of Smith-Lemli-Opitz syndrome. *Prenat Diagn* 2001;21:207–212.

RESOURCES
438, 462

128 Smith-Magenis Syndrome

Ann C.M. Smith, MA, DSc(Hon), and Brenda Finucane, MS

DEFINITION: Smith-Magenis syndrome (SMS), a microdeletion syndrome due to interstitial deletion of chromosome 17p11 (del 17p11.2), is associated with a distinct phenotypic pattern of physical, developmental delay/mental retardation, and behavioral features, including chronic sleep disturbance, stereotypies, and self-injury.

SYNONYMS: Interstitial deletion 17p11.2; Smith-Magenis chromosome region, SMS, del (17)(p11.2p11.2).

DIFFERENTIAL DIAGNOSIS: Prader-Willi syndrome; Down syndrome (in the newborn period); Velocardiofacial syndrome; Williams syndrome; Fragile X syndrome; Psychiatric diagnoses (DSM-IV) criteria resulting in dual diagnosis, including disorders of inattention (ADHD, ADD), pervasive developmental disorder (PDD), and/or obsessive compulsive disorder (OCD).

SYMPTOMS AND SIGNS: Craniofacial features include brachycephaly; midfacial hypoplasia; slight up-slanting, deep-set eyes; synophrys; short, full-tipped nose with reduced nasal height; micrognathia in infancy changing to relative prognathism with age; and a distinct appearance of the mouth, with fleshy upper lip with "tented" downturned appearance. Microcephaly occurs occasionally. Common features include infantile hypotonia with feeding difficulties and failure to thrive; developmental delays; mild to moderate psychomotor retardation; significant early expressive speech/language delay with/without associated hearing loss; ocular anomalies (nearsightedness/high myopia, microcornea, strabismus, and, less frequently, detached retina); middle ear and laryngeal anomalies; velopharyngeal insufficiency; persisting short stature; brachydactyly; scoliosis; and signs of peripheral neuropathy. The voice is often hoarse and low-pitched. Most affected persons have mild to moderate mental retardation. Neurobehavioral features include chronic sleep disturbance due to inverted circadian rhythm of melatonin, stereotypies, and self-injurious behaviors. Affected infants often have decreased vocalizations, babbling, and/or crying; happy, smiling, complacent dispositions; and generalized lethargy. Less variable features include cardiac defects; renal abnormalities, especially duplication of collecting system; low thyroxin levels; low immunoglobulins; seizures; abnormal electroencephalogram (EEG) without seizures; forearm abnormalities; and facial clefts.

ETIOLOGY/EPIDEMIOLOGY: Estimated to occur in 1 in 25,000 births, SMS been identified worldwide from a diversity of ethnic groups and occurs equally in both sexes. With few exceptions, cases occur sporadically, due to a *de novo* deletion of 17p11.2, thereby implying a low recurrence risk in future pregnancies.

DIAGNOSIS: The diagnosis of SMS requires confirmation of an interstitial deletion of chromosome 17p11.2 by standard G-banded analysis (550 band) and/or by fluorescence in situ hybridization analysis.

TREATMENT

Standard Therapies: A complete review of systems should be performed at the time of diagnosis. If not performed previously, echocardiography, renal ultrasonography, and ophthalmologic examination are indicated for baseline assessment. The following should be performed annually or as clinically indicated: otolaryngologic evaluation to assess and manage otitis media and other sinus abnormalities; audiologic assessment to monitor for conductive or sensorineural hearing loss. EEG should be performed in individuals who have clinical seizures to guide the choice of antiepileptic agent. For patients without seizures, EEG may be helpful to evaluate for possible subclinical events in which treatment may improve attention and/or behavior. Patients should be monitored for hypercholesterolemia and treated medically if indicated. From infancy on, referrals should be made for early intervention programs, followed by ongoing special education programs and vocational training in later years. Recommended therapies include speech/language, physical, and occupational, with emphasis on sensory integration. Use of psychotropic medication may show some benefit with respect to increasing attention and/or decreasing hyperactivity. Behavioral therapies play an integral role in behavioral management. Therapeutic management of the sleep disorder remains a challenge. Early reports of therapeutic benefit from melatonin are encouraging.

REFERENCES

Chen K-S, Potocki L, Lupski JR. The Smith-Magenis syndrome [del (17)p11.2]: clinical review and molecular advances. *Ment Retard Dev Disabil Res Rev* 1996;2:122–129.

Greenberg R, Lewis RA, Potocki L, et al. Multi-disciplinary clinical study of Smith-Magenis syndrome (deletion 17p11.2). *Am J Med Genet* 1996;62:247–254.

Potocki L, Glaze D, Tan DX, et al. Circadian rhythm abnormalities of melatonin in Smith-Magenis syndrome. *J Med Genet* 2000; 37:428–433.

Smith ACM, Dykens E, Greenberg F. The behavioral phenotype of Smith-Magenis syndrome (del 17p11.2). *Am J Med Genet* 1998;81:179–185.

Smith ACM, Dykens E, Greenberg F. Sleep disturbance in Smith-Magenis syndrome (del 17p11.2). *Am J Med Genet* 1998;81: 186–191.

Smith ACM, Gropman A. Smith-Magenis syndrome. In: Allanson J, Cassidy S, eds. *Clinical management of common genetic syndromes.* New York: Wiley-Liss, 2000.

Smith ACM, McGavran L, Robinson J, et al. Interstitial deletion of (17)(p11.2p11.2) in nine patients. *Am J Med Genet* 1986; 24:393–414.

RESOURCES
104, 401, 439

129 Sotos Syndrome

Juan Fernandez Sotos, MD

DEFINITION: Sotos syndrome is a genetic disorder characterized by excessive growth both prenatally and postnatally. Other features include a large dolichocephalic head, distinctive facial configuration, advanced bone age, and a nonprogressive neurologic disorder with mental retardation (Insert Fig. 38).

SYNONYM: Cerebral gigantism.

DIFFERENTIAL DIAGNOSIS: Mental retardation and overgrowth; Autosomal-dominant macrocephaly; Fragile X chromosome; Weaver syndrome; Beckwith-Wiedemann syndrome; Simpson-Golabi-Behmel syndrome; Marfan syndrome; Pituitary gigantism; Bannayan-Riley-Ruvalcaba syndrome.

SYMPTOMS AND SIGNS: The main clinical finding is prenatal and postnatal overgrowth. Growth velocity is particularly rapid in the first 3–4 years of life. The height increases to mean values of 3 SD and bone age is advanced by 2–4 years over chronologic age during childhood. Adult height usually exceeds the 50th percentile of the normal range, and some individuals may reach excessive adult heights. The craniofacial configuration is characteristic, with a prominent forehead and receding frontoparietal hairline in 96% of patients, dolichocephalic large head, hypertelorism, down-slanting of palpebral fissures, high narrow palate, and pointed chin. Premature eruption of teeth occurs in 60%–80% of patients. Delayed language development and mental deficiency are present in 80%–85% of patients. Seizures may occur in 30% of patients. Mildly enlarged ventricles and increased subarachnoid spaces are a frequent finding and usually require no treatment. Social difficulties and behavioral disorders in affected children are frequent.

ETIOLOGY/EPIDEMIOLOGY: The majority of cases is sporadic, but could be due to new mutations. Several families with members affected in two or three generations have been reported, suggesting autosomal-dominant inheritance. Deletions or point mutations of a single gene, *NSD1*, located at chromosome 5q35 have been identified in 24 of 42 sporadic cases, indicating that haploinsufficiency of *NSD1* is the major cause of Sotos syndrome. Other genetic abnormalities may be possible. The finding that all the *NSD1* mutations identified were either heterozygous or hemizygous is consistent with an autosomal-dominant condition in the majority of cases of Sotos syndrome. Males and females are affected equally. More than 300 cases have been reported and many more are known. It occurs in all ethnic groups and has been detected throughout the world.

DIAGNOSIS: There is no biochemical marker for the disease. The diagnosis is based on clinical grounds. The most characteristic manifestations are excessive growth and the craniofacial configuration. Without these signs, the diagnosis cannot be made. It is anticipated that future DNA studies of patients will permit a more certain diagnosis and delineation of the spectrum of the condition. The diagnostic tests are mainly to exclude other possibilities, such as fragile X by DNA analysis, a karyotype, serum growth hormone, and insulin-like growth factor type 1. MRI of the brain is helpful.

TREATMENT
Standard Therapies: The management of the mental retardation is no different than for any child with a mental deficiency. The excessive height usually is not a handicap for males. Girls with a predicted ultimate height in excess of 178 cm (5 feet 10 inches) may benefit from treatment with high doses of estrogen to curtail linear growth, as indicated for tall girls without the condition. Social and behavioral problems during childhood and immaturity in adulthood may benefit from psychological counseling. Other important concerns are the possibility of tumor development (<3.0%) and the risk of transmission. Because the evidence suggests that this is an autosomal-dominant disorder affecting males and females, the affected individual has a 50% risk of having affected children. Affected individuals are fertile. No evidence exists that life span is shortened.

Investigational Therapies: The molecular basis of the disease continues to be studied.

REFERENCES
Cole TRP. Sotos syndrome. In: Cassidy SB, Allanson JE, eds. *Management of genetic syndromes.* New York: Wiley-Liss, 2001:389–404.

Kurotaki N, Imaizumi K, Harada N, et al. Haploinsufficiency of *NSD1* causes Sotos syndrome. *Nat Genet* 2002;30:365–366.

Sotos JF. Overgrowth. Section V. Syndromes and other disorders associated with overgrowth. *Clin Pediatr* 1997;36:89–103.

Sotos JF, Dodge PR, Muirhead D, et al. Cerebral gigantism in childhood: a syndrome of excessively rapid growth and acromegalic features and a nonprogressive neural disorder. *N Engl J Med* 1964;271:109–116.

Zonana J, Sotos JF, Romshe CA, et al. Dominant inheritance of cerebral gigantism. *J Pediatr* 1977;91:251–256.

RESOURCES
418, 443, 444, 462

130   Split Hand/Split Foot Malformation

*Stavros Sifakis, MD,
and Petros Tsipouras, MD*

DEFINITION: The split hand/split foot malformation (SHFM) is characterized by variable defects of the hands and feet without involvement of ectodermally derived structures. The disorder typically manifests with absence of the central digital rays, a deep median cleft, and syndactyly of the remaining digits. It may be present as a distinct clinical entity (nonsyndromic SHFM) or may be a component of other syndromic entities (40% of cases).

SYNONYMS: Ectrodactyly; Ostrich foot; Lobster claw anomaly.

DIFFERENTIAL DIAGNOSIS: Ectrodactyly, ectodermal dysplasia, and cleft lip/palate syndrome; Limb-mammary syndrome; Acro-dermato-ungual-lachrymal-tooth syndrome; Ectodermal dysplasia, ectrodactyly, and macular dystrophy.

SYMPTOMS AND SIGNS: The functional effects of the manifestations of SHFM vary from mild to severe. The phenotypic severity of the upper extremities is greater when compared with that of the lower. The disorder is characterized by variability of clinical expression, both within and between affected families. In sporadic cases, single-limb involvement is common, whereas four-limb involvement is usually observed in families segregating SHFM. A subdivision of SHFM in two clinical types has been suggested on the basis of tibial aplasia/hypoplasia or absence thereof. Although the term SHFM implies the presence of a cleft in the affected limb, this is not a constant finding. A core of skeletal defects of the hands and feet in affected individuals has been identified: Monodactyly is the presence of a single digit, bidactyly refers to the classic "lobster claw" anomaly, and oligodactyly is the presence of three or more digits in the affected limb, frequently associated with a median cleft and soft tissue or bony syndactyly. A combination of these defects can exist in the same individual. Aplasia and/or hypoplasia of the phalanges, metacarpals, and metatarsals is usually present in the affected limbs. Triphalangeal thumb, clinodactyly, and poly-dactyly, although frequently observed in SHFM, appear to be nonspecific and not directly associated with the core phenotypic abnormalities of the disorder.

ETIOLOGY/EPIDEMIOLOGY: SHFM can occur either sporadically or as a familial trait, frequently displaying reduced penetrance. The disorder is genetically heterogenous; to date, four loci have been identified, three of which are inherited as autosomal-dominant traits and one as an X-linked trait. These loci have been designated SHFM1 (7q21–22), SHFM2 (Xq26), SHFM3 (10q24–25), and SHFM4 (3q27). The frequency is approximately 1 in 18,000 newborns.

DIAGNOSIS: The diagnosis is based on clinical manifestations present at birth. Radiographs may offer more descriptive information about the skeletal abnormalities. Syndromes that include SHFM as a component must be excluded.

TREATMENT
Standard Therapies: Surgical treatment of the congenital deformities could improve the function of the limb and its aesthetic appearance. Surgical strategies include early syndactyly release, pollicization, rotational osteotomy, and reconstruction of underdeveloped fingers. These plastic and reconstructive operations may have favorable results by improving function, especially in patients with minor defects.

REFERENCES
Ianakiev P, Kilpatrick MW, Toudjarska I, et al. Split-hand/split-foot malformation is caused by mutations in the p63 gene on 3q27. *Am J Hum Genet* 2000;67:59–66.

McKusick V. *Mendelian inheritance in man: a catalog of human genes and genetic disorders,* 12th ed. Baltimore: Johns Hopkins University Press, 1998.

Roelfsema NM, Cobben JM. The EEC syndrome: a literature study. *Clin Dysmorphol* 1996;5:115–127.

Spranger M, Schapera J. Anomalous inheritance in a kindred with split hand, split foot malformation. *Eur J Pediatr* 1988;147:202–205.

Zlotogora J. On the inheritance of the split hand/split foot malformation. *Am J Med Genet* 1994;53:29–32.

RESOURCES
60, 351

131   Sprengel Deformity

James R. Bowen, MD,
and Keti P. Tokmakova, MD

DEFINITION: Sprengel deformity is a congenital condition that arises from interruption of normal caudal migration of the scapula during embriologic development. The anomaly is manifested as elevation and medial rotation of the scapula, which is small with a distorted shape and size, and more cephalad than normal.

SYNONYMS: Congenital high scapula; Congenital undescended scapula; Scapula elevata.

DIFFERENTIAL DIAGNOSIS: Pterygium colli; Klippel-Feil syndrome.

SYMPTOMS AND SIGNS: The principal clinical feature is asymmetry of the neck and shoulder region caused by the upward and forward displacement of the scapula. The deformity is usually noticed at birth and progresses with growth. The level of the scapula in relation to the vertebral column varies with the severity of the condition. It may be situated from 1 to 12 cm higher than normal, averaging approximately 4 cm. On the affected side, the neck is full and short and the cervicoscapular line is diminished. The supraspinous portion of the scapula may be palpable in the supraclavicular area. The affected clavicle is often tilted obliquely upward and laterally at an angle of 25 degrees from the horizontal. The omovertebral structure may be palpable. Passive motion of the glenohumeral joint is usually within a normal range; however, the scapulocostal motion is restricted. Associated scoliosis and kyphosis are common, and torticollis may be present. Bilateral Sprengel deformities give the appearance of a very short, thick neck. Abduction is limited in both shoulders, and the cervical lordosis may be increased. The clavicle may be malformed or hypoplastic, or may fail to articulate with the acromion. The humerus may be shorter on the affected side. Associated congenital abnormalities include congenital scoliosis with hemivertebrae, Klippel-Feil syndrome, absent or fused ribs, diastematomyelia, renal abnormalities, spina bifida in the cervical region, syringomyelia, paraplegia, platybasia, situs inversus, and mandibulofacial dysostosis.

ETIOLOGY/EPIDEMIOLOGY: Various etiologic theories have been suggested, such as failure of descent, abnormal articulations with the vertebral column, defective musculature, and a "bleb theory" of atypical embryologic cerebrospinal fluid flow. Sprengel deformity usually occurs sporadically, but a few patients have an autosomal-dominant pattern of inheritance. The condition is seen in both sexes, with a female:male ratio of approximately 3:1. The left side is more often affected than the right, and the deformity may be bilateral.

DIAGNOSIS: Diagnosis is based on clinical and radiographic findings. The elevation of the scapula and its associated bony deformities are best visualized on anteroposterior radiographs of both shoulders with the arms at the sides. Radiographs with the shoulders in maximal active and passive abduction show the abnormally high position of the scapula and limited motion. Lateral radiographs of the cervical and dorsal spine and oblique and lateral radiographs of the scapula may demonstrate the omovertebral bone. CT has also been used to visualize the omovertebral bone and the abnormal scapula.

TREATMENT

Standard Therapies: The goals of treatment are to correct the deformity and improve function. In infants and young children, passive stretching and active exercises are performed to maintain strength and motion. If the deformity is disfiguring and the function of the shoulder is significantly impaired, operative intervention should be considered. Surgical options include detachment of the medial and superior scapular muscles, resection of the omovertebral structure, repositioning the scapula caudally, and reattaching the muscles to the lowered scapula. The best results are achieved with a modified Green and Woodward procedure.

REFERENCES

Borges JL, Shah A, Torres BC, et al. Modified Woodward procedure for Sprengel deformity of the shoulder: long-term results. *J Pediatr Orthop* 1996;16:508–513.

Cavendish ME. Congenital elevation of the scapula. *J Bone Joint Surg [Br]* 1972;54:395.

Cho TJ, Choi IH, Chung CY, et al. The Sprengel deformity: morphometric analysis using 3D-CT and its clinical relevance. *J Bone Joint Surg [Br]* 2000;82:711–718.

Pinsky HA, Pizzutillo PD, MacEwen GD. Congenital elevation of the scapula. *Orthop Trans* 1980;4:288–289.

Ross DM, Cruess RL. The surgical correction of congenital elevation of the scapula. *Clin Orthop* 1977;125:17.

RESOURCES
351, 449

132   Sturge-Weber Syndrome

Anne M. Comi, MD

DEFINITION: Sturge-Weber syndrome (SWS) is a neuro-cutaneous disorder characterized by the presence of a facial port-wine stain, a leptomeningeal angioma, and ocular abnormalities, most commonly glaucoma (Insert Fig. 39).

SYNONYMS: Flat facial hemangiomata; Meningeal hemangiomata with seizures; Sturge-Weber-Krabbe disease.

DIFFERENTIAL DIAGNOSIS: Isolated port-wine stain; Klippel-Trenaunay-Weber syndrome.

SYMPTOMS AND SIGNS: Typically occurring in childhood, the syndrome is characterized by a facial port-wine stain, seizures, and frequent neurologic deficits, including contralateral weakness, and homonymous hemianopsia. Progressive vision loss may result from glaucoma. Other possible signs and symptoms include hemiatrophy of weak limbs, eye enlargement in infancy, strokelike episodes and mental retardation, and soft tissue hypertrophy and blebbing of the port-wine stain.

ETIOLOGY/EPIDEMIOLOGY: SWS occurs sporadically, in all races and with equal frequency in both sexes. The incidence and prevalence are uncertain, because SWS is likely underdiagnosed. The cause is unknown, although it may result from a somatic mutation or injury affecting a subset of neural crest cells during the first trimester of fetal development.

DIAGNOSIS: Diagnosis depends on the finding of the facial port-wine stain, typically in the ophthalmic division of the fifth cranial nerve, in association with a leptomeningeal angioma, most commonly in the parietal-occipital region. A contrast-enhanced MRI is generally performed in infants with characteristic cutaneous findings. Absence of typical findings before 2 years of age does not rule out the disorder, and MRI may need to be repeated later. The typical leptomeningeal angioma may also be found without the associated port-wine stain. These individuals usually present with seizures and can manifest all the neurologic sequelae typical of SWS. In addition, ophthalmologic evaluation and close follow-up are essential to diagnose glaucoma, which can manifest at any time.

TREATMENT
Standard Therapies: Neurologic treatment of SWS includes standard anticonvulsant management of epilepsy and migraine prophylaxis with propanolol or verapamil. Hemispherectomy is used in the management of infants and children with refractory seizures, strokelike episodes, and progressive neurologic deficits. Laser treatments are central to the management of the facial port-wine stain and can minimize its functional and cosmetic disabilities. Management of glaucoma, if present, is divided between medical and surgical approaches. Medications include oral carbonic anhydrase inhibitors and topical b-blockers. Surgical interventions are often required, however, and include goniotomy, trabeculotomy, and laser trabeculoplasty.

Investigational Therapies: A small retrospective study indicated that aspirin may help minimize the progressive neurologic deficits frequently seen in SWS, but the efficacy and safety of aspirin requires further study. Numerous approaches to the treatment of the glaucoma associated with SWS are being studied, including augmentation of trabeculectomy with antimetabolite therapy, cryocoagulation of the ciliary body, and the use of glaucoma implants.

REFERENCES
Bodensteiner JB, Roach ES, eds. *Sturge-Weber syndrome.* Mt. Freedom, NJ: The Sturge-Weber Foundation, 1999.

Chapieski L, Friedman A, Lachar D. Psychological functioning in children and adolescents with Sturge-Weber syndrome. *J Child Neurol* 2000;15:660–665.

Kihiczak N, Schartz R, Jowiak S, et al. Sturge-Weber syndrome. *Pediatr Dermatol* 2000;65:133–136.

Sujansky E, Conradi S. Sturge-Weber syndrome: age at onset of seizures and glaucoma and the prognosis for affected children. *J Child Neurol* 1995;10:49–58.

RESOURCES
368, 450, 484

133   3-M Syndrome

*Susanne Schmandt, Dr Med,
and Phillip L. Pearl, MD*

DEFINITION: 3-M syndrome is an autosomal-recessive intrauterine growth retardation-malformation syndrome characterized by prenatal and postnatal proportionate growth retardation, slender ribs and long bones, tall vertebrae, facial dysmorphism, other minor anomalies, and normal intelligence.

SYNONYMS: Slender bone nanism; Three M slender boned dwarfism.

DIFFERENTIAL DIAGNOSIS: Russell-Silver syndrome; MULIBREY nanism; Dubowitz syndrome; Bloom syndrome; Dwarfism with gloomy face; Autosomal-dominant dwarfism with tall vertebral bodies; Floating harbor syndrome; Seckel bird-headed dwarfism; Fetal alcohol syndrome; Achondroplasia.

SYMPTOMS AND SIGNS: Neonates are typically not larger than 40 cm and have a low birth weight. Lips protrude and are fleshy; noses are small, upturned, and have a fleshy tip. The typical hatchet-shaped and triangular face with a flattened malar region and a pointed chin may not be recognized during the first years of life. Other features are dolichocephaly and relative macrocephaly, frontal bossing (becoming less obvious after childhood), broad forehead, thick eyebrows, long philtrum, high-set, square shoulders due to a short neck with prominent trapezius muscles and horizontally running clavicles, broad chest due to horizontally oriented ribs, mild pectus carinatum/excavatum, diastasis recti, hyperlordosis, prominent heels, pes planus, decreased extension at the elbows due to elbow dysplasia, joint hypermobility, dislocated hips and elbows, and winged scapulae. Signs of skeletal hypoplasia are slender ribs and long bones with narrow diaphyses as well as tall and foreshortened lumbar vertebral bodies (becoming more apparent with increasing age). Spina bifida occulta, small pelvis, short femoral necks, prominent talus,

and osteoporosis are often seen. Bone age is slightly retarded. Final height is only 120–130 cm. Except in a small minority of children, intelligence is normal. Sexual development is normal, and an unaffected offspring has been reported from an affected mother.

ETIOLOGY/EPIDEMIOLOGY: Joint laxity, dislocations, hernias, and a possible risk for aneurysms (1 case) suggest a generalized disorder of connective tissue (possibly type III collagen deficiency). With normal chromosomes, a gene mutation with possible expression in heterozygotes is assumed. Autosomal-recessive inheritance is likely because sex distribution in 30 reported cases is equal and there are no reports of affected individuals in more than one generation.

DIAGNOSIS: Diagnosis is made by clinical observation and aforementioned nonspecific radiographic findings.

TREATMENT
Standard Therapies: Treatment is symptomatic.

REFERENCES
Feldmann M, Gilgenkrantz S, Parisot S, et al. 3M dwarfism: a study of two further sibs. *J Med Genet* 1989;26:583–585.

Hennekam RC, Bijlsma JB, Spranger J. Further delineation of the 3-M syndrome with review of the literature. *Am J Med Genet* 1987;28:195–209.

Meo F, Pinto V, D'Addario V. 3-M syndrome: a prenatal ultrasonic diagnosis. *Prenat Diagn* 2000;20:921–923.

Miller JD, McKusick VA, Malvaux P, et al. The 3-M syndrome: a heritable low birthweight dwarfism. *Birth Defects Orig Art Ser* 1975;11:39–47.

Mueller RF, Buckler J, Arthur R, et al. The 3-M syndrome: risk of intracerebral aneurysm? *J Med Genet* 1992;29:425–427.

Van Goethem H, Malvaux P. The 3-M syndrome. A heritable low birthweight dwarfism. *Helv Paediatr Acta* 1987;42:159–165.

RESOURCES
96, 120, 351

134 Thrombocytopenia and Absent Radius Syndrome

Ron L. Ferguson, MD

DEFINITION: Thrombocytopenia and absent radius syndrome is a congenital syndrome characterized by hypomegakarocytic thrombocytopenia, bilateral absence of the radius leading to radial deviation of the hand, shortening of the ulna and occasionally of the humerus, and the presence of five digits on the hand, including a fully formed thumb with first metacarpal.

SYNONYMS: TAR syndrome; TARK4 syndrome.

DIFFERENTIAL DIAGNOSIS: Fanconi syndrome; Aase syndrome; Holt-Oram syndrome; Pseudothalidomide syndrome; Radial club hand.

SYMPTOMS AND SIGNS: At birth, the child has bilateral radial deviation of the hands on shortened forearms. The hands have five fingers, including fully formed thumbs with thumb metacarpals. The radius is completely absent radiographically, and the ulna is short. The humerus may also be short. Occasionally, the whole forearm and arm are absent, with the fully formed five-fingered hand attached to the shoulder girdle. Approximately 80% of these patients have congenital deformities of the lower extremities, including hip, knee, ankle, and foot abnormalities. Platelets counts are decreased, and the child may develop purpura, petechiae, and hemorrhage, including intracranial bleeding at or very shortly after birth. Anemia may be present, and the white blood cell count may be elevated. Also associated are congenital heart anomalies, lactose intolerance, excessive perspiration, pitting edema of the dorsum of the feet, and nevus flamus between the eyebrows. The natural history of the thrombocytopenia is to slowly resolve in the first decade of life with significant bleeding becoming unusual by age 2 years. During this time the platelet count slowly rises. The prognosis is good if the child does not have a significant problem before age 2.

ETIOLOGY/EPIDEMIOLOGY: Chromosomal analyses and gene testing have demonstrated no abnormality. An autosomal-recessive inheritance pattern was demonstrated in several families.

DIAGNOSIS: Diagnosis is based on the clinical findings. Any child with a bilateral radial club hand deformity and a five-fingered hand should have a platelet count at birth. Diagnosis may be made by ultrasonography *in utero* as early as 16 weeks of gestation, with cordocentesis demonstrating a low platelet count.

TREATMENT

Standard Therapies: Bleeding episodes are usually secondary to low platelet counts and can be treated with platelet transfusions. Surgery to reconstruct the upper extremity often requires centralization of the hand on the wrist. Reconstruction of the lower extremity deformities is variable. Surgery should not be undertaken until platelet counts have risen to the $50,000/mm^3$ range. The risks of early surgery must be weighed against the extent of disability caused by the congenital deformities. Qualitative platelet blockers (aspirin, antiinflammatory medications) should be avoided in these patients until their platelet counts are normal.

REFERENCES

Christensen CP, Ferguson RL. Lower extremity deformities associated with thrombocytopenia and absent radius syndrome. *Clin Orthop* 2000;375:202–206.

Goldberg, MJ. *The dysmorphic child: an orthopaedic perspective.* New York: Raven, 1986:302–306.

Hall JB, Levin J, Kuhn JP, et al. Thrombocytopenia with absent radius ('TAR'). *Medicine* 1969;48:411–439.

Schoenecker PL, Cone AK, Sedgwick WG, et al. Dysplasia of the knee associated with the syndrome of thrombocytopenia and absent radius. *J Bone Joint Surg [Am]* 1984;66:421–427.

Tongsong T, Sirichotiyakul S, Chanprapaph P. Prenatal diagnosis of thrombocytopenia-absent-radius (TAR) syndrome. *Ultrasound Obstet Gynecol* 2000;15:256–258.

RESOURCES

35, 113, 459

135 | Tooth Agenesis

Heleni Vastardis, DDS, DMSc

DEFINITION: Tooth agenesis is the most common anomaly of the human dentition. Tooth agenesis occurs in association with genetic syndromes or as an isolated sporadic or familial trait. More than 60 syndromes are associated with this condition, implying that common molecular mechanisms are responsible for tooth and other organ development. Agenesis of numerous teeth is commonly associated with specific abnormalities involving hair, skin, nails, and sweat glands, and particularly related to ectodermal dysplasia.

SYNONYMS: Several terms are used in the literature to describe numeric dental defects: "Oligodontia" is defined as agenesis of 6 or more permanent teeth. The term *anodontia* indicates complete absence of teeth. *Partial anodontia* is used synonymously with *oligodontia*. *Hypodontia*, besides describing the condition in which fewer than six teeth are absent, is also used to depict morphologic dental anomalies.

SYMPTOMS AND SIGNS: A close examination of the dental profile of individuals with tooth agenesis often shows aberrations in the overall rate of dental development, time and sequence of eruption, and the size and shape of the existing teeth. Unusual dental findings such as excessive spaces between erupted teeth, delayed eruption of maxillary lateral incisors, and/or prolonged retention of mandibular second primary molars could be indications of tooth agenesis warranting further investigation.

ETIOLOGY/EPIDEMIOLOGY: Primary dentition is less frequently affected (0.1%) than permanent dentition. In the permanent dentition, the incidence of tooth agenesis varies for different teeth; third molars are most frequently missing (30%), followed by mandibular second premolars (3.4%) and maxillary lateral incisors (2.2%). In the general caucasian population, the condition ranges from 1% to 9.6%; in the Japanese population, 6.6%–9.2%; and for the African-American population the reported incidence is 7.7%. The female:male ratio ranges from 3:2 for caucasians to 2:1 for African Americans. In primary dentition agenesis, the chance for permanent teeth to fail to develop is increased. The majority of persons with permanent tooth agenesis have intact primary dentition, suggesting different genetic mechanisms for the two sets of teeth. Although trauma, radiation, and systematic destruction of the developing tooth bud are likely causes in some cases, a considerable portion of all cases are inherited. Familial tooth agenesis is transmitted as an autosomal-dominant, -recessive, or X-linked condition. An autosomal-dominant form of tooth agenesis is caused by a missense mutation in the homeobox gene *MSX1*. An autosomal-recessive form of hypodontia has been linked to a region on chromosome 16q21.1. A frame shift mutation in the *PAX9* gene was associated with oligodontia in another family.

DIAGNOSIS: Diagnosis is based on dental history, clinical examination, and dental radiographs.

TREATMENT
Standard Therapies: Treatment of the tooth agenesis depends on the severity of the condition. It ranges from simple restorative modalities (e.g., recontouring of teeth, resin composite bonding, bleaching, veneers, crowns, dentures), to a single tooth implant, to a more involved treatment plan combining orthodontic and/or prosthodontic means.

Investigational Therapies: The creation of artificial tooth banks for transplantation purposes is being explored.

REFERENCES
Ahmad W, Brancolini V, ul Faiyaz MF, et al. A locus for autosomal-recessive hypodontia with associated dental anomalies maps to chromosome 16q12.1 [Letter]. *Am J Hum Genet* 1998;62:987–991.

Peck S, Peck L, Kataja M. Mandibular lateral incisor-canine transposition, concomitant dental anomalies and genetic control. *Angle Orthod* 1998;68:455–466.

Stockton DW, Das P, Goldenberg M, et al. Mutation of *PAX9* is associated with oligodontia. *Nat Genet* 2000;24:18–19.

Vastardis H. The genetics of human tooth agenesis: new discoveries for understanding dental anomalies. *Am J Orthod Dentofac Orthop* 2000;117:650–656.

Vastardis H, Karimbux N, Guthua SW, et al. A human *MSX1* homeodomain missense mutation causes selective tooth agenesis. *Nat Genet* 1996;13:417–421.

RESOURCES
320, 363

136   Townes-Brocks Syndrome

*Ave Maria Lachiewicz, MD,
and Christeen Hodge, MD*

DEFINITION: Townes-Brocks syndrome (TBS) is a multiple malformation syndrome. Characteristics are present at birth and vary from person to person. The most common characteristics include an absence of the anal opening and anomalies of the ears, hands, and feet. Hearing loss, malformations of the genital-renal system, craniofacial malformations, and mental retardation may also be present.

SYNONYMS: Imperforate anus with hand and foot anomalies; Deafness with imperforate anus and hypoplastic thumbs; Renal-ear-anal-radial [REAR] syndrome; Townes syndrome; Anus, hand, and ear syndrome.

DIFFERENTIAL DIAGNOSIS: VATER association; VACTERL with hydrocephalus; Baller-Gerold syndrome; Oculoauriculovertebral spectrum.

SYMPTOMS AND SIGNS: Imperforate anus is the most common, but other anal anomalies range from a skin-covered opening to more severe grades of imperforation. A variety of urogenital abnormalities has been associated with TBS. Ear anomalies commonly present include small ears with an overfolded superior helix and small antihelix, "satyr," or "lop" ears. Sensorineural hearing loss ranges from mild to profound and may be progressive. The hearing loss may also have a conductive component. The most common limb defects are a triphalangeal thumb and preaxial polydactyly with a well-formed or vestigial digit. Toe anomalies occur less frequently and include a short third toe/metatarsal, overlapping toes (usually the second and fourth overlap the third), syndactyly of the third and fourth toes, and an absent third toe. Mental retardation has been reported. Abnormalities of the heart, eye, and spine are infrequently observed.

ETIOLOGY/EPIDEMIOLOGY: TBS is an autosomal-dominant disorder that affects males and females equally. The specific features of the syndrome can differ among relatives. The minimal frequency of TBS is 1 case in every 250,000 live births. Eighteen different mutations in the *SALL1* gene located at 16q12.1 have been associated with TBS. Most of these are frameshift mutations, which result in premature termination of the *SALL1* protein. Some individuals have chromosome 16 abnormalities, and some have normal genetic studies.

DIAGNOSIS: Most individuals have at least two of the following characteristics: (a) anorectal malformation; (b) hand anomaly, usually involving the thumb; (c) ear malformation with possible sensorineural hearing loss; (d) a relative with the syndrome.

TREATMENT
Standard Therapies: Treatment of TBS often includes surgery for malformations. Specific conditions such as hearing loss or renal disease should be addressed. Genetic counseling for family members may be beneficial.

REFERENCES
Jones KL. *Smith's recognizable patterns of human malformation,* 5th ed. Philadelphia: WB Saunders, 1997:260–261.
Kohlhase J. *SALL1* mutations in Townes-Brocks syndrome and related disorders. *Hum Mutat* 2000;16:460–466.
McKusick VA. *Mendelian inheritance in man,* 12th ed. Baltimore: The Johns Hopkins University Press, 1998:163–164.
Powell CM, Michaelis RC. Townes-Brocks syndrome. *J Med Genet* 1999;36:89–93.
Townes PL, Brocks ER. Hereditary syndrome of imperforate anus with hand, foot, and ear anomalies. *J Pediatr* 1972;81:321–326.

RESOURCES
351, 354, 363

137   Treacher-Collins Syndrome

Eric A. Wulfsburg, MD

DEFINITION: Treacher-Collins syndrome is a genetic craniofacial syndrome characterized by malar hypoplasia, down-slanting palpebral fissures, mandibular hypoplasia, structural ear abnormalities, and deafness.

SYNONYMS: Mandibulofacial dysostosis; Franceschetti-Klein syndrome.

DIFFERENTIAL DIAGNOSIS: Miller syndrome; Nager syndrome; Other acrofacial dysostoses.

SYMPTOMS AND SIGNS: Treacher-Collins syndrome is an autosomal-dominant craniofacial syndrome with clinical variability that in the typical case is easily recognizable in the newborn period. Features affect only the head and face and include malar hypoplasia with absent or hypoplastic zygomatic arches, down-slanting palpebral fissures, and lower eyelid colobomas with partial to complete absence of the lower eyelashes. The external ears are typically malformed and may show severe microtia with atretic ear canals. Conductive deafness occurs in almost one half of patients. Mandibular hypoplasia may be severe and can be associated with cleft palate, macrostomia, feeding difficulties, and airway obstruction requiring tracheotomy. Approximately 25% of patients have growth of their scalp hair onto the lateral cheek. Intelligence is generally normal. Careful examination of parents and siblings is important, because wide variability exists in phenotype and only subtle features may be seen in mildly affected relatives.

ETIOLOGY/EPIDEMIOLOGY: This syndrome is the result of dominant mutations in the *TCOF1* gene located at chromosome 5q32-q33.1. Approximately 60% of cases are the result of new mutations. The incidence is approximately 1 in 10,000 to 20,000.

DIAGNOSIS: Observation of the typical features on careful craniofacial examination generally makes the diagnosis. Although Treacher-Collins syndrome is not a chromosomal syndrome, karyotyping is recommended to rule out similar appearing phenocopies. Consultation with a clinical geneticist to confirm the diagnosis is recommended. DNA mutation analysis may be available for clinical use in the future and would be of value in questionable cases and for prenatal diagnosis.

TREATMENT
Standard Therapies: Surgical treatment is best accomplished at a craniofacial center with multispeciality expertise in plastic surgery, otolaryngology, orthodontics, and dentistry. Radiography and three-dimensional CT are indicated in the presurgical evaluation of patients. Hearing augmentation requires consultation with an experienced otolaryngologist.

Investigational Therapies: New surgical procedures and hearing aid technologies are constantly being developed and make referral to a craniofacial team advisable.

REFERENCES
Marsh KL, Dixon MJ. Treacher-Collins syndrome. *Adv Otorhinolaryngol* 2000;56:53–59.
Posnick JC, Ruiz RL. Treacher-Collins syndrome: current evaluation, treatment, and future directions. *Cleft Palate Craniofac J* 2000;37:434.
Toriello HV. Treacher-Collins syndrome. *Ear Nose Throat J* 1999;78:752.

RESOURCES
96, 371, 468

138 Triploidy Syndrome–Partial Molar Pregnancy

Elizabeth I.O. Garner, MD,
Donald P. Goldstein, MD,
and Ross Stuart Berkowitz, MD

DEFINITION: Triploidy syndrome is an alternative term for partial mole, a subset of molar pregnancy that has been identified as a distinct entity from complete molar pregnancy.

SYNONYM: Partial hydatidiform mole.

DIFFERENTIAL DIAGNOSIS: Complete molar pregnancy; Hydropic changes of placenta.

SYMPTOMS AND SIGNS: The clinical presentation of partial mole is typically not as dramatic as that of complete mole. Excessive uterine enlargement is seen in only 4%–11% of patients with partial mole. Theca lutein ovarian cysts, hyperemesis, hyperthyroidism, and respiratory insufficiency are extremely rare. Preevacuation human chorionic gonadotropin (hCG) levels infrequently exceed 100,000 mIU/mL. Fetuses identified with partial moles generally have the features of triploidy, which include growth retardation and congenital malformations, including cleft palate, hydrocephalus, and syndactyly of the hands and feet. Triploid fetuses have been described with term delivery. Rapid deterioration after birth is the usual outcome, with the oldest known surviving nonmosaic patient living to 11 months.

ETIOLOGY/EPIDEMIOLOGY: Most partial moles are found on cytogenetic analysis to be triploid, having an extra haploid set of paternally derived chromosomes, the result of the fertilization of an apparently normal haploid ovum by two spermatozoa. The incidence of partial mole is approximately 1 in 700 pregnancies. In patients with a history of partial mole, the risk of repeat mole is approximately 1% in later gestations. After two molar gestations, this risk increases to approximately 20%.

DIAGNOSIS: The clinical diagnosis is most commonly incomplete or missed abortion. Careful pathologic review of chorionic tissues is therefore essential for the diagnosis of partial mole. Ultrasonography may contribute to the diagnosis. Histopathologically, partial moles show focal swelling of the chorionic villi, focal trophoblastic hyperplasia, and marked scalloping of the chorionic villi with stromal trophoblastic inclusions. Because triploid partial moles have a full complement of maternal chromosomes, identifiable fetal or embryonic tissue is often present. The extra set of paternal chromosomes may contribute to the focal trophoblastic hyperplasia, an absolute requirement for the diagnosis of partial mole.

TREATMENT
Standard Therapies: Treatment of partial mole involves evacuation of the uterus by means of dilation and curettage. Persistent gestational trophoblastic tumor, generally non-

metastatic and requiring chemotherapy, develops in 2%–4% of patients with partial mole. Despite this low risk of persistence, all patients with partial mole must be followed with hCG measurements to ensure complete sustained remission. Reliable contraception during the entire period of follow-up is strongly advised. Given that patients are at increased risk in future pregnancies, early ultrasonography and careful surveillance for suggestive symptoms is advised; however, women with partial molar pregnancy can usually expect normal fertility in subsequent pregnancies.

REFERENCES
Berkowitz RS, Goldstein DP. Recent advances in gestational trophoblastic disease. *Curr Opin Obstet Gynecol* 1998;10:61–64.
Berkowitz RS, Tuncer ZS, Bernstein MR, et al. Management of gestational trophoblastic diseases: subsequent pregnancy experience. *Semin Oncol* 2000;27:678–685.
Fine C, Bundy AL, Berkowitz RS, et al. Sonographic diagnosis of partial hydatidiform mole. *Obstet Gynecol* 1989;73:414–418.
Mittal TK, Vujanic GM, Morrisey BM, et al. Triploidy: antenatal sonographic features with postmortem correlation. *Prenat Diagn* 1998;18:1253–1262.
Vassilakos P, Riotton G, Kajii T. Hydatidiform mole: two entities. *Am J Obstet Gynecol* 1978;131:665–671.

RESOURCES
281, 476

139   Turner Syndrome

Adeline Vanderver, MD, and Phillip L. Pearl, MD

DEFINITION: Turner syndrome (TS) is a syndrome of gonadal dysgenesis with sex chromosome abnormalities in some or all cells, characterized most often by short stature, but with the potential to affect multiple organ systems. It is the most common sex chromosome abnormality in females.

SYNONYM: Ullrich-Turner syndrome.

DIFFERENTIAL DIAGNOSIS: Leri-Weill dyschondrosteosis; Noonan syndrome.

SYMPTOMS AND SIGNS: In the neonatal period and infancy, lymphedema of the hands and feet, nuchal folds or webbing, left-sided cardiac abnormalities, low hairline over the neck, low-set ears, or a small mandible are suggestive of

TS. In childhood, any of these physical findings in addition to cubitus valgus, stocky shieldlike chest, widespread nipples, nail hypoplasia, hyperconvex uplifted nails, multiple pigmented nevi, short fourth metacarpals, high-arched palate, short stature with declining growth velocity, markedly elevated levels of follicle-stimulating hormone (FSH), and chronic otitis media are suggestive. In adolescence, unexplained short stature, pubertal arrest, absence of breast development by age 13, or amenorrhea with elevated levels of FSH are suggestive. Overall, 23%–40% of patients have congenital heart defects. Systolic hypertension occurs in approximately 20% of patients. Aortic root dilatation occurs in some patients, and predisposes to aortic dissection. Congenital malformations of the urinary system may occur, most frequently rotational abnormalities and duplicated collecting systems. Primary autoimmune hypothyroidism occurs in 10%–30% of patients. Conductive hearing loss and sensorineural hearing loss are common. Chronic otitis media is common in young girls with TS and may contribute to hearing loss. Short stature may affect more than 95% of individuals. Gonadal failure occurs in 90% of individuals, although 30% will undergo pubertal development, albeit delayed and complicated by progressive ovarian failure. Osteopenia is common. No increase occurs in the prevalence of mental retardation, with the exception of patients with a small ring X chromosome that fails to undergo X inactivation.

ETIOLOGY/EPIDEMIOLOGY: The syndrome affects 1 in 2,000 to 5,000 live female births. The embryonal incidence is believed to be much higher, and it has been estimated that there is a high rate of spontaneous miscarriage with a survival to term in only approximately 1 of 100 fetuses with a 45,X abnormality. More than 50% of patients show a 45,X chromosome abnormality, with other genotypes including isochromosomes, deletions, rings, and translocations. More than half of patients have some degree of chromosomal mosaicism. A new gene, *SHOX* (short-stature homeobox containing gene), identified on Xp22 and Yp11.3, may be involved in growth regulation; haploinsufficiency of the *SHOX* gene may be responsible for the growth failure seen in TS.

DIAGNOSIS: Patients are defined as having TS if they meet the criteria of characteristic physical attributes in addition to the absence, complete or partial, of one copy of chromosome X in all or some cells. The syndrome may be discovered incidentally on prenatal evaluation. Postnatally, patients with suspected TS should have a peripheral blood karyotype perfomed, possibly supported by a second tissue analysis if initial testing is negative.

TREATMENT
Standard Therapies: Treatment is directed at optimizing growth and sexual development, as well as minimizing morbidity and mortality. Growth hormone (GH) therapy should be offered, with or without anabolic steroids, in the expectation of increasing final height. Orthopedic leg lengthening is a less used alternative. Estrogen therapy may be required to induce pubertal development, and should be coordinated with GH therapy to maximize growth and final height.

REFERENCES
Blaschke RJ, Rappold. *SHOX* in short stature syndromes. *Hormone Res* 2001;55:21–23.
Landin-Wilhelmsen K, Bryman I, Wilhelmsen L. Cardiac malformations and hypertension, but not metabolic risk factors, are common in Turner syndrome. *J Clin Endocrinol Metab* 2001; 86:4166–4170.
Practice Guidelines, the American Academy of Pediatrics Committee on Genetics. Health supervision for children with Turner syndrome. *Pediatrics* 1995;96:1166–1173.
Root AW, Kemp SF, Rundle AC, et al. Effect of long-term recombinant growth hormone therapy in children—the National Cooperative Growth Study, USA 1985–1994. *J Pediatr Endocrinol* 1998;11:403–412.
Saenger P, Wikland KA, Conway GS, et al. Recommendations for the diagnosis and management of Turner syndrome. *J Clin Endocrinol Metab* 2001;86:3061–3069.
Savendahl L, Davenport ML. Delayed diagnosis of Turner's syndrome: proposed guidelines for change. *J Pediatr* 2000;137: 455–459.

RESOURCES
362, 472, 473

---

140 Von Hippel-Lindau Disease

Virginia V. Michels, MD, and Vicki Couch, MS

DEFINITION: Von Hippel-Lindau disease (VHL) is a hereditary multisystem disorder characterized by benign and malignant tumors. Hallmark features include hemangioblastomas of the central nervous system (CNS), especially cerebellum and spinal cord, retinal angiomas, and renal cysts and renal cell carcinomas.

SYNONYMS: Hippel-Lindau syndrome; Lindau disease; Retinocerebellar angiomatosis; Angiomatosis retinae.

SYMPTOMS AND SIGNS: CNS hemangioblastomas are often multiple and most frequently found in the cere-bellum, spinal cord, and brainstem. The typical age of patients who present with CNS lesions is 25–40 years, although children or older adults may be affected. The lesions are benign, but may produce symptoms and signs due to size or location, including ataxia, slurred speech, nystagmus, headache, nausea, vertigo, and broad-based gait. Retinal angiomas may be present. These benign tumors, if untreated, may cause retinal detachment and hemorrhage, leading to blindness. Multiple renal cysts are common, frequently bilateral, and rarely cause renal impairment. Renal cell carcinoma is a leading cause of mortality in VHL. Pheochromocytomas may occur in young patients and are often bilateral and multiple. They may cause intermittent or sustained hypertension, episodic sweating, palpitations, and headaches, or may be asymptomatic. Pancreatic cysts are often multiple and rarely cause endocrine or exocrine insufficiency. Pancreatic islet cell cancer also can occur. Epididymal cysts and cystadenomas are relatively common in males. Some patients develop endolymphatic sac tumors, slow-growing, low-grade papillary adenocarcinomas that can cause hearing loss.

ETIOLOGY/EPIDEMIOLOGY: VHL is caused by mutations in the *VHL* gene (chromosomal locus 3p25-p26). It is an autosomal-dominant disorder. It is seen in all ethnic groups, and both sexes are affected equally. Approximately 80% of patients have an affected parent, whereas approximately 20% of patients have VHL due to a new mutation.

DIAGNOSIS: If there is a known family history of VHL, diagnosis is made based on the presence of a single retinal or cerebellar hemangioblastoma, renal cell carcinoma, or pheochromocytoma. In an isolated case, diagnosis of VHL can be made in a person who has two or more retinal or CNS hemangioblastomas or a single hemangioblastoma and a characteristic visceral tumor. Gene testing may be able to confirm a suspected diagnosis or make a diagnosis in an asymptomatic relative.

TREATMENT
Standard Therapies: Management is focused on surveillance of at-risk individuals, including children, for early detection and treatment of tumors. Screening includes annual eye examination with an indirect ophthalmoscope, beginning by age 2–5 years; annual blood pressure monitoring plus measurement of urinary catecholamines or plasma or urinary metanephrines, beginning by age 5 years; annual abdominal imaging by ultrasonography, beginning by age 11–12 years (or by CT or MRI beginning at age 20 years); and MRI with gadolinium of the brain and spine every 2 years, beginning by age 11–12 years. CNS lesions may require intervention by surgical resection or gamma knife surgery. Retinal hemangioblastomas may be treated using laser coagulation or cryotherapy. Renal cell carcinomas should be removed using nephron-sparing surgery when possible. Pheochromocytomas should be surgically removed, by adrenal-sparing surgery if appropriate. Pancreatic islet cell tumors can be excised surgically. Epididymal lesions generally do not require surgery. Consideration of the surgical removal of endolymphatic sac tumors must include discussion of the possible complication of deafness.

INVESTIGATIONAL THERAPIES: The VHL protein and other proteins, including vascular endothelial growth factor receptor, and their pathways may be a target for clinical trials.

REFERENCES
Couch V, Lindor NM, Karnes PS, et al. Von Hippel-Lindau disease. *Mayo Clin Proc* 2000;75:265–272.
McKusick VA, ed. Online Mendelian Inheritance in Man (OMIM) [database online]. Bethesda, MD: National Center for Biotechnology Information, National Library of Medicine; 2001. Entry no. 193300; last update 3/6/01.
Schimke RN, Collins D, Stolle CA. Von Hippel-Lindau syndrome. Seattle: GeneClinics, University of Washington; 2000. Last update 3/15/00. *www.geneclinics.org/profiles/vhl/details. html.*

RESOURCES
355, 368, 486

---

141   Weaver Syndrome

Thaddeus E. Kelly, MD, PhD

DEFINITION: Weaver syndrome is an autosomal-dominantly inherited overgrowth syndrome. Affected infants are long at birth and experience accelerated growth rates with advanced bone age. Joint contractures, especially camptodactyly, are common. Cognitive development may be delayed.

DIFFERENTIAL DIAGNOSIS: Acromegaly; Sotos syndrome; Marshall syndrome; Congenital adrenal hyperplasia (21 hydroxylase deficiency).

SIGNS AND SYMPTOMS: Infants have a normal birth weight but excessive length. Rate of growth is accelerated in the first few months of life and bone age is advanced. The forehead is broad and the ears are fleshy. The hands show contractural arachnodactyly and mobility of the elbows, hips, and knees is decreased . These children are heavy boned. There are no overt birth defects and general health is good, whereas cognitive development is usually delayed. Although reported cases have been sporadic, several families have been reported in which the findings in the affected parent were much less striking than in the affected child. The phenotype becomes less striking as affected individuals enter adulthood. Ultimate adult height is excessive, however, when compared with family members of normal stature.

ETIOLOGY/EPIDEMIOLOGY: Weaver syndrome has probably been unrecognized and underreported. Several published cases clearly established autosomal-dominant inheritance. Both sexes are affected equally .

DIAGNOSIS: The diagnosis is usually apparent by physical examination, but studies help confirm it. Bone age is advanced but not beyond the height age. Growth hormone and 17 hydroxy-progesterone levels are normal. The karyotype is normal. Films often show hypoplasia of one or more cervical vertebral bodies that may contribute to instability of the cervical spine. Among the less than 25 reported cases in the literature, three patients had embryonal tumors of different types.

TREATMENT
Standard Therapies: Treatment is supportive and symptomatic. The cervical spine may need to be stabilized. Physical therapy may help increase range of motion of the major joints. Affected adults have good general health without significant physical limitations. The prognosis for an affected child seems largely dependent on cognitive development, which should be closely monitored..

REFERENCES
Derry C, Temple IK, Venkat-Raman K. A probable case of familial Weaver syndrome associated with neoplasia. *J Med Genet* 1999;36:725–728.
Fryer A, Smith C, Rosenbloom L, et al. Autosomal dominant inheritance of Weaver syndrome. *Am J Med Genet* 1997;34: 418–419.
Greenberg F, Wasiewski W, McCabe ERB. Weaver syndrome: the changing phenotype in an adult. *J Med Genet* 1989;33:127–129.
Kelly TE, Alford BA, Abel M. Cervical spine anomalies and tumors in Weaver syndrome. *Am J Med Genet* 2000;95:492–495.
Muhonen MG, Menezes AH. Weaver syndrome and instability of the upper cervical spine. *J Pediatr* 1990;116:596–599.
Proud VK, Braddock SR, Cook L, et al. Weaver syndrome: autosomal dominant inheritance of the disorder. *Am J Med Genet* 1998;79:305–310.
Weaver DD, Graham CB, Thomas IT, et al. A new overgrowth syndrome with accelerated skeletal maturation, unusual facies, and camptodactyly. *J Pediatr* 1974;84:547–552.

RESOURCES
188, 488

142 Weill-Marchesani Syndrome

*Charles J. Anderson, MD,
and Nicole J. Anderson, MD*

DEFINITION: Weill-Marchesani syndrome is an inherited disease characterized by both skeletal and ocular manifestations. Skeletal manifestations include short stature and brachycephaly, short stubby hands and feet (brachydactyly), and limited joint mobility. The primary ocular manifestation is microspherophakia with long, loose, and degenerated zonular attachments to the lens. This leads to frequent lens subluxations or dislocations, which predispose patients to pupillary block glaucoma. (Insert Fig. 40).

SYNONYMS: Spherophakia-brachymorphia syndrome; Congenital mesodermal dystrophy; GEMSS syndrome (glaucoma, ectopia, microspherophakia, stiff joints, and short stature).

DIFFERENTIAL DIAGNOSIS: Marfan syndrome; Homocystinuria; Ehlers-Danlos syndrome; Osteogenesis imperfecta.

SIGNS AND SYMPTOMS: Characteristic physical features include short stature and small stubby fingers. In children, it is a leading cause of lens subluxation and glaucoma. Patients usually have lenticular myopia secondary to microsphermophakia. Ophthalmic examination may identify signs including dislocation, subluxation (usually downward), and cataractous changes of the crystalline lens. Patients may also have increased intraocular pressure and shallow anterior chamber angles from pupillary block glaucoma. Other ophthalmic signs include asymmetric axial lengths of the eye, iridonesis, pigmentary degeneration of the fundi, optic atrophy, and early vitreous liquefaction. With age, patients may experience stiffness and loss of flexibility in the joints. Patients generally have normal intelligence.

ETIOLOGY/EPIDEMIOLOGY: Weill-Marchesani syndrome was initially believed to be of autosomal-recessive inheritance. It is often incompletely recessive with partial expression in the heterozygote. More recently, an autosomal-dominant variant has been described.

DIAGNOSIS: The diagnosis is made on the presence of the characteristic clinical signs. No single test is available to confirm it. Family history and examination of other family members may be helpful.

TREATMENT
Standard Therapies: The disorder has no cure. Connective tissue disorders are treated with physical therapy and orthopedic treatments. Eye examinations with visual fields should be conducted at regular intervals at an early age to detect elevated intraocular pressure due to pupillary block, which can cause irreversible and sometimes asymptomatic visual loss. Treatment with mydriatic or miotic agents is controversial. Miotic agents (pilocarpine) cause ciliary body contraction and further loosening of the zonules, which causes forward lens movement, thus increasing pupillary block. Mydriatics may relieve the block, but also may cause lens dislocation into the anterior chamber. Long-term medical management of glaucoma has not been successful in these patients. A definitive or prophylactic YAG laser iridectomy may be indicated to treat or prevent closed-angle glaucoma. Subluxed and cataractous lenses are managed with complex lens extraction.

REFERENCES
Dietlein TS, Jacobi PC, Krieglstein GK. Ciliary body is not hyperplastic in Weill-Marchesani syndrome. *Acta Ophthalmol Scand* 1998;76:623–624.

Ereklioglu C, Hepsen IF, Hamdi ER. Weill-Marchesani syndrome in three generations. *Eye* 1999;13:773–777.

Groessl S, Anderson CJ. Capsular tension ring in a patient with Weill-Marchesani syndrome. *J Cataract Refract Surg* 1998;24: 1164–1165.

Ritch R, Wand M. Treatment of the Weill-Marchesani syndrome. *Ann Ophthalmol* 1981;13:665–667.

Wirtz MK, Samples JR, Kramer PL. Weill-Marchesani syndrome: possible linkage of the autosomal dominant form to 15q21.1. *Am J Med Genet* 1996;65:69–75.

RESOURCES
188, 288, 355

---

143   Weismann-Netter-Stuhl Syndrome

Adil Muhib Samara, MD, and Sandra R. Fernandes, MD

DEFINITION: Weismann-Netter-Stuhl syndrome is characterized by a general bilateral and symmetrical anterior bowing of the lower limbs. The bone radiographs usually show cortical thickening of the concave curvature and destruction of the trabeculae.

SYNONYM: Tibioperoneal toxopachyosteosis.

DIFFERENTIAL DIAGNOSIS: Paget disease; Rickets/osteomalacia; Congenital syphilis.

SYMPTOMS AND SIGNS: Bowed lower limbs, short stature, ambulation delay, family history, kyphoscoliosis, and facial dysmorphism are the most common clinical features. Characteristic radiologic findings are bilateral or unilateral bowing of the tibia and/or fibulae. Other bone deformities include bowing of the femur, low-set L5, sacrum horizontalization, squared pelvis, bowed or misshapen radium/ulna, coxa vara, genu varum, and abnormalities of the humeri and/or the ribs.

ETIOLOGY/EPIDEMIOLOGY: The disease may affect both genders and has been reported in whites, blacks, and Australian aborigines. The pathophysiology of the disease is unknown. Nevertheless, its occurrence has been reported in first-degree relatives and in monozygotic twins. Genetic disease with incomplete penetration is suggested by the uncommon family history for the disease. An HLA typing investigation was carried out in only 6 cases, showing the haplotype HLA-B27 and/or HLA-A3 in half of them. Only 14 cases in children have been reported.

DIAGNOSIS: Features helpful in making the diagnosis are symmetric anterior bowing of the tibia and fibula and cortical thickening of the concave surface of this curvature. These features are not found in Paget disease.

TREATMENT
Standard Therapies: There is no treatment for this disorder.

REFERENCES
Francis GL. The Weismann-Netter syndrome: a cause of bowed legs in childhood. *Pediatrics* 1991;88:334–337.

Norès JM, Monsegu MH, Masfrand V, et al. Identification and classification of tibioperoneal diaphyseal toxopachyosteosis (Weismann-Netter-Stuhl syndrome) based on two cases and a review of the literature. *Eur J Radiol* 1997;24:71–76.

Resnick D, ed. *Diagnosis of bone and joint disorders,* 2nd ed. Philadelphia: WB Saunders, 1988.

Robinow M, Johnson F. The Weismann-Netter syndrome. *Am J Med Genet* 1988;29:573–579.

Tieder M, Manor H, Peshin J, et al. The Weismann-Netter-Stuhl syndrome: a rare pediatric skeletal dysplasia. *Pediatr Radiol* 1995;25:37–40.

RESOURCES
188, 351

144   Werner Syndrome

Junko Oshima, MD, PhD,
and George M. Martin, MD

DEFINITION: Werner syndrome (WS) is a recessive genetic disorder characterized by features suggestive of accelerated aging (Insert Fig. 41).

SYNONYMS: Progeria of the adult; WRN mutation; Progeroid syndrome.

SIGNS AND SYMPTOMS: Patients with WS develop normally until the end of their first decade of life. The first symptom, often recognized retrospectively, is the lack of a growth spurt during the early teen years. Typically, symptoms start while patients are in their twenties and include gray hair, alopecia, hoarseness, and skin sclerosis, followed by bilateral ocular cataracts, type 2 diabetes mellitus, hypogonadism, skin ulcers, and osteoporosis in their thirties. Patients exhibit several forms of arteriosclerosis (hardening of the arteries), the most serious form of which is coronary atherosclerosis. The latter may lead to myocardial infarction, which together with cancer is the most common cause of death in these patients, typically at approximately age 50. The spectrum of cancers in WS is unusual in that it includes a large number of sarcomas and rare types of cancers. The osteoporosis is also unusual in that it especially affects the long bones. There are also characteristic osteolytic lesions of the distal joints of the fingers. Deep, chronic ulcers around the ankle are highly characteristic of the disorder. Some controversy exists concerning the degree to which the brain is involved. Although patients may have central nervous system complications of arteriosclerosis, they do not appear to be unusually susceptible to Alzheimer-type dementias.

ETIOLOGY/EPIDEMIOLOGY: Werner syndrome is caused by mutations at the *WRN* gene on chromosome 8. These result in the truncation of *WRN* gene products. Inheritance is autosomal recessive. The frequency of WS can be expected to vary as functions of the levels of consanguinity in populations. In the Japanese population, it may range from about 1 in 20,000 to 1 in 40,000, based on the frequencies of detectible heterozygous mutations. The prevalence in the U.S. population is unknown, but may be approximately 1 in 200,000. Men and women are affected equally.

DIAGNOSIS: Urinary hyaluronic acid is increased in most patients. The results of other standard laboratory tests are usually nonspecific. Diagnosis is based on the identification of the *WRN* mutations by molecular and genetic analyses.

TREATMENT
Standard Therapies: No specific treatments exist for WS. Helpful interventions include control of the diabetes, surgical treatment of ocular cataracts, prevention and treatment of skin ulcers, amelioration and treatment of atherosclerosis and its complications, and timely detection and treatment of malignancies.

REFERENCES
Epstein CJ, Martin GM, Schultz AL, et al. Werner's syndrome: a review of its symptomatology, natural history, pathologic features, genetics and relationships to the natural aging process. *Medicine* 1996;45:172–221.

Martin GM, Oshima J, Gray MD, et al. What geriatricians should know about the Werner syndrome. *J Am Geriatr Soc* 1999;47: 1136–1144.

McKusick VA, ed. *Mendelian inheritance in man.* Baltimore, MD: The Johns Hopkins University. Entry no. 277700; Last update of the online version (OMIM) 8/31/00.

Tollefsbol TO, Cohen HJ. Werner's syndrome: an underdiagnosed disorder resembling premature aging. *Age* 1984;7: 75–88.

RESOURCES
209, 210, 369

145   Williams Syndrome

Barbara R. Pober, MD, MPH

DEFINITION: Williams syndrome (WS) is a genetic disorder characterized by a broad array of medical and cognitive problems. Features found in more than 50% of patients include distinctive facial appearance, vascular stenoses, small physical size, mild mental retardation, and a characteristic personality/behavioral profile. Other common abnormalities include hypercalcemia, strabismus, hernias, joint contractures, small teeth, and malocclusion.

SYNONYMS: Williams-Beuren syndrome; Hypercalcemia with elfin facies.

DIFFERENTIAL DIAGNOSIS: Isolated supravalaortic stenosis; Noonan syndrome; Fetal alcohol syndrome; Velocardiofacial syndrome; Coffin-Lowry syndrome.

SIGNS AND SYMPTOMS: Most infants with WS are colicky, have difficulty feeding, and demonstrate poor weight gain. Facial features apparent in infancy include a flat nasal bridge, periorbital puffiness, full cheeks, and a small chin. Cardiovascular disease, most commonly supravalaortic stenosis and/or pulmonary stenoses, can present at birth; the onset of narrowing or progression of existing narrowing can also occur over time. Up to 50% of persons with WS develop hypertension during their lifetime. Other medical problems during early childhood may be hypercalcemia, recurrent ear infections, strabismus, small and malaligned teeth, constipation, gastroesophageal reflux, hypothyroidism, joint contractures, spinal curvature, and hypotonia. Older persons may develop diverticulosis, diverticulitis, hypertonia, hyperreflexia, and diabetes. Most patients have mild mental retardation. Patients demonstrate "scatter" in their cognitive profile, with a characteristic pattern of strengths and weaknesses. Relative strengths are language and memory skills; weaknesses manifest as poor visual spatial skills, limited abstract reasoning, and shortened attention span.

ETIOLOGY/EPIDEMIOLOGY: Williams syndrome is caused by deletion of 17 genes on chromosome 7q11.23. This deletion arises spontaneously in most cases. The prevalence of WS is estimated at ~1 in 20,000 births, and males and females are affected equally.

DIAGNOSIS: Florescent in *situ* hybridization confirms the diagnosis of WS in ~99% of cases; it demonstrates deletion of the elastin gene. Once the diagnosis of WS is established, a variety of laboratory tests to screen for potential medical problems are recommended.

TREATMENT
Standard Therapies: Therapies include monitoring for potential medical problems (such as cardiovascular disease, gastrointestinal problems, growth failure, etc.). Beneficial developmental interventions include speech therapy, physical therapy, occupational therapy, and special education instruction. Most persons with WS enjoy music and have a somewhat greater facility with it than would be expected based on their IQ; music therapy has been suggested, although not proven, to be beneficial both in relieving anxiety and enhancing learning.

Investigational Therapies: Research is focused on identifying the role of each of the 17 genes. Loss of the *LIMK1* gene has been implicated as the cause of the visuospatial problems in WS.

REFERENCES
Bellugi U, Wang P, Jernigan TL. Williams syndrome: an unusual neuropsychological profile. In: Browman SH, Grafam J, eds. *Atypical cognitive deficits in developmental disorders.* Hillsdale, NJ: Erlbaum, 1994:23–56.

Hallidie-Smith KA, Karas S. Cardiac anomalies in Williams-Beuren syndrome. *Arch Dis Child* 1988;63:809–813.

Morris CA, Demsey SA, Leonard CO, et al. Natural history of Williams syndrome: physical characteristics. *J Pediatr* 1988; 113:318–326.

Osborne L. Williams-Beuren syndrome: unraveling the mysteries of a microdeletion disorder. *Mol Genet Metab* 1999;67:1–10.

Pober BR, Dykens E. Williams syndrome: an overview of medical, cognitive, and behavioral features. *Psychiatr Clin North Am* 1996:929–943.

RESOURCES
196, 362, 393

146   Winchester Syndrome

*Manon Paquette, MS, DMD,
and Robert P. Langlais, DDS, MS*

DEFINITION: Winchester syndrome is a connective tissue disorder that has been traditionally classified as a mucopolysaccharidosis, in which acid mucopolysaccharides are stored in most tissues and excreted in large quantities in the urine. It has been suggested that Winchester syndrome be reclassified as a nonlysosomal storage disorder.

DIFFERENTIAL DIAGNOSIS: Juvenile rheumatoid arthritis (Still disease); Idiopathic multicentric osteolysis; Juvenile hyaline fibromatosis; Lipoid proteinosis (hyalinosis cutis et mucosae); Scheie syndrome; Farber disease.

SYMPTOMS AND SIGNS: Patients have short stature and are below the 3rd percentile for height and weight. Characteristic findings include coarse facial features, corneal opacifications, flat nose, recurrent purulent otitis media with possible perforation of the tympanic membrane and hearing loss, heart murmur, swollen joints, mild to severe arthralgias, and joint contractures with deformities. Examination of the mouth may show macroglossia, irregularly spaced teeth, supernumerary teeth, and gingival hypertrophy. Radiographs may show acrocephaly and other minor skull changes, temporomandibular joint arthritis, underdeveloped maxillary sinuses, and maxillary and mandibular hypoplasia. Additional radiographic findings include intraarticular and periarticular joint destruction simulating advanced rheumatoid arthritis, generalized osteoporosis and hypervascularity of the joints adjacent to bone undergoing resorption, ankylosis of some joints, and anterior beaking of the vertebrae in the cervical and lumbar spine. Subcutaneous nodules on the arms and thighs may appear leathery, hyperpigmented, and occasionally hypertrichotic and may be distributed over large areas of the body. Patients usually have normal mentation, but slight retardation has been reported.

ETIOLOGY/EPIDEMIOLOGY: The syndrome is inherited as an autosomal-recessive trait.

DIAGNOSIS: Diagnosis is frequently based on the clinical features, because other tests are often inconclusive. The latex fixation test and antinuclear antibody test are negative for rheumatoid factor. The biochemical findings from a 24-hour urine collection for urinary calcium, phosphorus, total protein, and mucopolysaccharide show a normal urinary mucopolysaccharide excretion and the presence of an abnormal oligosaccharide consisting of a trisaccharide containing one fucose and two galactoses. Skin biopsies obtained from the nodular leathery lesions show diffuse proliferation of fibroblasts deep into the dermis, extending into the subcutaneous adipose tissue. Absence of acid ceramidase in the leukocytes and the fibroblasts is expected. Exploration of the carpal area usually shows replacement of bone and cartilage by dense fibrocollagenous tissue, thinning of the cortex, and almost total absence of trabecular bone. Small and medium arterioles in this tissue undergo medial hypertrophy, which in many cases almost obliterates the lumen of the vessels.

TREATMENT

Standard Therapies: Treatment is usually symptomatic and includes medications such as nonsteroidal antiinflammatories, skeletal muscle relaxants, antibiotics and myringotomies for the ear infections, and orthopedic appliances and shoes. Other management protocols necessary for individual variations among patients are β-blockers and antiglaucoma medications.

REFERENCES

Dunger DB, Dicks-Mireaux C, O'Driscoll P, et al. Two cases of Winchester syndrome: with increased urinary oligosaccharide excretion. *Eur J Pediatr* 1987;146:615–619.

Hollister DW, Rimoin DL, Lachman RS, et al. The Winchester syndrome: a nonlysosomal connective tissue disease. *J Pediatr* 1974;84:701–709.

Hollister DW, Rimoin DL, Lachman RS, et al. The Winchester syndrome: clinical, radiographic and pathologic studies. *Birth Defects Orig Art Ser* 1974;10:89–100.

Prapanpoch S, Jorgenson RJ, Langlais RP, et al. Winchester syndrome. A case report and literature review. *Oral Surg Oral Med Oral Pathol* 1992;74:671–677.

Wallach J. *Interpretation of diagnostic tests,* 7th ed. Philadelphia: Lippincott Williams & Wilkins, 2000.

RESOURCE

351

147   Wolf-Hirschhorn Syndrome

Kurt Hirschhorn, MD

DEFINITION: Wolf-Hirschhorn syndrome (WHS) is a chromosomal disorder characterized by mental and growth retardation and abnormalities of the head, face, and internal organs.

SYNONYM: Chromosome 4p-.

DIFFERENTIAL DIAGNOSIS: Pitt-Rogers-Danks syndrome (allelic with WHS).

SYMPTOMS AND SIGNS: Patients with WHS are recognizable by the shape of their forehead (prominent glabella) and nose (beaked), giving the appearance of a Greek helmet. Many patients show defects of midline closure, including scalp defects, absent corpus callosum, severe midline cleft lip and palate, iris coloboma, hypospadias in males, sacral dimples, and diaphragmatic and umbilical hernia. They have severe growth retardation and moderate to severe mental retardation. Other facial aspects include a short philtrum, micrognathia, a carp-shaped mouth, low-set simple ears, hypertelorism, and downward-slanting palpebral fissures. Many patients have ventricular septal defects, renal hypoplasia, pulmonary isomerism, a common mesentery, delayed bone age, and various abnormal dermal ridges.

ETIOLOGY/EPIDEMIOLOGY: WHS is the result of a chromosomal deletion at 4p16.3 occurring either sporadically or, in approximately 20% of cases, as a result of a parental translocation including 4p. Multiple siblings have been described in the translocation cases. Males and females are affected with equal frequency.

DIAGNOSIS: In addition to the typical facial appearance, the diagnosis depends on chromosomal studies. G-banded chromosomes may show a reduction in the size of the short arm of chromosome 4. Occasionally the deletion is so small that it cannot be detected by banding studies alone and requires the use of fluorescent *in situ* hybridization using any of several available probes. The probes should cover the critical region of 165 kb, which includes two possible candidate genes whose absence may be responsible for the syndrome.

TREATMENT

Standard Therapies: Therapy is supportive, including speech therapy, special education, and parental counseling to help parents care for their affected children. Genetic counseling is essential, and chromosomal studies should be done on the parents to check for translocations. In familial cases, prenatal diagnosis is effective in determining the status of the fetus.

REFERENCES

Altherr MR, Bengtsson U, Elder FFB, et al. Molecular confirmation of Wolf-Hirschhorn syndrome with a subtle translocation of chromosome 4. *Am J Hum Genet* 1991;49:1235–1242.

Battaglia A, Carey JC, Cederholm P, et al. Natural history of Wolf-Hirschhorn syndrome: experience with 15 cases. *Pediatrics* 1999;103:830–836.

Hirschhorn K, Cooper HL, Firschein IL. Deletion of short arms of chromosome 4–5 in a child with defects of midline fusion. *Humangenetik* 1965;1:479–482.

McKusick VA, ed. *Online Mendelian Inheritance in Man (OMIM)* [database online]. Bethesda, MD: National Center for Biotechnology Information, National Library of Medicine; 2000. Entry no. 194190; last update 10/4/00.

Wolf U, Reinwein H, Porsch R, et al. Defizienz an den kurzen Armen eines Chromosoms Nr. 4. *Humangenetik* 1965;1:397.

Wright TJ, Ricke DO, Denison K, et al. A transcript map of the newly defined 165 kb Wolf-Hirschhorn syndrome critical region. *Hum Mol Genet* 1997;6:317–324.

RESOURCES

4, 495

148 Wolfram Syndrome

Timothy G. Barrett, MD, MB, PhD

DEFINITION: Wolfram syndrome is the inherited association of childhood-onset diabetes mellitus and progressive-onset optic atrophy.

SYNONYMS: DIDMOAD (diabetes insipidus, diabetes mellitus, optic atrophy, and deafness).

DIFFERENTIAL DIAGNOSIS: Thiamin-responsive megaloblastic anaemia, diabetes, and deafness; Mitochondrial diabetes and deafness.

SYMPTOMS AND SIGNS: Diabetes mellitus manifests at a median age of 6 years (range, 1 month to 16 years), often without ketonuria, and is insulin requiring. Optic atrophy manifests with loss of color vision and reduced visual acuity at 10 years (range, 1 month to 19 years), and progresses to perception of only light and dark in a median of 8 years. Cranial diabetes insipidus and sensorineural deafness manifest in two thirds of patients by 16 years (range, 2–39 years), but neither may produce symptoms. More than half of patients develop neuropathic bladder by 22 years (range, 10–44 years), and neurologic symptoms by 32 years (range, 5–44 years). These symptoms may include loss of taste and smell, ataxia, myoclonus, dysarthria, and psychiatric symptoms including endogenous depression and features of dementia such as short-term memory loss and disinhibition. Gastrointestinal dysmotility may also occur. Men are usually infertile, but affected women have had successful pregnancies. The median age of death is probably close to 40 years, and the oldest patient in a United Kingdom series was 49 years old. Deaths were due to intercurrent illness and apneas caused by central respiratory failure (underlying brainstem atrophy). There may be a milder subgroup of patients who are not severely affected and do not go on to develop all the symptoms.

ETIOLOGY/EPIDEMIOLOGY: Wolfram syndrome is inherited in an autosomal-recessive manner. The prevalence is believed to be approximately 1 in 500,000 children. The syndrome is usually due to mutations in the *WFS1* gene on chromosome 4p. This gene encodes a trans-

membrane protein of unknown function, but may be related to β-cell and neuron survival. All ethnic groups are affected.

DIAGNOSIS: The diagnosis is clinical and should be suspected in any child younger than 15 who develops diabetes mellitus and optic atrophy. Those with diabetes mellitus and insipidus, or diabetes and deafness, may have a separate syndrome. Mutation testing is available but may not alter management. The absence of a mutation does not rule out the diagnosis.

TREATMENT

Standard Therapies: Treatment is palliative. Multidisciplinary assessment is vital to manage the many facets of this condition. Almost all patients require replacement insulin. Cranial diabetes insipidus responds to intranasal or oral vasopressin. Approximately 25% of patients with hearing impairment benefit from hearing aids. Treatments for neuropathic bladder have included clean intermittent self-catheterization and ureterostomies. The advice of a urologist is essential. No treatment exists for optic atrophy. The relentless progression of the disease in most patients means that special educational and employment needs must be planned for in advance. Counseling and psychological support for both patients and their families is helpful.

REFERENCES

Barrett TG, Bundey SE, Macleod AF. Neurodegeneration and diabetes: UK nationwide study of Wolfram (DIDMOAD) syndrome. *Lancet* 1995;346:1458–1463.

Inoue H, Tanizawa Y, Wasson J, et al. A gene encoding a transmembrane protein is mutated in patients with diabetes mellitus and optic atrophy (Wolfram syndrome). *Nat Genet* 1998;20:143–148.

Khanim F, Kirk J, Latif F, et al. WFS1/Wolframin mutations, Wolfram syndrome, and associated diseases. *Hum Mutat* 2001;17:357–367.

Kinsley BT, Swift M, Dumont RH, et al. Morbidity and mortality in the Wolfram syndrome. *Diabetes Care* 1995;18:1566–1570.

RESOURCES

353, 355, 357

149   XLMR-Hypotonic Facies Syndrome

Fatima E. Abidi, PhD,
and Roger E. Stevenson, MD

DEFINITION: The syndrome is characterized by X-linked mental retardation with short stature, microcephaly, hypotonic facies with hypertelorism, small nose, open mouth and prominent lips, brachydactyly, genital anomalies, hypotonia, and in some cases, hemoglobin H inclusions in erythrocytes.

SYNONYMS: α-thalassemia mental retardation; Cerebro-faciogenital syndrome; ATR-X.

DIFFERENTIAL DIAGNOSIS: Coffin-Lowry syndrome; Some syndromes (Carpenter-Waziri syndrome; Holmes-Gang syndrome; Chudley-Lowry syndrome; Juberg-Marsidi syndrome; Smith-Fineman-Myers syndrome) are allelic to XLMR-hypotonic facies syndrome.

SYMPTOMS AND SIGNS: Most of the signs can be observed in infancy or early childhood because all milestones are delayed. Facial features include hypertelorism, epicanthal folds, flat nasal bridge, small triangular nose, anteverted nares, maxillary hypoplasia, open mouth with prominent lips, and widely spaced incisors. Minor anomalies of the skeleton may be observed: brachydactyly, tapering fingers, clinodactyly, digital contractures, overlapping digits, pes planus, varus and valgus foot deformations, kyphosis, scoliosis, pectus carinatum, and dimples over the lower spine. Short stature is seen in two thirds of patients. Most affected children have genital abnormalities, ranging from hypoplasia to ambiguous genitalia. Puberty is frequently delayed or arrested. Mental retardation is severe and speech is absent or severely limited.

ETIOLOGY/ EPIDEMIOLOGY: XLMR-hypotonic facies syndrome is an X-linked disorder mostly affecting males. The disease is due to mutation in the X-linked nuclear protein (*XNP*) gene located in Xq13.3. Female carriers are intellectually normal with no clinical manifestations. This is because marked skewing of X chromosome inactivation occurs in carrier females with preferential inactivation of the chromosome carrying the *XNP* mutation.

DIAGNOSIS: HbH inclusions may be found often by staining the erythrocytes with brilliant cresyl blue; however, the presence of these inclusions is variable and may be completely absent. Diagnostic confirmation depends on mutational analysis of the *XNP* gene. Identification of marked skewing (≥90:10) of the X-inactivation pattern in obligate carrier females may help.

TREATMENT

Standard Therapies: No curative treatment is available. Early educational intervention and physical therapy may have a positive impact on early developmental progress.

REFERENCES

Gibbons RJ, Brueton L, Buckle VJ, et al. The clinical and hematological features of X-linked α thalassemia/mental retardation syndrome (ATR-X). *Am J Med Genet* 1995;55:288–299.

Gibbons RJ, Higgs DR. Molecular-clinical spectrum of the ATR-X syndrome. *Am J Med Genet* 2000;97:204–212.

Gibbons RJ, Suthers GK, Wilkie AOM, et al. X-linked α-thalassemia/mental retardation (ATR-X) syndrome: localization to Xq12–21.31 by X-inactivation and linkage analysis. *Am J Hum Genet* 1992;51:1136–1149.

Stevenson RE, Schwartz CE, Schroer RJ. *X-linked mental retardation.* New York: Oxford University Press, 2000:385–388.

Villard L, Toutain A, Lossi A-M, et al. Splicing mutation in the *ATR-X* gene can lead to a dysmorphic mental retardation phenotype without α-thalassemia. *Am J Med Genet* 1996;58:499–505.

Weatherall DJ, Higgs DR, Bunch C, et al. Hemoglobin H disease and mental retardation. A new syndrome or a remarkable coincidence? *N Engl J Med* 1981;305:607–612.

RESOURCES

188, 351, 462

150 | Yunis-Varón Syndrome

Elisabeth Walch, MD,
and Christof Dame, MD

DEFINITION: Yunis-Varón syndrome (YVS) is an autosomal-recessive disorder associated with an extremely poor outcome due to the unique malformation of the skeletal and ectodermal system. This syndrome is classified with dysplasias with prominent membranous bone involvement.

DIFFERENTIAL DIAGNOSIS: Distal aphalangia; Cleidocranial dysplasia; Bone dysplasia; Osteochondrodysplasia; Storage disease; Pachygyria.

SYMPTOMS AND SIGNS: The most striking clinical features are bilaterally symmetric skeletal anomalies of hands and feet consisting of the agenesis of thumbs and halluces, distal aphalangia of fingers and toes, and agenesis/hypoplasia of both clavicles. Fingers and toes are short and pointed, sometimes with absence of nail formation. Clinical examination of the head often shows microcephaly, sparse hair, an abnormally soft skull, a wide anterior fontanelle, and diastasis of sutures. The typical facial dysmorphisms consist of hypoplastic facial bones, thin lips, a short upper lip, severe micrognathia and retrognathia, reduced nasolabial distance, labiogingival retraction, anteverted nostrils, dysplastic, low-set ears, prominent eyes, and cataracts. Skin features include redundant posterior neck skin, absent nipples, and sparse eyelashes and eyebrows. Associated genital malformations include hypospadia, bifid scrotum, undescended testes, and micropenis. Diminished fetal movement, spontaneous abortion, and intrauterine growth retardation during gestation also occur. Neonates have a generalized muscular hypotonia (floppy infant, rare spontaneous movements, shallow breathing, and decreased suck), often requiring tube feeding. Patients frequently suffer from cardiorespiratory insufficiency and may require mechanical ventilation. Most infants die in the first 4 months of life as a result of cardiorespiratory failure.

ETIOLOGY/EPIDEMIOLOGY: The disorder is inherited in an autosomal-recessive manner. A total of 18 cases, affecting both sexes equally, have been reported since the first description in 1980. The pathogenesis is unknown, but a metabolic disorder is suspected. Lysosomal storage phenomena and excretion of abnormal oligosaccharides have been reported.

DIAGNOSIS: The diagnosis is made on prenatal ultrasonography, which shows the characteristic symmetric skeletal anomalies of the hands and feet as well as central nervous system malformations. Radiologic examination verifies generalized osteopenia of the entire skeleton, severe ossification deficits of the calvaria, bilateral hypoplasia or agenesis of the clavicles, slender ribs, gracile long bones, and pelvic dysplasia. Pathologic bone fractures often occur. Ultrasonography in affected neonates may show associated diverse neurologic features, including hydrocephalus internus, agenesis of the corpus callosum, deep brain fissures, and Dandy-Walker malformation. Echocardiography may show concentric ventricular hypertrophy and cardiomegaly. A high turnover of bone-related proteins may be indicated by elevated procollagen I C-terminal peptide and urinary cross-linked N-telopeptides of type 1 collagen. Biochemical analysis of the urine may show elevated excretion of oligosaccharides. Histopathologic examination may show abnormal cortical architecture with pachygyria and polymicrogyria. Storage phenomena may be indicated by the accumulation of nonperiodic acid-Schiff material in nerve cells. Fibroblast cultures may be helpful in scientific analysis of intracytoplasmic vacuoles.

TREATMENT

Standard Therapies: Standard treatment is generally palliative. Due to a generalized hypotonia, tube feedings are required. Mechanical ventilation is often mandatory. Sequelae such as bone fractures can be treated with pain medication and, if necessary, by casting. Genetic counseling and prenatal ultrasonography are important for the index families because the risk for YVS in future pregnancies is 25%.

REFERENCES

Adès LC, Morris LL, Richardson M, et al. Congenital heart malformation in Yunis-Varón syndrome. *J Med Genet* 1993;30:788–792.

Garrett C, Berry AC, Simpson RH, et al. Yunis-Varón syndrome with severe osteodysplasty. *J Med Genet* 1990;27:114–121.

Hennekam RCM, Vermeulen-Meiers C. Further delineation of the Yunis-Varón syndrome. *J Med Genet* 1989;21:55–58.

Walch E, Schmitt M, Brenner R, et al. Yunis-Varón syndrome: evidence for a lysosomal storage disease. *Am J Med Genet* 2000;95:157–160.

Yunis E, Varón H. Cleidocranial dysostosis, severe micrognathism, bilateral absence of thumbs and first metatarsal bone, and distal aphalangia. *Am J Child* 1980;134:649–653.

RESOURCES

96, 149, 351, 357

6

Emerging/Infectious Diseases

1   Anthrax

*Kristy Murray Lillibridge, DVM,
and David Ashford, DVM, MPH, DSc*

DEFINITION: Anthrax occurs in both humans and animals and is caused by *Bacillus anthracis*, a gram-positive, spore-forming bacillus. In humans, the disease has three forms, which are based on route of infection: cutaneous, gastrointestinal, and inhalational.

SYNONYMS: Woolsorter disease; Malignant pustule; Siberian plague; Black baine; Ragpicker disease; Malignant edema.

DIFFERENTIAL DIAGNOSIS: Cutaneous: Plague; Tularemia; Staphylococcal disease; Herpes; Rat-bite fever; Leishmaniasis; Tropical ulcer; Mycobacterial disease; Syphilis. Gastrointestinal: Bacterial or parasitic dysentery. Inhalational: Hantavirus; Plague; Pneumonia; Influenza.

SYMPTOMS AND SIGNS: The most common form is cutaneous anthrax, which begins with a pruritic papule that enlarges and develops into an ulcer surrounded by vesicles, followed by formation of a characteristic black necrotic central eschar. The painless lesion is usually associated with local edema. If untreated, the fatality rate of cutaneous anthrax can reach 20%. Gastrointestinal anthrax can manifest as either intestinal or oropharyngeal disease. The symptoms for intestinal infection include fever, nausea, abdominal pain, vomiting, and anorexia, followed by hematemesis and bloody diarrhea, toxemia, shock, cyanosis, and death within 2–5 days. Symptoms for oropharyngeal illness include fever, sore throat, dysphagia, cervical lymphadenopathy, edema, tissue necrosis, toxemia, sepsis, and death. Inhalational anthrax may manifest as a biphasic illness, with the patient initially exhibiting 1–3 days of low-grade fever, malaise, dry cough, and substernal pressure, followed by sudden onset of high fever, dyspnea, stridor, dry cough, tachypnea, tachycardia, profuse diaphoresis, septic shock, and death within 1–2 days. After inhalation, spores are transported to the hilar and mediastinal lymph nodes, where they germinate and cause hemorrhagic necrosis and edema. Pleural effusions also occur. Meningitis may be a complication seen with all three forms of the disease.

ETIOLOGY/EPIDEMIOLOGY: *B. anthracis* spores are present in the soil and have worldwide distribution. Humans become infected after coming into contact with infected livestock animals or animal products. Cutaneous anthrax occurs after spores come in contact with exposed, broken skin; gastrointestinal anthrax occurs after ingestion of poorly cooked or raw contaminated meat from infected animals; and inhalational anthrax occurs after the inhalation of spores. There have been no confirmed cases of person-to-person transmission. Any suspected anthrax case in the United States warrants a rapid public health investigation and should be reported immediately to local public health authorities. *B. anthracis* is a potential agent of biological terrorism.

DIAGNOSIS: Cutaneous anthrax is diagnosed by clinical presentation, history of livestock or animal exposure, and detection of anthrax bacilli by gram-stained smears, IFA, or culture of vesicular fluid or exudate. Gastrointestinal anthrax is difficult to diagnose antemortem. Inhalational anthrax can be diagnosed by the characteristic radiographic finding of mediastinal widening combined with blood culture positive for *B. anthracis*.

TREATMENT
Standard Therapies: Intravenous penicillin G is the therapy of choice for all forms of anthrax. If antibiotic susceptibility testing identifies a penicillin-resistant strain, ciprofloxacin or doxycycline can be used as alternatives. Cutaneous lesions should not be excised, and topical therapy is not effective. Antimicrobial therapy is rarely successful for the gastrointestinal or inhalational forms of disease once symptoms have begun. With a known aerosol exposure to *B. anthracis* spores, prophylaxis with ciprofloxacin or doxycycline can be given to prevent anthrax. However, the effectiveness of postexposure prophylaxis has only been studied in laboratory animals. Anthrax vaccine can also be used in combination with antibiotics for postexposure prophylaxis if it is available.

REFERENCES
Ashford DA, Perkins B, Rotz LD. Use of anthrax vaccine in the United States. *MMWR* 2000;49:1–20.

Inglesby TV, Henderson DA, Bartlett JG. Anthrax as a biological weapon. *JAMA* 1999;281:1735–1745.

Lew DP. Bacillus anthracis (anthrax). In: Mandell GL, Bennett JE, Dolin R, eds. *Principles and practice of infectious diseases,* 5th ed. Philadelphia: Churchill Livingstone, 2000:2215–2220.

Penn CC, Klotz SA. Anthrax pneumonia. *Semin Respir Infect* 1997;12:28–30.

RESOURCES
89, 359

2   Botulism

Christopher R. Braden, MD

DEFINITION: Botulism is characterized by symmetric descending flaccid paralysis resulting from the effect of botulinum neurotoxin produced by *Clostridium botulinum*, a gram-positive, anaerobic, spore-forming coccus. Three clinical entities are generally recognized: food-borne, infant, and wound botulism. Because toxin-containing foods may place others at risk and because of the potential use of botulinum toxin as a biological weapon, any case of botulism is considered a public health emergency. State and local public health officials must be informed immediately if botulism is suspected.

DIFFERENTIAL DIAGNOSIS: Guillain-Barré syndrome (especially Miller-Fisher variant); Myasthenia gravis; Cerebral vascular accident.

SYMPTOMS AND SIGNS: Food-borne botulism may start with nausea, vomiting, and diarrhea. Paralysis may manifest within a few hours to days after exposure. The bulbar nerves are first affected, then the chest and extremities, with proximal and upper extremity weakness preceding distal and lower extremity weakness. Symptoms range from subtle motor weakness of the cranial nerves to rapid respiratory arrest and complete paralysis. Mental status and sensory pathways are unaffected. The clinical manifestations of wound botulism are similar to food-borne botulism. Infant botulism manifests as constipation followed by poor sucking, weak cry, lethargy, generalized weakness, and lack of muscle tone, most easily recognized as a floppy head.

ETIOLOGY/EPIDEMIOLOGY: *C. botulinum* is a common bacterium in soil. It causes food poisoning because its heat-resistant spores may survive food preservation methods and produce neurotoxin in anaerobic, low acid (pH > 4.6) conditions. Most cases in the United States are due to improperly home-processed foods. Ingestion of toxins allows their irreversible binding to the presynaptic motor nerve membrane, where they block the release of acetylcholine. Wound botulism is due to the proliferation and sporulation of *C. botulinum* in the wound, with the subsequent production and systemic absorption of toxin. Infant botulism is due to intestinal colonization with toxin-producing *C. botulinum* spores. There are seven serologically distinct types of botulinum toxin, designated A through G. Types A, B, and E cause disease in humans, although a few cases due to type F toxin have been reported. Type A toxin is the most common type in the United States, comprising about one half of cases. Type E toxin is most often associated with fish or marine animal sources. In

2000, 140 cases of botulism were reported from 29 states in the United States, of which 17 were food-borne, 104 were infant botulism, and 13 were wound botulism. Wound botulism has become more common; most cases have occurred among heroin users who injected the drug subcutaneously.

DIAGNOSIS: The diagnosis of botulism in patients with consistent symptoms and signs is aided by a history of recent consumption of suspicious foods. Immediate testing should include brain imaging studies and lumbar puncture; normal findings help exclude a cerebrovascular accident or space-occupying lesion and Guillain-Barré syndrome. Myasthenia gravis may be excluded with a normal edrophonium chloride test. Electromyographic studies in botulism show decreased amplitude of action potentials in involved muscle groups. Rapid repetitive electromyography (20–50 Hz) may show facilitation (i.e., increasing pattern of action potential amplitude). Testing serum, stool, culture samples, and associated foods for botulinum toxin confirms the diagnosis.

TREATMENT
Standard Therapies: Respiratory decompensation may occur rapidly; therefore, patients should be monitored in an intensive care unit with frequent evaluation of vital capacity. Prompt intubation and mechanical ventilation are warranted if vital capacity wanes. Surgical debridement is indicated for wound botulism, and antibiotic therapy should include agents with good anticlostridial activity, such as penicillin G or metronidazole. Intravenous equine antitoxin administered as early as possible in the course of illness is the only specific treatment available for food-borne and wound botulism. Antitoxin will not reverse established neurologic deficits, but will prevent the progression of disease, shorten the duration of ventilatory failure, and shorten the duration of hospitalization.

Investigational Therapies: Equine antitoxin is not recommended for infants. An investigational human-derived product is available under a treatment investigational new drug protocol.

REFERENCES
Hughes JM, Blumenthal JR, Merson MH, et al. Clinical features of type A and B food-borne botulism. *Ann Intern Med* 1981;95: 442–445.

Shapiro RL, Hatheway C, Swerdlow DL. Botulism in the United States: a clinical and epidemiologic review. *Ann Intern Med* 1998;129:221–228.

RESOURCES
89, 159, 359

3   Brucellosis

Kristy Murray Lillibridge, DVM, and David Ashford, DVM, MPH, DSc

DEFINITION: Brucellosis is a bacterial disease that may be transmitted to humans from domestic and wild animals or animal products. *Brucella* species are small, nonmotile, gram-negative coccobacilli.

SYNONYMS: Malta fever; Undulant fever; Mediterranean fever; Bang disease.

DIFFERENTIAL DIAGNOSIS: Infections and autoimmune diseases associated with fevers of unknown origin or chronic fatigue–like symptoms.

SYMPTOMS AND SIGNS: Symptoms of infection are nonspecific and include fever, sweats, malaise, headache, back pain, anorexia, fatigue, and weight loss. Fevers have variable durations and can exhibit irregular or intermittent patterns. The incubation period is usually 2–4 weeks after inoculation, but may be several months. Mild lymphadenopathy, splenomegaly, and hepatomegaly are occasionally reported. Anemia, leukopenia, and thrombocytopenia are commonly found. Rarely, endocarditis and central nervous system involvement occur.

ETIOLOGY/EPIDEMIOLOGY: *Brucella melitensis* subspecies *abortus*, *B. melitensis* subspecies *suis*, *B. melitensis* subspecies *canis,* and *B. melitensis* subspecies *melitensis* are zoonotic pathogens. Brucellosis has a worldwide distribution. In the United States, the disease has been dramatically reduced in domestic livestock and humans. Approximately 100 cases among humans are reported each year. Risk of disease is usually occupation related, with transmission occurring through cuts or abrasions in the skin after direct contact with diseased animals or their secretions, infected aerosols, accidental inoculation, or ingestion of raw milk or other unpasteurized dairy products. In the United States, any suspected case of brucellosis warrants a public health investigation and should be reported immediately to local public health authorities. *B. melitensis* subspecies *suis* and *B. melitensis* subspecies *melitensis* are potential biological terrorism agents.

DIAGNOSIS: Isolation and identification of a *Brucella* species from blood, bone marrow, or other tissues provides a definitive diagnosis. Prolonged isolation and a CO_2-enriched atmosphere with specialized media may be required for isolating the organism. In the absence of a positive culture, a serologic diagnosis can be made if there is evidence of an increasing titer on paired serum samples. A single, high-titer serologic result can be suggestive of the diagnosis. The standard serologic assay is a tube or microagglutination test.

TREATMENT

Standard Therapies: Doxycycline combined with streptomycin is the most effective treatment. Rifampin can be an alternative to streptomycin, but it is less efficacious. For pregnant women and children, doxycycline can be replaced with trimethoprim-sulfamethoxazole.

Investigational Therapies: The use of gentamicin instead of streptomycin is being explored.

REFERENCES

Acha PN, Szyfres B, eds. Brucellosis. *Zoonoses and communicable diseases common to man and animals.* Scientific publication no. 503. Washington, DC: World Health Organization, 1987:24–45.

Centers for Disease Control and Prevention. Summary of notifiable diseases, United States, 1996. *MMWR* 1996;45:26.

Centers for Disease Control and Prevention. Suspected brucellosis case prompts investigation of possible bioterrorism-related activity—New Hampshire and Massachusetts, 1999. *MMWR* 2000;49:509–512.

Coats ME. Brucellosis. In: Farris R, Newman E, Mahlow J, Nix B, eds. *Health hazards in veterinary practice,* 3rd ed. Austin: Texas Department of Health, 1995:15–17.

Young EJ. *Brucella* species. In: Mandell GL, Bennett JE, Dolin R, eds. *Principles and practice of infectious diseases,* 5th ed. Philadelphia: Churchill Livingstone, 2000:2386–2393.

RESOURCES

89, 159

4 Dengue Fever

John Mosely Hayes, DrPH, MSPH, MBA

DEFINITION: Dengue fever and its severe forms, dengue hemorrhagic fever (DHF) and dengue shock syndrome (DSS), are caused by any one of four closely related flaviviruses (Dengue-1, -2, -3, and -4) transmitted by mosquitoes. Lasting cross-protective immunity is specific to each serotype, so persons can have up to four dengue infections during their lifetimes.

SYNONYM: Breakbone fever.

DIFFERENTIAL DIAGNOSIS: (In increasing order of severity of manifestations) Influenza; Measles; Rubella; Malaria; Typhoid fever; Leptospirosis; Meningococcemia; Rickettsial infections; Bacterial sepsis; Viral hemorrhagic fevers.

SYMPTOMS AND SIGNS: Dengue fever is characterized by acute onset of high fever, frontal headache, retroorbital pain, myalgias, arthralgias, nausea, vomiting, and often maculopapular rash and hemorrhagic manifestations. Severity ranges from asymptomatic infections to fatal hypotensive and hemorrhagic disease. Hemorrhagic manifestations are usually skin hemorrhages (i.e., petechiae, purpura, or ecchymoses), but may also include epistaxis, bleeding gums, hematemesis, and melena. The acute phase of illness lasts approximately a week, whereas convalescence, characterized by weakness, malaise, and anorexia, may last 1–2 weeks. DHF may initially resemble dengue fever. As fever subsides, thrombocytopenia and hemoconcentration due to vascular plasma leakage may develop, resulting in circulatory failure and severe hemorrhage. Warning signs for DSS include severe abdominal pain, protracted vomiting, marked temperature change (from fever to hypothermia), or change in mental status (irritability or obtundation). DSS, which can lead to profound shock and death, can develop rapidly. Early signs include cold clammy skin, restlessness, rapid weak pulse, narrowing of pulse pressure, or hypotension. DHF and DSS can occur in both children and adults.

ETIOLOGY/EPIDEMIOLOGY: Dengue transmission requires (a) the vector mosquito (mainly the highly domesticated, daytime biting *Aedes aegypti*); (b) any one of the four dengue viruses; and (c) a human susceptible to the corresponding virus. Both sexes and all age groups are at risk. It is estimated that 2.5 billion persons live in dengue risk areas, and that each year tens of millions of dengue fever cases and hundreds of thousands of DHF cases occur. As the number of circulating dengue viruses in a population increases, so does the incidence of DHF. In locations

without experience in the management of DSS, the fatality rate may be greater than 10%.

DIAGNOSIS: Dengue fever can be effectively ruled out if the patient has not been in a dengue-endemic area, if symptoms have started more than 2 weeks after the patient left a dengue-endemic area, or if the fever lasts more than 2 weeks. Monitoring of blood pressure, hematocrit, platelet count, hemorrhagic manifestations, urinary output, and level of consciousness is crucial for early diagnosis and to guide treatment. The patient's deterioration between 3 and 6 days of illness, and the relationship of defervescence in conjunction with thrombocytopenia and plasma leakage are highly suggestive of DHF/DSS. Only virus isolation or specific antibody detection can provide unequivocal dengue diagnosis. Virus isolation is most often successful in serum specimens taken within 5 days after onset of symptoms and stored on dry ice, or, if to be delivered within 1 week, unfrozen in a refrigerator. For antibody detection, a serum sample taken 6 or more days after onset of symptoms is adequate (no refrigeration is required if the sample is delivered overnight).

TREATMENT

Standard Therapies: Aspirin should not be used due to its interference with platelet function. For pain and fever, acetaminophen preparations are preferred. Patients should be monitored closely. If treated early, DHF can be effectively managed by intravenous fluid replacement therapy. Intravenous fluid treatment should be adjusted using serial hematocrit, blood pressure, and urinary output data. Total fluid replacement in 24 hours should be approximately the volume required for maintenance, plus replacement of 5% of body weight deficit. Fluid should not be administered uniformly but based on close monitoring of urinary output and hematocrit readings. No preventive vaccine or specific antiviral agents are currently available.

REFERENCES

Gubler D, Kuno G, eds. *Dengue hemorrhagic fever.* New York: CAB International, 1997.
Kalayanarooj S, Vaughn DW, Nimmannitya S, et al. Early clinical and laboratory indicators of acute dengue illness. *J Infect Dis* 1997;176:313–321.
Rigau-Pérez JG, Clark GG, Gubler DJ, et al. Dengue and dengue haemorrhagic fever. *Lancet* 1998;352:971–977.
Vaughn DW, Green S, Kalayanarooj S, et al. Dengue in the early febrile phase; viremia and antibody response. *J Infect Dis* 1997;176:322–330.

RESOURCES

89, 359

5   Ebola and Other Viral Hemorrhagic Fevers

Scott A. Harper, MD, MPH, MSc, and Daniel G. Bausch, MD, MPH

DEFINITION: Viral hemorrhagic fever (VHF) refers to a severe disease syndrome caused by infection with RNA viruses from one of four families: Arenaviridae, Bunyaviridae, Filoviridae, and Flaviviridae. The VHF syndromes include Ebola hemorrhagic fever (HF), Marburg HF, Lassa fever, Rift Valley fever, Crimean-Congo HF, HF with renal syndrome, Argentine HF, Bolivian HF, Venezuelan HF, yellow fever, dengue HF, and hantavirus pulmonary syndrome.

DIFFERENTIAL DIAGNOSIS: Malaria; Typhoid fever; Bacillary dysentery; Bacterial sepsis; Septicemic plague; Leptospirosis; Borreliosis; Rickettsial diseases.

SYMPTOMS AND SIGNS: The incubation period for Ebola HF ranges from 3 to 21 days, with most patients presenting 5–10 days after infection. The initial presentation is usually nonspecific, including fever, malaise, myalgias, and headache, followed by gastrointestinal symptoms such as nausea, vomiting, and diarrhea. A fleeting maculopapular rash may be noted early in the course of the disease. Bleeding, most commonly from the mucosa or gastrointestinal tract, sometimes occurs. Patients with fatal cases usually exhibit rapid development of shock and increasing coagulopathy resulting in multiorgan system failure. Case-fatality ratios from the VHFs range from <5% to 90%, depending on the specific viral cause. Once recovered from acute disease, survivors are generally not infectious, with the exception of possible sexual transmission for as long as 3 months after the acute illness. Considerable differences may exist in incubation period, clinical syndrome, laboratory, and pathologic findings, depending on the specific virus causing the HF.

ETIOLOGY/EPIDEMIOLOGY: Although Ebola HF is limited to the African continent, VHFs occur worldwide. Most are zoonotic in nature and only occasionally infect humans. The reservoir for Ebola virus is unknown. Interhuman transmission occurs via direct contact with infected body fluids. A hallmark of Ebola HF is its propensity to cause nosocomial epidemics among health-care workers in settings where barrier nursing precautions are not strictly observed. Funeral rituals entailing touching of the corpse have also played a major role in transmission. Interhuman transmission has been noted in Marburg HF, Crimean-Congo HF, and Lassa fever.

DIAGNOSIS: Most VHFs are difficult to diagnose clinically; a high index of suspicion followed by prompt laboratory confirmation is imperative. Diagnostic tests for VHF agents are largely limited to reference laboratories with appropriate containment facilities. Enzyme-linked immunosorbent assay detection of antigen and IgM and IgG antibodies is the mainstay of diagnosis. Reverse transcription polymerase chain reaction and viral culture may also be used. Immunohistochemical detection of Ebola antigen in formalin-fixed tissues can be used for disease surveillance.

TREATMENT

Standard Therapies: Treatment is largely supportive, including maintenance of fluid balance with attention to renal, pulmonary, and cardiac function. Antibacterial and/or antiparasitic therapy may be indicated until the diagnosis can be confirmed or when secondary infection is suspected. Administration of the antiviral drug ribavirin should be considered in Lassa fever, Rift Valley fever, Crimean-Congo HF, and HF with renal syndrome, and is also likely effective in some South American HFs. An infectious disease specialist, local public health officials, and the CDC should be consulted as soon as the diagnosis is suspected.

Investigational Therapies: Convalescent serum has been tried in some VHFs, with variable results. Corticosteroids have been suggested for modification of the proinflammatory state present in many of the VHFs, as well as for replacement therapy in suspected adrenal gland necrosis, but clinical trials are needed.

REFERENCES

Centers for Disease Control and Prevention. Update: management of patients with suspected viral hemorrhagic fever—United States. *MMWR* 1995;44:475–479.

Centers for Disease Control and Prevention and World Health Organization. Infection control for viral hemorrhagic fevers in the African health care setting. Available at *www.cdc.gov/ncidod/dvrd/spb/mnpages/vhfmanual.htm.* Accessed 1998.

Peters CJ, LeDuc JW. An introduction to Ebola: the virus and the disease. *J Infect Dis* 1999;179(suppl 1):ix–xvi.

Peters CJ, Zaki SR. Overview of viral hemorrhagic fevers. In: Guerrant RL, Walker DH, Weller PF, eds. *Tropical infectious diseases: principles, pathogens, & practice,* 1st ed. Philadelphia: Churchill Livingstone, 1999:1182–1190.

RESOURCES

89, 359, 497

6   Ehrlichiosis

*Candace L. McCall, DVM, MPH,
and Christopher D. Paddock, MD*

DEFINITION: Ehrlichiae are small (0.5–1.5 μm) intracellular bacteria that primarily infect leukocytes, forming intracytoplasmic aggregates known as morulae. Human disease can be caused by several ehrlichial species, including three found in the United States: *Ehrlichia chaffeensis, E. phagoctyophila,* and *E. ewingii.*

SYNONYMS: Human ehrlichiosis; Human granulocytic ehrlichiosis (HGE); Human monocytic ehrlichiosis (HME).

DIFFERENTIAL DIAGNOSIS: Rocky Mountain spotted fever; Tularemia; Lyme disease; Relapsing fever; Colorado tick fever; Babesiosis; Enteroviral diseases; Leptospirosis; Gram-positive or gram-negative sepsis; Noninfectious hematologic syndromes.

SYMPTOMS AND SIGNS: Cases of human ehrlichioses in the United States share common symptoms, although they may vary in severity by etiologic agent. Early clinical presentation is generally nonspecific and may resemble various infectious and noninfectious acute febrile syndromes. After an incubation period of 5–10 days following a tick bite, the patient typically presents with fever, headache, and malaise. Other signs and symptoms, including gastrointestinal and upper respiratory manifestations, joint pain, confusion, and occasionally rash, may also occur. Patients with ehrlichiosis may develop severe manifestations if appropriate antibiotic treatment is delayed. Ehrlichiosis appears to increase in severity in persons older than 40 years. Severe ehrlichiosis may result in prolonged fever, acute renal failure, disseminated intravascular coagulopathy, meningoencephalitis, adult respiratory distress syndrome, or coma.

ETIOLOGY/EPIDEMIOLOGY: Ehrlichiosis is an emerging infectious disease that occurs worldwide. Ehrlichiae are transmitted by the bite of an infected tick, and most patients are infected in the spring and summer months. Mechanisms of transmission other than tick bites are uncommon. Perinatal transmission of HGE to an infant has been described. Because these bacteria infect leukocytes, transmission by blood transfusion may be possible. *E. ewingii* is the most recently discovered ehrlichia, and human infection with this organism occurs primarily in immunosuppressed persons.

DIAGNOSIS: Ehrlichial infections are difficult to diagnose, and the availability of confirmatory tests is relatively limited. Common clinical laboratory findings include leukopenia, thrombocytopenia, and elevated hepatic aminotransferase levels. Blood smears stained with Diff-Quick or Giesma stains may show morulae, providing a quick presumptive diagnosis. Antibody testing by indirect immunofluorescence assay or detection of ehrlichial DNA by polymerase chain reaction assay is most frequently used to confirm the diagnosis.

TREATMENT

Standard Therapies: Treatment decisions are based on epidemiologic and clinical findings. Therapy should be started promptly and should not be delayed while waiting for laboratory test results. Doxycycline or other tetracyclines are the treatments of choice. For most patients with mild or moderate disease, failure to improve clinically within 24–72 hours should prompt consideration of another diagnosis. Antibiotic therapy should be continued for at least 3 days after fever subsides and for a minimum of 7 days total. Standard duration is generally 10–14 days. If ehrlichiosis is severe or complicated, longer treatment courses may be required. Although clinical evidence is limited, rifampin has been used successfully in pregnant women with HGE.

REFERENCES

Bakken JS, Dumler JS. Ehrlichia species. In: Yu VL, Merigam TC, Barriere SL, eds. *antimicrobial therapy and vaccines.* Baltimore: Williams & Wilkins, 1999:546–551.

Buller RS, Arens M, Hmiel SP, et al. *Ehrlichia ewingii,* a newly recognized agent of human ehrlichiosis. *N Engl J Med* 1999;341: 148–155.

McQuiston JH, Paddock CD, Holman RC, et al. The human ehrlichioses in the United States. *Emerg Infect Dis* 1999;5: 635–642.

Walker DH, Dumler JS. Emergence of the ehrlichioses as human health problems. *Emerg Infect Dis* 1996;2:18–29.

RESOURCES

89, 359

7   Selected Encephalitides

Zoltan Kaliszky, MD, and William R. Tyor, MD

DEFINITION: Encephalitides are inflammations of the brain. Patients may present with altered level of consciousness, fever, headache, behavioral changes as well as seizures, and focal neurologic deficits. Important causes of viral encephalitis are herpes simplex virus type 1 (HSV-1) and Japanese encephalitis virus. Rasmussen encephalitis is a rare type.

SYNONYMS: For HSV-1 encephalitis: Acute necrotizing encephalitis; For Rasmussen encephalitis: Chronic focal encephalitis of Rasmussen; Rasmussen syndrome.

DIFFERENTIAL DIAGNOSIS: CNS infections caused by other viruses; Bacterial meningitis; Mycoplasma infection; Neurosyphilis; Fungal infections; Systemic lupus erythematosus; Sarcoidosis; Brain abscess; Acute disseminated encephalomyelitis; Drug toxicity or other CNS toxins; Metabolic disturbances; Vascular lesions; Tumor.

SYMPTOMS AND SIGNS: Typically, patients with HSV-1 encephalitis present with headache, nausea, vomiting, fever, altered mental status, seizures, and focal neurologic deficits. Altered mental status varies from subtle behavioral changes to coma. Occasionally, HSV-1 encephalitis is accompanied by a stiff neck or meningismus. Characteristically, HSV-1 causes asymmetric necrosis in the temporal lobes, orbital-frontal lobes, and the limbic system. Japanese encephalitis has an incubation period of 6–16 days, prodromal phase of 2–3 days, and acute phase of 2–4 days. After this, the stage of defervescence takes 7–10 days and the convalescent phase lasts for 4–7 weeks. In the prodromal phase, fever, headache, nausea and vomiting, and malaise predominate. The onset may be acute or subacute. The acute encephalitis phase can be manifested by seizures, changes in mental status, focal neurologic deficits including aphasia, hemiparesis, quadriparesis, segmental sensory disturbances, ataxia, cranial nerve palsies, and features of parkinsonism such as limb tremors and expressionless facies. Pathologically, the disease involves both the gray and white matter of the cerebral hemispheres, including the basal ganglia. The brainstem and cerebellum can also be involved. Histologically, the disease manifests with cerebral edema and capillary hemorrhages. Diffuse perivascular lymphocytosis and perivascular necrotic foci are also seen. Rasmussen encephalitis is a chronic inflammatory disease of the brain. Most frequently, affected individuals are 6–10 years old. Affected children typically develop focal seizures, limited to one hemisphere at onset. Seizures are often refractory to therapy and may be manifested by focal motor or sensorimotor symptoms. Epilepsia partialis continua can develop, which is often later associated with slowly progressive hemiplegia. Hemianopsia and intellectual deterioration may also occur. Pathologic changes of chronic inflammation are restricted to one hemisphere. Cerebral atrophy may be localized or involve the entire hemisphere.

ETIOLOGY/EPIDEMIOLOGY: Herpes simplex encephalitis caused by HSV-1 is the most frequent cause of acute sporadic encephalitis in the United States, with 250,000–500,000 cases per year. Japanese encephalitis is the most common mosquito-transmitted encephalitis in the world. The disease is most commonly found in China, Southeast Asia, the Indian subcontinent, the Philippines, New Guinea, the Island of Guam, and, more recently, Australia. The etiology of Rasmussen encephalitis is unknown. It may be viral, such as in Epstein-Barr virus and cytomegalovirus, or may have an autoimmune pathogenesis.

DIAGNOSIS: Diagnosis of HSV-1 encephalitis is based on the symptoms and signs of the encephalitis, imaging studies, and laboratory tests. Diagnosis of Japanese encephalitis is based on the clinical symptoms and signs, cerebrospinal fluid (CSF) analysis, which shows signs of viral infection, and serologic evidence within the CSF of anti-Japanese encephalitis virus IgM antibody. Diagnosis of Rasmussen encephalitis is based on the specific clinical picture and course, the electroencephalography findings, and the MRI results, which typically demonstrate diffuse atrophy of the involved hemisphere.

TREATMENT

Standard Therapies: Herpes simplex encephalitis is usually treated with acyclovir. If that is not successful, foscarnet can be used. Otherwise, therapy is supportive. Therapy for Japanese encephalitis is supportive. Formalin-inactivated vaccine is available for travelers and for endemic populations. Mosquito control remains the mainstay of prevention. Traditionally, the treatment of Rasmussen encephalitis has been the removal of the affected hemisphere; however, steroid treatment, plasmapheresis, and intravenous immunoglobulin may have some efficacy.

Investigational Therapies: Recombinant interferon-α is being investigated for treatment of Japanese encephalitis, as are isoquinolone compounds *in vitro* and monoclonal antibodies.

REFERENCES

Bradley WG, Daroff RB, Fenichel GM, et al. *Neurology in clinical practice*, 3rd ed, Vol. 2. Stoneham, MA: Butterworth-Heinemann, 2000:1353–1373.

Hinson KV, Tyor WR. Update on viral encephalitis. *Curr Opin Neurol* 2001;14:369–374.

Johnson RT. *Viral infections of the nervous system*. Philadelphia: Lippincott Raven, 1998.

Pellock JM, Dodson EW, Bourgeois Blaise FD. *Pediatric epilepsy,* 2nd ed. New York: Demos Medical, 2001:250–251.

Wyllie E. *The treatment of epilepsy*, 3rd ed. Philadelphia: Lippincott Williams & Wilkins, 2001:338–339.

RESOURCES

89, 359

---

8   Erysipelas

Tom Enta, MD

DEFINITION: Erysipelas is characterized by intense redness, swelling, and pain of the affected skin. The infection is most frequently found on the legs and, less often, on the face. The infection is sharply demarcated, extends peripherally, and often develops adenopathy. The patient may look ill and have increased temperature and elevated white blood cell count. The disease may subside without treatment, although extension may lead to cellulitis, fasciitis, septic shock, abscess formation, and gangrene.

SYNONYMS: St. Anthony's fire; Cellulitis phlegmon.

DIFFERENTIAL DIAGNOSIS: Herpes zoster; Acute contact dermatitis; Angioedema; Erysipeloid; Infection of the paranasal sinus with secondary inflammation of the facial bone.

SYMPTOMS AND SIGNS: The condition starts as a small break in the skin and at surgical sites. The area becomes red and edematous and extends. The elevated edge is raised from the surrounding normal skin. As the disease advances, blisters may develop. Petechiae and ecchymoses may develop in the more inflamed areas. As the condition subsides, the color becomes dull and the surface epidermis peels.

ETIOLOGY/EPIDEMIOLOGY: The causative organism is most often *Streptococcus pyogenes,* although other streptococci and staphylococci have been isolated. It was believed that the source of the skin infection was from the nasopharynx, but open wounds may be infected from a variety of sources. There is no great sex difference, and cases occur throughout the year.

DIAGNOSIS: A diagnosis of erysipelas is made by its characteristic clinical appearance of red swollen lesions with an advancing edge in the skin, often associated with fever, pain, and malaise. Bacteriologic isolation from the lesion and blood culture in the septic phase is not often positive. Detection of streptococci in a skin specimen with direct immunofluorescence gives better results. The white blood cell count may be elevated as the disease progresses. A skin biopsy will show considerable edema of the tissue with vascular dilatation and infiltration with streptococci.

TREATMENT

Standard Therapies: Penicillin has been the drug of choice. In patients with penicillin allergy, cephalothin may be used. Local treatment with cool tap water compresses reduces pain and swelling. Oral analgesics help pain and discomfort. Patients with severe cases must be carefully and closely observed. If the process is spreading rapidly, surgical intervention may be needed to remove large areas of skin and muscle. Erysipelas may recur in the same area. The chronically swollen lower limb is a vulnerable site, and attempts should be made to reduce the edema and improve the integrity of the skin. In patients with relapse, antimicrobial prophylaxis may be needed for a longer time, such as oral daily administration of penicillin for 1 year or longer.

REFERENCES

Chartier C, Grosshans E. Erysipelas: an update. 1996;35:779–781.

Guberman D, Gilead LT, Zlotogorski A, et al. Bullous erysipelas: a retrospective study of 26 patients. *J Am Acad Dermatol* 1999; 41:733–737.

Jorup-Ronstrom C. Epidemiological, bacteriological and complicating features of erysipelas. *Scand J Infect Dis* 1986;18:519–524.

Tsao H, Swartz MN, Weinberg AN, Johnson RA. Soft tissue infection—erysipelas, cellulitis and gangrenous cellulitis. In: *Fitzpatrick's dermatology in general medicine*, 5th ed. New York: McGraw-Hill, 1999:2216–2231.

RESOURCES

89, 359

9   Fascioliasis (Liver Fluke Disease)

Sandra M. O'Neill, RGN, BSc, PhD, and John P. Dalton, BSc, PhD

DEFINITION: Liver fluke disease is caused by infection with the parasitic worms of the genus *Fasciola*, of which *F. hepatica* (found in temperate climates) and *F. gigantica* (found in tropical climates) are the most common. The parasites migrate through the liver and take up residence in the bile ducts, where they cause lesions and chronic liver disease.

SYNONYMS: Fasciolosis; Fascioliasis.

DIFFERENTIAL DIAGNOSIS: Cholangitis; Cholecystitis; Bilharzia; Viral hepatitis.

SYMPTOMS AND SIGNS: The disease has three phases: acute, latent, and chronic. The acute phase begins approximately 4 days after infection and can last for 2–4 months. It is associated with fluke migration across the liver parenchyma. Symptoms include fever, abdominal pain with tender liver, gastrointestinal disturbances, and urticaria accompanied by bouts of bronchial asthma. The latent phase begins when mature flukes reach the bile duct; it can last for several months. Individuals in this phase are asymptomatic. The chronic phase can persist for several years. Symptoms include biliary colic, epigastric pain, fatty food intolerance, nausea, jaundice, pruritus, and right upper quadrant abdominal tenderness. Both the acute and chronic stages of disease are associated with hypereosinophilia, anemia, and abnormal liver function tests.

ETIOLOGY/EPIDEMIOLOGY: Transmission of liver fluke disease involves two hosts: a vector host, the aquatic mud snail, and a definitive mammalian host. After developmental stages within the snail, parasite larvae are released into water. These attach to vegetation and form cysts (metacercaria). Humans acquire infection after ingestion of aquatic plants or drinking water carrying metacercariae. Excystation occurs and the parasites migrate through the intestinal wall and enter the liver before moving into the bile ducts to complete their maturation. Mature liver flukes, measuring 10–25 mm in length and 3–5 mm in breath, lay eggs that are carried with the bile and then the feces onto pastures. The eggs hatch, releasing motile parasites (miracidia) that infect mud snails and thereby complete the cycle. Approximately 2.4 million people are infected with liver fluke disease worldwide, and a further 180 million are at risk for infection. The disease affects both sexes and all ages and is associated with morbidity but not mortality. It is highly prevalent in Ecuador, Peru, Bolivia, Chile, Iran, and Egypt. Sporadic (usually familial) outbreaks occur in countries such as Portugal, France, and Spain.

DIAGNOSIS: Liver fluke disease should be suspected if the patient recently spent time in a region where infection is prevalent in animals and/or humans. Patients usually report eating wild watercress, algae, or other aquatic plants. Acute and chronic infection can be confirmed by enzyme-linked immunosorbent assay that detects liver fluke–specific antibodies in sera. Parasite eggs are detected in the stool at the chronic stage of infection. They also may appear from ingested animal-contaminated food, but these are transitory and should not be confused with a genuine infection.

TREATMENT
Standard Therapies: Liver fluke disease can be successfully treated using triclabendazole.

REFERENCES
Dalton JP. *Fasciolosis.* Wallingford, UK: CABI Publishers, 1999.

Doherty JF, Price N, Moody AH, et al. Fascioliasis due to imported khat. *Lancet* 1995;345:462.

LaPook JD, Magun AM, Nickerson KG, et al. Sheep, watercress, and the Internet. *Lancet* 2000;356:218.

Loutan L, Bouvier M, Rojanawisut B, et al. Single treatment of invasive fasciliasis with triclabendazole. *Lancet* 1989;2:383.

O'Neill SM, Parkinson M, Strauss W, et al. Immunodiagnosis of *Fasciola hepatica* infection (fasciolosis) in a human population in the Bolivian Altiplano using purified cathepsin L1 cysteine proteinase. *Am J Trop Med Hyg* 1998;58:417–423.

RESOURCES
39, 89, 359

10 Hantavirus Pulmonary Syndrome

Joni C. Young, MS,
and Ali S. Khan, MD, MPH

DEFINITION: Hantavirus pulmonary syndrome (HPS) is a pan-American rodent-borne viral zoonosis. The disease is characterized by a nonspecific febrile prodrome, followed by severe respiratory compromise accompanied by shock that is often fatal. Persons are at risk for infection and developing disease 1–6 weeks after contact with infected rural rodents.

SYNONYMS: Hantavirus infection; Hantaviral disease; Hantavirus cardiopulmonary syndrome.

DIFFERENTIAL DIAGNOSIS: Pneumonias; Bacterial sepsis; Leptospirosis; Rickettsioses; Assorted hemorrhagic fevers indigenous to South America.

SYMPTOMS AND SIGNS: The prodromal phase includes fever, myalgia, malaise, headache, dizziness, and gastrointestinal symptoms; sore throat and coryza are generally absent. Cough develops late in the prodrome and heralds the cardiopulmonary phase, characterized by acute onset of severe noncardiogenic pulmonary edema and cardiac compromise. Chest radiographs depict bilateral interstitial pulmonary infiltrates, often resembling acute respiratory distress syndrome, oxygen saturation usually falls below 90%, and most patients require intubation. Classic features include thrombocytopenia, hemoconcentration, and left-shift white blood cell count; circulating immunoblasts are often noted. Manifestations of Central and South American disease may also include renal insufficency, conjunctival injection, head and neck suffusion, or frank hemorrhage. Asymptomatic and mild disease without hypoxia are increasingly reported.

ETIOLOGY/EPIDEMIOLOGY: In the United States, the major disease-causing hantavirus, family Bunyaviridae, is *sin nombre* virus, which has the nearly ubiquitous deer mouse as a reservoir. Disease should be suspected throughout the Western Hemisphere on the basis of identification of numerous other hantaviruses and their specific sigmodontine (New World mice and rats) rodent hosts. Since HPS was identified in 1993, more than 1,000 cases have been re-ported from nine countries. Human infection occurs primarily through aerosol inhalation of rodent urine, feces, or saliva. Rodent bites may also be a route of transmission. In South America, person-to-person transmission has been documented with Andes virus, and therefore appropriate precautions should be taken to avoid nosocomial transmission.

DIAGNOSIS: Diagnosis is by detection of IgM or IgG antibodies, particularly IgM during the acute phase of illness, by enzyme-linked immunosorbent assays. Immunohistochemical testing can be done on biopsy or postmortem specimens, and nucleic acid testing is available for virus characterization.

TREATMENT
Standard Therapies: Treatment is supportive and includes early intensive care with correction of pulmonary, hemodynamic, and electrolyte abnormalities. Fluids should be carefully monitored, and the early use of inotropic agents is advocated for shock.

Investigational Therapies: Intravenous ribavirin is being investigated in the United States and South America. Extracorporeal membrane oxygenation is also under investigation in the United States, as are high-dose steroids in South America.

REFERENCES
Chapman LE, Ellis BA, Koster FT, et al. Discriminators between Hantavirus-infected and -uninfected persons enrolled in a trial of intravenous ribavirin for presumptive hantavirus pulmonary syndrome. *Clin Infect Dis* 2002;34:293–304.
Duchin JS, Koster FT, Peters CJ, et al. Hantavirus pulmonary syndrome: a clinical description of 17 patients with a newly recognized disease. *N Engl J Med* 1994;330:949–955.
Kitsutani PT, Denton RW, Fritz CL, et al. Acute sin nombre hantavirus infection without pulmonary syndrome, United States. *Emerg Infect Dis* 1999;5:701–705.
Peters CJ, Khan, AS. Hantavirus pulmonary syndrome: the new American hemorrhagic fever. *Clin Infect Dis* 2002;34:1224–1231.

RESOURCES
39, 359, 497

11   Idiopathic Neonatal Hepatitis

Mary Elaine Patrinos, MD,
and Rosanne Harrigan, EdD, APRN-Rx

DEFINITION: The term *neonatal hepatitis* describes either a large group of intrahepatic cholestatic disorders due to a variety of causes or a specific disorder, idiopathic neonatal hepatitis (INH). INH is a diagnosis of exclusion and the most common cause of neonatal conjugated hyperbilirubinemia. Affected infants may be asymptomatic or present with jaundice, hepatomegaly, and failure to thrive.

SYNONYMS: Giant cell hepatitis; Neonatal hepatitis syndrome; Intrahepatic cholestasis.

DIFFERENTIAL DIAGNOSIS: Biliary atresia; α_1-antitrypsin deficiency; Choledochal cyst; Congenital syphilis; Disorders of bile acid synthesis; Galactosemia; Hereditary fructose intolerance; Hypopituitarism; Sepsis; Alagille syndrome; Progressive familial intrahepatic cholestasis; Congenital viral infections; Hemochromatosis.

SYMPTOMS AND SIGNS: Two categories of INH have been identified epidemiologically, a sporadic and a familial form. Affected infants are often of low birth weight. More than 50% develop jaundice within the first week of life. Acholic stools are uncommon, but may be present if the cholestasis is severe. Hepatomegaly and, occasionally, splenomegaly are present. Biochemical abnormalities include elevations in conjugated bilirubin, alkaline phosphatase, and serum bile acid levels. Coagulopathy may develop in affected individuals with a more fulminant course as a result of either vitamin K deficiency or decreased synthesis of clotting factors. The histopathology is heterogeneous, often demonstrating giant cells and extramedullary hematopoiesis. Other findings include a disarray of lobular architecture, hepatocellular swelling, focal hepatic necrosis, inflammatory infiltrates, and portal fibrosis. The prognosis is better for sporadic cases than the familial variety. Predictors of poor prognosis include prolonged severe jaundice, acholic stools, persistent hepatomegaly, and severe inflammation on biopsy. Septic complications may lead to decompensation.

ETIOLOGY/EPIDEMIOLOGY: The etiology is unknown. Idiopathic neonatal hepatitis occurs in 30%–40% of infants with neonatal cholestasis. The incidence appears to be higher in males than in females.

DIAGNOSIS: Evaluation of the infant with cholestasis includes observation of stool color, fractionated serum bilirubin, hepatocellular enzymes, albumin, prothrombin time, glucose, ammonia, bacterial cultures of blood and urine, VDRL test, assessment for other congenital viral infections, α_1-antitrypsin phenotype, metabolic screen, thyroid function studies, and sweat chloride. Ultrasonography, hepatobiliary scintigraphy, magnetic resonance cholangiography, and liver biopsy differentiate intrahepatic disorders from biliary atresia. Liver biopsy is the most reliable single test.

TREATMENT
Standard Therapies: Supportive treatment is the mainstay of therapy. Interventions include the use of medium-chain triglyceride-containing formulas, 2–4 times the recommended daily allowance of fat-soluble vitamins, cholestyramine, phenobarbital, and ursodeoxycholic acid for cholestatic pruritis. Liver transplantation is an option for infants who develop end-stage liver disease.

REFERENCES
Dellert SF, Balistreri WF. Neonatal cholestasis. In: Walker AW, Durie PR, Hamilton JR, et al., eds. *Pediatric gastrointestinal disease,* 3rd ed. Hamilton, Ontario, Canada: BC Decker, 2000:880–891.
Jaw TS, Kuo YT, Liu GC, et al. MR cholangiography in the evaluation of neonatal choestasis. *Radiology* 1999;212:249–256.
Nishinomiya F, Abukawa D, Takada G, et al. Relationships between clinical and histological profiles of non-familial idiopathic neonatal hepatitis. *Acta Paediatr Jap* 1996;38:242–247.

RESOURCES
39, 354, 174

12   Leptospirosis

*David A. Ashford, DVM, MPH, DSC,
and James J. Sejvar, MD*

DEFINITION: Leptospirosis is a widespread zoonotic disease caused by spirochetes of the genus *Leptospira*.

SYNONYMS: Weil disease; Fort Bragg fever; Autumnal fever; Canicola fever; Cane fever; Swamp fever; Mud fever; Nanukayami.

DIFFERENTIAL DIAGNOSIS: Malaria; Dengue fever; Yellow fever; Influenza; Scrub typhus; Acute hepatitis. Mimics most bacterial and viral diseases.

SYMPTOMS AND SIGNS: Clinical manifestations of leptospiral infection can vary widely; in 85%–90% of cases, however, it manifests as a self-limited acute febrile illness. Incubation is usually 5–14 days, but can range from 2 to 30 days. The illness generally begins abruptly with high, remittent fevers and headache. Chills, myalgias, and nonpurulent conjunctival injection are often seen. Muscle tenderness, especially in the calves and lumbar area, are distinguishing physical findings. Abdominal symptoms, including abdominal pain, nausea, vomiting, and diarrhea, occur in nearly 30% of patients. This acute febrile phase generally lasts 4–30 days. A delayed, immune-mediated phase of the illness can occur in up to 80% of patients. This is generally heralded by defervescence, and subsequent recurrence of fever. It is marked clinically by worsening headache, photophobia, muscle tenderness, and abdominal pain. Aseptic meningitis, with mild lymphocytic pleocytosis on cerebrospinal fluid (CSF) analysis, is common. Approximately 10%–15% of patients develop more severe disease, known as Weil disease, during the immune phase of the illness. Weil disease is marked by acute renal failure, sometimes requiring hemodialysis, liver failure with jaundice, and, more rarely, hemorrhagic pneumonitis and circulatory collapse.

ETIOLOGY/EPIDEMIOLOGY: Leptospirosis is found worldwide, but is more common in the tropics. Leptospires infect many wild and domestic animals, including rats, dogs, pigs, cattle, and horses. These animals can excrete leptospires in blood or materials of parturition, but environmental contamination more commonly occurs through infected urine. Humans can become infected by contact with tissues or fluids from infected animals or by contact with water or soil that has been contaminated by infected animals. Human-to-human transmission is rare.

DIAGNOSIS: The clinical symptoms of leptospirosis may be confused with many other causes of acute febrile illness, so it is important to consider leptospirosis in persons with appropriate travel or risk factor history. Leptospires can be isolated from blood, CSF, and urine during the first 7–10 days of illness, and from urine after days 10–14 of illness. The organism is fastidious and difficult to grow in culture, and as a result, the sensitivity of culture for diagnosis is low. The standard serologic assay for leptospirosis is the microscopic agglutination test. Several alternative, rapid diagnostic tests have been developed also, including an indirect hemagglutination assay, and two IgM indirect enzyme-linked immunosorbent assays.

TREATMENT
Standard Therapies: Prevention of leptospirosis has generally relied on using protective barriers such as wading boots and gloves, and avoiding high-exposure areas. Mild infections can be treated with oral doxycycline. More severe infections requiring hospitalization should be treated with intravenous penicillin; erythromycin may be used for penicillin-sensitive patients.

Investigational Therapies: Preexposure prophylaxis with oral doxycycline may reduce or prevent signs and symptoms. The potential benefits of preexposure chemoprophylaxis in individuals with identifiable, temporary high-risk exposure to leptospires are being assessed.

REFERENCES
Centers for Disease Control and Prevention. Outbreak of leptospirosis among white-water rafters—Costa Rica, 1996. *MMWR* 1997;46:577–579.
Seghal S, Sugunan A, Murhekar M, et al. Randomized controlled trial of doxycycline prophylaxis against leptospirosis in an endemic area. *Int J Antimicrob Agents* 2000;13:249–255.
Takafuji E, Kirkpatrick J, Miller R, et al. An efficacy trial of doxycycline chemoprophylaxis against leptospirosis. *JAMA* 1984; 310:497–500.
Tappero JW, Ashford DA, Perkins BA. Leptospirosis. In: Mandell GL, Bennet JE, Dolin R, eds. *Principles and practice of infectious diseases,* 5th ed. New York: Churchill-Livingstone, 2000: 2495–2501.

RESOURCES
89, 359, 497

13   Listeriosis

Christopher R. Braden, MD

DEFINITION: Listeriosis is an invasive infection caused by the motile gram-positive bacterium *Listeria monocytogenes.*

DIFFERENTIAL DIAGNOSIS: All causes of neonatal sepsis and meningitis, especially group B streptococcus infection; All causes of meningitis and encephalitis primarily affecting immunocompromised and elderly adults, including *Haemophilus influenzae, Streptococcus pneumoniae, Neisseria meningitidis,* and *Cryptococcus neoformans*; Acute febrile illnesses in pregnancy, including viral syndromes.

SYMPTOMS AND SIGNS: Clinical presentations of listeriosis in nonpregnant adults are typically sepsis, meningitis, or meningoencephalitis. Common symptoms of meningitis include fever, headache, malaise, ataxia, seizures, and altered mental status. Nuchal rigidity is less common compared with other bacterial meningitides, and encephalitis, especially rhomboencephalitis, is more common. Other clinical manifestations associated with *L. monocytogenes* infection include endocarditis, osteomyelitis, arthritis, pleuritis, endophthalmitis, and peritonitis. Infection during pregnancy is usually a self-limited illness of the third trimester, with a nonspecific acute febrile presentation possibly including myalgias, arthralgias, headache, and gastrointestinal symptoms. By contrast, fetal and neonatal infections are severe and frequently fatal, potentially causing preterm labor, amnionitis, spontaneous abortion, stillbirth, and early-onset sepsis. Late-onset disease presents as meningitis at one to several weeks of age.

ETIOLOGY/EPIDEMIOLOGY: *L. monocytogenes* is found in many environments, including soil and water. Factors that influence whether invasive disease occurs likely include the immune status of the host, virulence of the infecting strain of *L. monocytogenes,* and size of the inoculum. Among adults, those at highest risk for infection include pregnant women, immunocompromised persons, and the elderly. Infections in the fetus and newborn occur by transplacental transmission or possibly from environmental exposure to *L. monocytogenes* in the perinatal period. In adults, listeriosis is primarily a food-borne disease. Because maternal infection is rarely recognized, preventing fetal and neonatal infections depends on avoiding risky foods during pregnancy. The overall incidence of listeriosis in the United States is low, approximately 4 per million population; this is greater at the extremes of life. Infection by *L. monocytogenes* accounts for 20% of all cases of meningitis in both neonates and persons older than 60.

DIAGNOSIS: Diagnosis requires culture of *L. monocytogenes* from amniotic fluid, placenta, blood, cerebral spinal fluid, or affected organ systems. In severe early-onset neonatal sepsis, the organism may be identified by Gram stain of muconium. The isolation of *L. monocytogenes* from stool should be interpreted with caution because it may be present in the stool of healthy persons.

TREATMENT

Standard Therapies: To prevent food-borne listeriosis, all persons should observe safe food-handling precautions. Persons at high risk such as pregnant women and those with weak immune systems should also avoid soft cheeses and reheat leftover foods or ready-to-eat foods until steaming hot before eating. The treatment of choice for listeriosis is intravenous ampicillin. Many authorities recommend the addition of gentamicin. For persons intolerant to β-lactam antibiotics, trimethoprim-sulfamethoxizole is the best alternative.

REFERENCES

Centers for Disease Control and Prevention. Multistate outbreak of listeriosis—United States, 2000. *MMWR* 2000;49:1129–1130.

Gellin BG, Broome CV. Listeriosis. *JAMA* 1989;261:1313–1320.

Lorber B. Listeriosis. *Clin Infect Dis* 1997;24:1–11.

Schuchat A, Swaminathan B, Broome CV. Epidemiology of listeriosis. *Clin Microbiol Rev* 1991;4:169–183.

RESOURCES

89, 359, 497

14 Malaria

Timothy H. Holtz, MD, MPH

DEFINITION: Malaria is a parasitic infection caused by an intracellular protozoan. Malaria can cause high fevers, rigors, renal and pulmonary failure, coma, and sometimes death.

SYNONYMS: Ague; Quartan fever; Tertian fever.

SYMPTOMS AND SIGNS: Patients can present with a wide variety of symptoms and a broad spectrum of severity. Typical symptoms among nonimmune persons with malaria include spiking fever, rigors, chills, myalgias and arthralgias, headache, diarrhea, and vomiting. Cough and shortness of breath are common. When synchronous infections develop, each species of *Plasmodium* causes a characteristic pattern of periodic fever. The paroxysms of *P. vivax* and *P. ovale* malaria classically occur every 48 hours, whereas those of *P. malariae* occur every 72 hours; however, the classic presentation with predictably recurring fever and chills is highly variable and may not be seen. *P. falciparum* infections can feature a daily or irregular pattern of symptoms. Malaria with CNS symptoms can progress from fever with subtle mental status changes to coma within hours. Cerebral malaria is defined as unarousable coma not attributable to any other cause in a patient infected with *P. falciparum*. A patient with neurologic symptoms and malaria parasitemia, however, should be treated urgently as having cerebral malaria. Other acute complications include renal failure, hemolytic anemia, hypoglycemia, metabolic acidosis, thrombocytopenia, shock, and acute pulmonary edema. Uncomplicated malaria infection can progress to severe disease or death within hours. In patients who survive severe or complicated malaria, long-term sequelae can include permanent CNS deficits or lasting impairment of kidney function.

ETIOLOGY/EPIDEMIOLOGY: Malaria is caused by one or more of four species of an intracellular protozoan parasite, specifically *Plasmodium falciparum, P. vivax, P. ovale,* and *P. malariae.* Malaria is typically transmitted by the bite of an infective female *Anopheles* mosquito. Malaria transmission occurs primarily in tropical and subtropical regions in Sub-Saharan Africa, Central and South America, the Caribbean island of Hispaniola, the Middle East, the Indian subcontinent, Southeast Asia, and Oceania. Approximately 1,200 cases of malaria are reported in the United States each year, with 2–5 deaths annually. Most of the cases in the United States occur among travelers, immigrants, and refugees. A small number of malaria cases are acquired within the United States and its territories through congenital transmission, transmission through blood transfusion or organ donation, and, rarely, local transmission by anopheline mosquitoes.

DIAGNOSIS: Simple, direct microscopic examination of stained blood films is the most widely practiced and useful method for definitive diagnosis of malaria. Diagnosis can also be made through special staining, rapid antigen detection, and detection of parasite nucleic acid sequences through polymerase chain reaction.

TREATMENT
Standard Therapies: Patients infected with *P. vivax, P. ovale,* or *P. malariae,* and patients with uncomplicated *P. falciparum* infections acquired in areas where drug resistance has not been documented, should be treated with oral chloroquine. A 14-day course of primaquine should also be given to patients infected with *P. vivax* or *P. ovale* to eradicate dormant liver-stage parasites. The choice of treatment for uncomplicated *P. falciparum* infections acquired in areas where drug resistance has been documented is more difficult. Recommended regimens include a 3-day course of quinine combined with a 7-day course of tetracycline/doxycycline or a 3-day course of quinine combined with a single dose of sulfadoxine/pyrimethamine; a 3-day course of atovaquone/proguanil alone; or mefloquine alone. Halofantrine and artemisinin derivatives are effective, but are not available in the United States. Parenteral quinine/quinidine therapy in combination with doxycycline is recommended for falciparum malaria when there is a high-density infection or when the patient cannot take oral medication. Exchange transfusion may also be necessary.

Investigational Therapies: Tafenoquine and chlorproguanil/dapsone are in development stages.

REFERENCES
Barat LM, Zucker JR. Malaria. In: McMillan, JA, ed. *Oski's pediatrics,* 3rd ed. Philadelphia: Lippincott Williams & Wilkins, 1999:1177–1184.
Kachur SP, Bloland PB. Malaria. In: Wallace RB, ed. *Maxcy-Rosenau-Last's public health & preventive medicine,* 14th ed. Stamford, CT: Appleton & Lange, 1998:313–326.
Zucker JR, Campbell CC. Malaria: principles of prevention and treatment. *Infect Dis Clin North Am* 1993;7:547–567.

RESOURCES
89, 359, 497

15   Plague

Kristy Murray Lillibridge, DVM, and David Dennis, MD

DEFINITION: Plague is a zoonotic disease caused by infection with *Yersinia pestis* (*Yersinia pseudotuberculosis* subspecies *pestis*), a gram-negative, microaerophilic, bipolar staining bacillus.

SYNONYMS: Black death; La Peste; Pestilential fever.

DIFFERENTIAL DIAGNOSIS: For bubonic plague: Tularemia; Staphylococcal and streptococcal lymphadenitis; Cat scratch disease; Lymphatic filariasis. For pneumonic and septicemic plague: Tularemia; Other causes of life-threatening sepsis or pneumonia.

SYMPTOMS AND SIGNS: The most common clinical form is bubonic plague, which manifests as an acute febrile illness with chills, weakness, and headaches after 2–6 days of incubation. Shortly after disease onset, a bubo develops, which is characterized by intense pain and enlargement of one or more regional lymph nodes, especially those located in the groin, axilla, or neck. Pneumonic plague can occur as a secondary complication of bubonic plague, or as a primary inhalation form. Fever, cough, chest pain, and sputum production (occasionally bloody) are typically present. Septicemic plague can occur as a primary illness or secondary to bubonic or pneumonic plague. With all three forms of the illness, gastrointestinal symptoms such as nausea, vomiting, diarrhea, and abdominal pain occur and may result in delay of diagnosis. Fatality rates are high in the absence or delay of appropriate antimicrobial therapy, especially with the septicemic or pneumonic forms of illness. Plague meningitis is rare, and most often occurs approximately 1 week after inadequate treatment of bubonic plague.

ETIOLOGY/EPIDEMIOLOGY: Plague has a scattered worldwide distribution, with most cases occurring in developing countries, especially in Africa and Asia. Approximately 10 human cases occur per year in the United States, with most in southwestern states, where plague is endemic in the wild rodent population. In the United States, plague occurs when persons are bitten by infected rodent fleas, directly handle infected rodent or carnivore carcasses or tissues, or inhale respiratory secretions from infected domestic cats. Human-to-human transmission can occur when droplets are inhaled from a coughing patient. Any suspected plague case in the United States warrants a rapid public health investigation and should be reported immediately to local public health authorities. *Y. pestis* is considered a potential agent of biological terrorism.

DIAGNOSIS: Bacteria can be isolated and identified by culture as well as by direct fluorescence staining of a smear of a bubo aspirate, blood, sputum, or spinal fluid. A serologic diagnosis can be made in the absence of a positive culture if a fourfold increase or a single titer greater than 1:16 can be demonstrated.

TREATMENT
Standard Therapies: Early and effective antibiotic therapy is important in preventing death. Streptomycin is the treatment of choice; alternatives are gentamicin, tetracyclines, and chloramphenicol. Chloramphenicol is indicated for treating meningitis.

Investigational Therapies: Gentamicin and ciprofloxacin are being evaluated.

REFERENCES
Acha PN, Szyfres B, eds. Plague. In: *Zoonoses and communicable diseases common to man and animals.* Scientific publication no. 503. Washington, DC: World Health Organization, 1987: 131–140.
Butler T. *Yersinia* species, including plague. In: Mandell GL, Bennett JE, Dolin R, eds. *Principles and practice of infectious diseases,* 5th ed. Philadelphia: Churchill Livingstone, 2000: 2406–2414.
Campbell GL, Dennis D. Plague and other *Yersinia* infections. In: Braunwald E, Fauci A, Kasper D, et al., eds. *Harrison's principles of internal medicine,* 15th ed. New York: McGraw-Hill, 2001:993–1001.
World Health Organization. *Plague manual: epidemiology, distribution, surveillance and control.* Geneva, Switzerland: World Health Organization (WHO/CDS/CSR/CDC/99.2), 1999.

RESOURCES
89, 359, 497

16   Q Fever

Elena Kováčová, PhD,
and Jan Kazár, MD, DSc

DEFINITION: Q (query) fever is a zoonosis that occurs worldwide, except in New Zealand. It manifests mainly as atypical pneumonia or flulike illness, less often as hepatitis, isolated and/or prolonged fever, bone, exanthematous, or neurologic disease, and rarely as pericarditis and life-threatening myocarditis. Chronic Q fever manifests mostly as endocarditis; less frequent are infections of vascular grafts or aneurysms, chronic hepatitis, osteoarticular infections, and chronic pulmonary infections.

SYNONYM: *Coxiellosis* refers to infections of wild and domestic animals.

DIFFERENTIAL DIAGNOSIS: Pneumonia; Influenza; Brucellosis; Leptospirosis; Meningitis; Viral hepatitis; Dengue fever; Malaria; Other rickettsial infections.

SYMPTOMS AND SIGNS: After a 2- to 3-week incubation period, the onset is usually abrupt, with fever (up to 39°–40°C), fatigue, chills, and severe headache. Myalgia, sweats, cough, chest pain, sore throat, gastrointestinal symptoms, and skin rash may also be present. Findings include thrombocytopenia, anemia, altered liver functions, and elevated creatinine levels and erythrocyte sedimentation rate. Chronic Q fever occurs mostly in men older than 40 years who have underlying heart disease and/or impaired immunity. It manifests with fever, weakness, fatigue, weight loss, chills, anorexia, headache, myalgia, adenopathy, hepatosplenomegaly, purpuric rash, jaundice, dyspnea, pulmonary edema, angina pectoris, arrythmia, cardiac failure, palpitations, digital clubbing, hemorrhages, and embolization. Frequently, additional findings include thrombocytopenia; anemia; increased gammaglobulin, transaminase, and creatinine levels; rheumatoid factor; autoantibodies; and circulating immune complexes.

ETIOLOGY/EPIDEMIOLOGY: Infection is caused by an obligate intracellular parasite, *Coxiella burnetii*. It is transmitted vertically (in ticks) and horizontally (from ticks to wild and domestic animals). Cattle, sheep, and goats (less often cats and dogs) shedding the agent in their urine, feces, milk, and birth products are the most important source of human infection. Whereas wildlife Q fever is tick-borne, the human analogue is an airborne infection spread through the inhalation of contaminated aerosols originating from birth fluids and animal excretions or contaminated products. Under some conditions, it can be a wind-borne infection, and it could potentially be used as a biologic weapon. Q fever occurs more often in men than women.

DIAGNOSIS: Diagnosis is by microbiologic examination. *C. burnetii* can be isolated in laboratory animals, embryonated eggs, and in cell cultures (shell-vial method with centrifugation of the clinical specimen). Direct detection using immunoenzymatic and immunofluorescence assays with monoclonal antibodies has been employed with varying results; the more sensitive polymerase chain reaction is recommended. Serologic tests are easy to perform and inexpensive. The most common ones are complement fixation, microagglutination, enzyme-linked immunosorbent assay, and, as the method of choice, immunofluorescence.

TREATMENT
Standard Therapies: Tetracycline is replaced by other antibiotics. In acute Q fever, doxycycline and quinolones are commonly used. Erythromycin and cotrimexasole, as alternatives for pregnant women and children, are not reliable. In chronic Q fever, relapses occur on withdrawal of antibiotic therapy, so that combined regimens (e.g., doxycycline and chloroquine or doxycycline with ofloxacin) should be followed. Valve replacement is performed when hemodynamic failure occurs. Preventive measures consist of adequate disinfection and disposal of animal products of conception; strict hygiene procedures on goat, cattle, and sheep farms and in plants processing products of these animals; control of the import to and movement within countries of the domestic animals in question; and restriction of consumption of raw milk and raw milk products. Vaccination with an efficient phase I vaccine is recommended for all individuals at risk.

REFERENCES
Kazár J. Q fever—current concept. In: Raoult D, Brouqui P, eds. *Rickettsiae and rickettsial diseases at the turn of the third millennium.* New York: Elsevier, 1999:304–319.
Kováčová E, Kazár J. Rickettsial diseases and their serological diagnosis. *Clin Lab* 2000;46:239–245.
Maurin M, Raoult D. Q fever. *Clin Microbiol Rev* 1999;4:518–553.

RESOURCES
89, 359, 497

17   Rift Valley Fever

Anil A. Panackal, MD,
and Thomas G. Ksiazek, DVM, PhD

DEFINITION: Rift Valley fever (RVF) is a mosquito-borne zoonotic disease of domestic ungulates. Infection to humans is transmitted by mosquito bites and by contact with infected animals or their body fluids. Infection may not be apparent, but generally leads to self-limited febrile illness or mild hepatitis and, rarely, to more severe disease.

DIFFERENTIAL DIAGNOSIS: Crimean-Congo hemorrhagic fever; Dengue fever; Yellow fever; Lassa fever; Marburg disease; Ebola hemorrhagic fever; Al Khumrah hemorrhagic fever; Malaria; Leptospirosis; Viral hepatitides.

SYMPTOMS AND SIGNS: Although human infection is predominantly associated with a brief self-limited febrile illness, infection is classically characterized by complications such as retinitis, hemorrhagic fever, and encephalitis. After an incubation period of 2–5 days, infected individuals may develop a biphasic fever, malaise, anorexia, dizziness, myalgia, and varying degrees of hepatitis, including jaundice; most individuals recover after 2–7 days. Approximately half of patients with hemorrhagic syndrome die. Encephalitis, as manifested by fever, headache, disorientation or coma, focal signs, and convulsions, may develop 1–4 weeks after the acute illness fades. Severe retinal disease consists of bilateral macular hemorrhages, exudates, and infarction during the first 4 weeks after recovery.

ETIOLOGY/EPIDEMIOLOGY: A virus in the family Bunyaviridae, genus *Phlebovirus,* causes Rift Valley fever. The RVF virus is transmitted to humans primarily via mosquito bites during epidemics and epizootics during periods of heavy rainfall. Transovarial transmission is known to occur among floodwater *Aedes* mosquitoes, but many mosquito species have been implicated as secondary vectors. Domestic ungulates such as goats and sheep serve as amplifying hosts, and perinatal mortality and abortions are common during epizootics. Close contact with infected animals and animal body fluids is an important risk factor for RVF; infected animal blood and amniotic fluid has been reported to contain titers of 10^{10} infectious virus particles per milliliter. Laboratory infection is well documented among virologists who work with virus cultures. First described in Kenya in 1910, the disease has since been recognized in many African countries and in Saudi Arabia and Yemen.

DIAGNOSIS: RVF antigens or IgM antibodies to RVF virus can be detected by using enzyme-linked immunosorbent assays. Virus can be detected by isolation, or its nucleic acid amplified by reverse transcription polymerase chain reaction. Specific postmortem diagnosis can be established by immunohistochemical techniques on fixed tissues.

TREATMENT
Standard Therapies: Treatment is supportive. Although intravenous ribavirin has been shown to treat Lassa fever, hemorrhagic fever with renal syndrome, and Crimean-Congo hemorrhagic fever, its efficacy for the treatment of RVF has been demonstrated only in animal models. A formalin-inactivated vaccine (TSI-GSD 200), although not commercially available, is safe and effective; injections are given at days 0, 7, and 28 with a booster after 1 year, and this regimen has been shown to induce neutralizing antibodies.

Investigational Therapies: A live, attenuated vaccine, MP-12, is undergoing evaluation.

REFERENCES
Arthur RR. Rift Valley fever. In: Stickland GT, ed. *Hunter's tropical medicine and emerging infectious diseases.* Philadelphia: WB Saunders, 2000:253–255.

Centers for Disease Control and Prevention. Update: outbreak of Rift Valley fever—Saudi Arabia, August–November 2000. *MMWR* 2000;49:982–985.

Pittman PR, Liu CT, Cannon TL, et al. Immunogenicity of an inactivated Rift Valley fever vaccine in humans: a 12-year experience. *Vaccine* 1999;18:181–189.

Swanepoel R, Coetzer JAW. Rift Valley fever. In: Coetzer JAW, Thomson GR, Tustin RC, eds. *Infectious diseases of livestock.* Capetown, South Africa: Oxford University Press, 1994:688–717.

RESOURCES
89, 359, 497

18   TORCH Syndrome

Mark D.P. Davis, MD

DEFINITION: Several infections contracted *in utero* result in physical findings during the neonatal period that are similar and frequently indistinguishable clinically. Collectively, these infections are referred to as TORCH syndrome. Originally, the acronym *TORCH* referred to infection with *Toxoplasma gondii*, other agents, rubella virus, cytomegalovirus, or herpes simplex virus. This list is sometimes expanded to include other infections such as syphilis, varicella-zoster, parvoviral infection, hepatitis, and infection with human immunodeficiency virus.

DIFFERENTIAL DIAGNOSIS: Congenital syphilis; Neonatal bacterial sepsis; Listerial infection; Congenital leukemia; Pseudo-TORCH syndrome (Baraitser-Reardon syndrome).

SYMPTOMS AND SIGNS: TORCH syndrome may cause intrauterine growth retardation. In the neonate, congenital TORCH infection may be asymptomatic, but the following features may be observed: intracranial calcification and microcephaly, hydrocephalus, paraventricular calcification, sensorimotor deafness, maculopapular rash, petechiae, purpura, dermal erythropoiesis (with formation of "blueberry muffin" lesions), thrombocytopenia, generalized lymphadenopathy, limb atrophy and scarring (associated with fetal infection in the first or early second trimester), hepatosplenomegaly, icterus, hyperbilirubinemia, cardiac anomalies, conjunctivitis, and chorioretinitis.

ETIOLOGY/EPIDEMIOLOGY: In the United States, the incidence of congenital infection ranges from 1% of all births, or 40,000 newborns annually, for cytomegalovirus (CMV) to 6 cases of congenital rubella reported in 1987. Although rare, TORCH infections result in significant morbidity and mortality and should be diagnosed expeditiously when symptoms develop. Toxoplasmosis is caused by transmission of *T. gondii*, an intracellular parasitic protozoan acquired by the mother during gestation. Rubella is caused by the rubella virus, an RNA virus of the genus *Rubivirus* in the togavirus group. CMV infection is caused by transplacental transmission of cytomegalovirus, a DNA virus of the human herpesvirus group, which is ubiquitous. CMV infection also may be transmitted perinatally, through breast milk, or transfusion of CMV-infected blood. Herpes simplex viral infection is caused by the herpes simplex virus, a DNA virus of the herpesvirus group.

DIAGNOSIS: Diagnosis is confirmed by culture and identification of species-specific immunoglobulin M within the first 2 weeks of life. Histologic examination contributes to the diagnosis in infection with herpes simplex virus. CT and MRI scanning help to detect and differentiate intracranial infection. CT is useful primarily in those infections associated with intracranial calcification.

TREATMENT
Standard Therapies: Treatment for toxoplasmosis includes pyrimethamine with sulfadiazine or trisulfapyrimidine; primary infection during gestation is treated with spiramycin. Infants with symptomatic or asymptomatic congenital infection are treated with pyrimethamine and sulfadiazine for up to 1 year. Congenital infection with herpes simplex virus is treated with acyclovir. Varicella-zoster immunoglobulin is administered immediately if a maternal rash appears 5 days before to 2 days after birth. Treatment with acyclovir for varicella may be beneficial during pregnancy. Treatment is primarily supportive for congenital rubella or CMV infection.

Routine postexposure prophylaxis with immunoglobulin is not recommended for mothers exposed to rubella. Mothers not immune to rubella should be immunized after delivery, even if they are breast-feeding. Infant therapy is supportive care and isolation.

Investigational Therapy: The use of ganciclovir in CMV-infected newborns is being studied.

REFERENCES
Epps RE, Pittelkow MR, Su WP. TORCH syndrome. *Semin Dermatol* 1995;14:179–186.
Fine JD, Arndt KA. The TORCH syndrome: a clinical review. *J Am Acad Dermatol* 1985;12:697–706.
Sherman RA. Charts: the TORCH syndrome revisited. *Pediatr Infect Dis J* 1989;8:62–63.
TORCH syndrome and TORCH screening. *Lancet* 1990;335:1559–1561.

RESOURCES
89, 359, 368

19   West Nile Fever

Daniel A. Singer, MD

DEFINITION: West Nile fever describes the spectrum of disease caused by infection with the West Nile virus, a mosquito-borne flavivirus that can cause a range of clinical presentations from malaise and fever to encephalitis, coma, and death.

SYNONYMS: West Nile encephalitis; Kunjin fever.

DIFFERENTIAL DIAGNOSIS: All of the neurotropic viruses including St. Louis, western equine, eastern equine, Venezuelan equine, Powassan, and the California encephalitides; Herpesviruses; Enteroviruses; Toxic exposures.

SYMPTOMS AND SIGNS: West Nile virus infection is characterized by the abrupt onset of a febrile dengue-like illness. Patients frequently report headache, gastrointestinal distress, sore throat, myalgia, backache, arthralgia, and fatigue. A maculopapular rash or lymphadenopathy may be evident on physical examination. A small percentage of patients develop severe neurologic impairment, typically aseptic meningitis, encephalitis, or, rarely, anterior myelitis or encephalopolyradiculitis. The cerebrospinal fluid (CSF) usually shows elevated protein and pleocytosis in patients with neurologic illness. Marked muscle weakness may accompany neurologic manifestations. Severe West Nile encephalitis may progress to coma and death. Hepatitis, pancreatitis, and myocarditis can be associated with the infection. Most patients recover uneventfully and are immune to subsequent infections, probably for life. Those with neurologic manifestations are at risk for long-term sequelae. The case fatality rate in patients with neurologic disease is 10%–15%.

ETIOLOGY/EPIDEMIOLOGY: West Nile virus is typically acquired from the bite of an infected mosquito, although ticks may also transmit the disease. Birds are the primary reservoir for the virus, although many mammals are susceptible to infection. West Nile fever can occur as isolated cases or in an epidemic. The virus is found in Africa, Europe, the Middle East, West Asia, and Australia. The first report of West Nile virus in the Western Hemisphere was in 1999, when an epidemic occurred in New York City. Many states in the eastern United States have since reported cases.

Infection with West Nile virus can occur at any age, but severe neurologic illness occurs predominantly in the elderly and occasionally in young children.

DIAGNOSIS: The CDC established definitions for confirmed and probable cases of West Nile fever. Because there is wide cross-reactivity among members of the Japanese encephalitis serogroup, positive serologic results should be confirmed by a plaque reduction neutralization test (PRNT). A confirmed case of West Nile fever is defined as a clinically consistent case with at least one of the following: isolation of virus, detection of viral antigen, or viral genome products from tissue, blood, CSF, or other body fluid; demonstration of IgM antibody to West Nile virus in CSF by IgM-capture enzyme immunoassay (EIA); at least a fourfold serial change in PRNT antibody titer to West Nile virus in acute and convalescent serum or CSF samples; and demonstration of both West Nile virus–specific IgM (by EIA) and IgG (screened by EIA or hemagglutination-inhibition and confirmed by PRNT) antibody in a single serum specimen. A probable case is defined as a clinically compatible case that does not meet any of the previous laboratory criteria, plus at least one of the following: demonstration of serum IgM antibody against West Nile virus or demonstration of an elevated titer of West Nile virus–specific IgG antibody in convalescent-phase serum. West Nile fever can be ruled out by a negative test result for IgM antibody to West Nile virus in serum or CSF collected 8–21 days after onset of illness and/or a negative test result for IgG antibody to West Nile virus in serum collected ≥22 days after onset of illness.

TREATMENT

Standard Therapies: There is no vaccine. Prevention efforts should be directed toward reducing contact with mosquitoes. Treatment is supportive. Ribavirin has demonstrated activity against West Nile virus *in vitro*, but only at very high concentrations, and is unlikely to be useful.

REFERENCES

Centers for Disease Control and Prevention. Case definitions for infectious conditions under public health surveillance. *MMWR* 1997;46:12–13. Available at *www.cdc.gov/epo/dphsi/casedef/encephalitis_arboviral_current.htm*. Accessed June 20, 2001.

Centers for Disease Control and Prevention. Guidelines for surveillance, prevention, and control of West Nile virus infection—United States. *MMWR* 2000;49:25–28.

Hayes CG. West Nile fever. In: Monath TP, ed. *The arboviruses: epidemiology and ecology.* Vol. V. Boca Raton, FL: CRC Press, 1989:59–88.

Jordan I, Briese T, Fischer N, et al. Ribavirin inhibits West Nile virus replication and cytopathic effect in neural cells. *J Infect Dis* 2000;182:1214–1217.

RESOURCES
89, 359, 497

20 Whipple Disease

A. von Herbay, Dr Med, and M. Maiwald, Dr Med

DEFINITION: Whipple disease is a chronic infective disorder with a peculiar rod-shaped bacterium, *Tropheryma whippelii*. Infection usually involves the small intestine, but virtually any organ system may be infected.

DIFFERENTIAL DIAGNOSIS: Gluten-sensitive sprue; Giardiasis; Malignant lymphoma; Alzheimer disease; Multiple sclerosis.

SYMPTOMS AND SIGNS: Approximately two thirds of patients present with weight loss and diarrhea, and many also have crampy abdominal pain. Abdominal ultrasonography or CT usually shows mesenteric lymphadenopathy. Other common features include arthralgias, serous effusions, mediastinal or peripheral lymphadenopathy, skin hyperpigmentation, and fever. Laboratory examinations often show increased erythrocyte sedimentation rates, elevated stool fat contents, decreased serum carotene levels, decreased serum iron concentration, anemia, and decreased serum protein levels. Some patients develop neurologic or psychiatric symptoms, e.g., progressive impairment of memory or sleep, oculofacial myorhythmias, nystagmus, and gaze palsy.

ETIOLOGY/EPIDEMIOLOGY: The bacterium *T. whippelii* was identified in 1991/1992 on the basis of its rDNA sequence; it belongs to the actinomycetes. The natural habitats of this gram-positive bacterium are unknown, but an environmental source appears likely. A peroral route of infection is assumed. At the time of diagnosis, the mean age of patients is 56 years (range, 30–80 years). The male:female ratio is approximately 4:1. The incidence of the disease has been estimated to be 0.4 per million population per year (in Germany).

DIAGNOSIS: The standard diagnostic approach is to obtain mucosal biopsies from the small intestine. Even when the gross findings appear normal (in about 25% of patients), five biopsy particles should be taken from the distal duodenum as far as the endoscope can reach. Intestinal histology is diagnostic when numerous macrophages with periodic acid–Schiff (PAS) stain–positive granular particles are detected. These correspond to lysosomes filled with bacteria. Confirmation of diagnosis can be achieved either by electron microscopy or by polymerase chain reaction (PCR) analysis, which detects the DNA of *T. whippelii*. Positive PCR results are rare in patients without histologic features of Whipple disease.

TREATMENT
Standard Therapies: Antibiotic therapy to eradicate *T. whippelii* is curative. No evidence-based standard regimen is available. Therapy with tetracycline has a long-term, significant risk of clinical relapses, including those affecting the central nervous system. Trimethoprim-sulfamethoxazole is considered to be more effective because it penetrates the blood-brain barrier, but it does not reliably eradicate cerebral infections with *T. whippelii*. On an empiric basis, initial treatment is recommended with a third-generation cephalosporin, or penicillin G plus streptomycin, followed by trimethoprim-sulfamethoxazole.

Investigational Therapies: In a prospective study of the initial treatment of Whipple disease, patients have been randomized to either ceftriaxone or meropenem, followed by trimethoprim-sulfamethoxazole for 12 months. Experimental immunotherapy with interferon-γ was reported in a single case that was refractory to antibiotics.

REFERENCES
Dobbins WO III. *Whipple's disease.* Springfield, IL: Charles C Thomas, 1987.

Maiwald M, von Herbay A, Relman DA. Whipple's disease. In: Feldman M, Friedman LS, Sleisenger MH, eds. *Sleisenger &*

Fordtran's gastrointestinal and liver disease, 7th ed. Philadelphia: WB Saunders, 2001.

von Herbay A. Whipple's disease online. URL *www.Whipples
Disease.net.*

von Herbay A, Ditton HJ, Schuhmacher F, et al. Whipple's disease:
staging and monitoring by cytology and polymerase chain
reaction analysis of cerebrospinal fluid. *Gastroenterology* 1997;
113:434–441.

Whipple GH. A hitherto undescribed disease characterized
anatomically by deposits of fat and fatty acids in the intestinal
and mesenteric lymphatic tissues. *Johns Hopkins Hosp Bull*
1907;18:382–391.

RESOURCES

58, 89, 354

Endocrine Disorders

1   Achard-Thiers Syndrome

Catherine M. Gordon, MD, and Kelly Becker, BA

DEFINITION: Achard-Thiers syndrome occurs primarily in postmenopausal women and is characterized by type 2 (insulin-resistant) diabetes mellitus and signs of androgen excess.

SYNONYM: Diabetes of bearded women.

DIFFERENTIAL DIAGNOSIS: Polycystic ovary syndrome (PCOS); Type A syndrome; Type B syndrome; Adenoma-associated virilism of older women; Acquired adrenogenital syndrome; Empty sella syndrome; Diabetes (general).

SYMPTOMS AND SIGNS: The original description and usual emphasis in this syndrome is on the patient as a bearded woman with diabetes mellitus. In older women, the first clinical symptoms are often those associated with classic diabetes and may include abnormally high blood glucose due to the body's inability to utilize insulin properly. Affected individuals may also have abnormally high levels of glucose in the urine, frequent urination, excessive thirst and hunger, and weight loss. Other signs of the syndrome are directly due to the overproduction of androgens, and may include an increase in body hair, particularly on the face, chest, back, and other areas that normally have terminal hair; receding hairline; deepening of the voice; enlargement of the clitoris; infertility; and obesity. Typically, a detailed patient history shows the development of oligomenorrhea or amenorrhea soon after menarche, commonly followed by development of hirsutism and rapid weight gain. Many women with the disorder have acanthosis nigricans. The constellation of clinical androgen excess and hyperinsulinemia is now commonly identified earlier in a woman's life, typically during adolescence and young adulthood, as PCOS.

ETIOLOGY/EPIDEMIOLOGY: The morphology of these syndromes appears to be transmitted within families, and hyperandrogenism and insulin resistance also follow familial patterns. Approximately 50% of sisters of women with PCOS have some form of the syndrome. The exact mechanism of genetic transmission is unknown.

DIAGNOSIS: The diagnosis of Achard-Thiers syndrome should be suspected based on the clinical findings. Because affected women are hyperinsulinemic, a 2-hour oral glucose tolerance test shows abnormally elevated levels of glucose in the blood. Urinary excretion of 17-hydroxysteroids and 17-ketosteroids is within normal limits, even after corticotropin stimulation.

TREATMENT

Standard Therapies: Diabetes may be managed by diet and/or insulin or other medications, as required. Cosmetic measures (e.g., waxing, electrolysis) can be used to facilitate hair removal. For younger women with PCOS, treatment with an oral contraceptive is the most common therapy, whereas for postmenopausal women with Achard-Thiers syndrome, hormone replacement therapy is usually recommended. Antiandrogens have also been used.

Investigational Therapies: Insulin-sensitizing agents (i.e., metformin) are being investigated as a treatment for hyperandrogenism accompanying insulin resistance.

REFERENCES

Achard C, Thiers J. Le virilisme pilaire et son association a l'insuffisance glycolytique (diabete des femmes à barb). *Bull Acad Natl Med* 1921;86:51–64.

Dunaif A. Insulin resistance and the polycystic ovary syndrome: mechanism and implications for pathogenesis. *Endocr Rev* 1997;18:774–800.

Lubowe I. Achard-Thiers syndrome. *Arch Dermatol* 1971;103: 544–545.

Shore RN, DeCherney AH, Stein KM, et al. The empty sella syndrome: virilization in a 59-year old woman. *JAMA* 1974;227: 69–70.

Wilson JD, Foster DW, Kronenberg HM, et al. *Williams textbook of endocrinology,* 9th ed. Philadelphia: WB Saunders, 1998.

RESOURCES

32, 281, 365

2 Acromegaly

Robert D. Murray, MD,
and Shlomo Melmed, MD

DEFINITION: Acromegaly is the clinical consequence of chronic, excessive growth hormone (GH) production, usually the result of a benign hypersecreting tumor of the pituitary gland.

SYNONYM: Marie disease.

DIFFERENTIAL DIAGNOSIS: Multiple endocrine neoplasia type 1; McCune-Albright syndrome; Carney complex; Gigantism; Acromegaloidism.

SYMPTOMS AND SIGNS: Progression of the clinical features is insidious. The most characteristic features are the result of overgrowth of the soft tissues and cartilage. The bones of the jaw and skull are most typically affected, leading to bossing of the skull, prognathism, overbite of the jaw, separation and misalignment of the teeth, and broadening of the bridge of the nose. Additional features include thickening of the lips, enlargement of the tongue, large hands and feet, skin tags, seborrhea, hirsutism, and muscle weakness. Increased metabolic rate leads to excessive sweating and heat intolerance. As well as obvious somatic features, patients have organomegaly. Symptoms occurring as a direct result of tumor bulk include headaches and symptoms from pressure on surrounding structures. Expansion of the tumor superiorly may result in pressure on the optic chiasm with visual impairment. Lateral invasion of the tumor into the cavernous sinus may result in palsies of the third, fourth, or fifth cranial nerves. Complications of acromegaly include hypopituitarism, diabetes mellitus, hypertension, and osteoarthritis. Importantly, acromegaly is associated with a two-fold increase in mortality.

ETIOLOGY/EPIDEMIOLOGY: The prevalence is approximately 60 cases per million, with an incidence of approximately 4 cases per million. The frequency is equal in males and females. Acromegaly is the clinical consequence of chronic, excessive GH production. In more than 99% of patients, this results from a benign adenoma in the pituitary gland derived from the monoclonal expansion of a somatotroph cell. Approximately 40% of somatotrophinomas have a mutation in the *GNAS1* gene (*gsp* oncogene). Rarely, acromegaly may result from the ectopic secretion of "GH-releasing hormone" or GH from carcinoid tumors and tumors of the hypothalamus, pancreas, lung, and adrenal glands.

DIAGNOSIS: Diagnosis is generally made by recognition of the somatic features when the patient presents with an associated complication. Old photographs are often helpful to demonstrate changes in appearance over the years. The diagnosis is confirmed by demonstrating an elevated serum insulin-like growth factor type I (IGF-I) level (GH second messenger) for age and gender, and failure of GH to suppress below 1 ng/mL during an oral glucose tolerance test.

TREATMENT

Standard Therapies: Treatment is aimed at reducing tumor bulk, inhibiting further growth of the tumor, reducing GH and IGF-I levels, and restoring normal pituitary function. The mainstay of therapy is trans-sphenoidal adenomectomy. Although cure is less likely in patients with macroadenomas, surgery is essential when vision is compromised. Debulking large tumors and subsequently reducing GH levels makes the likelihood of controlling excess GH secretion by adjuvant therapy more effective. Pituitary irradiation is effective in controlling excessive GH secretion and inhibiting further tumor growth in most cases. Medical therapy has a role in patients for whom surgery is contraindicated; as primary therapy in patients with mild disease; as secondary therapy while waiting for pituitary irradiation to take effect; and after surgery that did not result in a cure. Medical therapy is primarily dependent on two classes of medication: dopaminergic agonists and somatostatin analogues.

Investigational Therapies: Pegvisomant, a genetically manipulated GH molecule that has been mutated to disable functional dimerization of the GH receptor, is being explored.

REFERENCES

Ben-Shlomo A, Melmed S. Acromegaly. *Endocrinol Metab Clin North Am* 2001;30:565–583.

Giustina A, Barkan A, Casanueva FF, et al. Criteria for cure of acromegaly: a consensus statement. *J Clin Endocrinol Metab* 2000;85:526–529.

Renehan AG, Bhaskar P, Painter JE, et al. The prevalence and characteristics of colorectal neoplasia in acromegaly. *J Clin Endocrinol Metab* 2000;85:3417–3424.

Swearingen B, Barker FG 2nd, Katznelson L, et al. Long-term mortality after transsphenoidal surgery and adjunctive therapy for acromegaly. *J Clin Endocrinol Metab* 1998;83: 3419–3426.

Trainer PJ, Drake WM, Katznelson L, et al. Treatment of acromegaly with the growth hormone-receptor antagonist pegvisomant. *N Engl J Med* 2000;342:1171–1177.

RESOURCES

79, 351, 393

3   ACTH Deficiency

Amy M. Connell, MD,
Arna Gudmundsdottir, MD,
and Udaya M. C. Kabadi, MD

DEFINITION: Isolated adrenocorticotropic hormone (ACTH) deficiency is a form of secondary adrenal insufficiency in which there is decreased synthesis and/or secretion of the pituitary hormone that regulates the release of cortisol from the adrenal gland.

SYNONYM: Secondary adrenal insufficiency; Secondary hypocortisolism.

DIFFERENTIAL DIAGNOSIS: Viral illness; Dehydration; Depression; Anorexia nervosa; Cancer; Acquired immunodeficiency syndrome; Tuberculosis.

SYMPTOMS AND SIGNS: Primary and secondary adrenal insufficiency may cause many of the same signs and symptoms including weakness, nausea, vomiting, diarrhea, dizziness, anorexia, fatigue, muscular weakening, myalgias, or arthralgia, and orthostasis. It may also manifest more acutely with volume depletion and hypotension. Additionally, screening laboratory tests may indicate the presence of hyponatremia, hyperkalemia, hypoglycemia, eosinophilia, mild normocytic normochromic anemia, and lymphocytosis. More specific manifestations such as mucocutaneous hyperpigmentation, darkening of scars or nipples, and salt craving frequently denote the presence of primary adrenal insufficiency. Because most causes of ACTH deficiency do not target this hormone alone, symptoms of deficiencies of other pituitary hormones may be evident, such as amenorrhea, erectile dysfunction, or lack of libido in both sexes because of decreased circulating gondadotropins, as well as symptoms of secondary hypothyroidism.

ETIOLOGY/EPIDEMIOLOGY: The etiology remains unknown in most cases of isolated ACTH deficiency, excluding the iatrogenic secondary adrenal insufficiency caused by chronic glucocorticoid administration. Causes such as tumor, hemorrhage, or granulomatous processes (sarcoidosis or histoplasmosis) of the pituitary leading to ACTH deficiency tend to destroy more of the gland and therefore affect the synthesis and release of other hormones as well. The possibility of an autoimmune disorder targeting the corticotrophs or the presence of ACTH-blocking antibodies must be considered. The incidence and prevalence are not clearly documented. The disorder has been described in both sexes.

DIAGNOSIS: Clinical features alone do not distinguish isolated ACTH deficiency from other causes of hypoadrenalism. The diagnosis is made by the demonstration of low cortisol production as assessed by 24-hour urinary free cortisol level with low plasma ACTH, absent or subnormal adrenal responses to stimulation of pituitary corticotrophs by vasopressin or corticoptropin-releasing hormone, as well as inhibited or occasionally intact adrenal responses to exogenous ACTH but always with subnormal basal and peak cortisol concentrations. A gold standard test for ACTH deficiency is insulin-induced hypoglycemia. To confirm the diagnosis of isolated ACTH deficiency, other anterior pituitary hormones, namely thyrotropin, PRL, luteinizing hormone, follicle-stimulating hormone, and growth hormone, must be normal. Once the diagnosis is established, MRI of the pituitary should be done to exclude a mass lesion, hemorrhage, or infiltrating lesion.

TREATMENT
Standard Therapies: Standard treatment involves appropriate glucocorticoid replacement. The dose of the steroid should be increased in the event of an illness or other physiologic stress. An identification bracelet or something similar indicating the presence of the disorder must always be on the person to alert attending personnel in case of an emergency. Mineralocorticoid replacement rarely may be necessary.

REFERENCES
Connell AM, Kabadi UM. Intractable nausea attributable to isolated renocorticotropic hormone: prompt resolution after administration of glucocorticoid. *Endocr Pract* 2000;6:375–378.
Dickstein G, Arad E, Schochves C. Low dose ACTH stimulation test. *Endocrinologist* 1997;7:285–293.
Oelkers W. Adrenal insufficiency. *N Engl J Med* 1996;335:1206–1212.
Stacpoole PW, Interlandi JW, Nicholson WE, et al. Isolated ACTH deficiency: a heterogeneous disorder. *Medicine* 1982;61:13–22.
Stren K, Grinspran, Billes BMK. Laboratory assessment of adrenal insufficiency. *J Clin Endocrinol Metab* 1994:79:923–931.

RESOURCES
79, 365

4 Adiposis Dolorosa

Rebecca B. Campen, MD

DEFINITION: Adiposis dolorosa is characterized by multiple, painful fatty lipomas that occur in adults. The lipomas are located primarily on the trunk and proximal extremities. Unlike ordinary lipomas, there is associated pain that can be severe and sometimes debilitating.

SYNONYM: Dercum disease.

DIFFERENTIAL DIAGNOSIS: Familial lipomatosis syndrome; Benign symmetric lipomatosis (Madelung disease); Gardner syndrome; Cowden disease; Proteus syndrome.

SYMPTOMS AND SIGNS: The typical patient is a middle-aged, obese woman with multiple, painful lipomas. Other members of the patient's family may be affected. The complaint of pain in the lipomas often appears out of proportion to physical findings. Pain can last for hours, can be paroxysmal or continuous, and worsens with movement. Adiposis dolorosa is often associated with emotional disturbances, generalized weakness, depression, and irritability. The condition can also be associated with early congestive heart failure, myxedema, arthralgias, paroxysmal flushing episodes, fine tremors, cyanosis, hypertension, headaches, and epistaxis.

ETIOLOGY/EPIDEMIOLOGY: Adiposis dolorosa occurs in both sexes but is more common in women. Most cases are sporadic. Hereditary forms have been reported that suggest autosomal-dominant transmission and variable expressivity. In cases of sporadic lipomas, molecular analysis suggests that a mutation lies on chromosome 12. The reason for pain in the lipomas is not understood. No abnormality has been found in the adipose tissue by light or electron microscopy, suggesting that pain may be due to stretching or pressure on nerves by the lipomas rather than neuromatous involvement in the tumors themselves.

DIAGNOSIS: The diagnosis should be suspected based on findings of multiple, painful fatty tumors. Biopsy should confirm that the tumors are lipomas. The lipomas of adiposis dolorosa are histologically indistinguishable from ordinary lipomas.

TREATMENT

Standard Therapies: Treatment is symptomatic and difficult. Pain can sometimes be relieved by analgesics, injection of steroids, or intravenous lidocaine. Treatment can also include liposuction or surgical excision, but lipomas often continue to develop in other areas.

Investigational Therapies: Interferon-α2b for pain relief is being explored.

REFERENCES

Berntorp E, Berntorp K, Brorson H, et al. Liposuction in Dercum's disease: impact on haemostatic factors associated with cardiovascular disease and insulin sensitivity. *J Intern Med* 1998;243:197–201.

Campen RC, Mankin H, Louis D, et al. Familial occurrence of adiposis dolorosa. *J Am Acad Dermatol* 2001;44:132–136.

Dercum FX. Three cases of a hitherto unclassified affection resembling in its grosser aspects obesity, but associated with special nervous symptoms—adiposis dolorosa. *Am J Med Sci* 1892;104:521–530.

Gonciarz A, Mazur W, Hartleb J, et al. Interferon alfa-2b induced long-term relief of pain in two patients with adiposis dolorosa and chronic hepatitis C. *J Hepatol* 1997;27:1141.

Juhlin L. Long-standing pain relief of adiposis dolorosa (Dercum's disease) after intravenous infusion of lidocaine. *J Am Acad Dermatol* 1986;15:383–385.

RESOURCES

131, 365

5 Congenital Adrenal Hyperplasia Due to 21-Hydroxylase Deficiency

Phyllis W. Speiser, MD

DEFINITION: Congenital adrenal hyperplasia (CAH) is a group of recessively inherited disorders caused by one of several enzyme deficiencies that impair the ability of the adrenal glands to produce corticosteroids. The most common disorder is due to steroid 21-hydroxylase (also termed 21-monooxygenase) deficiency.

SYNONYMS: Virilizing adrenal hyperplasia; Adrenogenital syndrome; Steroid hydroxylase deficiency.

DIFFERENTIAL DIAGNOSIS: 21-hydroxylase deficiency; 11-β hydroxylase deficiency; 3-β hydroxysteroid dehydrogenase deficiency; 17-α hydroxylase deficiency with or without 17,20-lyase deficiency; 17-β hydroxysteroid dehydrogenase deficiency; Corticosterone methyloxidase deficiency type II; Lipoid adrenal hyperplasia; Aromatase deficiency; Addison disease; Virilization due to endogenous or exogenous androgen excess; Hermaphroditism; Pseudohermaphroditism.

SYMPTOMS AND SIGNS: Infants often are listless, fail to gain weight, and vomit. Older children and adults who have not been adequately treated show symptoms similar to those of primary adrenal insufficiency, including muscle weakness, nausea, vomiting, anorexia, irritability, depression, hyperpigmentation, hypotension, lack of tolerance to cold temperatures, and the inability of the body to respond properly to stress. Newborn girls may have ambiguous external genitalia. Older girls or untreated women develop cystic ovaries, absent or irregular menses, hirsutism, and acne, and may be unable to conceive. Male infants with CAH due to 21-hydroxylase deficiency appear normal at birth; unrecognized sodium wasting is a potential cause of mortality. Children with undiagnosed non–sodium-wasting show signs of precocious puberty by 2–3 years. Unusually rapid growth, acne, voice deepening, enlargement of the phallus, pubic hair, and axillary hair may appear. Males may develop intratesticular adrenal nodules. Physical growth may be rapid in both sexes, but early bone fusion results in short stature.

ETIOLOGY/EPIDEMIOLOGY: The classic forms of CAH due to steroid 21-hydroxylase deficiency are most common and account for approximately 95% of cases. The incidence is 1 in 10,000 to 1 in 15,000 live births worldwide. There are geographically isolated areas with a much higher disease incidence, such as western Alaska and the is-

land of La Reunion. Males and females are equally affected, although males have a higher neonatal mortality rate because they seldom have physical signs of the disorder. The late-onset or mild form of CAH, nonclassic adrenal hyperplasia (NCAH), is more prevalent and affects approximately 1 in 30 Ashkenazi Jews and approximately 1 in 100 non-Jewish individuals.

DIAGNOSIS: The pathognomonic serum hormonal profile consists of high levels of androgens, including androstenedione and testosterone in girls and prepubertal boys, and high levels of 17-hydroxyprogesterone. If the diagnosis is suspected and basal hormone levels are not markedly elevated, a corticotropin stimulation test can be performed. Prenatal testing is available.

TREATMENT
Standard Therapies: Severely affected individuals must take oral corticosteroid drugs to correct hormonal deficiencies. The preferred glucocorticoid treatment is hydrocortisone in infants and children or prednisone in adolescents and adults. Parenteral hydrocortisone sodium succinate should be given if oral medication cannot be tolerated, or in preparation for surgery or other stressful procedures. Individuals affected with the nonclassic form of CAH may require glucocorticoid treatment only if they are symptomatic. Mineralocorticoid supplements in the form of fludrocortisone and extra dietary sodium chloride may be necessary to maintain proper sodium and water balance. Surgical reconstruction of the external genitalia of females may be necessary in some cases.

Investigational Therapies: Prenatal treatment of individuals at high risk for CAH with dexamethasone is available, and the long-term outcomes are being investigated. The relative effectiveness of a multidrug regimen for the routine postnatal treatment of CAH consisting of an antiandrogen, aromatase inhibitor, and reduced doses of glucocorticoid and mineralocorticoid is also being explored.

REFERENCES
Speiser PW, ed. *Endocrinol Metab Clin North Am* 2001;30.
Speiser PW, White PC. Congenital adrenal hyperplasia. *Endocr Rev* 2000;245–291.
Wilson JD, Foster DW, eds. *Textbook of endocrinology,* 9th ed. Philadelphia: WB Saunders, 1998:598–605.

RESOURCES
86, 281, 362

6   Primary Aldosteronism

Norman M. Kaplan, MD

DEFINITION: Primary aldosteronism is a cause of hypertension, often associated with hypokalemia. With newer diagnostic studies, it is being recognized more frequently at an earlier stage at which the serum potassium levels are not low. Most of the milder forms are caused by bilateral hyperplasia of the adrenal cortex; the more severe forms are usually caused by a solitary adenoma.

SYNONYM: Conn syndrome.

DIFFERENTIAL DIAGNOSIS: Liddle syndrome; Other forms of primary aldosteronism, including glucocorticoid-remediable aldosteronism, dexamethasone-suppressible hyperaldosteronism, and adrenal carcinomas; Secondary aldosteronism.

SYMPTOMS AND SIGNS: Hypertension is almost invariable and may be severe. If hypokalemia is not present, few if any specific symptoms are noted. If hypokalemia is present, weakness and polyuria may be noted.

ETIOLOGY/EPIDEMIOLOGY: There is no known cause of either solitary adenomas or bilateral adrenal hyperplasia. The latter condition can be secondary to excessive renin-angiotensin, as in renovascular hypertension. In contrast, renin-angiotensin levels are suppressed with primary mineralocorticoid excess associated with bilateral adrenal hyperplasia. Glucocorticoid-remediable aldosteronism is caused by an unequal crossover mutation between the genes encoding two adrenal enzymes. This results in the production of a chimeric gene that places aldosterone synthase expression under the regulatory control of corticotropin and in the production of 18-oxocortisol, which has mineralocorticoid effects.

DIAGNOSIS: If hypokalemia is present, other causes of potassium wastage must be excluded, including diuretic use or gastrointestinal losses. In the absence of hypokalemia, plasma levels of aldosterone (which are elevated) and renin activity (which is suppressed from the volume expansion and elevated blood pressure) should be measured. If plasma aldosterone is high and renin low, resulting in a high ratio, additional confirmation of primary aldosterone excess is best provided by failure to suppress either plasma or urine aldosterone levels by sodium loading. If aldosterone excess is proven, adrenal imaging (CT or MRI) will usually define the pathology. If the results of imaging are ambiguous, bilateral adrenal venous sampling may be required.

TREATMENT

Standard Therapies: Removal of solitary adenomas is best accomplished by laparoscopic adrenalectomy. If bilateral hyperplasia is seen, medical therapy with the aldosterone antagonist spironolactone should be provided. A diuretic may also be required, as may additional antihypertensive therapy.

REFERENCES

Dluhy RG, Lifton RP. Glucocorticoid-remediable aldosteronism. *J Endocrinol Metab* 1999;84:4341–4344.

Kaplan NM. Cautions over the current epidemic of primary aldosteronism. *Lancet* 2001;357:953–954.

Lim PCX, Young WF, MacDonald TM. A review of the medical treatment of primary aldosteronism. *J Hypertension* 2001;19:353–361.

Rossi GP, Sacchetto A, Chiesura-Corona M, et al. Identification of the etiology of primary aldosteronism with adrenal vein sampling in patients with equivocal computed tomography and magnetic resonance findings. *J Endocrinol Metab* 2001;86:1083–1090.

Stowasser M. Primary aldosteronism. *J Hypertension* 2001;19:363–366.

RESOURCES

281, 357, 365

---

7   Alström Syndrome

Jan D. Marshall, MS

DEFINITION: Alström syndrome is a genetic disorder traditionally defined by the following general profile: early pigmentary retinopathy that leads to childhood blindness, bilateral sensorineural hearing impairment, childhood obesity, Type 2 diabetes mellitus, dilated cardiomyopathy, and progressive renal failure.

SYNONYM: Alström-Halgren syndrome.

DIFFERENTIAL DIAGNOSIS: Bardet-Biedl syndrome; Laurence Moon syndrome; Usher syndrome; Leber congenital amaurosis.

SYMPTOMS AND SIGNS: Alström syndrome involves multiple organ systems with complex interactions. Considerable variability of phenotypic expression exists. A typical child with Alström syndrome presents in infancy with severe photodysphoria and nystagmus. By age 16 years, most are blind. Early in childhood, hearing appears normal, but within the first decade sensorineural hearing impairment is noted and bilateral hearing deficits evolve throughout the school-age years. Intelligence is normal, although early developmental milestones may be delayed in some children. Affected children typically have short, thick, wide feet and stubby fingers, but no polydactyly or syndactyly. Many children with Alström syndrome experience dilated cardiomyopathy (DCM) and subsequent heart failure either as infants or in adolescence. In infants, cardiac symptoms may precede vision defects, and most infants who survive appear to have a complete recovery by age 3 years. Several adolescent patients have had recurrent DCM. In the toddler years, obesity begins to develop, progressing to serious truncal obesity with a body mass index above the 90th percentile. Most children have normal height in the early years, but final height after puberty is often below the 50th percentile. Nearly all children are above the 95th percentile for weight. Obesity may moderate after puberty. Acanthosis nigricans is a frequent feature. Triglycerides are elevated. Insulin resistance and hyperinsulinemia eventually develop into type 2 diabetes mellitus during adolescence or early adulthood. It is not known how early affected children exhibit insulin resistance, but hyperinsulinemia has been reported in children as young as 4 years. Renal, hepatic, or cardiac dysfunction are typical in later years.

ETIOLOGY/EPIDEMIOLOGY: Alström syndrome is inherited in an autosomal-recessive fashion. The *ALMS1* gene on chromosome 2p13 has been identified. Alström syndrome occurs with increased frequency among ethnically isolated populations such as French Acadians and Pakistanis.

DIAGNOSIS: Alström syndrome is generally diagnosed on the basis of the clinical features. Delay of onset of some characteristic features (type 2 diabetes, cardiomyopathy, renal disease) makes differential diagnosis difficult, especially in young patients.

TREATMENT
Standard Therapies: There is no treatment. Clinical management of diabetes, hepatic, and cardiac complications should be implemented.

REFERENCES
Charles SJ, Moore AT, Yates JRW, et al. Alstrom's syndrome: further evidence of autosomal recessive inheritance and endocrinological dysfunction. *J Med Genet* 1990;27:590–592.
Collin GB, Marshall JD, Cardon LR, et al. Homozygosity mapping of Alström syndrome to chromosome 2p. *Hum Mol Genet* 1997;6:213–220.
Collin GB, Marshall JD, Ikeda A, et al. Mutations in *ALMS1* cause obesity, type 2 diabetes and neurosensory degeneration in Alström syndrome. *Nat Genet* 2002;31:74–78.
Marshall JD, Ludman MD, Shea SE, et al. Genealogy, natural history, and phenotypic features of Alström syndrome in a large Acadian kindred and three unrelated families. *Am J Med Genet* 1997;73:150–161.
Russell-Eggitt IM, Clayton PT, Coffey R, et al. Alström syndrome. Report of 22 cases and literature review. *Ophthalmology* 1998; 105:1274–1280.
Tremblay F, LaRoche RG, Shea SE, et al. Longitudinal study of the early electroretinographic changes in Alström's syndrome. *Am J Ophthalmol* 1993;115:657–665.

RESOURCES
220, 338, 355, 371

---

8   Androgen Insensitivity Syndrome

Bruce Gottlieb, PhD,
Lenore K. Beitel, PhD,
and Mark Trifiro, MD

DEFINITION: The androgen insensitivity syndrome (AIS) is a condition caused by mutations of the androgen receptor (AR) that typically includes feminization or undermasculinization of the external genitalia at birth, abnormal secondary sexual development in puberty, and infertility. (See also Partial Androgen Insensitivity Syndrome entry.)

SYNONYM: Testicular feminization (TFM).

DIFFERENTIAL DIAGNOSIS: Defects in testosterone biosynthesis; Feminization syndromes; Gonadal dysgenesis.

SYMPTOMS AND SIGNS: Androgen insensitivity syndrome can be subdivided into three phenotypes: complete androgen insensitivity syndrome (CAIS), partial androgen insensitivity syndrome (PAIS), and mild androgen insensitivity syndrome (MAIS). Individuals with CAIS (testicular feminization) have normal female external genitalia. They typically present either before puberty with inguinal masses that are subsequently identified as testes or at puberty with primary amenorrhea and sparse to absent pubic or axillary hair. Breasts and female adiposity develop normally. Sexual identity and orientation are female. Individuals with MAIS (undervirilized male syndrome) have unambiguously male external genitalia. They usually present with gynecomastia at puberty. They may have undermasculinization that includes sparse facial and body hair and small penis. Patients may be impotent, and spermatogenesis may be impaired.

ETIOLOGY/EPIDEMIOLOGY: Patients with androgen resistance have identifiable disease-causing mutations in the *AR* gene detected by direct sequencing of the gene. The frequency for CAIS and PAIS is estimated at 2–5 in 100,000. The frequency of MAIS has not been determined. The disorder is inherited in an X-linked recessive manner. Affected 46,XY individuals are infertile. Carrier women have a 50% chance of transmitting the *AR* gene mutation in each pregnancy.

DIAGNOSIS: The diagnosis of CAIS can be established by clinical and laboratory findings alone; the diagnosis of PAIS and MAIS may require a family history. The laboratory findings required include the following: 46,XY karyotype; evidence of normal or increased synthesis of testosterone by the testes; evidence of normal conversion of testosterone to dihydrotestosterone; evidence of normal or increased luteinizing hormone production by the pituitary gland; and evidence of deficient or defective androgen-binding activity of genital skin fibroblasts.

TREATMENT
Standard Therapies: The modalities of management—surgery, psychological support, and hormone replacement or supplementation—depend on the AIS phenotype. Genetic counseling is recommended, and prenatal testing should be considered if its availability can be confirmed. In CAIS, a common practice is to remove the testes after puberty when feminization of the affected individual is complete. Prepubertal gonadectomy is indicated if inguinal testes are physically or esthetically uncomfortable and if inguinal herniorrhaphy is necessary. In this event, estrogen replacement therapy is necessary to initiate puberty, maintain feminization, and avoid osteoporosis. Vaginal length may be sufficiently short to require dilation in an effort to avoid dyspareunia. Men with MAIS often require reduction mammoplasty for treatment of gynecomastia. A trial of androgen pharmacotherapy is recommended to attempt to improve virilization.

REFERENCES
Gottlieb B, Pinsky L, Beitel LK, et al. Androgen insensitivity. *Am J Med Genet* 1999;89:210–217.
Griffin JE, McPhaul MJ, Russell DW, et al. In: Scriver CR, Beaudet A, Sly W, et al., eds. *The metabolic and molecular bases of inherited diseases,* 8th ed. New York: McGraw-Hill, 2001:4117–4146.
Quigley CA, DeBellis A, Marscheke KB, et al. Androgen receptor defects: historical, clinical and molecular prospectives. *Endocr Rev* 1995;16:271–321.

RESOURCES
44, 338

---

9   Partial Androgen Insensitivity Syndrome

A.L.M. Boehmer, MD, PhD

DEFINITION: Partial androgen insensitivity syndrome (PAIS) is an X-linked recessive disorder of sexual differentiation in 46,XY individuals due to a defective androgen receptor. The phenotypic spectrum ranges from a female phenotype with labial fusion and enlarged clitoris to an otherwise normal male phenotype with azoospermia or oligospermia. All patients have testes and do not have a uterus.

SYNONYMS: Reifenstein syndrome; Lubs syndrome.

DIFFERENTIAL DIAGNOSIS: Dysgenetic male pseudohermaphroditism; 17-β hydroxysteroid dehydrogenase 3 deficiency; 5-α reductase 2 deficiency; 17,20 lyase deficiency; 3-β hydroxysteroid dehydrogenase deficiency.

SYMPTOMS AND SIGNS: Patients present in the neonatal period with labial fusion, enlarged clitoris, palpable inguinal swelling in a phenotypic girl, severe hypospadias in a boy, or an intersex phenotype. Primary amenorrhea in affected girls or undermasculinization, gynecomastia, and/or infertility in affected boys may be seen at puberty. 46,XY individuals with PAIS have testes, sometimes located in the abdomen or inguinal canals, which produce high levels of testosterone from the start of puberty through adulthood. High levels of luteinizing hormone are also found. Phenotypic boys with hypospadias develop gynecomastia during puberty. Facial hair is absent or sparse. Phenotypic female patients have a shallow vagina. A uterus is absent in all phenotypes and all patients are infertile.

ETIOLOGY/EPIDEMIOLOGY: Due to dysfunction of the receptor for testosterone, prenatal virilization and virilization at puberty is defective in affected 46,XY individuals. Depending on the degree of rest activity of the androgen receptor, virilization is nearly absent, decreased, or results in only azoospermia or oligospermia. Mutations in the androgen receptor gene, on chromosome Xq11-Xq12, can cause decreased numbers or qualitative defects of the receptors. No clear genotype/phenotype correlation exists. The minimal incidence of AIS (including patients with the complete androgen insensitivity syndrome) is 1 in 99,000.

DIAGNOSIS: Although one third of cases of AIS arise *de novo*, a positive family history for AIS may be helpful for diagnosis. The diagnosis is made based on a normal 46,XY karyotype, diminished virilization and the presence of normal appearing testis, absence of a uterus and fallopian tubes as established by ultrasonography, and normal androgen production. A human chorionic gonadotropin stimulation test may be used to test testicular function in prepubertal children. An SHBG suppression test enables the diagnosis in patients older than 1 year. The diagnosis is confirmed by identification of a causative mutation in the androgen receptor gene.

TREATMENT

Standard Therapies: Surgical reconstruction of the external genitalia including vaginal enlargement (if appropriate) is required. Because of the risk of further virilization or testicular neoplasm, gonadectomy is required in patients with a female phenotype. Male patients must be periodically monitored for testicular neoplasm. Prolonged high-dose androgen therapy increases masculinization in some patients. Psychological and genetic counseling should be offered to patients and their families.

REFERENCES

Boehmer ALM, Brinkmann AO, Bruggenwirth HT, et al. Genotype versus phenotype in families with androgen insensitivity syndrome. *J Clin Endocrinol Metab* 2001;86 (in press).

Boehmer ALM, Nijman JM, Lammers BAS, et al. Etiologic studies in severe or familial hypospadias. *J Urol* 2001;165:1246–1254.

Grumbach MM, Conte FA. Disorders of sexual differentiation. In: Wilson JD, Foster DW, Kronenberg HM, et al., eds. *Williams textbook of endocrinology,* 9th ed. Philadelphia: WB Saunders, 1998:1303–1425.

Quigley C, De Bellis A, Marschke K, et al. Androgen receptor defects: historical, clinical, and molecular perspectives. *Endocr Rev* 1995;16:271–321.

Slijper FME, Frets PG, Boehmer ALM, et al. Androgen insensitivity syndrome (AIS): emotional reactions of parents and patients to the clinical diagnosis of AIS and its confirmation by androgen receptor mutation analysis. *Horm Res* 2000;53: 9–15.

RESOURCES

44, 338

---

10   Asherman Syndrome

*Jeffrey Klein, MD,
and Mark V. Sauer, MD*

DEFINITION: Asherman syndrome (AS) is a condition in which partial or complete obliteration of the uterine cavity occurs secondary to intrauterine adhesions. It is most commonly observed secondary to endometrial trauma stemming from puerperal curettage, and may result in menstrual abnormalities, infertility, habitual abortion, and late gestational complications.

SYNONYMS: Intrauterine adhesions/synechiae; Amenorrhea traumatica-atretica.

DIFFERENTIAL DIAGNOSIS: Polycystic ovarian syndrome; Ovarian failure; Hypothalamic-pituitary dysfunction; Male factor infertility; Anovulation/oligoovulation; Diminished ovarian reserve; Tubal/pelvic factor infertility; Cervical incompetence; Müllerian anomalies; Fibroids; Genetic causes (e.g., parental translocation); Antiphospholipid antibody syndrome; Endometrial polyp; Submucous fibroid.

SYMPTOMS AND SIGNS: Women with AS may present with menstrual disturbances, infertility, habitual abortion, or other complications of pregnancy. Intrauterine adhesions may also be an incidental finding in an asymptomatic patient. The most common menstrual abnormalities are amenorrhea and hypomenorrhea, although patients may present with dysmenorrhea, oligomenorrhea, or even menometrorrhagia. Amenorrheic patients typically give a history of normal menses before the onset of AS, although primary amenorrhea is common in women with AS due to pelvic tuberculosis. A correlation exists between the extent of disease and the menstrual pattern. Amenorrheic patients typically have more extensive scarring and endometrial destruction, although mild adhesions at the level of the internal os may obstruct the egress of menstrual flow. Infertility and/or habitual abortion commonly occur in patients with AS, although the mechanism is uncertain. Among patients who achieve pregnancy, there is a higher incidence of a wide array of complications late in gestation, including placenta previa, placenta accreta, premature labor, and postpartum hemorrhage.

ETIOLOGY/EPIDEMIOLOGY: The disorder develops as a result of trauma to the endometrium. The gravid uterus is particularly prone to damage to the regenerative basalis layer of the endometrium at the time of curettage. In a large metanalysis of 1,856 cases of AS, pregnancy was a predisposing causal factor in 91% of cases. Postabortion curettage accounted for approximately two thirds of cases, with most occurring after missed abortions. The disorder has also been reported after cesarean section and evacuation of a molar pregnancy. AS has also occurred after trauma to the nonpregnant uterus (e.g., postmyomectomy, diagnostic curettage, and after cervical manipulations). Damage to the endometrial lining also results from tuberculosis and schistosomiasis infection. Although bacterial infection may result in adhesion formation in and around the fallopian tubes and pelvis, a direct connection between nontuberculous bacterial infection and AS has not been established.

DIAGNOSIS: The disorder should be suspected in patients with amenorrhea or hypomenorrhea, infertility, or habitual abortion after dilation and curettage of a puerperal uterus. Filling defects on hysterosalpingography in patients with AS are typically lacunar shaped, irregular, and persist in repeated films taken over time. Confirmation is made by hysteroscopy.

TREATMENT

Standard Therapies: Treatment consists of surgical excision followed by measures to prevent the formation of new adhesions. Blunt or sharp excision may be employed. Typically, this is performed under direct visualization at the time of hysteroscopy. After lysis of adhesions, the uterine walls are often splinted with an intrauterine device or balloon catheter to separate the raw surfaces and prevent readhesion. Many advocate administration of estrogen, with or without progestogen, for approximately 1 month to promote rapid regeneration of the endometrial lining. No consensus exists on the necessity of perioperative antibiotics and postoperative steroid treatment. Rarely, a patient may have extensive scarring of the internal os, precluding a vaginal approach to surgery. Exploratory laparotomy with hysterotomy and adhesiolysis from above may be done, although results are typically poor. Patients with AS caused by tuberculosis frequently have complete obliteration of the uterine cavity and are not candidates for surgical intervention.

REFERENCES

March CM. Acquired intrauterine adhesions: Asherman's syndrome. In: Adashi EY, Rock JA, Rosenwaks Z, eds. *Reproductive endocrinology, surgery, and technology.* New York: Lippincott-Raven, 1996:1475–1488.

Schenker JG, Margolioth EJ. Intrauterine adhesions: an updated appraisal. *Fertil Steril* 1982;37:593–610.

RESOURCE

55

---

11 Bartter Syndrome

*Denice M. Hodgson, MD,
Leonid V. Zingman, MD,
and Andre Terzic, MD, PhD*

DEFINITION: Bartter syndrome is composed of a group of similar conditions that share the characteristics of hypokalemic metabolic alkalosis, renal potassium and chloride wasting, hyperaldosteronism, and hyper-reninism without hypertension. The syndromes are renal tubular disorders that have been linked to mutations in the genes for several ion channels. The group can be divided into subgroups based on clinical presentation: classic Bartter, antenatal Bartter, and Gitelman syndromes. Subsets of the classic Bartter and antenatal Bartter groups have also been categorized based on genetic linkage to specific mutations: Bartter types I, II, and III.

SYNONYM: For antenatal Bartter syndrome: Hyperprostaglandin E2 syndrome.

DIFFERENTIAL DIAGNOSIS: Loop diuretic use (pseudo-Bartter syndrome); Thiazide diuretic use; Renal artery stenosis; Renin-secreting tumors; Conn syndrome; Adrenal hyperplasia; Cystic fibrosis; Bulimia; Nasogastric suction; Diarrheal disorders including laxative abuse.

SYMPTOMS AND SIGNS: Table 7.1 compares the clinical and laboratory findings of the three clinical variants of Bartter syndrome. Gitelman syndrome is generally the mildest of the variants and is more likely to present later in life, often in asymptomatic adults found to have hypokalemia on routine laboratory testing. Children are usually diagnosed after presenting with the symptoms listed in Table 7.1. Antenatal Bartter syndrome is the most severe. It usually manifests with polyhydramnios from intrauterine polyuria. Volume depletion and electrolyte abnormalities may be life threatening.

ETIOLOGY/EPIDEMIOLOGY: Prevalence is unknown. The inheritance pattern is not clearly established, but appears to be autosomal recessive. There is no racial, ethnic, or gender predilection. The clinical subgroups have been linked to gene mutations for the channel proteins listed in Table 7.1. The two different mutations of antenatal Bartter, in *NK2Cl* and *ROMK*, subdivide it into Bartter types I and II, respectively. The mutation in *ClCKb* found in a subset of patients with classic Bartter syndrome (those without nephrocalcinosis) is used to classify this group as Bartter type III.

DIAGNOSIS: Diagnosis is made on the basis of consistent history, physical examination, and laboratory testing. The following tests should be obtained: serum electrolytes, including magnesium, renin, and aldosterone levels; urine prostaglandin E2; and urine electrolytes. Antenatal Bartter syndrome can be diagnosed prenatally by the presence of polyhydramnios without fetal malformation and elevated amniotic fluid chloride and aldosterone. Molecular genetic evaluation can establish the diagnosis in atypical cases.

TREATMENT

Standard Therapies: In classic Bartter syndrome, potassium-sparing diuretics (spironolactone, amiloride, or tri-

TABLE 7.1

	Classic Bartter	Gitelman	Antenatal Bartter
Clinical features	■ Usually presents in infants ■ Polydipsia, polyuria, nocturia ■ ± Salt craving ■ ± Fatigue, muscle weakness; tetany is rare ■ Growth retardation ■ Developmental delay	■ Manifests in adults (often asymptomatic) and school-age children ■ Fatigue, muscle weakness, neuromuscular irritability (Chvostek and Trousseau signs, tremor, fasciculations, tetany) ■ ± Joint pain secondary to chondrocalcinosis	■ Prenatal presentation with polyhydramnios, premature delivery. In newborn: fever, volume depletion due to polyuria, vomiting, diarrhea. ■ Failure to thrive ■ Growth retardation ■ ± "Typical" facies: triangular face, prominent forehead, large eyes, protruding ears, drooping mouth ■ Nephrocalcinosis, osteopenia
Blood biochemistry	■ Moderate/severe hypokalemia ■ Metabolic alkalosis ■ Very high renin, aldosterone, angiotensin II ■ 20% have hypomagnesemia	■ Moderate/severe hypokalemia ■ Metabolic alkalosis ■ High renin, normal/high aldosterone ■ Marked hypomagnesemia	■ Severe electrolyte imbalance ■ Metabolic alkalosis ■ Slightly low to normal magnesium
Renal/urinary findings	■ High potassium and chloride excretion ■ High prostaglandin E2 ■ Normal-high calcium ■ Nephrocalcinosis uncommon	■ High potassium excretion ■ Normal prostaglandin E2 ■ Hypocalciuria (despite normocalcemia) ■ No nephrocalcinosis	■ High potassium and chloride excretion ■ Marked prostaglandin E2 ■ Severe hypercalciuria leading to nephrocalcinosis and osteopenia ■ Hyposthenuria
Ion channel mutation	■ Basolateral chloride channel (ClC-Kb = type III) of the thick ascending limb of loop of Henle	■ Thiazide-sensitive co-transporter (TSC or NaCl cotransporter or NCCT) of distal convoluted tubule	■ Apical bumetanide-sensitive cotransporter (BSC or NaK-2Cl or NKCC2 = type I) and inwardly rectifying potassium channel (ROMK = type II) both of thick ascending limb of loop of Henle

amterene) in conjunction with potassium supplementation have been associated with increased growth rates in children. Cyclooxygenase (COX) inhibitors may also be useful. Angiotensin-converting enzyme inhibitors can be beneficial; however, symptomatic hypotension is a limiting complication. In Gitelman syndrome, magnesium supplementation is usually required, which may also facilitate potassium supplementation. Because hyperprostaglandinuria is not a feature of Gitelman syndrome, COX inhibitors may be less effective or ineffective. In antenatal Bartter syndrome, the cornerstone of therapy is fluid and electrolyte replacement. COX inhibitors are not indicated antenatally because hyperprostaglandinuria is not yet a feature *in utero*. They may be beneficial in infants, but are associated with the development of necrotizing enterocolitis and decreased glomerular filtration rate and are not recommended in the first 4–6 weeks.

Investigational Therapies: COX-2 inhibitors are being explored for treatment of Bartter type II.

REFERENCES
Abraham MR, Jahangir A, Alekseev AE, et al. Channelopathies of inwardly rectifying potassium channels. *FASEB J* 1999;13:1901–1910.
Amirlak I, Dawson KP. Bartter syndrome: an overview. *Q J Med* 2000;93:207–215.
Guay-Woodford LM. Bartter syndrome: unraveling the pathophysiologic enigma. *Am J Med* 1998;105:151–161.
Kurtz I. Molecular pathogenesis of Bartter's and Gitelman's. *Kidney Int* 1998;54:1396–1410.
Simon DB, Bindra RS, Mansfield TA, et al. Mutations in the chloride channel gene, CLCNKB, cause Bartter's syndrome type III. *Nat Genet* 1997;17:171–178.

RESOURCES
365, 462

---

12   Carcinoid Syndrome

Richard R.P. Warner, MD

DEFINITION: Carcinoid syndrome is a disease consisting of a combination of symptoms, physical manifestations, and abnormal laboratory chemical findings caused by a carcinoid tumor.

SYNONYMS: Carcinoid cancer; Carcinoid disease; Functioning carcinoid; Carcinoid apudoma; Functioning argentaffinoma; Neuroendocrine tumor, carcinoid type.

DIFFERENTIAL DIAGNOSIS: VIPoma; Gastrinoma with Zollinger-Ellison syndrome; Medullary carcinoma of the thyroid; Hyperthyroidism; Pheochromocytoma; Cushing syndrome; Systemic mast cell disease; Crohn disease; Irritable bowel syndrome.

SYMPTOMS AND SIGNS: Symptoms include hot, red facial flushing, usually painless diarrhea, marked changes in blood pressure (usually hypotension), asthmatic-like wheezing, scarring of heart valves with congestive heart failure, weight loss and even malnutrition, dehydration, weakness, muscle and joint aching, and peptic ulcer. The acute occurrence of flushing, blood pressure changes, weakness, palpitations, faintness, and sometimes wheezing constitutes a carcinoid crisis that, when severe, may be life threatening. Not all of these features need be present in a carcinoid crisis or in the carcinoid syndrome.

ETIOLOGY/EPIDEMIOLOGY: The exact cause is unclear, but in approximately 4% of cases, the condition is inherited as a familial disease, sometimes as part of multiple endocrine neoplasia syndrome. These low-grade malignancies are slow growing and usually can produce hormonal chemical substances such as serotonin, bradykinin, and other peptides. When large amounts of these substances are released into circulation, the signs and symptoms of carcinoid syndrome appear. Only 20 new cases of clinically significant carcinoid tumors per 1 million of the U.S. population are diagnosed per year. Only approximately 20% of these patients exhibit the carcinoid syndrome. Males and females of all ages are equally affected, with the preponderance occurring in middle-aged individuals. All races may be affected, although there is a slightly increased prevalence in blacks.

DIAGNOSIS: In the past, measurement of 24-hour urinary excretion of 5-hydroxyindolacetic acid (5-HIAA), the metabolite of serotonin, in a patient on a low-serotonin diet was the main laboratory test used. It is still useful and will be clearly elevated in 75% of patients; however, blood chromogranin-A and serotonin levels are usually increased, even when 5-HIAA is normal. The combination of octreoscan with these tests is the best way to confirm the diagnosis, as well as indicate the presence of carcinoid tumors without the full syndrome. Usually the tumor and metastases also can be imaged by spiral CT with contrast or by other imaging techniques such as ultrasonography or

MRI of the abdomen and chest. Needle biopsy is useful to confirm the diagnosis when chemical tests are inconclusive or unavailable.

TREATMENT

Standard Therapies: Standard treatment is surgical when possible for total resection of tumor and for de-bulking metastatic carcinoid. Debulking of liver metas-tases can be done by surgical excision or by the newer techniques of cryoablation and radiofrequency ablation. Hepatic artery catheterization with injection of embolic inert particles alone or mixed with chemotherapy has been effective in many patients with liver metastases. Sys-temic chemotherapy is also used. Once tumors have been removed, periodic long-term surveillance is needed. Oc-treotide injections, either three or four subcutaneous in-jections per day or one long-acting intramuscular injec-tion every 3–4 weeks, are the mainstay of treatment. When combined with injection of low-dose interferon-α, the rate of tumor inhibition increases to more than 50%. Various nutritional products are available and may be useful, as may various antidiarrheal and anticholinergic medications. Adrenaline and adrenaline-like drugs should be avoided because of their provocative effect on the disorder.

Investigational Therapies: Researchers are exploring systemic injections of the radioisotope yttrium 90 at-tached to an analogue of octreotide and hepatic artery injections of ⁹⁰yttrium embedded in microscopic glass beads, as well as the use of thalidomide and other anti-cancer drugs.

REFERENCE

Jensen RG, Doherty GM. Carcinoid tumors and the carcinoid syndrome. In: DeVita VP Jr, Hellman S, Rosenberg SA, eds. *Cancer: principles and practice of oncology,* 6th ed. Phil-adelphia: Lippincott, Williams & Wilkins, 2001:1813–1833.

RESOURCES

85, 291

---

13   Cushing Syndrome

Michelle D. Johnson, MD, and Mary Lee Vance, MD

DEFINITION: Cushing syndrome results from excess cortisol production or steroid treatment for medical condi-tions such as asthma, arthritis, or lymphoma.

DIFFERENTIAL DIAGNOSIS: Pseudo-Cushing syn-drome (depression, alcoholism, anorexia nervosa).

SYMPTOMS AND SIGNS: Symptoms and signs include increased weight with truncal obesity, facial fullness, and proximal muscle wasting. Skin changes such as facial plethora, thinning of the skin with easy bruising, acne, hir-sutism, fungal infections, and characteristic purple striae typically found on the trunk are common. Women may have menstrual irregularities and men may have sexual dysfunction. Significant psychiatric problems include de-pression, mania, and psychosis. Hypertension, diabetes or glucose intolerance, and hyperlipidemia also occur. Pa-tients are at increased risk for osteoporosis and may present with unexplained fractures. The disorder is rare in children and causes linear growth failure with weight gain.

ETIOLOGY/EPIDEMIOLOGY: Corticotropin-releasing hormone (CRH), synthesized in the hypothalamus, stimu-lates the release of corticotropin (ACTH) from the anterior pituitary gland. Corticotropin stimulates the production of cortisol by the adrenal cortex. Cushing syndrome is divided into two categories: ACTH-dependent and ACTH-inde-pendent. Causes of the ACTH-dependent form include a pituitary adenoma, ectopic ACTH production, or rarely, ectopic CRH production. Causes of the ACTH-inde-pendent form include exogenous steroid treatment, an ad-renal adenoma, or adrenal carcinoma. The most common endogenous cause, approximately 60%–80% of cases, is a benign ACTH-secreting pituitary adenoma, specifically re-ferred to as Cushing disease. The incidence of pituitary-dependent Cushing disease ranges from 0.1 to 1.0 new cases per 100,000. Cushing disease is up to eight times more common in women than in men.

DIAGNOSIS: Evaluation for Cushing syndrome involves determination of increased cortisol production by screening and confirmatory tests and then identification of the cause. A common screening test is the 1 mg overnight dexamethasone suppression test. A better test is measure-ment of 24-hour urinary free cortisol (UFC). When UFC values are variable, the dexamethasone + CRH test distin-guishes between Cushing and pseudo-Cushing syndrome. Once excessive cortisol production is clearly established, additional tests are required to determine the cause. A low ACTH level indicates ACTH-independent Cushing syndrome, and an adrenal CT scan is indicated. If the ACTH level is high or inappropriately normal, either a 2-day or overnight high-dose dexamethasone suppression test is performed. Appropriate suppression of serum cortisol (overnight test) or UFC (2-day test) suggests a pituitary source, and a pituitary MRI study is indicated. Inferior petrosal sinus sampling with measurement of ACTH levels may be required.

TREATMENT

Standard Therapies: Treatment depends on the underlying cause. Initial treatment of choice for Cushing disease is transphenoidal resection of the pituitary adenoma by an experienced neurosurgeon. In specialized centers, immediate remission occurs in 80%–90% of patients. Patients will require hydrocortisone replacement after successful surgery until the hypothalamic–pituitary–adrenal axis recovers. If surgery is unsuccessful, pituitary irradiation is usually recommended. Conventional fractionated radiotherapy or a stereotactic method can be used. The beneficial effects of radiotherapy may take months to years. Hypercortisolism can be controlled with drugs such as ketoconazole that inhibit steroid synthesis and reduce cortisol production to normal while awaiting the effect of radiation.

REFERENCES

Boscaro M, Barzon L, Fallo F, et al. Cushing's syndrome. *Lancet* 2001;357:783–791.

Meir CA, Biller BMK. Clinical and biochemical evaluation of Cushing's syndrome. *Endocrinol Metabol Clin North Am* 1997;26:741–762.

Orth D. Medical progress: Cushing's syndrome. *N Engl J Med* 1995;332:791–803.

RESOURCES

126, 354, 362

---

14 Diabetes Insipidus

Debbie K. Song, BS,
and Eva L. Feldman, MD, PhD

DEFINITION: Diabetes insipidus (DI) refers to the passage of large volumes of dilute urine. The impaired urinary concentrating mechanism in DI may be due to a failure of adequate vasopressin secretion from the posterior pituitary in response to normal physiologic stimuli (central or neurogenic DI) or due to a partial or complete resistance and hence an impaired response of the distal renal tubule and collecting duct to vasopressin (nephrogenic DI).

DIFFERENTIAL DIAGNOSIS: Primary or psychogenic polydipsia; Drug-induced polydipsia associated with the use of thioridazine, chlorpromazine, and anticholinergic agents.

SYMPTOMS AND SIGNS: Clinical findings include polyuria, polydipsia, excessive thirst, nocturia, and nocturnal enuresis in children. Urine output volumes are generally in excess of 3 L/day. There is a risk of severe dehydration if the excreted water is not sufficiently replenished. Patients at risk for dehydration include those who are intubated, are comatose, or have injured hypothalamic thirst centers. The cardiovascular symptoms and signs of dehydration appear earliest and include orthostatic hypotension, tachycardia, narrowed pulse pressure, and poor peripheral perfusion. Other features of dehydration that may take more than 24 hours to manifest include weakness, psychic disturbances, fever, poor skin turgor, dry mucous membranes, decreased secretions, weight loss, metabolic acidosis, confusion, seizures, coma, and death.

ETIOLOGY/EPIDEMIOLOGY: Up to one third of central DI cases are idiopathic; identifiable causes of central DI include severe head trauma, pituitary or hypothalamic lesions secondary to surgical procedures, intracranial tumors, infiltrating infectious and/or autoimmune granulomatous processes, and vascular defects. Congenital central DI can be inherited in an autosomal-dominant fashion due to one of many identified mutations in the AVP-neurophysin gene. Familial hypopituitarism and septooptic dysplasia are also causes. Central DI can also be inherited as part of the autosomal-recessive Wolfram syndrome. Nephrogenic DI can be acquired in association with various tubulointerstitial renal diseases, electrolyte disorders such as hypokalemia or hypercalcemia, certain drug therapies (e.g., lithium), and pregnancy. A common metabolic cause is diabetes mellitus. Familial forms of nephrogenic DI may be inherited as an X-linked recessive trait involving mutations in the gene that encodes the antidiuretic (V_2) receptor or rarely as an autosomal-recessive trait caused by mutations in the water channel protein aquaporin 2.

DIAGNOSIS: A diagnosis of DI should be suspected in a patient with normal adrenal function who demonstrates hypotonic polyuria with a urine specific gravity less than 1.010, urine osmolality less than 300 mOsm/kg, and a urine output greater than 250 mL/h in adults or 3 mL/kg/h in children. A comparison of simultaneous urine and serum osmolalities can assist in distinguishing causes of hypotonic polyuria. To differentiate between central and nephrogenic DI, the response to a subcutaneous injection of vasopressin is monitored. If such diagnostic tests are equivocal, then a water deprivation test can be done to confirm the diagnosis. Additional diagnostic tests including hypertonic saline infusion, empiric trials with low-dose vasopressin, or more elaborate fluid deprivation tests may be required in patients with partial forms of central or nephrogenic DI.

TREATMENT
Standard Therapies: Treatment options for central DI depend on the severity of the vasopressin deficiency. Vasopressin replacement therapy in the form of a synthetic analogue, 1-desamino-8-D-arginine vasopressin, is preferred in cases of severe central DI, and may be administered by nasal insufflation, oral tablets, or parenteral injection. For patients with partial central DI who have some residual releasable vasopressin, oral therapy with chlorpropamide, clofibrate, or carbamazepine may be used. The withdrawal of certain drugs and the correction of metabolic and electrolyte disturbances that may underlie nephrogenic DI can in some cases reverse the renal resistance to vasopressin, although such normalization may take weeks. Otherwise, salt restriction is recommended to reduce solute load, and thiazide diuretics may be used in conjunction with potassium-sparing diuretics such as amiloride to decrease polyuria. New therapeutic approaches involving a combination of thiazide diuretics, indomethacin, and desmopressin may be useful.

REFERENCES
Baylis PH, Cheetham T. Diabetes insipidus. *Arch Dis Child* 1998;79:84–89.
Blevins LS, Wand GS. Diabetes insipidus. *Crit Care Med* 1992;20:68–79.
Reeves WB, Bichet DG, Andreoli TE. Posterior pituitary and water metabolism. In: Wilson JD, Foster DW, Kronenberg HM, Larsen PR, eds. *Williams textbook of endocrinology.* 9th ed. Philadelphia: WB Saunders, 1998:341–388.
Van't Hoff WG. Molecular developments in renal tubulopathies. *Arch Dis Child* 2000;83:189–191.

RESOURCES
132, 340, 353

15 Growth Hormone Deficiency

Robert D. Murray, MD
and Shlomo Melmed, MD

DEFINITION: Growth hormone (GH) is secreted from the anterior pituitary under control of the hypothalamus. In children, GH deficiency results in a reduction in height and growth velocity for age and pubertal stage. Adult GH deficiency is characterized by truncal adiposity, reduced lean body mass, osteopenia, an excess of adverse cardiovascular risk markers, insulin resistance, and impaired quality of life.

DIFFERENTIAL DIAGNOSIS: Constitutional delay of growth and puberty; Idiopathic short stature.

SYMPTOMS AND SIGNS: In children, the defining features are short stature and reduced growth velocity for age and pubertal stage. The impairment of growth velocity is proportional to the severity of GH deficiency. The presence of a GH gene deletion manifests before age 3 years with a height standard deviation score (SDS) of less than −3 and a growth velocity less than the 3rd percentile. In contrast, GH insufficiency presents at an older age with less growth retardation and a growth velocity of less than the 25th percentile. In addition, affected children can experience hypoglycemia during the neonatal period, have an increase in truncal fat mass, and immature facies, and males may have a small phallus. Bone age is delayed proportionally to the severity of GH deficiency. In adults, the syndrome is characterized by increased fat mass, especially truncal fat, reduced lean body mass, reduced muscle strength and exercise tolerance, osteopenia, an adverse lipid profile, insulin resistance, and reduced quality of life, particularly energy levels.

ETIOLOGY/EPIDEMIOLOGY: An estimated 10,000–15,000 children in the United States have pituitary dwarfism. Most cases of GH deficiency in childhood are "isolated-idiopathic." Known genetic causes include mutations in genes for specific transcription factors (*Pit1, Prop1*), the GH gene, the GH receptor, and the insulin-like growth factor type I (IGF-I) gene.

DIAGNOSIS: GH deficiency is sought in children with a height of less than −2 SDS with a growth velocity less than the 10th–25th percentile, where alternate diagnoses have been excluded. The diagnosis depends on GH stimulation tests. The insulin tolerance test is the mainstay for the diagnosis in both children and adults. In patients with severe GH deficiency, one provocative test is adequate; however, in patients with less severe GH deficiency, a positive test result should be confirmed with a second stimulation test.

TREATMENT

Standard Therapies: Replacement therapy uses recombinant human GH genetically bioengineered in *Escherichia coli.* Growth hormone replacement is self-administered as a subcutaneous injection before retiring at night in an attempt to best simulate normal physiology. GH has historically been discontinued after attainment of final height. With the recognition of the continued role of GH in adults, however, hormone replacement is continued in adulthood.

Investigational Therapies: A depot GH preparation is being investigated.

REFERENCES

Cutfield WS, Wilton P, Bennmarker H, et al. Incidence of diabetes mellitus and impaired glucose tolerance in children and adolescents receiving growth-hormone treatment. *Lancet* 2000; 355:610–613.

Drake WM, Howell SJ, Monson JP, et al. Optimizing GH therapy in adults and children. *Endocr Rev* 2001;22:425–450.

Murray RD, Shalet SM. Growth hormone: current and future therapeutic applications. *Expert Opin Pharmacother* 2000;1: 975–990.

Murray RD, Skillicorn CJ, Howell SJ, et al. Dose titration and patient selection increases the efficacy of GH replacement in GHD adults. *Clin Endocrinol* 1999;50:749–757.

Reiter EO, Attie KM, Moshang T Jr, et al. A multicenter study of the efficacy and safety of sustained release GH in the treatment of naive pediatric patients with GH deficiency. *J Clin Endocrinol Metab* 2001;86:4700–4706.

RESOURCES

188, 246, 362

---

16   HAIR-AN Syndrome

Kathleen B. Elmer, LtCol, USAF, MC, FS, MD,
and Rita M. George, MD

DEFINITION: The syndrome of hyperandrogenism, insulin resistance, and acanthosis nigricans (HAIR-AN syndrome) is a unique condition that affects women. The features of androgen excess include hirsutism and acne. Associated insulin resistance is often marked.

DIFFERENTIAL DIAGNOSIS: Cushing syndrome; Acromegaly; Congenital adrenal hyperplasia; Polycystic ovary syndrome; Type 2 diabetes; Obesity; Malignancy.

SYMPTOMS AND SIGNS: Usually the hyperandrogenic features and/or acanthosis nigricans (AN) are the presenting complaint. Women may seek medical attention for symptoms of masculinization such as hirsutism, increased muscle mass, androgenic alopecia, and menstrual irregularities. Symptoms may also include persistent acne. AN presents as velvety, hyperpigmented areas of skin. Although the entire skin surface may develop AN, the flexural surfaces such as the nape of the neck, antecubital fossae, and groin are more commonly involved. An unusual location or rapidly progressive presentation of AN may indicate an underlying malignancy, most commonly adenocarcinoma of the stomach. Patients should be screened for symptoms related to diabetes mellitus, such as polydipsia and polyuria.

ETIOLOGY/EPIDEMIOLOGY: Approximately 1%–3% of hyperandrogenic women are suspected of having HAIR-AN syndrome. Infrequently, females with autoimmune diseases such as Graves disease and Hashimoto thyroiditis have been diagnosed with this condition. Some consider this disorder to be a subphenotype of polycystic ovary syndrome in which relatively normal luteinizing hormone levels and severe insulin resistance occur. Missense mutations in portions of the insulin receptor are the most frequently cited abnormalities and may be the key to this disorder. For instance, insulin and insulin-like growth factor type I receptors are present on human keratinocytes and in the human granulosa cell compartment. Chronic hyperinsulinemia may cause both hyperandrogenism and AN through the binding of these receptors.

DIAGNOSIS: A thorough physical examination to ascertain the presence of androgenic features, diabetes, and AN should be performed. Laboratory testing should include a complete blood cell count, thyroid screen, serum prolactin, glucose, insulin, and electrolyte measurements. A lipid panel should be performed, because an elevated risk for coronary artery disease exists in women with hyperandrogenism. Due to the association of autoimmune abnormalities with certain types of insulin resistance, an antinuclear antibody test and erythrocyte sedimentation rate should be obtained. The total testosterone level should be checked. Depending on the degree of concern regarding an ovarian or adrenal abnormality, levels of 17α-hydroxyprogesterone, dehydroepiandrosterone sulfate, morning cortisol after low-dose dexamethasone, and luteinizing and follicle-stimulating hormones should be tested for. If an underlying cancer is suspected, studies to include abdominal/pelvic CT, MRI, and upper/lower endoscopy may be considered.

TREATMENT

Standard Therapies: Suppression of gonadotropins with estrogen-progesterone oral contraceptives will reduce ovarian androgen production. Weight loss by obese patients can improve insulin resistance. Antiandrogenic medications such as spironolactone may be needed. Insulin-sensitizing drugs such as metformin may also be required to combat insulin resistance. Hirsutism may be treated with finasteride.

Investigational Therapies: Insulin-sensitizing agents such as the thiazolidinediones, rosiglitazone, and pioglitazone are

relatively new drugs used to treat HAIR-AN syndrome. New generations of insulin sensitizers likely will be developed.

REFERENCES

Barbieri RL. Induction of ovulation in infertile women with hyperandrogenism and insulin resistance. *Am J Obstet Gynecol* 2000;183:1412–1418.
Barbieri RL. Hyperandrogenism, insulin resistance and acanthosis nigricans, 10 years of progress. *J Reprod Med* 1994;39:327–336.
Chang RJ, Katz SE. Diagnosis of polycystic ovary syndrome. *Endocrinol Metab Clin North Am* 1999;28:397–408.
Futterweit W. Polycystic ovary syndrome: clinical perspectives and management. *Obstet Gynecol Surv* 1999;54:403–413.
Gordon CM. Menstrual disorders in adolescents. Excess androgens and the polycystic ovary syndrome. *Pediatr Clin North Am* 1999;46:519–543.

RESOURCE
398

---

17 True Hermaphroditism

Thomas Moshang, Jr., MD

DEFINITION: The term *true hermaphroditism* does not define a single etiologic disorder but rather the pathologic findings of gonadal tissue containing both testicular and ovarian elements. The phenotype of a patient may be male, female, or ambiguous at birth.

SYNONYMS: Ovatestes; Mixed gonadal dysgenesis.

DIFFERENTIAL DIAGNOSIS: Congenital adrenal hyperplasia; Partial androgen insensitivity; 5α-reductase deficiency; Idiopathic ambiguous genitalia; Hypospadius.

SYMPTOMS AND SIGNS: The most common finding leading to the diagnosis is the birth of an infant with ambiguous genitals. However, most patients with true hermaphroditism are born with male or female genitals without apparent ambiguity, although there may be undescended testicles, hypospadias, or mild clitoromegaly with or without posterior labial fusion. Adolescent males with true hermaphroditism can present with pain in the testes (from small follicular cysts), gynecomastia, penile urethral bleeding (from a hemiuterus), or lack of pubertal changes. Adolescent females may present with virilization (in-

cluding clitoral enlargement), lack of breast development, or amenorrhea.

ETIOLOGY/EPIDEMIOLOGY: True hermaphroditism is relatively rare compared with the incidence of pseudohermaphroditism, accounting for less than 10% of the intersex cases. The development of ovatestes is associated with mosaic sex chromosome combinations (such as 45XO/46XY or 46XX/46XY and similar variations). However, most true hermaphrodites are 46XX without any evidence of the sex determining region of the Y chromosome (SRY). This finding suggests that the genetic determinants of the testicular tissue in many of the 46XX true hermaphrodites is either downstream of *SRY* or autosomal genes.

DIAGNOSIS: The diagnosis is a pathologic one; however, many biochemical and anatomic findings suggest the presence of gonads with combined elements of an ovary and testis. Ultrasonography may show the presence of a unicornate uterus, indicating the presence of müllerian inhibiting hormone from the contralateral gonad. The finding of significant testosterone levels in the newborn infant or older female is compatible with testicular tissue (as long as congenital adrenal hyperplasia is ruled out). Estradiol response to injections of human menopausal gonadotropins may detect the presence of ovarian tissue in true hermaphrodites, and MRI of the gonads may detect the presence of ovarian and testicular tissue.

TREATMENT

Standard Therapies: If no ambiguity exists, the gender of the child is not an issue. Problems occur when a child has ambiguous genitals. A number of activist organizations have expressed concern about surgical correction and gender assignment at the birth of children born with ambiguous genitalia, and one group has proposed not correcting the genitalia so that the child can later participate in gender assignment and surgical procedure. Because many affected children are 46XX and the ambiguous genitals are often severely undervirilized (i.e., slight clitoromegaly and fused posterior labia), surgery is used to reduce the clitoral size and vaginoplasty is performed. In 46XY true hermaphrodites, the hypospadius is corrected and testicular tissue is brought into the scrotum. Ovatestes are often removed. At adolescence, in affected children needing hormonal replacement, testosterone for males and estrogen for females is provided. These are initially given at low doses to mimic the normal progression of hormonal changes through the teenage years.

REFERENCES

Berkovitz GD, Seeherunvong T. Abnormalities of gonadal differentiation. *Baillieres Clin Endocrinol Metab* 1998;12:133–142.

Choi HK, Cho KS, Lee HW, et al. MR imaging of intersexuality. *Radiographics* 1998;18:83–96.

Damiani D, Fellous M, McElreavey K, et al. True hermaphroditism: clinical aspects and molecular studies in 16 cases. *Eur J Endocrinol* 1997;136:201–204.

Walker AM, Walker JL, Adams S, et al. True hermaphroditism. *J Paediatr Child Health* 2000;36:69–73.

RESOURCE

213

---

18 Hypophosphatasia

Jan C-C. Hu, BDS, PhD,
and James P. Simmer, DDS, PhD

DEFINITION: Hypophosphatasia is an inherited disease affecting skeletal mineralization that is manifested clinically as osteomalacia.

DIFFERENTIAL DIAGNOSIS: Hyperparathyroidism; Vitamin D–dependent rickets; Familial hypophosphatemia (vitamin D–resistant rickets); Localized juvenile periodontitis.

SYMPTOMS AND SIGNS: The symptoms of hypophosphatasia range from a subclinical reduction in serum alkaline phosphatase (ALP) activity to death *in utero* secondary to a complete absence of skeletal mineralization. The continuum of mineralization defects is classified by age of onset (in order of decreasing severity): perinatal, infantile, childhood, and adult. In perinatal hypophosphatasia, profound hypomineralization of the skeleton results in death either *in utero* or a few days after birth. Infantile hypophosphatasia manifests before age 6 months with rickets, rib fractures that predispose the patient to pneumonia, functional craniosynostosis with increased intracranial pressure, proptosis, papilledema, and brachycephaly. Elevated calcium levels may cause vomiting and nephrocalcinosis. Childhood hypophosphatasia in its mildest form (odontohypophosphatasia) only affects the teeth. The adult teeth are rarely affected, but the primary teeth can have varying degrees of cementum agenesis and premature exfoliation (around age 3) of fully rooted teeth. In more severe cases, skeletal deformities are apparent on radiographs, such as tongue-shaped radiolucencies at the ends of the long bones and a beaten copper appearance of the calvarium. Premature closure of cranial sutures can cause proptosis, elevated intracranial pressure, and brain damage. Adult hypophosphatasia is often diagnosed in middle age. Individuals may experience pain in the feet or thighs from recurrent metatarsal stress fractures or femoral pseudofractures, or in the joints from pseudogout.

ETIOLOGY/EPIDEMIOLOGY: Hypophosphatasia is caused by defects in the tissue-nonspecific alkaline phosphatase (*ALPL*) gene on chromosome 1p36-1p34. It has an incidence of 1 in 100,000 live births. Alkaline phosphatase is a cell surface tetramer that catalyzes the removal of phosphate from inorganic pyrophosphate (PPi), pyridoxil 5-phosphate (PLP), and phosphoethanolamine (PEA), but appears in serum as an active dimer. Each monomeric unit has catalytic activity. Hypophosphatasia is inherited in an autosomal-recessive pattern in more than 90% of cases. Dominant hypophosphatasia occurs when a mutant allele expresses an enzyme that reduces the activity of the wild-type protein associated with it in the *ALP* dimer or tetramer.

DIAGNOSIS: Perinatal hypophosphatasia shows marked hypomineralization of the skull and long bones on ultrasonography during the second or third trimester, whereas milder forms may show severe long bone bowing. In childhood and adult forms, laboratory tests show reduced fasting serum alkaline phosphatase activity and elevated serum PLP and urine PEA.

TREATMENT

Standard Therapies: There is no established medical treatment. Optimal orthopedic management of fractures is provided as needed.

REFERENCES

Mornet E. Hypophosphatasia: the mutations in the tissue-nonspecific alkaline phosphatase gene. *Hum Mutat* 2000;15:309–315.

Van Hoof V, De Broe M. Interpretation and clinical significance of alkaline phosphatase isoenzyme patterns. *Crit Rev Clin Lab Sci* 1994;31:197–293.

Whyte MP. Hypophosphatasia and the role of alkaline phosphatase in skeletal mineralization [Review]. *Endocr Rev* 1994; 15:439–461.

RESOURCES

196, 351, 498

19 Kallmann Syndrome

G. Eda Akbas, MD,
and Hugh S. Taylor, MD

DEFINITION: Kallmann syndrome (KS) is a genetically heterogeneous disorder characterized by idiopathic hypogonadotropic hypogonadism (IHH) due to gonadotropin-releasing hormone (GnRH) deficiency and by anosmia and hyposmia accompanied by olfactory bulb hypoplasia. In some cases, other anomalies, such as synkinesia and/or unilateral renal agenesis, may also be detected.

SYNONYMS: Idiopathic hypogonadotropic hypogonadism; Olfactogenital syndrome.

DIFFERENTIAL DIAGNOSIS: Functional GnRH deficiency; Delayed puberty; Septooptic dysplasia; Hypothalamic-pituitary mass lesions; Congenital adrenal hypoplasia.

SYMPTOMS AND SIGNS: Although hypogonadotropic hypogonadism and anosmia are the signature features, other somatic anomalies such as synkinesia or mirror movements of extremities, cerebellar syndrome, eye movement abnormalities, visual defects, midline facial defects (high-arched palate, labial or palatine cleft, dental agenesis), unilateral renal agenesis, and clubfoot may be present. There is a high incidence of synkinesia and renal agenesis in the X chromosome–linked form. Osteoporosis due to hypoestrogenism may occur.

ETIOLOGY/EPIDEMIOLOGY: Most patients present as sporadic cases. Kallman syndrome affects 1 boy out of 10,000; the prevalence in girls is 5–7 times lower. In the rare familial forms, three different modes of inheritance have been described: X chromosome linked, autosomal dominant, and autosomal recessive. The autosomal genes responsible for this condition remain unknown. Mutations in the Xp22.3 localized *KAL1* gene have been identified in the X chromosome–linked form. Although males with the syndrome have an X-linked recessive form of IHH accompanied by anosmia, no *KAL* gene mutations have been identified in females with IHH and anosmia, suggesting that other autosomal genes may be involved.

DIAGNOSIS: Most cases are diagnosed in adolescence, when an absence of spontaneous pubertal development is found concomitantly with a deficient sense of smell. Gonadotropin deficiency is defined by serum concentrations of luteinizing hormone of <4.0 mIU/L, follicle-stimulating hormone <5.0 mIU/L, testosterone <6.0 nM (males), and estradiol <100 pM (females). The diagnosis can be made only when a hypothalamic-pituitary mass lesion is ruled out by MRI and other pituitary dysfunctions are ruled out by normal serum concentrations of cortisol, free thyroxine, thyrotropin, and prolactin. Confirmation of the anosmia can be made through detailed questioning and smell perception tests. Rarely, the diagnosis can be made as early as infancy in the presence of cryptorchidism or micropenis.

TREATMENT

Standard Therapies: In female patients, induction of ovulation and resulting pregnancy can be accomplished by administration of exogenous gonadotropins. The use of pulsatile GnRH administration, with an average dose of 5 μg per pulse, has been successful in the activation of gonadotropin secretion and ovarian cyclicity. In male patients, long-term subcutaneous delivery of GnRH at 2-hour intervals has been successful in inducing puberty and stimulating sustained testosterone secretion and spermatogenesis, with the ability to impregnate in a limited number of cases. In patients who do not desire fertility, hormone replacement therapy is achieved by administration of exogenous sex steroids.

REFERENCES

Georgopoulos NA, Pralong FP, Seidman CE, et al. Genetic heterogeneity evidenced by low incidence of *KAL-1* gene mutations in sporadic cases of gonadotropin-releasing hormone deficiency. *J Clin Endocrinol Metab* 1997;82:213–217.

Layman LC. Genetics of human hypogonadotropic hypogonadism. *Am J Med Genet* 1999;89:240–248.

Legouis R, Hardelin J, Levilliers J, et al. The candidate gene for the X-linked Kallmann syndrome encodes a protein related to adhesion molecules. *Cell* 1991;67:423–435.

Seminara SB, Crowley WF Jr. Perspective: the importance of genetic defects in humans in elucidating the complexities of the hypothalamic-pituitary gonadal axis. *Endocrinology* 2001; 42:2173–2177.

Taylor HS, Block K, Bick DP, et al. Mutation analysis of the *EMX2* gene in Kallmann syndrome. *Fertil Steril* 1999;72:910–914.

RESOURCES

79, 368

20 Laron Dwarfism

Chandra Mosely, PhD, and John A. Phillips III, MD

DEFINITION: Laron dwarfism type I is an autosomal-recessive disorder caused by resistance to the action of growth hormone (GH) because of defects in the GH receptor (*GHR*) gene. Patients with Laron dwarfism type I have short stature, delayed bone age, and occasionally blue sclera and hip degeneration. They have low levels of insulin-like growth factor type I (IGF-I) despite having normal or increased levels of GH. The same phenotype, known as Laron dwarfism type II, may be caused by post-GHR defects.

SYNONYMS: Laron dwarfism type I: Laron syndrome; Pituitary dwarfism II; Growth hormone receptor dysfunction. Laron dwarfism type II: Laron syndrome type II; Laron syndrome due to postreceptor defect.

DIFFERENTIAL DIAGNOSIS: Isolated GH deficiency (IGHD).

SYMPTOMS AND SIGNS: Patients with Laron dwarfism have the clinical appearance of patients with IGHD, with severe growth retardation, delayed bone age, severely pinched facies, high-pitched voices, and small male genitalia. Males have delayed puberty. Birth weight and body proportions in children are normal, but birth length may be reduced. Motor development may be delayed, and some patients are mildly retarded. Teething and fontanelle closure are delayed. Patients with Laron dwarfism have small hands and feet and are obese with childlike body proportions. They may also have hip joint degeneration, limited elbow extensibility, and occasionally blue sclerae. In addition, patients with Laron dwarfism have several biochemical features. They may have spontaneous hypoglycemic episodes in infancy and usually have insulinopenia in response to glucose and arginine. Fasting plasma GH concentrations are usually elevated but may fluctuate from normal levels to more than 100 ng/mL in the same patient. Although GH levels are normal or increased in Laron dwarfism patients, IGF-I levels are low and, unlike those in GH-deficient patients, do not respond to GH administration. Serum levels of GH binding protein (GHBP), which is encoded by the *GHR* gene, are low in patients with Laron dwarfism type I but normal in patients with Laron dwarfism type II.

ETIOLOGY/EPIDEMIOLOGY: Laron dwarfism type I is inherited in an autosomal-recessive manner and caused by point mutations or deletions in the *GHR* gene, which is located on chromosome 5p13.1-p12. Laron dwarfism type II can be caused by IGF-I deletions or post-GHR defects. Although the first patients recognized with Laron dwarfism were all Asian Jewish, the disorder has since been described in other ethnic groups.

DIAGNOSIS: Laron dwarfism is characterized by clinical signs of GHD (short stature, decreased growth velocity, and delayed bone age) despite normal or increased plasma GH levels and low IGF-I levels that are unresponsive to exogenous GH. Laron dwarfism type I is also often characterized by low GHBP levels. Diagnosis of the disorder, however, should not be based on GHBP levels alone, because normal GHBP levels may be found in some patients.

TREATMENT

Standard Therapies: Replacement therapy with recombinant human IGF-I (rhIGF-I, somatomedin-1) has been shown to be effective in both type I and type II Laron dwarfism, because it stimulates growth, increases muscle and bone mass, and normalizes blood chemistry. Use of rhIGF-I may be beneficial as long-term replacement therapy for adult patients.

REFERENCES

Gastier JM, Berg MA, Vesterhus P, et al. Diverse deletions in the growth hormone receptor gene cause growth hormone insensitivity syndrome. *Hum Mutat* 2000;4:323–333.

Mauras N, Martinez V, Rini A, et al. Recombinant human insulin-like growth factor I has significant anabolic effects in adults with growth hormone receptor deficiency: studies on protein, glucose, and lipid metabolism. *J Clin Endocrinol Metab* 2000; 85:3036–3042.

Phillips JA III. Molecular biology of growth hormone receptor dysfunction. *Acta Paediatr Suppl* 1992;383:127–131.

Woods KA, Camacho-Hubner C, Barter D, et al. Insulin-like growth factor I gene deletion causing intrauterine growth retardation and severe short stature. *Acta Paediatr Suppl* 1997;423:39–45.

RESOURCES

188, 246, 351

---

21   Acquired Generalized Lipodystrophy

Abhimanyu Garg, MD

DEFINITION: Acquired generalized lipodystrophy (AGL) is characterized by generalized loss of subcutaneous fat during childhood or adolescence. Patients have severe insulin resistance, hyperinsulinemia, diabetes mellitus, hypertriglyceridemia, and low serum high-density lipoprotein (HDL) cholesterol concentrations.

SYNONYM: Lawrence syndrome.

DIFFERENTIAL DIAGNOSIS: Congenital generalized lipodystrophy; Neonatal progeroid syndrome (Wiedemann-Rautenstrauch syndrome); Severe weight loss due to malnutrition, famine, anorexia nervosa, malabsorption syndromes, uncontrolled diabetes mellitus, thyrotoxicosis, adrenocortical insufficiency, cancer cachexia, acquired immunodeficiency syndrome–associated wasting, and chronic infections.

SYMPTOMS AND SIGNS: Fat loss occurs from the face, neck, trunk, and extremities and sometimes affects the palms and soles. Fat loss occurs over several weeks or years. In some patients, subcutaneous nodular lesions precede the fat loss. Loss of fat results in prominence of superficial veins and muscles. Other features include acanthosis nigricans, hirsutism, and hepatomegaly due to fatty infiltration.

ETIOLOGY/EPIDEMIOLOGY: The disorder occurs three times more often in women than in men. Approximately 50 patients have been reported in all ethnicities. Some patients also have autoimmune diseases, such as childhood dermatomyositis. Subcutaneous nodular lesions show a mixed infiltrate of lymphocytes and mononuclear macrophages in adipose tissue suggestive of panniculitis. Autoantibodies against adipocyte membranes have been reported. This suggests the adipocyte loss in AGL could be immune-mediated.

DIAGNOSIS: Generalized lack of subcutaneous fat and extreme muscularity occurring during childhood is diagnostic. Histopathologic documentation of panniculitis preceding the onset of lipodystrophy supports the diagnosis. Presence of autoimmune diseases as well as low serum HDL cholesterol levels, hyperinsulinemia, and hypertriglyceridemia help to make the diagnosis.

TREATMENT

Standard Therapies: Cosmetic management involves facial reconstruction with free flaps, transposition of facial muscle, and silicone or other implants in the cheeks. Weight loss is effective in losing fat from areas of excess fat deposition. No specific treatment is available for acanthosis nigricans. The optimal diet for patients with lipodystrophy is not clear. Generally, a low-fat diet is recommended for patients with hypertriglyceridemia. Avoidance of weight gain and increased physical activity can reduce the risk of developing diabetes and dyslipidemia. Children with lipodystrophy should consume enough energy for growth and maturation. After onset of diabetes, hypoglycemic drugs should be used to control hyperglycemia. Hypertriglyceridemia can be controlled with fibrates, statins, and n-3 polyunsaturated fatty acids. Oral estrogens should be avoided in women because of the risk of exacerbation of hypertriglyceridemia. Recently, leptin replacement therapy was reported to dramatically improve hyperglycemia and hypertriglyceridemia, and reduce liver size in patients with AGL.

REFERENCES

Billings JK, Milgraum SS, Gupta AK, et al. Lipoatrophic panniculitis: a possible autoimmune inflammatory disease of fat. *Arch Dermatol* 1987;123:1662–1666.

Garg A. The lipodystrophies and other rare disorders of adipose tissue. In: Braunwald E, Fauci AS, Kasper DL, et al., eds. *Harrison's principles of internal medicine,* 15th ed. New York: McGraw-Hill, 2001:2316–2319.

Lawrence RD. Lipodystrophy and hepatomegaly with diabetes, lipemia, and other metabolic disturbances. *Lancet* 1946;1: 724–731.

Oral EA, Simha V, Ruiz E, et al. Leptin-replacement therapy for lipodystrophy. *N Engl J Med* 2002;346:570–578.

Seip M, Trygstad O. Generalized lipodystrophy, congenital and acquired (lipoatrophy). *Acta Paediatr Suppl* 1996;413:2.

RESOURCES

32, 354, 462

---

22 Acquired Partial Lipodystrophy

Abhimanyu Garg, MD

DEFINITION: Acquired partial lipodystrophy (APL) is characterized by loss of fat from the face, upper extremities, thoracic region, and upper abdomen that occurs during childhood or adolescence.

SYNONYMS: Barraquer-Simons syndrome; Progressive lipodystrophy.

DIFFERENTIAL DIAGNOSIS: Severe weight loss due to malnutrition, famine, anorexia nervosa, malabsorption syndromes, uncontrolled diabetes mellitus, thyrotoxicosis, adrenocortical insufficiency, cancer cachexia, acquired immunodeficiency syndrome–associated wasting, and chronic infections.

SYMPTOMS AND SIGNS: In most patients, onset occurs before age 16 years. Fat loss usually affects the face first and then the neck, shoulders, upper extremities, thoracic region, and upper abdomen. Fat loss usually occurs over months to several years. The hips and lower extremities are spared, and excess fat can accumulate there after puberty. Approximately one third of patients develop mesangiocapillary glomerulonephritis. Systemic lupus erythematosus has also been reported in a few patients. Patients with APL seldom develop insulin resistance.

ETIOLOGY/EPIDEMIOLOGY: Approximately 200 patients have been reported from all ethnicities. Women are affected three times as often as men. Most patients have serum immunoglobulin G, called complement 3 (C3) nephritic factor, and low serum C3 levels, suggesting activation of the alternative complement pathway. Adipocyte lysis in these patients may be related to the expression of complement proteins in adipocytes.

DIAGNOSIS: Gradual loss of subcutaneous fat from the upper body during childhood or adolescence sparing the lower limbs is diagnostic. Presence of serum C3 nephritic factor, low serum C3 levels, proteinuria, or mesangiocapillary glomerulonephritis helps to make the diagnosis.

TREATMENT

Standard Therapies: Cosmetic management involves facial reconstruction with free flaps, transposition of facial muscle, and silicone or other implants in the cheeks. Adipose tissue transplantation from the abdomen or hip to the face is successful in some patients. Weight loss is effective in losing fat from areas of excess fat deposition.

REFERENCES

Garg A. The lipodystrophies and other rare disorders of adipose tissue. In: Braunwald E, Fauci AS, Kasper DL, et al., eds. *Harrison's principles of internal medicine,* 15th ed. New York: McGraw-Hill, 2001:2316–2319.

Mathieson PW, Wurzner R, Oliveira DBG, et al. Complement-mediated adipocyte lysis by nephritic factor sera. *J Exp Med* 1993;177:1827–1831.

Poley JR, Stickler GB. Progressive lipodystrophy: a clinical study of 50 patients. *Am J Dis Child* 1963;106:66.

Sissons JGP, West RJ, Fallows J, et al. The complement abnormalities of lipodystrophy. *N Engl J Med* 1976;294:461–465.

RESOURCES

32, 354, 462

23 Congenital Generalized Lipodystrophy

Abhimanyu Garg, MD

DEFINITION: Congenital generalized lipodystrophy (CGL) is an autosomal-recessive disorder characterized by near total loss of body fat and a marked muscular appearance from birth. Patients have severe insulin resistance, hypertriglyceridemia, and fatty liver.

SYNONYM: Berardinelli-Seip syndrome.

DIFFERENTIAL DIAGNOSIS: Weidemann-Rautenstrauch syndrome (neonatal progeroid syndrome); Acquired generalized lipodystrophy; Werner syndrome.

SYMPTOMS AND SIGNS: Patients have extreme lack of body fat and marked muscularity. Children have accelerated growth, advanced bone age, voracious appetite, and increased metabolic rate. Other features include umbilical hernia or prominence, acanthosis nigricans, excessive body hair, hyperhidrosis, and acromegaloid features. Hepatomegaly due to fatty infiltration can lead to cirrhosis. Cardiomegaly occurs in some patients. Postpubertal women may have polycystic ovary syndrome. Focal lytic lesions have been noticed in axial skeleton in adults. Hyperinsulinemia occurs early, but diabetes mellitus appears during the pubertal years. Severe hypertriglyceridemia can lead to acute pancreatitis. Plasma leptin concentrations are low.

ETIOLOGY/EPIDEMIOLOGY: The prevalence is estimated to be fewer than 1 in 12 million people. Patients of all ethnicities are reported, but higher prevalence is noted among inbreeding communities. Recently, our group reported mutations in the *AGPAT2* gene encoding 1-acylglycerol-3-phosphate O-acyltransferase in patients with CGL linked to chromosome 9q34. AGPAT2 is the key enzyme involved in the biosynthetic pathways of triacylglycerol and glycerophospholipids from glycerol-3-phosphate in humans. Thus, mutations in *AGPAT2* may cause lipodystrophy by inhibiting triacylglycerol synthesis and storage in adipocytes. CGL may also be caused by mutations in another gene, called *BSCL2* (Berardinelli-Seip Congenital Lipodystrophy 2), which encodes a protein, seipin, of unknown function; thus, how *BSCL2* mutations cause CGL remains unclear. Therefore, at least two distinct mechanisms underlie extreme lack of adipose tissue in CGL patients.

DIAGNOSIS: Patients have a characteristic pattern of body fat loss, easily noted on MRI. They have a near total loss of metabolically active fat present in most of the subcutaneous areas, and intraabdominal, intrathoracic, and bone marrow regions, but preservation of mechanical fat present in the palms, soles, orbits, perineum, and periarticular regions.

TREATMENT

Standard Therapies: Cosmetic management involves facial reconstruction with free flaps, transposition of facial muscle, and silicone or other implants in the cheeks. No specific treatment is available for acanthosis nigricans. The optimal diet for patients with lipodystrophy is not clear. Generally, a low-fat diet is recommended for patients with hypertriglyceridemia. Avoidance of weight gain and increased physical activity can reduce the risk of developing diabetes and dyslipidemia. Children with lipodystrophy should consume enough energy for growth and maturation. After onset of diabetes, hypoglycemic drugs should be used to control hyperglycemia. Hypertriglyceridemia can be controlled with fibrates, statins, and n-3 polyunsaturated fatty acids. Oral estrogens should be avoided in women with lipodystrophies because of the risk of exacerbation of hypertriglyceridemia. Recently, leptin replacement therapy was reported to dramatically improve hyperglycemia and hypertriglyceridemia, and reduce liver size in patients with CGL.

REFERENCES

Agarwal AK, Arioglu E, de Almeida S, et al. *AGPAT2* is mutated in congenital generalized lipodystrophy linked to chromosome 9q34. *Nat Genet* 2002:31:21–23.

Chandalia M, Garg A, Vuitch F, et al. Postmortem findings in congenital generalized lipodystrophy. *J Clin Endocrinol Metab* 1995;80:3077–3081.

Garg A. The lipodystrophies and other rare disorders of adipose tissue. In: Braunwald E, Fauci AS, Kasper DL, et al., eds. *Harrison's principles of internal medicine*, 15th ed. New York: McGraw-Hill, 2001:2316–2319.

Garg A, Fleckenstein JL, Peshock RM, et al. Peculiar distribution of adipose tissue in patients with congenital generalized lipodystrophy. *J Clin Endocrinol Metab* 1992;75:358–361.

Garg A, Wilson R, Barnes R, et al. A gene for congenital generalized lipodystrophy maps to human chromosome 9q34. *J Clin Endocrinol Metab* 1999;84:3390–3394.

Magre J, Delepine M, Khallouf E, et al. Identification of the gene altered in Berardinelli-Seip congenital lipodystrophy on chromosome 11q13. *Nat Genet* 2001;28:365–370.

Oral EA, Simha V, Ruiz E, et al. Leptin-replacement therapy for lipodystrophy. *N Engl J Med* 2002;346:570–578.

RESOURCES

32, 354, 42

24 Familial Partial Lipodystrophy

Abhimanyu Garg, MD

DEFINITION: Familial partial lipodystrophies (FPL) are autosomal-dominant disorders, characterized by gradual loss of subcutaneous adipose tissue from the extremities and trunk. Affected individuals are predisposed to insulin resistance, diabetes, and dyslipidemia.

SYNONYM: Kobberling-Dunnigan syndrome.

DIFFERENTIAL DIAGNOSIS: Cushing syndrome; Multiple symmetric lipomatosis and truncal obesity.

SYMPTOMS AND SIGNS: Loss of fat results in excessive muscularity. In patients with FPL, Dunnigan variety (FPLD), excess fat may accumulate in the neck and face, resulting in a cushingoid appearance. Other features include mild to moderate insulin resistance, acanthosis nigricans, menstrual abnormalities, polycystic ovary disease, and fatty liver. Atherosclerotic vascular complications and acute pancreatitis are the major causes of morbidity and mortality. Compared with men who have FPLD, women with FPLD have increased prevalence of diabetes mellitus, hypertriglyceridemia, and low levels of high-density lipoprotein cholesterol.

ETIOLOGY/EPIDEMIOLOGY: The estimated prevalence rate is less than 1 in 15 million people. Most affected patients with FPLD have been white, but the disorder has been noted in African Americans and Asian Indians. Several missense mutations in the gene encoding the nuclear envelope protein lamin A/C on chromosome 1q21-22 have been found to be responsible for FPLD. Phenotypic heterogeneity has been reported related to the site of mutations. Mutations in the lamin A/C can result in adipocyte apoptosis and degeneration by disrupting nuclear function and thereby cause FPLD. Recently, mutation in PPARG (peroxisome proliferator-activated receptor-γ) gene was found in a patient with familial partial lipodystrophy who did not have the Dunnigan variety.

DIAGNOSIS: Affected women are more easily recognized than affected men. Lack of subcutaneous fat with associated muscular appearance, beginning at puberty, is diagnostic. MRI findings of lack of subcutaneous fat in the extremities and trunk but excess fat in intermuscular fasciae may be helpful for diagnosing FPLD. Analysis of mutations in the lamin A/C or PPARG genes can be confirmatory for FPLD or other variety of FPL, respectively.

REFERENCES

Agarwal AK, Garg A. A novel heterozygous mutation in peroxisome proliferator-activated receptor-γ gene in a patient with familial partial lipodystrophy. *J Clin Endocrinol Metab* 2002; 87:408–411.

Cao H, Hegele RA. Nuclear lamin A/C R482Q mutation in Canadian kindreds with Dunnigan-type familial partial lipodystrophy. *Hum Mol Genet* 2000;9:109–112.

Dunnigan MG, Cochrane MA, Kelly A, et al. Familial lipoatrophic diabetes with dominant transmission: a new syndrome. *Q J Med* 1974;49:33–48.

Garg A, Peshock RM, Fleckenstein JL. Adipose tissue distribution pattern in patients with familial partial lipodystrophy (Dunnigan variety). *J Clin Endocrinol Metab* 1999;84:170–174.

Peters JM, Barnes R, Bennett L, et al. Localization of the gene for familial partial lipodystrophy (Dunnigan variety) to chromosome 1q21–22. *Nat Genet* 1998;18:292–295.

Speckman R, Garg A, Du F, et al. Mutational and haplotype analyses in families with familial partial lipodystrophy (Dunnigan variety) reveal recurrent missense mutations in the globular C-terminal domain of lamin A/C. *Am J Hum Genet* 2000; 66:1192–1198.

RESOURCES

32, 354, 462

25 Polycystic Ovary Syndrome

Mazen Bisharah, MD,
and Togas Tulandi, MD

DEFINITION: Polycystic ovary syndrome (PCOS) is a clinical manifestation of hyperandrogenism and chronic anovulation in the presence of bilateral polycystic ovaries.

Three minimal criteria have been proposed: (a) menstrual irregularity; (b) evidence of hyperandrogenism clinically or biochemically; and (c) exclusion of other disease.

SYNONYMS: Stein-Leventhal syndrome; Hyperandrogenic chronic anovulation.

DIFFERENTIAL DIAGNOSIS: Idiopathic hirsutism; Congenital adrenal hyperplasia; Ovarian hyperthecosis; Ovarian or adrenal androgen secreting tumors; Exogenous androgen such as danazol or testosterone.

SYMPTOMS AND SIGNS: Signs and symptoms of PCOS may include menstrual disturbances from oligomenorrhea to amenorrhea, hirsutism, acne, male pattern balding or alopecia, increased muscle mass, deepening of the voice, clitoromegaly, anovulatory infertility, obesity, and glucose intolerance. Women with PCOS are at risk for the development of diabetes mellitus, hypertension, coronary artery disease, intravascular thrombosis, and endometrial cancer.

ETIOLOGY/EPIDEMIOLOGY: The cause is unknown; however, the main factor is a persistent anovulatory state. Other features are insulin resistance or hyperinsulinemia, androgen excess, and abnormal gonadotropin secretion. It is estimated that the incidence is 4%–7% of reproductive-aged women. Some evidence exists that PCOS is an inherited condition. The rates in mothers and sisters of women with PCOS are 24% and 32%, respectively.

DIAGNOSIS: The diagnosis depends on a combination of clinical, hormonal, and ultrasonographic findings. These include menstrual irregularities, hirsutism or hyperandrogenemia, luteinizing hormone:follicle stimulating hormone ratio of greater than 2:1, and polycystic ovaries on ultrasonography.

TREATMENT
Standard Therapies: The objectives are to induce ovulation in infertile women or to decrease manifestations of hyperandrogenism. Weight loss must be encouraged in all overweight patients to improve the menstrual pattern, hirsutism, and hyperinsulinism. Ovulation can be achieved with ovulation-inducing agents, including clomiphene cit-

rate, dexamethazone, and exogenous gonadotropin. In women with clomiphene resistance, laparoscopic ovarian drilling can be offered. Hirsutism can be treated with oral contraceptives, gonadotropin-releasing hormone agonists, or antiandrogens including cyproterone acetate, spironolactone, flutamide, finasteride, and glucocorticoids. Because antiandrogens inhibit only the growth of new hair, old hair can be removed mechanically with depilatory creams, shaving, plucking, bleaching, or electrolysis. Close long-term follow-up and screening for diabetes and cardiovascular disease are warranted.

Investigational Therapies: A promising treatment is the use of insulin-sensitizing agents, metformin or thiazolidinediones.

REFERENCES
Felemban A, Tan SL, Tulandi T. Laparoscopic treatment of polycystic ovaries with insulated needle cautery: a reappraisal. *Fertil Steril* 2000:73:266–269.
Futterweit W. Polycystic ovary syndrome: clinical perspectives and management. *Obstet Gynecol Surv* 1999;54:403–413.
Glueck CJ, Phillips H, Cameron D, et al. Continuing metformin throughout pregnancy in women with polycystic ovarian syndrome appears to safely reduce first trimester spontaneous abortion. *Fertil Steril* 2001;75:46–52.
Guzick D. Polycystic ovary syndrome: symptomatology, pathophysiology, and epidemiology. *Am J Obstet Gynecol* 1998;179 (suppl):89–93.
Kahsar-Miller MD, Nixon C, Boots LR, et al. Prevalence of polycystic ovary syndrome (PCOS) in first-degree relatives of patients with PCOS. *Fertil Steril* 2001;75:53–58.
Lobo RA, Carmina E. The importance of diagnosing the polycystic ovary syndrome. *Ann Intern Med* 2000;132:989–993.

RESOURCES
398, 496

---

26   Precocious Puberty

Jerrold S. Olshan, MD, and Alan H. Morris, MD

DEFINITION: Precocious puberty (PP) is the onset of secondary sexual characteristics in children at an age that is two standard deviations younger than the mean age of pubertal onset.

SYNONYMS: For central precocious puberty (CPP): True precocious puberty; Gonadotropin-dependent precocious puberty; Isosexual precocious puberty. For pseudoprecocious puberty: Gonadotropin-independent precocious puberty (GIPP).

DIFFERENTIAL DIAGNOSIS: Premature thelarche; Premature adrenarche; Premature pubarche; Premature menarche; Pseudoprecocious puberty (including peripheral precocious puberty, testotoxicosis, male-limited precocious puberty, congenital adrenal hyperplasia, adrenal or gonadal tumors); Exogenous sex steroid exposure; Hypertrichosis.

SYMPTOMS AND SIGNS: Secondary sexual characteristics include testicular enlargement ($\geq$4 mL) and/or pubic hair development in boys, and breast and/or pubic hair development in girls. Other signs suggestive of pubertal onset include acne, growth acceleration, voice changes, vaginal discharge or bleeding, and advanced skeletal maturation.

ETIOLOGY/EPIDEMIOLOGY: Pathologic CPP has an incidence of 1 in 5,000–10,000 children with a female:male ratio of greater than 20:1. Of girls with PP, 95% have idiopathic true PP, whereas more than 50% of boys have an identifiable etiology for PP. Central PP can be caused by CNS tumors and other CNS disorders, including hypothalamic hamartoma of the tuber cinereum, encephalitis, brain abscess, static encephalopathy, global delays, sarcoid or tubercular granuloma, head trauma, vascular lesion, cranial irradiation, and neurofibromatosis type 1. It can also follow the treatment of virilizing congenital adrenal hyperplasia or the treatment of other causes of GIPP, including gonadal, adrenal, ectopic, or exogenous sources of hormone production, and primary hypothyroidism. PP can also be the presenting sign of long-standing, untreated, primary hypothyroidism.

DIAGNOSIS: The criteria for the diagnosis and treatment of CPP need to be reached through a synthesis of clinical findings as well as laboratory evidence for activation of the hypothalamic–pituitary–gonadal axis. The gold standard for determination of pubertal gonadotropin secretion is the gonadotropin-releasing hormone (GnRH) stimulation test. In boys, serum testosterone levels are useful for the diagnosis of PP. Diagnostic studies including head MRI, pelvic ultrasonography, and skeletal age determination are frequently required in the workup of children with CPP.

TREATMENT

Standard Therapies: For PP, the aims of treatment are to arrest physical maturation, prevent early menarche, bring final adult height closer to genetic expectation, and allow normal psychosocial development. Treatment with potent, long-acting GnRH analogues has resulted in significant improvement in height in many, although not all, children with PP caused by both organic conditions and idiopathic CPP. In general, girls who progress rapidly through puberty need treatment, whereas girls who progress more slowly or have unsustained puberty will often do well without intervention.

Investigational Therapies: Aromatase inhibitors and tamoxifen are being investigated.

REFERENCES
Herman-Giddens ME, Slora EJ, Wasserman RC, et al. Secondary sexual characteristics and menses in young girls seen in office practice: a study from the Pediatric Research in Office Settings network. *Pediatrics* 1997;99:505–512.

Kaplowitz PB, Oberfield SE. Reexamination of the age limit for defining when puberty is precocious in girls in the United States: implications for evaluation and treatment. Drug and Therapeutics and Executive Committees of the Lawson Wilkins Pediatric Endocrine Society. *Pediatrics* 1999;104:936–941.

Lee PA. Central precocious puberty. An overview of diagnosis, treatment, and outcome. *Endocrinol Metab Clin North Am* 1999;28:901–918.

Palmert MR, Malin HV, Boepple PA. Unsustained or slowly progressive puberty in young girls: initial presentation and long-term follow-up of 20 untreated patients. *J Clin Endocrinol Metab* 1999;84:415–423.

RESOURCES
78, 362

---

27   Pseudohypoparathyroidism

Murat Bastepe, MD, PhD, and Harald Jüppner, MD

DEFINITION: The three major forms of pseudohypoparathyroidism (PHP) are PHP type Ia, PHP type Ib, and pseudo-PHP (pPHP). Other forms of PHP are classified as PHP type Ic and PHP type II. In addition, paternal uniparental isodisomy of chromosome 20q (patUPD20q) can lead to abnormalities similar to those observed in patients affected by PHP type Ib.

DIFFERENTIAL DIAGNOSIS: Hypoparathyroidism; Renal failure; Magnesium deficiency; Malabsorption; Seizure disorders.

SYMPTOMS AND SIGNS: PHP types Ia and Ib are characterized by end-organ resistance to parathyroid hormone (PTH), leading to hypocalcemia, hyperphosphatemia, and elevated PTH. The clinical symptoms in PHP types Ia and Ib are mainly the consequence of low blood calcium and can vary considerably. Additional end-organ resistance to other hormones, such as thyroid-stimulating hormone, gonadotropins, and calcitonin, can be present in PHP type Ia. This form is associated with Albright hereditary osteodystrophy (AHO), which includes round face, short-stature, brachydactyly, heterotopic ossifications, and often some degree of mental retardation. AHO is also present in pPHP, but patients do not show hormonal resistance. Hypocalcemia in PHP types Ia and Ib usually develops in the first years of life, but late-onset cases have been described. Besides the findings characteristic of AHO, clinical manifestations in these forms can include muscle cramps, tingling sensation, fatigue, tetany, or seizures. Symptoms and signs related to hypothyroidism and/or hypogonadism may also be observed in PHP type Ia.

ETIOLOGY/EPIDEMIOLOGY: PHP type Ia and pPHP are caused by heterozygous, inactivating mutations in the Gsα encoding exons of *GNAS1* (chromosome 20q13.3). PHP type Ia occurs only if the *GNAS1* mutation is inherited from a female carrier of the genetic defect. If the same mutation is inherited from a male carrier, the offspring is affected by pPHP. This unusual mode of inheritance for hormonal resistance is also observed for patients with PHP type Ib, which was genetically mapped to the *GNAS1* locus. Furthermore, a specific loss of methylation defect within this gene was identified in PHP type Ib patients; however, no mutation has been identified yet.

DIAGNOSIS: Low to normal blood calcium concentrations with elevated levels of serum phosphorous and PTH are the most common biochemical features of PHP types Ia and Ib. These abnormalities can be mild, however, and an elevated PTH can be the only initial laboratory evidence for PTH resistance. Patients with PHP type Ia may also show elevations in thyroid-stimulating hormone, gonadotropins, and calcitonin. Patients with PHP type Ia and pPHP, but not with PHP type Ib, present with AHO. In addition to the abnormalities in blood chemistries, individ-

uals affected by PHP types Ia and Ib show impaired urinary excretion of phosphate and blunted excretion of cAMP and phosphate after challenge with exogenous biologically active PTH (negative Ellsworth-Howard test). Basal ganglia calcifications can be detected even without detectable changes in blood calcium and phosphate.

TREATMENT
Standard Therapies: Treatment consists of 1,25(OH)$_2$D$_3$ and calcium salts (preferably calcium carbonate). If resistance toward other hormones, such as thyroid-stimulating hormone, is also present, treatment with thyroxine may be necessary.

REFERENCES
Bastepe M, Lane AH, Jüppner H. Paternal uniparental isodisomy of chromosome 20q (patUPD20q)—and the resulting changes in *GNAS1* methylation—as a plausible cause of pseudohypoparathyroidism. *Am J Hum Genet* 2001;68:1283–1289.
Jan de Boer SM, Levine MA. Pseudohypoparathyroidism: clinical, biochemical, and molecular features. In: Bilezikian JP, Markus R, Levine NA, eds. *The parathyroids: basic and clinical concepts.* New York: Academic, 2001:807–825.
Jüppner H, Schipani E, Bastepe M, et al. The gene responsible for pseudohypoparathyroidism type Ib is paternally imprinted and maps in four unrelated kindreds to chromosome 20q13.3. *Proc Natl Acad Sci USA* 1998;95:11798–11803.
Liu J, Litman D, Rosenberg M, et al. A *GNAS1* imprinting defect in pseudohypoparathyroidism type IB. *J Clin Invest* 2000;106:1167–1174.
Weinstein LS. Albright hereditary osteodystrophy, pseudohypoparathyroidism, and Gs deficiency. In: Spiegel AM, ed. *G proteins, receptors, and disease.* Totowa, NJ: Humana, 1998:23–56.

RESOURCES
354, 466

28 X-Linked Hypophosphatemic Rickets

Rohit Dwivedi, MD, and Michael J. Econs, MD

DEFINITION: X-linked hypophosphatemic rickets (XLH) is characterized by hypophosphatemia, growth retardation, low tubular reabsorption of phosphate, osteomalacia, and rickets in growing children.

SYNONYMS: X-linked hypophosphatemic osteomalacia; Vitamin D–resistant rickets.

DIFFERENTIAL DIAGNOSIS: Tumor-induced osteomalacia; Fanconi syndrome; Autosomal-dominant hypophosphatemic rickets; Hereditary hypophosphatemic rickets with hypercalciuria; Vitamin D–deficient rickets.

SYMPTOMS AND SIGNS: Low serum phosphate may be seen shortly after birth, but diagnosis is difficult during infancy. At the time of weight bearing, deviation from normal growth and progressive leg deformities may become evident. Some affected individuals have isolated hypophosphatemia; others have disabling bone disease. Clinical manifestations include short stature, bone pain, rickets with resultant lower extremity deformities, enthesopathy, and dental abscesses. Frontal bossing and spinal stenosis may occur. Weakness is not a predominant feature.

ETIOLOGY/EPIDEMIOLOGY: The disease is an X-linked dominant renal phosphate-wasting disorder with the responsible mutant gene located on chromosome Xp22.1. The gene has been designated *PHEX*, and it encodes a 749–amino acid protein that is a member of the M13 family of membrane-bound proteases. The etiology is not entirely clear, but it is possible that *PHEX* may serve a regulatory role in renal phosphate wasting, and it may degrade or inactivate a phosphaturic hormone, hypothetically termed phosphatonin. The prevalence is approximately 1 case per 20,000 individuals. Although the disease is completely penetrant, severity varies widely, even among members of the same family. The degree of hypophosphatemia is similar in males and females.

DIAGNOSIS: All persons with XLH have renal tubular phosphate wasting and resultant hypophosphatemia. Other findings are normal levels of calcium, normal-to-high parathyroid hormone, increased alkaline phosphatase, and inappropriately normal calcitriol values for the hypophosphatemia. Most affected children have radiographic evidence of rickets at the knee, but only half have radiographic evidence of rickets at the wrist. Rachitic changes on radiography include fraying, widening, and cupping of the metaphyseal ends of rapidly growing bones. Adults may also have radiographic abnormalities based on the severity of the disease, such as pseudofractures and enthesopathy. Bone biopsies show osteomalacia. Older patients often have osteoarthritis seen on radiography, particularly of the knee and ankle.

TREATMENT

Standard Therapies: Because the basic defect involves renal phosphate wasting, current therapy is generally with high-dose phosphate (1–3 g of elemental phosphorus per day in four doses) and calcitriol. Therapy is initiated in childhood and is labor intensive for the physician and the patient and is best done by someone who has experience treating hypophosphatemic patients. The objective of therapy in children is to correct or prevent deformity from rickets, enhance growth rate, and lessen bone pain. It is best to start at a low dose of calcitriol and phosphate (to avoid diarrhea from phosphate) and gradually increase therapy over several months. Typically, the patient is given 1 year of high-dose therapy and then switched to a long-term maintenance phase, which usually entails a lower dose of calcitriol, but little change in phosphate dosage. The major complications of therapy are nephrocalcinosis and secondary hyperparathyroidism. Nephrocalcinosis appears to be most correlated to phosphate doses. During the high-dose phase we generally monitor serum calcium, phosphorus, and creatinine, as well as urine calcium and creatinine monthly. Monitoring can be relaxed to every 3–4 months during maintenance phase of treatment. The dosage of calcitriol and phosphate is adjusted based on the laboratory results, although no attempt is made to normalize serum phosphorus concentrations. Treatment of adult patients is controversial; however, symptomatic adults may have clinical and histomorphometric improvement.

Investigational Therapies: Treatment with the PHEX enzyme and FGF23 receptor blockade is being explored.

REFERENCES

DiMeglio L, White KE, Econs MJ. Disorders of phosphate homeostasis. *Endocrinol Metab Clin North Am* 2000;29:591–609.

Econs MJ, McEnery PT. Autosomal dominant hypophosphatemic rickets/osteomalacia: clinical characterization of a novel renal phosphate wasting disorder. *J Clin Endocrinol Metab* 1997;82:674–681.

Glorieux, FH. Hypophosphatemic vitamin D resistant rickets. In: Favus MJ, ed. *Primer on the metabolic bone diseases and disorders of mineral metabolism.* Philadelphia: Lippincott Williams & Wilkins, 1999:328–331.

Tenenhouse HS, Econs MJ. Mendelian hypophosphatemias. In: Scriver CR, ed. *The metabolic and molecular bases of inherited disease.* New York: McGraw-Hill, 2001:5039–5068.

White KE, Jonsson KB, Carn G, et al. The autosomal dominant hypophosphatemic rickets (ADHR) gene is a secreted polypeptide overexpressed by tumors that cause phosphate wasting. *J Clin Endocrinol Metab* 2001;86:497–500.

RESOURCES

354, 362, 365, 498

29   Sheehan Syndrome

Mark E. Molitch, MD

DEFINITION: Sheehan syndrome refers to the development of pituitary necrosis within a few hours of delivery of a baby. The chronic form usually presents months to years later with symptoms of amenorrhea, fatigue, and cold intolerance. The less common, acute form usually presents with persistent postpartum hypotension, tachycardia, and failure to lactate.

SYNONYM: Postpartum hypopituitarism.

DIFFERENTIAL DIAGNOSIS: Hypopituitarism secondary to lymphocytic hypophysitis or pituitary adenoma; Postpartum thyroiditis with hypothyroidism; Hypoadrenalism.

SYMPTOMS AND SIGNS: The amount of pituitary necrosis and resultant hormone deficiency dictates the subsequent course of the disorder. Patients with the chronic form have lesser degrees of pituitary infarction and present from weeks to years after delivery. Amenorrhea and loss of libido are common, but subsequent spontaneous pregnancies can occur rarely. Cold intolerance, dry skin, and other symptoms may occur. A history of failure to lactate postpartum and some breast atrophy are common. Fatigue, loss of axillary and pubic hair, nausea, vomiting, abdominal pain, and diarrhea may occur. Patients sometimes remember transient polyuria and polydipsia after delivery, indicating transient diabetes insipidus (DI). In the less common, acute, potentially lethal form, usually <10% of normal pituitary tissue remains. Patients may present with persistent hypotension, tachycardia, failure to lactate, and hypoglycemia. Polyuria and polydipsia may also occur, indicating DI.

ETIOLOGY/EPIDEMIOLOGY: Antecedent hypotension and shock are usual findings, due to obstetrical hemorrhage and, occasionally, retained placenta. Pituitary ischemia and necrosis may be due to occlusive spasm of the arteries that supply the anterior lobe directly and the hypothalamic-pituitary stalk. Pregnancy-induced pituitary enlargement has also been implicated. The frequency is unknown, but 25% of women who die within 30 days of delivery show evidence of pituitary infarction.

DIAGNOSIS: The diagnosis should be considered and treatment started in patients with obstetric hemorrhage and a prolonged course of hypotension not responsive to appropriate blood product replacement even before the results of blood testing become available. Blood should be obtained for adrenocorticotropic hormone, cortisol, free thyroxine (T_4), thyrotropin (TSH), prolactin, growth hormone (GH), luteinizing hormone (LH), follicle-stimulating hormone (FSH), and estradiol basally. Adrenocorticotropic hormone and cortisol levels should both be low basally. Free T_4 levels are often low in the chronic form without an increase in TSH. Prolactin levels and GH levels will likely both be low. In most patients, estradiol, LH, and FSH levels are low. Dehydration testing and measurement of urine and serum osmolalities with concomitant measurement of plasma vasopressin using standardized protocols can be used to test for DI.

TREATMENT

Standard Therapies: In the acute form, initial treatment is with the equivalent of 100 mg of hydrocortisone given intravenously as a bolus followed by an additional 100–200 mg within the first 24 hours. Saline with 5%–10% dextrose is used for volume expansion after blood loss has been corrected. Once the various hormonal defects have been identified and the patient has been stabilized, chronic therapy can be started. Hydrocortisone or prednisone is used for glucocorticoid replacement. Thyroxine is given daily. Estrogen/progesterone can be replaced by oral contraceptives or menopausal-type regimens given continuously or cyclically. Patients with symptomatic DI may need treatment with desmopressin. Although GH therapy is FDA approved, its use is not universally accepted. Benefits of GH therapy include increased muscle mass, decreased fat mass, reduction in LDL cholesterol, increased bone mineralization, and an improved sense of well-being.

REFERENCES

Iwasaki Y, Oiso Y, Yamauchi K, et al. Neurohypophyseal function in postpartum hypopituitarism: impaired plasma vasopressin response to osmotic stimuli. *J Clin Endocrinol Metab* 1989; 68:560–565.

Ozbey N, Inanc S, Aral F, et al. Clinical and laboratory evaluation of 40 patients with Sheehan's syndrome. *Isr J Med Sci* 1994;30: 826–829.

Shahmanesh M, Ali Z, Pourmand M, et al. Pituitary function tests in Sheehan's syndrome. *Clin Endocrinol* 1980;12:303–311.

Sheehan HL, Davis JC. Pituitary necrosis. *Br Med Bull* 1968;24: 59–70.

30 Chronic Lymphocytic Thyroiditis

Noel R. Rose, MD, PhD,
and Patrizio Caturegli, MD

DEFINITION: Chronic lymphocytic thyroiditis is the most common cause of hypothyroidism in iodine-sufficient countries, accounting for more than 90% of noniatrogenic cases. It may take one of two forms: goitrous or atrophic. Both forms are characterized by the presence of thyroid autoantibodies in the serum and by varying degrees of thyroid dysfunction.

SYNONYMS: Hashimoto thyroiditis; Autoimmune thyroiditis; Chronic nonspecific thyroiditis; Struma lymphomatosa.

DIFFERENTIAL DIAGNOSIS: Thyroid cancer; Colloid goiter; Graves disease; Pituitary failure; Iatrogenic hypothyroidism; Nephrotic syndrome; Down syndrome.

SYMPTOMS AND SIGNS: The disorder is characterized by slow, progressive onset of classic signs of hypothyroidism, including increased fatigue and lethargy, cold intolerance, tendency for weight gain despite normal or reduced appetite, irregular menses, dry skin, brittle or reduced body and scalp hair, myxedema, bradycardia, pericardial effusion, depressed ventilatory drive, pleural effusion, sleep apnea, constipation, delayed tendon reflexes, muscle stiffness and cramps, memory loss, depression, and cerebellar ataxia. In children, growth velocity is reduced. Some patients present with goiter.

ETIOLOGY/EPIDEMIOLOGY: Chronic lymphocytic thyroiditis is the result of autoimmunity to antigens of the thyroid gland. It is 5- to 10-fold more prevalent in women, with a peak incidence at ages 50–60 years. The disease is due to a combination of genetic and exogenous factors. Among the latter, the best documented is iodine. Either high or low concentrations increase the incidence of thyroiditis. Thyroid autoimmunity is partly familial; up to 50% of first-degree relatives of patients with chronic thyroiditis have thyroid autoantibodies. Both hypothyroidism and hyperthyroidism can occur in the same family. A weak association exists with certain HLA haplotypes, especially B8 and DR3 with atrophic thyroiditis and DR5 with the goitrous form of disease. It is closely associated with Down syndrome and Turner syndrome.

DIAGNOSIS: An elevated thyrotropin (TSH) level together with a below normal thyroxine (T_4) level is diagnostic of primary hypothyroidism. Triiodothyronine (T_3) levels are usually not useful. Using the thyrotropin-releasing hormone stimulation test, the lack of a thyrotropin response indicates secondary hypothyroidism. Patients with pituitary failure as a cause of hypothyroidism usually show other signs of pituitary deficiencies, such as low follicle-stimulating hormone and luteinizing hormone levels. The presence of thyroid antibodies, mainly thyroperoxidase and thyroglobulin, strengthens the diagnostic suspicion of thyroiditis.

TREATMENT

Standard Therapies: Hypothyroidism is generally treated with levothyroxine. Levothyroxine doses must be closely monitored and adjusted during pregnancy, due to the increased production of thyroid-binding globulin and the requirement of euthyroidism for normal fetal brain development. Triiodothyronine treatment is useful in the short term for patients who have undergone thyroidectomy for thyroid cancer. Surgery may be needed in rare cases of compression of the trachea.

REFERENCES

Dayan CM, Daniels GH. Chronic autoimmune thyroiditis. *N Engl J Med* 1996;335:99–107.

Weetman AP. Autoimmune thyroid disease. In: Rose NR, Mackay IR, eds. *The autoimmune diseases*, 3rd ed. San Diego: Academic, 1998:405–430.

Witebsky E, Rose NR, Terplan K, et al. Chronic thyroiditis and autoimmunization. *JAMA* 1957;164:1439–1447.

RESOURCES

354, 466

31   Zollinger-Ellison Syndrome

Robert Jensen, MD

DEFINITION: Zollinger-Ellison syndrome is characterized by resistant peptic disease (ulcers, esophagitis) due to gastric acid hypersecretion caused by ectopic release of gastrin from a neuroendocrine tumor.

SYNONYM: Gastrinoma.

DIFFERENTIAL DIAGNOSIS: Idiopathic peptic ulcer disease; *Helicobacter pylori* infection; Antral G cell hyperplasia/hyperfunction; Gastric outlet obstruction; Retained gastric antrum; Gastric hyposecretory states.

SYMPTOMS AND SIGNS: The most common symptoms are abdominal pain, diarrhea, esophageal symptoms, nausea/vomiting, and bleeding. In 20%–25% of cases, multiple endocrine neoplasia type 1 (MEN1) (due to a defect in the *MEN1* gene on chromosome 11q13) with hyperparathyroidism are present. Prominent gastric folds occur in 30%–94% of cases.

ETIOLOGY/EPIDEMIOLOGY: The disease is a result of ectopic gastrin release by the neuroendocrine tumor. The incidence is 0.5–2 cases per million population per year.

DIAGNOSIS: Diagnosis is often delayed 5–6 years. Clinicians should suspect the diagnosis in patients who have ulcer disease that occurs with diarrhea, is resistant to treatment, presents without *H. pylori*, or is associated with endocrinopathies. The diagnosis requires demonstration of fasting hypergastrinemia when gastric acid is present (gastric pH <2.5).

TREATMENT

Standard Therapies: The two general problems that must be addressed are control of the gastric hypersecretion and treatment of the gastrinoma per se. For control of acid hypersecretion, the use of proton pump inhibitors is recommended. Tumor localization studies are essential, with at least CT and somatostatin receptor scintigraphy performed. If metastases to the liver and/or MEN1 are not present, surgical resection should be considered by a surgeon experienced in the treatment of this disease. In patients with progressive metastatic disease to the liver, treatment with octreotide is recommended as the first choice, followed by chemotherapy for resistant cases.

Investigational Therapies: The use of radiolabeled ([111]indium, [90]yttrium) somatostatin analogues to treat advanced metastatic disease is being studied, as is the treatment with long-acting somatostatin analogues combined with interferon-α.

REFERENCES

Alexander RA, Jensen RT. Pancreatic endocrine tumors. In: DeVita VT, Hellman S, Rosenberg SA, eds. *Cancer: principles and practice of oncology,* 7th ed. Philadelphia: Lippincott Williams & Wilkins, 2001:1788–1813.

Jensen RT. Gastrinoma. *Baillieres Clin Gastroenterol* 1996;10:555–766.

Jensen RT. Zollinger-Ellison syndrome. In: Doherty GM, Skogseid B, eds. *Surgical endocrinology: clinical syndromes.* Philadelphia: Lippincott Williams & Wilkins, 2001:291–344.

Norton JA, Fraker DL, Alexander HR, et al. Surgery to cure the Zollinger-Ellison syndrome. *N Engl J Med* 1999;341:635–644.

Roy P, Venzon DJ, Shojamanesh H, et al. Zollinger-Ellison syndrome: clinical presentation in 261 patients. *Medicine* 2000; 79:379–411.

RESOURCE

365

Gastroenterologic Disorders

1   Alagille Syndrome

Andrew E. Mulberg, MD,
and Alisha Rovner, BA

DEFINITION: Alagille syndrome (AGS) is an autosomal-dominant disorder defined by paucity of interlobular bile ducts with three to five of the following features: chronic cholestasis, cardiac disease (predominantly pulmonic stenosis), skeletal abnormalities, ocular abnormalities, and a characteristic facial phenotype. Less common clinical features include renal abnormalities, intracranial bleeding, and pancreatic insufficiency.

SYNONYMS: Syndromic bile duct paucity; Paucity of interlobular bile ducts; Arteriohepatic dysplasia; Watson-Alagille syndrome.

DIFFERENTIAL DIAGNOSIS: Biliary atresia.

SYMPTOMS AND SIGNS: Infants usually present with a history and physical examination consistent with the diagnosis of biliary atresia. Symptoms include jaundice, pale loose stools, and poor growth within the first 3 months of life. Extrahepatic manifestations of AGS in infancy are benign. After infancy, children with AGS have persistent jaundice, pruritus, xanthomas, and poor growth.

ETIOLOGY/EPIDEMIOLOGY: AGS is an autosomal-dominant disorder caused by a defect in *Jagged1*, located on chromosome 20, which encodes a ligand for the Notch signaling pathway. Notch mediates cell fate decisions during embryologic development. The mutation in *Jagged1*, inherited from a parent in approximately 50% of cases, can be identified in about 70% of individuals with AGS. The incidence of AGS is approximately 1 in 70,000 live births, with equal numbers of males and females. This number may be artificially low as a result of misdiagnosis. Outcome and prognosis are highly variable and related to the severity of hepatic or cardiac involvement.

DIAGNOSIS: The common laboratory abnormalities are elevations of serum bile acids, cholesterol, bilirubin, alkaline phosphatase, and GGT. Cholestasis resulting from extrahepatic causes can be differentiated by DISIDA scan. The distinctive histologic feature of AGS, intrahepatic bile duct paucity, may be absent the first 6 months of life. Bile duct paucity is defined as an average of up to 0.5 ducts per triad over 10 triads on liver biopsy. Cardiac findings include pulmonic artery stenosis, ventricular septal defect, atrial septal defect, and tetralogy of Fallot. A failure of the fusion of the anterior arches of the vertebrae, producing a butterfly appearance on radiography, is the most common skeletal abnormality. Many of the ocular abnormalities described in AGS are secondary to chronic vitamin deficiency. The primary defects include posterior embryotoxon (prominent Schwalbe's line), which can be identified in infants, and Axenfeld's anomaly. The typical facial appearance of AGS is a prominent forehead, hypertelorism, a straight nose, and a small, pointy chin, giving the face a triangular appearance.

TREATMENT

Standard Therapies: Treatment is based on trying to increase bile flow, relieve pruritus, optimize growth, and prevent fat-soluble vitamin deficiencies. Effective medications include ursodeoxycholic acid to increase bile flow and rifampin, Atarax, or Benadryl to treat itching. The skin should be kept hydrated with emollients, and fingernails must be trimmed. Fat malabsorption can be a result of liver and/or pancreatic dysfunction. Formulas with medium-chain triglycerides are often given to infants. If growth remains poor, nasogastric feedings or a gastrostomy tube may be necessary. Complications of fat-soluble vitamin deficiencies in children with AGS include vision problems (vitamin A), osteopenia with frequent fractures (vitamin D), ataxia and developmental delays (vitamin E), and coagulopathy (vitamin K). Fat-soluble vitamin levels (A, D, E) and PT/PTT should be checked every few months and supplemented accordingly. Children with AGS should be given the liquid form of vitamin E, d-α-tocopheryl polyethylene glycol 1,000 succinate (TPGS), to reverse or prevent vitamin E deficiency during childhood cholestasis and enhance the absorption of vitamin D. Only a minority of children with AGS requires liver transplantation. Indications for transplantation include progressive synthetic liver dysfunction, intractable pruritus, osteodystrophy, and massive variceal bleeding.

Investigational Therapies: The role of the pancreas in relation to poor growth and fat malabsorption in AGS is just starting to be explored. Pancreatic enzymes may play a role.

REFERENCES

Alagille D, Estrada A, Hadouchel M, et al. Syndromic paucity of interlobular bile ducts (Alagille syndrome or arteriohepatic dysplasia): review of 80 cases. *J Pediatr* 1987;110:195–200.

Emerick K, Rand E, Goldmuntz E, et al. Features of Alagille syndrome in 92 patients: frequency and relation to prognosis. *Hepatology* 1999;29:822–829.

Li L, Krantz ID, Den Y, et al. Alagille syndrome is caused by mutations in human *Jagged1*, which encodes a ligand for Notch1. *Nat Genet* 1997;16:243–251.

Rand L. Alagille Syndrome. In: Altschuler SM, Liacouras CA, eds. *Clinical pediatric gastroenterology*. New York: Churchill Livingston, 1998:309–313.

RESOURCES

14, 98, 354

---

2 Barrett Esophagus

Peter Higgins, MD, PhD, and Frederick K. Askari, MD, PhD

DEFINITION: Barrett esophagus is the presence of intestinal (columnar) epithelium in the lining of the esophagus above the gastroesophageal junction, in place of the normal squamous epithelium. It is a potentially precancerous lesion that can progress to adenocarcinoma.

SYNONYM: Intestinal metaplasia of the esophagus.

SYMPTOMS AND SIGNS: Barrett esophagus should be suspected in any patient with chronic (>8 years) gastroesophageal reflux symptoms. Patients with dysphagia are of particular concern, because this symptom could reflect a peptic stricture or adenocarcinoma of the esophagus. Patients with chronic gastroesophageal reflux disease (GERD) should have one endoscopic examination to rule out Barrett esophagus if comorbid illnesses permit. Endoscopy is essential because there are no clinical signs or symptoms that differentiate Barrett esophagus from GERD.

ETIOLOGY/EPIDEMIOLOGY: Metaplasia is believed to be a reaction to chronic acid exposure because columnar intestinal epithelium is more resistant to acid damage. The environmental/genetic alterations needed to change from squamous to columnar cells make these cells more susceptible to transformation to adenocarcinoma. Risk factors (beyond GERD) for Barrett include older age, male gender, caucasian or Hispanic ancestry, and smoking. In patients with Barrett esophagus, the risk of esophageal adenocarcinoma is increased 30-fold over the general population, to 0.5% per year. Among those referred for esophagogastroduodenoscopy for any reason, it is estimated that 1% will have Barrett esophagus. It develops in 10% of patients with erosive esophagitis and in 40% of those with esophageal strictures caused by acid reflux.

DIAGNOSIS: The diagnosis of Barrett esophagus requires both (a) endoscopic identification of extensions of red, salmon-colored, nonshiny mucosa up into the esophagus from the gastroesophageal junction and (b) histologic identification of biopsies of this mucosa as columnar epithelium, particularly if intestinal goblet cells are found. After diagnosis, the patient should have acid suppression with a proton pump inhibitor, then two sets of surveillance biopsies 3 months apart to rule out esophageal adenocarcinoma and to establish the level of dysplasia.

TREATMENT

Standard Therapies: The initial therapy for Barrett esophagus is aggressive control of acid reflux symptoms, initially with high-dose proton pump inhibitors, to reduce the stimulus for metaplasia and reduce reflux esophagitis. A surveillance program of esophagogastroduodenoscopy with biopsies, based on the level of dysplasia found on the first two sets of biopsies, should be initiated. A standard surveillance program for Barrett esophagus with no dysplasia is to proceed with surveillance biopsies every 2 years. If low-grade dysplasia is found, rebiopsy should be performed at 3 months to confirm, and if present, repeated at 6-month intervals. If the low-grade dysplasia remains stable over 1 year, then surveillance should be continued every year. If high-grade dysplasia is found, definitive therapy for high-grade dysplasia and adenocarcinoma is esophagectomy. One can also choose to postpone esophagectomy and proceed with surveillance biopsies for adenocarcinoma every 3 months, although this treatment is controversial.

Investigational Therapies: Several new endoscopic therapies are being developed, including laser therapy, plasma cautery, and photodynamic therapy.

REFERENCES

Schnell T, et al. High-grade dysplasia still is not an indication for surgery in patients with Barrett's esophagus. *Gastroenterology* 1998;114:G1149.

Spechler SJ. Barrett's esophagus. *Semin Gastrointest Dis* 1996;7:51.

Yamada T, Alpers DH, Laine L. *Textbook of gastroenterology.* Philadelphia: Lippincott Williams & Wilkins, 1999.

RESOURCES

135, 354

3 Biliary Atresia

Jorge A. Bezerra, MD

DEFINITION: Biliary atresia is an inflammatory and fibrosing disease of the hepatobiliary system, leading to the progressive obliteration of the extrahepatic bile ducts. As a consequence, bile flow into the intestine is severely impaired, and the infant develops jaundice, and often cirrhosis of the liver.

DIFFERENTIAL DIAGNOSIS: Neonatal hepatitis; α_1-antitrypsin deficiency; Cystic fibrosis; Septicemia; Galactosemia; Choledocal cyst.

SYMPTOMS AND SIGNS: The hallmark for biliary atresia is the development of jaundice in the first 2 months of life. Stools may be normally pigmented early in the course of the disease, but become progressively hypopigmented (acholic). Affected infants appear otherwise well, without fever or other symptoms; however, two clinical forms of biliary atresia can be diagnosed. In the first, jaundice develops earlier, usually in the first month of life; the infant may have a history of poor growth, and additional investigation reveals other associated malformations, such as cardiovascular defects, polysplenia, and situs inversus. This clinical form is termed "congenital" and occurs in 10%–35% of cases. The second form of biliary atresia, which has been arbitrarily named "acquired," is more common (65%–90% of cases) and develops in full-term infants of normal weight, growth, and development. Splenomegaly is a consistent finding in both forms of biliary atresia. In children diagnosed at later ages, malnutrition, diarrhea, and coagulopathy may be present. The existence of these signs reflects advanced liver disease.

ETIOLOGY/EPIDEMIOLOGY: Biliary atresia has an estimated incidence of 1 in 10,000 live births, is the single most common cause of pathologic neonatal jaundice, and accounts for 50%–60% of indications for liver transplantation in children worldwide. The etiology of biliary atresia is multifactorial. Pathogenesis results from the interaction among the following factors: (a) viral infection, (b) immunologic dysregulation, (c) defective embryogenesis of the biliary tract, (d) defect in fetal/prenatal circulation, and (e) environmental toxin exposure.

DIAGNOSIS: Biliary atresia should be considered in any infant with jaundice, hypopigmented stools, firm liver, and splenomegaly. Biochemical markers of liver injury show variable increases in serum aminotransferase, γ-glutamyl-transpeptidase, and alkaline phosphatase levels; the serum level of conjugated bilirubin is elevated. These markers may be helpful but are not diagnostic. Although endoscopic and imaging approaches have been used to assess patency of extrahepatic bile ducts, percutaneous liver biopsy has a high rate of diagnostic accuracy (~95%).

TREATMENT: The only therapeutic choice to relieve jaundice in affected infants is the Kasai portoenterostomy, a surgical procedure that establishes bile drainage by anastomosis of an intestinal conduit to the transected surface at the liver hilum in Roux-en-Y fashion. After portoenterostomy, attention is directed toward optimizing nutrition (25%–50% above usual caloric needs) and replacing fat-soluble vitamins. If portal hypertension develops, older infants are at risk for gastrointestinal hemorrhage. The success of Kasai portoenterostomy decreases with increasing patient age, with a success rate below 20% when surgery is performed after 3 months of age. Following successful biliary drainage, 60%–80% of affected children will require liver transplantation during their lifetime.

REFERENCES

Balistreri WF, Grand R, Hoofnagle JH, et al. Biliary atresia: current concepts and research directions. Summary of a symposium. *Hepatology* 1996;23:1682–1692.

Bates MD, Bucuvalas JC, Alonso MH, et al. Biliary atresia: pathogenesis and treatment. *Semin Liver Dis* 1998;18:281–293.

Ohi R. Biliary atresia: a surgical perspective. *Clin Liver Dis* 2000; 4:779–804.

Ryckman F, Fisher R, Pedersen S, et al. Improved survival in biliary atresia patients in the present era of liver transplantation. *J Pediatr Surg* 1993;28:382–385; discussion 386.

RESOURCES

39, 99, 365

4   Byler Disease

Inge-Merete Nielsen, MD,
and Hans R.L. Eiberg, MD

DEFINITION: Byler disease is a hereditary liver disease that causes jaundice, failure to thrive, dwarfism, severe pruritus, and early death.

SYNONYM: Progressive familial intrahepatic cholestasis.

DIFFERENTIAL DIAGNOSIS: Biliary atresia; Hepatitis.

SYMPTOMS AND SIGNS: Most infants with this disease show the first symptoms during the first or second months of life. They fail to thrive and become jaundiced. They have foul-smelling, greasy stools and bleeding episodes (e.g., nose bleeding) because of malabsorption of fat and the fat-soluble vitamin K. Later, the jaundice becomes more severe, especially during febrile illnesses. Affected children develop rickets because of malabsorption of vitamin D, and height for age is reduced (they become dwarfs). Severe pruritus is bothersome. The liver is enlarged, the abdomen is protuberant, and the extremities are thin. As the disease progresses, cirrhosis develops and ascites can be recognized. Most affected children die before age 10.

ETIOLOGY/EPIDEMIOLOGY: Byler disease/progressive familial intrahepatic cholestasis is inherited in an autosomal-recessive manner. The disease is due to a mutation in a gene (*FIC1*) located on chromosome 18q21. Several affected children have been described in two large kindreds (the Amish people and the Greenland Inuit people). It has also been described in several other ethnic groups, but only in sporadic cases or in a few siblings. The signs and symptoms differ a little in the described cases, which is believed to be due to different mutations in the gene.

DIAGNOSIS: The diagnosis should be suspected in infants who fail to gain weight and have pale, greasy, foul-smelling stools, conjugated hyperbilirubinemia, and an enlarged liver. The transaminases and alkaline phosphatases are elevated, the prothrombine clotting time is prolonged, and calcium is low. Ultrasonography shows an enlarged liver with patent hepatic and common bile ducts. Radionuclide hepatobiliary scintigraphy shows delayed excretion. Liver biopsy can show pseudoglandular transformation of hepatocytes, bile accumulation, and early in the disease course, discrete fibrosis, and later in the disease course, severe fibrosis.

TREATMENT

Standard Therapies: Only symptomatic treatment is possible. Because of the malabsorption of fat and fat-soluble vitamins, affected children should be given formula containing medium-chain triglycerides and extra vitamins A, D, E, and K. The amount of vitamins (oral or intramuscular) depends on the weight of the child and the severity of the symptoms. The serum levels of the vitamins should be monitored regularly to ensure adequate dosages. Calcium, phosphate, and zinc supplements may also be necessary. Cholestyramine, rifampin, ursodeoxycholic acid, or phenobarbital can be tried to relieve the severe pruritus in children with chronic cholestasis. Some children have had undergone transplantation with good results.

REFERENCES

Clayton RJ, Iber F, Ruebner BH, et al. Byler's disease: fatal familial intrahepatic cholestasis in an Amish kindred. *J Pediatr* 1965; 67:1025–1028.

Eiberg H, Nielsen I-M. Linkage of cholestasis familiaris groenlandica/Byler-like disease to chromosome 18. *Int J Circumpolar Health* 2000;59:57–62.

Klomp LW, Bull LN, Knisely AS, et al. A missense mutation in *FIC1* is associated with Greenland familial cholestasis. *Hepatology* 2000;32:1337–1341.

Nielsen I-M, Ornvold K, Jacobsen BB, et al. Fatal familial cholestatic syndrome in Greenland Eskimo children. *Acta Paediatr Scand* 1986;75:1010–1016.

RESOURCES

39, 98, 365

5   Caroli Disease

Vijay Poreddy, MD,
and Neil Kaplowitz, MD

DEFINITION: Caroli disease is characterized by congenital cystic dilatation of the intrahepatic biliary tree. Two distinct types exist: simple or with periportal fibrosis (congenital hepatic fibrosis), also called Caroli syndrome. The simple type (pure form) is rare and is characterized by segmental and saccular dilatation predisposing to bile stagnation, sludge and stone formation, cholangitis, and fatal sepsis. It is associated with medullary sponge kidney in 60%–80% and polycystic kidneys in up to 25% of cases. Caroli syndrome is more common and is associated with diffuse intrahepatic biliary dilatation, portal hypertension, and, eventually, liver failure. It is associated with polycystic kidneys in 40%–50% of cases but is not associated with medullary sponge kidney. Extrahepatic biliary cysts are seen in up to 50% of cases.

SYNONYM: Type V choledochal cyst.

DIFFERENTIAL DIAGNOSIS: Choledochal cyst; Polycystic liver; Hydatid cyst.

SYMPTOMS AND SIGNS: Clinical onset usually occurs during childhood. Infrequently, patients may be asymptomatic for the first 5–20 years and present with recurrent episodes of fever, chills, and abdominal pain as adults. The presence of jaundice is variable. The simple type is characterized frequently by stone formation, cholangitis, and hepatic abscess. Biliary infection and stones account for the usual presenting symptoms of fever and abdominal pain. Liver involvement may be limited to a single lobe or segment. Death is often due to septicemia. Other complications include secondary biliary cirrhosis, subphrenic abscess, and pericarditis. Patients with Caroli syndrome present in childhood with abnormalities related to hepatic fibrosis and portal hypertension, such as splenomegaly, hepatomegaly, esophageal varices, and gastrointestinal hemorrhage. Death is often related to complications of portal hypertension and liver failure. Cholangitis and biliary stone formation usually are absent. The most serious complication is cholangiocarcinoma, which has been postulated to occur due to prolonged exposure of ductal epithelia to high concentrations of unconjugated secondary bile acids. It develops in approximately 7% of cases, adenocarcinoma being the most common histologic type (70%–85%), and is seen with either type of Caroli disease.

ETIOLOGY/EPIDEMIOLOGY: The disease is inherited in an autosomal-recessive pattern, occurring with equal frequency in males and females. It is usually associated with autosomal-recessive polycystic kidney disease. Proposed mechanisms for bile duct malformation include neonatal occlusion of the hepatic artery, leading to bile duct ischemia and cystic dilatation; abnormal growth rate of the developing biliary epithelium and supporting connective tissue; and lack of normal involution of ductal plates that surround the portal tracts, resulting in epithelium-lined cysts that surround the portal triads.

DIAGNOSIS: A high index of suspicion is required. Liver biochemistry may be normal or show mild to moderate elevation of serum bilirubin, alkaline phosphatase, and aminotransferase levels. Liver synthetic function is well preserved. Liver biopsy in cases of congenital hepatic fibrosis reveals intrahepatic bile duct ectasia and proliferation with periportal fibrosis of varying degrees. Associated elevations in blood urea nitrogen and serum creatinine reflect underlying kidney disease. Ultrasonography, which is the best screening tool, and CT are of great value in demonstrating the cystic dilatation of intrahepatic bile ducts. Percutaneous or endoscopic cholangiography usually demonstrates a normal common bile duct with segmental, saccular dilatation of intrahepatic bile ducts.

TREATMENT: Management depends on the degree of involvement. Lobectomy usually is curative for segmental cystic disease confined to one lobe. For diffuse disease, Roux-en-Y hepaticojejunostomy with placement of transhepatic stents may be effective. Ursodeoxycholic acid therapy has been claimed to successfully dissolve intrahepatic stones. Chronic antibiotic therapy in multilobar disease may have some benefit. Liver transplantation is an option in patients with extensive disease, frequent complications, and poor quality of life. In patients with associated end-stage renal disease, both liver and kidney transplantation should be considered.

REFERENCES

Caroli J. Diseases of the intrahepatic biliary tree. *Clin Gastroenterol* 1973;2;147–161.

D'Agata I, Jonas M, et al. Combined cystic disease of the liver and the kidney. *Semin Liver Dis* 1994;14;215–228.

Lu S. Diseases of the biliary tree. In: Yamada T, ed. *Textbook of gastroenterology,* 3rd ed. Philadelphia: Lippincott Williams & Wilkins, 1999:2281–2325.

Ribeiro A, et al. Caroli syndrome in twin sisters. *Am J Gast-roenterol* 1996;91;1024–1026.

RESOURCES

39, 354

6   Crigler-Najjar Syndrome

Frederick K. Askari, MD, PhD

DEFINITION: Crigler-Najjar syndrome is characterized by the onset shortly after birth of severe chronic unconjugated hyperbilirubinemia in the absence of hemolysis.

SYNONYMS: Familial jaundice; Nonhemolytic unconjugated hyperbilirubinemia.

DIFFERENTIAL DIAGNOSIS: Gilbert syndrome; Dubin-Johnson syndrome; Chronic hemolysis.

SYMPTOMS AND SIGNS: The syndrome manifests at birth with a history and physical examination consistent with the diagnosis of chronic unconjugated hyperbilirubinemia. Symptoms include jaundice, icterus, and pale, clay-colored stools that persist after the first 3 weeks of life. Clinically, patients who cannot glucuronidate bilirubin are jaundiced and have unconjugated hyperbilirubinemia on laboratory examination of the serum. Syndrome type I is more severe and characterized by an inability to glucuronidate bilirubin, whereas type II is characterized by a partial defect in bilirubin conjugation. Patients with type I have no ability to conjugate bilirubin; therefore, a profound unconjugated hyperbilirubinemia leading to kernicterus and death often occurs in infancy or childhood. Chronic, unconjugated hyperbilirubinemia manifested as jaundice can lead to neurologic damage including ataxia, dystonia, or decreased mentation (bilirubin encephalopathy), which can lead to death from kernicterus if untreated.

ETIOLOGY/EPIDEMIOLOGY: Crigler-Najjar syndrome is an autosomal-recessive disorder caused by defects in the *UGT1* gene that is located on the telomeric end of chromosome 2. The frequency is estimated at approximately 1 in 750,000 live births, with equal numbers of males and females affected. The syndrome may be underrepresented due to misdiagnosis or underreporting. Outcome and prognosis are related to the severity of hyperbilirubinemia.

DIAGNOSIS: The diagnosis is made when a patient presents with persistent nonhemolytic unconjugated hyper-bilirubinemia shortly after birth. The common laboratory abnormalities are elevations of serum total bilirubin with predominance of the unconjugated fraction. No distinctive histologic feature is seen on liver biopsy. Neurologic findings may be present at the time of diagnosis.

TREATMENT

Standard Therapies: Treatment is based on trying to decrease bilirubin levels. The mainstay is aggressive phototherapy. The skin should be hydrated with emollients. Effective medications include phenobarbital for type II patients, oral calcium gluconate to bind intraluminal bilirubin, and intravenous hydration and albumin to decrease bilirubin levels during an acute crisis. Some patients have been managed with plasmapheresis. Indications to consider liver transplantation include severe refractory hyperbilirubinemia or the progression of neurologic damage.

Investigational Therapies: Experimental medical therapies include tin mesoporphyrin for the treatment of acute exacerbation. Other experimental therapies include hepatocyte transplantation, gene replacement therapy, and gene correction therapy.

REFERENCES

Arias IM, Gartner LM, Cohen M, et al. Chronic nonhemolytic unconjugated hyperbilirubinemia with glucuronosyltransferase deficiency. *Am J Med* 1969;47:395–409.

Askari FK, Hitomi E, Thiney M, et al. Retroviral mediated expression of HUG Br 1 in Crigler-Najjar syndrome type I human fibroblasts and correction of the genetic defect in Gunn rat hepatocytes. *Gene Ther* 1995;2:203–208.

Crigler JF, Najjar VA. Congenital familial nonhemolytic jaundice with kernicterus. *Pediatrics* 1952;10:169–170.

Ritter JK, Crawford JM, Owens IS. Cloning of two human liver bilirubin UDP-glucuronosyltransferase cDNAs with expression in COS-1 cells. *J Biol Chem* 1991;266:1043–1047.

Van der Veere CN, Sinaasappel M, et al. Current therapy for Crigler-Najjar syndrome type 1: report of a world registry. *Hepatology* 1996;24:311–315.

RESOURCES

39, 99, 354

7   Cronkhite-Canada Syndrome

Georg Oberhuber, MD

DEFINITION: Cronkhite-Canada syndrome is a non-hereditary adult gastrointestinal polyposis syndrome associated with skin hyperpigmentation, patchy vitiligo, alopecia, onychodystrophy, marked edema, tetany, glossitis, and cataracts.

SYNONYM: Canada-Cronkhite syndrome.

DIFFERENTIAL DIAGNOSIS: Juvenile polyps in the stomach, large bowel, and small bowel; Hyperplastic polyps in the stomach; Other diseases causing watery diarrhea and protein loss; Some presentations of celiac disease or infectious diseases; Presumed malignancy due to weight loss.

SYMPTOMS AND SIGNS: Patients with Cronkhite-Canada syndrome commonly present with diarrhea or protein-losing enteropathy, weight loss, abdominal pain, anorexia, weakness, hematochezia, vomiting, paresthesias, and xerostomia. The mortality rate is approximately 60%, with patients dying within months or years of the onset of symptoms. The prognosis is determined by the gastrointestinal loss of electrolytes and protein, and by the development of cachexia. Local complications include bleeding and prolapse of polyps. The polyps may show spontaneous regression. Approximately 15% of patients develop gastrointestinal carcinomas, frequently colorectal carcinomas.

ETIOLOGY/EPIDEMIOLOGY: The etiology is unknown. Infectious and immunologic causes have been hypothesized. Ultrastructural studies suggest that damage to the crypt epithelium results in leakage of fluid into the interstitium. Fewer than 200 cases have been published, most from Japan. The age of patients ranges from 30 to 90 years, although 80% are older than 50 years at the time of presentation. The disease has a slight male predominance. It does not appear to be inherited.

DIAGNOSIS: Physical findings include weight loss, hair loss, and dystrophy of the nails of both fingers and toes, including splitting, thinning, and partial separation from the nail bed. Laboratory investigations show hypoproteinemia, particularly hypoalbuminemia, hypocalcemia, hypomag-nesemia, anemia, occult blood in stool, and electrolyte deficiencies. Endoscopy of the upper and lower gastrointestinal tract shows multiple polyps in the stomach, jejunum, ileum, colon, and rectum. Sometimes polyps may occupy the entire mucosal surface of these sites. The polyp density is greatest in the stomach and colon, followed by the duodenum, ileum, and jejunum. The gross appearance of the polyps varies from diffuse mucosal micronodularity or granularity to gelatinous-appearing pedunculated polyps. Histologic examination shows polyps with a broad sessile base, expanded edematous lamina propria, and cystic glands with a normal-appearing epithelium lacking areas of dysplasia (i.e., intraepithelial neoplasia).

TREATMENT

Standard Therapies: Treatment includes substitution of electrolytes, protein, and vitamins. In some patients, parenteral nutrition is necessary. Corticosteroids may induce remission in some patients. Antibiotics (tetracycline) and ranitidine have been applied successfully. Surgery is necessary for complications induced by polyps or after the development of carcinoma.

Investigational Therapies: Various antibiotic regimens are being investigated.

REFERENCES

Burke AP, Sobin LH. The pathology of Cronkhite-Canada polyps. A comparison to juvenile polyposis. *Am J Surg Pathol* 1989; 13:940–946.

Cronkhite L, Canada W. Generalized gastrointestinal polyposis: an unusual syndrome of polyposis, pigmentation, alopecia, onychotrophia. *N Engl J Med* 1955;252:1011–1015.

Goto A. Cronkhite-Canada syndrome: epidemiological study of 110 cases reported in Japan. *Nippon Geka Hokan* 1995;64: 3–14.

Jenkins D, Stephenson PM, Scott BB. The Cronkhite-Canada syndrome: an ultrastructural study of pathogenesis. *J Clin Pathol* 1985;38:271–276.

Rappaport LB, Sperling HV, Stavrides A. Colon cancer in the Cronkhite-Canada syndrome. *J Clin Gastroenterol* 1986;8: 199–202.

RESOURCES

158, 364, 478

8 Small Bowel Diverticulosis

Madhusudhan R. Sanaka, MD,
and Edy E. Soffer, MD

DEFINITION: Small bowel diverticulosis is a disease of adults, usually associated with chronic abdominal pain, recurrent pseudoobstruction, bacterial overgrowth, and malabsorption.

DIFFERENTIAL DIAGNOSIS: Familial visceral myopathy; Familial visceral neuropathy; Inflammatory bowel disease; Scleroderma.

SYMPTOMS AND SIGNS: Small bowel diverticula (other than duodenal and Meckel diverticula) are most common in the proximal jejunum, but may extend into the ileum. They are false diverticula, usually multiple, and varying in size from a few millimeters to 10 cm. They may be asymptomatic or, more commonly, associated with symptoms consistent with intestinal dysmotility, such as chronic abdominal pain, early satiety and bloating, recurrent episodes of intestinal pseudoobstruction, or bacterial overgrowth. Malabsorption results from dysmotility, stasis, and bacterial overgrowth, which can also aggravate motor dysfunction. Rarely, small bowel diverticula can be associated with perforation, diverticulitis, hemorrhage, or obstruction.

ETIOLOGY/EPIDEMIOLOGY: Small bowel diverticulosis is an acquired condition of older adults. It is relatively uncommon, affecting both sexes with a prevalence of 0.3%–2.5%. Pathologic changes in the bowel include fibrosis of the smooth muscle or degeneration of the neurons and axons of the myenteric plexus. Small bowel diverticulosis is associated with abnormal small bowel manometric changes. It has been found in patients with established causes of intestinal dysmotility such as scleroderma and familial visceral myopathy or neuropathy. It is likely the result of those conditions, because small bowel diverticulosis can recur in uninvolved bowel after resection of the affected segment, with recurrence of symptoms.

DIAGNOSIS: Diagnosis is usually made by barium studies (Insert Fig. 42), which can show the presence of diverticulosis as well as changes suggestive of the underlying etiology, such as scleroderma. In cases of diverticulitis or bleeding, the diagnosis is often not suspected preoperatively; an indurated mass in the mesentery may be the only finding. Manometric studies of the small bowel can help determine the presence of dysmotility.

TREATMENT
Standard Therapies: Treatment for most patients is conservative: prokinetic agents, such as metoclopramide, and cyclic antibiotics. For bacterial overgrowth, broad-spectrum antibiotics such as ciprofloxacin or tetracycline alternatively in cycles of 1–2 weeks per month are useful. In patients with severe and persistent symptoms or complications such as ileus, bleeding, perforation, or volvulus, resection of the affected bowel is indicated. Diverticula may recur in the uninvolved segments after surgery.

REFERENCES
Akhrass R, Yaffe MB, Fischer C, et al. Small-bowel diverticulosis: perceptions and reality. *J Am Coll Surg* 1997;184:383–388.
de Lang DW, Cluysenaer OJ, Verberne GH, et al. Diverticulosis of the small bowel. *Ned Tijdschr Geneeskd* 2000;144:946–949.
Feldman M, Sleisenger MH, Scharschmidt BF, eds. *Sleisenger & Fordtran's gastrointestinal and liver disease,* 6th ed. Philadelphia: WB Saunders, 1998:315.
Kongara K, Soffer E. Intestinal motility in small bowel diverticulosis: a case report and review of literature. *J Clin Gastroenterol* 2000;30:84–86.

RESOURCES
135, 215, 354

9 Dubin-Johnson Syndrome

Michal Carmiel, MD,
and Paul D. Berk, MD

DEFINITION: Dubin-Johnson syndrome (DJS) is a benign liver disorder characterized by mild, predominantly conjugated hyperbilirubinemia that is due to impaired hepatobiliary transport of nonbile salt organic anions.

DIFFERENTIAL DIAGNOSIS: Rotor syndrome; Benign recurrent intrahepatic cholestasis; Cholestasis of pregnancy; Drug-induced cholestasis; Biliary tract obstruction.

SYMPTOMS AND SIGNS: Patients with DJS are usually asymptomatic, although upper abdominal discomfort may be reported. Hyperbilirubinemia and jaundice are typically noticed during intercurrent illness, pregnancy, or use of drugs that decrease hepatic excretion of organic anions (e.g., oral contraceptives). The syndrome usually is not observed before puberty, although cases have been described in neonates and infants. Pruritus is absent, and aside from jaundice, the physical examination is normal.

ETIOLOGY/EPIDEMIOLOGY: The syndrome has been described in all races and ethnic backgrounds and in both sexes. There is a particularly high prevalence (1:1,300) among Iranian Jews. Conjugated hyperbilirubinemia in DJS is due to impaired secretion of anionic bilirubin conjugates from hepatocytes into bile. The molecular basis of this disorder is absence of a functional multidrug resistance protein 2 (MRP2) from the apical membrane of the hepatocyte. Several mutations in the *MRP2* gene have been identified. The syndrome is inherited in an autosomal-recessive manner.

DIAGNOSIS: The diagnosis is based on phenotypic expression and biochemical data. Total serum bilirubin is typically 2–5 mg/dL (34–85μ*M*), of which more than 50% is conjugated. Over time, bilirubin levels can fluctuate widely between normal and values as high as 20–25 mg/dL (340–425 μ*M*). Iranian Jews with DJS frequently have prolonged prothrombin times. Hepatobiliary scintigraphy (HIDA scanning) may show rapid, intense, homogeneous accumulation of isotope within the liver and kidneys without visualization of the biliary tree. Late visualization of the gallbladder on HIDA scanning and nonvisualization during oral cholecystography are also typical of DJS. Abdominal CT in DJS may show increased liver density. Two tests in particular may yield data strongly suggestive of DJS. After intravenous administration of sulfobromophthalein (BSP), the dye initially disappears from serum at a normal rate, but then displays a characteristic increase in the serum BSP concentration at approximately 90 minutes after injection. Patients with DJS also have a diagnostic abnormality in urinary coproporphyrin excretion. Examination of hepatic tissue is also helpful in diagnosing DJS. Gross examination shows a liver that is intensely pigmented. On microscopic examination, lobular architecture is preserved, but there is a characteristic, intense accumulation of coarsely granular pigment, especially in the centrilobular zones.

TREATMENT

Standard Therapies: No specific treatment is indicated. The syndrome is generally considered to be a benign disorder requiring only reassurance of the patient and avoidance of invasive diagnostic procedures. Phenobarbital has been used in attempts to reduce the serum bilirubin, but the results have been highly variable.

REFERENCES

Berk PD, Noyer C. The familial conjugated hyperbilirubinemias. *Semin Liver Dis* 1994;14:386–394.

Berk PD, Wolkoff AW. Bilirubin metabolism and the hyperbilirubinemias. In: Braunwald EB, Fauci AS, eds. *Harrison's principles of internal medicine*, 15th ed. New York: McGraw-Hill, 2001:1715–1720.

Keitel V, Karterbeck J, Nies AT, et al. Impaired protein mutation of the conjugate export pump multidrug resistance protein 2 as a consequence of a deletion mutation in Dubin-Johnson syndrome. *Hepatology* 2000;32:1317–1328.

Paulusma CC, Kool M, Bosma PJ, et al. A mutation in the human canalicular multispecific organic anion transporter gene causes the Dubin-Johnson syndrome. *Hepatology* 1997;25:1539–1542.

Rubinstein ZJ, Seligsohn U, Modan M, et al. Hepatic computerized tomography in the Dubin-Johnson syndrome: increased liver density as a diagnostic aid. *Comput Rad* 1985;9:315–318.

RESOURCES

39, 299, 354

10 Giant Hypertrophic Gastritis

Juanita L. Merchant, MD, PhD

DEFINITION: Giant hypertrophic gastritis (GHG) is a general term for a collection of disorders resulting in large gastric folds due to infiltration of the gastric mucosa by inflammatory cells. Large folds may be caused by expansion of the epithelial cell compartment, expansion or infiltration of the lamina propria, e.g., by inflammatory cells, or diffuse disorders affecting both the mucosa and submucosa, e.g., granulomatous disorders and infiltrating malignancies.

SYNONYMS: Lymphocytic gastritis; Hypertrophic lymphocytic gastritis; Varioliform gastritis.

DIFFERENTIAL DIAGNOSIS: Celiac disease; Ménétrier disease; Hyperplastic gastropathy; Zollinger-Ellison syndrome; Protein-losing gastropathy; Foveolar hyperplasia; Lymphoma; Carcinoid; Carcinoma; Bacterial, viral, or fungal infections; Granulomatous disorders.

SYMPTOMS AND SIGNS: Patients with GHG present with epigastric pain, diarrhea, nausea, and vomiting. Weight loss and anorexia may occur. Endoscopic evaluation may show giant gastric folds with aphthous erosions. Gastrointestinal bleeding may also accompany the presentation. Hypoalbuminemia is a variable finding and is not a distinguishing feature because it is variably associated (20%–100%) with Ménétrier disease. Patients with hypoalbuminemia will also develop edema. The clinical and endoscopic manifestations of GHG are similar to Ménétrier disease; however, the distinguishing feature of GHG lies in the histopathology, which may show expansion of surface mucous or foveolar epithelial cells, but more characteristically will show massive lymphocytic infiltration of the lamina propria as well as intraepithelial lymphocytes.

ETIOLOGY/EPIDEMIOLOGY: The cause of GHG is unknown but may represent an exaggerated immune response to a dietary or microbial antigen or gastric irritant.

GHG and Ménétrier disease may be variants of the same disease. The male/female distribution is approximately equal. Little evidence has conclusively linked *Helicobacter pylori* infection to GHG; however, *H. pylori* is often associated with giant gastric folds. In cases where *H. pylori* can be documented, resolution of the clinical, endoscopic, and histologic abnormalities usually occurs using therapies directed toward eradication of the organism.

DIAGNOSIS: The diagnosis should be considered whenever an endoscopic finding of enlarged gastric folds is documented; however, the diagnosis is made by histopathologic examination.

TREATMENT
Standard Therapies: There are no standard therapies. If *H. pylori* colonization is documented, antibacterial therapy including colloidal bismuth subcitrate and a proton pump inhibitor should be instituted and symptoms followed. A repeat endoscopy with biopsies to obtain histopathologic documentation of resolution should be performed.

REFERENCES
Burdick SJ, Chung E, Tanner G, et al. Treatment of Ménétrier's disease with a monoclonal antibody against the epidermal growth factor receptor. *N Engl J Med* 2000;63:1697–1701.
Hayat M, Arora DS, Dixon MF, et al. Effects of *Helicobacter pylori* eradication on the natural history of lymphocytic gastritis. *Gut* 1999;45:495–498.
Hoat J, Hamichi L, Wallez L, et al. Lymphocytic gastritis: a newly described entity: a retrospective endoscopic and histological study. *Gut* 1988;29:1258–1264.
Müller H, Volkholz H, Stolte M. Healing of lymphocytic gastritis by eradication of *Helicobacter pylori*. *Digestion* 2001;63:14–19.
Wolfsen HC, Carpenter HA, Talley NJ. Ménétrier disease: a form of hypertrophic gastropathy or gastritis? *Gastroenterology* 1993;104:1310–1319.

RESOURCE
354

11 Eosinophilic Gastroenteritis

Adriaan C.I.T.L. Tan, MD, PhD

DEFINITION: Eosinophilic gastroenteritis is characterized by the triad of eosinophilic infiltration of segments of the gastrointestinal tract, peripheral eosinophilia, and abnormalities of gastrointestinal function (varying from dyspepsia and obstruction to diarrhea and ascites).

SYNONYMS: Allergic enteropathy; Allergic eosinophilic gastroenteropathy.

DIFFERENTIAL DIAGNOSIS: Parasitic diseases (e.g., roundworm infection, schistosomiasis); Vasculitis (polyarteritis nodosa, Churg-Strauss syndrome); Neoplastic diseases (small bowel lymphoma); Allergic disorders; Hypereosinophilic syndrome; Systemic mastocytosis; Inflammatory bowel disease; Eosinophilic granuloma.

SYMPTOMS AND SIGNS: Eosinophilic gastroenteritis may affect any part of the gastrointestinal tract from esophagus to rectum. Symptoms include abdominal pain, nausea, vomiting, diarrhea, and weight loss. The eosinophilic infiltration may involve one or more layers of the gastrointestinal wall. The clinical features depend on the layer and the location involved. Most commonly, the stomach wall and the small bowel are involved. Mucosal involvement leads to protein-losing enteropathy and malabsorption. Muscle layer involvement causes abdominal pain, vomiting, dyspeptic symptoms, and bowel obstruction. Subserosal involvement predominantly causes ascites with marked eosinophilia. Sometimes eosinophilic pleural effusion is present. Often, a family history of allergy is found.

ETIOLOGY/EPIDEMIOLOGY: The disease may occur at any age. It occurs in both sexes with a slight preponderance for the male. Approximately 250 cases have been described. Detailed prevalence is not known. The exact cause of the disease is uncertain. One hypothesis is that a type 1 hypersensitivity reaction to certain products results in mast cell degranulation. The products released (eosinophilic cationic protein, major basic protein, eosinophilic peroxidase), together with activation of tumor necrosis factor-α, lead to tissue inflammation.

DIAGNOSIS: In 80% of cases, peripheral blood eosinophilia is found. Malabsorption causes increased fat excretion, hypoalbuminemia, iron-deficiency anemia, and an abnormal D-xylose test result. Sometimes, a modestly elevated erythrocyte sedimentation rate and IgE (especially in children) are found. Barium studies can show irregular luminal narrowing (especially in the distal antrum and small bowel) mimicking malignancies. Endoscopic findings may show prominent mucosal folds, hyperemia, nodularity, erosions, or ulceration, or no abnormalities. Multiple endoscopic biopsy samples must be taken from both normal- and abnormal-appearing mucosa. Endoscopic biopsies can be nondiagnostic because of the patchy nature of the disease. A surgical full-thickness biopsy sample is sometimes necessary. In the biopsy specimen, at least 20 eosinophils per high-power field on microscopic examination are found.

TREATMENT

Standard Therapies: Corticosteroids (e.g., prednisone) may produce a rapid amelioration of symptoms. Although an allergic cause of the disease is controversial, therapy with sodium cromoglycate or ketotifen has been attempted with reasonable effect. In one case, montelukast (a leukotriene antagonist) had a beneficial effect. Elimination diets are often unsuccessful. Prognosis is favorable, but patients often have a chronic course with relapses and exacerbations. Maintenance therapy with prednisone or budesonide may be necessary.

REFERENCES

Kelly KJ. Eosinophilic gastroenteritis. *J Pediatr Gastroenterol Nutr* 2000;30(suppl):28–35.

Klein NC, Hargrove RL, Sleisenger MH, et al. Eosinophilic gastroenteritis. *Medicine* 1970;49:299–319.

Kravis LP, South MA, Rosenlund ML. Eosinophilic gastroenteritis in the pediatric patient. *Clin Pediatr* 1982;21:713–717.

Talley NJ, Shorter RG, Phillips SF, et al. Eosinophilic gastroenteritis: a clinicopathological study of patients with disease of the mucosa, muscle layer, and subserosal tissues. *Gut* 1990;31:54–58.

Tan ACITL, Kruimel JW, Naber THJ. Eosinophilic gastroenteritis treated with non-enteric-coated budesonide tablets. *Eur J Gastroenterol Hepatol* 2001;13:425–427.

RESOURCES

135, 354

12   Glucose-Galactose Malabsorption

Robert Prizont, MD

DEFINITION: Glucose-galactose malabsorption (GGM) is an autosomal-recessive disorder. The small intestinal brush border has an active cotransport system that facilitates sodium, glucose, galactose, and water absorption from the intestinal lumen into the cell and circulation. In GGM, mutational defects of the small intestinal cotransporter (*SGLT1*) occur. Brush border absorptive abnormalities result in osmotic, fermentative diarrhea.

SYNONYM: Familial glucose-galactose malabsorption and hereditary renal glycosuria.

DIFFERENTIAL DIAGNOSIS: Enteropathogenic, toxigenic, or rotavirus diarrheas; Enteropathy due to cow milk allergy; Primary lactase deficiency (rare); Congenital sodium and chloride diarrhea; Primary bile acid malabsorption.

SYMPTOMS AND SIGNS: Symptoms begin a few days after birth, when the newborn is exposed to lactose from milk. Profuse diarrhea, dehydration, hypernatremia, hyperchloremia, and metabolic acidosis ensue. Stools are loose or watery, with an acidic odor, and are positive for monosaccharides on dipstick test. Associated genetic abnormalities of a renal cotransport gene in the kidney (*SGLT2*) may lead to intermittent glycosuria. Additionally, renal stones have been reported in some patients. Deaths from dehydration or other complications have occurred. Discontinuation of oral feeding temporarily interrupts the diarrhea. Reinstatement of oral feeding based on regular protein-containing formulas may perpetuate the osmotic diarrhea, because most of these formulas contain varying amounts of glucose. In other cases, patients may grow up with manifestations of a chronic but intermittent diarrhea exacerbated by sugar-rich meals.

ETIOLOGY/EPIDEMIOLOGY: More than 40 cases have been reported. It is estimated there are 200 cases worldwide. Two thirds of patients are females. Parental consanguinity is common. The human gene *SGLT1* has been mapped to the long arm of chromosome 22 (22q1.3). Approximately 30% of patients are heterozygotes. Notably, mutations were also identified in some family members. Mutated *SGLT1* DNA sequence leads to amino acid substitutions and dysfunction of the transporter protein.

DIAGNOSIS: Oral tolerance load tests with glucose or galactose show an abnormal blood glucose curve with lack of a rise above the fasting blood glucose concentration, whereas an oral fructose tolerance load test shows a normal rise in blood glucose. Tissue obtained by small bowel biopsy exhibits normal small intestinal and villi architecture with normal lactase activity. A hydrogen breath test performed concomitantly with oral tolerance tests may aid in making the diagnosis.

TREATMENT
Standard Therapies: Discontinuation of breast- or bottle-feeding with replacement by liquid formulas containing sugar-free protein, lipids, and fructose improves the diarrhea and restores nutrition. Genetic counseling and testing of consanguineous couples may play an important role.

REFERENCES
Crane RK. The gradient hypothesis and other models of carrier mediated active transport. *Rev Physiol Biochem Pharmacol* 1977;78:101–159.

Hughes WS, Senior JR. The glucose-galactose malabsorption syndrome in a 23-year-old woman. *Gastroenterology* 1975;68: 142–145.

Lindquist B, Meeuwisse. Chronic diarrhea caused by monosaccharide malabsorption. *Acta Paediatr* 1962;51:674–685.

Schneider AJ, Kinter WB, Stirling CE. Glucose-galactose malabsorption. *N Engl J Med* 1966;274:305–312.

Wright EM, Martin MG, Turk E. Familial glucose-galactose malabsorption and hereditary renal glycosuria. In: Scriver CR, Braudet AL, Sly WS, et al., eds. *The metabolic and molecular bases of inherited disease*, 8th ed. New York: McGraw-Hill, 2001:4891–4908.

RESOURCES
135, 167, 354

13   Hepatorenal Syndrome

Jorge A. Marrero, MD

DEFINITION: Hepatorenal Syndrome (HRS) occurs in patients with chronic liver disease and advanced hepatic failure, and is characterized by impaired renal function and abnormalities in the arterial circulation and activity of the endogenous vasoactive systems. Renal vasoconstriction results in a low glomerular filtration rate (GFR). In the extrarenal circulation, a predominant arteriolar vasodilation yields arterial hypotension. HRS is classified clinically into two types. Type I displays a rapidly progressive reduction of renal function, defined as a doubling of initial serum creatinine to greater than 2.5 mg/dL or a 50% reduction of the initial 24-hour creatinine clearance to a level lower than 20 mL/min in less than 2 weeks. In type II, the renal failure does not have a rapidly progressive course.

DIFFERENTIAL DIAGNOSIS: Reversible prerenal azotemia, ongoing bacterial infection, drugs (i.e., NSAIDs, aminoglycosides, diuretics, etc.).

SYMPTOMS AND SIGNS: Many of the signs of hepatorenal syndrome are related to hepatic failure: ascites, jaundice, edema, and chronic liver disease. Most of the subjective symptoms reported by the patient are related to fluid overload as a result of abnormal sodium and water retention: abdominal pain, increased abdominal girth, and generalized edema. Patients are also prone to hepatic encephalopathy owing to hepatic failure, electrolyte imbalance, and renal failure.

ETIOLOGY/EPIDEMIOLOGY: HRS is the extreme expression of circulatory dysfunction occurring in patients with cirrhosis, owing to portal hypertension and hepatic failure. The most accepted theory for the development of HRS is peripheral arterial vasodilation. Patients with severe portal hypertension have arterial underfilling secondary to severe vasodilation of the splanchnic vascular bed. This arterial underfilling causes a decrease in effective arterial blood volume and results in activation of the vasoconstrictor systems, which do not affect the splanchnic area so the intense vasodilation persists. The renin-angiotensin systems and sympathetic systems are activated as part of the vasoconstrictor activation, and in turn lead to sodium retention and ascites. HRS develops as a result of renal ischemia due to the decreased effective arterial blood volume, and the renal vasodilator system (nitric oxide and prostaglandins) is unable to counteract the maximal activation of the vasoconstrictor systems. The reported incidence of HRS in patients with end-stage cirrhosis ranges from 7% to 15%. Predictive factors are sodium and water retention (indicated by a low urinary sodium of <5 mEq/L and dilutional hyponatremia), low mean arterial blood pressure, poor nutrition, reduced GFR, high plasma renin activity, and esophageal varices. Of note, the degree of liver failure assessed by the Child-Pugh classification does not correlate with the development of HRS. The overall survival is poor once HRS develops, with a 60% mortality at 2 weeks for type I patients.

DIAGNOSIS: The International Ascites Club has established criteria for the diagnosis of HRS. The major criteria are chronic or acute liver disease; a low GFR indicated by a creatinine of >1.5 mg/dL or a 24-hour creatinine clearance rate of <40 mL/min; absence of ongoing bacterial infectionand nephrotoxins; shock or gastrointestinal fluid losses; no improvement in renal function following diuretic withdrawal and expansion of plasma volume with 1.5 L isotonic saline; and proteinuria of <500 mg/dL with no ultrasonographic evidence of obstructive uropathy or parenchymal renal disease. The minor criteria are a urine volume of <500 mL/day, urine sodium <10 mEq/L, urine osmolality greater than plasma osmolality, and serum sodium concentration of less than 130 mEq/L. All major criteria are needed for the diagnosis, with the minor criteria providing additional supportive evidence.

TREATMENT

Standard Therapies: In general, the patient is in an intensive care unit for measurement of urine output, patient weight, blood pressure, evaluation and replacement of electrolytes, and the institution of emergent procedures such as dialysis. Liver transplantation offers the best treatment because it cures the diseased liver and the circulatory and renal dysfunction. The 5-year survival rate is about 70%. About 5% of patients progress to end-stage renal disease and require hemodialysis posttransplantation. Few patients with HRS receive liver transplants, because of the small donor pool and long waiting lists.

Investigational Therapies: A novel approach to the treatment of HRS has been the use of vasoconstrictors, to counteract severe vasodilatation in the splanchnic circulation. Ornipressin infusion has been studied in this regard. Another potential therapy is the transjugular intrahepatic portosystemic shunt (TIPS), but there has been little experience in HRS.

REFERENCES

Arroyo V, Gines P, Gerbes AL, et al. Definition and diagnostic criteria of refractory ascites and hepatorenal syndrome. *Hepatology* 1996;23:164.

Cardenas A, Uriz J, Gines P, et al. Hepatorenal syndrome. *Liver Transplant* 2000;6(suppl):63.

Gines P, Rodes J. Renal complications of cirrhosis. In: Schiff ER, Sorrell MF, Maddrey WC, eds. Schiff's diseases of the liver, 8th ed. Philadelphia: Lippincott-Raven, 1999:453–464.

RESOURCES

37, 39, 372

14 Hirschsprung Disease

Alberto Peña, MD, and Andrew R. Hong, MD

DEFINITION: Hirschsprung disease is a congenital condition in which a portion, or occasionally the whole, of the colon has no ganglion cells. This leads to a functional obstruction of the distal colon. The distal colon and rectum are always affected, but the proximal extent of involvement is variable. In the most common type, aganglionosis is present in the rectosigmoid colon. Above the aganglionic segment is a so-called transition zone, and then normal ganglionic bowel is seen. Characteristically, the aganglionic segment is not dilated, but the colon proximal to the aganglionic segment becomes gradually dilated, often reaching enormous proportions.

SYNONYMS: Congenital megacolon; Morbid megacolon.

DIFFERENTIAL DIAGNOSIS: Colonic atresia; Meconium plug syndrome; Meconium ileus; Ileal atresia; Necrotizing enterocolitis.

SYMPTOMS AND SIGNS: Patients with Hirschsprung disease characteristically do not pass meconium during the first 24 hours of life. Abdominal distention and vomiting may ensue, and the general condition of the patient may deteriorate. Examination of the rectum usually produces a characteristically explosive bowel movement that may temporarily alleviate the abdominal distention. Occasionally, the patient will develop foul-smelling watery diarrhea, distention, and symptoms of sepsis and toxemia, which signal the onset of enterocolitis.

ETIOLOGY/EPIDEMIOLOGY: The etiology is unclear. Arrested orocaudad migration of the ganglion cells is one theory. The condition occurs in approximately 1 in 4,000 newborns.

DIAGNOSIS: The primary diagnostic test is a contrast enema, which shows a normal caliber aganglionic segment of the colon beginning at the anus, followed proximally by a dilated colon with a transition zone in between. The diagnosis is confirmed by a suction rectal biopsy, which shows the characteristic lack of ganglion cells, increased activity of acetyl cholinesterase, and hypertrophic nerve trunks.

TREATMENT

Standard Therapies: Traditionally, patients are treated with a two-stage repair involving a diverting colostomy at the level of the transition zone, and then a later operation in which the aganglionic bowel is completely resected and the normal bowel is pulled down to the anus and sutured in place. It is becoming more common for pediatric surgeons to perform the primary repair during the newborn period without a protective colostomy. The complete operation has even been performed using a transanal approach, completely avoiding a laparotomy. Although the decreased morbidity of this approach is attractive, the long-term results are unknown.

Investigational Therapies: Current areas of research include investigations of the genetic defects associated with Hirschsprung disease.

REFERENCES

Harrison MW, Deitz DM, Campbell JR, et al. Diagnosis and management of Hirschsprung's disease. A 25-year perspective. *Am J Surg* 1986;152:49–56.

Klein MD, Coran AG, Wesley JR, et al. Hirschsprung's disease in the newborn. *J Pediatr Surg* 1984;19:370–374.

Puri P. Hirschsprung's disease: clinical and experimental observations. *World J Surg* 1993;17:374.

Rescorla FJ, Morrison AM, Engles D, et al. Hirschsprung's disease. Evaluation of mortality and long-term function in 260 cases. *Arch Surg* 1992;127:934–941.

Soper RT. Surgery for Hirschsprung's disease. *AORN J* 1968;8:69.

Teitelbaum DH, Qualman SJ, Caniano DA. Hirschsprung's disease. Identification of risk factors for enterocolitis. *Ann Surg* 1988;207:240.

RESOURCES

202, 354, 408

15   Intestinal Lymphangiectasia

Anne B. Ballinger, MD

DEFINITION: In intestinal lymphangectasia (IL), blockage or dilatation of lymphatic vessels occurs with associated loss of lymphatic fluid into the gastrointestinal (GI) tract. This loss results in a protein-losing enteropathy, leading to hypoalbuminemia and hypogammaglobulinemia. In addition, lymphocytes are depleted into the GI tract, resulting in immunodeficiency.

SYNONYMS: Primary IL; Waldmann syndrome; Yellow nail syndrome.

SYMPTOMS AND SIGNS: In general, the earlier the onset, the more severe the disease. If primary IL is apparent in the neonatal period or within the first few months of life, it is characterized by massive edema, diarrhea, malabsorption, and, at times, overwhelming infection. If it manifests in early childhood, the edema and GI symptoms may occur in association with a negative effect on growth and sexual development. If onset is in adolescence or early adulthood, it is associated with chronic edema, and other symptoms, which may include abdominal pain and excessive fatigue. Edema is mostly asymmetric and may be associated with chylous fluid accumulation within body cavities. Over time, peripheral lymphatic abnormalities may lead to stasis dermatitis and peripheral ulcers. Central lymphatic abnormalities may lead to formation of chylous ascites. Diarrhea is seen in a minority of patients. Clinical fat malabsorption and abdominal pain also may occur. Other symptoms include tetany secondary to hypocalcemia, growth retardation, and recurring thrombotic episodes. Significant loss of albumin leads to a hypoproteinemic state. Fatigue may be persistent and often severe. Other manifestations of lymphatic and/or connective tissue dysplasia may be evident, such as lymphangiomas or other vascular tumors. Occasional patients may exhibit yellow nail syndrome.

ETIOLOGY/EPIDEMIOLOGY: The etiology of primary IL is idiopathic. The occurrence of IL may be due to abnormal development of lymphatic structures. No increased incidence is seen between gender or ethnic groups, and there is no inherited prevalence. Lymphangectasia may also occur as a result of lymphatic obstruction or elevated lymphatic pressure. Many disorders may lead to secondary IL; the etiology and incidence are specific to each primary disorder.

DIAGNOSIS: The disease should be suspected in any patient with a combination of edema, hypoalbuminemia, and lymphocytopenia. In primary IL, one finds asymmetric edema as well as the possible occurrence of lymphangiomas, whereas in secondary IL, one finds the symptoms and signs of the underlying condition. Laboratory abnormalities may include hypocalcemia. Steatorrhea may be demonstrable on a fecal fat collection, and protein malabsorption is evident by a fecal α_1-antitrypsin excretion. Radiographic studies include barium series. Other diagnostic tests include biopsy of the small intestinal mucosa and endoscopy.

TREATMENT

Standard Therapies: In primary IL, treatment is mainly symptomatic and aims to reduce the fat load on the blocked lymphatics by means of a low-fat, high-protein medium-chain triglyceride diet. Other symptomatic measures include the judicious use of diuretics with the addition of albumin infusions. In some patients, improvement has occurred after local resection of the affected portion of the bowel. Additional therapy has been the use of octreotide (somatostatin analogue). Technetium scintography can identify specific localized lymphatic abnormalities in a particular segment of the bowel and thus make surgical treatment possible. In some cases, secondary IL is associated with a treatable primary condition, which offers the possibility of complete disease resolution.

REFERENCES

Ballinger AB, Farthing MJ. Octreotide in the treatment of intestinal lymphangectasia. *Eur J Gastroenterol Hepatol* 1998;10: 699–702.

Bhatnagor A, Kashyap R, Chavhan UP, et al. Diagnosing protein-losing enteropathy. A new approach using Tc-99m human immunoglobulin. *Clin Nucl Med* 1995;20:969–972.

Broder S, Cullihan TR, Jaffe ES, et al. Resolution of longstanding protein-losing enteropathy in a patient with intestinal lymphangectasia after treatment for malignant lymphomas. *Gastroenterology* 1981;80:166–168.

Puri AS, Aggarwal R, Gupta RK, et al. Intestinal lymphangectasia; evaluation by CT and scinitography. *Gastrointest Radiol* 1992; 17:119–121.

Saverymutto SH, Peters AM, Lavender JP, et al. Detection of protein losing enteropathy by ^{111}In-transferrin scanning. *Eur J Nucl Med* 1983;8:40–41.

RESOURCES

310, 354

16   Intestinal Pseudoobstruction in Adults

*Madhusudhan R. Sanaka, MD,
and Edy E. Soffer, MD*

DEFINITION: Chronic intestinal pseudoobstruction (CIP) is a disorder of gastrointestinal (GI) motility characterized by symptoms of intestinal obstruction without a true mechanical obstruction of the intestine.

SYNONYMS: Pseudoobstruction; Chronic idiopathic intestinal pseudoobstruction.

DIFFERENTIAL DIAGNOSIS: Intestinal obstruction; Cyclic vomiting syndrome; Irritable bowel syndrome; Inflammatory bowel disease.

SYMPTOMS AND SIGNS: CIP causes chronic recurrent symptoms suggestive of intestinal obstruction. As implied by the prefix *pseudo-*, symptoms occur in the absence of an obstruction. It may affect any part of the GI tract, locally or diffusely from esophagus to colon. Symptoms may include dysphagia and heartburn, early satiety, nausea and vomiting, bloating, abdominal distention and discomfort, and constipation. Predominant involvement of the small intestine causes poor transit of intestinal contents and bacterial overgrowth leading to steatorrhea and diarrhea. Symptoms may lead to decreased food intake, weight loss, and malnutrition. Physical findings may include abdominal distention, succussion splash, hypertympanic note on percussion, and cachexia in severe cases.

ETIOLOGY/EPIDEMIOLOGY: CIP is a rare disorder that may develop at any age. Symptoms result from abnormal gut motility caused by various disorders affecting visceral smooth muscle, enteric or extrinsic nerves of the gut, or hormones that together control and coordinate GI motility. In adults, CIP is seen commonly secondary to systemic diseases such as scleroderma, diabetes, amyloidosis, and paraneoplastic syndromes, especially small cell lung carcinoma. It can also be seen with narcotic and anticholinergic drug usage and various types of familial visceral myopathies and neuropathies.

DIAGNOSIS: Diagnosis is made by a combination of history, physical findings, laboratory tests, radiologic tests, and scintigraphic and manometric assessment of GI motility and transit. Plain abdominal films may show

bowel loops distended with air, which may be mistaken for mechanical bowel obstruction. Barium contrast studies of the entire GI tract must be done to rule out mechanical obstruction. Antroduodenal manometry, GI transit studies, and intestinal biopsy are useful to confirm the diagnosis. Manometry can detect abnormal patterns of contractions and may provide information regarding whether the underlying process is myopathic or neuropathic. Transit studies are noninvasive and help determine the presence, severity, and location of the gut segment involved. Full-thickness bowel biopsy can provide the most definitive information, particularly if elaborate evaluation of the enteric nerves, pacemaker cells, and neurotransmitters is performed.

TREATMENT

Standard Therapies: Management of CIP is mainly supportive. The goal of treatment is to reduce symptoms and to restore and maintain adequate nutrition. Dietary measures include low-fat, low-lactose, and low-residue, soft to liquid diet with polypeptides or hydrolyzed proteins and supplemental minerals and vitamins. Broad-spectrum antibiotics such as doxycycline, ciprofloxacin, and metronidazole are useful to treat the bacterial overgrowth. Prokinetic agents such as metoclopramide, erythromycin, and octreotide may be beneficial in some patients, but, overall, they have limited usefulness. If these conservative measures fail, a jejunostomy tube can be placed for venting as well as for tube feeding. Total parenteral nutrition (TPN) is used for patients who cannot maintain adequate nutrition with other methods. Ablative surgery has a limited role in CIP, and may be helpful with localized disease such as megaduodenum, or when the colon is selectively involved. Small intestinal transplantation is a life-saving alternative for patients who cannot tolerate TPN.

REFERENCES
Camilleri M, Coulie B. Intestinal pseudo-obstruction. *Ann Rev Med* 1999;50:37–55.
Di Lorenzo C. Pseudo-obstruction: current approaches. *Gastroenterology* 1999;116:980–987.
Grant D. Intestinal transplantation: 1997 report of the international registry. Intestinal transplant registry. *Transplantation* 1999;67:1061–1064.
Messing B, Lemann M, Landais P, et al. Prognosis of patients with nonmalignant chronic intestinal failure receiving long-term home parenteral nutrition. *Gastroenterology* 1995;108:1005–1010.

RESOURCES
61, 202, 354

17   Intestinal Pseudoobstruction (Pediatric Presentation)

Paul E. Hyman, MD,
and Manu Sood, MD

DEFINITION: Chronic intestinal pseudoobstruction is a severe, disabling disorder marked by repetitive episodes or continuous signs of bowel obstruction, including radiographic evidence of dilated bowel with air-fluid levels, in the absence of a fixed lumen-occluding lesion. Pseudoobstruction can present throughout life.

SYNONYMS: Chronic idiopathic intestinal pseudoobstruction (CIIP); Pseudointestinal obstruction syndrome; Pseudoobstruction syndrome.

DIFFERENTIAL DIAGNOSIS: Mechanical intestinal obstruction; Paralytic ileus; Irritable bowel syndrome; Aerophagia; Hypokalemia; Drug toxicity such as from anticholinergics and opiates; Pediatric condition falsification; Visceral pain-associated disability syndrome.

SYMPTOMS AND SIGNS: Over 50% of pediatric patients develop symptoms as neonates. Those less severely affected can present months later with constipation or diarrhea, vomiting, and failure to thrive. About 40% of the patients with congenital disease also have intestinal malrotation; about 25% have urinary bladder involvement. Nearly 75% of pediatric patients complain of abdominal distention and vomiting; 60% describe constipation, intermittent abdominal pain, and poor weight gain; and one third complain of diarrhea. Twenty percent of pediatric patients with neuropathic and 80% of those with myopathic pseudoobstruction have associated urinary tract and bladder involvement. In most children with congenital disease, the clinical course has an illness plateau with intermittent increases in acuity. Triggers for acute decompensation include intercurrent infections, general anesthesia, psychological stress, and poor nutrition. Nonspecific radiographic signs include intestinal obstruction with air-fluid levels, and dilated stomach, small intestine, and colon. Stasis of the contrast material in the affected loop may be prolonged, so evacuation or water-soluble contrast should be planned.

ETIOLOGY/EPIDEMIOLOGY: Pseudoobstruction may occur as a disease of smooth muscle, enteric nerves, or interstitial cells of Cajal, or secondary to inflammation or toxins. Most congenital forms are sporadic, possibly new mutations, and usually occur without a family history. At times, pseudoobstruction results from familial inherited disease. Both autosomal-recessive and -dominant patterns of inheritance have been reported in myopathic and neuropathic pseudoobstruction. *In utero* exposure to toxins has been associated with the neuropathic forms. Children with chromosomal abnormalities may suffer from pseudoobstruction or neuropathic constipation. Acquired pseudoobstruction may be a complication of infection from cytomegalovirus or Ebstein-Barr virus, or from autoimmune disease of enteric neurons or muscles. Mucosal inflammation causes abnormal motility, so patients with celiac disease, Crohn disease, and chronic enterocolitis develop dilated bowel and symptoms.

DIAGNOSIS: Intestinal pseudoobstruction is a clinical diagnosis based on symptoms of bowel obstruction in the absence of an anatomic lesion. Manometric studies should be used to evaluate strength and coordination of contractions and relaxation in the esophagus, gastric antrum, small intestine, and colon. Abnormalities on manometry of the small bowel and colon usually correlate with the clinical severity of the disease, and help in treatment planning. Quantitative culture of duodenal fluid or the breath hydrogen test can diagnose bacterial overgrowth in dilated small bowel loops.

TREATMENT
Standard Therapies: One third of patients require parenteral nutrition; one third require tube feeding. Continuous feeding by a gastrostomy or jejunostomy should be initiated if bolus feeding fails. Nutrition must be adequate to optimize gut neuromuscular function. Mineral oil, polyethelene glycol, suppositories, and/or enemas are used to treat constipation. Bowel decompression is used for acute abdominal pain. For chronic visceral pain, low-dose tricyclic antidepressants and gabapentin may help; narcotics disrupt motility. Cisapride increases intestinal contractions and improves symptoms in a minority of patients. Combined erythromycin and octreotide improve bowel motility. Bacterial overgrowth may be treated with antibiotics or probiotics. A gastrostomy decompresses the bowel during acute episodes and is useful for enteral feeding during plateaus in disease. Ileostomy or colostomy is often necessary to decompress bowel and begin enteral feeding. With irreversible intestinal failure and recurrent sepsis secondary to bacterial translocation, total enterectomy may be necessary. For life-

threatening intestinal pseudoobstruction, intestinal transplantation is a high-risk procedure with potential for cure.

REFERENCE

Hyman PE. Chronic intestinal pseudo-obstruction. In: Wyllie R, Hyams S, eds. *Pediatric gastrointestinal disease pathophysiology diagnosis management*, 2nd ed. Philadelphia: WB Saunders, 1999.

RESOURCES

61, 192, 354

---

18 Jejunal Atresia

Kavita S. Reddy, MD

DEFINITION: Jejunal atresia is the most common cause of bowel obstruction in the newborn. It can be classified into four different types: type 1 accounts for approximately 20% of cases and consists of a membrane or diaphragm with the bowel wall in continuity; type 2 is a single atresia with discontinuity of the bowel wall in 35% of the defects; type 3 multiple atresia accounts for approximately 5% of cases; and type 4 is found in 35% of the defects and involves either both ends of the bowel in blind loops accompanied by a small mesenteric defect or extensive mesenteric defect resulting in loss of blood supply to the distal bowel.

SYNONYMS: Christmas tree syndrome; Maypole or apple-peel syndrome.

DIFFERENTIAL DIAGNOSIS: Cystic fibrosis.

SYMPTOMS AND SIGNS: Bilious vomiting, epigastric distention, and absence of stools in the neonatal period are common symptoms.

ETIOLOGY/EPIDEMIOLOGY: Between 1968 and 1995, the birth prevalence of isolated jejunal atresia in the Metropolitan Atlanta Congenital Defects Program was 1.3 in 10,000 live births. Obliteration of the superior mesenteric artery may be the underlying cause for this malformation. Familial cases of jejunal atresia suggest a genetic cause with an autosomal-recessive mode of inheritance. Discordance in the type of jejunal atresia in monozygotic twins supports an environmental etiology. Males and females are affected equally.

DIAGNOSIS: Due to agenesis of the mesentery, the distal small bowel comes straight off the cecum and twists around the marginal artery, resembling a maypole. Radiography of the abdomen show a high jejunal occlusion, malrotation, microcolon, and coiled or spiral-like terminal ileum. At laparotomy, the jejunum ends blindly in a dilated proximal loop, 3–4 cm beyond the ligament of Treitz. The bowel is incompletely rotated and is foreshortened, with a large mesentric gap, precariously supplied in retrograde fashion by anastomotic arcades from a mesenteric artery. Prenatal ultrasonographic testing should be offered to families with a previous child with jejunal atresia. Sonographic findings of a high intestinal obstruction and a triple bubble sign indicate jejunal atresia.

TREATMENT

Standard Therapies: Jejunal atresia is usually corrected surgically.

Investigational Therapies: A surgical method of wing-shaped end-to-end anastomosis between a dilated proximal and diminutive distal bowel is being investigated.

REFERENCES

Imaizumi K, Kimura J, Masuno M, et al. Apple-peel intestinal atresia associated with balanced reciprocal translocation t(2;3)(q31.3;p24.2)mat. *Am J Med Genet* 1999;87:434–435.

Kato T, Hebiguchi T, Yoshino H, et al. Wing-shaped end-to-end anastomosis for the treatment of high jejunal atresia. *Tohoku J Exp Med* 2000;192:119–126.

Matsumoto Y, Komatsu K, Tabata T. Jejuno-ileal atresia in identical twins: report of a case. *Surg Today* 2000;30:438–440.

Roberts HE, Cragan JD, Cono J, Khoury MJ, Weatherly MR, Moore CA. Increased frequency of cystic fibrosis among infants with jejunoileal atresia. *Am J Med Genet* 1998;78:446–449.

Tongsong T, Chanprapaph P. Triple bubble sign: a marker of proximal jejunal atresia. *Int J Gynaecol Obstet* 2000;68:149–150.

Yamanaka S, Tanaka Y, Kawataki M, et al. Chromosome 22q11 deletion complicated by dissecting pulmonary arterial aneurysm and jejunal atresia in an infant. *Arch Pathol Lab Med* 2000;124:880–882.

19   Mesenteric Panniculitis

Philip M. Ginsburg, MD, and Eli D. Ehrenpreis, MD

DEFINITION: Mesenteric panniculitis is a condition in which the fatty tissue within the abdominal cavity becomes thickened and inflamed. This poorly understood disease actually represents a spectrum of conditions that characterize a continuum that starts with fatty degeneration, then progresses to inflammation and eventual fibrosis of the mesentery.

SYNONYMS: Mesenteric lipodystrophy; Liposclerotic mesenteritis; Mesenteric lipogranuloma; Retractile mesenteritis; Sclerosing mesenteritis; Mesenteric fibromatosis (desmoid).

DIFFERENTIAL DIAGNOSIS: Primary or metastatic neoplasm; Granulomatous infection; Omental torsion, infarction, or hemorrhage; Pancreatitis; Inflammatory pseudotumor; Inflammatory bowel disease; Retroperitoneal fibrosis; Systemic panniculitis; Weber-Christian disease.

SYMPTOMS AND SIGNS: Frequent symptoms include intermittent crampy abdominal pain, bloating, anorexia, nausea/vomiting, early satiety, weakness/malaise, and either diarrhea or constipation. An abdominal mass is palpable in more than 50% of cases and is frequently the presenting complaint. In general, patients are asymptomatic or have only subtle nonspecific gastrointestinal and constitutional complaints for months or even years until the diagnosis is made. Rarely, patients present with an acute abdomen or intestinal obstruction.

ETIOLOGY/EPIDEMIOLOGY: Fewer than 300 cases of idiopathic mesenteric panniculitis and its associated conditions have been reported. It is likely underdiagnosed and underreported, so adequate clinical and epidemiologic data are lacking. It is twice as common in males and has been reported to predominate in whites. Usually occurring during the fifth and sixth decades of life, the condition has been described in every age group. The etiology is unknown, but the underlying pathogenesis in idiopathic cases is most likely autoimmune, although infections, drugs, ischemia, trauma, and prior surgery have also been suggested as causative factors.

DIAGNOSIS: The diagnosis is suggested based on characteristic clinical symptoms and physical examination findings in the setting of a negative evaluation for more common diagnoses. Many cases are incidentally discovered at laparotomy or after a routine radiographic study shows a characteristic mesenteric mass. A surgically obtained tissue sample is required for definitive diagnosis and to rule out other conditions such as neoplasm or infection.

TREATMENT
Standard Therapies: There is no uniformly recognized standard therapy. Initial therapy usually involves empiric corticosteroids directed at an inflammatory component, but long-term use is problematic. Surgical excision or debulking is occasionally attempted with little success. Surgical bypass or resection is reserved for refractory obstructive symptoms.

Investigational Therapies: The use of antiinflammatory, immunosuppressive, cytotoxic, and hormonal medications is being investigated, including azathioprine, cyclophosphamide, tamoxifen, and progesterone. The use of antibiotics, colchicine, and radiation is also being explored, as is thalidomide therapy.

REFERENCES
Durst AL, Freund H, Rosenmann E, et al. Mesenteric panniculitis: review of the literature and presentation of cases. *Surgery* 1977;81:203–211.
Emory TS, Monihan JM, Carr NJ, et al. Sclerosing mesenteritis, mesenteric panniculitis and mesenteric lipodystrophy: a single entity? *Am J Surg Pathol* 1997;21:392–398.
Koornstra JJ, van Olffen GH, van Noort G. Retractile mesenteritis: to treat or not to treat. *Hepatogastroenterology* 1997;44: 408–410.
Mazure R, Marty PF, Niveloni S, et al. Successful treatment of retractile mesenteritis with oral progesterone. *Gastroenterology* 1998;114:1313–1317.
Sabate JM, Torrubia S, Maideu J, et al. Sclerosing mesenteritis: imaging findings in 17 patients. *AJR* 1999;172:625–629.

RESOURCES
135, 354

20   Microvillus Inclusion Disease

Nigel L. Kennea, MB, BChir, MRCP

DEFINITION: Microvillus inclusion disease is a familial enteropathy of unknown etiology. It causes severe watery diarrhea beginning in the first few days of life. Affected infants are generally unable to absorb enteral feeds and thus require long-term intravenous nutrition. This condition is often fatal, although intestinal transplantation has been used with success in a few patients.

SYNONYM: Congenital microvillus atrophy.

DIFFERENTIAL DIAGNOSIS: Congenital chloride diarrhea; Congenital sodium diarrhea.

SYMPTOMS AND SIGNS: Infants with microvillus inclusion disease have intractable watery diarrhea, which usually manifests soon after birth. The diarrhea is largely secretory, but often worsens with malabsorption when the infant is fed. This condition leads to severe, life-threatening dehydration if not recognized early. The prognosis is very poor. If affected infants survive the initial presentation, they are generally unable to absorb full enteral feeding and require intravenous hydration and total parenteral nutrition (TPN). In addition to problems of fluid balance and nutrition, they are prone to the complications of long-term TPN, particularly cholestatic liver disease and long-line sepsis.

ETIOLOGY/EPIDEMIOLOGY: This is a familial enteropathy. Some researchers have suggested the disease has an autosomal-recessive mode of inheritance. The true prevalence is unknown, but less than 100 cases have been reported. The cause is unknown, although it may result from an inborn error of brush border construction and differentiation, leading to aberrant assembly of components of the enterocyte surface membrane.

DIAGNOSIS: Diagnosis is made with small bowel biopsy. On light microscopy there is severe villus atrophy (without crypt hyperplasia) with an accumulation of periodic acid-Schiff–positive material in the epithelium. On electron microscopy of the biopsy, characteristic membrane-bound inclusions are seen with an increase in secretory granules. Prior to biopsy, all causes of infantile diarrhea and malabsorption (including infection and specific malabsorptive syndromes) should be ruled out, although such conditions usually manifest with less severe diarrhea.

TREATMENT
Standard Therapies: Treatment is initially supportive with the need to manage large fluid and electrolyte loss with appropriate intravenous therapy. Subsequently, nutrition is provided by long-term TPN. Some infants can tolerate small volumes of enteral feeding. Trials of treatments with elemental diets and various drug regimens have been unsuccessful. This condition has been treated by small bowel transplantation or a combination of liver and small bowel transplantation.

REFERENCES
Cutz E, Rhoads JM, Drumm B, et al. Microvillus inclusion disease: an inherited defect of brush-border assembly and differentiation. *N Engl J Med* 1989;320:646–651.

Davidson GP, Cutz E, Hamilton JR, et al. Familial enteropathy: a syndrome of protracted diarrhea from birth, failure to thrive, and hypoplastic villus atrophy. *Gastroenterology* 1978;75:783–790.

Oliva MM, Perman JA, Saavedra JM, et al. Successful intestinal transplantation for microvillus inclusion disease. *Gastroenterology* 1994;106:771–774.

Phillips AD, Jenkins P, Raafat F, et al. Congenital microvillus atrophy: specific diagnostic features. *Arch Dis Child* 1985;60:135–140.

RESOURCES
354, 365

21   Peutz-Jeghers Syndrome

Carol Burke, MD

DEFINITION: Peutz-Jeghers syndrome (PJS) is a dominantly inherited gastrointestinal polyposis syndrome characterized by multiple hamartomatous polyps throughout the gastrointestinal tract and by pigmented macules on the skin or mucous membranes. These patients have increased risk of cancer within and outside the GI tract.

SYNONYM: Familial hamartomatous polyposis.

SYMPTOMS AND SIGNS: Gastrointestinal polyps, called hamartomas, are the most problematic aspect of PJS, occurring most often in the small intestine, then the colon and stomach. Patients may experience abdominal pain or gastrointestinal bleeding (either obvious, occult, or associated with iron-deficiency anemia) owing to the polyps. Intussusception or obstruction from the polyps may result in abdominal pain, distension, nausea, and emesis. By the age of 20, almost half of PJS patients require surgery for bowel blockage. The pigmented macules, usually present in infancy or childhood, occur on the lips, in the mouth, or around the eyes and nose, as well as around the anus, or on the hands and feet. They may fade with age.

ETIOLOGY/EPIDEMIOLOGY: PJS is a dominantly inherited syndrome due to genetic alterations on chromosome 19. The mutation in the *LKB1* or *STK11* gene seems to result in a predisposition to both benign and cancerous tumors. The incidence in the United States is 1 in 100,000. PJS patients have a 50% chance of passing on the mutated gene to their offspring, or it may be sporadic. Gene testing for PJS is not now commercially available. It should be done only in consultation with a genetic counselor who is an expert in PJS. The mutation is found in up to 50% of affected patients, and if so, all "at-risk" relatives may have genetic testing. If the gene test result is positive or the family mutation is unknown, regular checkups of all affected and at-risk relatives is essential to prevent symptoms and cancer. PJS patients have an increased risk for cancer both within and outside of the GI tract. Colorectal cancer occurs in approximately 38%, pancreas in 35%, stomach in 27%, small intestine in 13%, and esophagus in 3%. Breast cancer occurs in 55%, ovarian and lung in 20%, and unusual tumors may occur in the testicles or ovaries (sex cord tumors with annular tubules) about 13% of the time.

DIAGNOSIS: PJS is diagnosed when the freckles are noticed or hamartomas are found in the intestinal tract. Since PJS is hereditary, first-degree relatives should undergo endoscopic and radiologic testing.

TREATMENT

Standard Therapies: Regular examinations help to prevent intestinal obstruction/intussusception and cancer. Upper endoscopic evaluation of the small intestine is recommended. Most PJS polyps are in the jejunum, so enteroscopy is favored. Small bowel radiography or enteroclysis can visualize the distal jejunum and ileum. Any large (>1 cm) polyps should be removed during enteroscopy to minimize the risk for symptomatic disease. If large distal polyps are detected on radiography, intraoperative enteroscopic removal should be considered. The age to begin screening and the frequency of examinations depend on family history and symptoms. The guidelines are as follows: (a) Evaluate the small intestine every 2–3 years or when symptoms of abdominal pain, nausea, or vomiting occur; (b) perform a colonoscopy every 1–3 years; (c) conduct the following examinations as applicable: annual Pap smear with pelvic examination and transvaginal ultrasonography beginning in the teen years; breast examinations beginning by the age of 20 and yearly mammograms beginning at 30; and testicular examinations starting by the age of 20. If other cancers are prominent in a family, directed checks of the organs should be offered to the affected or at-risk family members. All PJS patients should be enrolled in an inherited colorectal cancer registry.

REFERENCES

Giardiello FM, Brensinger JD, Tersmette A, et al. Peutz-Jeghers syndrome, and risk of cancer. A meta-analysis with recommendations for surveillance [Abstract]. *Gastroenterology* 1999;116:411.
Hemminki A, Markie D, Tomlinson I, et al. A serine/threonine kinase gene defective in Peutz-Jeghers syndrome. *Nature* 1998;391:184–187.
Kuwada S, Burt R. The clinical features of the hereditary and nonhereditary polyposis syndromes. *Surg Oncol Clin North Am* 1996;5:553–568.
McGarrity T, Kulin H, Zaino R. Peutz-Jeghers syndrome. *Am J Gastroenterol* 2000;95:596–604.

RESOURCES
208, 354, 379

22   Familial Adenomatous Polyposis

Carol Burke, MD

DEFINITION: Familial adenomatous polyposis (FAP) is a dominantly inherited syndrome resulting in polyposis throughout the gastrointestinal tract. Hundreds to thousands of precancerous adenomas develop in the colon, often beginning in puberty. All patients with FAP develop colorectal cancer, usually by the age of 40, unless the colon is removed.

SYNONYMS: Adenomatous polyposis coli (APC); Aattenuated familial adenomatous polyposis (fewer than 100 colorectal polyps, occurring 10–15 years later than FAP); Gardner syndrome (if extraintestinal manifestations occur); Turcot syndrome (if malignant brain tumor is present).

SYMPTOMS AND SIGNS: Approximately 80% of FAP patients also develop upper gastrointestinal polyps. These may be few or numerous, carpeting the stomach or duodenum. In the stomach, they are usually fundic gland polyps and do not require special treatment. Duodenal adenomas are the same type as found in the colon and may become cancerous, particularly around the papilla. Rarely, cancers of the liver (hepatoblastoma) or thyroid occur. Outside the intestinal tract, the most common benign tumors include osteomas (usually on the skull, jaw, or long bones), epidermoid cysts, lipomas, or fibromas. Other signs include supernumerary teeth or congenital hypertrophy of the retinal epithelium. About 12% of FAP patients develop a fibrous tumor within the abdominal cavity or on the abdominal wall (called a desmoid). Desmoids are not cancerous but rarely can grow and strangle the intestines, resulting in death. Polyps in the colon may not produce symptoms until they are numerous, large, or become cancerous. Advanced polyposis or cancer may include a change in bowel habit, gastrointestinal bleeding, either occult or obvious, or an unexplained iron deficiency anemia, abdominal pain, fatigue, or weight loss.

ETIOLOGY/EPIDEMIOLOGY: FAP results from a mutation in the *APC* gene on the long arm of chromosome 5 (5q). The gene is inherited in about 70% of cases. Patients with sporadic FAP have a 50% chance of passing the mutated gene to their children. Incidence in the United States is approximately 1 in 10,000.

DIAGNOSIS: A detailed family history should reveal the dominantly inherited pattern of colorectal cancer. A patient with a sporadic mutation may not have a family history. Gene testing should be performed only by a genetic counselor expert in FAP. The test for the *APC* mutation is commercially available and has an accuracy of 80%. If the mutation is found, family members should be tested. Any person with a positive test result or whose family mutation is not known should undergo surveillance, which includes a yearly flexible sigmoidoscopy or colonoscopy beginning in puberty. The diagnosis may also be made by endoscopic

findings, most often in conjunction with a known family history.

TREATMENT

Standard Therapies: The patient should be referred to a colorectal surgeon if adenomas are detected. Surgical options include a subtotal colectomy and ileorectal anastomosis or an ileal-pouch anal anastomosis. Upper endoscopic surveillance with a forward- and side-viewing endoscope should be done at the time of colectomy and every 3 years thereafter. The side-viewing scope is necessary to visualize the papilla, which should be sampled for biopsy, even if normal, because adenomatous changes may not be grossly apparent. Fundic gland polyps do not require removal. Any adenoma detected in the stomach should be completely excised. Surgical intervention for duodenal adenomas is rarely required but should be made with the assistance of FAP specialists if there is a worrisome histologic or morphologic change. Sulindac and Sulindac sulfone have induced the regression of existing polyps and decreased new polyp formation. Neither is currently FDA approved. Celecoxib is approved by the FDA for the treatment of colon polyps in patients with FAP. FAP patients may be enrolled in an inherited colorectal cancer registry.

REFERENCES

Burke C, van Stolk R, Arber N, et al. Exisulind prevents adenoma formation in familial adenomatous polyposis (FAP) [Abstract]. *Gastroenterology* 2000;118:657.

Giardello FM, et al. The use and interpretation of commercial APC testing for familial adenomatous polyposis. *N Engl J Med* 1997;336:823–827.

Giardiello FM, Hamilton SR, Krush AJ, et al. Treatment of colonic and rectal adenomas with sulindac in familial adenomatous polyposis. *N Engl J Med* 1993;328:1313–1316.

Guillem JG, Smith AJ, Calle JP, et al. Gastrointestinal polyposis syndromes. *Curr Prob Surg* 1999;36:217–323.

Steinbach G, Lynch PM, Phillips, et al. The effect of celecoxib, a cyclooxygenase-2 inhibitor, in familial adenomatous polyposis. *N Engl J Med* 2000;342:1946–1952.

RESOURCES

176, 379, 448

23   Ruvalcaba-Myhre-Smith Syndrome

Paul H. Parker, MD,
Michael J. Nowicki, MD,
and Phyllis R. Bishop, MD

DEFINITION: Ruvalcaba-Myhre-Smith syndrome is a syndrome consisting of macrocephaly, pigmented macules on the penis, developmental delay, and intestinal polyps.

SYNONYM: Bannayan-Riley-Ruvalcaba syndrome (see entry on Dysmorphic Disorders).

DIFFERENTIAL DIAGNOSIS: Intestinal ganglioneuromatosis; Juvenile polyposis; Peutz-Jeghers syndrome; Cowden syndrome.

SYMPTOMS AND SIGNS: The classic triad consists of macrocephaly, pigmented macules on the penis, and intestinal polyposis. Additional features may include developmental delay, Hashimoto thyroiditis, hypotonia, myopathy, long-chain hydroxyacyl-coenzyme A dehydrogenase deficiency, carnitine deficiency, café-au-lait spots, lipomas, hemangiomas, and ocular findings (prominent corneal nerves, prominent Schwalbe lines, and pseudopapilledema). Hamartomatous intestinal polyps are found in 45% of cases and are typically located in the terminal ileum and colon. These usually manifest as painless rectal bleeding in childhood. Although malignant transformation has not been described, there has been a report of adenomatous changes in 20% of these polyps.

ETIOLOGY/EPIDEMIOLOGY: The disorder is inherited in an autosomal-dominant manner and primarily affects men. The condition has been linked to a locus on chromosome 10 and probably arises from germline mutations in the *PTEN* phosphatase gene at that locus.

DIAGNOSIS: The diagnosis is based on the clinical features. Endoscopic removal of hamartomatous polyps of the bowel confirms the diagnosis in patients with rectal bleeding.

TREATMENT
Standard Therapies: There is no specific therapy for the underlying disorder. Investigations for, and removal of, all intestinal polyps are recommended.

REFERENCES
Bishop PR, Nowicki MJ, Parker PH. What syndrome is this? *Pediatr Dermatol* 2000;17:319–321.
Burt RW. Polyposis syndromes. In: Yamada T, Alpers DH, Laine L, et al., eds. *Atlas of gastroenterology,* 2nd ed. Philadelphia: Lippincott Williams & Wilkins, 1999:395–402.
Coyle WJ, Ryan MT, Nowicki MJ. Adenomatous changes in the hamartomatous polyps of the Ruvalcaba-Myhre-Smith syndrome. *J Clin Gastroenterol* 1998;26:85–87.
Diliberti JH, Weleber RG, Dudden S. Ruvalcaba-Myhre-Smith syndrome: a case with probable autosomal dominance inheritance and additional manifestations. *Am J Med Genet* 1983;15: 491–494.

RESOURCES
352, 354

24   Sucrase-Isomaltase Deficiency

Debra G. Silberg, MD, PhD

DEFINITION: Congenital sucrase-isomaltase deficiency (CSID) is an autosomal-recessive genetic disorder caused by abnormalities in the intestinal brush border enzyme, sucrase-isomaltase, resulting in malabsorption and diarrhea.

DIFFERENTIAL DIAGNOSIS: Lactase deficiency; Milk or soy protein allergy; Cystic fibrosis; Secondary disaccharidase deficiency; Celiac disease.

SYMPTOMS AND SIGNS: The clinical presentation of CSID is variable and depends on the activity of sucrase-isomaltase and the amount and timing of the introduction of sucrose in the diet. Infants can present with watery diarrhea and failure to thrive. Breast-feeding protects infants from developing symptoms until sucrose is added to the diet. When sucrose is the major carbohydrate constituent in formula, the potential exists for osmotic diarrhea, dehydration, electrolyte imbalance, and, if prolonged, malnutrition. Formulas with glucose polymers can also result in diarrhea. After infancy, the diet is more complex, containing increasing quantities of sucrose and starch. Children with CSID can present with chronic or intermittent diarrhea associated with abdominal distention, cramping, and failure to thrive; however, some individuals with mild to no symptoms may present as adults with a diagnosis of irritable bowel syndrome.

ETIOLOGY/EPIDEMIOLOGY: The disease is inherited in an autosomal-recessive manner. It is caused by mutations in the sucrase-isomaltase gene, which is located on chromosome 3q25-26. The gene produces the small intestinal brush border enzyme sucrase-isomaltase. The enzyme consists of two subunits: sucrase, which digests sucrose, maltose, and maltotriose, and isomaltase, which digests maltose and isomaltose. As many as five different alterations of the enzymes lead to changes in the processing, transport, and membrane insertion of the enzyme. The prevalence of CSID is estimated at ≤0.2% of North Americans, predominantly caucasians, with an increased rate in Greenland, Alaskan, and Canadian Inuits.

DIAGNOSIS: The diagnosis should be suspected in infants and children with chronic diarrhea of unclear etiology. Patients with CSID are often initially misdiagnosed. Screening tests that support the diagnosis include (a) stool pH <6 with reducing substances detected after hydrolysis; (b) abnormal sucrose hydrogen breath test result; and (c) abnormal sucrose tolerance test result with a normal glucose tolerance test result. The definitive diagnosis is determined by a biopsy from the third portion of the duodenum or proximal jejunum assayed for quantitative disaccharidase activity. Sucrase should be profoundly reduced or absent, with a moderate decrease in maltase, a reduction of isomaltase, and normal lactase activity. The mucosa of the small intestine should be normal to eliminate secondary causes such as celiac sprue.

TREATMENT

Standard Therapies: Dietary counseling should be obtained for patients and their families to be aware of the foods that contain the substrates for sucrase-isomaltase. Sacrosidase, a β-fructofuranoside fructohydrolase, from *Saccharomyces cerevisiae*, has sucrase activity and can be taken orally with meals to prevent the gastrointestinal symptoms in patients with CSID. One half of the sacrosidase dose is ingested after beginning a meal and the other portion halfway through the meal to allow patients to consume a near normal diet. Sacrosidase does not replace the contribution of isomaltase.

REFERENCES

Antonowicz I, Lloyd-Still JD, Khaw KT, et al. Congenital sucrase-isomaltase deficiency. Observations over a period of 6 years. *Pediatrics* 1972;49:847–853.

Baudon JJ, Veinberg F, Thioulouse E, et al. Sucrase-isomaltase deficiency: changing pattern over two decades. *J Pediatr Gastroenterol Nutr* 1996;22:284–288.

Jacob R, Zimmer KP, Schmitz J, et al. Congenital sucrase-isomaltase deficiency arising from cleavage and secretion of a mutant form of the enzyme. *J Clin Invest* 2000;106:281–287.

Treem WR. Congenital sucrase-isomaltase deficiency. *J Pediatr Gastroenterol Nutr* 1995;21:1–14.

Treem WR, McAdams L, Stanford L, et al. Sacrosidase therapy for congenital sucrase-isomaltase deficiency. *J Pediatr Gastroenterol Nutr* 1999;28:137–142.

RESOURCES

109, 35

9

Hematologic/Oncologic Disorders

1   Abetalipoproteinemia

Jahangir Iqbal, PhD,
Reuven Yakubov, BA,
and M. Mahmood Hussain, PhD,
Lic Med, FAHA

DEFINITION: Abetalipoproteinemia is an autosomal-recessive disorder characterized by the absence of apolipoprotein B (apoB)-containing lipoproteins in the plasma.

SYNONYMS: Low-density β-lipoprotein deficiency; Bassen-Kornzweig syndrome.

DIFFERENTIAL DIAGNOSIS: Hypobetalipoproteinemia; Chylomicron retention disease; Celiac disease.

SYMPTOMS AND SIGNS: Infants usually present with diarrhea, vomiting, and abdominal swelling. The disease is usually misdiagnosed as celiac disease, which has similar symptoms. Steatorrhea and poor weight gain are observed in infancy due to fat malabsorption. Plasma lipid levels are very low. Patients have mild to moderate anemia, usually with mild hemolysis. Plasma levels of lipid-soluble vitamins also are extremely low. During the first 10–20 years of life, the vitamin E deficiency results in neurologic complications such as loss of deep-tendon reflexes, and cerebellar signs such as dysmetria, ataxia, and spastic gait. By the third or fourth decade, untreated patients show severe ataxia and spasticity. These severe effects on the central nervous system are the ultimate cause of death in most patients, which often occurs by the fifth decade. Vitamin A deficiency results in a progressive pigmented retinopathy, characterized as an atypical retinitis pigmentosa. The first ophthalmic symptoms are decreased night and color vision. The retinitis pigmentosa usually begins at about age 10. In untreated patients, daytime visual acuity usually deteriorates to virtual blindness by the fourth decade. Vitamin K levels are also low and cause elevated prothrombin time and delayed coagulation.

ETIOLOGY/EPIDEMIOLOGY: Abetalipoproteinemia is an autosomal-recessive disease caused by mutations in the gene encoding for the 97-kDa subunit of microsomal triglyceride transfer protein (MTP). Mutations result in loss of *in vitro* lipid transfer activity in the liver and intestinal microsomes. The lack of MTP activity leads to the absence of apoB in plasma because apoB is not properly lipi-dated and undergoes rapid presecretory degradation. To date, approximately 100 isolated cases from many parts of the world have been reported with a sex ratio of 1:1. Approximately one third of reported cases were due to consanguineous marriages.

DIAGNOSIS: Diagnosis is based on the measurement of lipid and apoB levels in the plasma, determination of red blood cell morphology, and eye examination. Lipid levels are extremely low. ApoB-containing lipoproteins (chylomicrons, very low density lipoproteins, and low-density lipoproteins) are not detectable in plasma. Acanthocytosis of red blood cells is also a diagnostic feature of the disease. Signs of fat-soluble vitamin deficiency such as retinitis pigmentosa are common.

TREATMENT
Standard Therapies: The symptoms of fat malabsorption can be largely eliminated by avoiding fat, particularly long-chain saturated fatty acids, in the diet. A lipid-poor diet permits normal absorption of carbohydrates and proteins and eliminates digestive intolerance. Administration of pharmacologic doses of fat-soluble vitamins is helpful: oral administration of 5–10 mg/day of vitamin K can normalize the prothrombin time. Plasma levels of vitamin A can be increased to the normal range by supplementing 25,000 IU daily or every other day. Vitamin E deficiency can be corrected by feeding 150–200 mg/kg per day of vitamin E.

Investigational Therapies: Gene therapy is being explored.

REFERENCES
Berriot-Varoqueaux N, Aggerbeck LP, Samson-Bouma M, et al. The role of the microsomal triglygeride transfer protein in abetalipoproteinemia. *Ann Rev Nutr* 2000;20:663–697.

Grant CA, Berson EL. Treatable forms of retinitis pigmentosa associated with systemic neurological disorders. *Int Ophthalmol Clin* 2001;41:103–110.

Kane JP, Havel RJ. Disorders of the biogenesis and secretion of lipoproteins containing the B apolipoproteins. In: Scriver CR, Beaudet AL, Sly WS, et al., eds. *The metabolic and molecular bases of inherited disorders.* New York: McGraw-Hill, 1995: 1853–1885.

Triantafillidis JK, Kottaras G, Sgourous S, et al. A-beta-lipoproteinemia: clinical and laboratory features, therapeutic manipulations, and follow-up study of three members of a Greek family. *J Clin Gastroenterol* 1998;26:207–211.

RESOURCES
109, 342, 354

2   Adenoid Cystic Carcinoma

Christopher A. Moskaluk, MD, PhD

DEFINITION: Adenoid cystic carcinoma (ACC) is an uncommon form of malignant neoplasm that arises within secretory glands, most commonly the major and minor salivary glands of the head and neck. Other possible sites of origin include the trachea, lacrimal gland, breast, skin, and vulva. This neoplasm is defined by its distinctive histologic appearance.

DIFFERENTIAL DIAGNOSIS: Benign mixed tumor; Mucoepidermoid carcinoma; Polymorphous low-grade adenocarcinoma; Basaloid squamous carcinoma.

SYMPTOMS AND SIGNS: Symptoms and signs depend largely on the site of origin of the tumor. Early lesions of the salivary glands manifest as painless masses of the mouth or face, usually growing slowly. Advanced tumors may manifest with pain and/or nerve paralysis, for this neoplasm has a propensity to invade peripheral nerves. Tumors of the lacrimal gland may manifest with proptosis and changes in vision. Adenoid cystic carcinoma arising in the tracheobronchial tree may manifest with respiratory symptoms, whereas tumors arising in the larynx may lead to changes in speech.

ETIOLOGY/EPIDEMIOLOGY: Most individuals are diagnosed with the disease in the fourth through sixth decades of life, but a wide age range has been reported, including pediatric cases. The female:male ratio is approximately 3:2. No strong genetic or environmental risk factors have been identified. Damage to the DNA genome occurs in the development of ACC, as it does in all cancers studied to date. Various studies have shown chromosomal abnormalities and genetic deletions occurring in samples of ACC. Some evidence exists that the p53 tumor suppressor gene is inactivated in advanced and aggressive forms of this neoplasm. Otherwise, the specific molecular abnormalities that underlie this disease process are unknown.

DIAGNOSIS: The diagnosis is made by histologic analysis of a biopsy or resection specimen of a tumor mass. The three major variant histologic growth patterns of ACC are cribriform, tubular, and solid. The solid pattern is associated with a more aggressive disease course. No serum markers exist for this neoplasm. Recurrences are usually identified by radiographic imaging techniques, such as CT.

TREATMENT
Standard Therapies: Surgical resection, whenever possible, is the mainstay therapy. Many centers advocate postoperative radiotherapy to help limit local failure. A few specialized centers offer neutron beam therapy, which may be more effective. No chemotherapy is effective for metastatic and/or unresectable ACC, although some patients may receive palliation.

Investigational Therapies: The effects of relatively new chemotherapeutic drugs (paclitaxel, gemcitabine), alone or in combination with other drugs, in the control of metastatic or locally recurrent ACC are being studied.

REFERENCES
Ellis G, Auclair P. *Tumors of the salivary glands,* 3rd ed. Fascicle 17. Washington, DC: Armed Forces Institute of Pathology, 1996.
Fordice J, Kershaw C, el-Naggar A, et al. Adenoid cystic carcinoma of the head and neck. Predictors of morbidity and mortality. *Arch Otolaryngol Head Neck Surg* 1999;125:149–152.
Spiers A, Esseltine D, Ruckdeschel J, et al. Metastatic adenoid cystic carcinoma of salivary glands: case reports and review of the literature. *Cancer Control* 1996;3:336–342.

RESOURCES
10, 83, 379

3   Congenital Afibrinogenemia

Marguerite Neerman-Arbez, PhD

DEFINITION: Congenital afibrinogenemia, the most severe form of fibrinogen deficiency, is characterized by the complete absence of fibrinogen.

DIFFERENTIAL DIAGNOSIS: Hypofibrinogenemia; Dysfibrinogenemia; Hypodysfibrinogenemia.

SYMPTOMS AND SIGNS: Umbilical cord hemorrhage is often the first sign of the disorder; gum bleeding, epistaxis, menorrhagia, gastrointestinal bleeding, and hemarthrosis occur with varying intensity, and spontaneous intracerebral bleeding and splenic rupture can occur as well.

ETIOLOGY/EPIDEMIOLOGY: Congenital afibrinogenemia is inherited in an autosomal-recessive manner and has an estimated prevalence of approximately 1 to 2 in 1 million. As with other autosomal-recessive diseases, the condition is clinically significant only when two alleles are mutated, in homozygosity or compound heterozygosity; both sexes are affected. The disease is caused by mutations in either of the three fibronogen genes, *FGG, FGA,* or *FGB*, clustered on the long arm of human chromosome 4 (region 4q28-31). Many families with this disorder have been studied, allowing the identification of numerous causative mutations; researchers have found that most cases are due to null mutations in the *FGA* gene (>80% of patients studied).

DIAGNOSIS: The diagnosis is made following measurement of fibrinogen levels in patient plasma using standard laboratory analyses such as Clauss (clottable fibrinogen) and radial immunodiffusion, rocket immunoelectrophoresis, and nephelometry. Because the disease locus is known, precise moleclar diagnosis at the DNA level can be made, as can prenatal diagnosis.

TREATMENT
Standard Therapies: Treatment consists of plasma-derived fibrinogen preparations administered either prophylactically (every 2–4 weeks) or on demand, e.g., after trauma or before surgery.

REFERENCES
Lak M, Keihani M, Elahi F, et al. Bleeding and thrombosis in 55 patients with inherited afibrinogenaemia. *Br J Haematol* 1999;107:204–206.
Neerman-Arbez M. State of the art: the molecular basis of inherited afibrinogenaemia. *Thromb Haemost* 2001;86:154–163.
Neerman-Arbez M, Honsberger A, Antonarakis SE, et al. Deletion of the fibrinogen alpha-chain gene (*FGA*) causes congenital afibrinogenemia. *J Clin Invest* 1999;103:215–218.
Online Mendelian Inheritance in Man: *www.ncbi.nlm.nih.gov/omim/*.
Rabe F, Salomon E. Ueber-faserstoffmangel im Blute bei einem Falle von Hämophilie. *Arch Intern Med* 1920;95:2–14.

RESOURCES
302, 357

4 X-Linked Agammaglobulinemia

Roger H. Kobayashi, MD

DEFINITION: X-linked agammaglobulinemia is a chromosomal disorder restricted to B lymphocytes, characterized by recurrent sinopulmonary and gastrointestinal infections within the first 2 years of life.

SYNONYM: Bruton agammaglobulinemia.

DIFFERENTIAL DIAGNOSIS: AIDS; Hyper-IgM syndrome; CVID.

SYMPTOMS AND SIGNS: Children with X-linked agammaglobulinemia typically present within the first year of life with respiratory tract infections caused by encapsulated pyogenic bacteria, e.g., *Streptococcus pneumonia* and *Haemophilus influenzae*. Gastrointestinal infections are also common. These infections are persistent despite appropriate therapy, occur in multiple locations, and are unusually severe. Skin infections (pyoderma) and systemic infections (sepsis, meningitis, septic arthritis) are less common. Complications are not associated with viral infections except with enteroviral infections, which may cause chronic meningoencephalitis, dermatomyositis-like syndrome, or hepatitis. Occasionally, patients may have septic arthritis or chronic arthritis. No striking characteristics are apparent on physical examination except for the paucity of lymphoid tissue, i.e., markedly hypoplastic tonsils and lymph nodes.

ETIOLOGY/EPIDEMIOLOGY: Mutations of the B cell–specific tyrosine kinase *Btk* gene, located on the long arm of X chromosome at Xq22, result in developmental arrest of B-cell maturation and function. Only males are affected and more than 1,000 cases have been reported or are known to exist. Carrier detection is available.

DIAGNOSIS: Quantitative immunoglobulin levels (IgG, IgM, IgA) are markedly decreased. IgG levels are typically below 100 mg/dL, but rarely may be as high as 300 mg/dL.

Characteristically, there is a failure to produce functional antibodies. Natural antibodies such as isohemagglutinins are reduced or absent, as are antibody responses to childhood vaccines such as tetanus, diphtheria, *H. influenzae* type B, or *Pneumococcus*. B-lymphocytes and plasma cells are absent in peripheral blood and tissues. Lymphocyte subsets as determined by monoclonal antibody staining (anti-CD19, anti-CD20) are diminished. *Btk* gene analysis is diagnostic. The latter two tests may also be used in the neonatal period or in the months shortly thereafter for diagnosis at a time when maternally acquired antibodies may obscure immunoglobulin levels.

TREATMENT

Standard Therapies: Replacement of immunoglobulin is mandatory. Immune globulin is given intravenously or, less commonly, by slow, subcutaneous infusion. Intramuscular gammaglobulin is rarely used because of the difficulty in achieving high serum IgG levels and the discomfort associated with it. Appropriate institution of antibiotics is important and prevents complications. Live viral vaccines (especially polio vaccine) are contraindicated.

Investigational Therapies: Various pharmaceutical companies are conducting B-cell growth or activation studies.

REFERENCES

Buckley RH, Schiff R. The use of intravenous gammaglobulin in immunodeficiency diseases. *N Engl J Med* 1991;325:110–117.

Huston DP, ed. Diagnostic laboratory immunology. *Immunol Allergy Clin North Am* 1994;14:199–481.

Lederman HM, Weinkelstein JA. X-linked agammaglobulinemia: an analysis of 96 patients. *Medicine* 1985;64:145–156.

Rosen FS, Cooper MD, Wedgwood RJ. The primary immunodeficiencies. *N Engl J Med* 1984;310:235–242, 300–310.

Stiehm ER, ed. *Immunologic disorders in infants and children,* 4th ed. Philadelphia: WB Saunders, 1996:1084.

RESOURCES

193, 218, 359

5   Acquired Agranulocytosis

Yoriko Saito, MD

DEFINITION: Acquired agranulocytosis encompasses a large group of acquired conditions characterized by a decreased peripheral granulocyte count with an absolute neutrophil count (ANC) of less than 1,500/mm³.

SYNONYM: Acquired or secondary neutropenia.

DIFFERENTIAL DIAGNOSIS: Aplastic anemia; Hypocellular form of myelodysplastic syndrome; Preleukemia/leukemia; Fanconi anemia; Paroxysmal nocturnal hemoglobinuria; Ethnic/benign familial neutropenia; Kostmann syndrome/infantile agranulocytosis; Myelokathexis/neutropenia with tetraploid nuclei; Cyclic neutropenia; Schwachman-Diamond-Oski syndrome; Chediak-Higashi syndrome; Reticular dysgenesis; Dyskeratosis congenital.

SYMPTOMS AND SIGNS: The range of presentation is varied, from patients who are completely asymptomatic to patients who have recurrent and severe systemic infections. Patients with neutropenia associated with marrow failure or exhaustion caused by bone marrow transplantation, cancer chemotherapy, or other medications, and with pure white cell aplasia, are at high risk for overwhelming bacterial sepsis. The types of infections in neutropenic patients depend on the degree and chronicity of the neutropenia as well as the nature of the associated diseases. Patients receiving suppressive chemotherapy are particularly at risk for bacterial sepsis and fungal infections. Viral and parasitic infections are less commonly found unless dysfunction of cell-mediated immunity is coexistent, such as in AIDS. Patients with less severe chronic neutropenia may present with recurrent sinusitis, stomatitis, perirectal infection, or gingivitis, usually without systemic septic manifestations.

ETIOLOGY/EPIDEMIOLOGY: Acquired agranulocytosis can present in any age group and in both sexes (Table 9.1). The overall annual risk for agranulocytosis is 3.4 per 1 million in an ambulatory population from Israel, Europe, and the northeast United States, with approximately 72% of all cases in the United States attributed to medications (Table 9.2).

DIAGNOSIS: In an asymptomatic patient, close observation for several weeks is appropriate, particularly in young children, where the most common neutropenias are benign. A detailed history of medication use must be taken.

TABLE 9.1	Etiologies of Acquired Agranulocytosis
Peripheral destruction of neutrophils	■ Autoimmune neutropenia associated with systemic lupus erythematosus, rheumatoid arthritis/Felty, Sjögren, Graves, lymphoproliferative disease ■ Cold antibodies (infectious mononucleosis, *M. pneumoniae*) ■ Isoimmune neonatal neutropenia ■ Chronic benign neutropenia and chronic benign neutropenia of infancy and childhood (immune-mediated)
Bone marrow suppression/ ineffective hematopoiesis	■ Nutritional deficiency (folate, B_{12}, copper) ■ Pure white cell aplasia associated with thymoma ■ Neutropenia in infants of hypertensive mothers
Peripheral margination of neutrophils	■ Neutrophil activation by means of complement in hemodialysis, membrane oxygenators, burns, transfusion-related acute lung injury (TRALI)
Multifactorial	■ Drug-induced ■ Associated with viral (varicella, measles, rubella, hepatitis A/B, infectious mononucleosis, influenza, cytomegalovirus, parvovirus B19, Kawasaki), bacterial and other infections (*S. aureus*, brucellosis, rickettsia, *M. tuberculosis*) ■ Systemic sepsis ■ HIV/AIDS ■ Bone marrow transplantation ■ Graft-versus-host disease

The presence of recurrent infections suggests more significant neutropenia and may warrant a bone marrow examination. If neutropenia is persistent after several weeks of observation, a search for underlying disorders such as autoimmune diseases or lymphoproliferative disease may be considered.

TREATMENT

Standard Therapies: The major goal of therapy is the management of infectious complications (empiric broad-coverage antibiotics for patients with chemotherapy or other drug-induced or severe infection-associated neutropenia, and management of recurrent nonsystemic infections in less severe chronic neutropenia). All patients with chronic neutropenia should receive routine preventive dental care. Corticosteroids and intravenous IgG have been effective in some cases of immune-mediated neutropenia. Recombinant granulocyte colony-stimulating factor has been shown to correct neutropenia in cyclic neutropenia, severe infantile agranulocytosis, and AIDS-associated neu-

TABLE 9.2	Medications Implicated in Acquired Agranulocytosis

- Marrow-suppressive chemotherapeutic agents
- Dipyrone
- Mianserin
- Sulfasalazine
- Cotrimoxazole
- Antiarrhythmic agents (procainamide, tocanamide, amiodarone, aprindine)
- Digoxin
- Dipyridamole
- Propranolol
- Benzodiazepines
- Barbiturates
- Gold compounds
- Penicillins (amoxycillin, benzylpenicillin, azlocillin, phenethicillin, cloxacillin)

- Thiouracil derivatives (methythiouracil, propylthiouracil)
- Phenylbutazone
- Cimetidine, ranitidine
- Penicillamine
- Diclofenac
- Carbamazepine
- Angiotensin-converting enzyme inhibitors (captopril, enalapril)
- Hydrochlorothiazide with potassium-sparing diuretic
- Indomethacin
- Cephalosporins (cephalexin, cephazolin, cefuroxime, cefitaxime, cephradine)
- Oxyphenbutazone
- Nitrofurantoin
- Salicylic acid derivatives

- Clozapine
- Carbimazole
- Sulfonylurea derivatives (tolbutamide, glibenclamide)
- Methyldopa
- Thiamazole
- Aminoglutethimide
- Ibuprofen
- Pentazocine
- Levamisole
- Promethazine
- Chloramphenicol
- Paracetamol and combination preparations
- Perazine
- Mebhydrolin
- Imipramine

tropenia. Granulocyte transfusions may be used in neutropenic patients with life-threatening bacterial and fungal infections after a trial of conventional therapies. Although the definitive therapy for drug-induced neutropenia is the withdrawal of the offending drug, this is not always practical. When there is no therapeutic alternative, a patient without infectious complications and ANC greater than 500–700/mm^3 may be maintained on the putative causative medication with close observation.

Investigational Therapies: Several cytokines and chemokines are being explored.

REFERENCES

Dale DC. Immune and idiopathic neutropenia. *Curr Opin Hematol* 1998;5:33.

Evans RH, Scadden DT. Haematological aspects of HIV infection. *Clin Haematol* 2000;13:215.

Sievers EL, Dale DC. Non-malignant neutropenia. *Blood Rev* 1996;10:95.

van der Klauw MM, Wilson JH, Stricker BH. Drug-associated agranulocytosis: 20 years of reporting in the Netherlands (1974–1994). *Am J Hematol* 1998;57:206.

RESOURCES
318, 343, 357

6   Ameloblastoma

Barry Steinberg, MD, DDS, PhD, and Mary Stavropoulos, DDS

DEFINITION: Ameloblastomas are tumors that are derived from odontogenic epithelium. They are primarily found in the jawbones but, in rare (1%) cases, they can be found peripherally. Those located in the jawbones can be unicystic but more commonly are solid or multicystic. The unicystic lesions are seen in a younger age group, with most appearing within the first two decades of life. The more common multicystic ameloblastoma occurs in a wider range of ages.

DIFFERENTIAL DIAGNOSIS: Myxomas; Keratocysts; Hemangiomas; Aneurysmal bone cysts; Giant cell lesions, calcifying; Epithelial odontogenic tumors; Ameloblastomic fibromas.

SYMPTOMS AND SIGNS: The clinical findings are non-specific. The patient may present with swelling. Rarely, there may be nasal obstruction with tumors involving the maxilla. Pain and neurologic changes would be atypical findings. Ameloblastomas are slow growing and locally invasive. Often, they are present as fortuitous findings on routine dental examinations and/or radiographs; however, sometimes they are missed or neglected and the patient presents later with massive swelling. Radiographically, ameloblastomas can be seen as unilocular and, more often, multilocular radioluscencies. The latter is often described as having a "soap bubble" appearance. Roots of adjacent teeth may be resorbed and the borders of the lesion can be irregular.

ETIOLOGY/EPIDEMIOLOGY: Ameloblastoma has no gender or ethnic predilection. The cells may be derived from the dental lamina, lining of odontogenic cysts, cell rests of the enamel organ, or from oral mucosal basal cells. No genetic or environmental influences on the development of these lesions are known.

DIAGNOSIS: Diagnosis is made by biopsy and histologic evaluation of the suspected lesion. CT scans are helpful in delineating the size and location of the tumor and in treatment planning.

TREATMENT
Standard Therapies: Treatment is surgical. The procedure depends on whether the lesion is unicystic or multicystic. The rarer unicystic ameloblastoma has a much lower recurrence rate compared with the multicystic form and can be treated by enucleation (removal of tumor) followed by curettage of surrounding bone. Multicystic lesions have a much higher recurrence rate and may require more aggressive excisions. Other factors that impact on surgical planning include anatomic location, patient age, and degree of cortical bone loss. The inferior border of the mandible should be preserved if at all possible. Children who will have adequate follow-up may be treated less aggressively. Lesions of the posterior maxilla and mandible should be treated more radically because recurrence into the adjacent soft tissue in these regions makes definitive therapy of the recurrence a challenge. In general, multicystic ameloblastomas are resected with wide margins, giving consideration to the patient's age and potential resulting deformity. Chemotherapy and radiation therapies have little role in the management of ameloblastomas. Reconstruction (particularly of larger mandibular defects) can be done with

bone grafts. Some surgeons may elect to do this at the time of resection.

REFERENCES

Feinberg SE, Steinberg B. Surgical management of ameloblastoma: current status and review of the literature. *Oral Surg Oral Med Oral Pathol Oral Radiol* 1996;81:383–388.

Posnick JC. Clinically aggressive (locally persistent) nonmetastasizing and premalignant head and neck tumors of childhood. In: Posnick JC, ed. *Craniofacial and maxillofacial surgery in children and young adults.* Philadelphia: WB Saunders, 2000: 678–682.

Waldron CA. Odontogenic cysts and tumors. In: Neville BW, Damm DD, Allen CM, et al., eds. *Oral and maxillofacial pathology.* Philadelphia: WB Saunders, 1995:512–520.

Williams TP. Management of ameloblastoma: a changing perspective. *J Oral Maxillofac Surg* 1993;51:1064–1070.

RESOURCES

30, 373

7 Acquired Aplastic Anemia

Neal Young, MD

DEFINITION: Acquired aplastic anemia is a bone marrow failure syndrome defined by pancytopenia with a very fatty, even empty, bone marrow.

DIFFERENTIAL DIAGNOSIS: Fanconi anemia (constitutional aplastic anemia); Myelodysplasia; Rare variants of leukemia; Myelofibrosis.

SYMPTOMS AND SIGNS: Symptoms are due to anemia, leukopenia, and thrombocytopenia. Most patients present with complaints secondary to bleeding or oxygen deprivation. Thrombocytopenia typically results in mucocutaneous hemorrhage manifested as petechiae, epistaxis, gingival oozing, and menorrhagia. Cardiovascular symptoms may predominate in the older, severely anemic patient, but more frequent are fatigue, lassitude, and shortness of breath. Infection is rare, but serious bacterial infections and ultimately progressive fungal disease are the most serious complications of pancytopenia. Physical examination is remarkable only for ecchymoses, petechiae, and pallor. Lymphadenopathy and splenomegaly are not present.

ETIOLOGY/EPIDEMIOLOGY: Most patients are older children, adolescents, or young adults. There is no gender preference. Aplastic anemia has an incidence of 2 in 1 million in Europe and Israel, but the rate is two- to threefold higher in Asia and probably other parts of the developing world, for reasons that are unclear.

DIAGNOSIS: Pancytopenia in an otherwise healthy young person suggests aplastic anemia. A bone marrow biopsy is required to establish acellularity; leukemia and other invasive processes can be excluded on the aspirate smear. The prognosis is determined quantitatively by the degree of pancytopenia; patients with <200 neutrophils/mL have an especially poor prognosis.

TREATMENT

Standard Therapies: Most aplastic anemia probably results from immunologic (autoimmune) destruction of hematopoietic cells by T-lymphocytes. Effective therapy is provided either by hematopoietic stem cell transplantation or immunosuppression. Bone marrow transplantation from a histocompatible sibling is the treatment of choice in children and younger patients, especially if neutropenia is severe. For most other patients, immunosuppression and bone marrow transplantation provide roughly equivalent outcomes. Immunosuppression is usually a combination of antithymocyte globulin with cyclosporine. The 5-year survival rate for severe aplastic anemia treated with either stem transplantation or immunosuppression is 70%–80%. In aplastic anemia, hematopoietic growth factors or corticosteroids are not indicated and may be dangerous. Transfusion therapy and the treatment of severe infections is best managed by hematology or oncology specialists.

REFERENCES

Ball SE. The modern management of severe aplastic anaemia. *Br J Haematol* 2000;110:41–53.

Young NS. Acquired aplastic anemia. In: Young NS, ed. *Bone marrow failure syndromes.* Philadelphia: WB Saunders, 2000:1–46.

Young NS, Alter BP, eds. *Aplastic anemia acquired and inherited.* Philadelphia: WB Saunders, 1993.

RESOURCES

50, 356

8 Diamond-Blackfan Anemia

Blanche P. Alter, MD, MPH

DEFINITION: Diamond-Blackfan anemia (DBA) is congenital pure red cell aplasia.

SYNONYMS: Blackfan-Diamond anemia; Congenital hypoplastic anemia; Chronic congenital aregenerative anemia; Hereditary red cell aplasia; Congenital erythroid hypoplasia; Erythrogenesis imperfecta; Chronic idiopathic erythroblastopenia with aplastic anemia (type Josephs-Diamond-Blackfan); Aase syndrome.

DIFFERENTIAL DIAGNOSIS: Acquired pure red cell aplasia; Transient erythroblastopenia of childhood (TEC); Parvovirus B19 infection; Fanconi anemia; Aplastic anemia; Autoimmune hemolytic anemia.

SYMPTOMS AND SIGNS: Pallor, lassitude, and even congestive heart failure may occur, due to severe anemia. Approximately 30% of patients are diagnosed in the first 3 months of life, 90% in the first year. One third have physical anomalies, such as abnormal thumbs, characteristic facies, or short neck; short stature is common. A substantial risk exists for the development of myelodysplastic syndrome or acute myeloid leukemia, as well as selected solid tumors such as osteosarcomas.

ETIOLOGY/EPIDEMIOLOGY: There are at least three different gene loci for DBA. Approximately 20% have mutations at 19q13 in RPS19, which are inherited in an autosomal dominant manner. The molecular mechanism is not known. Males and females are affected equally, and all racial and ethnic groups have been reported. Diamond-Blackfan anemia is estimated to occur in 5 to 10 per 1million live births.

DIAGNOSIS: Patients with DBA have a macrocytic anemia, with reticulocytopenia and marrow erythroblastopenia. White blood cells and platelets are usually normal. Bone marrow examination distinguishes the red cell underproduction in this condition from erythroid hyperplasia in hemolytic anemias. Erythroid vacuoles and nuclear inclusions suggest parvovirus. Red cell adenosine deaminase is elevated in most patients.

TREATMENT

Standard Therapies: More than half of patients respond to treatment with prednisone. Patients who do not respond to steroids can be transfused with leukocyte-depleted, irradiated, packed red blood cells. Iron overload requires chelation with parenteral desferrioxamine. Remissions occur in approximately 25% of patients, both prednisone-responsive and those solely transfused. Stem cell transplant (with bone marrow or cord blood) is an option for patients with an HLA-matched sibling donor.

Investigational Therapies: Researchers are investigating stem cell transplant for DBA from alternative donors.

REFERENCES
Alter BP, Young NS. The bone marrow failure syndromes. In: Nathan DG, Orkin SH, eds. *Nathan and Oski's hematology of infancy and childhood*, 5th ed. Philadelphia: WB Saunders, 1998:237–335.

Draptchinskaia N, Gustavsson P, Andersson B, et al. The gene encoding ribosomal protein S19 is mutated in Diamond-Blackfan anaemia. *Nat Genet* 1999;21:169–175.

McKusick VA, ed. Online Mendelian Inheritance in Man (OMIM). Baltimore, MD: The Johns Hopkins University. Entry no. 205900; last update 7/27/2000.

Willig TN, Niemeyer CM, Leblanc T, et al. Identification of new prognosis factors from the clinical and epidemiologic analysis of a registry of 229 Diamond-Blackfan anemia patients. *Pediatr Res* 1999;46:553–561.

Willig TN, Perignon JL, Gustavsson P, et al. High adenosine deaminase level among healthy probands of Diamond Blackfan anemia (DBA) cosegregates with the DBA gene region on chromosome 19q13. *Blood* 1998;92:4422–4427.

RESOURCES
133, 134, 356

9 Fanconi Anemia

Blanche P. Alter, MD, MPH

DEFINITION: Fanconi anemia (FA) is an inherited auto-somal-recessive disorder with a high frequency of aplastic anemia, often associated with characteristic birth defects.

SYNONYMS: Estren-Dameshek anemia; Constitutional aplastic anemia type I and II; Fanconi pancytopenia; Aplastic anemia with congenital anomalies; Congenital pancytopenia.

DIFFERENTIAL DIAGNOSIS: Acquired aplastic anemia; Dyskeratosis congenital; Amegakaryocytic thrombocytopenia; Thrombocytopenia absent radii; Bloom syndrome; Seckel syndrome; Dubowitz syndrome.

SIGNS AND SYMPTOMS: Bruising, pallor, or infection may be the first signs of bone marrow failure. Hematologic changes such as thrombocytopenia, followed by macrocytic anemia and neutropenia, occur at a median age of 6.5 years in males and 8 years in females. Approximately 75% of patients with FA have birth defects, including short stature, café-au-lait spots and hyper- or hypopigmentation, abnormal thumbs and radial rays, structural renal anomalies, microcephaly, microphthalmia, hearing defects, and others. There is a high risk of development of myelodysplastic syndrome and acute myeloid leukemia, as well as specific solid tumors (particularly oropharyngeal, esophageal, vuland cervical, and liver neoplasias).

ETIOLOGY/EPIDEMIOLOGY: Inheritance is autosomal recessive. At least seven complementation groups have been identified, with six genes mapped and cloned. Affected patients are homozygotes or double heterozygotes for mutations of FA genes in the same complementation group. The heterozygote frequency ranges from approximately 1 in 100 to 1 in 300, depending on the population, with the expected number of new cases estimated to be 1 in 40,000 to 1 in 360,000 live births. The male:female ratio is 1.2:1 in the more than 1,000 cases reported in the literature. All racial and ethnic groups have been reported.

DIAGNOSIS: Cytopenias in a child with characteristic morphologic abnormalities strongly suggest the diagnosis, but patients with FA are definitively diagnosed by the presence of increased chromosome breaks and rearrangements in peripheral blood T-lymphocytes cultured with DNA cross-linking agents such as diepoxybutane or mitomycin C (MMC), and/or by increased numbers of cells arrested in cell cycle at G2/M. Genotyping may be done with retroviral transduction of cells with candidate genes, with the end point of the assay being correction of sensitivity to MMC. Within complementation groups, common mutations are investigated first, followed by complete sequencing as needed. Complete assessment of the hematologic status requires blood counts, bone marrow examinations, and marrow cytogenetics.

TREATMENT

Standard Therapies: The management of FA requires a multidisciplinary team of subspecialists, including hand surgeons, nephrologists, urologists, gastroenterologists, and endocrinologists. Treatment is indicated when the patient's platelet count is <30,000/mm³, hemoglobin <8 g/dL, and/or neutrophils <500/mm³. Hematopoietic stem cell (bone marrow, cord blood, or peripheral blood) transplantation is recommended if there is an HLA-matched sibling donor. Medical treatment of anemia (with some effect on platelets) consists of androgens (usually oxymetholone) with or without prednisone, and/or granulocyte colony-stimulating factor specifically for neutropenia. Supportive care includes transfusion of leukocyte-depleted, irradiated, packed red blood cells or platelets and antibiotics. Hand surgery can be performed to correct thumb abnormalities.

Investigational Therapies: Alternative donor transplantation is high risk and reserved for patients with acute leukemia, clinical myelodysplastic syndrome, or refractory aplastic anemia. Improved stem cell transplantations are being evaluated, and gene therapy trials are being developed. Researchers are also studying genotype/phenotype and predictors of leukemia and solid tumors.

REFERENCES
Alter BP, Young NS. The bone marrow failure syndromes. In: Nathan DG, Orkin SH, eds. *Nathan and Oski's hematology of infancy and childhood,* 5th ed. Philadelphia: WB Saunders, 1998:237–335.

D'Andrea AD, Grompe M. Molecular biology of Fanconi anemia: implications for diagnosis and therapy. *Blood* 1997;90:1725–1736.

Joenje H, Levitus M, Waisfisz Q, et al. Complementation analysis in Fanconi anemia: assignment of the reference FA-H patient to group A. *Am J Hum Genet* 2000;67:759–762.

McKusick VA, ed. Online Mendelian Inheritance in Man (OMIM). Baltimore MD: The Johns Hopkins University. Entry no. 227650; last update 9/25/2000.

RESOURCES
201, 356

10   Autoimmune Hemolytic Anemias

Lawrence D. Petz, MD

DEFINITION: Autoimmune hemolytic anemias (AIHA) are a group of disorders characterized by anemia resulting from a shortened red blood cell lifespan that is caused by autoantibodies. Autoimmune hemolytic anemias are divided into three categories depending on the characteristics of the autoantibodies: warm antibody AIHA, cold agglutinin syndrome, and paroxysmal cold hemoglobinuria.

DIFFERENTIAL DIAGNOSIS: Iron deficiency anemia; Aplastic anemia; Anemia of chronic disease; Megaloblastic anemia; Anemia associated with marrow infiltration; Thalassemia; Hemoglobinopathies; Enzyme deficiencies; Paroxysmal nocturnal hemoglobinuria; Microangiopathic hemolytic anemia.

SYMPTOMS AND SIGNS: Individuals with anemia of any cause may have fatigue, shortness of breath, and palpitations. Clinical manifestations of hemolytic anemia are pallor, jaundice, and splenomegaly. In individuals with mild anemia, these findings may be absent and, in such cases, diagnosis is dependent on laboratory findings.

ETIOLOGY/EPIDEMIOLOGY: Autoimmune hemolytic anemia is likely caused by a breakdown in the mechanisms that normally prevent an individual from forming antibodies against his or her own normal tissues. How this happens is unknown, and probably varies among the various types of AIHA. The prevalence of AIHA of all categories is about 1 in 25,000 individuals overall, and 1 in 41,000 for the warm antibody type. There is a general increase in incidence throughout life, with a significant rise occurring in individuals older than 50 years. The disorder is more common in females, with a male:female ratio of about 1:1.3.

DIAGNOSIS: The patient's history and physical examination may suggest a hemolytic anemia, but usually the manifestations are nonspecific and the diagnostic workup involves a laboratory evaluation of anemia. Laboratory indications of hemolysis are sought by tests that yield evidence of increased hemoglobin breakdown and of bone marrow regeneration. A positive direct antiglobulin test indicates that the hemolysis is caused by autoantibodies. Determining the characteristics of antibodies in the patient's serum by specialized laboratories distinguishes between warm antibody AIHA, cold agglutinin syndrome, and paroxysmal cold hemoglobinuria.

TREATMENT

Standard Therapies: The initial therapy for patients with autoimmune hemolytic anemia of warm antibody type should be corticosteroids. If remission cannot be maintained on low doses, alternative treatment is indicated because of the side effects of long-term corticosteroid treatment. Splenectomy should be considered in patients who do not respond to corticosteroids because it has the potential for complete and long-term remission. A syndrome of overwhelming postsplenectomy infection (OPSI) may occur, however, which has high morbidity and mortality. Other therapies that have been used with modest success are high-dose intravenous immunoglobulin, plasma exchange, danazol, and immunosuppressive drugs such as azathioprine, cyclophosphamide, and cyclosporine. Therapy for cold agglutinin disease is generally less effective and consists of avoidance of exposure to severe cold and the use of chlorambucil. Corticosteroids and splenectomy are not as commonly effective as they are in warm antibody AIHA. Plasma exchange offers a modest degree of temporary benefit in some patients with cold agglutinin syndrome. Paroxysmal cold hemoglobinuria generally subsides spontaneously, but is often treated with corticosteroids during an acute hemolytic episode. Transfusions should be provided for all patients when necessary. Transfused red blood cells generally survive as well as the patient's own and provide temporary benefit while other therapy is taking effect.

REFERENCES

Dacie JV. The auto-immune haemolytic anaemias. In: *The haemolytic anaemias,* 3rd ed. London: Churchill Livingstone, 1992. Vol. 3.

Engelfriet CP, Overbeeke MA, dem Borne AE. Autoimmune hemolytic anemia. *Semin Hematol* 1992;29:3–12.

Petz LD. Blood transfusion in hemolytic anemias. *Immunohematology* 1999;15:15–23.

Petz LD, Catlett JP, Lessin LS. Hemolytic anemias. In: Kelly WN, ed. *Textbook of internal medicine.* New York: Lippincott-Raven, 1997:1454–1472.

RESOURCES

27, 357

11 Cold Hemolytic Anemia Syndromes

Kenneth M. Algazy, MD

DEFINITION: Cold hemolytic anemia syndromes are autoimmune disorders caused by antibodies that bind to red blood cells (RBCs) at temperatures less than 37°C. The two major types are based on the type of antibody present: agglutinins and hemolysins (Donath-Landsteiner antibody). Acute cold agglutinin syndrome is more common and accounts for approximately one third of all autoimmune hemolytic anemias. The syndrome of paroxysmal cold hemoglobinuria (PNH) due to hemolysins is rare. Hemolysis from cold-reacting antibodies occurs less commonly than warm antibody–induced hemolysis, but a greater possibility exists of precipitating complement activation, which can induce intravascular red cell destruction.

SYNONYMS: Cold agglutinin disease; Cryopathic hemolytic syndromes.

DIFFERENTIAL DIAGNOSIS: Warm autoimmune hemolytic anemias; Hereditary hemolytic anemias; Paroxysmal nocturnal hemoglobinuria; Hemoglobinopathy-associated hemolytic anemias.

SYMPTOMS AND SIGNS: The patient presents with chronic hemolysis, with or without jaundice, or episodes of acute fulminant hemolysis induced by a decrease in body temperature. The presence of cold-reacting hemolysis should be suspected if the patient develops acrocyanosis, skin necrosis (rare), hemolysis, or simply anemia during recovery from an infection. Numbness or occasionally pain may accompany the color changes (Raynaud phenomena), and, rarely, trophic changes and even gangrene of extremities have been reported. Splenomegaly may be present depending on the etiology. Laboratory findings demonstrate anemia, evidence of reticulocytosis, mild indirect hyperbilirubinemia (less than 3.5 mg/dL), hemoglobinemia if intravascular hemolysis, low or absent haptoglobulin levels, and chronic low-grade hemoglobinuria and hemosiderinuria. The cold agglutinin titer may range from 1:1,000 to 1:1,000,000, usually in the range of 1:25,000; the blood bank can demonstrate greater reactivity in the cold. The direct antiglobulin test result will be positive; sometimes, normal donor type-specific RBCs will react more vigorously with the patient's serum because the patient's RBC receptors are already tightly bound with antibody.

ETIOLOGY/EPIDEMIOLOGY: Chronic idiopathic cold agglutinin disease occurs primarily in the elderly, with a peak incidence in the seventh and eighth decades of life. Occasionally, younger adults and even children can develop cold agglutinins. Most cold agglutinins can be identified in the blood bank as IgM with either big I or little i antigen specificity. Malignant clones of lymphoid cells (lymphomatous malignancy) or simply antigenically stimulated B-lymphocytes produce the antibodies. Infectious agents can complex with I/i antigens to cause antibody production. These disorders can also appear as a cold agglutinin disease due to a monoclonal proliferation of B cells or can appear as paroxysmal cold hemoglobinuria secondary to certain viruses in children or syphilis (congenital or tertiary).

TREATMENT

Standard Therapies: Because the antibodies react preferentially in the cold, the hallmark of therapy is to keep the patient warm. Transfusion with cross-matched RBCs should be undertaken only if the patient develops severe anemia and/or the threat of cardiovascular compromise. Neither splenectomy nor the use of steroids is effective therapy for chronic cold agglutinin disease. For severe chronic hemolysis secondary to cold agglutinin disease, chlorambucil or cyclophosphamide has been used to decrease antibody production. In dire circumstances, plasma exchange can be used to remove the offending antibody, as long as the blood as well as the patient can be maintained at 37°C. Treatment with interferon-α may also be useful.

REFERENCE

Beutler E, Lichtman MA, Coller BS, et al., eds. *Williams hematology*, 6th ed. New York: McGraw-Hill, 2000.

RESOURCES

27, 356, 357

12   Congenital Nonspherocytic Hemolytic Anemia

Pamela S. Becker, MD, PhD

DEFINITION: Congenital nonspherocytic hemolytic anemia is a group of inherited hemolytic anemias characterized by early destruction of red blood cells in the circulation due to defects in the red cell enzymes. Of the several types of enzyme deficiencies, the most common is glucose-6-phosphate dehydrogenase (G6PD) deficiency.

SYNONYMS: Congenital hemolytic anemia; Glucose 6-phosphate dehydrogenase deficiency; Pyruvate kinase (PK) deficiency.

DIFFERENTIAL DIAGNOSIS: Hexokinase deficiency; Glucosephosphate isomerase deficiency; Phosphofructose kinase deficiency; Aldolase deficiency; Triosephosphate isomerase deficiency; Pyrimidine nucleotidase deficiency; Adenosine deaminase excess; Glutathione synthetase deficiency; Glutathione reductase deficiency; Acquired hemolytic anemia.

SYMPTOMS AND SIGNS: Most patients with G6PD deficiency have anemia and symptoms only after exposure to certain oxidant drugs or chemicals, but some have variants that have ongoing chronic hemolysis. The other enzyme deficiencies are associated with variable degrees of chronic hemolytic anemia. Symptoms include pallor and fatigue. At times of infection or stress (e.g., pregnancy), the anemia can worsen and be accompanied by jaundice. Severely affected patients may have chronic jaundice. Other symptoms include neonatal jaundice, gallstones by the teenage years, and enlargement of the spleen. Some infections, such as one type of parvovirus, B19, can lead to aplastic crisis, characterized by lack of red cell production and, consequently, profound anemia for a period of approximately 10 days. Signs include pale conjunctivae, icteric sclerae, palpable splenomegaly, and gallstones seen on ultrasonographic examination.

ETIOLOGY/EPIDEMIOLOGY: G6PD deficiency is X-linked recessive, and PK deficiency is autosomal recessive. The pathogenesis of these forms of hemolytic anemia is related to enzyme deficiency related to defects in the glycolytic pathway, the pentose phosphate pathway, nucleotide, or glutathione metabolism. It is the most common disorder of red cell metabolism, affecting more than 200 million people worldwide. The incidence varies among different ethnic groups, affecting 12% of African American males, 35% of those living at low altitude in Sardinia, 20%–32% in lowland Greece, 14% in Cambodia, 5.5% in China, and 2.6% in India. Of the enzyme deficiencies in the glycolytic pathway, the most common is PK deficiency. PK deficiency occurs worldwide, with a prevalence for heterozygosity of approximately 1% in the United States. The gene for G6PD is located on the X chromosome, band Xp28, and the PK gene is located on chromosome 1q21.

DIAGNOSIS: Laboratory evaluation includes a complete blood count, peripheral blood smear, reticulocyte count, serum total and direct bilirubin, and lactate dehydrogenase (LDH). The hemoglobin and hematocrit values are mildly to moderately decreased. The peripheral blood smear may show specific features for certain enzyme deficiencies: for example, bite cells or blister cells for G6PD deficiency, and echinocytes for PK deficiency. The reticulocyte count and index are elevated, as are the indirect bilirubin and LDH. The specific enzyme assays are diagnostic for each disorder. Abdominal ultrasonography demonstrates the presence of gallstones and splenomegaly. After splenectomy, the reticulocyte count in patients with PK deficiency can rise as high as 40%–70%.

TREATMENT

Standard Therapies: The standard treatment is folic acid replacement, so that adequate stores will be available to maintain increased red cell production. Red cell transfusions may be needed for profound anemia during aplastic crisis, or on a chronic basis for the rare, severe forms. For severe neonatal jaundice, exchange transfusion may be required. Splenectomy can greatly ameliorate the symptoms of chronic hemolytic anemia. Cholecystectomy is often required to ameliorate symptoms related to gallstones. Patients with iron overload may also require treatment with chelating agents.

Investigational Therapies: Studies of gene transfer are currently under investigation.

REFERENCES

Luzzatto L, Mehta A. Glucose 6-phosphate dehydrogenase deficiency. In: Scriver CR, Beaudet A, Sly W, et al., eds. *The metabolic and molecular bases of inherited disease,* 7th ed. New York: McGraw-Hill, 1995:3367–3398.

Tanaka KR, Paglia DE. Pyruvate kinase and other enzymopathies of the erythrocyte. In: Scriver CR, Beaudet A, Sly W, et al., eds.

The metabolic and molecular bases of inherited disease, 7th ed. New York: McGraw-Hill, 1995:3485–3511.

RESOURCES

50, 356

13   Hereditary Spherocytic Hemolytic Anemia (Hereditary Spherocytosis)

Pamela S. Becker, MD, PhD

DEFINITION: Hereditary spherocytosis (HS) is an inherited hemolytic anemia characterized by aberrant red cell shape. The cells are more susceptible to damage and have a short survival due to destruction, largely in the spleen.

SYNONYMS: Spherocytosis; Spherocytic hemolytic anemia.

DIFFERENTIAL DIAGNOSIS: Autoimmune hemolytic anemia; Hereditary stomatocytosis; ABO incompatibility in the neonate.

SYMPTOMS AND SIGNS: Symptoms include pallor and fatigue related to anemia. With infection or stress (e.g., pregnancy), the anemia can worsen and can be accompanied by jaundice. Other symptoms include neonatal jaundice, gallstones by the teenage years, and enlargement of the spleen. Some infections, such as one type of parvovirus, B19, can lead to aplastic crisis, characterized by lack of red cell production and, consequently, profound anemia for approximately 10 days, until the red cell production recovers. Signs include pale conjunctivae, icteric sclerae, palpable splenomegaly, and gallstones seen on ultrasonography. Severe forms can be associated with chronic jaundice and transfusion-dependent anemia.

ETIOLOGY/EPIDEMIOLOGY: The typical, common form is autosomal dominant, although there are rare occurrences of autosomal-recessive forms. Pathogenesis is based on red cell membrane loss, leading to reduced membrane surface area and, consequently, conversion of the classic biconcave shape to that of a sphere. Most cases of the autosomal-dominant form are due to ankyrin defects, including point mutations, truncations, and gene deletions. Ankyrin deficiency leads to loss of spectrin; therefore, HS usually has a combined ankyrin and spectrin deficiency. The gene for ankyrin is located on chromosome 8p11.2, for alpha spectrin on chromosome 1q22-q25, for beta spectrin on chromosome 14q23-q24.2, and for protein 4.2 on chromosome 15q15-q21. Autosomal-dominant HS is the most common hemolytic anemia in the Northern European population, with an incidence of approximately 1 in 5,000. It is less common in other races and ethnic groups.

DIAGNOSIS: Laboratory evaluation includes a complete blood count, peripheral blood smear, reticulocyte count, serum total and direct bilirubin, and lactase dehydrogenase (LDH). The hemoglobin and hematocrit values are mildly to moderately decreased, the mean corpuscular volume slightly decreased, and the mean corpuscular hemoglobin concentration slightly elevated. The peripheral blood smear shows variable spherocytes and microspherocytes, as well as polychromatophils and acanthocytes. In the autosomal-recessive form, poikilocytes and schistocytes may also be present. The reticulocyte count and index are elevated, as are the indirect bilirubin and LDH. The definitive assay for spherocytosis is the osmotic fragility test. The test does not distinguish autoimmune hemolytic anemia from hereditary spherocytosis, so a direct and indirect antiglobulin (Coombs) test is necessary to exclude autoimmune hemolytic anemia. Abdominal ultrasonography demonstrates the presence of gallstones and splenomegaly.

TREATMENT

Standard Therapies: The standard treatment is folic acid replacement, so that adequate stores will be available to maintain increased red cell production. Red cell transfusions may be needed for times of profound anemia during aplastic crisis, or on a chronic basis for the severe forms. For severe neonatal jaundice, exchange transfusion may be required. If patients have moderate to severe anemia and/or chronic jaundice, splenectomy will usually nearly eliminate the symptoms of the autosomal-dominant condition and improve the symptoms in the more severe recessive forms. Cholecystectomy is often required to ameliorate the symptoms related to the gallstones.

Investigational Therapies: Subtotal splenectomy and gene transfer are under investigation.

REFERENCES

Becker PS, Lux SE. Hereditary spherocytosis and hereditary elliptocytosis. In: Scriver CR, Beaudet A, Sly W, et al., eds. *The metabolic and molecular bases of inherited disease,* 7th ed. New York: McGraw-Hill, 1995:3513–3560.

Bolton-Maggs PH. The diagnosis and management of hereditary spherocytosis. *Baillieres Best Pract Res Clin Haematol* 2000;13: 327–342.

Gallagher PG, Forget BG. Hematologically important mutations: spectrin and ankyrin variants in hereditary spherocytosis. *Blood Cells Mol Dis* 1998;24:539–543.

RESOURCES

27, 356

---

14 Warm Antibody Hemolytic Anemia

Lawrence D. Petz, MD

DEFINITION: Warm-reactive autoimmune hemolytic anemia (AIHA) due to IgM antibodies is a form of autoimmune hemolytic anemia caused by IgM autoantibodies directed against red cell membrane antigens with maximal activity at 37 °C (warm-reactive).

SYNONYMS: Warm autoimmune hemolytic anemia secondary to IgM autoantibodies; Warm-reactive AIHA secondary to IgM.

DIFFERENTIAL DIAGNOSIS: Cold agglutinin disease or AIHA due to cold-reactive IgM; Autoimmune hemolytic anemia due to IgG; Hereditary spherocytosis; Clostridial sepsis; Early stages of Wilson disease; Hyperlipoproteinemic liver disease.

SYMPTOMS AND SIGNS: Patients present with pallor and anemia secondary to red blood cell hemolysis. Hemoglobinuria, hemoglobinemia, and occasionally icterus develop if hemolysis is brisk. Patients with high titer, complete warm-reactive AIHA from IgM antibodies have clinical features related to *in vivo* agglutination. Severe red blood cell agglutination can compromise perfusion diffusely and lead to infarction involving virtually any organ. For example, patients may have skin mottling, painful acrocyanosis, and skin necrosis that results from red cell agglutination in the cutaneous capillaries. Hemodynamic decompensation occurs with hemagglutination in the pulmonary vascular bed and heart. Symptoms may mimic a pulmonary embolism. Infarction and ultimately tissue necrosis may also involve the brain, kidney, or liver.

ETIOLOGY/EPIDIMIOLOGY: Autoimmune hemolytic anemia is caused by autoantibodies directed against red blood cell membranes. In adults, AIHA is often associated with an underlying autoimmune disease, such as systemic lupus erythematosis. Most commonly, AIHA occurs in middle-aged and older individuals, with a peak incidence at 50 years. Most cases of AIHA can be separated into two groups based on thermal amplitude. The annual incidence of AIHA is estimated to be 1 in 80,000 persons, although most of these cases are IgG-mediated warm-reactive AIHA or, less commonly, IgM-mediated cold-reactive AIHA. In unusual cases, AIHA is caused by warm-reactive IgM autoantibodies.

DIAGNOSIS: For most cases of AIHA, the direct antiglobulin test or Coombs test is diagnostic, although the red cell agglutination in warm-reactive, IgM-mediated AIHA may preclude testing with the Coombs reagent. To define the antibody, further serologic studies are required. A reducing agent that inactivates IgM by breaking disulfide bonds but does not affect IgG antibodies, DTT, can be used to distinguish IgM from IgG antibodies. Radioimmune antiglobulin test can also be used to determine if antibody is bound to the red cell membrane. To define the red cell antigen recognized by the antibody, patient serum can be reacted with high-frequency, antigen-negative red cells. Thermal amplitude studies are used to define the optimal binding temperature of the antibody.

TREATMENT

Standard Therapies: Therapy has included supportive measures with packed red blood cell transfusions. If patients have hemodynamic instability and respiratory failure, pressor support and mechanical ventilation may be necessary. In an effort to limit the antibody, immunosuppressive therapies have been tried, including cytoxan, mycophenolate, and cyclosporine A. Red cell exchanges, plasmapheresis, and erythrocytopheresis have been used to remove circulating antibodies. Corticosteroid therapy is typically initiated to decrease the antibody production. Although aggressive immunosuppressive therapy has been used, all previously reported cases of high-titer, complete, warm-reactive, IgM-mediated AIHA have been fatal.

Investigational Therapies: Treatment with Rituximab may be beneficial, but further studies are needed.

REFERENCES

Friedmann AM, King K, Shirey S, et al. Fatal autoimmune hemolytic anemia in a child due to warm-reactive IgM. *J Pediatr Hematol Oncol* 1998;20:502–505.

McCann EL, Shirey RS, Kickler TS, et al. IgM autoagglutinins in warm autoimmune hemolytic anemia: a poor prognostic feature. *Acta Haematol* 1992;88:120–125.

Salama A, Mueller-Eckhardt C. Autoimmune haemolytic anaemia in childhood associated with non-compliment binding IgM atoantibodies. *Br J Haematol* 1987;65:67–71.

Shirey RS, Kickler TS, Bell W, et al. Fatal immune hemolytic anemia and hepatic failure associated with warm-reacting IgM autoantibody. *Vox Sang* 1987;52:219–222.

RESOURCES

27, 50, 356

15 Sickle Cell Anemia

Garrett E. Bergman, MD

DEFINITION: Sickle cell anemia is a severe chronic hemolytic anemia usually manifested in childhood, characterized by abnormally shaped red blood cells, reticulocytosis, and recurrent episodes of "crises" of pain, primarily in bone, muscle, or the abdomen.

DIFFERENTIAL DIAGNOSIS: Aplastic anemia; Thalassemia major; Other hemolytic anemias.

SYMPTOMS AND SIGNS: Infants, generally older than 3 months and toddlers may present with the unique hand-foot syndrome of sickle cell anemia: painful, generally symmetric swelling of the dorsum of the hands and/or feet, associated with a chronic hemolytic anemia. Growth retardation in early childhood is common. The initial presentation may be sudden and unexpected overwhelming sepsis, primarily from encapsulated organisms (*Haemophilus influenza* and *Streptococcus pneumoniae*). This catastrophic event is secondary to functional asplenia. Older children and adults have recurrent episodes of vasoocclusive or "painful crises" involving the muscles and bones of the arms, legs, abdomen, and back. Osteomyelitis also occurs more frequently in patients with sickle cell anemia. Children and adults may develop severe cerebrovascular strokes from occlusion of the major blood vessels in and around the brain. Hepatosplenomegaly may be seen early in life, but by age 5 or 6 years the spleen is not palpable. The acute chest syndrome, with severe chest pain and infiltrates on chest films, is believed to be due to combined infection and microinfarctions. Common complications include gallstones, aregenerative or aplastic crises, and iron overload.

ETIOLOGY/EPIDEMIOLOGY: A single genetic amino acid substitution of valine for glutamic acid at the number 6 position in the β chain of the hemoglobin molecule alters its intramolecular configuration and renders it susceptible to "sickling," a form of protein denaturation. The abnormal hemoglobin is called sickle hemoglobin. Cells containing a high enough concentration of sickle hemoglobin can undergo internal polymerization, under certain conditions of deoxygenation, and deform the shape of the red cell. These sickled cells are much less flexible and unable to traverse the microvascular bed; they occlude small vessels through the body and cause acute painful local anoxia and chronic organ damage in virtually all organs. The gene is inherited in an autosomal-recessive manner, with males and females affected equally. The gene is a common mutant, prevalent in Central Africa, the Middle East, the Mediterranean, and in parts of India. African Americans have a gene incidence of approximately 8%, leading to an incidence of the homozygous disease state of approximately 1 in 580 newborns.

DIAGNOSIS: The diagnosis can be suspected in the presence of a chronic hemolytic anemia by the direct observation of sickle cells upon microscopic examination of the peripheral blood. Sickle hemoglobin-containing red blood cells can be induced to develop sickle forms in a simple test called a sickle cell preparation. Diagnosis is confirmed by hemoglobin electrophoresis.

TREATMENT

Standard Therapies: Aggressive general supportive therapy for any of the protean complications is mandatory. There is no curative therapy, and there is no proven medication that can decrease the symptoms or consequences of chronic disease. Patients should probably be treated with supplemental oral folic acid to avoid an aregenerative crisis. Early in life, affected children should receive vaccinations for *H. influenza* and *S. pneumoniae* to diminish the risk of sudden overwhelming sepsis. Daily oral antibiotic prophylaxis (e.g., amoxicillin) against these organisms has been recommended until school age or even later. In only occasional and selected patients, or in all patients for certain serious complications such as strokes, a regimen of chronic red blood cell transfusion is indicated. Any chronic transfusion program must be coupled with an aggressive iron-chelation regimen to prevent iron overload–related multiorgan damage. Intermittent painful crises must be treated with adequate analgesic medications, including narcotics. Possible precipitating events should be sought and, if identified, treated aggressively. Patients will often need adequate and careful rehydration during any crisis. Oral administration of hydroxyurea has been useful in some cases to diminish the frequency of painful vasoocclusive episodes; the long-term value of this therapy is uncertain.

Investigational Therapies: Bone marrow transplantation is being explored.

REFERENCES

Lukens JN. Hemoglobinopathies S, C, D, E, and O and associated diseases. In: Lee GR, Foerster J, Lukens JN, et al., eds. *Wintrobe's clinical hematology,* 10th ed. Baltimore: Williams & Wilkins, 1999.

Platt OS, Dover GJ. Sickle cell disease. In: Nathan DG, Orkin SH, eds. *Nathan and Oski's hematology of infancy and childhood,* 5th ed. Philadelphia: WB Saunders, 1998.

RESOURCES

357, 435

16 X-linked Sideroblastic Anemia

Masayuki Yamamoto, MD, PhD, and Hideo Harigae, MD, PhD

DEFINITION: X-linked sideroblastic anemia (XLSA) is an inherited disease linked to a deficiency in erythroid-specific 5-aminolevulinate synthase (ALAS-E).

DIFFERENTIAL DIAGNOSIS: Idiopathic hemochromatosis; Pearson syndrome; Secondary drug-induced sideroblastic anemia; Primary acquired sideroblastic anemia; Autosomally inherited sideroblastic anemia; XLSA with cerebellar ataxia; Copper deficiency; Zinc overload.

SYMPTOMS AND SIGNS: Patients exhibit various grades of anemia. The severe form can be recognized in newborns and during infancy by symptoms of anemia, namely, pale skin and growth retardation. Patients with mild disease may reach adulthood without showing any symptoms of anemia. After middle age, patients exhibit symptoms of hemochromatosis, such as liver cirrhosis, glucose intolerance, renal failure, congestive heart failure, and arrhythmias.

ETIOLOGY AND EPIDEMIOLOGY: Associated with ALAS-E deficiency, XLSA is inherited in an X-chromosome linked fashion. Females are rarely affected. The disease is due to a mutation in the *ALAS-E* (*ALAS2*) gene, which is located on chromosome Xp11.21. No apparent deviation has been observed among ethnic groups.

DIAGNOSIS: The anemia is hypochromic and microcytic. In most carrier females, red cell histograms are biphasic. In severe cases, deformity of red cells is prominent, showing anisocytosis, poikilocytosis, and target cells. The levels of serum iron and ferritin are high, with an increased saturation level of transferrin. The cellular composition of bone marrow is sometimes hyperplastic, with the erythroid series being dominant. Ring sideroblasts are observed in more than 15% of nucleated cells. The activity of 5-aminolevulinate synthase in bone marrow is low, and the level of ALA is decreased. A definite diagnosis can be made based on the detection of a mutation in the coding region of the *ALAS-E* gene. Mutations are frequently detected in exons 5 and 9.

TREATMENT

Standard Therapies: Alterations in the ALAS-E protein structure, caused by mutation, can impair the binding ability of pyridoxal 5'-phosphate cofactor. Oral administration of pyridoxine may restore the activity and improve anemia. Patients who are refractory to pyridoxine treatment require blood transfusion as an alternative treatment. For mild cases, phlebotomy may be an effective remedy for depleting iron levels. For severe and rapidly progressing cases, stem cell transplantation should be encouraged.

REFERENCES

Cotter PD, May A, Fitzsimons EJ, et al. The molecular biology and pyridoxine responsiveness of X-linked sideroblastic anaemia. *Haematologica* 1998;83:56–70.

Furuyama K, Fujita H, Nagai T, et al. Pyridoxine refractory X-linked sideroblastic anemia caused by a point mutation in the erythroid 5-aminolevulinate synthase gene. *Blood* 1997;90: 822–830.

Gonzalez MI, Caballero D, Vazquez L, et al. Allogeneic peripheral stem cell transplantation in a case of hereditary sideroblastic anaemia. *Br J Haematol* 2000;109:658–660.

Urban C, Binder B, Hauer C, et al. Congenital sideroblastic anemia successfully treated by allogeneic bone marrow transplantation. *Bone Marrow Transplant* 1992;10:373–375.

Yamamoto M, Nakajima O. Animal models for X-linked sideroblastic anemia. *Int J Hematol* 2000;72:157–164.

17 X-Linked Sideroblastic Anemia and Cerebellar Ataxia (XLSA/A)

Roland Lill, MD, and Gyula Kispal, MD

DEFINITION: XLSA/A (OMIM 301 310) is a recessive disorder characterized by onset in infantile or early childhood of nonprogressive spinocerebellar ataxia and mild anemia with hypochromia and microcystosis. The disorder is associated with diminished tendon reflex, incoordination, elevated free erythrocyte protoporphyrin, normal parenchymal iron stores, and irresponsiveness to pyridoxine supplementation. These latter criteria and the neurologic symptoms distinguish the disorder from the more common X-linked sideroblastic anemia.

SYNONYMS: Sideroblastic anemia; Spinocerebellar ataxia.

DIFFERENTIAL DIAGNOSIS: X-linked sideroblastic anemia; Iron deficiency anemia.

SYMPTOMS AND SIGNS: Affected patients are born at low birth weight (~2.5 kg). Infants exhibit mild postnatal growth retardation and substantially impaired gross motor and cognitive development; however, patients are without sensory loss or mental retardation and exhibit normal intelligence. In some cases, affected family members show mild spasticity. Selective cerebellar hypoplasia is evident on CT. Patients are anemic with hypochromic (MCH) and microcytic (MCV) erythrocytes. Blood film examination shows Pappenheimer bodies. Red cell precursors contain sideroblasts, i.e., mitochondria with granular deposits of iron. Bone marrow examination reveals ring sideroblasts, indicating increased erythrocyte iron. Serum contains normal or only slightly elevated levels of ferritin, whereas soluble transferrin receptor (sTfR) concentrations are elevated significantly (30–50 μg/L). Total erythrocyte protoporphyrin is increased (20 μM). The normal synthesis of heme by incorporation of ferrous iron into protoporphyrin seems to be defective. This last step of heme biosynthesis is catalyzed by ferrochelatase in the mitochondrial matrix. The effect on heme biosynthesis is not directly linked to the function of protein mutated in XLSA/A, the mitochondrial ABC transporter ABC7.

ETIOLOGY/EPIDEMIOLOGY: XLSA/A is inherited in an X-linked recessive manner. The disease is due to mutations in the ABC transporter ABC7 (ABCB7 according to nomenclature by *www.humanabc.org*). The *ABC7* gene is located on chromosome Xq13. The ABC7 protein is a constituent of the mitochondrial inner membrane and performs a crucial function in the export from mitochondria of an (unknown) component required for the maturation of cytosolic iron-sulfur (Fe-S) proteins, a process that is indispensable for a eukaryotic cell. The prevalence is not known because only a few cases have been examined.

DIAGNOSIS: The diagnosis is based on the presence of a mild anemia, which sometimes can be overlooked. The disorder is associated with spinocerebellar ataxia. Males with early-onset ataxia should receive a hematologic evaluation, including a blood film and serum iron status. A bone marrow examination should be performed, if abnormal blood count indices, increased concentrations of free erythrocyte protoporphyrin, and increased sTfR are detected. It reveals a large number of immature red cells with intramitochondrial iron surrounding the nucleus (ring sideroblasts). Diagnosis can be ascertained by sequencing the *ABC7* gene.

TREATMENT

Standard Therapies: The disorder is not responsive to treatment with pyridoxal phosphate, unlike other forms of XLSA. The favorable long-term prognosis of the spinocerebellar syndrome calls for early physical, occupational, and speech therapy and appropriate educational placement.

Investigational Therapies: Iron supplementation may have adverse effects, underlining the importance of differentiation of XLSA/A from other iron deficient anemias.

REFERENCES

Allikmets R, Raskind WH, Hutchinson A, et al. Mutation of a putative mitochondrial iron transporter gene (*ABC7*) in

X-linked sideroblastic anemia and ataxia (XLSA/A). *Hum Mol Genet* 1999;8:743–749.

Bekri S, Kispal G, Lange H, et al. Human *ABC7* transporter: gene structure and mutation causing X-linked sideroblastic anemia with ataxia (XLSA/A) with disruption of cytosolic iron-sulfur protein maturation. *Blood* 2000;96:3256–3264.

Csere P, Lill R, Kispal G. Identification of a human mitochondrial ABC transporter, the functional orthologue of yeast Atm1p. *FEBS Lett* 1998;441:266–270.

Kispal G, Csere P, Prohl C, et al. The mitochondrial proteins Atm1p and Nfs1p are required for biogenesis of cytosolic Fe/S proteins. *EMBO J* 1999;18:3981–3989.

Pagon RA, Bird TD, Detter JC, et al. Hereditary sideroblastic anemia: an X-linked recessive disorder. *J Med Genet* 1985;22:267–273.

Raskind WH, Wijsman E, Pagon RA, et al. X-linked sideroblastic anemia and ataxia: linkage to phosphoglycerate kinase at Xq13. *Am J Hum Genet* 1991;48:335–341.

18 Hereditary Angioedema

Gavin M. Joynt, MB, BCh, and Anthony M.H. Ho, MSc, MD

DEFINITION: Hereditary angioedema is characterized by recurrent, circumscribed, nonpitting, subepithelial edema involving primarily the extremities, larynx, face, and gut.

SYNONYMS: Hereditary angioneurotic edema; Congenital C1 esterase inhibitor deficiency.

DIFFERENTIAL DIAGNOSIS: Acquired C1 esterase inhibitor deficiency; Angiotensin-converting enzyme inhibitor–induced angioedema; Allergic angioedema; Histamine-induced angioedema; Idiopathic angioedema.

SYMPTOMS AND SIGNS: Angioedema describes deep swelling of the dermis. Lesions usually involve a subcutaneous site (the face or one limb) and are well-circumscribed, nonerythematous, and resolve without sequelae. Pain, urticaria, and pruritis are unusual. Visceral involvement, a consequence of edema in the submucosa and serosa of the bowel wall, results in symptoms ranging from nausea and vomiting to severe colic, sometimes followed by watery diarrhea. Pharyngeal involvement is characterized by progressive symptoms of throat discomfort, dysphagia, dysphonia, and stridor that are accompanied by swelling of the epiglottis, vocal folds, and/or surrounding laryngeal structures. Lesions may extend into the larger bronchi. Death by asphyxiation can occur. Most symptoms last 1–4 days without therapy, and most patients have one or more attacks per month, although episodes can be separated by periods of remission ranging from days to years.

ETIOLOGY/EPIDEMIOLOGY: The incidence is approximately 1 in 50,000 to 1 in 150,000 and the disease can affect any age group. The gene for C1 esterase inhibitor has been mapped to chromosome 11. The genetic defect is a consequence of many different mutations and is usually transmitted as an autosomal-dominant trait with high penetrance. Approximately 20% of patients have spontaneous mutations. The result is either a deficiency of C1 inhibitor protein (type I) or normal levels of dysfunctional inhibitor in serum (type II).

DIAGNOSIS: Diagnosis relies on a history of episodic angioedema. Trauma, surgery, and emotional stress may precipitate acute episodes. During an episode, serum CH50, C2, and C4 are low, but the C3 level is normal. During remission, CH50 and C2 are usually normal but C4 remains low in 80%–85% of cases. A low (<30%–50% of normal) immunoassayed level of serum C1 inhibitor confirms the diagnosis (type I). In 15% of affected patients, the immunoassayed C1 inhibitor is normal but a bioassay shows low C1 inhibitor activity (type II).

TREATMENT

Standard Therapies: Acute attacks do not usually respond to epinephrine, antihistamines, or corticosteroids. Prevention of asphyxiation from laryngeal swelling requires expert emergency airway management and concurrent intravenous administration of C1 inhibitor concentrate. If not available, fresh frozen plasma may be useful to replace C1 inhibitor levels. Urgent tracheal intubation or cricothyroidotomy/tracheostomy may be needed if the process is rapidly progressive or nonresponding. Abdominal symptoms are generally treated supportively, sometimes with narcotics. Cutaneous symptoms may take longer to respond. Reduction in the frequency and severity of attacks can be achieved with stanozolol. Prophylaxis with androgens is problematic, especially in children. Side effects may limit use, and liver enzymes should be checked at least every 6 months. Antifibrinolytics, such as aminocaproic or tranexamic acid, are less effective. Patients requiring surgery, particularly dental surgery, are at high risk for developing laryngeal angioedema. Treatment with danazol or stanozolol 5–7 days preoperatively, and C1 inhibitor concentrate or fresh frozen plasma 24 hours before the operation, is recommended. Angiotensin-converting enzyme inhibitors may elevate kinin levels and should be avoided.

REFERENCES

Donaldson VH, Evans RR. A biochemical abnormality in hereditary angioneurotic edema: absence of serum inhibitor of C1-esterase. *Am J Med* 1963;35:37–44.

Frank MM, Gelfand JA, Atkinson JP. Hereditary angioedema: the clinical syndrome and its management. *Ann Intern Med* 1976; 84:580–593.

Niels JF, Weiler JM. C1 esterase inhibitor deficiency, airway compromise, and anesthesia. *Anesth Analg* 1998;87:480–488.

Nielsen EW, Gran JT, Straume B, et al. Hereditary angio-oedema: new clinical observations and autoimmune screening, complement screening and kallikrein-kinin analyses. *J Intern Med* 1996;239:119–130.

Waytes AT, Rosen FS, Frank MM. Treatment of hereditary angioedema with a vapor-heated C1 inhibitor concentrate. *N Engl J Med* 1996;334:1630–1634.

RESOURCES

175, 356

---

19 | Congenital Antithrombin III Deficiency

Marilyn Manco-Johnson, MD

DEFINITION: Because antithrombin III (AT III) limits blood coagulation, congenital antithrombin III deficiency is characterized by a marked tendency toward venous or arterial thrombosis. The three recognized forms of the disorder are classic AT III deficiency and two variants, AT III-1a and AT III-1b.

SYMPTOMS AND SIGNS: Patients usually have the first episode of thrombosis between the ages of 10 and 35. Precipitating events include surgery, pregnancy, childbirth, trauma, or use of oral contraceptives. Because pregnancy and estrogen use are significant risk factors, women tend to develop thromboses at an earlier age than men. Approximately 40% of patients with congenital AT III deficiency develop pulmonary embolisms. Embolisms also commonly occur in the veins deep in the legs and pelvic region, the more superficial veins in the legs, and the mesenteric veins. Edema is common in affected legs and pelvic areas. Clots that form in the heart may result in thromboembolism to other organs, such as the brain or kidneys.

ETIOLOGY/EPIDEMIOLOGY: Congenital AT III deficiency is inherited as an autosomal-dominant gene. In the classic form of the disorder, an insufficient amount of antithrombin is produced in the liver. In the variant forms, AT III-1a and AT III-1b, both normal and abnormal AT III are produced but interact so that inhibition of normal antithrombin results. The disease is estimated to occur in approximately 1 in 3,000 to 1 in 5,000 individuals.

DIAGNOSIS: Diagnosis of AT III is confirmed by the blood AT III assay. Any individual with a history of venous thromboembolism before the age of 40 should be evaluated for AT III deficiency even if the blood level is normal. Patients who have any of the following characteristics should be screened for AT III deficiency: a family history of thrombosis, a thrombosis before age 35, recurrence of thrombosis even with heparin therapy, deep vein thrombosis early in pregnancy, or loss of large amounts of protein in the urine. Studies suggest that early diagnosis and treatment may reduce the incidence of thrombosis.

TREATMENT

Standard Therapies: The goal of treatment is to prevent thrombosis, primarily through the use of oral anticoagulants, such as coumadin drugs, heparin, and intravenous concentrated AT III. The orphan drug Thrombate III (Bayer Corporation) is now a standard therapy. When the risk of thrombosis is high, as during pregnancy or with surgery, AT III replacement therapy is particularly important. AT III should also be replaced to help dissolve blood clots after thrombosis has occurred. Heparin and AT III replacement can cause bleeding, so the therapy must be carefully monitored. AT III can also increase the patient's risk of developing hepatitis, because it is derived from pooled plasma. Women who are prone to this disorder should refrain from taking estrogen. A drug known as AT nativ (Kabivitrum) has been approved as a treatment for congenital AT III deficiency. The use of anticoagulants may prevent recurrences.

Investigational Therapies: AT III replacement is under development. Human AT III is being investigated to determine its safety and efficacy in preventing or arresting episodes of thrombosis in patients with congenital AT III deficiency, especially those who have suffered trauma or are about to undergo surgery or childbirth.

REFERENCES

Bick RL. Hypercoagulability and thrombosis. *Hematol Oncol Clin North Am* 1992;6:1421–1431.

Grewal HP. Congenital antithrombin III deficiency causing mesenteric venous infarction: a lesson to remember: a case history. *Angiology* 1992;43:618–620.

McKusick VA. *Mendelian inheritance in man*, 10th ed. Baltimore: The Johns Hopkins University Press, 1992:87–92.

Montague M. Pregnancy and thrombophilia in women with congenital deficit of antithrombin III, protein C, protein S or plasminogen: analysis of 39 cases. *Med Clin* 1993;100:201–204.

Tabemero MD, et al. Incidence and clinical characteristics of hereditary disorder associated with venous thrombosis. *Am J Hematol* 1991;36:249–254.

Wyngaarden JB, et al., eds. *Cecil textbook of medicine*, 19th ed. Philadelphia: WB Saunders, 1992:1011–1012.

RESOURCES

27, 356

20 Banti Syndrome

P. Aiden McCormick, MD, FRCP

DEFINITION: The name Banti syndrome is an old descriptor for cases of portal hypertension and splenomegaly in the absence of significant hepatic disease or portal or hepatic venous thrombosis.

SYNONYMS: Idiopathic portal hypertension; Noncirrhotic portal fibrosis.

DIFFERENTIAL DIAGNOSIS: Cirrhosis; Portal vein thrombosis; Hemolytic anemia; Hematologic malignancy; Nodular regenerative hyperplasia; Partial nodular transformation of liver; Early primary biliary cirrhosis; Hepatic sarcoidosis; Venooclusive disease of liver.

SYMPTOMS AND SIGNS: Individuals with Banti syndrome usually present in adulthood with portal hypertension and splenomegaly. The disease is usually asymptomatic; bleeding from esophageal or gastric varices may be the first sign. Liver function is well preserved, and jaundice, ascites, and encephalopathy are rare. The liver may be normal sized or slightly enlarged. If arsenical intake is implicated, palmar skin keratosis and melanosis may be present.

ETIOLOGY/EPIDEMIOLOGY: Banti syndrome is relatively common in parts of India and Japan, but rare in Western countries. Arsenic intake has been implicated; the condition has been reported in patients taking long-term arsenical preparations such as Fowler solution for psoriasis. Increased arsenic levels are present in drinking water in some countries and may contribute to regional differences in incidence. Cases have occurred in patients taking long-term azathioprine, particularly after kidney transplantation, and workers exposed to vinyl chloride have developed idiopathic portal hypertension as well as angiosarcoma. The precise mechanisms for splenomegaly and portal hypertension are not fully understood. Increased resistance to portal venous flow through the liver is probably the most important factor, although increased splenic blood flow may also play a role.

DIAGNOSIS: The diagnosis should be suspected if splenomegaly and portal hypertension exist in the presence of a near normal liver biopsy and patent portal and splenic veins.

TREATMENT
Standard Therapies: If an etiologic factor such as arsenic or azathioprine is identified, the exposure should be stopped. The main clinical problem is bleeding esophageal or gastric varices. Because liver function is usually well preserved, the prognosis for bleeding is more favorable than when hepatic cirrhosis is present. Treatment is the same as for other causes of portal hypertension. If large varices are identified before bleeding occurs, prophylactic β-blockade or endoscopic banding should be considered. Active bleeding may be treated with vasoconstrictor drugs and/or endoscopic sclerotherapy or banding as appropriate. With resistant or recurrent bleeding, transjugular shunt or surgical shunt may be necessary.

REFERENCES

Lorenz R, Brauer M, Classen M, et al. Idiopathic portal hypertension in a renal transplant patient after long-term azathioprine therapy. *Clin Invest* 1992;70:152–155.

Mazumder DN, Das Gupta J, Santra A, et al. Chronic arsenic toxicity in west Bengal—the worst calamity in the world. *J Ind Med Assoc* 1998;96:4–7.

Nevens F, Fevery J, Van Steenbergen W, et al. Arsenic and noncirrhotic portal hypertension. A report of eight cases. *J Hepatol* 1990;11:80–85.

Ohnishi K, Saito M, Sato S, et al. Portal hemodynamics in idiopathic portal hypertension (Banti's syndrome). Comparison with chronic persistent hepatitis and normal subjects. *Gastroenterology* 1987;92:751–758.

Thomas LB, Popper H, Berk PD, et al. Vinyl-chloride-induced liver disease. From idiopathic portal hypertension (Banti's syndrome) to angiosarcomas. *N Engl J Med* 1975;292:17–22.

RESOURCES

39, 354

---

21 Bernard-Soulier Syndrome

A. Koneti Rao, MD

DEFINITION: Described first in 1948, the Bernard-Soulier syndrome is an inherited platelet bleeding disorder characterized by thrombocytopenia, giant platelets, and an abnormality in platelet–vessel wall interaction owing to a deficiency in the platelet membrane glycoprotein (GP) Ib-V-IX complex.

DIFFERENTIAL DIAGNOSIS: Congenital thrombocytopenia; Autoimmune thrombocytopenia; May-Hegglin anomaly; Gray platelet syndrome.

SIGNS AND SYMPTOMS: Patients have mucocutaneous bleeding, including purpura, epistaxis, gingival bleeding, and menorrhagia. Bleeding into joints or deep visceral hematomas are uncommon. Severity of symptoms is highly variable from easy bruising to recurrent and severe spontaneous bleeding starting from birth. Intensity of manifestations may vary among affected family members. The physical examination is otherwise unremarkable. These patients do not have splenomegaly.

ETIOLOGY/EPIDEMIOLOGY: Bernard-Soulier syndrome is inherited as an autosomal-recessive trait. No prevalence data are available. Platelets are deficient in platelet membrane GPIb, GPIX, and GPV, which exist as a complex. GPIb is a platelet receptor for von Willebrand factor (vWF). Following injury to the blood vessel, platelets adhere to the subendothelium by binding of vWF to platelet GPIb. This process (adhesion) is impaired in Bernard-Soulier syndrome. The syndrome arises owing to mutations in the genes governing GPIb (which consists of two peptides, GPIbα and GPIbβ) and GPIX.

DIAGNOSIS: Most patients have moderate thrombocytopenia (50,000–100,000/μL) with large platelets on the pe-

ripheral smear. Bleeding time is prolonged, with normal prothrombin time and activated partial thromboplastin time. In platelet aggregation studies, the responses to ADP, epinephrine, and collagen are normal. Characteristically, platelet agglutination by ristocetin is absent or decreased, and this is not corrected by normal plasma. Plasma levels of factor VIII and vWF factor are normal. The diagnosis is confirmed by demonstrating that platelet GPIb is decreased on platelets. Heterozygotes have normal platelet counts and platelet function, but their platelets may be abnormally large. They have intermediate concentrations of GPIb-IX-V complex on platelets.

TREATMENT

Standard Therapies: Platelet transfusions are indicated for control of clinically significant bleeding manifestations and in relation to surgical procedures. Some patients may develop antibodies to GPIb following platelet transfusions, and these antibodies may compromise the efficacy of subsequent platelet transfusions. Splenectomy or corticosteroids are not indicated in these patients. Administration of desmopressin may be beneficial in controlling bleeding manifestations in some patients.

Investigational Therapies: Recombinant factor VIIa is under investigation.

REFERENCES

George JN, Nurden AT. Inherited disorders of the platelet membrane: Glanzmann thrombasthenia, Bernard-Soulier syndrome, and other disorders. In: Colman RW, Hirsh J, Marder VJ, et al., eds. *Hemostasis and thrombosis. Basic principles and clinical practice.* Philadelphia: JB Lippincott, 2001:921–943.

Lopez JA, Andrews RK, Afshar-Kharghan V, et al. Bernard-Soulier syndrome. *Blood* 1998;91:4397–4418.

RESOURCES

73, 357

22 Chédiak-Higashi Syndrome

Laurence A. Boxer, MD

DEFINITION: Chédiak-Higashi syndrome (CHS) is an autosomal-recessive disorder characterized by increased susceptibility to infection due to defective degranulation of neutrophils, mild bleeding diathesis, partial oculocutaneous albinism, progressive peripheral neuropathy, and a tendency to develop a life-threatening lymphoma-like syndrome.

SYNONYMS: Béguez-César disease; Chédiak-Higashi anomaly; Chédiak-Steinbrinck-Higashi syndrome.

DIFFERENTIAL DIAGNOSIS: Other genetic forms of partial albinism; Acute and chronic myelogenous leukemias.

SYMPTOMS AND SIGNS: Patients with CHS have light skin and silvery hair. They frequently complain of solar sensitivity and photophobia. Other symptoms and signs vary considerably, but frequent infections and neuropathy are common. The infections involve the mucous membranes, skin, and respiratory tract. Affected children are susceptible to gram-positive and gram-negative bacteria and fungi, most commonly *Staphylococcus aureus*. The neuropathy may be central and motor in type, and ataxia may be a prominent feature. Neuropathy often begins in the teenage years and becomes the most prominent problem. Patients with CHS may have prolonged bleeding times with normal platelet counts, resulting in impaired platelet aggregation associated with a platelet storage pool disorder. Natural killer cell function is also impaired, leading to inability on the part of the patient to contain Epstein-Barr virus. When patients are infected with Epstein-Barr virus, they are susceptible to entering the accelerated phase of the disorder characterized by marked enlargement of the liver, spleen, and lymph nodes.

ETIOLOGY/EPIDEMIOLOGY: The syndrome is inherited in an autosomal-recessive pattern. It is caused by a mutation in the gene for CHS located on chromosome 1q42-q44. The gene encodes a cytosolic protein named lysosomal-trafficking regulator, which has structural features homologous to a vacuolar sorting protein, termed VPS15 yeast. This CHS protein is believed to be associated with vacuolar transport in the Golgi apparatus or molecular sorting in endosomes.

DIAGNOSIS: The diagnosis is established by finding large inclusions in all nucleated blood cells. These can be seen on Wright-stained blood films, but are accentuated in the cells of the myeloid series by a peroxidase stain.

TREATMENT
Standard Therapies: Treatment is generally supportive. High doses of ascorbic acid improve the clinical status of some patients in the stable phase. It has been shown *in vitro* to correct the chemotactic defect. Although the efficacy of the vitamin is controversial, given its safety, it is reasonable to administer ascorbic acid to all patients. The only curative therapy for the accelerated phase is bone marrow transplantation from an HLA-compatible donor or unrelated donor compatible at the D locus. Stem cell transplantation reconstitutes normal hematopoietic and immunologic functions and corrects the natural killer cell deficiency; however, it does not correct or prevent the peripheral neuropathy, although it may benefit the central neuropathy.

REFERENCES
Boxer LA, Smolen JE. Neutrophil granule constituents and their release in health and disease. *Hematol Oncol Clin North Am* 1988;2:101–134.
Haddad E, LeDeist F, Blanche S, et al. Treatment of Chediak-Higashi syndrome by allogenic bone marrow transplantation. Report of 10 cases. *Blood* 1995;85:3328–3333.
Nagle DL, Karim EA, Woolf EA, et al. Identification and mutation analysis of the complete gene for Chediak-Higashi syndrome. *Nat Genet* 1996;14:307–311./REF}

RESOURCES
218, 321, 359

23   Chylomicron Retention Disease

Reuven Yakubov, BA,
Jahangir Iqbal, PhD,
and M. Mahmood Hussain, PhD, Lic Med

DEFINITION: Chylomicron retention disease is an autosomal-recessive disorder characterized by the selective absence of the apolipoprotein (apo) B48-containing lipoproteins, chylomicrons, in the plasma. This results in fat malabsorption with the consequences of steatorrhea, hypolipidemia, vitamin A and E deficiency, slight acanthocytosis, mental and growth retardation, and nervous system disorders.

SYNONYM: Anderson disease.

DIFFERENTIAL DIAGNOSIS: Abetalipoproteinemia; Hypobetalipoproteinemia.

SYMPTOMS AND SIGNS: Patients usually present in early infancy with steatorrhea and growth and mental retardation. Neurologic signs, such as the loss of deep tendon reflexes, are variable and not as severe as in abetalipoproteinemia and hypobetalipoproteinemia. Furthermore, acanthocytosis and retinitis pigmentosa are seldom seen in chylomicron retention disease.

ETIOLOGY/EPIDEMIOLOGY: The molecular and genetic mechanisms responsible for the disease are unknown; however, the disease may be related to defects in chylomicron secretion.

DIAGNOSIS: Diagnosis is based on the determination of plasma lipid and apoB levels and microscopic analysis of intestinal biopsies. Low plasma levels of apoB100 and absence of apoB48 are diagnostic features. In addition, low plasma cholesterol levels (<75 mg/dL), half the normal low-density lipoprotein levels, and normal plasma triglycerides (TG) are observed. The lack of postprandial rise in plasma TG levels is characteristic. Intestinal biopsy shows normally structured villi that contain abnormal enterocytes loaded with lipid droplets. Endoscopy shows a snowy white epithelium.

TREATMENT
Standard Therapies: A low-fat diet supplemented with lipid-soluble vitamins A and E and essential fatty acids should be implemented as early as possible, to allow the patient a return of normal growth and abatement of gastrointestinal symptoms. Patient compliance with the dietary regimen is vital; departure from the low-fat diet results in rapid relapse and recurrence of symptoms.

REFERENCES
Dannoura AH, Berriot-Varoqueaux N, Amati P, et al. Anderson's disease: exclusion of apolipoprotein and intracellular lipid transport genes. *Arterioscler Thromb Vasc Biol* 1999;19:2494–2508.
Kane JP, Havel RJ. Disorders of the biogenesis and secretion of lipoproteins containing the B apolipoproteins. In: Scriver CR, Beaudet AL, Sly WS, et al., eds. *The metabolic and molecular bases of inherited disorders.* New York: McGraw-Hill, 1995: 1853–1885.
Levy E. The genetic basis of primary disorders of intestinal fat transport. *Clin Invest Med* 1996;19:317–324.
Levy E, Chouraqui JP, Roy CC. Steatorrhea and disorders of chylomicron synthesis and secretion. *Pediatr Clin North Am* 1988; 35:53–67.

RESOURCES
354, 359, 462

24   Ewing Sarcoma of Bone

Jon Trent, MD, PhD

DEFINITION: Ewing sarcoma (ES) of bone is a malignant tumor in the Ewing family of tumors (ES of bone, extraosseous ES, and primitive neuroectodermal tumors).

The tumor most commonly arises from the bones of the pelvis/sacrum, proximal extremity, or distal extremity. Rarely, ES may arise from other bones or soft tissue.

SYNONYM: Ewing tumor.

DIFFERENTIAL DIAGNOSIS: Osteosarcoma; Chondrosarcoma; Osteochondromas; Lymphoma; Medulloblastoma; Small cell carcinoma; Neuroblastoma.

SYMPTOMS AND SIGNS: Individuals with ES often experience tumor-associated pain and swelling, fever, anemia, and abnormally increased levels of circulating white blood cells (leukocytosis). Ewing sarcoma can be associated with preexisting skeletal abnormalities (such as enchondromas and aneurysmal bone cysts) and genitourinary abnormalities (such as hypospadias and duplicate collecting systems).

ETIOLOGY/EPIDEMIOLOGY: Ewing sarcoma affects males more often than females and usually develops when a person is between the ages of 10 and 20 years. The exact cause is unknown. Earlier trauma to the area of involvement is sometimes a preceding factor.

DIAGNOSIS: Diagnosis is made by histopathology. The *MIC2* gene product (CD99) is a surface protein found on most ES and its presence may aid in diagnosis. Ewing sarcoma tends to metastasize to the lungs and/or bones; therefore, radiographic evaluation generally includes chest radiography, CT of the chest, and a bone scan. Plain films, CT, and/or MRI of the primary tumor may be helpful in defining the extent of soft tissue involvement, determining bone marrow invasion, and in planning surgical therapy. Some clinicians perform a bone marrow biopsy to evaluate whether the tumor has metastasized to the bone marrow. The most common sites of marrow metastases are the vertebral bodies; a screening MRI of the entire spine is the most sensitive test to detect bone marrow involvement.

TREATMENT

Standard Therapies: The optimal treatment approach is systemic chemotherapy with surgery or radiotherapy as an adjunct for local control. Surgery alone offers long-term survival rates of less than 10% due to occult but aggressive metastatic disease. It is used as an adjuvant for local control, often with an attempt at limb preservation. Radio-therapy offers excellent local control, but no prospective studies have been done to compare it with surgery. Radiation therapy alone gives local control of 44%–86% with a long-term survival rate of 16%–25%. Multimodality therapy provides an overall survival rate of approximately 56% at longer than 3 years. Most studies give 12–18 months of chemotherapy with 3–6 cycles before local therapy. Total duration of chemotherapy can now be shorter (often less than 12 months) because of dose-intensive therapy with the use of marrow-stimulating growth factors.

Investigational Therapies: The drug gemcitabine has shown activity in soft tissue sarcomas and is currently available at M.D. Anderson Cancer Center for patients with advanced ES and other bone tumors. The drug liposomal N-acetylglucosiminyl-N-acetylmuramly-L-Ala-D-isoGln-L-Ala-glycerolidpalmitoyl (ImmTher) has received an orphan drug designation for its use in the treatment of ES, but more studies are needed to determine its long-term safety and effectiveness. Various combinations of chemotherapeutic agents, total body irradiation, and stem cell transplantation are being evaluated as effective therapy for high-risk ES.

REFERENCES

Bacci G, et al. Long-term results in 144 localized Ewing's sarcoma patients treated with combined therapy. *Cancer* 1989;63:1477–1486.

Behrman RE, ed. *Nelson textbook of pediatrics,* 15th ed. Philadelphia: WB Saunders, 1996.

Buyse, ML, ed. *Birth defects encyclopedia.* Boston: Blackwell Scientific, 1990.

Devita VT Jr, Hellman S, Rosenberg SA, eds. *Cancer: principles and practice of oncology,* 6th ed. Philadelphia: Lippincott Williams & Wilkins, 2001.

Isselbacher AB, et al., eds. *Harrison's principles of internal medicine,* 13th ed. New York: McGraw-Hill, 1994.

RESOURCES

30, 83, 35, 379

---

25   Factor IX Deficiency

*Guy Young, MD,
and Diane J. Nugent, MD*

DEFINITION: Factor IX deficiency is an inherited bleeding disorder caused by a diminished or absent amount of factor IX, an important protein in the hemostatic system.

SYNONYMS: Hemophilia B; Christmas disease.

DIFFERENTIAL DIAGNOSIS: Factor VIII deficiency (hemophilia A).

SYMPTOMS AND SIGNS: The lack of factor IX leads to impaired thrombus formation and thus prolonged and often severe bleeding from various sites. Patients with factor IX deficiency are categorized as having severe disease if they have less than 1% factor IX activity, moderate with 1%–5% activity, and mild with 5%–15% activity. Severe factor IX deficiency leads to spontaneous hemorrhage, with the most common sites being joints and mucous membranes. Bleeding, however, can occur from anywhere, including the central nervous system, deep muscles, retroperitoneum, and visceral organs. Patients with moderate hemophilia occasionally have spontaneous hemorrhage; more often, however, they have significant bleeding after minor trauma. Patients with a mild deficiency bleed only after trauma, but the severity is out of proportion to the level of trauma. All patients with hemophilia have excessive bleeding after invasive procedures, no matter how minor, and require prophylactic therapy even for immunizations. Inadequately treated joint bleeding leads to chronic arthropathy, which results in severe joint dysfunction.

ETIOLOGY/EPIDEMIOLOGY: Factor IX deficiency is an X-linked recessive disorder caused by various mutations in the gene for factor IX. It occurs in 1 of 30,000 males, with the severe form accounting for most patients. All ethnic groups are affected equally. Female carriers of factor IX deficiency may be symptomatic due to nonrandom X chromosome inactivation. They have a phenotype similar to mild hemophilia.

DIAGNOSIS: Factor IX deficiency should be suspected in any male with prolonged or unusual bleeding symptoms. Common presentations in infancy include prolonged bleeding after circumcision or heel sticks, swelling after immunizations, and a known history of hemophilia in maternal relatives. Beyond infancy, patients may present with joint hemorrhages, mucous membrane bleeding, or excessive bleeding after trauma. A coagulation evaluation should be undertaken, including a platelet count, prothrombin time, and activated partial thromboplastin time

(aPTT). Patients with factor IX deficiency will have a prolonged aPTT. With this finding, specific factor assays should be done for factors VIII and IX. The patient has hemophilia B if the factor IX activity is less than 15%.

TREATMENT

Standard Therapies: The treatment is replacement of factor IX by concentrates in the form of either recombinant protein or plasma-derived protein. The major benefit of recombinant factor IX is the low risk of viral transmission. Patients with severe factor IX deficiency may receive either prophylactic or on-demand therapy. Those who have intracranial hemorrhage or recurrent joint hemorrhage should receive prophylactic therapy. Patients with mild to moderate hemophilia generally receive only on-demand therapy because they bleed less frequently and are less likely to develop chronic joint disease. All invasive procedures require replacement of factor IX before the procedure.

Investigative Therapies: Gene therapy is being researched.

REFERENCES

Aledort LM. Issues in making therapeutic choice: recombinant and/or human-derived products. *Haemophilia* 2001;7:89–90.

Chuah MK, Collen D, Vanden Driessche T. Gene therapy for hemophilia. *J Gene Med* 2001;3:3–20.

Kasper CK. Protocols for the treatment of haemophilia and von Willebrand disease. *Haemophilia* 2000;6(suppl):84–93.

Mannucci P, Tuddenham EG. The hemophilias—from royal genes to gene therapy. *N Engl J Med* 2001;344:1782–1784.

White G, Shapiro A, Ragni M, et al. Clinical evaluation of recombinant factor IX. *Semin Hematol* 1998;35(suppl 2): 33–38.

RESOURCES

302, 357

---

26   Factor XII Deficiency

Robert W. Colman, MD

DEFINITION: Factor XII (FXII) deficiency is an abnormality in a plasma protein inherited as an autosomal-recessive trait. The trait is characterized by a prolonged activated partial thromboplastin time (aPTT) in the absence of an associated clinical bleeding disorder.

SYNONYM: Hageman trait.

DIFFERENTIAL DIAGNOSIS: Prekallikrein deficiency; High molecular weight kininogen deficiency.

SYMPTOMS AND SIGNS: In patients with congenital FXII deficiency, there is probably an increased incidence of venous thromboses and acquired thrombotic disorders, such as myocardial infarction and rethrombosis of coronary arteries after thrombolytic therapy.

ETIOLOGY/EPIDEMIOLOGY: FXII is coded for by a single gene of 12 kb that maps to chromosome 5, comprising 13 introns and 14 exons. Most Hageman trait plasma lacks both functional and antigenic (CRM-) FXII. Immunoreactive FXII cross-reacting material (CRM+) has been recognized in three patients who lack functional FXII activity. Individual patients of Swiss, Asian, and Italian extraction are noted to have decreased levels of FXII. The molecular basis of several types of CRM–FXII has been elucidated. In one family, a T-to-C transition leads to a transversion of the transcription initiator site. In a second family, a splice site mutation in the FXII gene results in a truncated transcript and a lack of circulatory FXII protein. Defects in the light chain of FXII result in disorders of the enzymatic activity of the protein.

DIAGNOSIS: In patients with prolonged aPTT who have no history of a bleeding disorder, the most likely diagnosis is the acquired condition of a lupus anticoagulant, part of the antiphospholipid syndrome. Therefore, this syndrome should be ruled out by specific tests incriminating an antibody to phospholipid–plasma protein complexes. If the results of these tests are negative, assays for FXII, pyruvate kinase, and HK as well as factor XI should be performed.

TREATMENT
Standard Therapies: No treatment is required in the asymptomatic individual. If FXII deficiency is associated with deep venous thrombosis, anticoagulation with warfarin or low molecular weight heparin is indicated. The anticoagulant should be extended for at least 6 months and possibly indefinitely.

REFERENCES
Bradford HN, Pixley RA, Colman RW. Human factor XII binding to the GP Ib-IX-V complex inhibits thrombin-induced platelet aggregation. *J Biol Chem* 2000;275:22756–22763.

Cool DE, MacGillivray RT. Characterization of the human blood coagulation factor XII gene. Intron/exon gene organization and analysis of the 5'-flanking region. *J Biol Chem* 1987;262:13662–13673.

Halbmayer WM, Mannhalter C, Feichtinger C, et al. The prevalence of factor XII deficiency in 103 orally anticoagulated outpatients suffering from recurrent venous and/or arterial thromboembolism. *Thromb Haemost* 1992;68:285–290.

Samuel M, Pixley RA, Villanueva MA, et al. Human factor XII (Hageman factor) autoactivation by dextran sulfate: circular dichroism, fluorescence, and ultraviolet difference spectroscopic studies. *J Biol Chem* 1992;267:19691–19697.

RESOURCES
302, 356

---

27 Glanzmann Thrombasthenia

*W. Beau Mitchell, MD,
and Deborah L. French, PhD*

DEFINITION: Glanzmann thrombasthenia is an inherited bleeding disorder caused by defects in the platelet membrane receptor αIIbβ3, which results in a lifelong mucocutaneous bleeding diathesis of variable severity.

DIFFERENTIAL DIAGNOSIS: von Willebrand disease; Mild factor VIII or factor IX deficiency; Immune thrombocytopenia; Afibrinogenemia; Dysfibrinogenemia; Hermanski-Pudlak syndrome; Bernard-Soulier syndrome; Chédiak-Higashi syndrome; Wiskott-Aldrich syndrome; Gray platelet syndrome; Hypersplenism; Cardiac disease; Liver disease; Renal disease.

SYMPTOMS AND SIGNS: Most patients are diagnosed before age 5, many at birth or in infancy. Epistaxis, purpura, and gingival bleeding are the most common symptoms, and may be more pronounced in children. Spontaneous petechiae are rare except in the newborn period, where they may represent an exaggeration of the normal newborn petechiae observed after birth trauma. Epistaxis is the most common form of bleeding and may be life threatening. In adolescent and adult women, menorrhagia is common and may be severe, particularly at menarche. Gastrointestinal bleeding and hematuria may occur, but are less common. Other types of bleeding are uncommon, and spontaneous hemorrhage is rare. Hemarthroses and intracranial hemorrhages have been reported, but are usually associated with trauma. Bleeding after trauma or minor surgery can be severe, and patients are frequently diagnosed after circumcision or tooth extraction. Parturition and postpartum bleeding may be severe, and the risk extends for at least 2 weeks postpartum. Most patients will at some point experience bleeding severe enough to require red cell and/or platelet transfusions.

ETIOLOGY/EPIDEMIOLOGY: This autosomal-recessive disease results from mutations in the genes encoding either the αIIb or β3 integrin subunits. Approximately 60 patients have been reported. Many additional cases have likely gone unreported or undiagnosed. The disease is more common in populations with a high degree of intra-group marriage, such as in the Middle East, India, and France.

DIAGNOSIS: Patients have normal platelet counts and morphology; normal prothrombin time, partial thromboplastin time, and coagulation factor levels; and markedly prolonged bleeding times. Platelet aggregation is normal in response to ristocetin but absent or severely diminished in response to adenosine diphosphate, collagen, epinephrine, and other agonists. Clot retraction may be absent, decreased, or normal, depending on the nature of the defect. Heterozygous carriers usually have no clinical symptoms.

TREATMENT
Standard Therapies: Acute severe hemorrhage is usually controlled by platelet transfusion, but may require red cell transfusion. Iron deficiency is common due to chronic blood loss, particularly from gingival bleeding. Patients should maintain good dental hygiene and receive iron sup-

plementation as needed. Platelets should be given before any invasive procedure and continued until the wound has healed. Mechanical packing and cauterization of mucosal vessels may be required for severe epistaxis. Tranexamic acid and epsilon aminocaproic acid may help to control minor bleeding, and can be given as an adjunct to platelets for tooth extraction. Using hormonal therapy to induce amenorrhea may eliminate menorrhagia.

Investigational Therapies: Recombinant factor VIIa has been reported to be effective in treating bleeding, but it has a potential thrombotic risk. A few patients received allogeneic bone marrow transplants for severe, recurrent bleeding and were cured of disease.

REFERENCES
Bellucci S, Damaj G, Boval B, et al. Bone marrow transplantation in severe Glanzmann's thrombasthenia with antiplatelet alloimmunization. *Bone Marrow Transplant* 2000;25:327–330.
Coller BS, French DL. Hereditary qualitative platelet disorders. In: Beutler E, Lichtman MA, Coller BS, et al., eds. *Williams hematology,* 6th ed. New York: McGraw-Hill, 2001:1551–1581.
French DL, Coller BS. Hematologically important mutations: Glanzmann thrombasthenia. *Blood Cells Mol Dis* 1997;23: 39–51.
George JN, Caen JP, Nurden AT. Glanzmann thrombasthenia: the spectrum of clinical disease. *Blood* 1990;75:1383–1395.

RESOURCES
357, 359

---

28 | Glioblastoma Multiforme

*Mustafa Saad, MD,
and Adnan I. Qureshi, MD*

DEFINITION: Glioblastoma multiforme is the most malignant and rapidly growing category of astrocytomas.

SYNONYM: Grade 4 astrocytoma.

DIFFERENTIAL DIAGNOSIS: Other intracranial neoplasm including metastatic lesion; Brain abscess; Tuberculoma; Toxoplasmosis; Stroke.

SYMPTOMS AND SIGNS: The clinical presentation of glioblastoma multiforme is similar to that of other brain tumors except that the onset and progression are more

acute because of its rapid growth. The duration of symptoms is relatively short, ranging from weeks to a few months. Depending on the site, glioblastoma produces symptoms by a combination of compression, infiltration, vascular compression, and increase in intracranial pressure. These include headaches, vomiting, drowsiness, lethargy, seizures, focal neurologic deficits, and mental state changes. The headaches classically occur more at awakening, change with posture, and are accompanied by nausea and vomiting. Mostly, however, they are nonspecific and difficult to differentiate from chronic tension headaches. Bilateral papilledema is present in 25% of cases. Other signs of increased intracranial pressure, such as changes in temperature, blood pressure, pulse, or respiratory rate, are usually present only in the terminal stages of the disease.

ETIOLOGY/EPIDEMIOLOGY: Glioblastoma multiforme is the most common form of glial tumor and is responsible for most of the 12,000 brain tumor–associated deaths that occur in the United States annually. Glioblastoma multiforme tends to occur mainly in an older age group, with peak incidence in the sixth decade. They are more common in whites as compared to other races and have a male:female ratio of 1.5:1. There is an increased incidence of these tumors in patients with neurofibromatosis, tuberous sclerosis, Turcot syndrome, and Li-Fraumani syndrome, in addition to an increased incidence in certain families. The role of environmental factors in their pathogenesis is unknown, with the strongest association found with ionizing radiation given in childhood.

DIAGNOSIS: A brain tumor should be considered in any patient older than 40 years with recent onset of persistent headaches, vomiting, seizures, or focal cerebral deficits. Fundoscopy should be performed to look for papilledema. Diagnosis is done by means of CT or MRI. Chest radiography should also be ordered to look for a likely source of metastasis, if a secondary metastatic lesion is suspected. Histologic diagnosis is usually carried out after surgical resection of the tumor.

TREATMENT

Standard Therapies: There is no curative treatment. The various treatment modalities are used to help provide a better quality and prolongation of life. Standard treatment for newly diagnosed patients involves maximum feasible resection of the tumor, followed by limited field radiation therapy, with adjuvant chemotherapy using any of the nitrosourea agents. The median survival time is 10 months, compared with 4 months in those who are not treated. Supporting therapy includes glucocorticoids for cerebral edema, anticonvulsants for seizures, and anticoagulants for venous thromboembolic disease. Patients with neurologic deficits may require physical, occupational, and speech therapy.

Investigational Therapies: These include immunotherapy involving interferons, interleukins, activated killer cells to destroy the tumor cells, gene therapy to produce defective viruses that home in and destroy tumor cells, and other ways of inhibiting the growth factor and angiogenesis involved in the growth of brain tumors.

REFERENCES

Davis FG, McCarthy BJ. Epidemiology of brain tumors. *Curr Opin Neurol* 2000;13:635–640.
Hildebrand J, Dewitte O, Dietrich PY, et al. Management of malignant brain tumors. *Eur Neurol* 1997;38:238–253.
Wen PY, Fine HA, Black PM, et al. High-grade astrocytomas. *Neurol Clin* 1995;13:875–900.

RESOURCES

30, 352

---

29 Glucose-6-Phosphate Dehydrogenase Deficiency

Theresa W. Gauthier, MD, and Martha H. Manar, MD

DEFINITION: Glucose-6-phosphate dehydrogenase (G6PD) deficiency is a disorder of the red blood cells. Many different mutations of the enzyme occur and are known by such names as G6PD A-, G6PD Mediterranean, and G6PD Union deficiencies.

DIFFERENTIAL DIAGNOSIS: Unstable hemoglobin syndromes; Hereditary nonspherocytic hemolytic anemia due to pyruvate kinase deficiency; Glucose-phosphate isomerase deficiency; Hexokinase deficiency.

SYMPTOMS AND SIGNS: Mild forms of G6PD deficiency, such as G6PD A- deficiency, are characterized by hemolytic anemia on exposure to oxidizing drugs including primaquine, furadantin, and diaminodiphenylsulphone. In these forms, young erythrocytes generally have normal or near-normal G6PD activity and the hemolytic anemia is self-limited. With severe forms, such as G6PD Mediterranean deficiency, even young red cells are severely deficient. Many infectious diseases can also trigger hemolytic anemia in the G6PD-deficient patient. In some forms, ingestion of fava beans will produce hemolytic anemia. The most serious clinical consequence of G6PD deficiency, which affects only a small subset of G6PD-deficient newborns, is neonatal jaundice, which can lead to kernicterus. These are usually infants who have also inherited the UDPGT1 promoter mutation that causes Gilbert disease. The common (polymorphic) forms of G6PD deficiency are associated with hemolytic anemia only in the presence of stress such as drug administration or infection, but some less common variants are functionally so severe that they are associated with chronic hemolysis. These are designated as class I variants, and the clinical syndrome is hereditary nonspherocytic hemolytic anemia.

ETIOLOGY/EPIDEMIOLOGY: The gene encoding G6PD is located on the X chromosome, and the disorder is transmitted in a sex-linked fashion. Males are fully affected; females possess a mosaic of red cells, some normal and some deficient. The ratio of deficient to normal cells varies markedly in heterozygotes. More than 100 mutations of G6PD have been characterized at the DNA level, and many more have been described as being distinct on the basis of their biochemical characteristics. The prevalence of G6PD mutations and the type of mutation found varies among populations. In the Mediterranean region, G6PD Mediterranean deficiency is the most common variant and has a gene frequency that varies from less than 1% to more than 50%. Among African Americans, the gene frequency of G6PD A- deficiency is approximately 0.11.

DIAGNOSIS: Diagnosis is easily established on blood samples from males using enzyme assay or a screening test. In mild variants, however, the residual cells after a hemolytic episode may have normal or near normal enzyme activity. Sequencing of the G6PD gene is the most accurate way of establishing a diagnosis in heterozygous females.

TREATMENT

Standard Therapies: If the hemolytic anemia is drug induced, the drug should be discontinued. Generally, no therapy is needed, but blood transfusion may be required in the treatment of severe hemolytic episodes. Vitamin E has been used in chronic nonspherocytic hemolytic anemia due to G6PD deficiency, but not with uniform or convincing success. Splenectomy sometimes helps. Infants with neonatal icterus should be treated with phototherapy and/or exchange transfusion.

REFERENCES
Beutler E. Glucose-6-phosphate dehydrogenase (G6PD) deficiency. *N Engl J Med* 1991;324:169–174.
Beutler E. G6PD: population genetics and clinical manifestations. *Blood Rev* 1996;10:45–52.
Beutler E. Glucose-6-phosphate dehydrogenase deficiency and other red cell enzyme abnormalities. In: Beutler E, Lichtman MA, Coller BS, et al., eds. *Williams hematology.* New York: McGraw-Hill, 2001:527–545.
Beutler E, Vulliamy T. Hematologically important mutations: glucose-6-phosphate dehydrogenase. *Blood Cells Mol Dis.* 2002; 28:93–103.
Fiorelli G, Martinez DM, Cappellini MD. Chronic nonspherocytic haemolytic disorders associated with glucose-6-phosphate dehydrogenase variants. *Baillieres Clin Haematol* 2000; 13:39–55.

RESOURCES
58, 109, 365

---

30 Chronic Granulomatous Disease

Mary Dinauer, MD, PhD

DEFINITION: Chronic granulomatous disease (CGD) is an inherited immunodeficiency characterized by serious, recurrent bacterial and fungal infections and episodes of granulomatous inflammation. Symptoms usually begin in infancy or childhood. The disorder results from defects in the production of oxidants by neutrophils and other phagocytic leukocytes, leading to abnormalities in host defense and inflammation.

SYNONYMS: Chronic dysphagocytosis; Granulomatosis, chronic, familial; Granulomatosis, septic, progressive; Fatal granulomatous disease of childhood; Congenital dysphagocytosis.

DIFFERENTIAL DIAGNOSIS: Leukocyte adhesion deficiency; Wegener's granulomatosis; Sarcoidosis.

SYMPTOMS AND SIGNS: CGD is characterized by repeated bacterial and fungal infections that can involve the skin, lymph nodes, lungs, liver, or bones. Perirectal infections or brain abscesses can also occur. Infections are commonly due to *Staphylococcus aureus* as well as gram-negative bacteria (including *Serratia marscesans* and *Burkholderia cepacia*), *Nocardia,* and fungal species such as *Aspergillus* that normally do not cause infections. Some patients also develop granulomatous inflammation, possibly involving the skin; gastrointestinal tract, which can result in gastric outlet obstruction or colitis-like symptoms; or genitourinary tract, which can lead to obstruction. Granulomas are also seen in sites of chronic bacterial or fungal infection. Poor growth and an enlarged liver or spleen can occur. Blood analysis often shows signs of chronic inflammation, with leukocytosis and hypergammaglobulinemia. Symptoms usually begin in infancy or childhood, but some individuals with milder forms of the disease are well until their teens or even adulthood.

ETIOLOGY/EPIDEMIOLOGY: Prevalence is estimated at 1 in 250,000 individuals from all ethnic groups. Four subgroups exist, resulting from genetic defects in any one of four subunits of leukocyte enzyme known as the NADPH oxidase that generates superoxide during the respiratory burst. About two thirds of patients have an X-linked recessive form of CGD; therefore, many of the affected patients are male. The remaining patients have autosomal-recessive forms of CGD. In most cases of X-linked CGD, there is a male family history.

DIAGNOSIS: The diagnosis is established by laboratory testing for neutrophil respiratory burst oxidant production. This test is available at many regional medical centers caring for children with immunodeficiencies or at certain reference laboratories. Commonly used methods include the nitroblue tetrazolium (NBT) slide test (which should be done on a freshly drawn blood sample), a flow cytometric assay using dihydrorhodamine (DHR), or chemiluminescence.

TREATMENT
Standard Therapies: Treatment consists of prophylactic antibiotic therapy, such as trimethoprim and sulfamethoxazole. Corticosteroid drugs may be of benefit for granulomatous complications. Prophylactic Actimmune (interferon-γ) (Genentech) is also recommended and is given by intramuscular injection thrice weekly. Acute infections are treated aggressively; other treatment is symptomatic and supportive. With current management, most patients survive through at least early adulthood. Genetic counseling is recommended for patients and their families.

Investigational Therapies: The National Institutes of Health/National Institute of Allergy and Infectious Diseases (NIH/NAID) is conducting a clinical trial using a nonmyeloablative allogeneic bone marrow transplant protocol, open to children with a history of at least two serious infections and an HLA-identical sibling. Preliminary clinical studies on the use of gene therapy for treatment of CGD have been undertaken by the NIH/NAID and Indiana University School of Medicine.

REFERENCES
Mckusick VA, ed. Online Mendelian Inheritance in Man (OMIM). Johns Hopkins University. Entry no. 306400; last update 4/2/99.
Malech HL, Maples PB, Whiting-Theobold N, et al. Prolonged production of NADPH oxidase-corrected granulocytes after gene therapy for chronic granulomatous disease. *Proc Natl Acad Sci USA* 1997;94:12133–12138.
Sechler JM, et al. Recombinant human interferon-gamma reconstitutes defective phagocyte function in patients with chronic granulomatous disease in childhood. *Proc Natl Acad Sci USA* 1988;85:4874–4878.
Segal BH, et al. Genetic, biochemical, and clinical features of chronic granulomatous disease. *Medicine (Baltimore)* 2000;79:170–200.
Winkelstein JA, et al. Chronic granulomatous disease. Report on a national registry of 368 patients. *Medicine (Baltimore)* 2000;79:155–169.

RESOURCES
105, 193, 359

---

31   Hereditary Hemochromatosis

Richard L. Nelson, MD

DEFINITION: Hereditary hemochromatosis (HH) is an inherited, autosomal-recessive disease characterized in homozygotes by increased absorption of dietary iron, with consequent iron deposition in many organs, including the skin, joints, liver, pancreas, and heart. This iron buildup is toxic to many tissues and eventually results in arthritis, cirrhosis, diabetes, or heart failure.

SYNONYMS: Bronze diabetes; Iron overload.

SYMPTOMS AND SIGNS: No symptoms are specific to hemochromatosis, but rather of the aforementioned diseases arising from iron overload.

ETIOLOGY/EPIDEMIOLOGY: HH is believed to be the most prevalent recessive genetic disorder in the Western world. The gene responsible for the most prevalent form of HH, the *HFE* gene, produces a protein that binds β2-microglobulin. The *C282Y* mutation of the *HFE* gene is the one most commonly associated with clinical HH. The prevalence of HH *C282Y* homozygotes, reported to be 0.005%, is higher in Celtic populations and lower in African-American and Hispanic populations.

DIAGNOSIS: The demonstration of elevated serum ferritin levels and high transferrin saturation, particularly in the presence of end-organ toxicity consistent with the disorder, suggests the diagnosis, which is confirmed by genetic analysis.

TREATMENT

Standard Therapies: The therapy is a course of iron depletion, with frequent blood donation, until the serum ferritin level declines to a range of 10–20 ng/mL, and is kept below 50 ng/mL in follow-up. This goal is maintained by occasional phlebotomy, especially in men and postmenopausal women. The ideal time to initiate therapy is before the appearance of established HH-related diseases, especially cirrhosis and diabetes.

Investigational Therapies: Research is being done on the efficacy of dietary therapy of HH: iron chelation with tannins (tea) and phytates (fiber).

REFERENCES

Barton JC, McDonnell SM, Adams PC, et al. Management of hemochromatosis. *Ann Intern Med* 1998;129:932–939.

Burke W, Thomson E, Khoury M, et al. Hereditary hemochromatosis: gene discovery and its implications for population-based screening. *JAMA* 1998;280:172–178.

Conroy-Cantilena C. Phlebotomy, blood donation and hereditary hemochromatosis. *Transfer Med Rev* 2001;15:136–143.

Feder JN, Tsuchihashi Z, Irrinki A, et al. The hemochromatosis founder mutation in HLA-H disrupts beta2-microglobulin interaction and cell surface expression. *J Biol Chem* 1997;272:14025–14028.

Nelson RL, Persky V, Davis FG, et al. Is hereditary hemochromatosis a balanced polymorphism? *Hepatogastroenterology* 2001;48/38:523–526.

Steinberg KK, Cogswell ME, Chang JC, et al. Prevalence of C282Y and H63D mutations in the hemochromatosis (HFE) gene in the United States. *JAMA* 2001;285:2216–2222.

RESOURCES

36, 173, 365

---

32   Paroxysmal Cold Hemoglobinuria

Natalie D. Depcik-Smith, MD, and Mark E. Brecher, MD

DEFINITION: Paroxysmal cold hemoglobinuria (PCH) is a hemolytic anemia characterized by an autoantibody of the IgG subtype with affinity for cold temperatures directed toward the patient's red blood cells.

SYNONYM: Donath-Landsteiner hemolytic anemia.

DIFFERENTIAL DIAGNOSIS: Idiopathic (primary) cold agglutinin disease; Secondary cold agglutinin disease; Chronic cold agglutinin disease; Warm–antibody autoimmune hemolytic anemia; Myoglobinuria; Paroxysmal nocturnal hemoglobinuria.

SYMPTOMS AND SIGNS: Children and adults present with hemoglobinuria, jaundice, and pallor. Fever and abdominal pain are also common. Due to the transient nature of the disease in children, most are in the recovery phase of the illness at the time of presentation. Both children and adults are anemic at onset to varying degrees, with hemoglobins ranging from 25 to 125 g/L (mean, 68 g/L). The hemoglobin level often drops precipitously during an acute attack.

ETIOLOGY/EPIDEMIOLOGY: Most cases of PCH involve children and are self-limited, following a viral illness. The incidence has been reported as 2%–5% of all cases of autoimmune hemolytic anemia but more than 50% of all immune hemolytic syndromes diagnosed in children. In adults, the disease runs a more chronic, relapsing course. Earliest reports of the disease had identified PCH following infection with *Treponema pallidum*, the agent of syphilis. With the dramatic decline in the prevalence of syphilis, PCH in adults has declined and the current understanding of the adult form of the disease is less clear. No known genetic, sex, or racial risk factors exist, although the disease has been reported in families. Incidence is approximately equal in men and women.

DIAGNOSIS: The peripheral blood smear should be reviewed in cases of suspected hemolytic anemia. Red blood cell morphology is usually normal, but polychromasia and red cell fragmentation is infrequently seen. Spherocytosis and red cell rosetting around neutrophils (Insert Fig. 43) with erythophagocytosis (Insert Fig. 44) may be a clue to underlying PCH. The gold standard for diagnosis is the Donath-Landsteiner test. The direct antiglobulin test for complement is usually positive, but is not as specific as the Donath-Landsteiner test.

TREATMENT

Standard Therapies: Strict avoidance of cold temperatures is the most important prophylactic measure for the prevention of hemolysis. In general, cross-matching of blood can be accomplished. When transfusion is necessary due to severe anemia, it should not be delayed. Survival of the transfused red cells is likely similar to that of the patient's own cells. Use of a blood warmer during transfusion is particularly important. Splenectomy (in adult, relapsing cases) has met with mixed success. Corticosteroid therapy is not effective in PCH. Most cases terminate spontaneously and only require supportive therapy for a few days to weeks after onset.

REFERENCES

Depcik-Smith ND, Escobar MA, Ma AD, et al. RBC rosetting and erythophagocytosis in adult paroxysmal cold hemoglobinuria. *Transfusion* 2001;41:163.

Gottshe B, Salama A, Mueller-Eckhardt C. Donath-Landsteiner autoimmune hemolytic anemia in children: a study of 22 cases. *Vox Sang* 1990;58:281–286.

Heddle NM. Acute paroxysmal cold hemoglobinuria. *Trans Med Rev* 1989;3:219–229.

Hernandez JA, Steane SM. Erythophagocytosis by segmented neutrophils in paroxysmal cold hemoglobinuria. *Am J Clin Pathol* 1984;6:787–788.

Packman CH, Leddy JP. Cryopathic hemolytic syndromes. In: Beutler E, Lichtman MA, Collier BS, et al., eds. *Williams hematology*, 6th ed. New York: McGraw-Hill, 2001:649–653.

RESOURCES

27, 359

---

33   Paroxysmal Nocturnal Hemoglobinuria

Charles J. Parker, MD

DEFINITION: Paroxysmal nocturnal hemoglobinuria (PNH) is an acquired disease that arises as a result of a somatic mutation of the *PIG-A* gene. The primary clinical manifestation of this deficiency is intravascular hemolysis resulting in hemoglobinuria.

DIFFERENTIAL DIAGNOSIS: Antibody-mediated hemolytic anemias, especially paroxysmal cold hemoglobinuria.

SYMPTOMS AND SIGNS: Hemoglobinuria is the presenting symptom in approximately 25% of patients, but essentially all patients have laboratory evidence of ongoing hemolysis. The failure to compensate adequately for the hemolysis is due to underlying bone marrow dysfunction that is an important component of the disease. The disorder arises out of the setting of bone marrow failure syndromes, particularly aplastic anemia. Thus, in addition to anemia with evidence of hemolysis, patients with PNH usually have leukopenia, thrombocytopenia, or both. Another important clinical manifestation is thrombophilia. Female patients with PNH are at increased risk for thrombosis during pregnancy and the puerperium. When closely questioned, many patients with PNH complain of painful or difficult swallowing.

ETIOLOGY/EPIDEMIOLOGY: The disorder is not inherited and results from a somatic mutation affecting a primitive hematopoietic stem cell. The prevalence appears to be in the range of 1 case per $0.5–1.0 \times 10^6$ population. It has been described in all ages and many racial groups. It occurs in all parts of the world, but the incidence may be increased in regions where aplastic anemia is more common (e.g., the Far East and Indochina). There may be a slight female predominance.

DIAGNOSIS: The disease is diagnosed most frequently in adults in the fourth and fifth decades, but has been reported in all age groups ranging from children younger than 10 years to elderly adults. The disorder should be suspected in patients with unexplained symptoms or signs of chronic intravascular hemolysis, including hemoglobinuria, hemosiderinuria, and a markedly elevated serum lactate dehydrogenase. These findings coexisting with evidence of bone marrow failure (e.g., thrombocytopenia, leukopenia, or both) suggest PNH arising in the setting of aplastic anemia. The diagnosis of PNH is made by flow cytometry.

TREATMENT

Standard Therapies: Patients should take folate supplements. Serum ferritin should be determined, and supplemental iron given to iron-deficient patients. In some patients, the hemolysis of PNH is ameliorated by prednisone. Some responding patients require maintenance doses of steroids. An every-other-day schedule (not to exceed 15 mg) is favored to diminish the complications of long-term steroid use. If daily steroids are required, the dose should not exceed 10 mg. Few therapeutic options exist for steroid nonresponders. Allogeneic bone marrow transplantation can be curative but is usually reserved for patients with bone marrow failure and those with recurrent life-threatening thromboembolic disease. Thromboses should be managed with standard anticoagulant therapy, and thrombolytic therapy has been advocated for Budd-Chiari syndrome in the acute setting. Affected females who become pregnant should receive prophylactic heparin through the puerperium.

Investigational Therapies: The benefit of prophylactic coumadin in patients with no history of thromboembolic disease is being studied.

REFERENCES

Parker CJ, Lee GR. Paroxysmal nocturnal hemoglobinuria. In: Lee GR, Foerster J, Greer J, et al., eds. *Wintrobe's clinical hematology*, 10th ed. Baltimore: Williams & Wilkins, 1998:1264–1288.

Rosse WF. Paroxysmal nocturnal hemoglobinuria as a molecular disease. *Medicine* 1997;76:63–93.

Young NS, Moss J. *PNH and the GPI-linked proteins.* San Diego: Academic, 2000.

RESOURCES

350, 359

34   The Hemophilias

Margaret W. Hilgartner, MD

DEFINITION: The hemophilias are a group of bleeding disorders classified by coagulation factor deficiencies.

DIFFERENTIAL DIAGNOSIS: Deficiency of the other coagulation proteins; Platelet and thrombocytopenic abnormalities; Thrombophilic disorders.

SYMPTOMS AND SIGNS: The severity of factor VIII and IX disorders is defined by the degree of clotting factor deficiency in the patient's plasma. The normal plasma range is 50%–120% of each of these factors. Severe disease is found in those with less than 1% plasma level, moderate disease in those with 2%–10%, and mild disease in those with 10%–40%. Patients with severe disease have spontaneous bleeding beginning in early childhood, primarily into their joints, and leading to severe chronic arthopathy of most major joints by adulthood. The carrier female may have clotting factor levels in the range of mild disease, may bruise easily, and have menorrhagia. Patients with severe factor XI deficiency are not prone to spontaneous bleeding, even though their plasma level of factor XI may be very low.

ETIOLOGY/EPIDEMIOLOGY: Hemophilia A (factor VIII deficiency) occurs primarily in males, in 1 in 10,000 live male births, and is transmitted by females. Hemophilia B (factor IX deficiency) occurs in 1 in 750,000 births, again primarily in the male and transmitted by the female. A specific defect exists at a different gene on the X chromosome for each disorder. Hemophilia C (factor XI deficiency) occurs in 5.5%–8.0% of Ashkenazi Jews and in 1in 20,000 births among other ethnic groups in both males and females. Four mutations may account for this deficiency. Deficiencies of factors VIII and IX are the most common and potentially severe diseases.

DIAGNOSIS: The diagnosis of a bleeding disorder with either factor VIII or IX deficiency may be suspected when a baby has bleeding from the umbilical cord, routine heel stick, excessive bruising in the neonatal period, following circumcision, or later with bleeding into the knees or elbows when crawling. The activated partial thromboplastin time is markedly prolonged for factor VIII and IX deficiency but not for factor XI deficiency. The diagnosis of factor XI deficiency is usually made later in life when the patient may have bleeding with oral surgery or bleeding of the mucous membrane. The genotype is important in determining whether the patient may bleed with a low plasma factor level. Homozygotes may have more severe bleeding with trauma or surgery than the heterozygote patient.

TREATMENT

Standard Therapies: Treatment is based on replacement of the missing clotting factor. Concentrates of all three factors derived from normal human plasma are available for infusion, as are replacements of factors VIII and IX made by recombinant technology. The preferred treatment is to administer, by repeated infusions, specific recombinant clotting factors two to three times weekly to prevent bleeding episodes. Persons with moderate and mild disease require treatment for each bleeding episode sufficient to control bleeding and to allow for the 3–5 days necessary for healing to occur. If the patient has repeated bleeding into one joint, prophylactic treatment may be indicated. Several alternative therapies are available for patients with moderate and mild factor VIII disease, including desmopressin and amicar, an antifibrinolytic agent. Bleeding in the patient with factor XI deficiency requires the infusion of fresh frozen plasma. Some patients may require repeated infusions for trauma-induced bleeding and surgery.

Investigational Therapies: Experimental therapy using gene replacement for both factor VIII and IX deficiency is being explored.

REFERENCES

Bolton-Maggs P. *Factor XI deficiency and its management: treatment of hemophilia.* Montreal, Quebec, Canada: World Federation of Hemophilia, 1999:1–16.

DiMichele D, Neufield E. Hemophilia: a new approach to an old disease. *Hematol Clin North Am* 1998;12:1315–1344.

Forbes CD, Aledort LM, Madhok R, eds. *Hemophilia.* New York: Chapman & Hall, 1997.

Seligsohn U. Factor XI deficiency. *Thromb Hemost* 1993;70:68–71.

RESOURCES

302, 357

35 Hermansky-Pudlak Syndrome

William A. Gahl, MD, PhD

DEFINITION: Hermansky-Pudlak syndrome (HPS) is an autosomal-recessively inherited disorder characterized by oculocutaneous albinism and a bleeding tendency due to absent platelet dense bodies. Some patients also have pulmonary fibrosis or granulomatous colitis.

DIFFERENTIAL DIAGNOSIS: Oculocutaneous albinism; Ocular albinism; Chédiak-Higashi disease; Platelet storage pool deficiency.

SYMPTOMS AND SIGNS: The oculocutaneous albinism of HPS is variable in degree, but manifests with congenital nystagmus and decreased visual acuity varying from 20/50 to 20/400. Hair, skin, and eyes (irides) are hypopigmented compared with other family members. Iris transillumination and a pale retina are other signs related to albinism. Patients also present with bleeding due to impairment of platelet aggregation. Mucous membranes and soft tissue bleeds include bruising at the time of ambulation, frequent hematomas of unknown origin, heavy menstrual periods, and epistaxis. Prolonged bleeding can occur after tooth extraction, childbirth, and minor surgery. The platelet count, coagulation factors, prothrombin time, and partial thromboplastin time are normal; the bleeding time is often prolonged. Patients with a subtype due to mutations in the *HPS1* or *HPS4* gene are at increased risk for developing pulmonary fibrosis. Symptoms include shortness of breath, fatigue, and cough. Approximately 15% of patients have a granulomatous colitis resembling Crohn disease. Symptoms include cramping and bloody diarrhea. Occasionally, cardiac and renal involvement occurs.

ETIOLOGY/EPIDEMIOLOGY: The disorder can be caused by mutations in at least four genes: *HPS1, ADTB3A, HPS3,* and *HPS4*. All types of HPS are inherited in an autosomal-recessive fashion, and both genders are equally affected. There is a concentration of approximately 450 patients in northwest Puerto Rico with the same mutation in the *HPS1* gene, and a smaller group of patients in central Puerto Rico, each having an identical mutation in *HPS3*. Outside of Puerto Rico, the incidence of all types of HPS is probably in the range of 1 in 1 million live births.

DIAGNOSIS: Absence of platelet dense bodies on wet-mount electron microscopy in a patient with some degree of hypopigmentation makes the diagnosis. The absence of giant intracellular granules should be documented to rule out Chédiak-Higashi disease. Oculocutaneous albinism is diagnosed by demonstrating horizontal nystagmus and decreased visual acuity, as well as abnormal optic nerve fiber decussation on measurement of visual evoked potentials. Bleeding diathesis can be documented by demonstrating a lack of a secondary aggregation response by platelets, as well as absent dense bodies. A high-resolution CT chest scan should be performed in patients with restrictive lung disease. For patients with gastrointestinal symptoms, a colonoscopy can help confirm the diagnosis of granulomatous colitis.

TREATMENT

Standard Therapies: For oculocutaneous albinism, sun avoidance to prevent skin cancers is the most important intervention. In general, corrective lenses are not helpful. For the bleeding diathesis, intravenous DDAVP (1-desamino-8-D-arginine vasopressin) can be used prior to minor surgical procedures, and topical thrombin and gelfoam can also retard bleeding. For major surgery and profuse bleeding, platelet transfusions are indicated. No therapy exists for the pulmonary fibrosis, but the granulomatous colitis appears to respond to agents that treat Crohn disease, e.g., steroids or tumor necrosis factor-α inhibitors.

Investigational Therapies: Pirfenidone, an investigational antifibrotic agent, is being studied to treat the pulmonary fibrosis of HPS. Lung transplantation has not been performed.

REFERENCES
Brantly M, Avila NA, Shotelersuk V, et al. Pulmonary function and high resolution CT findings in patients with an inherited form of pulmonary fibrosis, Hermansky-Pudlak syndrome, due to mutations in *HPS-1. Chest* 1999;117:129–136.

Gahl WA, Brantly M, Kaiser-Kupfer MI, et al. Genetic defects and clinical characteristics of patients with a form of oculocutaneous albinism (Hermansky-Pudlak syndrome). *N Engl J Med* 1998;338:1258–1264.

Huizing M, Anikster Y, Gahl WA. Hermansky-Pudlak syndrome and related disorders of organelle formation. *Traffic* 2000;1: 823–835.

Shotelersuk V, Gahl WA. Hermansky-Pudlak syndrome: models for intracellular vesicle formation. *Mol Genet Metab* 1998;65:85–96.

Witkop CJ, Babcock MN, Rao GHR, et al. Albinism and Hermansky-Pudlak syndrome in Puerto Rico. *Bol Asoc Med P Rico-Agosto* 1990;82:333–339.

RESOURCES
180, 286, 362

---

36 Langerhans Cell Histiocytosis

Kenneth L. McClain, MD, PhD

DEFINITION: Langerhans cell histiocytosis (LCH) is a nonmalignant proliferation of Langerhans cells (LCs). Children and adults may have LCH in skin, bones, lymph nodes, brain, lung, liver, spleen, and bone marrow (see also Hemophagocytic Histiocytosis entry).

SYNONYMS: Histiocytosis-X; Eosinophilic granuloma; Hand-Schuller-Christian syndrome; Letterer-Siwe disease.

DIFFERENTIAL DIAGNOSIS: Candida infection; Neuroblastoma; Leukemia; Tuberculosis; Ewing sarcoma; Bone cyst; Lymphoma; Storage disease; Portal hypertension; Infiltrative disease of the bone marrow; Congenital cysts.

SYMPTOMS AND SIGNS: Infants often present with an extensive seborrhea-like rash on the scalp, an erythematous papular rash, or deep ulcerative lesions in the groin. Some have purplish brown lesions 3–6 mm in diameter. Marked hypertrophy of the gingiva with early eruption of teeth occurs. Infiltration of the liver and spleen results in massive organomegaly. Liver dysfunction causes hypoproteinemia with edema and ascites. Lymph nodes in the cervical, axillary, and inguinal areas are most often affected, but mediastinal nodes may enlarge, causing wheezing and respiratory compromise. Lung involvement results in tachypnea and pneumothoraces. Bone marrow infiltration causes pancytopenia, but thrombocytopenia is often the most obvious problem, with bleeding and anemia that may be exacerbated by hypersplenism. Bone lesions in children or adults present as painful lesions. For children the skull is most often affected, followed by long bones of the upper and lower extremity, ribs, and spine. Adults have many more lesions in the mandible and maxilla. Pulmonary involvement is more prevalent in adults. Many adult female patients have ulcerative lesions in the genital tract or groin. Both children and adults may initially present with diabetes insipidus. Patients with cerebellar involvement present with ataxia. Cerebral infiltrations of several types may lead to headaches and behavior changes.

ETIOLOGY/EPIDEMIOLOGY: The etiology is unknown. The disorder occurs in approximately 5 children and 2–3 adults per million population. Several cytokines are expressed at higher levels in the LCs and surrounding lymphocytes. An underlying immune defect is the likely cause of disease, but no specific gene mutations or chromosomal abnormalities have been identified. Patients with LCH have a higher incidence of malignancy, either before or after diagnosis.

DIAGNOSIS: Diagnosis is made by radiography of the skull; a complete skeletal bone survey and bone scan; chest radiography; complete blood count and differential; erythrocyte sedimentation rate; liver function tests, including AST, ALT, bilirubin, and alkaline phosphatase; electrolytes; and urinalysis. CT of the skull is indicated if mastoids are involved. With pulmonary disease, high-resolution CT is indicated, and with brain involvement, MRI is indicated. For diabetes insipidus, a water deprivation test or serum and urine osmolality should be performed.

TREATMENT

Standard Therapies: Treatments vary depending on the extent of disease and involve chemotherapy with prednisone, vinblastine sulfate (Velban) with or without 6-mercaptopurine, and methotrexate. Patients with liver, spleen, lung, or bone marrow involvement are considered to be at higher risk for not responding to therapy. Patients with lesions in multiple bones or more than one risk organ have an excellent chance for responding to combination chemotherapy. If a patient does not respond to the standard therapy by the 6th week (or 12th week for a partial response), they should be changed to the salvage therapy (2-CdA/Ara-C) on the LCH-S protocol. A separate protocol exists for following and treating patients with central nervous system involvement.

Investigational Therapies: Anticytokine therapy is being investigated.

REFERENCES

Baugartner I, von Hochstetter A, Baumert B, et al. Langerhans cell histiocytosis in adults. *Med Pediatr Oncol* 1997;28:9–14.

Bhatia S, Nesbit ME, Egeler RM, et al. Epidemiology study of Langerhans cell histiocytosis in children. *J Pediatr* 1997;130: 774–784.

Egeler RM, Favara BE, van Meurs M, et al. Differential *in situ* cytokine profiles of Langerhans-like cells and T cells in Langerhans cell histiocytosis: abundant expression of cytokines relevant to disease and treatment. *Blood* 1999;94:4195–4201.

Geissman G, Lepelletier Y, Fraitag S, et al. Differentiation of Langerhans cells in Langerhans cell histiocytosis. *Blood* 2001; 97:1241–1248.

McClain KL. Histiocytic disorders. In: Haskell CM, ed. *Cancer treatment*, 5th ed. Philadelphia: WB Saunders, 2001:1236–1244.

RESOURCES

183, 357

---

37   Hyper-IgM Syndrome

Roger H. Kobayashi, MD

DEFINITION: Hyper-IgM syndrome is a primary immunodeficiency disease characterized by recurrent, severe bacterial or opportunistic infections, typically within the first 2 years of life.

SYNONYMS: Immunoglobulin deficiency with increased IgM; X-linked hyper-IgM syndrome.

DIFFERENTIAL DIAGNOSIS: AIDS; X-linked agammaglobulinemia; Combined variable immunodeficiency (CVID).

SYMPTOMS AND SIGNS: As with most primary immunodeficiencies, recalcitrant infections occur early in life. However, unlike X-linked agammaglobulinemia, lymphoid hyperplasia is common and, although bacterial infections predominate, *Pneumocystis carinii* pneumonia may be the initial presenting infection. Gastrointestinal infections and malabsorption are common and occasionally severe. Neutropenia is commonly observed. The X-linked form of the disease may be associated with persistent stomatitis or oral ulcers. Bacterial cholangitis may be a life-threatening complication. Autoimmune cytopenias and thyroid disease can be seen, and anemia associated with chronic Parvovirus B19 infection has been reported. Arthritis and malignancies also occur with increased frequency in these patients.

ETIOLOGY/EPIDEMIOLOGY: X-linked transmission is most common; therefore, most cases occur in males. The occurrence of the disease in women suggests autosomal-recessive or -dominant inheritance in some cases. In the X-linked form, the defect lies in the T cell, which fails to express the activation protein, CD40 ligand, necessary for signaling B-lymphocytes to switch production from IgM to other immunoglobulin types. Rarely, it may be the failure of the B-lymphocyte (CD40 receptor defect) to appropriately receive the T-cell signal.

DIAGNOSIS: Serum IgG and IgA are markedly decreased with concomitant normal or elevated levels of serum IgM (polyclonal elevation). Neutropenia occurs in more than 50% of patients, and anemia is common. Peripheral B-lymphocyte numbers are normal, but T cells characteristically fail to express CD40 ligand on their surfaces. Antibody function of the non-IgM classes is diminished. More than 20 separate point mutations that cause CD40 ligand to be defectively expressed have been described.

TREATMENT

Standard Therapies: As with other hypogammaglobulinemias, infusion of intravenous immune globulin (IVIG) at 400 mg/kg/dose every 3–4 weeks results in a marked decrease in infections. Trough levels of serum IgG are maintained above 500 mg/dL. IgM levels may normalize and, in some cases, neutropenia may improve, but persistent cases require granulocyte colony-stimulating factor. In some cases, malabsorption may be severe, requiring total parenteral nutrition. Infants are especially prone to *Pneumocystis* pneumonia, mandating trimethoprim-sulfamethoxazole prophylaxis. All patients with anemia should be evaluated for parvovirus B19 infection by polymerase chain reaction and treated with high-dose IVIG 2,000 mg/kg divided over 1–2 days. Sclerosing cholangitis is a major complication requiring subspecialty management.

Investigational Therapies: Studies evaluating agents that activate the B-cell CD40 receptor are ongoing. Gene therapy is also being investigated.

REFERENCES

Allen RC, Armitage RJ, Conley ME, et al. CD40 ligand gene defects responsible for X-linked hyper-IgM syndrome. *Science* 1993;259:990–993.

Hayward AR, Levy J, Pacchem F, et al. Cholangiopathy and tumors of the pancreas, liver and biliary tree in boys with X-linked immunodeficiency with hyper-IgM. *J Immunol* 1997; 158:977–983.

Levy J, Espanol-Boren T, Thomas C, et al. Clinical spectrum of X-linked hyper-IgM syndrome. *J Pediatr* 1997;130:47–54.

Notarangelo LD, Duse M, Ugazio AG. Immunodeficiency with hyper-IgM (HIM). *Immunodeficiency Rev* 1992;3:101–122.

Seyama K, Kobayashi RH, Hasle H, et al. Parvovirus B19-induced anemia as the presenting manifestation of X-linked hyper-IgM syndrome. *J Infect Dis* 1998;178:318–324.

RESOURCES

27, 356, 359

---

38   Large Granular Lymphocyte Leukemia

William J. Hogan, MD, MRCPI, and Ayalew Tefferi, MD

DEFINITION: Large granular lymphocyte (LGL) leukemia is a chronic disorder characterized by clonal large granular lymphocytes.

SYNONYMS: LGL lymphoproliferative disease (LGL-LPD); T-cell chronic lymphocytic leukemia; Chronic T-cell lymphocytosis; T-suppressor cell leukemia; T-lymphoproliferative disease.

DIFFERENTIAL DIAGNOSIS: Other low-grade lymphoproliferative disorders; Reactive lymphocytosis; Viral infections.

SYMPTOMS AND SIGNS: Patients with LGL leukemia may present with a combination of fatigue and constitutional symptoms, cytopenias, hepatosplenomegaly, and bone marrow infiltration. Approximately one fourth of patients are asymptomatic at diagnosis. Anemia is noted in half of patients. Oval macrocytosis is present in some patients. Severe neutropenia (<500/mL) may be noted and may be associated with recurrent infections and mouth sores. Thrombocytopenia may be present and is generally mild. Patients with LGL lymphoproliferative disorders frequently have humoral immune abnormalities, including positive test results for rheumatoid factor, antinuclear antibodies, and polyclonal hypergammaglobulinemia. Rheumatoid arthritis, vasculitic syndromes, or splenomegaly may also be present.

ETIOLOGY/EPIDEMIOLOGY: The mean age at diagnosis is 60 years, with a slight male gender predilection. The cause is unknown, but findings from various studies suggest that a retrovirus or homologous protein may be implicated in the pathogenesis of the disease.

DIAGNOSIS: Diagnosis depends on the combination of the described clinical features, supported by blood cell morphology, immunophenotyping, and gene rearrangement studies. The diagnosis should be considered in patients with chronic or cyclic neutropenia, pure red cell aplasia, or rheumatoid arthritis associated with increased numbers of LGL cells. A substantial proportion of patients do not have elevated total lymphocyte counts and patients with less than 2000 LGL/μL (the traditional threshold for diagnosis) may have disease requiring therapy. Flow cytometry in conjunction with morphology is helpful in making the diagnosis of LGL leukemia.

TREATMENT

Standard Therapies: Individualization of therapy is particularly important in this disorder. Therapy is often supportive. Significant cytopenias as a result of pure red cell aplasia, hemolysis, or multilineage aplasia may warrant specific therapy. Additional indications for therapy may include neutropenia with recurrent infections, symptomatic splenomegaly, or rheumatoid arthritis. If evidence of significant hemolysis exists, corticosteroids may be the intervention of choice. In patients with pancytopenia, immunosuppression with antithymocyte globulin or cyclosporine may be helpful. Cyclophosphamide may also be useful, particularly in patients with pure red cell aplasia, as it can reduce the long-term toxicity of chronic corticosteroid therapy.

Investigational Therapies: Methotrexate is being investigated.

REFERENCES
Brouet JC, Sasportes M, Flandrin G, et al. Chronic lymphocytic leukaemia of T-cell origin. Immunological and clinical evaluation in eleven patients. *Lancet* 1975;2:890–893.

Dhodapkar MV, Li CY, Lust JA, et al. Clinical spectrum of clonal proliferations of T-large granular lymphocytes: a T-cell clonopathy of undetermined significance. *Blood* 1994;84: 1620–1627.

Lamy T, Loughran TP Jr. Current concepts: large granular lymphocyte leukemia. *Blood Rev* 1999;13:230–240.

Loughran TP Jr, Kidd PG, Starkebaum G. Treatment of large granular lymphocyte leukemia with oral low-dose methotrexate. *Blood* 1994;84:2164–2170.

Tefferi A, Li CY, Witzig TE, Dhodapkar MV, et al. Chronic natural killer cell lymphocytosis: a descriptive clinical study. *Blood* 1994;84:2721–2725.

RESOURCES
241, 242, 357

---

39 Lymphangioleiomyomatosis

Arnold S. Kristof, MD, FRCPC, and Joel Moss, MD, PhD

DEFINITION: Lymphangioleiomyomatosis (LAM) is a disease of abnormal smooth muscle proliferation in the lung, abdominal organs, and axial lymphatics. It occurs primarily in women of childbearing age and involves the formation of abdominal angiomyolipomas as well as cystic pulmonary lesions that cause recurrent pneumothoraces and chronic respiratory failure.

DIFFERENTIAL DIAGNOSIS: Tuberous sclerosis complex; Emphysema; Eosinophilic granuloma; Sarcoidosis; Diffuse pulmonary lymphangiomatosis; Cystic fibrosis; Asthma.

SYMPTOMS AND SIGNS: LAM is most often diagnosed in patients who present with progressive dyspnea or recurrent pneumothoraces. Patients may experience chronic cough, wheezing, and hemoptysis, as well as symptoms related to chylous ascites or pleural effusions. Angiomyolipomas and axial lymphatic masses, which frequently involve the kidneys, may give rise to flank pain, hematuria, and, rarely, abdominal hemorrhage. Engorgement of the lymphatics (e.g., lymphangioleiomyoma) can result in lower extremity swelling. Physical examination of the lung most commonly shows crackles; wheezing occurs in some patients. Dullness to percussion and decreased breath sounds are present in patients with chylothorax. Abdominal masses may be palpated in patients with angiomyolipomas and lymphangioleiomyomas.

ETIOLOGY/EPIDEMIOLOGY: Approximately 400 cases of LAM are reported in the United States; the true incidence is unknown. Lung cysts characteristic of LAM occur in approximately 30% of patients with tuberous sclerosis complex (TSC), suggesting a common etiology. Unlike TSC, LAM is not inherited, and specific genetic mutations have not been described.

DIAGNOSIS: Characteristic thin-walled cysts seen on high-resolution chest CT are consistent with LAM. Angiomyolipomas seen on abdominal imaging support the diagnosis. The gold standard is open lung, transbronchial, or angiomyolipoma biopsy with histopathologic evidence of proliferation of abnormal smooth muscle cells that are immunoreactive with a monoclonal antibody, HMB45. Chest radiography shows increased interstitial markings with preserved lung volumes. Pulmonary function testing demonstrates an obstructive ventilatory abnormality with superimposed restriction in 20% of patients. A significant bronchodilator response may be detected in 25% of patients. The diffusion capacity is commonly decreased disproportionately to abnormalities in spirometry or lung volumes, and correlates inversely with disease severity.

TREATMENT
Standard Therapies: Dyspnea and cough are treated symptomatically. Patients with a significant bronchodilator response on pulmonary function testing may benefit from inhaled bronchodilators and/or corticosteroids. Supplementary oxygen should be administered as required. Recurrent pneumothorax and chylous effusions may warrant chemical pleurodesis. The use of talc should be avoided, because patients may ultimately require lung transplantation.

Reduced dietary intake of triglycerides in patients with chylous effusions has not been shown to be beneficial. Because LAM is strongly associated with osteoporosis, bone density should be measured in all patients, and any bone density loss should be treated aggressively with bisphosphonates in conjunction with calcium and vitamin D supplementation. Surgical resection of abdominal angiomyolipomas should be considered in patients with unrelenting pain or hemorrhage. Because LAM occurs primarily in women of childbearing age, the mainstay of treatment has been the use of agents or procedures that reduce estrogen levels. No controlled trials have shown that exogenous progesterone, androgens, or bilateral oophorectomy have an effect on survival or preservation of lung function.

REFERENCES
Kalassian KG, Doyle R, Kao P, et al. Lymphangioleiomyomatosis: new insights. *Am J Respir Crit Care Med* 1997;155:1183–1186.
Kitaichi M, Nishimura K, Itoh H, et al. 1995. Pulmonary lymphangioleiomyomatosis: a report of 46 patients including a clinicopathologic study of prognostic factors. *Am J Respir Crit Care Med* 1995;151:527–533.
Moss J. LAM and other diseases characterized by smooth muscle proliferation. In: Lenfant C, ed. *Lung biology in health and disease.* New York: Marcel Dekker, 1999.

RESOURCES
40, 229, 357

40   Hereditary Lymphedema

Joseph L. Feldman, MD

DEFINITION: Hereditary (primary) lymphedema is developmental dysplasia of the lymph circulatory system, resulting in the accumulation of protein-rich fluid in the interstitium and peripheral edema.

SYNONYMS: Nonne-Milroy disease or congenital lymphedema; Meige disease or lymphedema praecox (if onset is before age 35); Lymphedema tarda (onset after age 35).

DIFFERENTIAL DIAGNOSIS: Lipedema; Venous insufficiency; Phlebothrombosis; Myxedema; Tumor obstructing lymph flow.

SYMPTOMS AND SIGNS: Signs include swelling of all or a segment of a limb, usually unilateral. Hereditary lymphedema usually is first noticed distally but can involve the adjacent trunk, including the genitalia. Congenital lymphedema is present at birth and can affect more than one limb and the face. Meige disease usually occurs around the time of puberty and onset can be gradual or sudden. Trauma, infection, or pregnancy can precipitate the edema. Pitting edema may be present in early, nonfibrotic lymphedema. Chronic lymphedema is nonpitting and fibrotic with thickened cutaneous folds. Stemmer sign may be present. The patient may have limb tightness, heaviness, and restricted joint movement.

ETIOLOGY/EPIDEMIOLOGY: Hereditary lymphedema can be inherited in different ways. Milroy and Meige diseases are familial and dominantly inherited in some families. A lymphedema gene has been localized to the bottom of human chromosome 5 (vascular endothelial growth factor–C receptor). Four other lymphedema-causing genetic changes have been identified. The estimated occurrence of primary lymphedema is 1 in 6,000. The distribution is reported to be 87% in women and 13% in men. Associated developmental disorders may include Klippel-Trenaunay-Weber syndrome, Turner XO syndrome, Noonan syndrome, and lymphedema-hypoparathyroid syndrome. Lymphostatic enteropathy due to intestinal lymphangiectasis has been observed with Noonan syndrome and Nonne-Milroy disease.

DIAGNOSIS: The history and physical examination usually confirm the diagnosis. Lymphoscintigraphy is the imaging examination of choice. Direct lymphography is invasive and rarely used due to complications caused by the contrast agent. Venous ultrasonography or venography can rule out phlebothrombosis as the cause of limb edema. MRI can detect tissue edema, lymphoceles, and fibrosis.

TREATMENT
Standard Therapies: Complex decongestive therapy is the preferred treatment for lymphedema. It includes manual lymph decongestive massage, compression bandaging with short stretch elastic bandages, exercises, and instruction in self-care. Sequential intermittent compression pumps are used occasionally to treat nonfibrotic lymphedema and never as the sole modality of treatment. Rehabilitation therapy is necessary in cases of severe lymphedema resulting in impairment of the activities of daily living. Peripheral lymphedema is more severe in overweight individuals; they should follow a reducing diet and exercise program. Diuretics can be of short-term benefit in early, nonfibrotic lymphedema, but cause concentration of os-

motically active interstitial proteins and, in the long term, aggravate lymphedema. Emotional support should be available to patients because they may experience embarrassment, anger, anxiety, and depression. Surgical treatment—debulking or microlymphatic anastomoses—is rarely effective.

REFERENCES

Consensus Document of the ISL Executive Committee. The diagnosis and treatment of peripheral lymphedema. *Lymphology* 1995;28:113–117.

Ferrell RE, Levinson KL, Esman JH, et al. Hereditary lymphedema: evidence for linkage and genetic heterogeneity. *Hum Mol Genet* 1998;7:2073–2078.

Greenlee R, Hoyme H, Witte M, et al. Developmental disorders of the lymphatic system. *Lymphology* 1993;26:156–168.

Ko DSC, Lerner R, Klose G, et al. Effective treatment of lymphedema of the extremities. *Arch Surg* 1998;133:452–458.

Weissleder H, Schuchhardt C. *Lymphedema—diagnosis and therapy.* Cologne, Germany: Viavital Verlag, 2001.

RESOURCES

310, 311, 356

---

41   Hemophagocytic Lymphohistiocytosis

Kenneth L. McClain, MD, PhD

DEFINITION: Hemophagocytic lymphohistiocytosis (HLH) is an aggressive proliferation of macrophages that causes fevers, organomegaly, pancytopenia, coagulopathy, liver failure, and central nervous system symptoms.

SYNONYMS: Familial hemophagocytic lymphohistiocytosis; Familial erythrophagocytic lymphohistiocytosis; Viral-associated hemophagocytic syndrome.

DIFFERENTIAL DIAGNOSIS: Sepsis; Leukemia; Fever of unknown origin.

SYMPTOMS AND SIGNS: Patients present with high fevers, maculopapular rash, failure to thrive, hepatosplenomegaly, lymphadenopathy, cytopenias, coagulopathy, elevated liver function test results, and high serum ferritin.

ETIOLOGY/EPIDEMIOLOGY: The disease most often affects infants from birth to 18 months, but older children and adults are also affected. In Sweden, the incidence is estimated to be 1.2 children per million per year or 1 in 50,000 live births. The male:female ratio is nearly equal. It is likely that many children go undiagnosed. Among the infections associated with HLH are Epstein-Barr virus, cytomegalovirus, parvovirus, herpes simplex, varicella-zoster virus, and measles, fungal and bacterial. HLH has been found in patients with lupus, arthritis, immune deficiencies, and malignancies. Familial cases may represent as many as 50% of all cases and are frequently associated with parental consanguinity. There is no way to distinguish between familial or sporadic cases based on any laboratory test or clinical feature. Markedly elevated levels of several cytokines in the blood cause HLH. Among these are interferon-γ, tumor necrosis factor-α, interleukin-10, and interleukin-12, as well as elevated levels of interleukin-2 receptor. Patients have markedly decreased or absent natural killer cell function and the test serves as a surrogate marker for disease susceptibility. Natural killer dysfunction is associated with a defect in the perforin gene on chromosome 10. The connection between these defects and the disease is still being investigated.

DIAGNOSIS: Specific criteria for diagnosis include the following: fever, peaks above 38.5 °C for 7 days or more; splenomegaly, more than 3 cm below costal margin; cytopenias affecting two or more lineages; hemoglobin less than 90 g/L; platelets less than 100×10^9/L; neutrophils less than 1.0×10^9/L; coagulopathy with markedly prolonged prothrombin time/partial thromboplastin time; fibrinogen less than 1.5 g/L or less than 3 SD; and hypertriglyceridemia (fasting level greater than 2 m*M*) and/or hyperferritinemia (>1,000 ng/mL). The key diagnostic finding, hemophagocytosis by macrophages in the bone marrow, lymph nodes, or spleen, is present in 80% of patients.

TREATMENT

Standard Therapies: Treatment by the Histiocyte Society HLH-94 protocol includes induction with dexamethasone and etoposide (VP-16), followed by continuous cyclosporine with pulses of dexamethasone and VP-16 for 1 year. This therapy may be sufficient for children older than 4 years, but bone marrow transplantation provides the best overall cure rate, above 60%. It is critical that all patients be registered on this protocol so advances in the cure and understanding of HLH can be made. Use of immunosuppressive agents, antiviral drugs, or steroids alone have not been as successful as the HLH-94 protocol, and the use of these is discouraged.

REFERENCES
Arico M, Janka G, Fischer A, et al. Hemophagocytic lymphohistiocytosis. Report of 122 children from the International
Registry. *Leukemia* 1996;10:197–203.
Esumi N, Ikushima S, Hibi S, et al. High serum ferritin level as a
marker of malignant histiocytosis and virus-associated hemophagocytic syndrome. *Cancer* 1988;61:2071–2076.
Haddad E, Sulis M-L, Jabado N, et al. Frequency and severity of
central nervous system lesions in hemophagocytic lymphohistiocytosis. *Blood* 1997;89:794–800.

Henter J-I, Elinder G, Söder O, et al. Hypercytokinemia in familial hemophagocytic lymphohistiocytosis. *Blood* 1991;78:2918–
2922.
Stepp SE, Dufourcq-Lagelouse R, Le Deist F, et al. Perforin gene
defects in familial hemophagocytic lymphohistiocytosis.
Science 1999;286:1957–1959.

RESOURCES
183, 357

42   Angioimmunoblastic Lymphadenopathy-Type T-Cell Lymphoma

John W. Sweetenham, MD

DEFINITION: Angioimmunoblastic T-cell lymphoma
(AIL) is a subtype of peripheral T-cell non-Hodgkin lymphoma (NHL). Characteristic presenting features include
generalized, low-volume lymphadenopathy, hepatosplenomegaly, skin rashes, and polyclonal hypergammaglobulinemia, associated with marked constitutional symptoms
including fevers, night sweats, and arthralgias.

SYNONYMS: Angioimmunoblastic lymphadenopathy
with dysproteinemia; Immunoblastic lymphadenopathy;
Lymphogranulomatosis X.

DIFFERENTIAL DIAGNOSIS: Other forms of NHL,
particularly indolent lymphomas and primary cutaneous
T-cell lymphoma.

SYMPTOMS AND SIGNS: The median age of onset is
approximately 60–65 years. Typical presenting symptoms
include marked constitutional symptoms such as night
sweats, fevers, and weight loss. A history of generalized
pruritis and pruritic skin rashes is common. Other
common presenting symptoms include lymphadenopathy, which is usually low volume, hepatosplenomegaly,
the presence of pleural effusions, ascites, peripheral
edema, and a polyclonal hypergammaglobulinemia. Mediastinal lymphadenopathy is common. Autoimmune phenomena such as mild arthritis, Coombs-positive hemolytic anemia, rheumatoid factor, cryoglobulins, and
circulating immune complexes are also common. Most
patients have stage III or IV disease at presentation.

ETIOLOGY/EPIDEMIOLOGY: The disorder is a subtype
of NHL, constituting less than 1% of all cases. The etiology
is unknown, although an association with Epstein-Barr
virus has been reported.

DIAGNOSIS: The diagnosis of AIL is made by biopsy of
an affected lymph node or involved extranodal site.

TREATMENT
Standard Therapies: Optimal therapy is poorly defined.
Various approaches have included the use of corticosteroids alone, single-agent chemotherapy, and multiagent
combination chemotherapy. The most widely reported
chemotherapy regimen is COPBLAM/IMVP16 (cyclophosphamide, vincristine, bleomycin, adriamycin, procar-
bazine, prednisone, ifosfamide, methotrexate, etoposide).
Reported median overall survivals for patients with AIL
are between 6 and 18 months. Long-term (>5 years)
disease-free survival is reported in only 20%–30% of
patients.

Investigational Therapies: Experimental therapies have
included cyclosporine A and interferon.

REFERENCES
Ganesan TS, Dhaliwal HS, Dorreen MS, et al. Angioimmunoblastic lymphadenopathy: a clinical, immunological
and molecular study. *Br J Cancer* 1987;55:437–442.
Pautier P, Devidas A, Delmer A, et al. Angioimmunoblastic-like T-
cell non-Hodgkin's lymphoma: outcome after chemotherapy
in 33 patients and review of the literature. *Leuk Lymphoma*
1999;32:545–552.
Schlegelberger B, Zwingers T, Hohenadel K, et al. Significance of
cytogenetic findings for the clinical outcome in patients with

T-cell lymphoma of angioimmunoblastic lymphadenopathy type. *J Clin Oncol* 1996;14:593–599.

Siegert W, Nerl C, Agthe A, et al. Angioimmunoblastic lymphadenopathy (AILD)-type T-cell lymphoma: prognostic impact of clinical observations and laboratory findings at presentation. *Ann Oncol* 1995;6:659–664.

Steinberg AD, Seldin MF, Jaffe ES, et al. Angioimmunoblastic lymphadenopathy with dysproteinemia. *Ann Intern Med* 1988; 108:575–584.

RESOURCES

27, 30, 352

---

43 Mantle Cell Lymphoma

Jorge Romaguera, MD

DEFINITION: Mantle cell lymphoma is an uncontrolled growth of lymphocytes that normally reside in the mantle zone of the germinal follicle.

DIFFERENTIAL DIAGNOSIS: Follicular indolent lymphoma; Small lymphocytic lymphoma.

SYMPTOMS AND SIGNS: Signs of mantle cell lymphoma include enlarged nodes in the neck and groin and under the arms. Drenching sweats, fevers, more than 10% weight loss, diarrhea, gastrointestinal bleeding, or abdominal pain occur in 10% of patients.

ETIOLOGY/EPIDEMIOLOGY: Mantle cell lymphoma accounts for 8% of all non-Hodgkin lymphomas. It occurs more frequently in males, by a 3:1 ratio. The median age at diagnosis is 61 years. In 90%–100% of patients, the disease is in the advanced stages at presentation. The cause is not known.

DIAGNOSIS: Biopsy of enlarged lymph nodes is strongly recommended. Nodal distribution of the characteristic cell can be nodular or diffuse. This cell is of intermediate size and stains positive for CD5/CD19 (coexpression) and FMC-7, but negative for CD23. A chromosomal translocation juxtaposes the cyclin D1 oncogene located on 11q23 to the active 14q32 area and overproduces the cyclin D1 protein (a cell cycle regulator). Cyclin D1 immunohistochemical stains are positive.

TREATMENT

Standard Therapies: There are no standard therapies. Response to cyclophosphamide, doxorubicin, vincristine, and prednisone is poor. The complete response rate is 21%, with the median duration of response 10 months, and median survival 3 years. Autologous stem cell transplantation is not effective as salvage therapy. The best responses have been seen with aggressive, intense frontline chemotherapy with high-dose cyclophosphamide, total body irradiation, and autologous stem cell transplantation (100% complete response, 73% event-free survival at 2 years). The best results for relapsed/resistant disease are achieved with intense chemotherapy followed by allogeneic stem cell transplantation. Monoclonal antibody therapy seems to be effective and promising.

Investigational Therapies: For initial therapy, fractionated cyclophosphamide, doxorubicin, vincristine, and dexamethasone, alternating with high-dose methotrexate/cytarabine and rituximab in each cycle, are being investigated. For patients who have relapsed, allogeneic stem cell transplantation with nonmyeloblative chemotherapy is being studied.

REFERENCES

Foran JM, Cunningham D, Coiffer B, et al. Treatment of mantle cell lymphoma with Rituximab (chimeric monoclonal anti-/CD20 antibody): analysis of factors associated with response. *Ann Oncol* 2000;11(suppl 1):177.

Khouri I, Lee MS, Romaguera J. Allogeneic hematopoietic transplantation for mantle cell lymphoma: molecular remissions and evidence of graft-vs-malignancy. *Ann Oncol* 2000.

Khouri IF, Romaguera J, Kantarjian H, et al. Hyper-CVAD and high dose methotrexate/cytarabine followed by stem cell transplantation: an active regimen for aggressive mantle cell lymphoma. *J Clin Oncol* 1998;16:3803.

Romaguera J, Dang N, Hagemeister FB, et al. Preliminary report of Rituximab with intensive chemotherapy in untreated aggressive mantle cell lymphoma. *Blood* 2000;96:11.

RESOURCES

241, 251, 352

44   X-Linked Lymphoproliferative Syndrome

Roger H. Kobayashi, MD

DEFINITION: X-linked lymphoproliferative (XLP) syndrome is an X-linked disease in which young males are exquisitely susceptible to overwhelming Epstein-Barr virus (EBV) infections.

SYNONYMS: Duncan disease; Purtilo syndrome; Fatal infectious mononucleosis syndrome.

DIFFERENTIAL DIAGNOSIS: Hypogammaglobulinemia; Malignant lymphoma; Aplastic anemia; Hemophagocytic syndrome.

SYMPTOMS AND SIGNS: Patients appear normal until they contract EBV infection, developing one or more of the following manifestations: fatal infectious mononucleosis, malignant lymphoma, hypogammaglobulinemia, or aplastic anemia. In the fulminant infectious mononucleosis form, high fever, massive hepatosplenomegaly, elevated white cell count with atypical lymphocytosis, and elevated immunoglobulins are presenting findings. As the disease rapidly progresses, pancytopenia with massive bone marrow infiltration ensues. Those who survive develop lymphoma, bone marrow failure, or combined immunodeficiency. Virtually all patients die, and no patient has survived past 40 years of age. Just before death, marrow failure and histiocytic hemophagocytosis are seen. As many as one third of patients may present with hypogammaglobulinemia before EBV infection. Rarely, lymphoma, agammaglobulinemia, or aplastic anemia may be the initial presenting feature.

ETIOLOGY/EPIDEMIOLOGY: XLP disease occurs from a defect in the *SH2D1A* gene located at Xq25 of the long arm of the X chromosome. This gene encodes for a small protein that may be important in signal transduction in activated T-lymphocytes. This defect allows for uncontrolled proliferation of EBV-infected B cells.

DIAGNOSIS: The clinical diagnosis depends on characteristic findings, together with a positive family history. A positive family history includes two or more maternally related males with XLP presentation after an EBV infection or a maternally-related male from an XLP family with genetic linkage to the XLP locus. A positive family history with low serum IgG and/or elevated IgA or IgM is suggestive but requires genetic studies. Absent or poor anti-EBNA response after EBV infection is also suspicious and should be followed up with genetic studies. Similarly, findings of histiocytic hemophagocytosis after EBV infection warrant genetic evaluation.

TREATMENT
Standard Therapies: Treatment is with histocompatible bone marrow transplantation. High-dose intravenous immune globulin (IVIG) together with interferon-α or interferon-γ have been tried in the fulminant phase with poor results. High-dose IVIG or methylprednisolone together with VP-16 (etoposide) have been used successfully in several children with the fulminant form, allowing for subsequent bone marrow transplantation. In XLP-identified patients without prior EBV infection, IVIG has been used prophylactically; the benefits are unproven, however, because several patients subsequently developed overwhelming EBV infection and died.

Investigational Therapies: Prophylaxis with EBV vaccine has been considered.

REFERENCES
Nicholsk E, Harkin DP, Levitz S, et al. Inactivating mutations in an *SH2* domain-encoding gene in X-linked lymphoproliferative syndrome. *Proc Natl Acad Sci USA* 1998;95:13765–13770.
Pracher E, Panzer-Grumayer ER, Zoubek A, et al. Successful bone marrow transplantation in a boy with X-linked lymphoproliferative syndrome and acute severe infectious mononucleosis. *Bone Marrow Transplant* 1994;13:655–658.
Purtilo DT. X-linked lymphoproliferative syndrome: an immunodeficiency disorder with acquired agammaglobulinemia fatal infectious mononucleosis or malignant lymphoma. *Arch Pathol Med* 1981;105:119–121.
Sullivan JL, Byron KS, Brewster FE, et al. X-linked lymphoproliferative syndrome: natural history of the immunodeficiency. *J Clin Invest* 1983;71:1765–1770.
Woda BA, Sullivan JL. Reactive histiocytic disorders. *Am J Clin Pathol* 1993;99:459–463.

RESOURCES
193, 352, 359

45 Lynch Syndromes

Henry T. Lynch, MD

DEFINITION: Lynch syndromes I and II account for approximately 5%–8% of all colorectal cancer (CRC) patients. Lynch syndrome I is an autosomal-dominantly inherited disease that predisposes to site-specific CRC with an early age of onset (~44 years), proximal predominant location of CRC (~70% proximal to the splenic flexure), and a statistically significant excess of synchronous and metachronous CRCs. Lynch syndrome II shows these same features but, in addition to CRC, there is a statistically significant excess of carcinomas of the endometrium, ovary, stomach, small bowel, hepatobiliary system, and transitional cell carcinomas of the ureter and renal pelvis. Sebaceous adenomas and carcinomas and multiple keratoacanthomas occur in the Muir-Torre syndrome variant.

SYNONYM: Hereditary nonpolyposis colorectal cancer (HNPCC).

DIFFERENTIAL DIAGNOSIS: All diseases associated with hereditary CRC. Familial adenomatous polyposis (FAP) can be excluded because of its profuse colonic adenomas, but the attenuated variant of FAP with an *APC* germline mutation is included. Other related disorders include: Familial CRC clusters; Hereditary hamartomatous polyposis syndromes; Ashkenazi *I1307K* mutation; Turcot syndrome; Familial CRC; Inflammatory bowel disease.

SYMPTOMS AND SIGNS: Symptoms and signs are those of each Lynch syndrome cancer. Pathology findings of CRC show a tendency toward a solid growth pattern, which accounts for the high frequency of poorly differentiated carcinomas, wherein these tumors resemble the "undifferentiated carcinoma" and the "medullary carcinoma" that have been described. These tumors appear to have a better prognosis than more typical types of CRC. Tumors contain the host-lymphoid response, namely, the Crohn-like reaction, peritumoral lymphocytic infiltrations, and tumor-infiltrating lymphocytes.

ETIOLOGY/EPIDEMIOLOGY: Causal germline mutations have been implicated in the DNA mismatch repair genes *MLH1, MSH2, MSH6, PMS1,* and *PMS2,* the most common being *MLH1* and *MSH2.* All racial and ethnic groups are at risk.

DIAGNOSIS: The syndrome should be suspected in patients with early age of onset of CRC and the integral cancers in the Lynch syndrome II variant, particularly when these appear to cluster within first- and second-degree relatives of the affected proband (revised Amsterdam criteria). An annual colonoscopy (because of accelerated carcinogenesis) is indicated because of excess of proximal CRC, in which a third of these tumors occur in the cecum. Screening for carcinoma of the endometrium includes transvaginal ultrasonography of the endometrium and the ovaries, endometrial aspiration, and CA 125 for ovaries. Ovarian screening has limitations, however.

TREATMENT

Standard Therapy: Standard therapy for CRC and integrally associated cancers is usually undertaken. Because of lifetime vulnerability of the entire colonic mucosa, a subtotal colectomy for initial CRC is recommended, with annual endoscopic evaluation of the remaining rectal-sigmoid area. Prophylactic colectomy is an option, particularly for carriers of mismatch repair gene mutations with early adenoma occurrence, poor compliance for full colonoscopy, or intense fear of CRC. Prophylactic hysterectomy and bilateral salpingo-oophorectomy is an option for women with germline mutations who have completed their families.

Investigational Therapies: Chemoprevention, including celecoxib, is being studied.

REFERENCES

Jessurun MR, Manivel JC. Cecal, poorly differentiated adenocarcinomas, medullary-type [Abstract]. *Mod Pathol* 1992;5:43.

Lynch HT, de la Chapelle A. Genetic susceptibility to non-polyposis colorectal cancer. *J Med Genet* 1999;36:801–818.

Lynch HT, Shaw MW, Magnuson CW, et al. Hereditary factors in cancer: study of two large Midwestern kindreds. *Arch Intern Med* 1966;117:206–212.

Vasen HFA, Watson P, Mecklin J-P, et al., ICG-HNPCC. New clinical criteria for hereditary nonpolyposis colorectal cancer (HNPCC, Lynch syndrome) proposed by the International Collaborative Group on HNPCC. *Gastroenterology* 1999;116:1453–1456.

Watson P, Lin K, Rodriguez-Bigas MA, et al. Colorectal carcinoma survival among hereditary nonpolyposis colorectal cancer family members. *Cancer* 1998;83:259–266.

46   Mastocytosis

Cem Akin, MD, PhD,
and Dean D. Metcalfe, MD

DEFINITION: Mastocytosis is characterized by the presence of increased numbers of mast cells in tissues, most commonly in the skin, bone marrow, spleen, liver, lymph nodes, and the gastrointestinal tract.

DIFFERENTIAL DIAGNOSIS: Idiopathic flushing, angioedema and/or anaphylaxis; Carcinoid syndrome; Pheochromocytoma; Leukemias; Lymphomas; Reactive mast cell hyperplasia.

SYMPTOMS AND SIGNS: Whereas cutaneous mastocytosis is the most common presentation in children, systemic (bone marrow) involvement is often encountered in adult-onset disease. Urticaria pigmentosa is the most common skin manifestation. The lesions may be pruritic. Infants and young children may experience idiopathic bullous eruptions over involved areas. Less common patterns of skin disease include diffuse cutaneous mastocytosis, telangiectasia macularis eruptive perstans, and mastocytomas. Most patients, in addition to the skin lesions, may variably demonstrate one of the following findings: ulcer disease, malabsorption, diarrhea, bone marrow pathology (mast cell aggregates), osteoporosis or osteosclerosis, hepatosplenomegaly, lymphadenopathy, soft tissue pain, fatigue, flushing and systemic anaphylaxis. Some forms of mastocytosis may be associated with a hematologic disorder such as myelodysplastic syndromes or myeloproliferative disorders. Mast cell leukemia is rare and is diagnosed by the presence of large numbers of mast cells in the peripheral blood.

ETIOLOGY/EPIDEMIOLOGY: Mastocytosis affects approximately equal numbers of males and females. The disease can occur at any age, although childhood-onset disease usually starts before age 6 months. Adult-onset mastocytosis appears to be a clonal neoplastic disorder of the hematopoietic stem cell. Somatic gain-of-function mutations in c-*kit*, the gene encoding the receptor for stem cell factor, have been detected in lesional skin in most adult patients and a few children. The cause of most cases of typical childhood-onset mastocytosis is unknown.

DIAGNOSIS: The diagnosis is suspected based on the presence of typical skin lesions and confirmed by biopsy. In some individuals with no skin lesions, a bone marrow biopsy demonstrating characteristic mast cell aggregates surrounded by a mononuclear infiltrate is diagnostic. Bone marrow biopsy and aspirate is recommended for patients with adult-onset disease and for children only if they have hepatosplenomegaly, lymphadenopathy, or peripheral blood abnormalities. Flow cytometric analysis of the bone marrow aspirate shows mast cells with surface CD2 and CD25 in most patients with systemic mastocytosis. A complete blood count, routine chemistry, liver function, and coagulation tests should be obtained in virtually every patient. An elevated baseline serum or plasma tryptase level (usually >20 ng/mL), considered to be a surrogate marker of total body mast cell numbers, may be helpful in diagnostic evaluation.

TREATMENT

Standard Therapies: Management of mastocytosis is aimed at controlling symptoms. H1 histamine receptor blockers are used to reduce pruritus and flushing. H2 antihistamines are useful in controlling symptoms due to gastric acid hypersecretion. Oral cromolyn sodium may help lessen gastrointestinal pain and cramping. Corticosteroids are used to control symptoms such as diarrhea with malabsorption and ascites. Topical corticosteroids or psoralen-UV-A treatment may result in temporary fading of the urticaria pigmentosa lesions. Epinephrine is used to treat episodes of vascular collapse. Patients with mastocytosis and an associated hematologic disorder should be treated for the specific hematologic disease. Interferon-α2b has been used with mixed success in patients with advanced bone marrow mastocytosis.

Investigational Therapies: Therapies under investigation include bone marrow transplantation and the use of tyrosine kinase inhibitors, targeting the mutated c-*kit* gene product.

REFERENCES

Akin C, Schwartz LB, Kitoh T, et al. Soluble stem cell factor receptor (CD117) and IL-2 receptor alpha chain (CD25) levels in the plasma of patients with mastocytosis: relationships to disease severity and bone marrow pathology. *Blood* 2000;96:1267–1273.

Escribano L, Orfao A, Diaz-Agustin B, et al. Indolent systemic mast cell disease in adults: immunophenotypic characterization of bone marrow mast cells and its diagnostic implications. *Blood* 1998;91:2731–2736.

Longley BJ Jr, Metcalfe DD, Tharp M, et al. Activating and dominant inactivating c-KIT catalytic domain mutations in distinct clinical forms of human mastocytosis. *Proc Natl Acad Sci USA* 1999;96:1609–1614.

Metcalfe DD, Soter NA, eds. Mast cell disorders. *Hematol Oncol Clin North Am* 2000;14:497–701.

Valent P, Horny H-P, Escribano L, et al. Diagnostic criteria and classification of mastocytosis: a consensus proposal. *Leuk Res* 2001;25:603–625.

RESOURCES

259, 351

47   May-Hegglin Anomaly

Michael J. Kelley, MD

DEFINITION: May-Hegglin anomaly is an inherited platelet condition characterized by thrombocytopenia, giant platelets, and leukocyte inclusions.

SYNONYM: Macrothrombocytopenia with leukocyte inclusions.

DIFFERENTIAL DIAGNOSIS: Sebastian syndrome; Idiopathic thrombocytopenia; Fechtner syndrome; Epstein syndrome; Bernard-Soulier syndrome; Gray platelet syndrome.

SYMPTOMS AND SIGNS: May-Hegglin anomaly is usually discovered incidentally when a platelet count is performed. Bleeding complications are generally mild. Approximately one third to one half of patients have symptoms including easy bruising, hypermenorrhagia, and postoperative hemorrhage. Exsanguination has not been reported. Many persons with the anomaly have had normal childbirth and surgery without complications. There are no distinctive physical findings.

ETIOLOGY/EPIDEMIOLOGY: May-Hegglin anomaly is inherited as an autosomal-dominant condition. The disorder is associated with mutations of the nonmuscle myosin heavy-chain type A (MYH9) gene on chromosome 22q. Prevalence is estimated at approximately 1 in 500,000. The anomaly is increasingly recognized since the widespread availability of electronic particle counters for automated platelet counting. May-Hegglin anomaly occurs in most caucasian and Asian ethnic groups, but rarely, if at all, in Africans. The features of May-Hegglin anomaly are present at birth.

DIAGNOSIS: Clinically, the platelet count is usually 40,000–80,000/μL but can be as low as 5,000/μL or nearly normal. The platelet number is underestimated by counting in electronic particle counters compared with manual counting using a hemocytometer, because many platelets may be above the size cutoff used for platelets. The mean platelet volume is usually greater than normal but can be normal if the electronic particle counter does not count the larger platelets. Hemoglobin indices and leukocyte count are normal. The peripheral blood smear is characteristic for giant platelets, large platelets, low to normal platelet estimate, and large distinctive azurphilic inclusions in leukocytes. Normal renal and auditory functions are typical and distinguish May-Hegglin anomaly from Fechtner and Epstein syndrome. Each neutrophil typically has at least one inclusion, as do many of the other granulocytes and monocytes. Immunohistochemical analysis of peripheral blood smears may show altered localization of nonmuscle myosin heavy-chain type A. Toxic granulations are absent. Bleeding time, platelet aggregation studies, and coagulation studies are normal. Ultrastructural analysis of leukocytes by electron microscopy shows the inclusions to be parallel bundles of filaments with characteristics of intermediate filaments. Genetic analysis is possible; penetrance is apparently complete with no phenocopies other than Sebastian syndrome, which is identical except for variant leukocyte inclusions.

TREATMENT
Standard Therapies: Most patients require no treatment and have normal life spans. For patients with significant hemorrhage, platelet transfusions are the treatment of choice. Other etiologies for hemorrhage should be considered. Treatment with corticosteroids, immunoglobulins, and splenectomy has not been effective.

REFERENCES
Greinacher A, Bux J, Kiefel V, et al. May-Hegglin anomaly: a rare cause of thrombocytopenia. *Eur J Pediatr* 1992;151:668–671.

Greinacher A, Mueller-Eckhardt C. Hereditary types of thrombocytopenia with giant platelets and inclusion bodies in the leukocytes. *Blut* 1990;60:53–60.

Kelley MJ, Jawien W, Ortel TL, et al. Mutation of MYH9, encoding non-muscle myosin heavy chain, in May-Hegglin anomaly. *Nat Genet* 2000;26:108–110.

May-Hegglin/Fechtner Syndrome Consortium. Mutations in *MYH9* result in the May-Hegglin anomaly, and Fechtner and Sebastian syndromes. *Nat Genet* 2000;26:103–105.

Noris P, Spedini P, Belletti S, et al. Thrombocytopenia, giant platelets, and leukocyte inclusion bodies (May-Hegglin anomaly): clinical and laboratory findings. *Am J Med* 1998;104: 355–360.

Pecci A, Noris, P, Invernizzi R, et al. Immunocytochemistry for the heavy chain of the non-muscle myosin IIA as a diagnostic tool for MYH9-related disorders. *Br J Hematol* 2002;117:164–167.

RESOURCES
357

---

48   Medulloblastoma

Corey Raffel, MD, PhD

DEFINITION: Medulloblastoma is a rapidly growing tumor, made up of small round cells with little cytoplasm, which occurs in the cerebellum of children. Mitotic activity is high and neuroblastic or glial differentiation may be seen.

SYNONYM: Primitive neuroectodermal tumor (PNET).

DIFFERENTIAL DIAGNOSIS: Ependymoma; Pilocytic astrocytoma; Astrocytoma; Choroid plexus papilloma; Choroid plexus carcinoma.

SYMPTOMS AND SIGNS: Symptoms often include those of raised intracranial pressure. Because the tumor often fills the fourth ventricle, cerebrospinal fluid circulation is obstructed and hydrocephalus results. Symptoms of elevated intracranial pressure include headache, vomiting, and, less often, diplopia. Signs of elevated intracranial pressure include papilledema and paresis of extraocular muscles. Children with medulloblastoma often have evidence of cerebellar dysfunction. Symptoms include difficulty walking and poor balance. Signs include truncal ataxia and, less often, appendicular ataxia. In infants the only sign may be an abnormally rapid rate of head growth. Rarely, a patient will present obtunded, from severe hydrocephalus.

ETIOLOGY/EPIDEMIOLOGY: The cause is unknown. The tumor occurs most often in children (80% of patients are younger than 15 years of age), with a median age at diagnosis of 6 years. It is more common in boys than girls, with a 2:1 male predominance. The incidence is approximately 5 cases per million population younger than 15 years.

DIAGNOSIS: The diagnosis of medulloblastoma should be considered in any child with the symptoms and signs previously mentioned. Workup includes MRI of the head before and after administration of gadolinium-based contrast material. The tumor appears as a bright, contrast-enhancing mass that arises in the roof of the fourth ven-tricle and usually fills the ventricle. The enhancement is usually homogeneous. There may be cystic areas in the tumor. If MRI is unavailable, CT before and after the administration of intravenous iodine-based contrast material may be used. On CT, the mass appears to attenuate radiographs more than the surrounding cerebellum. Again, contrast enhancement is usually bright and relatively homogeneous. If the patient is not severely obtunded from hydrocephalus, MRI of the entire spine should also be performed to look for cerebrospinal fluid dissemination of the tumor.

TREATMENT

Standard Therapies: Standard therapy for medulloblastoma includes surgical resection and radiation therapy. Gross total removal of tumor improves outcome; however, if the tumor is invading the floor of the fourth ventricle, it should be left in place, because attempted removal virtually guarantees severe neurologic sequelae. Adjuvant radiation therapy is usually given in 180 rad fractions. A total dose of 3,600 rad to the neuraxis with a tumor boost to 5,400 rad is standard. Because the effects of craniospinal radiation therapy to the child's brain are devastating, chemotherapy has been added in an attempt to decrease the dose of irradiation. Platinum-based chemotherapy has been shown to improve the outcome in children with high-risk disease. Five-year survival for optimally treated normal-risk patients is approximately 65%; for optimally treated high-risk patients, 5-year survival is less than 20%.

REFERENCES

Chintagumpala M, Berg S, Blaney SM. Treatment controversies in medulloblastoma. *Curr Opin Oncol* 2001;13:154–159.

Greenberg HS, Chamberlain MC, Glantz MJ, et al. Adult medulloblastoma: multiagent chemotherapy. *Neurooncology* 2001; 3:29–34.

Newton HB. Review of the molecular genetics and chemotherapeutic treatment of adult and paediatric medulloblastoma. *Expert Opin Invest Drugs* 2001;10:2089–2104.

Packer RJ, Cogen P, Vezina G, et al. Medulloblastoma: clinical and biological aspects. *Neurooncology* 1999;1:139–151.

Reddy AT. Advances in biology and treatment of childhood brain tumors. *Curr Neurol Neurosci Rep* 2001;1:137–143.

RESOURCES

30, 290, 352

49 Melanoma

Jonathan J. Lewis, MD, PhD

DEFINITION: Melanoma is a type of skin cancer that results from the malignant transformation of the normal melanocytes or pigment cells found in the skin.

DIFFERENTIAL DIAGNOSIS: Benign nevus; Dysplastic mole; Seborrheic keratoses; Squamous and basal carcinoma.

SYMPTOMS AND SIGNS: Patients usually present with a pigmented lesion of the skin that has undergone recent change. These lesions typically have irregular borders, an irregular surface, and irregular colors, which may range from pink to blue to brown to black. Late symptoms may include itchiness and bleeding. Any of these changes in a nevus is a sign that it may be undergoing a malignant transformation. In 5%–10% of cases, melanoma arises from other sites, including the oral cavities, nasal sinuses, genitalia, and rectum. Melanoma may also occur in the uveal tract and the retina of the eye. In all these sites, it presents as a pigmented lesion.

ETIOLOGY/EPIDEMIOLOGY: Individuals of Celtic ancestry have the highest risk for developing melanoma. Men develop melanoma slightly more frequently than women. In women, melanomas occur more commonly on the lower extremities, whereas in men they occur more commonly on the trunk, head, and neck. A primary cause of melanoma is believed to be sun exposure, and that both UVA and UVB are carcinogenic. At highest risk are people with fair complexions who have had intermittent sun exposure and a history of severe sunburns. The incidence of melanoma in the United States is 40,000 per year, of whom 7,400 will die from it.

DIAGNOSIS: Careful and thorough examination of the skin is crucial. Any pigmented lesion that is irregular or that has a diameter of more than 6 mm and elevation should arouse suspicion. To make the diagnosis, a full-thickness biopsy should be performed. An excisional biopsy can be done on small lesions, whereas for large lesions a punch biopsy through the representative area or areas can be performed. A shave biopsy should not be done, as it does not allow adequate assessment of the depth of the lesion, which is crucial in diagnosis and staging. The diagnosis is then based on examination under the microscope, best done by a dermatopathologist. Once the diagnosis is established, careful examination and evaluation of the draining lymph nodes and other sites of metastases should be performed.

TREATMENT

Standard Therapies: Standard treatment is a wide local excision. When indicated, a sentinel lymph node biopsy should be performed; most appropriately in patients with intermediate-thickness melanomas. Systemic therapy in the adjuvant setting for high-risk lesions can be useful. One current standard of care includes the use of interferon. Once metastatic, several systemic agents may be used, including the chemotherapy agent dacarbazine and the biologic agent interleukin-2.

Investigational Therapies: Vaccines are being evaluated; different approaches include some that use the antibody arm and others that use the T cell arm of the immune system.

REFERENCES

Belli F, Rivoltini L, Lewis JJ, et al. Vaccination of metastatic melanoma patients with autologous tumor-derived heat shock protein peptide-complex-96 (Oncophage): clinical and immunological findings. *J Clin Oncol* 2002 (in press).

Kelley MC, Ollila DW, Morton DL. Lymphatic mapping and sentinel lymphadenectomy for melanoma. *Semin Surg Oncol* 1998;14:283–290.

Kirkwood JM, Strawdeerman MH, Ernstoff MS, et al. Interferon alfa-2b adjuvant therapy of high-risk resected cutaneous melanoma: The Eastern Cooperative Oncology Group Trial EST 1684. *J Clin Oncol* 1996;14:7–17.

Nestle FO, Alijagic S, Gilliet M, et al. Vaccination of melanoma patients with peptide- or tumor lysate-pulsed dendritic cells. *Nat Med* 1998;4:328–332.

Rosenberg SA, Yang JC, White DE, et al. Durability of complete responses in patients with metastatic cancer treated with high-dose interleukin-2: identification of the antigens mediating response. *Ann Surg* 1998;228:307–319.

RESOURCES

30, 352, 437

50   Mycosis Fungoides

John A. Zic, MD

DEFINITION: Mycosis fungoides is the most common variant of the primary cutaneous T-cell lymphomas, characterized by the indolent onset of red patches of skin in sun-protected areas, which may progress to thick plaques, tumors, and/or total body erythroderma.

SYNONYM: Mycosis fungoides of Alibert and Bazin.

DIFFERENTIAL DIAGNOSIS: Large plaque parapsoriasis; Adult T-cell leukemia/lymphoma; Sezary syndrome; Allergic contact dermatitis; Eczematous dermatitis; Psoriasis; Tinea corporis.

SYMPTOMS AND SIGNS: The classic presentation is a middle-aged to older adult with an asymptomatic eruption of large (>5 cm), pink to red, scaly flat patches on the thighs or buttocks of several years' duration. Often, the patient has been misdiagnosed with eczema or psoriasis. Low- to midpotency topical steroids stabilize the condition temporarily over a period of years. The patches ultimately evolve into thin elevated plaques. Skin biopsy shows an atypical lymphocytic infiltrate. On average, most patients have the eruption for 6–10 years before the diagnosis is established. Patients with less than 10% of their body surface covered with patches or plaques and no extracutaneous involvement have a normal life expectancy with treatment. Approximately 1 in 10 early-stage patients will progress to more advanced stages. Thick plaques may ulcerate, forming tumors, and total body erythema may evolve. Blood involvement is not uncommon in advanced patients. Regional peripheral lymphadenopathy is the most common extracutaneous finding, followed by metastasis to bone marrow, lung, and liver. Patients with large, often ulcerated, tumors or erythroderma have a poor prognosis, with a median survival of approximately 30 months. Most advanced-stage patients die of sepsis due to *Staphylococcus*.

ETIOLOGY/EPIDEMIOLOGY: The etiology and risk factors are unknown. One theory is that activated T cells destined for the skin undergo malignant transformation and proliferation. Approximately 1,000 new cases are diagnosed in the United States each year, and approximately 10,000 to 15,000 Americans are affected. The male:female ratio is 2:1, and twice as many blacks are diagnosed as whites.

DIAGNOSIS: Multiple punch biopsies of the skin are required to make the diagnosis. Pathologists experienced with the disease should evaluate the specimens. Occasionally, T-cell receptor gene rearrangement studies are helpful in establishing the diagnosis. Routine chemistries and a manual complete blood count and differential should be obtained. CT scans are helpful only in patients with tumors, erythroderma, or widespread disease.

TREATMENT
Standard Therapies: Patients in the early stage of disease with only skin involvement are treated with topical nitrogen mustard, topical carmustine, topical bexarotene gel, and phototherapy. Patients with progressive disease may be treated with psoralen-UVA phototherapy alone or with subcutaneous interferon, total skin or localized electron beam radiotherapy, oral bexarotene, photopheresis, and methotrexate. Patients in advanced stages may receive intravenous denileukin diftitox, single agent chemotherapy, and combination chemotherapy.

Investigational Therapies: Peripheral blood stem cell transplantation is being explored.

REFERENCES
Siegel RS, Pandolfino T, Guitart J, et al. Primary cutaneous T cell lymphoma: review and current concepts. *J Clin Oncol* 2000; 18:2908–2925.

Willemze R, Kerl H, Sterry W, et al. EORTC classification for primary cutaneous lymphomas: a proposal from the cutaneous lymphoma study group of the EORTC. *Blood* 1997;90:354–371.

Zic JA, Salhany KE, Greer JP, et al. Cutaneous T-cell lymphoma: mycosis fungoides and Sezary syndrome. In: Lee GR, Foerster J, Greer JP, et al., eds. *Wintrobe's clinical hematology*, 10th ed. Baltimore: Williams & Wilkins, 1998.

RESOURCES
82, 273

51   Multiple Myeloma

Morie A. Gertz, MD

DEFINITION: Multiple myeloma is a malignancy of plasma cells that infiltrates the bone marrow. The clinical manifestations are bone disease characterized by lytic destruction, pathologic fractures, and diffuse osteoporosis. Anemia due to progressive bone marrow replacement is common, and patients may develop renal insufficiency related to the production of excessive immunoglobulin light chains, toxic to the renal tubules.

SYNONYMS: Plasma cell myeloma; Myeloma.

DIFFERENTIAL DIAGNOSIS: Metastatic malignancy to bone; Normochromic normocytic anemia; Renal insufficiency of an indeterminate origin.

SYMPTOMS AND SIGNS: The most common presenting symptoms are fatigue, due to anemia, secondary to progressive infiltration of the bone marrow, and bone pain. Typically, the pain involves the spine. Patients may have associated pathologic fractures of multiple ribs. Skeletal destruction may occur in any bone. Radiography of the calvarium generally demonstrates lytic lesions.

ETIOLOGY/EPIDEMIOLOGY: No specific etiology has been identified, although there is an increased incidence of multiple myeloma in individuals exposed to ionizing radiation. Only 1% of patients have such a history. No familial or inherited predisposition to this disorder has been recognized. The male:female ratio is 55:45. The incidence is 4 per 100,000 per year. The disease is seen in 13,800 patients per year in the United States and constitutes 1% of all cancer and 10% of hematologic cancers. It is twice as common in blacks as whites. The median age at diagnosis is 62 years.

DIAGNOSIS: The diagnosis requires bone marrow aspiration and biopsy demonstrating more than 10% plasma cells in the bone marrow. Appropriate staging procedures include a radiograph of the entire skeleton, searching for fractures or lytic disease. Laboratory testing includes measurement of hemoglobin, renal function, blood calcium level, and uric acid. The hallmark of multiple myeloma is the detection of a monoclonal protein (M protein) in the serum or urine. The source of the protein is the malignant plasma cell in the bone marrow.

TREATMENT

Standard Therapies: Occasional patients will be diagnosed without symptoms present, and may be observed for the development of symptomatic disease. For patients with solitary plasmacytomas, radiation therapy suffices. For patients who cannot be treated with localized radiation, systemic chemotherapy is the treatment of choice. High-dose chemotherapy followed by stem cell transplantation is appropriate treatment for suitably selected patients. For patients who are not candidates for stem cell transplantation, lower intensity chemotherapy regimens, including alkylating agent–based regimens and the use of high-dose corticosteroids, can produce clinically important and durable responses.

Investigational Therapies: The role of nonmyeloablative donor transplantation for treatment and the exact role of antiangiogenesis agents are being investigated, as is whether bisphosphonates have an antitumor effect in this disorder. The optimal conditioning regimens for autologous stem cell transplant are also being explored.

REFERENCES

Chen MG, Gertz MA. Multiple myeloma and other plasma cell neoplasms. In: Gudnerson LL, Tepper JE, eds. *Clinical radiation oncology.* New York: Churchill Livingstone, 2000:1189–1202.

Gertz MA, Lacy MQ. Bone marrow transplant for multiple myeloma. *Cancer Res Ther Control* 1999;9:297–302.

Greipp PR. Plasma cell disorders. In: Kelley WN, et al., eds. *Textbook of internal medicine,* 3rd ed. Philadelphia: Lippincott-Raven, 1997:1400–1405.

Vesole DH. Bone marrow and stem cell transplantation for multiple myeloma. *Cancer Treat Res* 1999;99:171–194.

RESOURCES

207, 241, 350

52 Nezelof Syndrome

Richard A. Insel, MD,
Blake G. Scheer, MD,
and Alan P. Knutsen, MD

DEFINITION: Nezelof syndrome is associated with severe T-cell immunodeficiency, normal or increased immunoglobulin level, and decreased antibody function. It is considered a form of severe combined immunodeficiency (SCID), although it is not considered a distinct genetic type per se, but may be a clinically less severe form of the disease.

SYNONYMS: Thymic dysplasia with normal immunoglobulins; Cellular immunodeficiency with abnormal immunoglobulin synthesis; Combined immunodeficiency with predominant T-cell defect.

DIFFERENTIAL DIAGNOSIS: Severe combined immunodeficiency; Acquired immunodeficiency syndrome.

SYMPTOMS AND SIGNS: Patients with Nezelof syndrome have symptoms similar to patients with SCID, but at times these may be milder and may present later in infancy. Recurrent infections occur in infancy or childhood and may be associated with failure to thrive and chronic diarrhea and malabsorption. These may include oral candidiasis that is recalcitrant to therapy, infection with *Pneumocystis carinii*, recurrent bronchopulmonary infections, and bacterial otitis media, severe measles or varicella, or other opportunistic infections.

ETIOLOGY/EPIDEMIOLOGY: The genetic abnormality is unknown but the disorder arises as a variant form of SCID. Deficiency of the enzyme adenosine deaminase, which causes SCID, is responsible for some cases. The disorder may show an autosomal-recessive inheritance. Affected siblings in a kinship may show variation in the degree of T-cell and B-cell immunodeficiency.

DIAGNOSIS: The diagnosis should be suspected based on decreased CD3 total and CD4 helper T-lymphocytes, decreased T-cell function, and normal to increased immunoglobulin levels. Some immunoglobulin classes such as IgM may be at a normal level, with others such as IgG marginally decreased. At times, increased IgE levels are observed. Antibody responses to immunization are decreased. Lymphopenia may be present.

TREATMENT
Standard Therapies: Treatment is bone marrow transplantation from a histocompatible HLA-identical sibling. If such a donor is not available, transplantation should be performed with a T-cell depleted marrow from a haploidentical half-matched family member or an HLA-matched unrelated donor.

REFERENCES
Gosseye S, Nezelof C. T system immunodeficiencies in infancy and childhood. *Pathol Res Pract* 1981;17:975–977.
Hong R. Disorders of the T-cell system. In: Stiehm ER, ed. *Immunologic disorders in infants & children*, 4th ed. Philadelphia: WB Saunders, 1996.
Miller ME, Schieken RM. Thymic dysplasia. A separate entity from Swiss agammaglobulinemia. *Am J Med Sci* 1967;253: 741–750.

RESOURCES
193, 218, 359

53 Islet Cell Tumors of the Pancreas

Terry C. Lairmore, MD

DEFINITION: Islet cell tumors are derived from neuroendocrine cells that populate the endocrine pancreas during embryologic development. Neuroendocrine tumor (NET) is a more appropriate term that encompasses neoplasms of the pancreatic islet cells, carcinoid tumors, and neoplasms arising in the dispersed system of APUD cells.

SYNONYMS: Pancreatic islet cell tumors; Neuroendocrine tumors of the pancreas.

DIFFERENTIAL DIAGNOSIS: Reactive hypoglycemia; Factitious hypoglycemia; Renal failure.

SYMPTOMS AND SIGNS: The symptoms and signs of NET of the pancreas and gastrointestinal (GI) tract result from the specific hormone product secreted or the local effect of the tumor mass. The following symptoms and signs are categorized according to the specific hormone oversecreted: *insulinoma*, confusion and bizarre behavior associated with fasting, need for frequent sugar intake, weight gain; *gastrinoma* (Zollinger-Ellison syndrome [see also under Endocrine Disorders]), reflux esophagitis, secretory diarrhea, abdominal pain; *pancreatic polypeptide*, no known symptoms or signs; *vasoactive-intestinal peptide*, secretory diarrhea, hypokalemia, achlorhydria; and *glucagonoma*, hyperglycemia, migratory erythematous rash, and hypoaminoacidemia.

ETIOLOGY/EPIDEMIOLOGY: Islet cell tumors of the pancreas occur with an estimated frequency of 1–2 per million population. Sporadic insulinomas and gastrinomas have no known sex or ethnic predilection. Neuroendocrine tumors of the pancreas and GI tract also occur in association with several hereditary endocrine cancer syndromes. These include multiple endocrine neoplasia type 1 and von Hippel-Lindau syndrome.

DIAGNOSIS: In general, radiographic tests are not indicated until the biochemical diagnosis is established. Zollinger-Ellison syndrome is diagnosed by the finding of an inappropriately elevated fasting serum gastrin level in association with gastric acid hypersecretion. The diagnosis is confirmed by an abnormal secretin stimulation test. Insulinoma is best diagnosed during a supervised fast with the measurement of plasma levels of glucose, insulin, and C-peptide at frequent intervals. Sulfonylureas should also be measured to exclude the surreptitious administration of oral hypoglycemic drugs, and antiinsulin antibodies should be measured to exclude exogenous insulin administration.

TREATMENT

Standard Therapies: Functional neuroendocrine tumors or those that carry a significant risk of malignancy should be surgically removed. This consists of complete exposure of the pancreas, intraoperative ultrasonography, and inspection and palpation of the gland by an experienced endocrine surgeon. Small, circumscribed, likely benign tumors are enucleated. Major pancreatic resection (distal pancreatectomy, pancreaticoduodenectomy) is appropriate for large, multiple, or malignant tumors.

REFERENCES

Lairmore TC, Chen VY, DeBenedetti MK, et al. Duodeno-pancreatic resections in patients with multiple endocrine neoplasia type 1. *Ann Surg* 2000;231:909–919.

Moley JF, Lairmore TC, Phay JE. Hereditary endocrinopathies. *Curr Probl Surg* 1999;36:653–764.

Norton JA. Neuroendocrine tumors of the pancreas and duodenum. *Curr Probl Surg* 1994;31:11–164.

Norton JA, Cromack DT, Shawker TH, et al. Intraoperative ultrasonographic localization of islet cell tumors. *Ann Surg* 1988;207:160–168.

Yim JH, Siegel BA, DeBenedetti MK, et al. Prospective study of the utility of somatostatin-receptor scintigraphy in the evaluation of patients with multiple endocrine neoplasia type 1. *Surgery* 1998;124:1037–1042.

RESOURCES

30, 82, 354

54   Pheochromocytoma

William M. Manger, MD, PhD

DEFINITION: Pheochromocytoma, a neuroendocrine tumor, secretes catecholamines (mainly epinephrine and norepinephrine, rarely dopamine) that cause sustained and/or paroxysmal hypertension and a large variety of manifestations. Of these tumors, 98% occur in the abdomen (90% in the adrenal medulla) or pelvis, <2% in the chest, and <0.1% on the neck or base of the skull. About 20% are familial, usually occur in the adrenal medulla, and are often bilateral. About 10% are malignant, but these cannot be differentiated from benign tumors except by evidence of metastatic or invasive lesions.

SYNONYM: Paraganglioma, when occurring in extra-adrenal sites.

DIFFERENTIAL DIAGNOSIS: Neurogenic hypertension (the most common); All hypertension of uncertain cause; Anxiety; Panic attacks; Hyperthyroidism; Paroxysmal tachycardia; Hyperdynamic β-adrenergic circulatory state; Menopause; Vascular headache; Coronary insufficiency syndrome; Acute hypertensive encephalopathy; Intracranial lesions; Autonomic hyperreflexia; Diencephalic seizure; Toxemia of pregnancy (or eclampsia with convulsions); Carcinoid; Familial dysautonomia; Acrodynia; Neuroblastoma; Ganglioneuroblastoma; Ganglioneuroma;

Adrenal medullary hyperplasia; Clonidine withdrawal; Baroreflex failure; Factitious (induced by certain drugs); Hypoglycemia; Reaction to monoamine oxidase inhibitors; Fatal familial insomnia.

SYMPTOMS AND SIGNS: Symptoms and signs result mainly from hemodynamic and metabolic effects of excess circulating catecholamines; numerous peptides may be secreted by these tumors and cause clinical manifestations. Most frequent symptoms are severe headache and inappropriate generalized sweating and palpitations (with or without tachycardia). Other manifestations include anxiety, tremulousness, nausea, vomiting, chest and abdominal pain, weight loss, constipation, diarrhea, paresthesias, pallor, rarely flushing, hypertensive retinopathy, and fever. Paroxysmal attacks usually occur one or more times weekly and last less than 15 minutes. Arrhythmias are frequent, and occasionally catecholamine cardiomyopathy occurs. Approximately 50% of affected persons have sustained hypertension; others have paroxysmal hypertension, and a few remain normotensive. Familial pheochromocytoma may be associated with multiple endocrine neoplasia (MEN), von Hippel-Lindau disease (VHL), carotid body or multiple paragangliomas, and neurofibromatosis type-1. Coexistence of pheochromocytoma with medullary thyroid carcinoma (MTC) or C-cell hyperplasia and sometimes with parathyroid neoplasms and hyperplasia constitutes MEN type-2a. Coexistence of pheochromocytoma with MTC, mucosal neuromas, thickened corneal nerves, alimentary tract ganglioneuromatosis, and sometimes a marfanoid habitus constitutes MEN type-2b. Hyperparathyroidism occurs in about 50% of patients with type 2-a, but rarely in type-2b. Pheochromocytomas coexist in about 14% of patients with VHL disease, which is characterized by hemangioblastoma of the central nervous system and retinal angioma. Renal and pancreatic cysts, renal carcinoma, and cystadenoma of the epididymis may coexist.

ETIOLOGY/EPIDEMIOLOGY: The etiology is unknown. There is no sex predilection in adults, but before puberty it is more common in boys. Tumors may occur at any age, with the highest frequency in the fourth and fifth decades. About 20% of pheochromocytomas are familial with an autosomal dominant inheritance and are due to genetic mutations: *RET* protooncogene on chromosome 10 for MEN type-2a and 2b syndromes, on chromosome 3p for VHL, on chromosome 11q for carotid body and multiple paragangliomas, and on chromosome 17q for neurofibromatosis. Familial tumors are usually bilateral but also may be multicentric.

DIAGNOSIS: The diagnosis must be made or excluded definitively, because if unrecognized, pheochromocytoma will nearly always result in the patient's death. Measurement of plasma catecholamines or 24-hour urinary total metanephrines is favored for screening patients, because they detect pheochromocytoma in more than 95% of cases, and invariably detect those with sustained hypertension due to circulating catecholamines. Drugs that interfere with tests (e.g., labetalol, catecholamines, L-dopa, tricyclic antidepressants, phenoxybenzamine, busparone, and some vasodilators) must be avoided. Differentiation between neurogenic hypertension and pheochromocytoma with mildly elevated plasma catecholamines may be made with the clonidine suppression test, which decreases catecholamines to normal levels if elevations are not due to pheochromocytoma. When diagnosis has been established biochemically, tumor localization is required. Usually, this can be done by CT scan or MRI.

TREATMENT
Standard Therapies: Ninety percent of pheochromocytomas are successfully removed by surgery. Preoperative α- and β-adrenergic blockade may be needed to control hypertension and arrhythmias, respectively. Many tumors can be removed by laparoscopy. Multiple or large (>8cm) tumors may require a transperitoneal approach, or special surgery may be needed if the tumor is in the chest, neck, or base of skull. With familial disease, coexisting thyroid and parathyroid lesions are treated after pheochromocytoma excision. Chemotherapy and radiotherapy may be helpful in managing malignant pheochromocytomas; adrenergic blockers and metyrosine may control manifestations of hypercatecholemia.

REFERENCES
Bravo EL, Gifford RW Jr., Manger WM. Adrenal medullary tumors: pheochromocytoma. In: Mazzaferri EL, Samaan NA, eds. *Endocrine Tumors*. Oxford, Blackwell Scientific Publications; 1993:426–447.

Manger WM, Gifford RW, Jr. *Clinical and Experimental Pheochromocytoma*. 2nd ed. Oxford, Blackwell Science; 1996.

Manger WM, Gifford RW Jr. Pheochromocytoma: a clinical overview. In: Laragh JH, Brenner BM. *Hypertension: Pathophysiology, Diagnosis, and Management*. 2nd ed. New York: Raven Press; 1995:2225–2244.

RESOURCES
30, 82, 281

55 Polycythemia Vera

*Kenneth M. Algazy, MD,
and Garrett E. Bergman, MD*

DEFINITION: Polycythemia vera (PV) is a clonal neoplastic disorder characterized by an increased production and circulating numbers of all three blood elements, RBCs, white blood cells and platelets. Patients may develop symptoms of hyperviscosity and thrombotic complications, secondary to their very high red blood cell (RBC) count and marked thrombocytosis. After a few to 20 or more years, the disease "burns out," the bone marrow becomes fibrotic, and the patient's picture may mimic that of myelofibrosis, with splenomegaly, extramedullary hematopoiesis, and transfusion dependency.

SYNONYMS: Polycythemia vera; Polycythemia rubra vera.

DIFFERENTIAL DIAGNOSIS: One must distinguish PV from secondary polycythemia, or more accurately secondary erythrocytosis, a physiologic reaction rather than a neoplastic reaction. In secondary erythrocytosis, the RBC number and mass are increased either as a response to hypoxia or due to aberrant production of or enhanced response to erythropoietin. Generally the white blood cells and platelets are present in normal numbers; often underlying pulmonary or cardiac disease is evident, or a tumor (renal, cerebral) secreting erythropoietin is discovered. Rare familial forms of secondary erythrocytosis can be attributed to increased sensitivity to erythropoietin or to abnormal high-oxygen affinity variants of hemoglobin. High-altitude erythrocytosis should be considered if the patient has been living at above 3,000 meters. So-called "stress polycythemia" is due to a contracted blood volume (with a total normal number of circulating RBCs).

SYMPTOMS AND SIGNS: This disorder is usually insidious in onset, generally appearing first in the sixth or seventh decade of life. It may be discovered serendipitously on routine testing, or the patient may complain of headache, weakness, pruritis, dizziness, or sweating; or a thrombotic event may be the presenting symptom. About one third of patients develop thrombotic complications, notably cerebrovascular accident, myocardial infarction or angina, and spontaneous deep vein thrombosis or pulmonary embolus; even mesenteric artery thrombosis and Budd-Chiari syndrome (hepatic vein thrombosis) have been noted in some series of patients. From the rapid turnover of blood-forming elements in the marrow, high serum uric acid levels and complicating gout have been observed. Severe pruritis can be aggravated by a hot shower, and may be secondary to the release of histamine from increased numbers of mast cells in the skin. Easy bruising or gum bleeding has also been frequently observed in these patients.

ETIOLOGY/EPIDEMIOLOGY: PV is caused by a malignant transformation of a single progenitor cell that proliferates in the bone marrow, at a variable rate, eventually to become the predominant hematopoietic precursor cell. At diagnosis, about one fourth of patients have an abnormal karyotype, and this percentage increases as the disease progresses, but there does not seem to be a strong familial predisposition. The incidence may be slightly higher among Ashkenazic Jews of Northern European ancestry than in the general population, where the incidence has varied from 5 to 20 per million people.

DIAGNOSIS: The diagnosis of PV should be suspected whenever a patient presents for care with any of the above signs or symptoms and a hematocrit above 50%. The classic presentation of full-blown disease is one of erythrocytosis, leukocytosis, thrombocytosis and splenomegaly; early on, patients may have only some of these findings. All three blood cell lines are increased in number; absolute neutrophilia is very common. Occasional neutrophil precursors (metamyelocytes, myelocytes) are present in the peripheral blood. Increased numbers of basophils are commonly seen. Blood levels of vitamin B_{12} and uric acid are usually increased above normal. Platelet counts commonly are above 600,000/mm³ and above 1,000,000/mm³ in 10% of patients. Arterial partial pressure of oxygen (PaO_2) is decreased, as low as 65 torr, with normal or near normal oxygen saturation values. Splenomegaly develops later in the course of the disease when extramedullary hematopoiesis occurs, due to myelofibrosis. In secondary erythrocytosis, only the red cell number is increased; the neutrophil and platelet counts are generally normal, unless underlying infection is present (e.g., in chronic lung disease). Measurement of total red cell mass, while diagnostically useful, is difficult and expensive.

TREATMENT
Standard Therapies: There are two stages of PV requiring different treatment approaches. In the first, or "plethoric"

phase, problems relate to the increased circulating red cell mass: thromboses (cerebrovascular, cardiac, mesenteric), possible hyperviscosity (headache), and bleeding (mucous membrane). The therapeutic goal is to reduce the hematocrit, by repeated phlebotomy. About 500 mL of whole blood (less for patients weighing <50 kg , or with cardiac disease) are removed by venesection every 2–4 days to maintain the hematocrit at <50%. This is repeated periodically until iron-deficiency anemia develops, limiting the autonomous generative capability of the marrow. Once iron deficiency develops, the patient's hematocrit and hyperviscosity can be controlled. Phlebotomy alone will effectively control the hematocrit level and concomitant symptoms but not leukocytosis, thrombocytosis, pruritis, or hyperuricemia (and gout). Additional treatments in the "plethora phase" suppress the bone marrow production of all cellular elements: when bleeding or thrombotic complications have occurred or are threatened (platelet count over 800,000/mm³), myelosuppression is given in the form of hydroxyurea, busulfan, chlorambucil, or radioactive phosphorus (^{32}P). Hydroxyurea is easy to administer, short acting, and therefore safe for long-term suppressive therapy. Busulfan, chlorambucil, and ^{32}P are also effective for long-term control, but appear to carry a greater risk of inducing a leukemic transformation of PV. Anagrelide is useful for prevention of thrombotic complications from extreme and uncontrolled thrombocytosis. Pruritis is not generally affected by phlebotomy or myelosuppression until remission is induced; antihistamines are not effective, but UV light treatments with psoralens and interferon-α may help some patients. In the "spent phase" of PV, the marrow is "burned out" and the spleen markedly enlarges to make blood cells. The treatment of PV at this stage is symptomatic. Paradoxically, repeated blood transfusions may be required to support the RBC count of the patient. Thrombocytopenia may become severe and symptomatic. Splenectomy should be considered at that point, when transfusion requirements become great, or if the enlarged spleen becomes very uncomfortable to the patient. In 1986 the Polycythemia Vera Study Group reported that the median survival from diagnosis was 13.9 years for patients receiving phlebotomy alone, and 11.8 years for those treated with ^{32}P. Causes of death were attributed to thrombotic complications in 31%, and leukemia eventually developed in 19%.

Investigational Therapies: Interferon could be considered for cases difficult to control by other means. Bone marrow transplantation has been used with success on a few occasions. It should only be considered for end-stage, "burned out" cases, extremely difficult to manage in other ways.

56 Pseudomyxoma Peritonei

Paul H. Sugarbaker, MD

DEFINITION: Pseudomyxoma peritonei is characterized by the accumulation of mucus and tumors composed of mucus-secreting epithelial cells throughout the peritoneal space.

SYNONYMS: Jelly belly; Mucinous peritoneal carcinomatosis; Perforated appendiceal cystadenoma or cystadenocarcinoma; Appendiceal cancer.

DIFFERENTIAL DIAGNOSIS: Peritoneal mesothelioma; Ovarian cancer; Serous papillary cancer of the peritoneum; Malignant peritoneal effusions from gastric cancer; Colon cancer or small bowel adenocarcinoma; Ascites from any cause.

SYMPTOMS AND SIGNS: A common symptom in a male is mucoid fluid diagnosed at the time of a hernia repair for either an inguinal or umbilical hernia. A common symptom in a female is a cystic ovarian mass, usually on the right, but often bilateral. In both males and females, appendicitis often calls attention to the disease at the time of appendectomy. Another common symptom is gradually expanding abdominal girth. Infertility may also occur. Some patients with no specific symptoms have had a CT scan that shows the characteristic distribution of mucinous fluid and tumor throughout the abdomen and pelvis.

ETIOLOGY/EPIDEMIOLOGY: Most patients have an appendiceal adenoma or mucinous carcinoma that has perforated the appendix and caused a release of the tumor cells into the free peritoneal cavity. Rarely, a mucinous adenocarcinoma of the small bowel, of the large bowel, or of the gallbladder will perforate and become widely distributed on the peritoneal surfaces. The mucinous tumor cells in copious mucoid fluid do not invade the peritoneal surfaces as most cancers would; they distribute themselves in a characteristic fashion throughout the abdominal and pelvic space. They accumulate in areas where the peritoneal fluid is absorbed. The incidence of the disease is the same in males and females. However, the manifestations of early disease are unique in women. Ovulation causes a sticky ovarian surface with blood clot present at the site of the Graafian follicle. Tumor cells adhere and then progress at this site to cause a multicystic ovary, in which the cysts are filled by mucoid fluid.

DIAGNOSIS: The diagnosis may be obtained through biopsy or by definitive findings on CT scan of the abdomen and pelvis. Minimally invasive procedures are preferred to establish a diagnosis because tumor cell implantation at the site of surgical trauma is a consistent finding. If the diagnosis is made at the time of exploratory surgery, appendectomy should be performed; mucoid fluid should be obtained for histopathologic and cytologic examination, and the abdomen then closed for definitive treatment at a pseudomyxoma peritonei referral center.

TREATMENT
Standard Therapies: The curative approach, which cures approximately 75% of patients, depends on combined treatment strategies. First, a cytoreductive approach is used to remove visible tumor. Step 2 involves intraperitoneal chemotherapy with mitomycin C used at the time of sur-

gery while the abdomen is still open. In the postoperative period, the same series of tubes and drains is used to administer 5 days of intraperitoneal chemotherapy with 5-fluorouracil. If the disease recurs, second-look surgery is indicated. Reoperative surgery, in patients who show a small volume of recurrent disease, has a 75% cure rate.

REFERENCES
Esquivel J, Sugarbaker PH. Elective surgery in recurrent colon cancer with peritoneal seeding: when to and when not to operate [Editorial]. *Cancer Ther* 1998;1:321–325.
Esquivel J, Sugarbaker PH. Clinical presentation of pseudomyxoma peritonei syndrome. *Br J Surg* 2000;87:1414–1418.
Ronnett BM, Shmookler BM, Sugarbaker PH, et al. Pseudomyxoma peritonei: new concepts in diagnosis, origin, nomenclature, relationship to mucinous borderline (low malignant potential) tumors of the ovary. In: *Anatomic pathology.* Chicago: ASCP Press, 1997:197–226.
Sugarbaker PH. Results of treatment of 385 patients with peritoneal surface spread of appendiceal malignancy. *Ann Surg Oncol* 1999;6:727–731.
Sugarbaker PH, Ronnett BM, Archer A, et al. Pseudomyxoma peritonei syndrome. *Adv Surg* 1997;30:233–280.

RESOURCES
30, 352, 397

57 Acquired Pure Red Cell Aplasia

Neal Young, MD

DEFINITION: Acquired pure red cell aplasia (PRCA) is a hematologic disease in which only erythrocyte production is affected. Typical patients have severe, transfusion-dependent anemia with the absence of reticulocytes in the peripheral blood and of erythroid precursor cells in the bone marrow.

DIFFERENTIAL DIAGNOSIS: Diamond-Blackfan anemia (constitutional pure red cell aplasia); Transient erythroblastopenia of childhood; Transient aplastic crisis; Myelodysplasia; Large granular lymphocytic leukemia.

SYMPTOMS AND SIGNS: Patients present with symptoms of anemia. In younger patients, fatigue and lassitude, dyspnea on exertion, and tinnitus are most frequent; new-onset or worsening angina may occur in the older individual. Physical examination shows only pallor. Lym-

phadenopathy and splenomegaly suggest alternative diagnoses.

ETIOLOGY/EPIDEMIOLOGY: Usually, older individuals are affected, but there is no gender preference. A clear viral etiology—chronic B19 parvovirus—accounts for a significant minority of cases. In others, the disease is idiopathic but probably has an immunologic pathophysiology, with T cell–mediated suppression of erythropoiesis. In a third group, PRCA is associated with myelodysplasia, and there may be cytogenetic abnormalities of the bone marrow such as 5q-. Pure red cell aplasia also accompanies chronic lymphocytic leukemia.

DIAGNOSIS: The morphologic diagnosis rests on the typical appearance of the bone marrow with absent erythroid precursors. With parvovirus infection, pathognomonic giant erythroblasts may occur. In myelodysplasia, other bone marrow abnormalities may be observed, such as hypogranulated myeloid precursor cells or micromegakaryocytes. Chronic parvovirus infection is suggested by evidence of immunodeficiency—congenital, acquired (AIDS), or iatrogenic (immunosuppressive drugs or chemotherapy)—and is diagnosed by the finding of viral DNA in blood, usually in the absence of specific antibodies to B19. Research laboratories can establish the presence of inhibitory lymphocytes.

TREATMENT

Standard Therapies: Administration of commercially available immunoglobulin can ameliorate or cure parvovirus infection by replacing absent neutralizing antibodies to the virus. For immunologically mediated pure red cell aplasia, immunosuppressive agents usually are used in sequence (e.g., a course of corticosteroids followed by cyclosporine, antithymocyte globulin, azathioprine, or cyclophosphamide) until a response is observed. Treatment of underlying chronic lymphocytic leukemia may also improve PRCA. Most patients can be expected to respond to some form of appropriate therapy; in the minority who prove refractory, blood can be replaced by transfusion, usually two units of packed red cells every 2 weeks. Transfusion should be to levels adequate for normal activity. Chronic transfusions should be accompanied by iron chelation therapy with desferioxamine to avoid secondary hemochromatosis.

REFERENCES

Fisch P. Pure red cell aplasia [Review]. *Br J Haematol* 2000;111: 1010–1022.

Kang EM, Tisdale JT. Pure red cell aplasia. In: NS Young, ed. Bone marrow failure syndromes, 1st ed. Philadelphia: WB Saunders, 2000:135–155.

RESOURCES

27, 50, 356

---

58   Henoch-Schönlein Purpura

Frank T. Saulsbury, MD

DEFINITION: Henoch-Schönlein purpura (HSP) is an acute small vessel vasculitis that primarily affects children. The dominant clinical manifestations are purpura, arthritis, abdominal pain, gastrointestinal bleeding, and nephritis. The clinical features are a consequence of widespread leukocytoclastic vasculitis subsequent to IgA deposition in vessel walls.

SYNONYM: Anaphylactoid purpura.

DIFFERENTIAL DIAGNOSIS: Necrotizing vasculitides; IgA nephropathy.

SYMPTOMS AND SIGNS: Cutaneous purpura concentrated on the legs and buttocks is a constant feature. The purpuric lesions may be preceded briefly (generally <24 hours) by urticarial or maculopapular lesions. The characteristic rash consists of crops of palpable purpura 2–10 mm in diameter. Arthritis occurs in approximately 75% of patients, and commonly involves the knees and ankles. The arthritis may be acutely painful and incapacitating, but it is self-limited and nondeforming. Gastrointestinal involvement occurs in 50%–75% of patients. Colicky abdominal pain, vomiting, and bleeding are the dominant features. Rare gastrointestinal complications include intussusception and massive gastrointestinal bleeding. Nephritis occurs in 40% of patients. The clinical hallmark of HSP nephritis is hematuria. Although microscopic hematuria is a constant feature, 25% of patients with nephritis have gross hematuria. Proteinuria occurs in conjunction with hematuria in two thirds of patients. Nephritis may become chronic. Approximately 30%–50% of patients have persistent microscopic hematuria or proteinuria in long-term follow-up, but only approximately 1% of patients progress to end-stage renal disease. Otherwise, HSP is an acute, self-limited illness that generally lasts 2–4 weeks. One third of patients experience recurrence of symptoms, usually within 4 months of the original episode.

ETIOLOGY/EPIDEMIOLOGY: The etiology of HSP is unknown, but it is clear that IgA1 but not IgA2 plays a pivotal role in the immunopathogenesis of HSP. The reasons for the exclusive involvement of IgA1 are unknown, but defective glycosylation of IgA1 may contribute to this phenomenon. Henoch-Schönlein purpura is the most common acute vasculitis affecting children, with an incidence of approximately 10 cases per 100,000 children per year. The mean age of patients is 6 years; 90% are younger than 10 years. Boys are affected slightly more often. Most patients present in the fall and winter months, and HSP often follows a respiratory infection. Anecdotal reports have implicated a wide variety of pathogens, but no single pathogen has emerged as a dominant etiologic agent. However, preceding or concomitant group A beta hemolytic streptococcal infection is present in a substantial minority of patients.

DIAGNOSIS: Diagnosis is based on the presence of typical clinical manifestations. Serum IgA concentrations are increased in 50% of patients, but there is no diagnostic laboratory test for HSP. Laboratory studies are useful only to exclude other conditions that resemble HSP.

TREATMENT
Standard Therapies: Corticosteroids are effective in treating arthritis and abdominal pain, but no evidence exists that they have any effect on the purpura, duration of the illness, or frequency of recurrences. Patients with severe nephritis should receive high-dose intravenous methylpred-

nisolone followed by oral corticosteroids plus an immunosuppressive agent, either azathioprine or cyclophosphamide.

Investigational Therapies: Dapsone, plasmapheresis, and factor XIII infusions are being studied in patients with prolonged or severe HSP.

REFERENCES
Allen DM, Diamond LK, Howell DA. Anaphylactoid purpura in children (Schönlein-Henoch syndrome). *Am J Dis Child* 1960;99:833–854.
Saulsbury FT. Henoch-Schönlein purpura in children: report of 100 patients and review of the literature. *Medicine* 1999;78: 395–409.
Saulsbury FT. Henoch-Schönlein purpura. *Curr Opin Rheum* 2001;13:35–40.

RESOURCES
27, 357, 396

---

59   Idiopathic Thrombocytopenic Purpura

Kenneth M. Algazy, MD

DEFINITION: Idiopathic thrombocytopenic purpura is an autoimmune destruction of platelets producing thrombocytopenia.

SYNONYMS: Autoimmune thrombocytopenic purpura; Acute thrombocytopenic purpura; Chronic idiopathic thrombocytopenic purpura.

DIFFERENTIAL DIAGNOSIS: Thrombotic thrombocytopenic purpura; Anticardiolipin syndrome; Thrombocytopenia associated with other hematologic disorders; Drug-induced thrombocytopenia; Heparin-induced thrombocytopenia; Henoch-Schönlein purpura; Other vascular purpuras.

SYMPTOMS AND SIGNS: The disease can be seen in an acute state in children. This state appears to follow a viral infection and is generally self-limiting. The platelet count will return to normal even when no therapeutic intervention is attempted. In the adult form, it can occur either by itself or as part of a collagen vascular disease such as systemic lupus erythematosus. In both children and adults, the disease presents as petechiae, purpura, or bleeding from mucous membranes such as the oral or nasal epithelium. Petechiae and purpura are most prominent in the lower extremities.

ETIOLOGY/EPIDEMIOLOGY: The disorder is caused by antibodies directed against various portions of the platelet. The antibodies can be the result of induction by an acute viral illness or by a collagen vascular process. This condition can be seen as an initial or later symptom of HIV disease.

DIAGNOSIS: The diagnosis is based on the presence of thrombocytopenia with generally normal hemoglobin and white count with no evidence of recent new drug use and possibly after an innocuous upper respiratory tract infection. The platelet count can be reduced to any value lower than normal or lower than the patient's baseline value. An HIV test should be done in all patients presenting with thrombocytopenia to rule out an associated HIV infection.

TREATMENT
Standard Therapies: Standard therapy, in the pediatric and adult age range, involves the use of steroids. Prednisone can be used. In children, frequently the thrombocytopenia is simply observed. Either initially or shortly after steroids have been given, if the platelet response is not adequate, intravenous immunoglobulins can be administered. If the patient continues to require higher doses of steroids than deemed advisable or if immunoglobulins have to be continuously repeated, splenectomy can be effective in inducing remissions. In patients who are Rh(D)-positive, anti-D can be administered, which is much less expensive than intravenous immunoglobulins and almost as effective. Additionally, if anti-D is repeated for several months,

the disease may go into spontaneous remission, whereas with immunoglobulin therapy, sustained remissions are infrequent.

Investigational Therapies: Various therapeutic interventions have been suggested. Immunosuppressive agents such as cyclophosphamide, azathioprine, 6-mercaptopurine, vincristine, danazol, interferon, and cyclosporine have been considered. In addition, abnormal B-cell production of immunoglobulins can be challenged by adding rituximab. Colchicine has also been found to be effective by some and, in addition, in unusual circumstances, platelets can be loaded with chemotherapeutic agents such as vin-

blastine to produce destruction of reticuloendothelial cells that are responsible for platelet destruction.

REFERENCES

Blanchette V, Freedman J, Garvey B. Management of chronic immune thrombocytopenia purpura in children and adults. *Semin Hematol* 1998;35:36–51.

Scaradavou A, Woo B, Woloski BMR, et al. Intravenous anti-D treatment of immune thrombocytopenia purpura: experience in 272 patients. *Blood* 1997;89:2689–2700.

RESOURCES

216, 357, 396

---

60 Thrombotic Thrombocytopenic Purpura and Hemolytic Uremic Syndrome of Adults

Kenneth M. Algazy, MD

DEFINITION: Thrombotic thrombocytopenic purpura and hemolytic uremic syndrome of adults are characterized by a reduction in the platelet count due to consumption related to widespread thromboses.

SYNONYM: Moschcowitz disease.

DIFFERENTIAL DIAGNOSIS: Idiopathic thrombocytopenic purpura; Heparin-induced thrombocytopenia; Vasculitis.

SYMPTOMS AND SIGNS: The disease is characterized by a classic pentad of features. These include microangiopathic hemolytic anemia, thrombocytopenic purpura, neurologic symptoms, renal disease, and fever. Thrombotic thrombocytopenic purpura usually occurs in previously healthy individuals, but the syndrome is also associated with other disorders. It can be found in association with infections, some of the newer antiplatelet agents, cancer, collagen vascular diseases, pregnancy, and HIV disease. The disorder can also be seen in non-Hodgkin lymphoma.

ETIOLOGY/EPIDEMIOLOGY: These disorders appear to be due to either an inhibitor of von Willebrand factor–cleaving protease or the constitutional deficiency of this protease.

DIAGNOSIS: The diagnosis is suggested by thrombocytopenia in the presence of the aforementioned clinical situ-

ations. The characteristic morphologic picture is of fragmentation of red cells seen on the peripheral blood smear. The presence of fragmented red cells in association with symptoms and signs, particularly the pentad mentioned previously, secure the diagnosis.

TREATMENT

Standard Therapies: Plasma infusion and exchange effectively decreases the presence of an inhibitor and replaces the inhibited or absent protease, and therefore can be curative. In refractory patients, the many manipulations that have been used to treat the disorder include splenectomy, steroids, immunosuppression, vincristine, immunoabsorption, and intravenous immunoglobulins.

Investigational Therapies: Eventually, the protease will be efficiently prepared, and rather than exchanging plasma, administration of the protease may treat the disease.

REFERENCES

Furlan M, Robles R, Galbusera M. Von Willebrand factor–cleaving protease in thrombotic thrombocytopenic purpura and the hemolytic uremic syndrome. *N Engl J Med* 1998;339: 1578–1594.

Kwaan HC, Soff GA. Management of thrombotic thrombocytopenic purpura and hemolytic uremic syndrome. *Semin Hematol* 1997;34:159–166.

RESOURCE

357

61 Shwachman-Diamond Syndrome

Susan F. Burroughs, MD

DEFINITION: Shwachman-Diamond syndrome (SDS) is an inherited disorder characterized by absolute requirements of pancreatic acinar and bone marrow dysfunction. Patients may have pancreatic insufficiency with malabsorption and intermittent or persistent cytopenias, most commonly neutropenia. Other supportive features include short stature, skeletal changes, and liver abnormalities.

SYNONYMS: Shwachman syndrome; Shwachman-Bodian syndrome; Shwachman-Diamond-Oski syndrome; Lipomatosis of pancreas, congenital; Pancreatic insufficiency and bone marrow dysfunction.

DIFFERENTIAL DIAGNOSIS: Cystic fibrosis; Pearson marrow-pancreas syndrome; Congenital neutropenia (Kostmann's syndrome); Johanson-Blizzard syndrome; Metaphyseal chondroplasia (McKusick type).

SYMPTOMS AND SIGNS: Individuals with SDS typically have one to several of the following: signs and symptoms of fat malabsorption, short stature, delayed puberty, skeletal changes including rib cage abnormalities and metaphyseal dysostosis, pallor, fatigue, bleeding, and frequent infections. Less frequently, they may have psychomotor delay, hypotonia, liver, skin, and dental abnormalities, endocardial fibrosis, renal tubular acidosis and diabetes mellitus. Symptoms of fat malabsorption may improve with age, because some patients have improvement in pancreatic function. Pancytopenia may develop due to bone marrow failure with aplastic anemia or myelodysplastic syndrome, and it may evolve into acute myeloid leukemia.

ETIOLOGY/EPIDEMIOLOGY: The cause of this syndrome is unknown, although it is a congenital disorder with what appears to be autosomal-recessive inheritance, affecting males and females in a ratio of approximately 1.7:1. The location and nature of the genetic defect are the subject of intensive research efforts, and the gene has been mapped to a centromeric region of chromosome 7. Due to the lack of a specific diagnostic test and variability in severity of the syndrome, estimates of the incidence of this disorder have ranged from 1 in every 20,000 to 1 in every 200,000 births.

DIAGNOSIS: The diagnosis of pancreatic acinar dysfunction may be made by the pancreatic stimulation test or by indirect indicators of pancreatic acinar dysfunction (72-hour fecal fat and/or serum trypsinogen). A sweat test can rule out cystic fibrosis. Imaging tests of the pancreas (CT, MRI, or ultrasonography) can be used to document fatty infiltration or atrophy of the pancreas. Documentation of cytopenias should show persistent or intermittent abnormalities, including an absolute neutrophil count less than 1,500/mm³ and/or hemoglobin, hematocrit, or platelet count less than the age-related normal range. A bone marrow biopsy and aspirate with cytogenetics may be used to document cellularity, dysplastic changes, and the presence of any clonal abnormalities such as monosomy 7 or 7q-. Radiography may be used to document skeletal abnormalities.

TREATMENT

Standard Therapies: Pancreatic enzyme replacement therapy and fat-soluble vitamins (A, D, E, and K) are the main treatment for pancreatic insufficiency. High-calorie and/or high-protein diets, prophylactic antibiotics, and transfusions are sometimes used. Growth factors (e.g., granulocyte colony-stimulating factor) have been used to stimulate neutrophil production. Their use may be best limited to short-term courses, as long-term safety in SDS has not been firmly established. Frequent preventive dental care, special services for developmental delays and genetic counseling may be of benefit.

Investigational Therapies: Chemotherapy and bone marrow or peripheral stem cell transplantation are used for the treatment of bone marrow failure syndromes. Several research projects are evaluating the pancreatic acinar cell defect, bone marrow dysfunction and predilection to malignancy, and the genetic basis of SDS. Others are studying bone marrow aspirates and biopsies with cytochemical and immunohistochemical stains and flow cytometry for early identification and characterization of the myelodysplastic changes in SDS patients.

REFERENCES

Durie PR. Inherited causes of exocrine pancreatic dysfunction. *Can J Gastroenterol* 1997;11:145–152.

Ginzberg H, Shin J, Ellis L, et al. Segregation analysis in Shwachman-Diamond syndrome: Evidence for recessive inheritance. *Am J Hum Genet* 2000;66:1413–1316.

Mack DR, Forstner GG, Wilschanski M, et al. Shwachman Syndrome: exocrine pancreatic dysfunction and variable phenotypic expression. *Gastroenterology* 1996;111:1593–1602.

Popovic M, et al. Refined mapping of the Shwachman-Diamond syndrome locus at 7p12-q11. *Am J Hum Genet* 2000;67(suppl 2):321.

Smith OP, Hunn IM, Chessels JM, et al. Haematological abnormalities in Shwachman-Diamond syndrome. *Br J Haematol* 1996;94:279–284.

RESOURCES

318, 357, 434

62   Hereditary Hemorrhagic Telangiectasia

Alan E. Guttmacher, MD,
and Jamie E. McDonald, MS

DEFINITION: Hereditary hemorrhagic telangiectasia (HHT) is a multisystem vascular dysplasia characterized by the presence of multiple arteriovenous malformations (AVMs) that lack intervening capillaries and result in direct connections between arteries and veins.

SYNONYM: Osler-Weber-Rendu (OWR) disease.

DIFFERENTIAL DIAGNOSIS: von Willebrand disease; Ataxia-telangiectasia; CREST syndrome; Hereditary benign telangiectasia; Chronic liver disease.

SYMPTOMS AND SIGNS: Most patients have recurrent epistaxis. Telangiectases of the face, oral cavity, or hands may develop. Telangiectases can occur in the gastrointestinal (GI) tract, most commonly in the stomach and proximal small intestine. Epistaxis and/or GI bleeding can cause mild to severe anemia. Pulmonary AVMs have been reported in 33% of patients and cerebral AVMs in 11%. Spinal AVMs are less common. Hepatic AVMs also occur; although also apparently less common, their frequency is unknown. Any AVM can manifest as hemorrhage. Pulmonary AVMs can lead to transient ischemic attacks, embolic stroke, or cerebral abscess. Migraine headache, polycythemia, and hypoxemia with cyanosis and clubbing of the nails also may be complications. Hepatic AVMs can cause high-output heart failure or portal hypertension. Cerebral AVMs may cause seizure or cerebral hemorrhage.

ETIOLOGY/EPIDEMIOLOGY: This is an autosomal-dominant disorder. Hereditary hemorrhagic telangiectasia type 1 is caused by a mutation in the endoglin gene; HHT type 2 is caused by a mutation in the activin receptor gene *ALK1*. The ethnic and geographic distribution is wide; the incidence in North America is approximately 1 in 10,000.

DIAGNOSIS: The diagnosis is considered definite when three or more of the following criteria are present, and possible or suspected when two of the criteria are present: recurrent spontaneous epistaxis; multiple telangiectases at characteristic sites, including face, lips, oral cavity, and fingers; one or more visceral AVMs (pulmonary, cerebral, hepatic, spinal) or GI telangiectases (with or without bleeding); and family history of HHT. Only limited laboratory genetic testing is available.

TREATMENT

Standard Therapies: Management includes treatment of identified complications such as nosebleeds, GI bleeding, anemia, and AVMs, as well as surveillance for undiagnosed AVMs. All patients should have a brain MRI with and without gadolinium to screen for cerebral AVM once at any age; and, starting at 10 years of age, some combination of contrast echocardiography, chest CT, or chest radiography and arterial blood gas determination to screen for pulmonary AVM approximately every 5 years. For pulmonary AVMs with feeding vessels that exceed 3 mm, transcatheter embolotherapy with detachable balloons or stainless-steel coils is the treatment of choice. Cerebral AVMs greater than 1 cm in diameter are usually treated, if feasible, using neurovascular surgery, embolotherapy, and/or stereotactic radiosurgery. If nosebleeds are not adequately controlled by humidification and daily application of nasal lubricants by the patient, laser ablation or skin grafting may be the most effective interventions. Endoscopic applications of a heater probe, bicap, or laser are the mainstays of treatment for symptomatic GI bleeding. Treatment for cardiac failure or liver failure secondary to hepatic AVMs is problematic.

REFERENCES

Guttmacher AE, Marchuk DA, White RI. Hereditary hemorrhagic telangiectasia. *N Engl J Med* 1995;333:918–924.

Plauchu H, de Chadarevian JP, Bideau A, et al. Age-related clinical profile of hereditary hemorrhagic telangiectasia in an epidemiologically recruited population. *Am J Med Genet* 1989;32: 291–297.

Shovlin CL, Guttmacher AE, Buscarini E, et al. Diagnostic criteria for hereditary hemorrhagic telangiectasia (Rendu-Osler-Weber Syndrome). *Am J Med Genet* 2000;91:66–67.

Shovlin CL, Letarte M. Hereditary haemorrhagic telangiectasia and pulmonary arteriovenous malformations: issues in clinical management and review of pathogenic mechanisms. *Thorax* 1999;54:714–729.

RESOURCES

181, 356

63 Thalassemia Major

John N. Lukens, MD

DEFINITION: Thalassemia major is a severe hemolytic anemia caused by mutations involving the α-globin or the β-globin genes of hemoglobin. Blood transfusions are required for growth and long-term survival.

SYNONYM: Cooley anemia.

DIFFERENTIAL DIAGNOSIS: Pyruvate kinase deficiency; Hereditary spherocytosis; Hereditary pyropoikilocytosis; Sickle cell anemia.

SYMPTOMS AND SIGNS: Because α-globin is a component of both fetal and adult hemoglobins, thalassemia major due to α-globin gene mutations is characterized by anemia from birth. Anemia due to β-thalassemia variants becomes apparent only as Hgb F is replaced by Hgb A during the first several months of life. Once manifest, anemia in both α- and β-thalassemia major is attended by pallor, intermittent jaundice, an expanding abdominal girth (due to splenomegaly), and failure to thrive. In the absence of transfusions, the hemoglobin concentration falls to 3–5 g/dL. By 1 year of age, growth retardation is prominent, the head is large with frontal bossing, and the cheekbones are prominent, tending to obscure the base of the nose and to accentuate prominence of the upper teeth (thalassemic facies). In the untreated patient, death usually occurs by age 5 years. A comprehensive chronic transfusion program facilitates growth and prevents skeletal complications. If measures to limit iron overload are not stringent, however, affected individuals are at risk for death from hepatic fibrosis and myocardial hemosiderosis during the second decade of life.

ETIOLOGY/EPIDEMIOLOGY: Approximately 300 different thalassemia mutations exist. α-Globin gene mutations are seen primarily in individuals of South East Asian and African origins, whereas β-globin gene mutations are seen chiefly in individuals of Mediterranean and Middle Eastern descent. Patients with thalassemia major are homozygous or (more often) doubly heterozygous for mutant genes. Each parent has a single mutant gene (thalassemia minor).

DIAGNOSIS: α-Thalassemia major (also known as Hgb H disease) should be suspected at birth in Asian infants with severe microcytic, hypochromic anemia. The diagnosis is confirmed by the electrophoretic demonstration of Hgb Bart's (in the neonatal period) or Hgb H (after the first months of life). Because of differences in gene mutations, African Americans are not at risk for α-thalassemia major. β-Thalassemia major also is characterized by severe microcytic, hypochromic anemia. Its onset is delayed until after the first 6 months. Red cell morphologic changes are prominent, with nucleated forms, anisocytosis, poikilocytosis, target cells, and basophilic stippling. The diagnosis is confirmed by hemoglobin electrophoresis. Hgb F is the major hemoglobin (70%–95%), Hgb A is absent or greatly decreased, and Hgb A_2 is normal or increased.

TREATMENT

Standard Therapies: Management should be orchestrated by a center having experience with chronic transfusion therapy. Transfusions are started when the hemoglobin falls below 7 g/dL or when growth deviates from the norm. The hemoglobin is maintained above 10 g/dL with a mean hemoglobin of 12 g/dL. Splenectomy may be required for an increasing transfusion requirement. Iron chelation with daily infusions of deferoxamine is started after the first 10–20 transfusions or when the serum ferritin reaches 1,000 ng/mL. Because of the demands of chronic transfusion therapy and the lethal potential of iron overload, allogeneic stem cell transplantation is indicated for patients with HLA-matched family members. Transplantation should be done before the patient is 16 years of age and is most successful if done before the onset of hepatomegaly, portal fibrosis, and iron overload.

Investigational Therapies: Pharmacologic reactivation of γ-globin synthesis with hydroxyurea appears to have benefited some but not most patients.

REFERENCES

Lucarelli G, Galimberti M, Polchi P, et al. Marrow transplantation in patients with thalassemia responsive to iron chelation therapy. *N Engl J Med* 1993;329:840–844.

Lukens JN. The thalassemias and related disorders. In: Lee GR, Foerster J, Lukens J, et al., eds. *Wintrobe's clinical hematology,* 10th ed. Baltimore: Williams & Wilkins, 1999:1405–1448.

Olivieri NF. Medical progress: the β-thalassemias. *N Engl J Med* 1999;341:99–109.

RESOURCES

118, 357, 435

64 Thalassemia Minor

John N. Lukens, MD

DEFINITION: Thalassemia minor is a disorder of hemoglobin synthesis characterized by a mild microcytic, hypochromic anemia.

SYNONYM: Thalassemia trait.

DIFFERENTIAL DIAGNOSIS: Iron deficiency anemia; Anemia of chronic disease.

SYMPTOMS AND SIGNS: Individuals with thalassemia minor have no symptoms attributable to the disorder and no abnormal physical findings. The anemia is insufficient to produce pallor. The disorder is suspected because of an abnormal hemogram or detected through family studies done to characterize symptomatic anemia in a relative.

ETIOLOGY/EPIDEMIOLOGY: Thalassemia minor is the most common genetic disorder worldwide. It is due to mutations involving the α-globin or β-globin genes of hemoglobin. α-Globin gene mutations occur primarily in individuals of Southeast Asian or African origins, whereas β-globin mutations had their origins in the Mediterranean basin. Because of global migrations and ethnic intermarriage, however, most individuals with thalassemia minor in North America are unaware of ancestral roots in areas of the world having high prevalence rates of thalassemia.

DIAGNOSIS: Anemia is mild or absent. The red blood cell (RBC) count is elevated, the mean corpuscular volume (MCV) and the mean corpuscular hemoglobin (MCH) are low (mean values 65 fL and 20 pg, respectively), and the mean corpuscular hemoglobin concentration (MCHC) is normal or only slightly decreased (mean value 31 g/dL RBC). RBC morphology is characterized by target cells and basophilic stippling. Iron deficiency also is associated with low values for MCV, MCH, and MCHC. The two disorders can be differentiated by considering the RBC indices in the context of anemia. Differences in hemogram profiles have made it possible to develop several discriminative functions to distinguish between the two disorders. In the simplest of these, the MCV is divided by the RBC count. A value less than 13 is indicative of thalassemia minor, whereas a value greater than 13 is in keeping with iron deficiency. The diagnosis of α-thalassemia minor can be confirmed by the electrophoretic demonstration of an increase in hemoglobin A_2 (3.4%–8%). There is no readily available test for β-thalassemia minor. This disorder is suspected in the presence of erythrocytosis and a modest decrease in MCV and MCH in the absence of iron deficiency or an abnormal hemoglobin electrophoretic pattern.

TREATMENT
Standard Therapies: No treatment is necessary or indicated. Therapeutic iron should be avoided unless iron deficiency is documented biochemically, as iron absorption is increased. Although rare, iron overload due to long-term iron administration has been described.

REFERENCES
Lukens JN. The thalassemias and related disorders. In: Lee GR, Foerster J, Lukens J, et al., eds. *Wintrobe's clinical hematology,* 10th ed. Baltimore: Williams & Wilkins, 1999:1405–1448.
Mentzer WC. Differentiation of iron deficiency from thalassemia trait. *Lancet* 1973;1:882.

RESOURCES
118, 356, 435

65 Idiopathic Thrombocytosis

Kenneth M. Algazy, MD

DEFINITION: Idiopathic thrombocytosis is characterized by elevation of platelet counts primarily but also potential elevation of white cells in the setting of a myeloproliferative disorder. Although the elevated platelets are the hallmark of the condition, the disorder frequently involves other cell lines. This is a clonal myeloproliferative disorder that can progress to an acute leukemia.

SYNONYMS: Essential thrombocytosis; Essential thrombocythemia.

DIFFERENTIAL DIAGNOSIS: Secondary thrombocytosis in the postsplenectomy state; Active collagen vascular disease; Other myeloproliferative disorders such as polycythemia vera and chronic myelogenous leukemia.

SYMPTOMS AND SIGNS: The presentation is clinically heterogeneous. Two thirds of patients with essential primary thrombocytosis are asymptomatic. One third present with complications that include thrombosis and/or bleeding in the cerebral, myocardial, and peripheral arterial circulation as well as deep vein thrombosis and pulmonary emboli. The bleeding can be manifested by gastrointestinal, skin, and mucous membrane hemorrhaging. Platelet counts are elevated above normal. The spleen may be enlarged and the patient frequently has iron deficiency anemia due to chronic gastrointestinal bleeding.

ETIOLOGY/EPIDEMIOLOGY: The disorder is caused by a clonal proliferation of bone marrow stem cells that are closest to the platelet. These megakaryocyte-related stem cells appear to be autonomous and may be associated with clonal abnormalities that also involve the erythroid and myeloid line.

DIAGNOSIS: The diagnosis is made by finding an elevated platelet count with hemorrhagic and thrombotic complications or simply found on a routine complete blood cell count. To secure the diagnosis, other causes of thrombocytosis should be ruled out such as rheumatoid arthritis; malignancies of the stomach, ovary, and lung; chronic myelogenous leukemia; and polycythemia rubra vera. In addition, iron deficiency anemia alone, without idiopathic thrombocytosis, can have an elevated platelet count and under these circumstances the diagnosis may not be apparent until iron has been replenished.

TREATMENT

Standard Therapies: The standard therapy is hydroxyurea, which is frequently sufficient to control the disease for extended periods in most patients. When this fails, anagrelide can be administered. This agent will control the platelet count but has side effects of fluid retention as well as not lasting for a prolonged period so that administration must occur on a regular basis, two to three times daily. Interferon-α has proven to be valuable but produces flulike side effects for the initial weeks of administration. Antiplatelet agents are controversial because some patients affected with this disorder have more of a problem with bleeding than they do with thromboses. An older form of therapy is the use of either busulfan or radiophosphorus. Both of these treatments should be reserved for the very elderly because receiving these drugs for any prolonged period of time can be associated with an increased incidence of leukemic conversion.

Investigational Therapies: Tyrosine kinase inhibitors, similar to those used in chronic myelogenous leukemia, may be used in the future.

REFERENCES

Buss DH, Cashell AW, O'Connor ML, et al. Occurrence, etiology, and clinical significance of extreme thrombocytosis: a study of 280 cases. *Am J Med* 1994;96:247–253.

Cortelazzo S, Finazzi G, Ruggeri M, et al. Hydroxyurea for patients with essential thrombocythemia and a high risk of thrombocytosis. *N Engl J Med* 1995;332:1132–1126.

RESOURCES

356, 396

---

66 | Twin-Twin Transfusion Syndrome

Ruben A. Quintero, MD

DEFINITION: Twin-twin transfusion syndrome (TTTS), a condition that occurs in approximately 10% of monochorionic twins, is believed to result from uneven exchange of blood between two fetuses through a common placenta.

SYNONYMS: Fetofetal transfusion; Chorioangiopagus twins.

DIFFERENTIAL DIAGNOSIS: Selective growth retardation of a monochorionic twin; Premature rupture of membranes of twin A; Anhydramnios from renal anomaly in one twin.

SYMPTOMS AND SIGNS: While pregnant, the mother may experience rapid increase of abdominal girth, back pain, vaginal spotting, overt signs of preterm labor, premature rupture of membranes, or miscarriage. A woman may also be asymptomatic and diagnosed only during a routine ultrasonographic examination.

ETIOLOGY/EPIDEMIOLOGY: Vascular communications are present in virtually 100% of monochorionic placentas. If the direction or number of communications is greater from one twin to the other, a net flow of blood occurs from one twin (donor) to the other twin (recipient), causing TTTS. Evenly developed vascular communications may also produce TTTS if unrelated hemodynamic decompensation of one fetus, as in congenital heart disease, occurs. The increased blood flow to the recipient twin results in polyuria and polyhydramnios. Decreased cardiac contractility, tricuspid valve regurgitation, reverse flow in the ductus venosus, pulsatile venous flow (PUVF), hydrops, and fetal death may ensue. The decreased blood flow to the donor twin results in anuria, oligohydramnios, and entrapment within its sac (stuck twin). Absent or reverse end-diastolic velocity in the umbilical artery, PUVF, and death may also occur.

DIAGNOSIS: The diagnosis of TTTS is made by ultrasonography as follows: polyhydramnios in the recipient twin (maximum vertical pocket >8 cm) and simultaneous oligohydramnios in the donor twin (maximum vertical pocket <2 cm) in a sonographically established monochorionic twin gestation.

TREATMENT
Standard Therapies: Serial amniocentesis is used to relieve the polyhydramnios. Data suggest that this may be effective in early stages of the disease, but less so in more advanced cases. Another therapy is occlusion of the placental vascular communications by means of endoscopic fetal surgery, which stops any further blood exchange between the fetuses, halting the disease. Outcomes appear to be independent of disease severity. Umbilical cord occlusion by means of endoscopic surgery or by ultrasonography to interrupt blood exchange between the twins may also be used, but because this results in the death of one of the fetuses, it is used only in the most advanced stages of the disease.

REFERENCES
Baldwin V. *Pathology of multiple pregnancy.* New York: Springer-Verlag, 1994.

De Lia J, Cruiskshank D, Keye W. Fetoscopic neodymium: yttrium-aluminum-garnet laser occlusion of placental vessels in severe twin-twin transfusion syndrome. *Obstet Gynecol* 1990;75:1046–1053.

Hecher K, Plath H, Bregenzer T, et al. Endoscopic laser surgery versus serial amniocenteses in the treatment of severe twin-twin transfusion syndrome. *Am J Obstet Gynecol* 1999;180:717–724.

Quintero R, Morales W, Allen M, et al. Staging of twin-twin transfusion syndrome. *J Perinatol* 1999;19:550–555.

Quintero R, Morales W, Mendoza G, et al. Selective photocoagulation of placental vessels in twin-twin transfusion syndrome: evolution of a surgical technique. *Obstet Gynecol Surv* 1998;53 (suppl):97–103.

RESOURCES
474, 475

---

67   Wegener Granulomatosis

John H. Stone, MD, MPH

DEFINITION: Wegener granulomatosis (WG) is a multiorgan system inflammatory illness associated with granulomatous inflammation and vasculitis.

SYNONYMS: Wegener disease; Pathergic granulomatosis.

DIFFERENTIAL DIAGNOSIS: Polyarteritis nodosa; Microscopic polyangiitis; Churg-Strauss syndrome; Henoch-Schönlein purpura; Systemic lupus erythematosus; Lymphoma; Lymphomatoid granulomatosis; Mycobacterial and deep fungal infections; Sarcoidosis; Goodpasture syndrome.

SYMPTOMS AND SIGNS: Symptoms include fatigue, fever, and weight loss. Scleritis, orbital pseudotumor with proptosis, conjunctivitis, and dacrocystitis may occur. Serous otitis media with conductive hearing loss and granulomatous inflammation in the middle ear, as well as nasal bleeding and crusting, nasal septal perforation, and "saddle-nose" deformity may occur. Other symptoms include pan-sinusitis with bony erosions and subglottic stenosis. In the lungs, there may be pulmonary nodules and cavities (Insert Figs. 45 and 46), alveolar hemorrhage caused by pulmonary capillaritis, nonspecific infiltrates, brochiolitis obliterans with organizing pneumonia, and, rarely, bronchocenteric lesions leading to bronchial stenosis. There may be mesenteric vasculitis with gastrointestinal hemorrhage, as well as migratory arthritis, often involving the large joints of the lower extremities. Skin may show a palpable purpura, cutaneous ulcerations, and nodules over the elbows that may mimic rheumatoid nodules. Vasculitic neuropathy of the peripheral nerves may be present. Meningeal involvement by granulomatous inflammation, leading to a chronic meningitis presentation, can also occur.

ETIOLOGY/EPIDEMIOLOGY: The cause of WG is unknown. In Western countries, most cases occur in whites, and the disease is believed to be less common among blacks; however, the disease is known to occur in all races. Typically, patients with WG are middle-aged, but the disease also occurs in the elderly and (rarely) in children. The gender distribution is approximately equal, with perhaps a slight male predominance.

DIAGNOSIS: Because of the numerous mimickers of WG among infectious, malignant, and other types of disorders, confirmation of the diagnosis by biopsy of an involved tissue is critical. Lung biopsies are most likely to yield all three typical histopathologic features (granulomatous inflammation, necrosis, and vasculitis), and pulmonary lesions are often amenable to biopsy through thoracoscopic procedures, which have less morbidity than open-lung biopsies. Kidney biopsies that show segmental, necrotizing glomerulonephritis (often with crescents) may also be diagnostic of WG in the setting of other findings, e.g., clinical or radiologic evidence of nasal, sinus, or lung involvement, or serologic evidence of antineutrophil cytoplasmic antibodies. The finding of granulomatous inflammation is unusual in the kidneys in WG, but glomerulonephritis is the renal equivalent of small vessel vasculitis.

TREATMENT

Standard Therapies: Treatment is based on the concepts of "severe" and "limited" disease. Severe WG is any form of organ involvement that poses an immediate threat either to the patient's life or to a vital organ; limited WG is any form of the disease that does not pose such a threat. Severe WG requires treatment with a combination of oral daily cyclophosphamide and high doses of corticosteroids. Limited disease may be treated with methotrexate in lieu of cyclophosphamide. In both severe and limited disease, long-term therapy for months to years is typically required. In the case of severe disease, however, attempts should be made to switch cyclophosphamide to either methotrexate or azathioprine after 3–6 months, assuming that the underlying disease appears controlled, to avoid some of the side effects of cyclophosphamide. Steroids should be tapered and discontinued by 6 months, if possible, and all WG patients treated with the combination of steroids and a cytotoxic agent should be treated with prophylaxis against *Pneumocystis carinii* pneumonia.

REFERENCES

Hoffman GS, et al. Wegener's granulomatosis: an analysis of 158 patients. *Ann Intern Med* 1992;116:488–498.

Hoffman GS, Specks U. Anti-neutrophil cytoplasmic antibodies. *Arthritis Rheum* 1998;41:1521–1537.

Regan MJ, Hellmann DB, Stone JH. Treatment of Wegener's granulomatosis. *Rheum Dis Clin North Am* 2001;27:863–886.

RESOURCES

37, 357, 490

Inborn Errors of Metabolism

1   Glutaric Acidemia Type I

Stephen I. Goodman, MD,
and Frank E. Frerman, PhD

DEFINITION: Glutaric acidemia type I (GAI) is a recessively inherited inborn error characterized clinically by an extrapyramidal movement disorder that appears in early childhood and biochemically by increased amounts of glutaric and 3-hydroxyglutaric acids in urine.

SYNONYMS: Glutaric acidemia type I; Glutaric aciduria; Glutaric aciduria type I.

DIFFERENTIAL DIAGNOSIS: Static cerebral palsy.

SYMPTOMS AND SIGNS: Patients often have macrocephaly at birth but are otherwise normal, and then suddenly develop hypotonia, dystonia, and athetosis after 4 months to 4 years. A few patients with enzyme deficiency do not develop neurologic manifestations.

ETIOLOGY/EPIDEMIOLOGY: The disease is caused by a deficiency in glutaryl-CoA dehydrogenase (GCD), a mitochondrial enzyme that converts glutaryl-CoA, an intermediate in the oxidation of lysine, hydroxy lysine, and tryptophan, to crotonyl-CoA and carbon dioxide. A large number of different GCD mutations have been found, and there is no one common mutant allele except in inbred populations such as the Old Order Amish of Lancaster County, Pennsylvania, and the Island Lake Indians of Manitoba, Canada.

DIAGNOSIS: CT and MRI of the brain show large subarachnoid spaces with frontal and temporal cortical atrophy. Urine organic acid analysis shows increased glutaric and 3-hydroxyglutaric acids; this may be consistent, intermittent (occurring only during catabolic episodes), or (rarely) absent. Demonstrating deficiency of GCD in leukocytes or cultured fibroblasts or, in some patients, by mutation detection, makes a definitive diagnosis. Prenatal diagnosis may be established by showing increased glutaric acid in amniotic fluid, by enzyme assay in cultured amniocytes or chorionic villus samples, and, in appropriate instances, by mutation detection.

TREATMENT

Standard Therapies: Treatment after the onset of neurologic disease is not effective. Treatment of asymptomatic patients with carnitine, riboflavin, and a low lysine and tryptophan diet, and preventing catabolism during intercurrent illness with fluids, electrolytes, and glucose, may prevent the development of acute striatal necrosis.

REFERENCES

Goodman SI, Frerman FE. Organic acidemias due to defects in lysine oxidation: 2-ketoadipic acidemia and glutaric academia. In: Scriver CR, Beaudet AL, Valle D, et al., eds. *The metabolic and molecular bases of inherited disease,* 8th ed. New York: McGraw-Hill, 2001:2195–2204.

Hauser SE, Peters H. Glutaric aciduria type I: an underdiagnosed cause of encephalopathy and dystonia-dyskinesia syndrome in children. *J Paediatr Child Health* 1998;34:302–304.

Superti-Furga A, Hoffmann GF. Glutaric aciduria type I (glutaryl-CoA-dehydrogenase deficiency): advances and unanswered questions. Report from an international meeting. *Eur J Pediatr* 1997;15:6821–6828.

RESOURCES

109, 336, 382

2   Glutaric Acidemia Type II

Stephen I. Goodman, MD,
and Frank E. Frerman, PhD

DEFINITION: Glutaric acidemia type II (GAII) is a recessively inherited inborn error characterized clinically by hypoketotic hypoglycemia and metabolic acidosis and biochemically by the excretion of metabolites of the substrates of eight mitochondrial acyl-CoA dehydrogenases. Patients may also accumulate and excrete sarcosine (N-methylglycine).

SYNONYMS: Glutaric aciduria type II; Severe multiple acyl-CoA dehydrogenase deficiency; Ethylmalonicadipic aciduria or mild multiple acyl-CoA dehydrogenase deficiency.

DIFFERENTIAL DIAGNOSIS: Other disorders of fatty acid oxidation including deficiency of VLCAD (very long chain acyl-CoA dehydrogenase) and CPT (carnitine palmitoyltransferase) II deficiency.

SYMPTOMS AND SIGNS: Patients with severe disease usually present in infancy with hypotonia, cardiomyopathy, hypoglycemia, metabolic acidosis, and the smell of sweaty feet. They may also have congenital anomalies, including large and cystic kidneys, facial dysmorphism, and anomalies of the external genitalia. Patients with less severe disease may present in childhood or adulthood with hypoketotic hypoglycemia or cardiomyopathy, and have variable courses.

ETIOLOGY/EPIDEMIOLOGY: In some patients, GAII is caused by deficiency of electron transfer flavoprotein (ETF), and in others by a deficiency of ETF-ubiquinone oxidoreductase (ETF-QO), or ETF dehydrogenase. No reliable data exist regarding the incidence of the disease.

DIAGNOSIS: Urine organic acid analysis usually shows increased isovalerylglycine and ethylmalonic, glutaric, and 2-hydroxyglutaric acids, and the acylcarnitine profile shows carnitine esters of several short, medium, and long-chain acids, and glutaric acid. Amino acid analysis often shows increased sarcosine in serum and urine, particularly in patients with later onset. Definitive diagnosis is made by demonstrating abnormalities of ETF or ETF-QO antigens or activity in cultured fibroblasts. Prenatal diagnosis may be established by showing increased glutaric acid in amniotic fluid or acylcarnitine esters in maternal urine and, in appropriate cases, by demonstrating large cystic fetal kidneys by ultrasonography.

TREATMENT

Standard Therapies: Acute disease is treated with fluid and electrolytes, and glucose to control hypoglycemia. Long-term treatment involves administration of riboflavin and carnitine, but this is often ineffective.

REFERENCES

Frerman FE, Goodman SI. Defects of electron transfer flavoprotein and electron transfer flavoprotein-ubiquinone oxidoreductase: glutaric acidemia type II. In: Scriver CR, Beaudet AL, Valle D, et al., eds. *The metabolic and molecular bases of inherited disease,* 8th ed. New York: McGraw-Hill, 2001: 2357–2365.

RESOURCES

109, 336, 382

---

3   Isovaleric Acidemia

Susan C. Winter, MD, FAAP, FCMG, and Neil R.M. Buist, MB, ChB

DEFINITION: Isovaleric acidemia is an inherited disorder of isovaleryl CoA dehydrogenase that converts isovaleryl CoA to 3-methylcrotonyl CoA, intermediates in the catabolism of the amino acid, leucine.

SYNONYMS: Isovaleric aciduria; Isovaleryl CoA dehydrogenase deficiency.

DIFFERENTIAL DIAGNOSIS: All organic acidurias; Disorders of branched chain amino acid metabolism; Urea cycle defects; Mitochondrial electron transport chain defects; Other disorders associated with abnormal body odor.

SYMPTOMS AND SIGNS: Neonates or infants with isovaleric acidemia usually present with vomiting, hypotonia, lethargy or coma, respiratory distress caused by metabolic acidosis, and later, failure-to-thrive, developmental delay, and sometimes pancreatitis. During crises, an odor of sweaty feet is characteristic. Acute life-threatening ketoacidotic episodes often occur with even minor catabolic stress such as a viral illness. Neurologic sequelae include ataxia, dystonia, tremor, and seizures. Laboratory tests show ketoacidosis, hyperammonemia, elevated liver enzymes, neutropenia, thrombocytopenia, anemia, low free carnitine, and elevated acyl-carnitines in blood and urine. Hyperglycemia can be present with massive ketosis and can be misdiagnosed as diabetes mellitus. Pancreatitis can be a recurrent complication.

ETIOLOGY/EPIDEMIOLOGY: Isovaleryl CoA dehydrogenase deficiency is inherited in an autosomal-recessive manner. The enzyme has been mapped to chromosome 15q14-q15.

DIAGNOSIS: During crises, the odor is characteristic. Elevations of isovaleric acid, isovalerylglycine, and 3-hydroxyisovaleric acid are detected by urine organic acids studies. Newborn screening by tandem mass spectrometry shows typical elevation of isovaleryl-carnitine. Diagnosis is confirmed by enzyme analysis in cultured skin fibroblasts or leukocytes; prenatal diagnosis is available.

TREATMENT

Standard Therapies: Dietary restriction of protein intake is necessary, and use of a low leucine medical food is helpful. L-carnitine at 100–300 mg/kg/day orally or intravenously and glycine at 250 mg/kg/day orally are given. Aggressive therapy of infections and catabolic events includes hemodialysis for overwhelming acidosis or coma.

REFERENCES

Gilbert-Barness E, Barness LA. *Metabolic diseases: foundations of clinical management, genetics, and pathology.* Natick, MA: Eaton Publishing, 2000:81–83.

Mohsen AW, Anderson BD, Volchenboum SL, et al. Characterization of molecular defects in isovaleryl-CoA dehydrogenase in patients with isovaleric academia. *Biochemistry* 1998; 37:10325–10335.

Scriver CR, Beaudet AL, Sly WS, et al., eds. *The metabolic and molecular bases of inherited disease*, 8th ed. New York: McGraw-Hill, 2001.

RESOURCES

58, 109, 382

---

4 Propionic Acidemia

Susan C. Winter, MD, FAAP, FCMG, and Neil R. M. Buist, MD, ChB

DEFINITION: Propionic acidemia is an inherited disorder of propionyl CoA carboxylase, which converts propionyl CoA to methylmalonyl CoA.

SYNONYM: Propionic aciduria.

DIFFERENTIAL DIAGNOSIS: Other organic acidurias; Disorders of branched chain amino acid catabolism; Urea cycle defects; Biotinidase deficiency and disorders of mitochondrial electron chain transport.

SYMPTOMS AND SIGNS: Neonates or infants with propionic acidemia present with vomiting, hypotonia, lethargy or coma, failure to thrive, developmental delay, respiratory distress due to metabolic acidosis, and, occasionally, pancreatitis. Neurologic complications include cerebral atrophy, mental retardation, dystonia, and seizures. In older children and adults being treated, fatal cardiomyopathy often occurs. Acute life-threatening ketoacidotic episodes often occur with or without even minor catabolic stress such as a viral illness. Laboratory tests show ketoacidosis, hyperammonemia, elevated liver enzymes, neutropenia, thrombocytopenia, anemia, low free carnitine, and elevated acyl-carnitines in blood and urine.

ETIOLOGY/EPIDEMIOLOGY: Propionyl CoA carboxylase deficiency is inherited in an autosomal-recessive manner. The enzyme consists of an α subunit encoded on chromosome 13 and a β subunit encoded on chromosome

3. Biotin is the cofactor and binds to the α subunit. Propionyl-CoA combines with carnitine, which becomes depleted as the metabolite is excreted in the urine.

DIAGNOSIS: Elevations of propionic acid, 3 hydroxypropionate, methyl citrate, and tigylglycine are detected by urine organic acids studies. Newborn screening by tandem mass spectrometry shows typical elevation of propionyl-carnitine. All forms can be diagnosed by enzyme analysis in cultured skin fibroblasts; prenatal diagnosis is available.

TREATMENT

Standard Therapies: Treatment consists of dietary restriction of the precursor amino acids isoleucine, valine, methionine, and threonine. Biotin therapy is generally of little help. L-carnitine 100–300 mg/kg/day either orally or intravenously is useful. Aggressive therapy of infections and catabolic events including hemodialysis for overwhelming acidosis or coma is recommended.

Investigational Therapies: Liver transplantation should be curative but persistence of the enzyme defect in other tissues may not make this an ideal treatment and it is being investigated.

REFERENCES

Gilbert-Barness E, Barness LA. *Metabolic diseases, foundations of clinical management, genetics, and pathology.* Natick, MA: Eaton Publishing, 2000:87–88.

McKusick VA, ed. Online Mendelian Inheritance in Man, OMIM [database online]. Bethesda, MD: National Center for Biotechnology Information, National Library of Medicine, 2000. MIM# 232000.

Scriver CR, Beaudet AL, Sly WS, et al., eds. *The metabolic and molecular bases of inherited disease*, 8th ed. New York: McGraw-Hill, 2001.

RESOURCES
109, 354, 382

5 The Methylmalonic Acidemias

Susan C. Winter, MD, FAAP, FCMG, and Neil R.M. Buist, MB, ChB

DEFINITION: The methylmalonic acidemias (MMA) are a group of at least eight different inborn errors of metabolism that affect the conversion of methylmalonyl-CoA to succinyl-CoA, resulting in accumulation of methylmalonic acid in blood and increased excretion in the urine. The most common is due to deficiency of the enzyme methylmalonyl-CoA mutase; the others involve the metabolism or transport of vitamin B_{12}.

SYNONYMS: Methylmalonic aciduria; Methylmalonyl-CoA mutase deficiency; Adenosylcobalamin deficiency (CblA, CblB); Combined adenosylcobalamin and methylcobalamin deficiency (CblC, CblD, CblF); Methylcobalamin deficiency (CblE, CblG).

DIFFERENTIAL DIAGNOSIS: Other organic acidurias; Disorders of branched chain amino acid catabolism; Urea cycle defects; Disorders of mitochondrial electron chain transport.

SYMPTOMS AND SIGNS: The mutase deficiencies manifest in neonates or infants with vomiting, hypotonia, lethargy or coma, failure to thrive, developmental delay, and respiratory distress. Acute life-threatening ketoacidotic episodes often occur with or even without minor catabolic stress such as viral illness. Laboratory tests generally show ketoacidosis, hyperammonemia, elevated liver enzymes, neutropenia, thrombocytopenia, anemia, low free carnitine, and elevated acyl-carnitines in blood and urine; occasionally pancreatitis is seen. In older children and adults on treatment, renal failure can occur. Methylmalonic acidemias due to abnormalities of cobalamin metabolism (CblA, Cb1B, Cb1C, Cb1D, and Cb1F) can present in a similar way to mutase deficiency or with milder symptoms and signs. CblE and Cb1G present with neurologic problems including developmental delay, seizures, blindness, altered tone, nystagmus, and ataxia. Cerebral atrophy and megaloblastic anemia usually occur.

ETIOLOGY/EPIDEMIOLOGY: All forms of MMA are rare and, with one possible exception, inherited as autosomal-recessive traits. Methylmalonyl-CoA mutase is located on chromosome 6p21. CblD may be X-linked, because only males have been described with the disease. Metabolites combine with carnitine, which becomes deficient as body stores are depleted and lead to disturbed CoA metabolism

DIAGNOSIS: Diagnosis is made by demonstration of elevation of methylmalonic acid in serum or urine with propionic acid and hydroxypropionate also elevated. Newborn screening by tandem mass spectrometry shows typical elevation of propionyl-carnitine. All forms can be demonstrated by enzyme analysis in cultured skin fibroblasts; prenatal diagnosis is available.

TREATMENT
Standard Therapies: Dietary restriction of precursor amino acids (isoleucine, valine, methionine, and threonine) is indicated. Cobalamin therapy, preferably with hydroxycobalamin 1–2 mg/day, is advised. L-carnitine at 100–300 mg/kg/day orally or intravenously also has been used.

REFERENCES
Gilbert-Barness E, Barness LA. *Metabolic diseases, foundations of clinical management, genetics, and pathology.* Natick, MA: Eaton Publishing, 2000:81–83.
Scriver CR, Beaudet AL, Sly WS, et al., eds. *The metabolic and molecular bases of inherited disease,* 8th ed. New York: McGraw-Hill, 2001.

RESOURCES
109, 354, 382

6 X-Linked Adrenoleukodystrophy

Hugo W. Moser, MD

DEFINITION: X-linked adrenoleukodystrophy (X-ALD) is a progressive disorder that involves the nervous system and the adrenal cortex. It must be distinguished from neonatal adrenoleukodystrophy, which is distinct with respect to clinical features, genetic defect, and mode of inheritance.

SYNONYMS: Schilder disease; Addison-Schilder disease.

DIFFERENTIAL DIAGNOSIS: Addison disease; Attention deficit disorders; Brain tumors; Autism; Asperger syndrome; Multiple sclerosis; Spastic paraparesis; Psychosis; Other leukodystrophies; Alzheimer disease.

SYMPTOMS AND SIGNS: The symptoms and signs vary widely. Approximately 40% of patients have the childhood or adolescent cerebral forms, which manifest most commonly between ages 4 and 8 years. First symptoms resemble those of attention deficit disorder or a psychological disorder. These are followed by more serious disturbances of behavior, cognition, coordination, visuomotor coordination, hearing, and vision, and may lead to severe generalized neurologic disability within 2–4 years and death at varying intervals thereafter. Approximately 40%–45% of male patients have the adrenomyeloneuropathy (AMN) phenotype, which affects the spinal cord mainly. In males it occurs in young adulthood as a slowly progressive paraparesis, impaired sphincter control, and sensory disturbances that involve the legs mainly, and it progresses over decades. Approximately 25% of patients with AMN also develop cerebral involvement. Of male patients, 70% have primary adrenocortical insufficiency (Addison disease). In 10%–20% of male patients, adrenal insufficiency is the only clinical manifestation. Most of these patients, however, develop evidence of AMN in adulthood. Approximately 50% of women who are heterozygous for X-ALD in middle age or later develop a syndrome that resembles AMN but is usually milder. Addison disease and cerebral involvement are present in approximately 1% of heterozygous women.

ETIOLOGY/EPIDEMIOLOGY: The disease results from defects in the gene *ABCD1*, which is located on Xq28. It codes for ALDP, a peroxisomal membrane protein. The deficiency of ALDP leads to the accumulation of very long chain fatty acids (VLCFA), particularly in the nervous system and the adrenal cortex, and also in plasma. The disease affects 1 in 21,000 males, and the combined frequency of affected males and females in the general population is estimated to be 1 in 16,800. It has been described in all ethnic groups. Mode of inheritance is X-linked recessive.

DIAGNOSIS: Demonstration of increased levels of VLCFA in plasma is the most frequently used diagnostic procedure. It is reliable for the identification of affected males, but 15% of heterozygous women have normal levels. Exclusion of heterozygote status requires mutation analysis. The diagnosis should be suspected particularly in the following clinical settings: Addison disease of unexplained etiology; progressive behavioral disturbances and cognitive deficits in boys and adolescents; and progressive spastic paraparesis in men and women.

TREATMENT

Standard Therapies: Seventy percent of male patients have primary adrenocortical insufficiency that responds fully to adrenal steroid replacement therapy. This therapy does not appear to alter neurologic progression. Bone marrow transplantation should be considered for patients in the early stages of the childhood or adolescent cerebral phenotype.

Investigational Therapies: Therapies being investigated include dietary therapy with a mixture of glyceryl trioleate and glyceryl trierucate, as well as lovastatin and 4 phenylbutyrate.

REFERENCES

Bezman L, Moser AB, Raymond GV, et al. Adrenoleukodystrophy: incidence, new mutations and results of extended family screening. *Ann Neurol* 2001;49:512–517.

Kemp S, Pujol A, Waterham HR, et al. X-linked adrenoleukodystrophy mutation database: role in diagnosis and clinical correlations. *Hum Mutat* 2001;18:499–515.

Moser HW, Smith KD, Watkins PA, et al. X-linked adrenoleukodystrophy. In: Scriver CR, Beaudet AL, Sly WS, et al., eds. *The metabolic and molecular bases of inherited disease,* 8th ed. New York: McGraw-Hill, 2001:3257–3301.

Pai GS, Khan M, Barbosa E, et al. Lovastatin therapy for X-linked adrenoleukodystrophy: clinical and biochemical observations on twelve patients. *Mol Genet Metabol* 2000;69: 312–322.

Shapiro E, Krivit W, Lockman L, et al. Long-term effect of bone-marrow transplantation for childhood-onset cerebral adrenoleukodystrophy. *Lancet* 2000;356:713–718.

RESOURCES

109, 351, 354

7   Alkaptonuria

*Wendy J. Introne, MD,
and William A. Gahl, MD, PhD*

DEFINITION: Alkaptonuria is an inborn error of metabolism due to deficiency of homogentisate 1,2-dioxygenase, an enzyme in the tyrosine degradation pathway. Homogentisic acid accumulation results in urine that turns dark upon standing, progressive joint destruction, and pigment deposition in connective tissues.

SYNONYM: Ochronosis.

DIFFERENTIAL DIAGNOSIS: Ankylosing spondylitis; Quinacrine ingestion; Minocycline ingestion.

SYMPTOMS AND SIGNS: Infants with alkaptonuria may have urine that turns dark upon oxidation or black-stained cloth diapers upon washing with soap. Other symptoms begin in the second or third decades of life and progress slowly. Dark pigmentation of the sclera occurs midway between the pupil and the inner and outer canthi at the insertion of the rectus muscles. Cartilage in the ear becomes blue or brown, thickened, and irregular. By middle age, pigmentation of tendons may be visible, particularly in the hands, as well as pigmentation along the lateral aspects of the fingers and in the web between the thumb and second digit. Perspiration may also be ochronotic, and patients may report stained clothing in the axillary region. All patients develop arthritis, which can be severe and disabling. Back pain is usually the first symptom. Degeneration of the intervertebral discs results in narrowed joint spaces and calcification by age 40–50 years. Eventually, the vertebrae may fuse. All of the other large joints can be affected. Hip, knee, and shoulder replacements are common, and most patients have had at least one joint replaced by age 50–60 years. Alkaptonuria is sometimes diagnosed intraoperatively based on the finding of ochronotic cartilage, bone, and supporting connective tissue. Other complications of alkaptonuria include ochronotic heart valves, particularly the aortic valve. Initial thickening leads to calcification, stenosis and/or insufficiency, and valve replacement. Kidney and prostate stones are also common.

ETIOLOGY/EPIDEMIOLOGY: Alkaptonuria is inherited in an autosomal-recessive manner. The disease is the result of a mutation in the homogentisate 1,2-dioxygenase gene, which is located on chromosome 3q21-23. The prevalence is estimated at 1 in 250,000. All ethnic groups are affected, with pockets of increased frequency in Slovakia, the Dominican Republic, and Germany.

DIAGNOSIS: The diagnosis should be suspected based on the findings of black urine or characteristic radiographic changes in the spine. Vastly increased homogentisic acid (gram quantities) in the urine makes the diagnosis. Homogentisic acid level is determined with urine organic acid analysis.

TREATMENT
Standard Therapies: Treatment is generally palliative. For pain control, antiinflammatories are tailored to individual patients. Occasionally, stronger pain medications such as narcotics are required. Joint and aortic valve replacements also provide symptomatic relief, and subacute bacterial endocarditis prophylaxis is usually warranted for the valvular involvement. Large doses of vitamin C and restriction of dietary protein have not proven efficacious, and severe dietary restrictions are difficult to maintain.

Investigational Therapies: Treatment with 2-(2-nitro-4-trifluoromethylbenzoyl)-1,3-cyclohexanedione (NTBC, nitisinone) is being investigated.

REFERENCES
Anikster Y, Nyhan WL, Gahl WA. NTBC in alkaptonuria. *Am J Hum Genet* 1998;63:920–921.
La Du BN. Alkaptonuria. In: Scriver CR, Beaudet A, Sly W, et al., eds. *The metabolic and molecular bases of inherited disease,* 8th ed. New York: McGraw-Hill, 2001:2109–2123.
O'Brien WM, La Du BN, Bunim JJ. Biochemical, pathologic, and clinical aspects of alcaptonuria, ochronosis and ochronotic arthropathy. *Am J Med* 1963;34:813–838.
Ptacin M, Sebastian J, Banrah VS. Ochronotic cardiovascular disease. *Clin Cardiol* 1985;8:441–445.

8   Aspartylglucosaminuria

Neil R.M. Buist, MB, ChB,
and Susan C. Winter, MD, FAAP, FCMG

DEFINITION: Aspartylglucosaminuria is caused by a deficiency of the enzyme aspartylglucosaminidase in lysosomes, and is classified as one of the lysosomal storage diseases.

DIFFERENTIAL DIAGNOSIS: Mucopolysaccharidoses; Oligosacharidoses; Costello syndrome.

SYMPTOMS AND SIGNS: Patients appear normal for several months after birth and then present with recurrent infections, diarrhea, and hernias. Later, subtle facial dysmorphism emerges with gradual coarsening of the features similar to, but less overt than, those seen in Hurler and Hunter syndromes. Mild macroglossia, hoarse voice, and hepatomegaly are common, and crystal-like lens opacities have been reported. After several years, mild dysostosis multiplex and developmental delay are noted, followed by gradual developmental regression.

ETIOLOGY/EPIDEMIOLOGY: This is an autosomal-recessively inherited disorder of lysosomal catabolism with the gene localized to 4q32-q33. Most cases have been reported in Finland, where a single mutation explains more than 90% of cases.

DIAGNOSIS: The diagnosis is made by identification of aspartylglucosamine and other mucopolysaccharide derivatives in urine. The enzyme can be quantitated in leukocytes, cultured fibroblasts, and amniocytes, making prenatal diagnosis possible. Electron microscopy shows intralysosomal accumulations in tissues; but it cannot be used for a definitive diagnosis.

TREATMENT
Standard Therapies: No known treatment for this disorder exists.

Investigational Therapies: Bone marrow transplantation is being tried in many different lysosomal storage diseases and may be attempted for this disorder.

REFERENCES
McKusick VA, ed. Online Mendelian Inheritance in Man, OMIM [database online]. Bethesda, MD: National Center for Biotechnology Information, National Library of Medicine, 2000. MIM# 208400.
Scriver CR, Beaudet AL, Sly WS, et al., eds. *The metabolic and molecular bases of inherited disease,* 8th ed. New York: McGraw-Hill, 2000.
Tollersrud OK, et al. Aspartylglucosaminuria in northern Norway: a molecular and genealogical study. *J Med Genet* 1994;31: 360–363.

RESOURCES
58, 314, 364

9   Carnitine Deficiency Syndromes

Susan C. Winter, MD, FAAP, FCMG,
and Neil R.M. Buist, MB, ChB

DEFINITION: Carnitine transporter deficiency is an autosomal-recessive genetic disorder in which blood carnitine levels are very low.

SYNONYMS: Primary carnitine deficiency (Carnitine transporter deficiency); Secondary carnitine deficiency; Systemic carnitine deficiency; Muscular carnitine deficiency; Carnitine insufficiency.

DIFFERENTIAL DIAGNOSIS: Organic acidurias; Disorders of branched chain amino acid catabolism; Urea cycle defects; Disorders of mitochondrial electron chain transport; Fatty acid oxidation defects; Carnitine palmitoyl transferase I and II deficiency; Carnitine translocase deficiency.

SYMPTOMS AND SIGNS: Carnitine deficiency results in altered mitochondrial fat metabolism to energy. Progressive muscle weakness, hypotonia, failure to thrive, cardiomyopathy, encephalopathy ranging from lethargy to coma, and hepatic dysfunction with hyperammonemia and hypoketotic hypoglycemia (Reye syndrome) are seen. Severe deficiencies associated with organic acidurias can result in death if left untreated.

ETIOLOGY/EPIDEMIOLOGY: True primary carnitine deficiency is due to a recessively inherited genetic deficiency of the carnitine membrane transporter. All other forms of carnitine deficiency are secondary to other pathology. When carnitine deficiency is detected, it is imperative to find the primary cause, and treat both the deficiency and the primary pathology.

DIAGNOSIS: Carnitine deficiency can be confirmed with measurement of carnitine levels in blood or tissue (muscle or liver). Because most body carnitine is located in the muscle, muscle measurement is most accurate but it is difficult to obtain. Therefore, assay of plasma free and acyl carnitine is the most useful study, and deficiency is defined as a free level below 20 μM. An acyl/free ratio is useful in determining the etiology as well as the insufficiency state. If the ratio is greater than normal (0.4), there may be an increased organic acid accumulation and an insufficiency of free carnitine to support the metabolic demand for excretion of metabolites. Measurement of organic acids in urine, acyl-carnitine derivatives in blood, or urinary acyl-glycine derivatives often show the primary metabolic disorder.

TREATMENT
Standard Therapies: Carnitine is available in an oral and intravenous form and should be used to treat any patient with a deficiency. Oral carnitine absorption is poor (approximately 25%); in the acutely ill patient with life-threatening metabolic decompensation, intravenous carnitine should be used. Treatment should be continued for life for all patients with primary carnitine deficiency and with secondary carnitine deficiency due to inborn errors of metabolism. In all other causes of secondary carnitine deficiency, treatment should continue for as long as the primary pathology persists.

REFERENCES

Gilbert-Barness E, Barness LA. *Metabolic diseases, foundations of clinical management, genetics, and pathology.* Natick, MA: Eaton Publishing, 2000.

McKusick VA, ed. Online Mendelian Inheritance in Man, OMIM [database online]. Bethesda, MD: National Center for Biotechnology Information, National Library of Medicine, 2000. MIM #212140, 212160.

Scriver CR, Beaudet AL, Sly WS, et al., eds. *The metabolic and molecular bases of inherited disease,* 8th ed. New York: McGraw-Hill, 2000.

RESOURCES
58, 158, 365

---

10   Carnitine Palmitoyl Transferase I Deficiency

Neil R.M. Buist, MB, ChB, and Susan C. Winter, MD, FAAP, FCMG

DEFINITION: Carnitine palmitoyl transferase I (CPTI) deficiency is an autosomal-recessively inherited condition affecting an enzyme that is most active in liver, heart, and muscle. CPTI is one of several enzymes required for the transport of fatty acids bound to carnitine into mitochondria for the generation of energy.

SYNONYMS: Carnitine palmitoyltransferase I deficiency; CPT deficiency, hepatic, type I.

DIFFERENTIAL DIAGNOSIS: Reye syndrome; Defects of energy generation such as defects of carbohydrate catabolism, fatty acids and carnitine, and the electron transport chain.

SYMPTOMS AND SIGNS: Classically, infants present from birth through early childhood with hypoglycemia, hypoketosis, coma, hepatomegaly, and hepatocellular dysfunction (Reye syndrome). Persistent neurologic damage, probably due to hypoglycemia, frequently occurs. Heart and muscle involvement is rarely of significance; kidney involvement can cause renal tubular malabsorption (Fanconi syndrome). Symptoms may lessen with age.

ETIOLOGY/EPIDEMIOLOGY: Carnitine palmitoyl transferase I deficiency is inherited in an autosomal-recessive manner. The gene is located on chromosome 11q13. Long-chain fatty acids are the predominant fuel for aerobic metabolism. They enter mitochondria attached to carnitine by a transport system that is composed of carnitine translocase, CPTI, and CPTII. In the absence of sufficient long-chain fatty acids to support adenosine triphosphate and phosphocreatinine synthesis, glucose and medium-chain fatty acids become other available fuels. Thus, the most metabolically active tissues are most susceptible to damage. The enormous relative size of the liver and its high metabolic requirements in infancy ensure that the liver becomes the first and major target organ for metabolic decompensation. The hypoketosis develops from failure to import fatty acids for catabolism and the hypoglycemia reflects increased dependency on other fuels.

DIAGNOSIS: Definitive diagnosis is by enzyme assay in muscle, liver, or cultured skin fibroblasts.

TREATMENT
Standard Therapies: Treatment consists of aggressive management of liver disease and all potential catabolic events such as viral infections or anorexia from any cause. High glucose intake and a high-carbohydrate and low-fat diet supplemented with medium-chain triglycerides is critical. Carnitine may be tried.

Investigational Therapies: Liver transplantation should cure all tendency to hypoglycemia; the long-term consequences of the defect in other tissues is unknown.

REFERENCES
Falik-Borenstein ZC, et al. Brief report: renal tubular acidosis in carnitine palmitoyltransferase type I deficiency. *N Engl J Med* 1992;327:2427.
McKusick VA, ed. Online Mendelian Inheritance in Man, OMIM [database online]. Bethesda, MD: National Center for Biotechnology Information, National Library of Medicine, 2000. MIM# 255120.
Scriver CR, Beaudet AL, Sly WS, et al., eds. *The metabolic and molecular bases of inherited disease,* 8th ed. New York: McGraw-Hill, 2000.

RESOURCES
58, 158, 364

11   Carnitine Palmitoyl Transferase II Deficiency

*Neil R.M. Buist, MB, ChB,
and Susan C. Winter, MD, FAAP, FCMG*

DEFINITION: Carnitine palmitoyl transferase II (CPTII) deficiency is an autosomal-recessively inherited condition affecting an enzyme that is most active in the muscle, heart, and liver. CPTII is one of several enzymes required for transport of fatty acids bound to carnitine across the mitochondrial membrane delivered for energy metabolism. The disorder exists in an infantile "hepatic" form and an adult "myopathic" form.

DIFFERENTIAL DIAGNOSIS: Reye syndrome; Defects of energy generation including defects of carbohydrate catabolism, fatty acids and carnitine, and the electron transport chain; McArdle syndrome; Disorders of the electron transport chain; Other intermittent myopathies (e.g., alcohol or drug induced).

SYMPTOMS AND SIGNS: Classically, infants present from birth or later with hypoglycemia, hypoketosis, coma, hepatomegaly with fatty infiltration, and hepatocellular dysfunction (Reye syndrome). Cardiomyopathy and cardiac arrhythmias, encephalopathy, and death in infancy may occur if the disorder is untreated. Adults present with muscle pains and cramps that are induced by exercise or reduced caloric intake. This can progress to rhabdomyolysis, myoglobinuria, and consequent renal tubular failure. The greater the provocative stress, the greater the risk for profound muscle damage. The heart and liver remain unaffected.

ETIOLOGY/EPIDEMIOLOGY: Carnitine palmitoyl transferase II deficiency is inherited in an autosomal-recessive manner with the gene localized to 1p32. Different mutations of the same gene are responsible for the infantile and adult presentations.

DIAGNOSIS: Definitive diagnosis in infants is by enzyme assay in muscle, liver, or cultured skin fibroblasts. In adults, diagnosis is confirmed by enzyme assay in muscle or cultured skin fibroblasts.

TREATMENT
Standard Therapies: In infants, aggressive therapy with glucose, carnitine, and medium-chain triglycerides should be attempted. Adults must learn to titrate their activity to their exercise tolerance to minimize muscle damage. Continuous intake of glucose during exercise may improve function but will not maximize it. Dietary supplementation with medium-chain triglycerides should be used, and some clinicians recommend a trial of carnitine as well. Liver transplantation in infants seems contraindicated because the heart is a major target organ.

REFERENCES
McKusick VA, ed. Online Mendelian Inheritance in Man, OMIM [database online]. Bethesda, MD: National Center for Biotechnology Information, National Library of Medicine, 2000. MIM #600650.
Scriver CR, Beaudet AL, Sly WS, et al., eds. *The metabolic and molecular bases of inherited disease,* 8th ed. New York: McGraw-Hill, 2000.
Videen JS, Haseler LJ, Karpinski NC, et al. Noninvasive evaluation of adult onset myopathy from carnitine palmitoyl transferase

II deficiency using proton magnetic resonance spectropscopy. *J Rheumatol* 1999;26:1757–1763.

RESOURCES

58, 158, 364

12 Carnosinemia

Steven M. Willi, MD

DEFINITION: Carnosinemia is an autosomal-recessive disorder caused by a deficiency in the enzyme carnosinase. It usually manifests in the first year of life with neurologic defects.

SYNONYMS: Carnosinase deficiency; Carnosinuria; Hyper-beta carnosinemia; Homocarnosinemia.

DIFFERENTIAL DIAGNOSIS: Juvenile amaurotic idiocy; Urea cycle defects; Phenylketonuria; Other inborn errors of amino acid metabolism.

SYMPTOMS AND SIGNS: Several patients with this disorder have been asymptomatic. When symptoms are present, they vary widely and can include myoclonic and/or absence seizures, psychomotor retardation, spastic paraparesis, hypotonia, tremor, mental retardation, retinitis pigmentosa, peripheral sensory neuropathy, optic atrophy, neurosensory hearing loss, progressive childhood dementia, nonspecific electronencephalographic abnormalities, and attention deficit disorder. No correlation between the severity of neurologic abnormalities and residual carnosinase activity is known. No definite conclusions can be drawn about the relationship between serum carnosinase deficiency and the neurologic defects.

ETIOLOGY/EPIDEMIOLOGY: Carnosinemia is inherited in an autosomal-recessive pattern and in one patient was linked to a deletion in the long arm of chromosome 18 at the position q21.3. Only 24 cases have been described worldwide.

DIAGNOSIS: Carnosinemia should be suspected in patients with hypercarnosinuria and anserinuria. The diagnosis is confirmed by the presence of low carnosinase activity. The carrier state is characterized by intermediate serum carnosinase activity, hypercarnosinuria, and a normal phenotype.

TREATMENT
Standard Therapies: A carnosine/anserine-free (i.e., vegan) diet has been used.

Investigational Therapies: Growth hormone therapy is being investigated.

REFERENCES
Cohen M, Hartlage PL, Krawiecki N, et al. Serum carnosinase deficiency: a non-disabling phenotype? *J Ment Defic Res* 1985;29:383–389.

Gjessing LR, Lunde HA, Morkrid L, et al. Inborn errors of carnosine and homocarnosine metabolism. *J Neural Transm* 1990;29(suppl):91–106.

Lenney JF, Peppers SC, Kucera CM, et al. Homocarnosinosis: lack of serum carnosinase is the defect probably responsible for elevated brain and CSF homocarnosine. *Clin Chim* 1983; 132:157–165.

Perry TL, Hansen S, Tischler B, et al. Carnosinemia. A new metabolic disorder associated with neurologic disease and mental defect. *N Engl J Med* 1967;277:1219–1227.

Willi SM, Zhang Y, Hill JB, et al. A deletion in the long arm of chromosome 18 in a child with serum carnosinase deficiency. *Pediatr Res* 1997;41:210–213.

RESOURCES
58, 109, 462

13   Human Cytochrome Oxidase Deficiency

*Pranesh Chakraborthy, MD,
Annette Feigenbaum, MD,
and Brian Robinson, PhD*

DEFINITION: Cytochrome oxidase (COX) deficiency refers to a group of genetic diseases with variable clinical features. COX may be isolated or part of a broader respiratory chain or mitochondrial dysfunction, e.g., mtDNA depletion syndrome.

SYNONYM: Complex IV deficiency.

SYMPTOMS AND SIGNS: Patients with isolated COX deficiency can present in several ways. Leigh syndrome (LS) can be caused by isolated COX deficiency or by other respiratory chain defects and pyruvate metabolism defects. The neurologic findings are variable, with myopathy and brainstem dysfunction prominent. Feeding difficulties and failure to thrive are common, and seizures may occur. Affected children may experience progressive or intermittent neurologic deterioration often related to an intercurrent illness. Death usually results from infection, aspiration, brainstem dysfunction causing recurrent cardiorespiratory collapse, or overwhelming acidosis. Fatal infantile COX deficiency is characterized by myopathy and renal tubular dysfunction, as well as episodic severe lactic acidosis. French Canadian LS is clinically similar to LS, but usually has a later age of onset and age of death. Death usually results from decompensation leading to pulmonary edema and overwhelming acidosis. With reversible "benign" infantile COX deficiency, infants present with very severe clinical features, but spontaneously clinically recover with normalization of COX activity in affected tissues. Infantile cardiomyopathy and hypotonia manifest in early infancy and are characterized by severe myopathy, lactic acidosis, hypertrophic cardiomyopathy, and early death. Renal tubulopathy with leukoencephalopathy manifests in infancy or early childhood with ataxia, weakness, seizures, lactic acidosis, and proximal renal tubular dysfunction. It is associated with COX deficiency in muscle, lymphocytes, and skin fibroblasts. Hepatopathy and encephalopathy is a rare syndromic combination in which COX deficiency is due to mutations in the *SCO1* gene.

ETIOLOGY/EPIDEMIOLOGY: Isolated COX deficiency is usually inherited as an autosomal-recessive condition caused by mutations in the genes responsible for COX assembly. Some rare mtDNA mutations also may cause isolated COX deficiency.

DIAGNOSIS: A defect in mitochondrial metabolism is suggested by elevated blood, cerebrospinal fluid, or brain lactate concentrations; the symmetric brainstem and basal ganglia lesions of LS are suggested by MRI and abnormal brainstem auditory evoked potentials. The diagnosis is made by demonstrating deficient enzyme activity and/or protein in one or more tissues, e.g., on skin and muscle biopsy analyzed in an accredited laboratory. The COX deficiency can be detected on analysis of muscle or kidney tissue but usually not on brain, liver, or skin fibroblast culture analysis. DNA studies may delineate the defect more specifically and can be used for prenatal diagnosis.

TREATMENT

Standard Therapies: The treatment is symptomatic and supportive. A mitochondrial "cocktail" is sometimes used: combinations of antioxidants such as vitamins C and E, pharmacologic doses of vitamin K, cofactors such as riboflavin and succinic acid, and carnitine.

REFERENCES

Robinson BH. Human cytochrome oxidase deficiency. *Pediatr Res* 2000;48:581–585.

Tritschler HJ, Bonilla E, Lombes A, et al. Differential diagnosis of fatal and benign cytochrome c oxidase-deficient myopathies of infancy: an immunohistochemical approach. *Neurology* 1991;41:300–305.

von Kleist-Retzow JC, Cormier-Daire V, de Lonlay P, et al. A high rate (20%–30%) of parental consanguinity in cytochrome-oxidase deficiency. *Am J Hum Genet* 1998;63:428–435.

RESOURCES

58, 364, 478

14 Long-Chain Acyl-CoA Dehydrogenase Deficiency

Simon Eaton, PhD

DEFINITION: All patients originally classified as having a deficiency in long-chain acyl-CoA dehydrogenase (LCAD) have in fact been found to have a deficiency in a related but distinct enzyme, very-long-chain acyl-CoA dehydrogenase (VLCAD).

DIFFERENTIAL DIAGNOSIS: See very-long-chain acyl-CoA dehydrogenase.

SYMPTOMS AND SIGNS: There have been no proven human deficiencies of this enzyme, because all those originally classified as LCAD deficient are in fact VLCAD deficient. A mouse model of LCAD deficiency suggests that the symptoms and signs would be similar to VLCAD deficiency. However, other investigators have suggested that the LCAD enzyme is more important in the metabolism of polyunsaturated fatty acids.

ETIOLOGY/EPIDEMIOLOGY: The etiology is unknown.

DIAGNOSIS: The diagnosis of LCAD deficiency would be expected to be made on the basis of laboratory tests for fatty acid oxidation disorders, e.g., a controlled fast with measurements of ketone bodies, glucose, insulin, and acylcarnitine esters.

REFERENCES

Kurtz DM, Rinaldo P, Rhead WJ, et al. Targeted disruption of mouse long-chain acyl-CoA dehydrogenase gene reveals crucial roles for fatty acid oxidation. *Proc Natl Acad Sci USA* 1998;95:15592–15597.

Le WP, Abbas AS, Sprecher H, et al. Long-chain acyl-CoA dehydrogenase is a key enzyme in the mitochondrial beta-oxidation of unsaturated fatty acids. *Biochim Biophys Acta* 2000; 1485:121–128.

Yamaguchi S, et al. Identification of very-long-chain acyl-coa dehydrogenase-deficiency in 3 patients previously diagnosed with long-chain acyl-coa dehydrogenase-deficiency. *Pediatr Res* 1993;34:111–113.

15 Medium-Chain Acyl-CoA Dehydrogenase Deficiency

Charles R. Roe, MD

DEFINITION: Medium-chain acyl-CoA dehydrogenase (MCAD) deficiency is an autosomal-recessive disorder of mitochondrial fatty acid oxidation. Medium-chain length acyl-CoA and free acid compounds accumulate and are associated with hypoglycemia, seizures, coma, and occasionally, sudden death.

DIFFERENTIAL DIAGNOSIS: Carnitine palmitoyltransferase I and II; Carnitine acylcarnitine translocase; Very-long-chain acyl-CoA dehydrogenase; L-3-hydoxy-acyl-CoA dehydrogenase; Trifunctional protein; Short-chain acyl-CoA dehydrogenase; Glutaric aciduria type II.

SYMPTOMS AND SIGNS: Clinical presentation is typical of Reye syndrome. It often begins with nausea and vomiting associated with even mild infection and proceeds to somnolence and decreased responsiveness due to accumulation of encephalopathic medium-chain length fatty acids. This is followed by hypoglycemia and often seizures. Without appropriate intervention, it can proceed to death. The clinical presentation can vary remarkably in the same family from being asymptomatic to Reye syndrome to sudden death due to cerebral edema and herniation. A simple episode of otitis media or mild gastroenteritis can lead to sudden death in affected children. Severe episodes can lead to significant neurologic sequelae such as seizure disorder developmental losses.

ETIOLOGY/EPIDEMIOLOGY: The disorder is inherited in an autosomal-recessive manner and is due to mutations in the nuclear gene for mitochondrial MCAD. Of affected individuals, 90% carry a common DNA mutation (K304E or A985G[cDNA]). The highest incidence is noted in families of Northern European origin; it is seen rarely in those of Oriental, Spanish, Italian, African, or Native American origins.

DIAGNOSIS: The single most specific test is blood acyl-carnitine analysis. Direct enzyme analysis for MCAD activity is available from skin fibroblasts. Urine organic acid analysis often shows nonspecific dicarboxylic aciduria. DNA mutation analysis may be helpful but the 20% incidence of compound heterozygotes decreases the specificity of this test. Postmortem evaluation for MCAD is suggested by the presence of hepatic steatosis usually in combination with cerebral edema. Diagnosis can be done by acylcarnitine analysis of blood usually saved for toxicology analysis. This can also be done on fresh frozen liver.

TREATMENT
Standard Therapies: Many children have died while waiting for the results of laboratory tests including blood glucose. In emergencies, a glucose test by Accu-Chek should be done immediately, and a 10% glucose infusion should be initiated in any obtunded child at the same time. Intravenous L-carnitine (30 mg/kg) as a bolus along with the same amount in the 24-hour fluids is also highly recommended, if available, to conjugate and facilitate the excretion of the toxic medium-chain length fatty acids. The goal of urgent therapy is to control endogenous lipolysis while providing adequate glucose (and insulin as needed). Chronic treatment includes a reasonably low-fat (high carbohydrate) diet, frequent feeding, and avoidance of fasting.

Often, a secondary deficiency of L-carnitine can be corrected by supplementation.

REFERENCES
Boles RG, et al. Retrospective biochemical screening of fatty acid oxidation disorders in postmortem livers of 418 cases of sudden death in the first year of life. *J Pediatr* 1998;132:924–933.
Iafolla AK, et al. Medium-chain acyl-coenzyme A dehydrogenase deficiency: clinical course in 120 affected children. *J Pediatr* 1994;124:409–415.
Roe CR, Ding JH. Mitochondrial fatty acid oxidation disorders. In: Scriver CR, Beaudet A, Sly W, et al., eds. *The metabolic and molecular bases of inherited disease,* 8th ed. New York: McGraw-Hill, 2001:2297–2326.
Roe CR, Millington DS, Maltby DA, et al. Recognition of medium-chain acyl-CoA dehydrogenase deficiency in asymptomatic siblings of children dying of sudden infant death or Reye-like syndromes. *J Pediatr* 1986;108:13.
Tanaka K, et al. A survey of the newborn populations in Belgium, Germany, Poland, Czech Republic, Hungary, Bulgaria, Spain, Turkey, and Japan for the G985 variant allele with haplotype analysis at the medium-chain acyl-CoA dehydrogenase gene locus: clinical and evolutionary considerations. *Pediatr Res* 1997;41:201–209.

RESOURCES
58, 158, 382, 478

16 Short-Chain Acyl-CoA Dehydrogenase Deficiency

Jerry Vockley, MD, PhD

DEFINITION: Short-chain acyl-CoA dehydrogenase (SCAD) deficiency is a disorder of fatty acid catabolism (mitochondrial β-oxidation). The clinical findings are variable, ranging from severe, neonatal acidosis to mild developmental delay with hypotonia.

DIFFERENTIAL DIAGNOSIS: Oxidative phosphorylation defects; Ethylmalonic aciduria/encephalopathy syndrome.

SYMPTOMS AND SIGNS: Clinical findings include episodes of intermittent metabolic acidosis, neonatal hyperammonemic coma, neonatal acidosis with hyperreflexia, multicore myopathy, infantile onset lipid storage myopathy with failure to thrive, and hypotonia. A variety of clinical findings has been reported in patients homozygous for one of two polymorphic variants in the SCAD gene, most frequently hypotonia and developmental delay. Most people homozygous for one of the polymorphisms,

however, are clinically well. The full clinical spectrum of this deficiency, and the clinical relevance of the common polymorphisms, remains to be defined.

ETIOLOGY/EPIDEMIOLOGY: The deficiency is caused by mutations in the *SCAD* gene leading to deficiency of SCAD activity. The *SCAD* gene is located in the terminal region of the long arm of chromosome 12. A variety of molecular defects has been identified. No good estimates of true deficiency are available. The common 625G→A polymorphism has an allele frequency of 0.26 in a European population.

DIAGNOSIS: Diagnosis of SCAD deficiency in the appropriate clinical setting should be suspected on the basis of elevated EMA excretion in urine. Patients with this finding should have DNA analysis for the common polymorphisms. If these are not identified, or if EMA excretion exceeds 25–30 mmol/mmol creatinine, additional enzymatic evaluation is warranted. Because SCAD activity is too low to reliably measure in fibroblasts by most assay methods, it should be determined in muscle. The presence of the common polymorphisms generally leads to reduction of muscle SCAD activity to 50%–67% of normal; rarely, patients with no other identifiable mutations have had complete loss of activity.

TREATMENT

Standard Therapies: Treatment for SCAD deficiency has largely been dietary, consisting of reduction of fat intake to 25% of calories from fat, with smaller, more frequent meals to avoid reliance on β-oxidation. In episodes of acute metabolic acidosis, intravenous hydration with a solution containing 10% glucose should be used to reestablish an anabolic state, followed by reintroduction of the patient's usual diet. Routine supplementation with carnitine is not likely to be of use chronically, although short-term use in acute crises may be warranted.

Investigational Therapies: The treatment of β-oxidation defects with the fatty acylglycerol triheptanoic acid is being investigated.

REFERENCES

Corydon M, Vockley J, Rinaldo R, et al. Role of common gene variations in the molecular pathogenesis of short-chain acyl-CoA dehydrogenase deficiency. *Pediatr Res* 2001;49:18–23.

Corydon MJ, Gregersen N, Lehnert W, et al. Ethylmalonic aciduria is associated with an amino acid variant of short chain acyl-coenzyme A dehydrogenase. *Pediatr Res* 1996;39:1059–1066.

Gregersen N, Andresen BS, Bross P. Prevalent mutations in fatty acid oxidation disorders: diagnostic considerations. *Eur J Pediatr* 2000;159(suppl):213–218.

Gregersen N, Winter VS, Corydon MJ, et al. Identification of four new mutations in the short-chain acyl-CoA dehydrogenase (SCAD) gene in two patients: one of the variant alleles, 511CÆT, is present at an unexpectedly high frequency in the general population, as was the case for 625GÆA, together conferring susceptibility to ethylmalonic aciduria. *Hum Mol Genet* 1998;7:619–627.

Matern D, Hart P, Murtha A, et al. Acute fatty liver of pregnancy associated with short-chain acyl-coenzyme A dehydrogenase deficiency. *J Pediatr* 2001;xx:585–588.

RESOURCES

58, 158, 354, 382

17 Very-Long-Chain Acyl-CoA Dehydrogenase Deficiency

Simon Eaton, PhD

DEFINITION: Very-long-chain acyl-CoA dehydrogenase (VLCAD) deficiency is a disorder affecting oxidation of fatty acids. Inability to use fats as a fuel results in muscle pains, heart problems, and low blood glucose due to overdependence on carbohydrates. The disorder is very severe in newborns and milder in children and adults.

DIFFERENTIAL DIAGNOSIS: Carnitine palmitoyl transferase II deficiency; Short-chain acyl-CoA dehydrogenase deficiency; Systemic carnitine deficiency; Carnitine-acyl-carnitine translocase deficiency; Long-chain 3-hydroxy-acyl-CoA dehydrogenase deficiency.

SYMPTOMS AND SIGNS: In neonates and infants, signs include metabolic crises/coma due to low blood glucose levels, especially precipitated by illness/fasting, congestive heart failure and cardiac arrest, hypotonia, and hepatic dysfunction. In older children and adults, signs include rhabdomyolysis induced by fasting or physical exercise, leading to myoglobinuria.

ETIOLOGY/EPIDEMIOLOGY: The disease is caused by lack of an enzyme involved in the use of fatty acids as a fuel. This results in very low blood glucose levels and problems in tissues that use fat as a preferred fuel (e.g., muscle, the heart). Epidemiology is not known but many different mutations in the *VLCAD* gene have been described. There is no particularly common mutation, so it is difficult to estimate prevalence in the general population.

DIAGNOSIS: The diagnostic tests are those of fatty acid oxidation disorders, i.e., measurement of nonesterified fatty acids, ketone bodies, glucose in plasma, and dicarboxylic acids in urine. The method of choice for diagnosis is acyl-carnitine analysis of blood spots, enabling differential diagnosis with other fatty acid oxidation disorders.

TREATMENT

Standard Therapies: As with all fatty acid oxidation disorders, avoidance of fasting, especially during illness, is essential. During an episode, intravenous 10% glucose should be given. A low-fat diet enriched in medium-chain fatty acids and uncooked cornstarch at night (to release carbohydrates slowly throughout the night) is also recommended. Carnitine has been given, but can cause accumulation of acyl-carnitine esters.

REFERENCES

Andresen BS, Olpin S, Poorthuis BJHM, et al. Clear correlation of genotype with disease phenotype in very-long-chain acyl-CoA dehydrogenase deficiency. *Am J Hum Genet* 1999;64:479–494.

Mathur A, Sims HF, Gopalakrishnan D, et al. Molecular heterogeneity in very-long-chain acyl-CoA dehydrogenase defi-ciency causing pediatric cardiomyopathy and sudden death. *Circulation* 1999;99:1337–1343.

Saudubray JM, Martin D, Delonlay P, et al. Recognition and management of fatty acid oxidation defects: a series of 107 patients. *J Inherit Metab Dis* 1999;22:488–502.

Wanders RJA, Vreken P, denBoer MEJ, et al. Disorders of mitochondrial fatty acyl-CoA beta-oxidation. *J Inherit Metab Dis* 1999;22:442–487.

RESOURCES

58, 158, 354, 382

---

18   Familial Dysbetalipoproteinemia

Pierre N.M. Demacker, PhD, and Anton F.H. Stalenhoef, MD, PhD

DEFINITION: Familial dysbetalipoproteinemia (FD) is an inherited disease of the lipoprotein metabolism characterized by increased levels of plasma lipids due to accumulation of β very-low-density lipoproteins (β-VLDL).

SYNONYMS: Type III hyperlipoproteinemia; Remnant removal disease.

DIFFERENTIAL DIAGNOSIS: Combined hyperlipidemia.

SYMPTOMS AND SIGNS: Plasma of these patients usually is yellow colored, not clear, and has some fluorescence. Yellow deposits in the creases of the palms are also typically seen, as are tuberoeruptive xanthomas of the elbows and tuberous xanthomas of the digits. Further clinical findings include both peripheral vascular and coronary artery disease. This syndrome presents together with other metabolic disorders such as glucose intolerance and obesity.

ETIOLOGY/EPIDEMIOLOGY: Familial dysbetalipoproteinemia is usually inherited as a recessive disorder with the apo E-2 as the mutant apolipoprotein that differs from the wild-type apo E (apo E-3) by a single amino acid substitution (arginine is exchanged by cysteine). In most patients with isolated apo E-2 homozygosity (approximately 98%), no hyperlipidemia is present. Full expression of FD requires overproduction of VLDL by additional genetic and environmental factors, including weight, hypothyroidism, diabetes, increased age, and low-estrogen conditions. If these secondary factors are predominant, typically increased β-VLDL concentrations can already be observed in heterozygotes for the apo E-2 genotype (E-4/2 and E-3/2).

The disorder is usually expressed in men in early adulthood, in women after menopause. The prevalence of the homozygous apo E-2/2 fenotype varies between 0.7% and 3% in different populations throughout the world; of these, approximately 2% of patients acquire hyperlipidemic FD. Its frequency in the population is approximately 1 in 5,000.

DIAGNOSIS: A strong relationship exists between plasma lipids and body weight variation or diet composition in the preceding days. A presumptive diagnosis is made by demonstrating fasting hyperlipidemia in combination with a VLDL-chol to plasma triglyceride ratio greater than 0.69 (on a mM base) or broad β-lipoprotein on electrophoresis. A definitive diagnosis can be established by documenting the E-2/2 pattern of apo E on isoelectric focusing or by genotyping.

TREATMENT

Standard Therapies: Treatment should be started immediately after definitive diagnosis to avoid further clinical complaints. The standard therapy is weight reduction by an isocaloric diet and increased exercise. In most cases, plasma lipids then approach normal limits. Further decrease of plasma lipids can be attained by treatment with a fibrate or a statin.

REFERENCE

Mahley RW, Rall SC Jr. Type III hyperlipoproteinemia (dysbetalipoproteinemia): the role of apolipoprotein E in normal and abnormal lipoprotein metabolism. In: Scriver CR, Beaudet AL, Sly WS, et al., eds. *The metabolic base of inherited disease*. Vol 2. New York: McGraw-Hill, 1995:1953–1973.

RESOURCES

35, 309, 357

19 Erdheim-Chester Disease

Robert D. Shamburek, MD

DEFINITION: Erdheim-Chester disease (ECD) is a rare non-Langerhans cell histiocytic disorder of unknown cause characterized by heterogeneous systemic manifestations that usually affects adults. It is microscopically characterized by lipid-laden foamy macrophages, chronic inflammatory cells, and varying degrees of fibrosis.

SYNONYMS: Lipogranulomatosis; Lipoid granulomatosis.

DIFFERENTIAL DIAGNOSIS: Langerhans cell histiocytosis; Gaucher disease; Niemann-Pick disease; Acute monocytic leukemia; Histiocytic lymphoma; Malignant histiocytosis; Paget disease; Sarcoidosis.

SYMPTOMS AND SIGNS: The clinical spectrum of Erdheim-Chester disease ranges from asymptomatic tissue infiltration to fulminant multiorgan failure. Clinical manifestations vary considerably and depend on the location and degree of histiocytic infiltration. Clinical features most frequently include lower extremity bone pain, xanthelasma and periorbital xanthomata, exophthalmos, and diabetes insipidus. Other sites of involvement include bone, skin, retroorbital, lung, central nervous system, pituitary gland, retroperitoneum, and pericardium. Almost two thirds of patients are symptomatic at diagnosis. Bone pain in the knees, shins, and ankles is the most common presenting complaint. Constitutional symptoms include weakness and weight loss. Polyuria and polydipsia can be profound in cases with primary diabetes insipidus. Retroorbital infiltrates result in exophthalmos, leading to visual impairment and potentially loss of vision. Dyspnea is an early symptom of diffuse interstitial lung diseases. Neurologic symptoms are less frequent but include gait disturbance and seizure caused by xanthogranulomatous infiltrate of the meninges, brainstem, and cerebellum. Hydronephrosis leading to renal failure occurs occasionally due to retroperitoneal and ureteral involvement. Despite the presence of cutaneous xanthoma, plasma lipids are usually normal.

ETIOLOGY/EPIDEMIOLOGY: Erdheim-Chester disease is believed to be a noninherited disorder of middle-aged patients, with a slight male preponderance. The clinical course is characterized by a slow progressive multiorgan dysfunction determined by the location and extent of involvement. More than half of patients die within 2–3 years after diagnosis, mainly due to renal, pulmonary, and cardiac failure. Spontaneous resolution can occur, but the natural history of ECD is poorly understood.

DIAGNOSIS: Definitive diagnostic criteria have not been established, but clinical, radiologic, and pathologic findings are helpful in establishing a diagnosis. Symmetric long bone pain with associated osteosclerotic lesions, xanthomata around the eyelids, exophthalmos, and/or diabetes insipidus are suggestive of the disease. The diagnosis is confirmed by tissue biopsies that contain histiocytes with non-Langerhans cell features. Sites to biopsy typically include the most accessible such as the tibia, xanthomata, lung, and retroperitoneal tissue. Plain radiography is most helpful in the diagnosis and classically shows symmetric sclerotic and lytic lesions of the metaphyses and diaphyses with sparing of the epiphyses. The long bones of the legs and arms are typically involved, with the axial skeleton spared except for the mandible. The distal femur and proximal tibia are the most frequently affected sites. Bone scintigraphy complements plain radiography, often showing other subclinical sites. CT and MRI scans are useful in defining central nervous system, ocular, pulmonary, abdominal/retroperitoneal, and bony lesions.

TREATMENT

Standard Therapies: No effective treatments are proven. Systemic corticosteroids, azathioprine, cyclosporine, interferon-α2a, chemotherapy, and radiation therapy have been used with disappointing results. Diabetes insipidus responds well to therapy with vasopressin. Renal stents and percutaneous nephrostomy have been used to preserve renal function. Palliative surgical debulking procedures have been tried on ocular and retroperitoneal lesions.

REFERENCES

Shamburek RD, Brewer HB Jr, Gochuico BR. Erdheim-Chester disease: a rare multisystem histiocytic disorder associated with interstitial lung disease. *Am J Med Sci* 2001;321:66–75.

Veyssier-Belot C, Cacoub P, Caparros-Lefebvre D, et al. Erdheim-Chester disease: clinical and radiologic characteristics of 59 cases. *Medicine* 1996;75:157–169.

RESOURCES

138, 351, 368

20   Fabry Disease

Robert J. Desnick, MD, PhD

DEFINITION: Fabry disease is an inborn error of glycosphingolipid catabolism caused by deficient activity of the lysosomal enzyme, α-galactosidase A (α-Gal A), resulting in the progressive accumulation of globotriaosylceramide (GL-3) and related glycosphingolipids in the plasma and tissue lysosomes throughout the body.

SYNONYMS: Anderson-Fabry disease; Angiokeratoma corporis diffusum universale; Hereditary dystopic lipidosis; GLA deficiency; Ceramide trihexosidase deficiency.

DIFFERENTIAL DIAGNOSIS: Fucosidosis; Sialidosis; Adult-type α-galactosidase deficiency; Aspartylglucosaminuria; Adult-onset α-galactosidase B deficiency; α-mannosidase deficiency; Rheumatoid arthritis; Erythromelalgia; Raynaud syndrome.

SYMPTOMS AND SIGNS: Fabry disease has a classic form and a cardiac variant. The classic phenotype is most common; however, the milder cardiac variant, which presents later in life and primarily affects the cardiovascular system, might be underdiagnosed. In classically affected males who have essentially no α-Gal A activity, clinical onset usually occurs in childhood or adolescence with periodic crises of severe pain in the extremities that are usually triggered by exercise, fatigue, emotional stress, or rapid changes in temperature and humidity; the appearance of vascular cutaneous lesions; hypohidrosis; and characteristic corneal and lenticular opacities. With advancing age, progressive GL-3 accumulation in the microvasculature leads to renal failure, cardiac involvement, and cerebrovascular disease. Classically affected males also may have gastrointestinal, auditory, pulmonary, and other manifestations. Males affected with the cardiac variant phenotype are essentially asymptomatic during most of their lives. They may have cardiomegaly, typically involving the left ventricular wall and interventricular septum, and electrocardiographic abnormalities consistent with a cardiomyopathy. They also have mild to moderate proteinuria, but do not develop renal failure.

ETIOLOGY/EPIDEMIOLOGY: Fabry disease is inherited as an X-linked recessive trait, and is due to mutations in the α-Gal A gene, located at Xq22.1. The incidence is approximately 1 in 40,000 males; it has been reported in patients from most ethnic, racial, and demographic groups.

DIAGNOSIS: Fabry disease should be considered in males and females who report periodic crises of acroparesthesias, angiokeratomas, hypohidrosis, characteristic corneal and lenticular opacities, strokes, or renal insufficiency of unknown etiology. The most reliable method for the diagnosis of affected males is the determination of α-Gal A activity in plasma and/or isolated leukocytes. Affected males with classical Fabry disease will have essentially no α-Gal A activity, whereas those with cardiac variants have residual activity (<10% of normal). Molecular genetic testing and the identification of a mutation in a male's α-Gal A gene provides additional confirmation of the diagnosis. Demonstration of significantly decreased α-Gal A activity in plasma and/or isolated leukocytes is diagnostic in females.

TREATMENT
Standard Therapies: Prophylactic administration of low maintenance dosages of diphenylhydantoin or carbamazepine provides pain relief by reducing the frequency and severity of the periodic crises of pain and constant discomfort. Treatment of the cardiac, pulmonary, and cerebrovascular manifestations is nonspecific and symptomatic. Because renal insufficiency is the most frequent and serious complication in classically affected patients, chronic hemodialysis and/or renal transplantation can be live-saving procedures.

Investigational Therapies: Enzyme replacement with α-Gal A is being investigated.

REFERENCES
Desnick RJ, Ioannou YA, Eng CM. α-galactosidase A deficiency: Fabry disease. In: Scriver CR, Beaudet AL, Sly WS, et al., eds. *The metabolic and molecular bases of inherited diseases*, 8th ed. New York: McGraw-Hill, 2001:3733–3774.

Eng CM, Banikazemi M, Gordon R, et al. A phase 1/2 clinical trial of enzyme replacement in Fabry disease: pharmacokinetic, substrate clearance, and safety studies. *Am J Hum Genet* 2001;68:711–722.

Eng CM, Guffon N, Wilcox WR, et al. Safety and efficacy of recombinant human a-galactosidase A replacement therapy in Fabry disease. *N Engl J Med* 2001;345:9–16.

von Scheidt W, Eng CM, Fitzmaurice TF, et al. An atypical variant of Fabry's disease with manifestations confined to the myocardium. *N Engl J Med* 1991;324:395.

RESOURCES
58, 148, 314

21 Farber Disease

Hugo Moser, MD

DEFINITION: Farber disease is an inborn error of metabolism caused by a deficiency of the lysosomal enzyme acid ceramidase. This leads to the accumulation of ceramide and is associated with characteristic symptoms and progressive tissue damage, particularly in the joints, liver, lung, and nervous system.

SYNONYMS: Farber lipogranulomatosis; Acid ceramidase deficiency.

DIFFERENTIAL DIAGNOSIS: Juvenile rheumatoid arthritis; Sarcoidosis; Multicentric reticulohistiocytosis; Neuronal storage diseases, such as GM gangliosidosis and Tay-Sachs disease.

SYMPTOMS AND SIGNS: The most common phenotype has features that are so characteristic diagnosis can be made at a glance. These include painful swelling of the joints, particularly the interphalangeal, metacarpal, ankle, wrist, knee, and elbow; palpable subcutaneous nodules in relation to the affected joints and over pressure points; and a hoarse cry that may progress to aphonia. Symptoms usually first appear between ages 2 weeks and 4 months. Other features are poor weight gain, intermittent fever, and respiratory difficulties. The disease is progressive and often leads to death in 2–3 years. Liver and spleen often are moderately enlarged, and there may be moderate lymphadenopathy. Nervous system involvement includes hypotonia and muscular atrophy, psychomotor retardation, seizures, and impaired vision. Eye examination may show a diffuse grayish opacification of the retina with a cherry red center. Less frequent neonatal, juvenile, and adult forms of the disease have also been described.

ETIOLOGY/EPIDEMIOLOGY: The disease is inherited in an autosomal-recessive manner. The basic abnormality is the deficiency of the enzyme acid ceramidase. The gene that codes for this enzyme is located on chromosome 8. Eleven mutations in the gene have been identified. The enzyme defect leads to an accumulation of ceramide within the lysosome, which leads to an inflammatory reaction particularly in the joints and subcutaneous tissues and damages the larynx, lung, and heart valves. Ceramide also accumulates in the nerve cells, which damages the function of peripheral nerves and may cause seizures and progressive loss of psychomotor function. Approximately 100 patients have been described among all ethnic groups.

DIAGNOSIS: Diagnosis in patients with the classic phenotype can be made on the basis of clinical findings and is confirmed by the demonstration of acid ceramidase deficiency in white blood cells or cultured skin fibroblasts. Prenatal diagnosis is achieved by demonstrating acid ceramidase deficiency in cultured amniocytes or chorion villus cells. Carriers show reduced enzyme activity, but mutation analysis is the most reliable method for the identification of heterozygous carriers. Although the diagnosis in patients with the classic phenotype can be made relatively easily, it is frequently missed in patients with milder phenotypes, in whom subcutaneous nodules may not be prominent.

TREATMENT
Standard Therapies: Therapy is supportive, with emphasis on maintenance of joint mobility, prevention of contractures, and relief of pain and inflammatory response. Laryngeal involvement may require tracheostomy. Great care has to be taken to avoid pulmonary aspiration.

Investigational Therapies: Bone marrow transplantation is being investigated.

REFERENCES
Bar J, Linke T, Ferlinz K, et al. Molecular analysis of acid ceramidase deficiency in patients with Farber disease. *Hum Mutat* 2001;17:199–209.
Chatelut M, Feunteun J, Harzer K, et al. A simple method for screening for Farber disease on cultured skin fibroblasts. *Clin Chim Acta* 1996;245:61–71.
Li C-M, Park J-H, He X, et al. The human acid ceramidase gene (ASAH): structure, chromosomal location, mutation analysis and expression. *Genomics* 1999;62:223–231.
Moser HW, Linke T, Fensom AH, et al. Acid ceramidase deficiency: Farber lipogranulomatosis. In: Scriver CR, Beaudet AL, Sly WS, et al., eds. *The metabolic and molecular bases of inherited disease*, 8th ed. New York: McGraw-Hill, 2001: 3573–3588.
Yeager AM, Armfield Uhas K, Coles CD, et al. Bone marrow transplantation for infantile ceramide deficiency. *Bone Marrow Transplant* 2000;26:357–363.

RESOURCES
58, 109, 351

22   Hereditary Fructose Intolerance

Neil R. M. Buist, MB, ChB,
and Susan C. Winter, MD, FAAP, FCMG

DEFINITION: Hereditary fructose intolerance is an inherited disorder of carbohydrate metabolism associated with liver and kidney damage, due to a deficiency of the enzyme fructose-1-phosphate aldolase.

SYNONYMS: Fructosemia; Fructose-1-phosphate aldolase deficiency; Fructose-1,6-bisphosphate aldolase b deficiency; Aldolase b deficiency; Aldob deficiency; Aldolase b, fructose-bisphosphate.

DIFFERENTIAL DIAGNOSIS: Tyrosinemia; Galactosemia; Infectious hepatitis; Byler disease; Fructose 1,6-bisphosphatase deficiency.

SYMPTOMS AND SIGNS: Patients are asymptomatic until the first time they ingest fructose. Even 1–2 teaspoons of applesauce or juice provoke symptoms, which start with vomiting or food refusal and are followed rapidly by symptomatic hypoglycemia that may provoke seizures or even brain damage. These acute attacks occur with each exposure to fructose. Chronic consumption leads to failure to thrive, progressive liver damage, cirrhosis, or liver failure. Concomitant renal damage leads to generalized tubular dysfunction (the renal Fanconi syndrome). Symptoms rapidly disappear when fructose is strictly withdrawn and even major liver damage can totally reverse. The symptoms recur at any age; however, older patients develop a lifelong aversion to fruit and sweet tastes and so avoid most crises.

ETIOLOGY/EPIDEMIOLOGY: Fructosemia is inherited as an autosomal-recessive trait; incidence is 1 in 20,000 to 1 in 100,000. The enzyme defect is in the anaerobic catabolic pathway from glucose to pyruvate. The gene is located at 9q22.3. Fructose-1-phosphate is acutely toxic to liver and kidney cells and interferes with glucose homeostasis.

DIAGNOSIS: A history of acute episodes coinciding with initiating fructose ingestion is highly characteristic. Abnormal liver function tests including clotting factors, associated with food-induced hypoglycemia, together with the urine findings typical of the renal Fanconi syndrome are strong confirmatory findings. Provocative fructose challenges are dangerous. Enzyme assay must be performed on liver tissue. Mutation analysis of DNA can be informative, in which case prenatal diagnosis can be done.

TREATMENT
Standard Therapies: Standard treatment is immediate, rigid, and lifelong dietary exclusion of all sources of fructose. Symptoms dissipate within 1–2 days of starting the diet, and liver and kidney damage may totally resolve within a month. Liver transplantation would be curative but is not indicated except in cases of advanced liver failure.

REFERENCES
Ali M, Rellos P, Cox TM. Hereditary fructose intolerance. *J Med Genet* 1998;35:353–365.
McKusick VA, ed. Online Mendelian Inheritance in Man, OMIM [database online]. Bethesda, MD: National Center for Biotechnology Information, National Library of Medicine, 2000. MIM# 229600.
Scriver CR, Beaudet AL, Sly WS, et al., eds. *Metabolic and molecular basis of inherited disease*, 8th ed. New York: McGraw-Hill, 2001.

RESOURCES
109, 178, 354

23   Fructosuria

Neil R.M. Buist, MB, ChB,
and Susan C. Winter, MD, FAAP, FCMG

DEFINITION: Fructosuria is characterized by urinary excretion of fructose after ingestion, and is caused by a deficiency of the enzyme hepatic fructokinase.

SYNONYMS: Essential fructosuria; Hepatic fructokinase deficiency; Benign fructosuria; Levulosuria.

SYMPTOMS AND SIGNS: There are no symptoms or signs; the condition is benign.

ETIOLOGY/EPIDEMIOLOGY: Fructosuria is inherited as an autosomal-recessive trait localized on 2p23.3–2p23.2.

DIAGNOSIS: Fructose is a "reducing sugar" that gives an abnormal reaction when urine is tested with Clinitest (Ames). It does not react with glucose oxidase tests (such as Clinistix). Fructose can be identified by chromatography of urine.

TREATMENT
Standard Therapies: No treatment is required.

REFERENCES
McKusick VA, ed. Online Mendelian Inheritance in Man, OMIM [database online]. Bethesda, MD: National Center for Biotechnology Information, National Library of Medicine, 2000. MIM# 229800.
Scriver CR, Beaudet AL, Sly WS, et al., eds. *The metabolic and molecular bases of inherited disease,* 8th ed. New York: McGraw-Hill, 2000.

RESOURCES
109, 364

---

24   Fucosidosis

Gregory A. Grabowski, MD

DEFINITION: Fucosidosis is an inborn error of metabolism resulting from the deficiency of α-L-fucosidase, a lysosomal enzyme in the glycoprotein degradation pathway. Accumulation of α-fucosyl oligosaccharides and polypeptides in tissues and bodily fluids leads to mental retardation, neurologic deterioration, coarsening of the facies, growth retardation, skeletal disease, and other manifestations of the fucosidosis variants.

DIFFERENTIAL DIAGNOSIS: α- and β-mannosidosis; Aspartylglucosaminuria; Mucopolysaccharidosis types I H and II; Fabry disease.

SYMPTOMS AND SIGNS: The two major phenotypes are type I, a severe infantile form, and type II, a less severe later onset form. The differences between I and II are not distinct and may represent a continuum. In type I fucosidosis, psychomotor retardation, coarse facies, growth retardation, dysostosis multiplex, and neurologic deterioration occur within the first year of life. The presence of hepatosplenomegaly, seizures, enlargement of the heart, and propensity to infections is less characteristic. Sweat chloride concentration is increased. The less severe variant, type II, has onset of psychomotor retardation and the other findings of type I disease between ages 12 and 24 months and is more slowly progressive. These patients survive longer, have sweat chloride values that are closer to normal, and have distinctive skin lesions termed angiokeratoma. In addition, patients may have anhidrosis. Patients with type I fucosidosis die within the first few years of life, whereas those with type II can survive into the third and fourth decades. In both variants, the radiographic and clinical features of dysostosis multiplex are relatively mild, and the phenotype is dominated by progressive neurologic abnor-malities. These findings include spasticity, tremors, mental retardation, hypertonia, and occasionally dystonia.

ETIOLOGY/EPIDEMIOLOGY: Fucosidosis is inherited as an autosomal-recessive trait. The disease is caused by mutations in the α-L-fucosidase gene that maps to human chromosome 1p34. A pseudogene is present on chromosome 2q31-q32. Frequency estimates suggest an incidence of less than 1 in 200,000 live births. All ethnic groups are involved. Consanguinity in families with fucosidosis is high. A genetic isolate is present in Italy.

DIAGNOSIS: The diagnosis should be suspected if skeletal disease during the first year of life is accompanied by neurologic findings and mental retardation. The finding of angiokeratoma and anhidrosis in combination with neurologic deterioration in the first decade of life should prompt a workup. Vacuolated lymphocytes in the peripheral blood or bone marrow storage cells suggest a storage disease. Similar storage cells are found in several organs including the epithelial cells of sweat glands and endothelial cells of blood vessels. The diagnosis is directly established by the demonstration of the isolated deficiency of α-L-fucosidase in cells and bodily fluids. Additional confirmatory studies can be accomplished by mutation identification in the α-L-fucosidase gene, and the presence of fucosyl glycopeptides and oligosaccharides in bodily fluids.

TREATMENT
Standard Therapies: Treatment is generally palliative. Families identified at risk for fucosidosis type I should be provided with a variety of reproduction options.

Investigational Therapies: For later-onset fucosidosis, bone marrow transplantation with histocompatible bone marrow is being investigated.

REFERENCES
Galluzzi P, Rufa A, Balestri P, et al. MR brain imaging of fucosidosis type I. *Am J Neuroradiol* 2001;22:777–780.

Miano M, Lanino E, Gatti R, et al. Four-year follow-up of a case of fucosidosis treated with unrelated donor bone marrow transplantation. *Bone Marrow Transplant* 2001;27:747–751.

Thomas GH. Disorders of glycoprotein degradation: α-mannosidosis, β-mannosidosis, fucosidosis, and sialidosis. In: Scriver CR, Beaudet A, Valle D, et al., eds. *The metabolic and molecular bases of inherited disease,* 8th ed. New York: McGraw-Hill, 2001:3507–3534.

Willems PJ, Gatti R, Darby JK, et al. Fucosidosis revisited: a review of 77 patients. *Am J Med Genet* 1991;38:111–131.

RESOURCES

58, 314, 368

---

25 Galactosemia

Gerard T. Berry, MD

DEFINITION: Hereditary galactosemia is an inborn error of metabolism due to deficiency of galactose-1-phosphate uridyltransferase (GALT), one of three enzymes in the galactose pathway. Galactose-1-phosphate accumulation results in damage to brain, liver, gastrointestinal, erythroid, and kidney tissues and could potentially lead to *Escherichia coli* sepsis and death.

SYNONYM: Transferase deficiency galactosemia.

DIFFERENTIAL DIAGNOSIS: ABO or Rh incompatibility with jaundice and hemolytic anemia; Neonatal hepatitis; Encephalitis.

SYMPTOMS AND SIGNS: With the advent of newborn screening for galactosemia, many patients are asymptomatic when diagnosed. The disease can be devastating even in the first 1 or 2 weeks of life because of *E. coli* sepsis. The most common initial clinical sign is poor growth. Vomiting and poor feeding also occur in most patients. Jaundice may be present in the first few weeks of life and persist. While on lactose, many infants with galactosemia present in the first 2–3 weeks with only poor feeding and growth, jaundice, and mild irritability or lethargy. With continual ingestion, a multiorgan toxicity syndrome ensues, associated with liver disease that may progress to cirrhosis with portal hypertension, splenomegaly, ascites, renal tubular dysfunction, sometimes the full-blown renal Fanconi syndrome, anemia primarily due to decreased red blood cell (RBC) survival, lethargy, and brain edema associated with a bulging fontanel. Cataracts may also occur. After initiation of a lactose-free diet in the newborn period, usually the problems related to liver and kidney disease, anemia, and brain edema disappear unless severe organ damage such as hepatic cirrhosis has occurred. Most infants begin to grow and develop at a normal rate. Even prospectively treated patients, however, may manifest long-term complications such as speech defects, delays in language acquisition, learning problems, and, in most females, hypergonadotropic hypogonadism.

ETIOLOGY/EPIDEMIOLOGY: Galactosemia is inherited in an autosomal-recessive manner. The disease is due to a mutation in the *GALT* gene, which is located on chromosome 9p13. The prevalence is estimated at 1 in 35,000 to 1 in 60,000. All ethnic groups are affected, with increased frequency in individuals of northern European ancestry.

DIAGNOSIS: The deficiency of the enzyme GALT may be detected in RBCs in patients with the most common forms of galactosemia. Newborn screening programs in various states use either an enzymatic and/or a metabolite screening method. When metabolites are assayed, the level of galactose-1-phosphate or total galactose and galactose-1-phosphate in RBCs are usually measured. Most of the gene defects that produce galactosemia are known; therefore, some patients or siblings may be screened for the disease or for being a carrier by genotype analyses.

TREATMENT

Standard Therapies: Standard therapy is a lactose-restricted diet, which is life-long.

REFERENCES
Berry GT, Nissim I, Lin Z, et al. Endogenous synthesis of galactose in normal man and patients with hereditary galactosemia. *Lancet* 1995; 346:1073–1074.

Berry GT, Singh RH, Mazur AT, et al. Galactose breath testing distinguishes variant and severe galactose-1-phosphate uridyltransferase genotypes. *Pediatr Res* 2000;48:323–328.

Elsas LJ, Lai K. The molecular biology of galactosemia [Review]. *Genet Med* 1998;1:40–48.

Holton JB, Walter JH, Tyfield LA. Galactosemia. In: Scriver CR, Beaudet AL, Sly WS, et al., eds. *The metabolic and molecular bases of inherited disease,* 8th ed. Vol. 1. New York: McGraw-Hill, 2001.

Tyfield L, Reichardt J, Fridovich-Keil J, et al. Classical galactosaemia and mutations at the galactose-1-phosphate uridyl transferase (GALT) gene [Review]. *Hum Mutat* 1999;13:417–430.

RESOURCES

98, 166, 354

26 Gaucher Disease

Roscoe O. Brady, MD

DEFINITION: Gaucher disease is caused by a deficiency of the enzyme glucocerebrosidase, resulting in the accumulation of toxic quantities of the glycolipid glucocerebroside throughout the body. In a few patients, this lipid also accumulates in the brain.

SYNONYM: Sphingolipidosis 1.

DIFFERENTIAL DIAGNOSIS: Niemann-Pick disease; Pompe disease; Hurler disease.

SYMPTOMS AND SIGNS: Virtually all patients have hematologic abnormalities consisting of anemia, thrombocytopenia, and leukopenia. The spleen and liver are often enlarged, and skeletal damage that causes deformities and easy fractures of bones such as hips and vertebrae is frequently observed. Most patients have no brain involvement and are classified as having type 1 Gaucher disease. A few patients (type 2) have early onset of organomegaly along with severe brain damage and early death. Patients with type 3 have neurologic problems that begin in childhood such as difficulty in moving their eyes in the horizontal plane, and some of these also have progressive myoclonic epilepsy.

ETIOLOGY/EPIDEMIOLOGY: Gaucher disease is the most prevalent hereditary metabolic storage disorder. It is an autosomal-recessive disorder occurring with equal frequency in both sexes. It is caused by mutations in the glucocerebrosidase gene that is located on chromosome 1. It is the most common genetic disorder of persons of Ashkenazic Jewish descent, the incidence among whom may be as high as 1 in 800 births. There are approximately 7,500 patients with Gaucher disease in the United States.

DIAGNOSIS: Gaucher disease should be suspected in patients with unexplained anemia and easy bruising, particularly if they have enlargement of the spleen and liver and fractures. The diagnosis can be confirmed by measuring acid beta-glucosidase activity in homogenates of white blood cells or cultured skin fibroblasts. Additional laboratory abnormalities include elevation of acid phosphatase, angiotensin-converting enzyme, and chitotriosidase in the serum.

TREATMENT

Standard Therapies: Enzyme replacement therapy (ERT) is effective for patients with type 1 disease (Insert Fig. 47). Anemia and thrombocytopenia are improved; hepatosplenomegaly is greatly reduced, and the skeletal damage is ameliorated. These systemic manifestations also improve with ERT in patients with type 2 and type 3 disease. The effect of ERT on the horizontal eye movements in patients with type 3 disease is variable, and no improvement occurs in myoclonic seizures. It does not reverse the brain damage in patients with type 2 disease.

Investigational Therapies: Bone marrow transplantation (BMT) can cure patients with type 1 disease. Because of the effectiveness of enzyme replacement therapy, BMT is rarely performed. Compounds that block the formation of glucocerebroside (substrate depletion) are being explored for use in conjunction with ERT. Gene therapy is also being explored.

REFERENCES

Barton NW, Brady RO, Dambrosia JM, et al. Replacement therapy for inherited enzyme deficiency—macrophage-targeted glucocerebrosidase for Gaucher's disease. *N Engl J Med* 1991; 324:1464–1470.

Brady RO, Kanfer JN, Shapiro D. Metabolism of glucocerebrosides. II. Evidence of an enzymatic deficiency in Gaucher's disease. *Biochem Biophys Res Commun* 1965;18:221–225.

Grabowski GA, Barton NW, Pastores G, et al. Enzyme therapy in Gaucher disease Type 1: comparative efficacy of mannose-terminated glucocerebrosidase from natural and recombinant sources. *Ann Intern Med* 1995;122:33–39.

Kampine JP, Brady RO, Kanfer JN, et al. The diagnosis of Gaucher's disease and Niemann-Pick disease using small samples of venous blood. *Science* 1967;155:86–88.

Schneider EL, Ellis WG, Brady RO, et al. Infantile (Type II) Gaucher's disease: *in utero* diagnosis and fetal pathology. *J Pediatr* 1972;81:1134–1139.

RESOURCES

300, 368, 462

27   Glut-1 Deficiency Syndrome

Juan Pascual, MD, PhD,
Kris Engelstad, BS,
and Darryl C. De Vivo, MD

DEFINITION: Glut-1 deficiency syndrome (Glut1-DS) is an inborn disorder of metabolism that results in impaired neurologic development (cognitive and motor), along with epilepsy that can be resistant to anticonvulsant drugs.

SYNONYMS: Glucose transporter defect; Glucose transporter protein syndrome (GTPS); De Vivo disease.

DIFFERENTIAL DIAGNOSIS: Other (non–Glut1-DS) forms of neonatal convulsions; Medically refractory epilepsy; Hypoglycemic encephalopathy; Opsoclonus-myoclonus; Spastic ataxia; Acquired microcephaly and hypoglycorrhachia (low cerebrospinal fluid [CSF] glucose).

SYMPTOMS AND SIGNS: Infants commonly develop symptoms before the sixth month of life, typically in the form of seizures or abnormal movements. These early manifestations are characterized by any of the following: unexplained apnea and cyanosis, forced eye or head deviation, head thrusts, opsoclonus-myoclonus, and other abnormal, brief, rapid, and forced repetitive limb movements. In older children, the seizures evolve into astatic, atypical absence and generalized tonic-clonic epilepsy. A variable degree of cognitive, verbal, and motor delay is observed in all patients, along with acquired microcephaly. Hypotonia, spasticity, slurring of speech, improvement with carbohydrate intake, and ataxia are frequently observed.

ETIOLOGY/EPIDEMIOLOGY: The syndrome may appear sporadically as the result of individual mutations or may be inherited in an autosomal-dominant fashion. It is transmissible from either parent and affects males and females with equal frequency. The disease is caused by insufficient glucose availability to the brain as a result of re-duced function of the glucose transporter type 1, due to a variety of different mutations in the glucose transporter type 1 gene, located on chromosome 1. The prevalence is unknown. The disease has no racial or geographic predilection.

DIAGNOSIS: The diagnosis is suspected when clinicians encounter early onset of seizures, poorly controlled epilepsy despite the trial of several medications, acquired microcephaly, and developmental delays not otherwise explained. Confirmatory diagnosis includes a CSF/blood glucose ratio of less than 0.35 (both samples must be drawn simultaneously), with absolute CSF glucose values of less than 40 mg/dL. CSF lactate is never elevated.

TREATMENT

Standard Therapies: A ketogenic diet has proven successful in the treatment of both infants and children. Ketones derived from the fat in the diet effectively replace glucose as the source of fuel for the brain. Seizure cessation is achieved in most cases, often without the use of antiepileptic medications. Improvement of other manifestations of the disease appears to be less satisfactory. Barbiturates (phenobarbital) and caffeine should be avoided, as they directly inhibit the transporter Glut-1.

REFERENCES

Brockmann, Wang D, Korenke CG, et al. Autosomal dominant Glut-1 deficiency syndrome and familial epilepsy. *Ann Neurol* 2001;50:476–485.

De Vivo DC, Trifiletti RR, Jacobson RI, et al. Defective glucose transport across the blood-brain barrier as a cause of persistent hypoglycorrhachia, seizures, and developmental delay. *N Engl J Med* 1991;325:703–709.

Seidner G, Alvarez MG, Yeh JI, et al. GLUT-1 deficiency syndrome caused by haploinsufficiency of the blood-brain barrier hexose carrier. *Nat Genet* 1998;18:188–191.

Wang D, Kranz-Eble P, De Vivo DC. Mutational analysis of *GLUT1* (*SLC2A1*) in Glut-1 deficiency syndrome. *Hum Mutat* 2000;16:224–231.

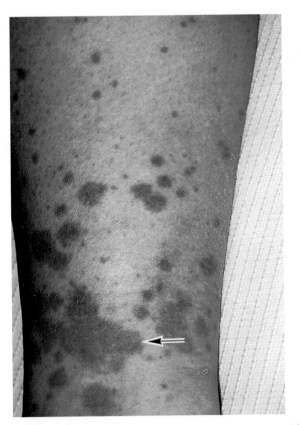

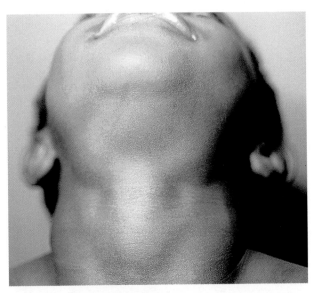

FIGURE 3 Bilateral enlargement of the submandibular glands.

FIGURE 1 The typical palpable purpura lesion in a patient with type II cryoglobulinemia. (Reprinted from Shakil AO, Di Bisceglie AM. *N Engl J Med* 1994; 331:1624; with permission.)

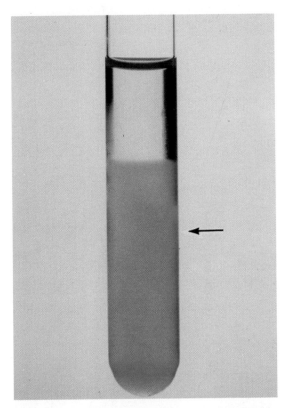

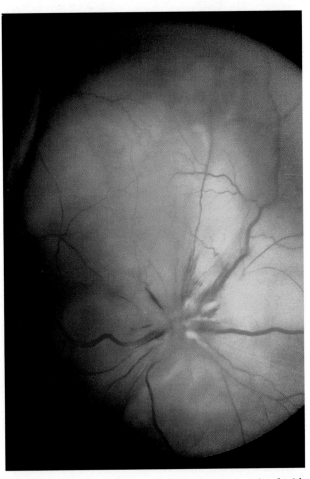

FIGURE 2 Serum of a patient with type II cryoglobulinemia after 48 hours at 4°C. Cryoglobulins are shown before centrifugation. (Reprinted from Shakil AO, Di Bisceglie AM. *N Engl J Med* 1994; 331:1624; with permission.)

FIGURE 4 Fundus showing retinal detachment associated with VKH syndrome.

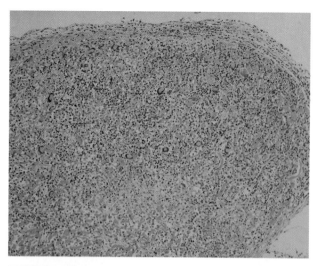

FIGURE 5 Idiopathic giant cell myocarditis. Multinucleated giant cells are seen interspersed with a diffuse inflammatory infiltrate and extensive myocyte necrosis (hematoxylin and eosin, original magnification ×25).

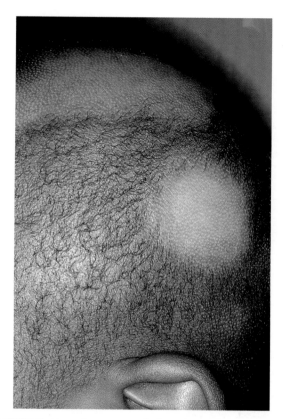

FIGURE 7 Alopecia areata and alopecia totalis are different extents of the same condition. Alopecia totalis involves the entire head. Alopecia universalis the whole body.

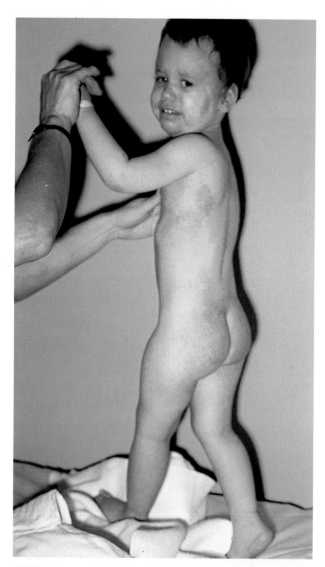

FIGURE 6 Acrodermatitis enteropathica is a congenital inability to absorb zinc.

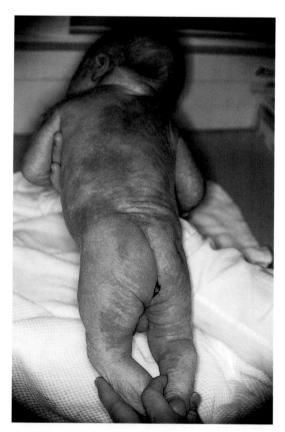

FIGURE 8 Congenital phlebectasia, a rare condition also known as cutis marmorata telangiectatica congenita.

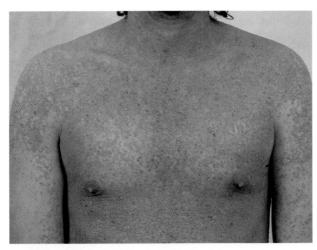

FIGURE 9 Patient with Darrier disease.

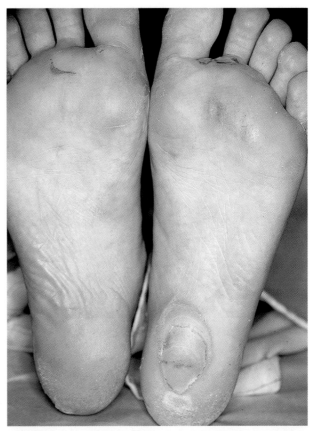

FIGURE 12 Weber-Cockayne is a type of epidermolysis bullosa simplex in which blisters appear late in the teenage years (recurrent epidermolysis bulosa of the hands and feet).

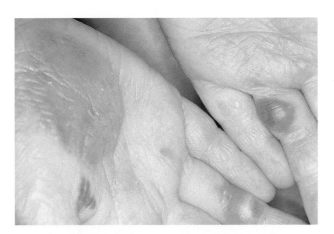

FIGURE 10 Epidermolysis bullosa dermolytic, recessive type (EBD-r) (sometimes called recessive epidermolysis bullose dystrophica, REBS, of Hallipeau).

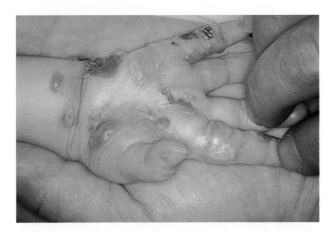

FIGURE 11 Epidermolysis bullosa of the Herlitz type (EB-Herlitz, blister within the d-e junction, otherwise knows as litalis).

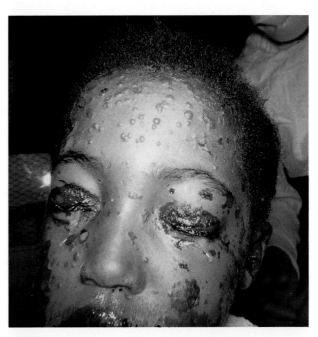

FIGURE 13 Erythema multiforme in a child, from live measles vaccine.

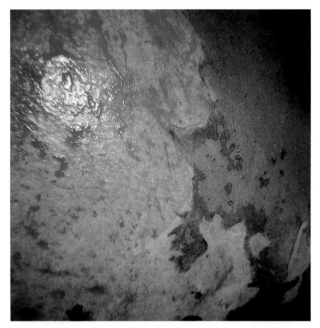

FIGURE 14 Toxic epidermal necrolysis.

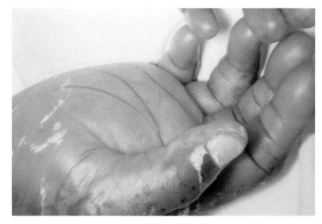

FIGURE 16 Erythema multiforme.

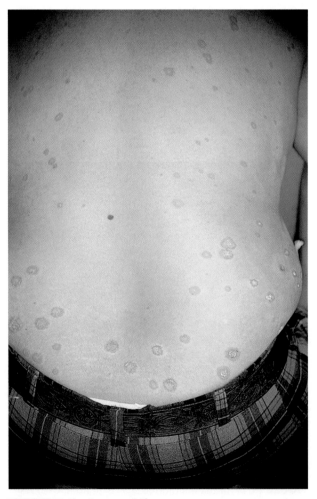

FIGURE 15 Erythema multiforme.

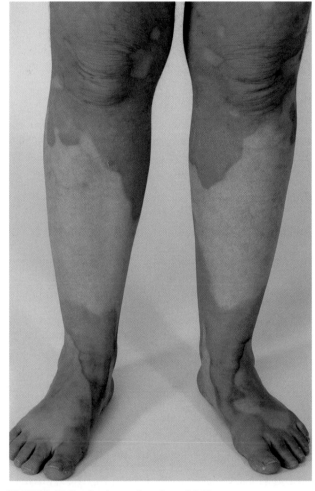

FIGURE 17 Erythrokeratodermia variabilis.

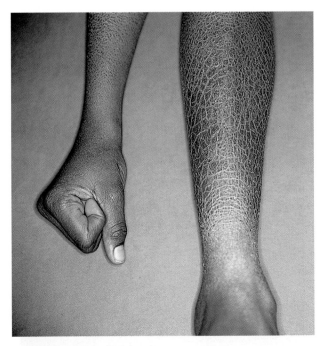

FIGURE 18 X-linked ichthyosis.

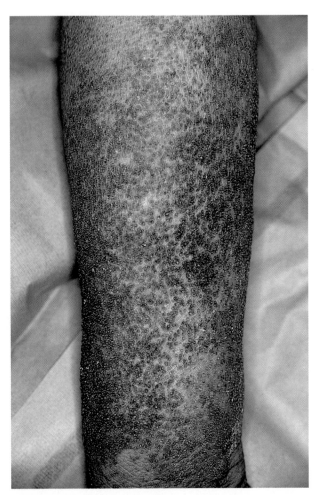

FIGURE 20 Ichthyosis and deafness is part of the KID (keratosis, ichthyosis, and deafness) syndrome.

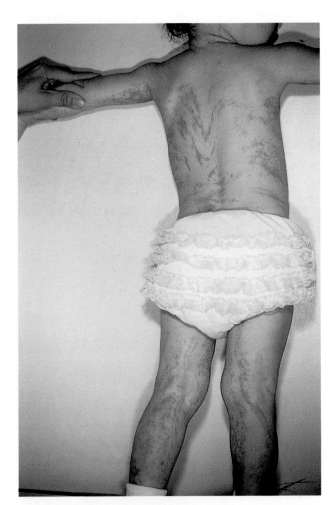

FIGURE 19 Incontinentia pigmenti.

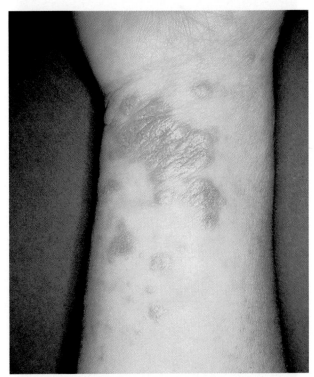

FIGURE 21 Lichen planus.

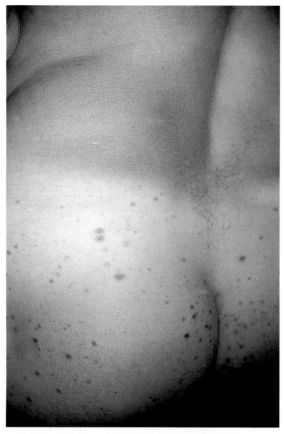

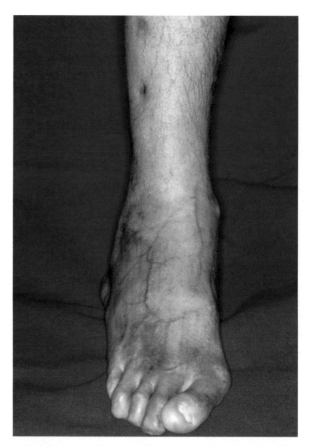

FIGURE 22 Pityriasis lichnoides et varioliformis acuta of Mucha and Haberman. The sun-exposed area is improved from the UV light.

FIGURE 24 Atrophic and wrinkled hyperpigmented skin on the right foot; the veins are shining through. Note onychodystrophy of the great toe and anonychia of the remaining toes.

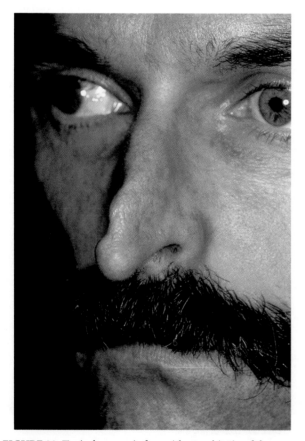

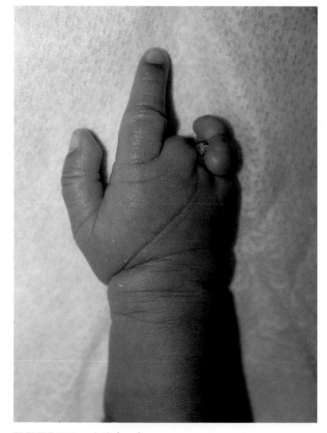

FIGURE 23 Typical acrogeric face with atrophic tip of the nose.

FIGURE 25 Amniotic bands.

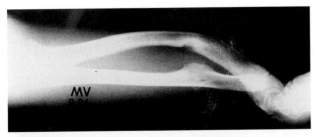

FIGURE 26 Anteroposterior radiograph of the forearm in a 14-year-old boy demonstrating a large distal ulna exostosis with shortening and radial bowing. The radial head is located but there is disruption of the normal alignment of the wrist.

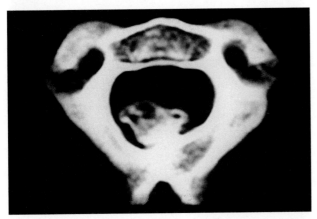

FIGURE 27 Computed tomography through the second cervical vertebrae demonstrating a large intraspinal exostosis in an 8-year old boy.

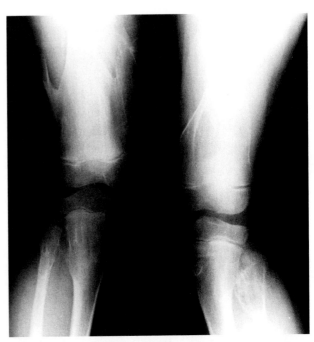

FIGURE 29 Standing anteroposterior radiograph of the knees in a 12-year-old boy. Observe the numerous exostoses and the genu valgum of the distal femur and proximal tibia, particularly on the left.

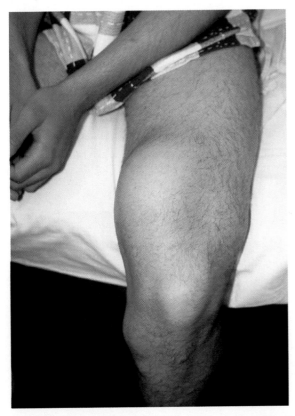

FIGURE 28 Clinical photograph of the left knee demonstrating a large exostosis involving the medial aspect of the distal femur. Smaller lesions can be seen about the proximal tibia.

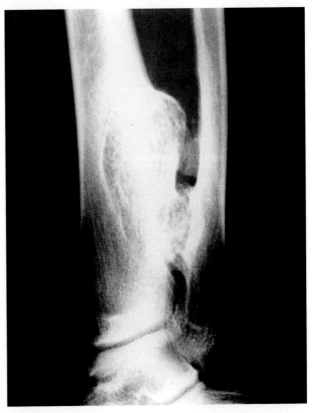

FIGURE 30 Radiograph of the right ankle demonstrating exostoses, bowing of the fibular, and valgus or lateral tilt to the ankle joint.

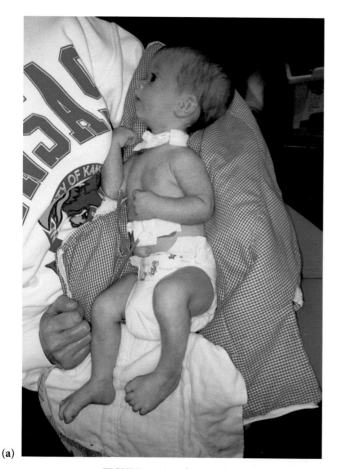

(a)

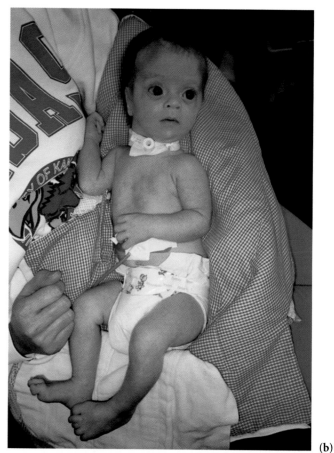

(b)

FIGURE 31 A and B: A male patient with Marshall-Smith syndrome at the age of 2 years and 3 months.

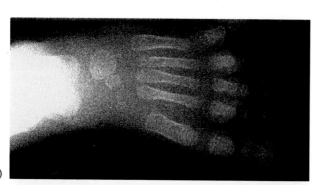

(a)

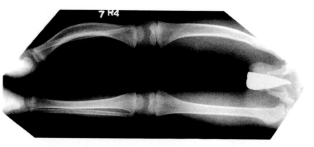

FIGURE 33 The ribs appear ribbon-like and somewhat twisted. The vertebral bodies are relatively tall. The pelvis is narrow with flared iliac wings.

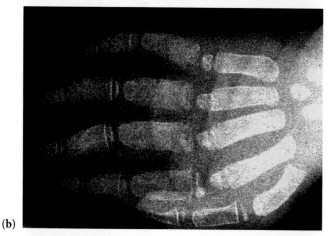

(b)

FIGURE 32 Hand (A) and foot radiographs (B) of a 1-month-old patient with Marshall-Smith syndrome showing advanced bone maturation.

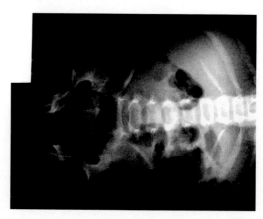

FIGURE 34 There is moderate to severe apex anterolateral bowing of the right tibia and mild apex lateral bowing of the right femur with flaring of the metaphysis.

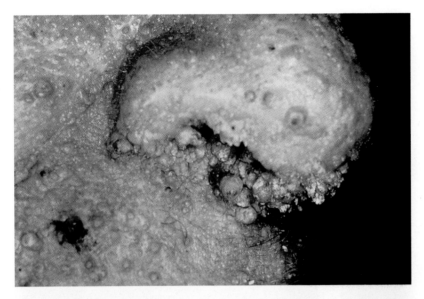

FIGURE 35 Cowden syndrome tumors (trichofolliculomas) associated with thyroid and breast tumors. First noted in Rachael Cowden, and in her progeny.

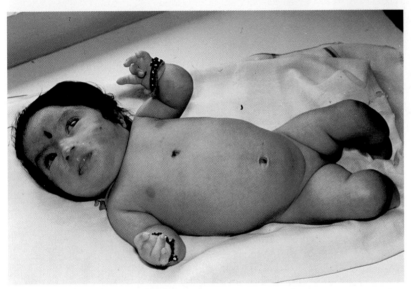

FIGURE 36 An infant at 1 month of age with Roberts syndrome. Note the rudimentary upper and lower limbs with short neck.

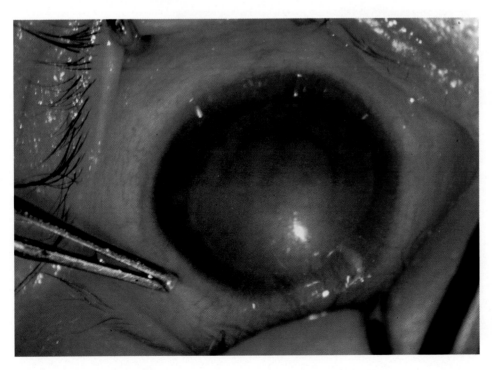

FIGURE 37 Right eye showing superficial corneal scar with vascularization.

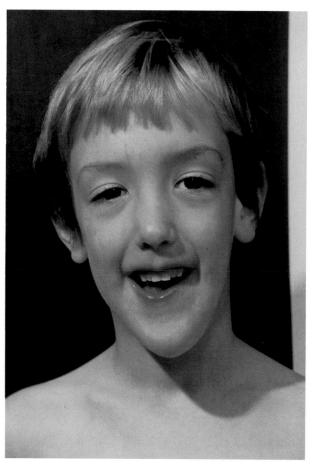

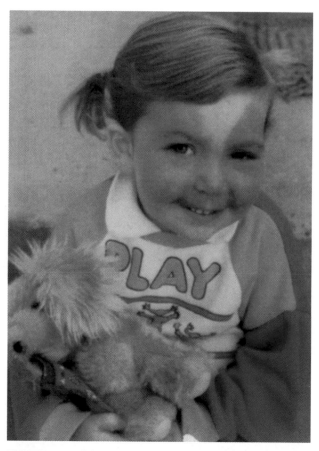

FIGURE 39 A child with Sturge-Weber syndrome.

FIGURE 38 A girl 4 years 8 months of age with Sotos syndrome. Height was 124 cm (height age 7 years 7 months) and weight was 35.2 kg (weight age 7 years 9 months). Bone age was 4 years 10 months. Note the characteristic features: large head, frontal bossing, hypertelorism, down-slanting of palpebral fissures, pointed chin, and large ears.

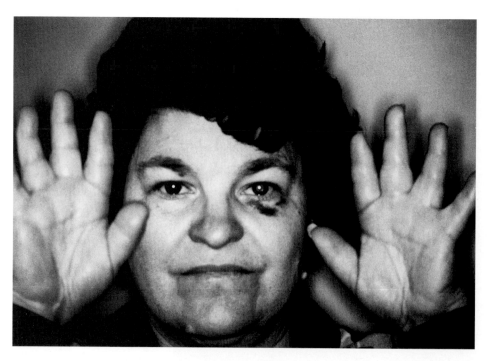

FIGURE 40 Patient with Weill-Marchesani syndrome.

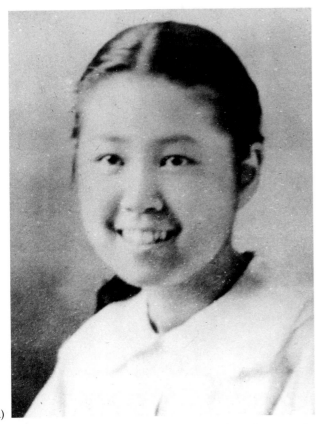

(a)

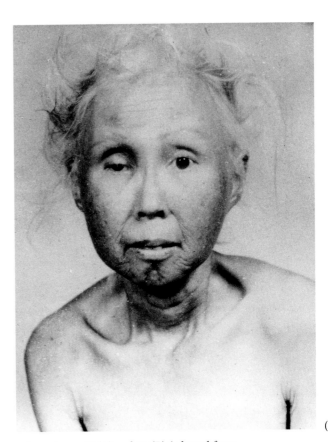

(b)

FIGURE 41 Japanese-American Werner syndrome patient at ages 15 (**A**) and 48 (**B**) (adapted from *Medicine* 1966;177:221; with permission).

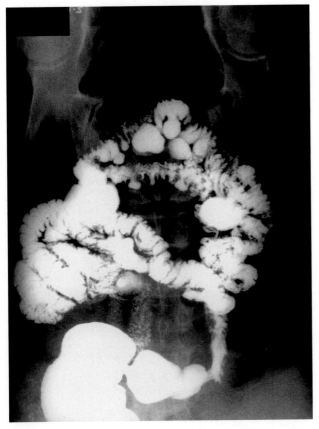

FIGURE 42 Barium study of the small bowel showing scattered diverticula.

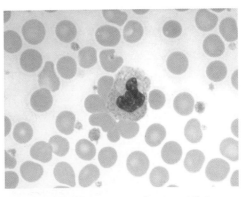

FIGURE 43 Red cell rosetting around neutrophils in paroxysmal cold hemoglobinuria.

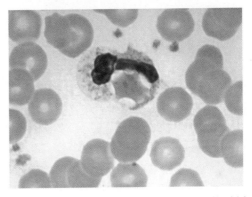

FIGURE 44 Erythrophagocytosis in paroxysmal cold hemoglobinuria.

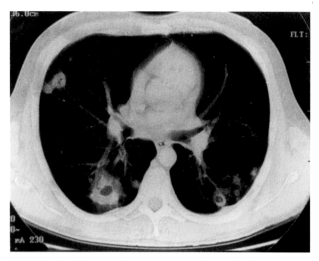

FIGURE 45 CT scan of the chest in a patient with Wegener granulomatosis. The scan reveals multiple pulmonary nodules, primarily in the periphery of both lungs. Many of the lesions are cavitary.

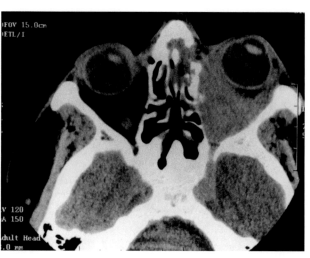

FIGURE 46 CT scan of the orbits in a patient with Wegener granulomatosis. The scan shows an orbital mass (pseudotumor) behind the left eye, causing mild proptosis and a substantial visual field defect.

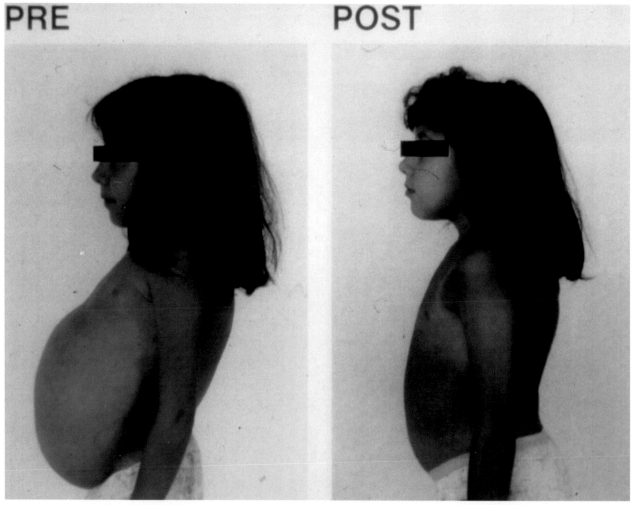

(a)

(b)

FIGURE 47 Reduction of hepatosplenomegaly in an eight year-old patient with Gaucher disease before (pre) and after 26 months (post) of enzyme replacement therapy.

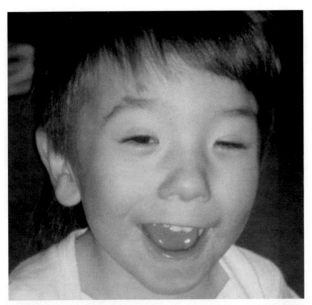

FIGURE 48 Infant with maternal phenylketonuria syndrome. Note the epicanthal folds, maxillary hipoplasia, flattened nasal bridge, upturned nose, elongated philtrum, thin upper lip, and micrognathia, indistinguishable from fetal alcohol syndrome.

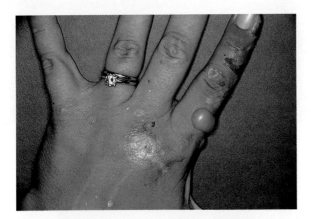

FIGURE 49 The hand of a patient with porphyria cutanea tarda.

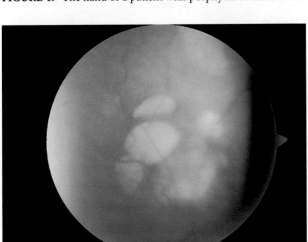

FIGURE 50 In a patient with Aicardi syndrome the chorioretinal lesions vary in size and may be unilateral or bilateral. Note white lacunae with minimal pigmentation at the borders. The lesions appear to cluster around the disc and decrease in size and number as one approaches the periphery of the fundus.

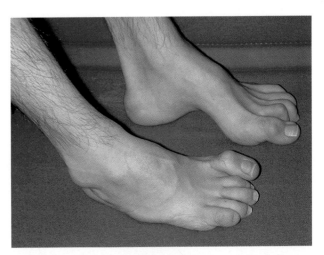

FIGURE 51 Feet of a patient with Charcot-Marie-Tooth disease.

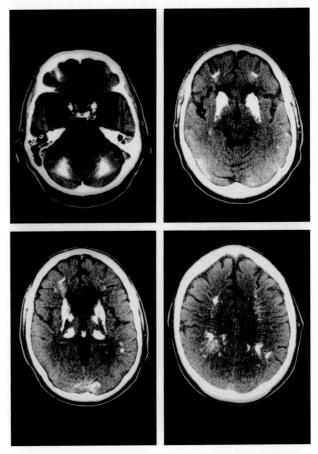

FIGURE 52 Noncontrast CT scan showing bilateral symmetric calcification involving basal ganglia, dentate nucleus, thalamus, and white matter in Fahr disease (bilateral striopallidodentate calcinosis). (Reprinted from *Parkinsonism Rel Disord* 2001;7:269–295; with permission.)

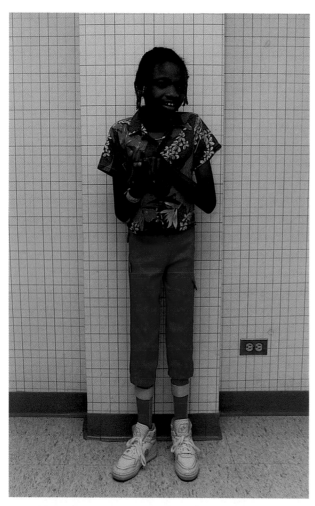

FIGURE 53 Patient with Rett syndrome.

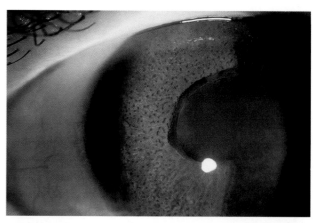

FIGURE 54 Cogan-Reese syndrome. Note pedunculated pigmented nodules on iris, atrophic stroma, and ectropion uveae.

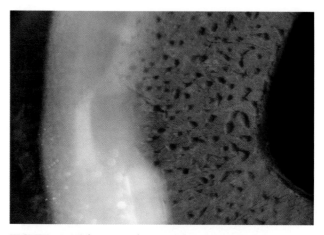

FIGURE 55 High power of iris nodules.

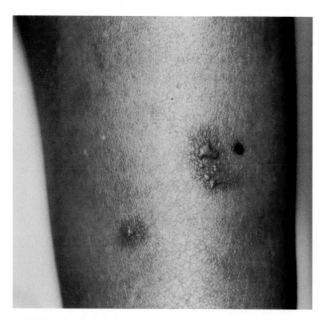

FIGURE 56 Cutaneous vasculitis in a patient with Churg-Strauss syndrome. The photograph shows purpuric macules with a bullous component. Biopsy revealed leukocytoclastic vasculitis with eosinophilic predominance, strongly consistent with Churg-Strauss syndrome. The patient also had asthma, glomerulonephritis, and digital ischemia.

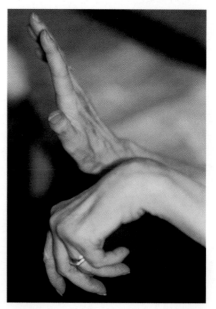

FIGURE 57 Vasculitis neuropathy related to Churg-Strauss syndrome. The photograph depicts a patient who has an inability to extend her left hand because of a left wrist drop caused by mononeuritis multiplex. Extension of the right hand is also diminished because of involvement on that side. Mononeuritis multiplex, a common complication of systemic vasculitis, occurs with a high frequency in Churg-Strauss syndrome.

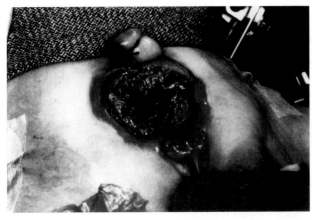

FIGURE 58 Male exstrophy. Notice the excellent size of the bladder template and the reasonably good size of the phallus.

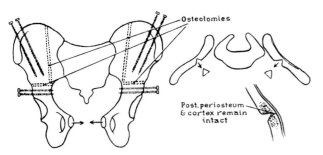

FIGURE 59 Combined transverse anterior innominate and anterior vertical iliac osteotomy with pin placement and preservation of the posterior periosteum and cortex. (Reprinted from *J Urol* 1997;155: 670; with permission.)

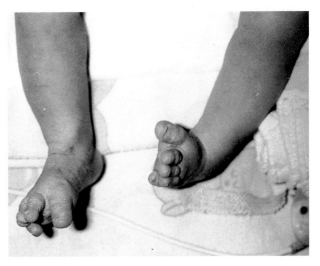

FIGURE 61 Left rigid clubfoot with flexion contracture of great toes in a patient with Antley-Bixler syndrome.

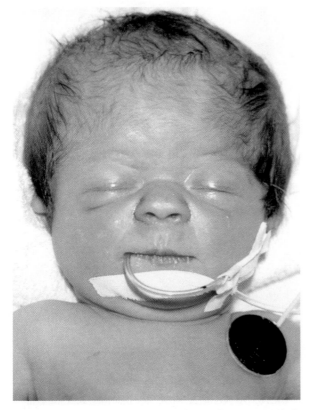

FIGURE 60 An infant with Antley-Bixler syndrome. Frontal view showing a newborn with low-set displastic ears, depressed nasal bridge, and midface hypoplasia.

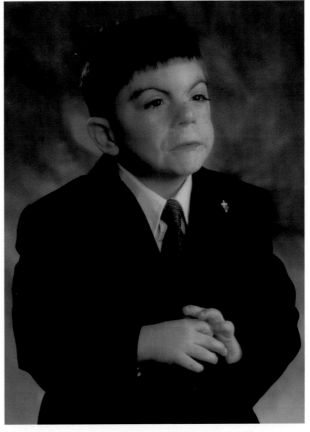

FIGURE 62 Photograph of a boy with Cornelia de Lange syndrome.

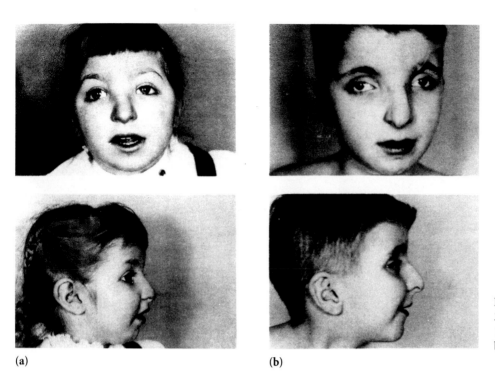

FIGURE 63 A: Patient 1, a 3.5-year-old girl, when seen in 1957. B: Patient 2, a 7-year-old boy, when evaluated in 1958.

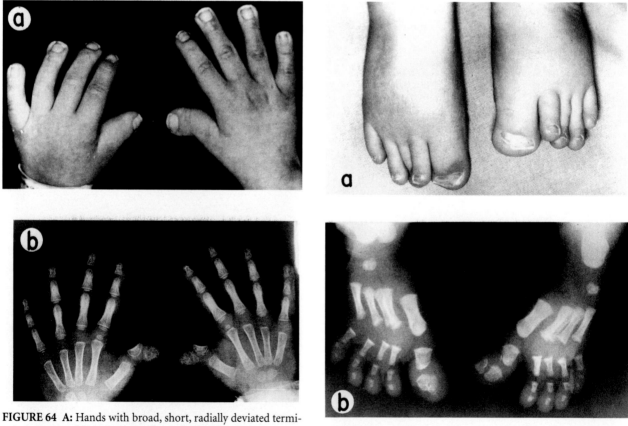

FIGURE 64 A: Hands with broad, short, radially deviated terminal phalanges of thumbs. B: Radiograph of hands with triangular appearance of proximal phalanx of thumb responsible for angulation deformity.

FIGURE 65 A: Feet with broad, flat first toes. B: Radiograph of feet with duplication of distal phalanx of first toe and deformity of proximal phalanx.

28   Glutathione Synthetase Deficiency

Zheng-Zheng Shi, MD,
Geetha M. Habib, MD,
and Michael W. Lieberman, MD

DEFINITION: Glutathione synthetase deficiency is an inborn error of glutathione (GSH) metabolism characterized in its severe form by 5-oxoprolinuria, metabolic acidosis, hemolytic anemia, and central nervous system damage.

SYNONYMS: 5-oxoprolinuria; Pyroglutamic aciduria.

DIFFERENTIAL DIAGNOSIS: 5-oxoprolinuria due to 5-oxoprolinase deficiency; Hemolytic anemia due to glucose-6-phosphate dehydrogenase deficiency.

SYMPTOMS AND SIGNS: There are two forms of GSH synthetase deficiency. The milder form affects only erythrocytes, manifesting mild hemolytic anemia with or without splenomegaly. The severe form is generalized: most patients show symptoms of metabolic acidosis, hemolytic anemia, and 5-oxoprolinuria during the neonatal period. In approximately two thirds of these patients, neurologic symptoms such as convulsions and retarded psychomotor development may also be present or may develop later in life. Severely affected patients may also develop recurrent bacterial infection. Some patients die from infections and acidosis in the neonatal period or during childhood. Adult patients may also die from progressive central nervous system damage. Children or adults who survive are usually stable; however, during episodes of gastroenteritis and other infections, they may become critically ill. Neurologic complications include mental retardation, learning difficulties, and muscular hypotonia or hypertonia.

ETIOLOGY/EPIDEMIOLOGY: Glutathione synthetase deficiency is an inherited autosomal-recessive disorder. The gene encoding GSH synthetase is located on chromosome 20q11.2. Missense mutations, deletion, and splicing errors have been identified in this single-copy gene in patients with GSH synthetase deficiency. Data on prevalence in the general population are not available. To date, more than 40 patients with GSH synthetase deficiency have been documented worldwide. Of these, 4 were mildly affected; the rest had the more severe form.

DIAGNOSIS: The diagnosis should be suspected in a newborn with severe metabolic acidosis and hemolytic anemia. Urinary excretion of 5-oxoproline should be measured by gas chromatography-mass spectrometry. Almost all patients, including those who are mildly affected, have elevated 5-oxoprolinuria. Decreased GSH synthetase activity in erythrocytes, leukocytes, or cultured skin fibroblasts confirms the diagnosis. Reduced GSH in erythrocytes and/or fibroblasts is supportive of the diagnosis.

TREATMENT

Standard Therapies: Treatment includes correction of acidosis, supplementation of vitamin E and/or C, and avoidance of drugs known to precipitate hemolytic crises in glucose-6-phosphate dehydrogenase deficiency. After initial correction of acidosis by parenteral administration of sodium bicarbonate, patients can be maintained on oral sodium bicarbonate or citrate.

Investigational Therapies: Therapeutic trials include administration of GSH substitutes such as N-acetyl cysteine and GSH esters to elevate tissue GSH levels.

REFERENCES

Larsson A, Anderson ME. Glutathione synthetase deficiency and other diseases of the γ-glutamyl cycle. In: Scriver CR, Beaudet AL, Sly WS, et al., eds. *The metabolic and molecular bases of inherited disease,* 8th ed. New York: McGraw-Hill, 2001: 2205–2216.

Ristoff E, Mayatepek E, Larsson A. Long-term clinical outcome in patient with glutathione synthetase deficiency. *J Pediatr* 2001 (in press).

Shi ZZ, Habib GM, Rhead WJ, et al. Mutations in the glutathione synthetase gene cause 5-oxoprolinuria. *Nat Genet* 1996;13: 361–365.

RESOURCES

109, 368, 462

29   Type 0 Glycogen Storage Disease

*David A. Weinstein, MD, MMSc,
Dwight D. Koeberl, MD, PhD,
and Joseph I. Wolfsdorf, MB, BCh*

DEFINITION: Type 0 glycogen storage disease (GSD0) is caused by a deficiency in hepatic glycogen synthase, an enzyme critical for normal glycogen synthesis. There is a marked decrease in glycogen stores, resulting in fasting hypoglycemia and postprandial hyperglycemia.

SYNONYM: Hepatic glycogen synthase deficiency.

DIFFERENTIAL DIAGNOSIS: Fructose 1-phosphate aldolase deficiency (fructose intolerance); GSD-I; Hypoglycemia.

SYMPTOMS AND SIGNS: Fasting ketotic hypoglycemia develops on cessation of nighttime feeding. Early in infancy, children are usually asymptomatic, but weaning from overnight feeds is difficult. During gastrointestinal illness or periods of poor enteral intake, children may become lethargic and usually the hypoglycemia is an incidental finding. Growth throughout childhood may be mildly delayed, but most children remain developmentally normal. Results of the physical examination are usually normal, with no hepatomegaly. Hyperglycemia and hyperlacticacidemia occur after meals, particularly in the morning, and may lead to confusion with early diabetes.

ETIOLOGY/EPIDEMIOLOGY: The disorder is inherited in an autosomal-recessive manner and is a result of mutations in the *GYS2* gene located on chromosome 12p12.2. Although only 15 cases have been described, evidence exists that the disease is underdiagnosed. The disorder affects both genders equally, and cases have been described from Eastern Europe, Western Europe, North America, and South America.

DIAGNOSIS: The diagnosis should be considered in any child with ketotic hypoglycemia who has a history of needing frequent meals or snacks. Monitoring shows a unique metabolic disturbance characterized by alternating fasting hypoglycemia and hyperketonemia followed by hyperglycemia and hyperlacticacidemia with feeding. A liver biopsy shows hepatocytes that contain only small amounts of glycogen with moderate steatosis. Mutation analysis likely will replace liver biopsy as the gold standard for confirmation of the diagnosis.

TREATMENT
Standard Therapies: The goal of treatment is to prevent hypoglycemia by avoiding fasting. Frequent meals and snacks can be given every 3–4 hours during the day. Uncooked cornstarch (2 g/kg) will prevent hypoglycemia overnight. As carbohydrates are preferentially shunted to lactic acid, a diet with an increased amount of protein is recommended.

REFERENCES
Aynsley-Green A, Willianson DH, Gitzelmann R. Hepatic glycogen synthetase deficiency. Definition of syndrome from metabolic and enzymatic studies on a 9-year-old girl. *Arch Dis Child* 1999;52:573–579.
Gitzelmann R, Spycher MA, Feil F, et al. Liver glycogen synthase deficiency: a rarely diagnosed entity. *Eur J Pediatr* 1996;155:561–567.
Ohro M, Bosshard NU, Buist NR, et al. Mutations in the liver glycogen synthase gene in children with hypoglycemia due to glycogen storage disease type 0. *J Clin Invest* 1998;102:507–515.

30   Type I Glycogen Storage Disease

*David A. Weinstein, MD, MMSc,
Dwight D. Koeberl, MD, PhD,
and Joseph I. Wolfsdorf, MB, BCh*

DEFINITION: Type I glycogen storage disease (GSD I) is caused by deficiency of glucose-6-phosphatase (G6Pase) activity, which catalyzes the synthesis of glucose from glucose-6-phosphate. Impairment of this enzyme causes an inability to maintain normal glucose homeostasis as it catalyzes the final step in both glycogenolysis and gluconeogenesis. Glycogenolysis results in hyperlacticacidemia, hyperuricemia, and hyperlipidemia. Two principal subtypes exist: Type Ia - G6Pase deficiency and Type Ib - deficiency of the G6P transporter, which results in the failure of G6P to get to the enzyme in the endoplasmic reticulum.

SYNONYM: Von Gierke disease.

DIFFERENTIAL DIAGNOSIS: Fructose 1-phosphate aldolase deficiency (fructose intolerance), GSD I through VII.

SYMPTOMS AND SIGNS: Severe hypoglycemia develops within 3–4 hours after a meal. Symptomatic hypoglycemia may appear soon after birth, but most children do not present until age 3–6 months when feeds are being spaced. The disorder occasionally is diagnosed on a routine physical exam after hepatomegaly and a protuberant abdomen are noted. Often, however, children are diagnosed during an evaluation for tachypnea, seizures, lethargy, developmental delay, or failure to thrive. Long-term complications of GSD I include hepatic adenomas, focal segmental glomerulosclerosis, renal tubular dysfunction, nephrocalcinosis, nephrolithiasis, and osteoporosis. Type 1b has all of the aforementioned manifestations with the addition of neutropenia and inflammatory bowel disease.

ETIOLOGY/EPIDEMIOLOGY: Type I glycogen storage disease is inherited in an autosomal-recessive manner and is the result of mutations in the G6PC gene located on chromosome 17q21. The overall incidence is estimated to be 1 in 200,000 births. Approximately 60 mutations exist from all around the world, but the highest incidence is in the Ashkenazi Jewish population.

DIAGNOSIS: The simplest means of determining the probable enzymatic defect in a child suspected of having a glycogenosis is to obtain serial measurements of metabolites (glucose, lactate, and ketones) during a fasting study. A fasting study in GSD I will result in ketotic hypoglycemia with a progressive lactic acidosis, and glucagon (30 μg/kg) will fail to elicit a glucose response after hypoglycemia occurs. Glucagon may exacerbate the acidosis, and the testing should be performed under close observation. An assay of G6Pase activity on a liver biopsy has been the primary method of confirming the diagnosis. Differentiation between the types requires an analysis of G6Pase activity in both intact and fully disrupted microsomes. In type Ib, G6Pase activity is normal when the assay is performed on previously frozen tissue that disrupts the microsomal membrane. In patients with a classic phenotype for GSD I, mutation analysis can now be used to confirm the diagnosis instead of a liver biopsy.

TREATMENT

Standard Therapies: Treatment consists of providing a continuous dietary source of glucose to prevent blood glucose from falling below the threshold for glucose counter-regulation. Glucose delivery in infants is usually achieved with frequent feeds during the day and continuous feeds at night through a nasogastric or gastrostomy tube. Cornstarch can be used starting at age 6–12 months as a method of glucose delivery, which allows feeds to be spaced and glucose fluctuations to be minimized. Cornstarch doses and spacing of feeds should be individualized based on results of periodic metabolic evaluations and glucose monitoring. If fasting is required or if gastrointestinal illness does not allow adequate intake of carbohydrate, intravenous glucose should be administered using 10% dextrose at 1–1.25 times the estimated hepatic production rate to ensure euglycemia and minimize lactic acidosis. Restriction of galactose, fructose, sucrose, and lactose is critical, as these sugars cannot be converted to glucose and will exacerbate the metabolic derangements. Neutropenia in type 1b responds well to G-CSF therapy, and the associated inflammatory bowel disease responds to conventional therapy.

REFERENCES

Rake JP, ten Berge AM, Visser G, et al. Glycogen storage disease type 1a: recent experience with mutation analysis, a summary of mutations reported in the literature, and a newly developed diagnostic flow chart. *Eur J Pediatr* 2000;159: 322–330.

Wolfsdorf JI, Crigler JF Jr. Effect of continuous glucose therapy begun in infancy on the long-term clinical course of patients with type 1 glycogen storage disease. *J Pediatr Gastroenterol Nutr* 1999;29:136–143.

Wolfsdorf JI, Holm IA, Weinstein DA. Glycogen storage diseases: phenotypic, genetic, and biochemical characteristics, and therapy. *Endocrinol Metab Clin North Am* 1999;28: 801–823.

RESOURCES

56, 109, 364

31   Type II Glycogen Storage Disease

David A. Weinstein, MD, MMSc, Dwight D. Koeberl, MD, PhD, and Joseph I. Wolfsdorf, MB, BCh

DEFINITION: Type II glycogen storage disease (GSD II) is caused by deficiency of the lysosomal enzyme, acid-α-glucosidase (GAA). Glycogen accumulation in lysosomes occurs in all tissues, although primarily in skeletal muscle and heart. All forms of GSD II share the presence of myopathy, and most patients have elevations of creatine kinase.

SYNONYMS: Acid-maltase deficiency; Pompe disease.

DIFFERENTIAL DIAGNOSIS: Noonan syndrome.

SYMPTOMS AND SIGNS: A spectrum of severity of clinical presentations ranges from infantile hypotonia and progressive cardiac hypertrophy to adult-onset proximal weakness and muscle atrophy. Patients with the most severe phenotype, infantile-onset, present with hypotonia, feeding difficulties, macroglossia, hepatomegaly, and rapidly progressive hypertrophic cardiomyopathy. In severe GSD II, death by age 1 year by cardiorespiratory failure is expected. Patients with juvenile-onset GSD II usually present after age 2 years with difficulty walking and delayed motor milestones. Progressive weakness, swallowing difficulty, and death from respiratory failure in the second decade occur. Patients with adult-onset GSD II present between the second and seventh decades of life with proximal muscle weakness, sometimes manifesting as exercise intolerance and orthopnea. Death from complications of respiratory failure occurs in adult-onset GSD II. Cardiomegaly is uncommon in juvenile and adult-onset GSD II.

ETIOLOGY/EPIDEMIOLOGY: Acid-α-glucosidase deficiency is caused by mutations in the *GAA* gene on human chromosome 17q25. A common splice-site mutation in intron 1 accounts for approximately 50% of mutant alleles in adult-onset GSD II among caucasian populations. Two different, common mutations cause infantile-onset GSD II among Taiwanese populations (asp645glu) and African-American patients (arg854x). The severity of GSD II correlates with the amount of residual GAA activity in muscle, from less than 1% in infantile, to 1%–10% in juvenile, and more than 10% of normal activity in adult-onset GSD II.

The true incidence of GSD II is unknown, but estimates range from 1 in 40,000 to 1 in 100,000.

DIAGNOSIS: Glycogen storage disease type II should be considered in infants with hypotonia and/or hypertrophic cardiomyopathy, and in older individuals with proximal muscle weakness with or without respiratory failure, especially if creatine kinase is elevated. Muscle biopsy shows vacuoles that stain positively with periodic acid-Schiff, and elevated glycogen content. Electromyographic abnormalities include pseudomyotonic discharges and irritability, with variable abnormalities in different muscles in later-onset GSD II. The diagnosis is confirmed by GAA analysis in cultured patient fibroblasts, muscle tissue, or carefully isolated lymphocytes. More than 40 different mutations have already been defined in GSD II, limiting the usefulness of gene sequencing for diagnostic purposes.

TREATMENT
Standard Therapies: Hypoglycemia is absent in GSD II because the defect is isolated to the lysosomes with no abnormalities in the metabolism of cytosolic glycogen. A high-protein diet has had some benefits in patients with late-onset disease.

Investigational Therapies: Enzyme replacement with recombinant human GAA is being investigated, as is gene therapy with adenoviral vectors.

REFERENCES
Amalfitano A, Bengur AR, Morse RP, et al. Recombinant human acid α-glucosidase enzyme therapy for infantile glycogen storage disease type II: results of phase I/II clinical trial. *Genet Med* 2001;3:132–138.

Hirschhorn R, Reuser AJJ. Glycogen storage disease type II: acid α-glucosidase (acid maltase) deficiency. In: Scriver CR, Beaudet AL, Sly WS, Valle D, eds. *The metabolic and molecular bases of inherited disease*, 8th ed. New York: McGraw-Hill, 2001:3389–3420.

Van den Hout H, Reuser AJJ, Vulto AG, et al. Recombinant human α-glucosidase from rabbit milk in Pompe patients. *Lancet* 2000;356:397–398.

RESOURCES
8, 56, 109, 364

32   Type III Glycogen Storage Disease

David A. Weinstein, MD, MMSc,
Dwight D. Koeberl, MD, PhD,
and Joseph I. Wolfsdorf, MB, BCh

DEFINITION: Type III glycogen storage disease (GSD III) is caused by deficiency of glycogen debrancher enzyme. Although the terminal chains of glycogen can be broken down normally, glycogenolysis is arrested when the outermost branch points are reached. Abnormal glycogen accumulates in affected tissues. The two main subtypes are defined by the location of the defect. Type IIIA accounts for 85% patients and is due to a generalized defect involving both the liver and muscle. Type IIIB is limited to the liver only.

SYNONYMS: Debrancher enzyme deficiency; Cori disease; Forbes disease.

DIFFERENTIAL DIAGNOSIS: Glucose intolerance; Glucose-6-phosphatase deficiency; Glucose-6-phosphate dehydrogenase deficiency; GSD-I, GSD-II, GSD-IV through VII; Hepatic carcinoma, primary; Hepatic cysts; Hepatic failure; Hypoglycemia.

SYMPTOMS AND SIGNS: Clinical symptoms depend on tissue involvement. Patients with hepatic involvement may be indistinguishable in infancy from patients with GSD I, and typically have hepatomegaly and ketotic hypoglycemia. Because the outer chains of glycogen can be degraded and normal gluconeogenesis can occur, the hypoglycemia typically improves with age. A variable myopathy can occur, which is usually minimal in childhood, but can become prominent in adulthood. Associated laboratory studies include a profound elevation of serum transaminases (often worse than in GSD I), elevated creatine kinase concentrations, and hyperlipidemia. Long-term complications include short stature, idiopathic hypertrophic cardiomyopathy, cardiac dysfunction, and hepatic adenomas.

ETIOLOGY/EPIDEMIOLOGY: Although the overall incidence of GSD III is approximately 1 in 100,000 live births, it is unusually frequent among North African Jews in Israel (prevalence 1 in 5,400 with a carrier prevalence of 1 in 35). It is inherited in an autosomal-recessive manner, and is a result of mutations in the debrancher gene, which has been localized to chromosome 1p21.

DIAGNOSIS: A fasting study results in ketotic hypoglycemia without the hyperlacticacidemia associated with GSD I. Glucagon fails to elicit a response when given after a fast, but a glycemic response will occur if given after a carbohydrate-rich meal. Definitive diagnosis depends on demonstration of abnormal glycogen on biopsy of the liver and muscle along with demonstration of abnormal enzyme activity. Definitive subtyping depends on both liver and muscle biopsies as a normal creatine kinase concentration cannot rule out muscle involvement. Assessment of enzyme activity in skin fibroblasts or lymphocytes can be used as a screen, but the tests cannot be used for subtyping and may not be definitive.

TREATMENT
Standard Therapies: As with GSD I, continuous glucose delivery is required to maintain blood sugars above 70 mg/dL. After infancy, uncooked cornstarch (1.75 g/kg) given every 6 hours usually will maintain normoglycemia, improve growth, and improve laboratory abnormalities. Patients do not need to restrict dietary intake of fructose or galactose, but a diet high in protein may be beneficial.

REFERENCES
Coleman RA, Winter HS, Wolf B, et al. Glycogen debranching enzyme deficiency: long-term study of serum enzyme activities and clinical features. *J Inherit Metab Dis* 1992;15:869–881.
Gremse DA, Buculas JC, Balistreri WF. Efficacy of cornstarch therapy in type III glycogen storage disease. *Am J Clin Nutr* 1990;52:671–674.
Shen J, Bao Y, Liu HM, et al. Mutations in exon 3 of the glycogen debranching enzyme gene are associated with glycogen storage disease type III that is differentially expressed in liver and muscle. *J Clin Invest* 1996;98:352–357.

RESOURCES
56, 58, 364

33 Type IV Glycogen Storage Disease

David A. Weinstein, MD, MMSc,
Dwight D. Koeberl, MD, PhD,
and Joseph I. Wolfsdorf, MB, BCh

DEFINITION: Glycogen storage disease type IV (GSD IV) is caused by a deficiency in branching enzyme activity, an enzyme critical to the synthesis of normal glycogen. As a result, abnormal, unbranched glycogen accumulates in liver with accompanying progressive liver cirrhosis.

SYNONYMS: Amylopectinosis; Andersen disease.

DIFFERENTIAL DIAGNOSIS: Cardiomyopathy, dilated; Galactose-1-phosphate uridyltransferase deficiency (galactosemia); Hemochromatosis, neonatal; Hydrops fetalis; Tyrosinemia.

SYMPTOMS AND SIGNS: Patients with GSD IV frequently present during infancy with hepatosplenomegaly and failure to thrive. Hypoglycemia is unusual in GSD IV until cirrhosis is advanced. The typical clinical course is progressive liver cirrhosis with portal hypertension, esophageal varices, and ascites, culminating in death by age 5 years. An alternative presentation manifests as neuromuscular involvement with hypotonia and muscular atrophy in infancy, followed by early death. Childhood-onset GSD IV may present as myopathy or cardiomyopathy. Adult-onset central and peripheral nervous system involvement may be accompanied by accumulation of unbranched glycogen in neuronal tissue (polyglucosan body disease).

ETIOLOGY/EPIDEMIOLOGY: The disorder is inherited in an autosomal-recessive manner, and mutations in the branching enzyme gene on chromosome 3p14 have been implicated in all forms of GSD IV. A missense mutation al-

tered tyrosine 329 to serine (*Y329S*) and was associated with partial branching enzyme activity and a mild, nonprogressive clinical course. The *Y329S* mutation was also found in Ashkenazi Jewish patients with adult-onset polyglucosan disease. By contrast, a 210-nucleotide deletion abolished branching enzyme activity and was associated with the fatal, neonatal neuromuscular form of GSD IV.

DIAGNOSIS: The diagnosis of GSD IV is established by demonstration of abnormal glycogen and the demonstration of branching enzyme deficiency in liver, muscle, leukocytes, erythrocytes, or fibroblasts. Patients have 1%–10% of normal branching enzyme activity. In adult polyglucosan body disease, the enzyme deficiency can only be detected in leukocytes or in a nerve biopsy.

TREATMENT
Standard Therapies: No specific treatment is effective. If hypoglycemia is present, correction of that symptom can improve the clinical picture.

REFERENCES
Bao Y, Kishnani P, Wu J-Y, et al. Hepatic and neuromuscular forms of glycogen storage disease type IV caused by mutations in the same glycogen-branching enzyme gene. *J Clin Invest* 1996;97:941–948.
Chen Y-T. Glycogen storage diseases. In: Scriver CR, Beaudet AL, Sly WS, et al., eds. *The metabolic and molecular bases of inherited disease.* New York: McGraw-Hill, 2001:1521–1551.
Matern D, Starzl T, Arnaout W, et al. Liver transplantation for glycogen storage disease types I, II, and IV. *Eur J Pediatr* 1999; 158(suppl 2):43–48.

RESOURCES
56, 109, 365

34 Type V Glycogen Storage Disease

David A. Weinstein, MD, MMSc,
Dwight D. Koeberl, MD, PhD,
and Joseph I. Wolfsdorf, MB, BCh

DEFINITION: Glycogen storage disease type V (GSD V) is caused by a deficiency of muscle phosphorylase, an en-

zyme essential to the first step in glycogen breakdown. The release of energy from stored glucose in muscle is severely impaired with resultant exercise intolerance.

SYNONYM: McCardle disease.

DIFFERENTIAL DIAGNOSIS: Glycogen storage disease type VII; Mitochondrial myopathy; Phosphoglycerate kinase deficiency; Phosphoglycerate mutase deficiency; Phosphofructokinase deficiency; Lactate dehydrogenase deficiency.

SYMPTOMS AND SIGNS: Patients with GSD V present with exercise intolerance with muscle cramping, typically in the second or third decade. Approximately half of patients experience myoglobinuria with dark-colored urine after muscle breakdown. Renal failure frequently follows myoglobinuria. Whereas vigorous exercise precipitates symptoms, mild exercise is typically well tolerated. A "second wind" phenomenon after brief rest is frequently reported. Serum creatine kinase is often elevated at rest. Uric acid may be elevated, and gout is seen occasionally. Rarely, infantile involvement may occur with progressive hypotonia, muscle weakness, and respiratory insufficiency.

ETIOLOGY/EPIDEMIOLOGY: The disorder is inherited in an autosomal-recessive manner, and mutations in the muscle phosphorylase gene on chromosome 11q13 have been reported. Rare families have been reported with multigenerational GSD V inheritance in an apparently autosomal-dominant pattern, and the genetic factors underlying this phenomenon have yet to be defined. Another gene codes for liver-specific phosphorylase, and the presence of this alternative phosphorylase in liver explains the lack of hypoglycemia in GSD V. Two common mutations are found in caucasian (R49X) and Japanese (a single codon deletion in exon 17) patients.

DIAGNOSIS: The diagnosis of GSD V is likely if the ischemic forearm test demonstrates the absence of an elevation in lactate (in response to vigorous arm muscle contraction while an arm tourniquet is in place). Alternatively, mutation analysis of the muscle phosphorylase gene may demonstrate the underlying gene defect. The demonstration of muscle phosphorylase deficiency in a flash-frozen muscle biopsy can also confirm the diagnosis.

TREATMENT
Standard Therapies: Avoidance of vigorous exercise generally prevents symptoms. Aerobic exercise can improve exercise tolerance, as can glucose or fructose ingestion. Vitamin B_6 has been shown to decrease muscle cramping and increase muscle endurance in some patients. A high-protein diet has been beneficial for some individuals.

REFERENCES
Chen Y-T. Glycogen storage diseases. In: Scriver CR, Beaudet AL, Sly WS, et al., eds. *The metabolic and molecular bases of inherited disease.* New York: McGraw-Hill, 2001:1521–1551.
DiMauro S, Bruno C. Glycogen storage diseases of muscle. *Curr Opin Neurol* 1998;11:477–484.

RESOURCES
56, 109, 354

---

35 Types VI and IX Glycogen Storage Disease

*David A. Weinstein, MD, MMSc,
Dwight D. Koeberl, MD, PhD,
and Joseph I. Wolfsdorf, MB, BCh*

DEFINITION: Glycogen storage disease type VI (GSD VI) and type IX (GSD IX) both result in a reduction in liver phosphorylase activity that catalyzes the rate-limiting step during glycogenolysis. Glycogen storage disease type VI is the result of a deficiency of the phosphorylase enzyme, whereas GSD IX is the result of a deficiency of the associated kinase that activates the enzyme.

SYNONYMS: For type VI: Hepatic glycogen phosphorylase deficiency; Hers disease. For type IX: Phosphorylase kinase deficiency.

DIFFERENTIAL DIAGNOSIS: For type VI: Fructose 1-phosphate aldolase deficiency (fructose intolerance); GSD 0 though GSD III.

SYMPTOMS AND SIGNS: Fasting ketotic hypoglycemia, which is generally milder than GSD I and GSD III, is the cardinal symptom of this heterogeneous group of disorders. Hepatomegaly and short stature are common but may be of variable severity. Mild hyperlipidemia and increased serum transaminases can occur, but lactic acid and uric acid concentrations are normal. Muscle involvement can occur with hypotonia, myoglobinuria, and muscle weakness. Rarely, these disorders can be associated with a proximal renal tubular acidosis, neurologic abnormalities, and cirrhosis. A severe cardiac-specific phosphorylase kinase variant, which can lead to cardiac failure, has also been reported.

ETIOLOGY/EPIDEMIOLOGY: GSD VI has a higher prevalence in the Mennonite population. It is inherited as an autosomal-recessive disorder with the gene localized to 14q21-22. GSD IX can be both X-linked or inherited as an autosomal-recessive disorder, because multiple genes are involved in forming the large four-subunit enzyme. Overall, GSD IX occurs in approximately 1 in 100,000 births and accounts for approximately 25% of all GSDs.

DIAGNOSIS: It is possible to diagnose glycogen phosphorylase deficiency by assaying the activity of the enzyme in leukocytes and erythrocytes. Because there are liver, muscle, heart, and brain isoforms of this enzyme, the diagnosis can be missed when a blood assay is used. Definitive diagnosis requires demonstration of abnormal enzyme activity from biopsies of affected tissues. Mutation analysis likely will become the standard for diagnosis of GSD VI and the X-linked variant of GSD IX, but will unlikely be able to fully rule out GSD IX because of the multiple genes involved in synthesizing the phosphorylase kinase protein.

TREATMENT

Standard Therapies: The prognosis for these disorders is excellent, and most patients do not require specific treatment except for avoidance of fasting and routine consumption of a bedtime snack. In the unusual patient with overnight hypoglycemia, uncooked cornstarch (2 g/kg) given at bedtime prevents nocturnal hypoglycemia.

REFERENCES

Elpeleg ON. The molecular background of glycogen metabolism disorders. *J Pediatr Endocrinol Metab* 1999;12:363–379.

Nakai A, Shigematsy Y, Takano T, et al. Uncooked cornstarch treatment for hepatic phosphorylase kinase deficiency. *Eur J Pediatr* 1994;153:581–583.

Williams PJ, Gerver WJM, Berger R, et al. The natural history of liver glycogenosis due to phosphorylase kinase deficiency: a longitudinal study of 41 patients. *Eur J Pediatr* 1990;149:268–271.

RESOURCES

56, 58, 109, 364

36   Type VII Glycogen Storage Disease

*David A. Weinstein, MD, MMSc,
Dwight D. Koeberl, MD, PhD,
and Joseph I. Wolfsdorf, MB, BCh*

DEFINITION: Glycogen storage disease type VII (GSD VII) is caused by a deficiency of muscle phosphofructokinase, an enzyme essential to the glycolytic pathway. The use of carbohydrates for energy in muscle is severely impaired with resultant exercise intolerance.

SYNONYMS: Muscle phosphofructokinase deficiency; Tauri disease.

DIFFERENTIAL DIAGNOSIS: Glycogen storage disease type V.

SYMPTOMS AND SIGNS: Patients with GSD VII present with exercise intolerance with childhood onset, often accompanied by muscle cramping and myoglobinuria. The attacks may feature nausea and vomiting. Exercise intolerance is exacerbated by carbohydrate consumption. A com-

pensated hemolytic anemia causes an elevation of serum bilirubin and the reticulocyte count. Uric acid is usually elevated. Rarely, infantile involvement may occur with progressive hypotonia, muscle weakness, and death. A late-onset variant affects middle-aged adults and causes only muscle weakness.

ETIOLOGY/EPIDEMIOLOGY: The disorder is inherited in an autosomal-recessive manner, and mutations in the muscle phosphofructokinase gene on chromosome 12 have been reported. Ashkenazi Jewish patients carry two common mutations, including an exon 5 defect that accounts for approximately 68% of mutations in this population. A child with early-onset rhabdomyolysis and myoglobinuria was found to have phosphofructokinase deficiency and a more common enzyme defect, adenylate deaminase deficiency.

DIAGNOSIS: The diagnosis of GSD VII can be accomplished routinely by muscle biopsy and enzyme analysis. Alternatively, deficiency of the M subunit of phosphofructokinase can be demonstrated in red blood cells. Among the Ashkenazi Jewish population, molecular diagnosis of causative mutations provides an alternative approach.

TREATMENT
Standard Therapies: Avoidance of vigorous exercise can prevent muscle cramping and rhabdomyolysis. A patient with the infantile variant responded to a ketogenic diet.

REFERENCES
Chen Y-T. Glycogen storage diseases. In: Scriver CR, Beaudet AL, Sly WS, et al., eds. *The metabolic and molecular bases of inherited disease.* New York: McGraw-Hill, 2001:1521–1551.

DiMauro S, Bruno C. Glycogen storage diseases of muscle. *Curr Opin Neurol* 1998;11:477–484.

RESOURCES
56, 58,109, 364

---

37   Congenital Disorders of Glycosylation

Marc C. Patterson, MD

DEFINITION: The congenital disorders of glycosylation (CDG) are a family of diseases in which the number and length of oligosaccharides attached to asparagine residues in proteins (N-linkage) are reduced. The most frequent phenotype recognized, CDG 1a, is associated with deficient activity of phosphomannomutase, characterized by olivopontocerebellar hypoplasia, demyelinating peripheral neuropathy, cutaneous lipoatrophy and lipohypertrophy, severe cerebellar ataxia and developmental delay, and multiple organ system dysfunctions. At least 10 additional enzyme deficiencies have been recognized.

SYNONYMS: Jaeken disease; Phosphomannomutase 2 deficiency (CDG-Ia); Phosphomannose isomerase deficiency (CDG-Ib); *hALG6* deficiency (CDG-Ic); *hALG3* deficiency (CDG-Id); Dolichol-phosphate mannose synthase-1 deficiency (CDG-Ie); Mannose-P-dolichol utilization defect 1(CDG-If), *hALG12* deficiency (CDG-Ig), *MGAT2* deficiency (CDG-IIa); Glucosidase I deficiency (CDG-IIb); GDP fucose transporter defect (CDG-IIc; LAD II); β*GALT1* deficiency (CDG-IId); Defects of N-glycan synthesis; Carbohydrate-deficient glycoprotein syndrome; Disialotransferrin developmental deficiency syndrome.

DIFFERENTIAL DIAGNOSIS: Alpha-1 antitrypsin deficiency; Hereditary fructose intolerance; Galactosemia; Inborn errors of bile acid metabolism; Peroxisomal disorders; Sphingolipidoses; Fatty acid oxidation defects; Congenital coagulation deficiencies; Homocystinuria; Hyperinsulinemic hypoglycemia; Cerebral palsy; Urea cycle defects; Organic acidurias; Respiratory chain disorders; Ataxia telangiectasia; Other hereditary ataxias; Refsum disease; Abetalipoproteinema.

SYMPTOMS AND SIGNS: Neonates with CDG 1a may have low muscle tone, abnormal rolling eye and head movements, and depressed reflexes. Feeding problems with failure to thrive, as well as episodes of liver dysfunction, unexplained coma, susceptibility to infections, nephrotic syndrome, cardiac hypertrophy, and/or pericardial effusions and abnormal blood clotting may occur in infancy. Children often have fat pads above the buttocks, a "cellulite" appearance to the skin, inverted nipples, and mild facial dysmorphism with large, soft ears. Up to 20% of affected children die in infancy and early childhood. Those who survive develop slowly, and most have microcephaly and an IQ less than 60. Older children may develop visual loss secondary to retinitis pigmentosa, strokelike episodes and seizures, often in the context of intercurrent infections, and progressive peripheral neuropathy. Most never walk unassisted and are wheelchair dependent. Hypogonadism and premature aging are frequent in adults. With the exception of CDG1b, the less common forms of CDG have primary neurologic abnormalities, of varying severity, without the typical cerebellar atrophy. In CDG1b, hypoglycemia, hepatic dysfunction, coagulopathies, and protein-losing enteropathy dominate the phenotype.

ETIOLOGY/EPIDEMIOLOGY: All forms of CDG are inherited as autosomal-recessive traits, causing impaired function of enzymes involved in the process of n-glycosylation. Most cases of CDG1a have been reported from Europe, but there may be an ascertainment bias. Several hundred patients with CDG1a have been recognized worldwide, but the true prevalence is unknown. The other forms of CDG have been recognized in only a handful of kindreds.

DIAGNOSIS: Abnormalities are common in many laboratory tests that assay glycoproteins (hormones, coagulation factors, thyroid studies); carbohydrate-deficient transferrin is the most widely used screening test. Definitive diagnosis requires enzyme assay. Molecular analysis is available on a clinical basis for *PMM2* (CDG-Ia) and in research laboratories for the less common subtypes.

TREATMENT

Standard Therapies: Enteral or parenteral feeding support may be required in infancy. Antiepileptic drugs may be useful in children with frequent seizures, and some children have overt hypothyroidism requiring replacement therapy. The protean nature of CDG requires the involvement of appropriate subspecialists, particularly in neurology, hematology, endocrinology, and gastroenterology. General supportive care involving a multidisciplinary team is important, as is family support through counseling and support groups.

Investigational Therapies: Oral mannose supplementation is being investigated.

REFERENCES

Aebi M, Hennet T. Congenital disorders of glycosylation: genetic model systems lead the way. *Trends Cell Biol* 2001;11:136–141.

Babovic-Vuksanovic D, Patterson MC, Schwenk WF, et al. Severe hypoglycemia as a presenting symptom of carbohydrate-deficient glycoprotein syndrome. *J Pediatr* 1999;135:775–781.

Dennis JW, Warren CE, Granovsky M, et al. Genetic defects in N-glycosylation and cellular diversity in mammals. *Curr Opin Struct Biol* 2001;11:601–607.

Jaeken J, Matthijs G. Congenital disorders of glycosylation. *Annu Rev Genom Hum Genet* 2001;2:129–151.

RESOURCES

351, 368, 463

---

38   Hartnup Disease

*Neil R.M. Buist, MB, ChB, DCH,
and Susan C. Winter, MD, FAAP, FCMG*

DEFINITION: Hartnup disease is caused by a hereditary defect in the transport and uptake of neutral amino acids in the small intestine and renal tubules.

SYMPTOMS AND SIGNS: Most patients are asymptomatic; their condition is detected only if their urine is subjected to amino acid chromatography as is done for newborn screening in some centers. The neutral amino acids comprise several essential amino acids, including threonine, the branched chain amino acids, methionine, phenylalanine, and tryptophan. Malabsorption of all of these occurs in the gut, and more are lost in urine through impaired tubular reabsorption. A low protein intake can result in overt deficiency of tryptophan, which can cause pellagra-like symptoms of dermatitis and central nervous system problems of cerebellar ataxia and emotional lability, and if untreated, retardation of growth and development. Maternal Hartnup disease is benign.

ETIOLOGY/EPIDEMIOLOGY: The disorder is inherited in an autosomal-recessive manner. The alpha-neutral amino acid transport in the intestine and renal tubule is affected and the gene is located on chromosome 11q13.

DIAGNOSIS: The condition is diagnosed by the unique pattern of amino acids in the urine. Indicanuria is usual through intestinal conversion from the malabsorbed tryptophan. Oral amino acid tolerance tests show diminished absorption, but these tests are not needed to confirm a diagnosis.

TREATMENT

Standard Therapies: Therapy in well-nourished patients without symptoms is not necessary. When nutrition is marginal, a small protein supplement is advisable along with extra nicotinamide.

REFERENCES

McKusick VA, ed. Online Mendelian Inheritance in Man, OMIM [database online]. Bethesda, MD: National Center for Biotechnology Information, National Library of Medicine, 2000. MIM# 234500.

Scriver CR, Beaudet AL, Sly WS, et al., eds. *The metabolic and molecular bases of inherited disease,* 8th ed. New York: McGraw-Hill, 2001.

RESOURCES

109, 365, 462

39   Histidinemia

Neil R.M. Buist, MB, ChB, and Susan C. Winter, MD, FAAP, FCMG

DEFINITION: Histidinemia is caused by a deficiency of the enzyme histidase, which results in the accumulation of histidine and several of its metabolites in blood and urine.

SYNONYMS: Histidase deficiency; Hyperhistidinemia; Histidine-ammonia-lyase (HAL) deficiency; HAS deficiency.

DIFFERENTIAL DIAGNOSIS: No other conditions are likely to be confused with histidinemia

SYMPTOMS AND SIGNS: For more than 20 years, histidinemia was believed to be associated with mental retardation, often accompanied by a speech disorder. Results from newborn screening in Japan showed that most patients are completely normal. Maternal histidinemia is also considered benign.

ETIOLOGY/EPIDEMIOLOGY: Histidinemia is an autosomal-recessively inherited trait located on 12q22-q23. Incidence is believed to be 1 in 20,000 to 1 in 50,000.

DIAGNOSIS: Newborn screening, once commonplace, has been discontinued. Diagnosis is made by detection of elevated histidine levels in blood with excretion of several histidine metabolites in urine. The enzyme can be assayed in cultured skin fibroblasts.

TREATMENT
Standard Therapies: No treatment is needed. A low-histidine diet was recommended in the past, but this is no longer advocated.

REFERENCES
McKusick VA, ed. Online Mendelian Inheritance in Man, OMIM [database online]. Bethesda, MD: National Center for Biotechnology Information, National Library of Medicine, 2000. MIM# 235800.
Scriver CR, Beaudet AL, Sly WS, et al., eds. *The metabolic and molecular bases of inherited disease,* 8th ed. New York: McGraw-Hill, 2001.

RESOURCES
58, 109, 364

40   Homocystinuria

Olaf Bodamer, MD, PhD

DEFINITION: Homocystinuria is an inborn error of sulfur amino acid metabolism. It is caused by a deficiency of cystathionine β-synthase (CBS), which leads to elevated levels of homocystine and methionine and decreased levels of cystathionine and cystine in body fluids. Homocystinuria also occurs in disorders of folate and cobalamin metabolism.

SYNONYMS: Homocystinemia; Cystathionine β-synthase deficiency.

DIFFERENTIAL DIAGNOSIS: Marfan syndrome; Disorders of folate and cobalamin metabolism including homocystinuria due to N(5,10)-methylentetrahydrofolate reductase deficiency; Renal insufficiency; Bacterial contamination of urine in cystathioninuria.

SYMPTOMS AND SIGNS: Clinical presentation varies depending on the presence and anatomic distribution of thromboembolic events or on the presence of pyridoxine responsiveness. Symptoms may include downward-oriented ectopia lentis with iridodonesis; myopia, which may precede ectopia lentis; skeletal deformities including genu valga, pes cavus, pectus excavatum, and carinatum; vascular disease with life-threatening thromboembolic events; malar flush; and osteoporosis. Ectopia lentis is striking and typically presents in most patients at age 10. It may be the only symptom at presentation. Developmental delay and mental retardation are also common. About one third of patients have normal intelligence. Psychiatric abnormalities may include behavioral abnormalities, schizophrenia, depression, or personality disorders. A subgroup of patients is responsive to pyridoxine (vitamin B$_6$), and they may have milder or fewer symptoms.

ETIOLOGY/EPIDEMIOLOGY: Homocystinuria is secondary to deficiency of CBS, the enzyme that catalyzes the condensation of homocysteine and serine to form cystathionine. The gene encoding CBS has been cloned, and many mutations causing CBS deficiency have been identified. The deficiency is inherited as an autosomal-recessive trait. Recurrence risk for future pregnancies after giving birth to an affected child is 25%. There is no sex preference. Estimated overall frequency of CBS deficiency is 1 in 200,000 to 300,000 newborns.

DIAGNOSIS: Measurement of plasma amino acids including homocysteine and homocystine is used to make the diagnosis. Methionine levels are typically elevated in most patients, accompanied by low cystine levels. Urinary levels of homocystine can be measured alternatively. Urinary excretion of homocystine is also identified by nitroprusside tests; however, nitroprusside tests may yield false-positive results when other disulfides are present. Enzymatic and molecular tests are available to confirm, and for prenatal diagnosis. Additional investigations such as skeletal films, brain MRI, and slit-lamp eye examination may be indicated. Some states have neonatal screening programs for homocystinuria based on the detection of elevated plasma methionine levels.

TREATMENT
Standard Therapies: Dietary therapy with methionine restriction may prevent many complications in patients unresponsive to pyridoxine when employed shortly after birth. A trial with pyridoxine is indicated in all patients with homocystinuria to identify those who are responsive to it. Doses have ranged from 100 to 1,200 mg/day but should be determined individually; peripheral neuropathy may be a side effect of larger doses. Folate supplement should be given to avoid deficiency. Betaine may be beneficial in patients who are unresponsive to pyridoxine. Particular care should be taken when patients with CBS deficiency undergo surgery, because the frequency of postoperative thromboembolic complications may be increased.

REFERENCES
Homocystinuria. Online Mendelian Inheritance in Man, OMIM [database online; *http://www.ncbi.nlm.nih.gov*]. Bethesda, MD: National Center for Biotechnology Information, National Library of Medicine, 2000. MIM# 236200.

Mudd SH, et al. The natural history of homocystinuria due to cystathionine beta-synthase deficiency. *Am J Hum Genet* 1985;37:1–31.

Nyhan WL, Ozand PT. Homocystinuria. In: Nyhan WL, Ozand PT, eds. *Atlas of metabolic diseases.* London: Chapman & Hall, 1998:126–132.

RESOURCES
58, 109, 354

---

41   Type IV Hyperlipidemia

Paul N. Hopkins, MD, MSPH

DEFINITION: Type IV hyperlipidemia is a descriptor for elevated plasma triglycerides without elevated low-density lipoprotein (LDL) cholesterol. Only very-low-density lipoproteins (VLDL) are elevated with no fasting chylomicronemia. Type IV is one of the three phenotypes (along with types IIa and IIb) that are used to define familial combined hyperlipidemia. Familial hypertriglyceridemia may be defined as multiple cases of type IV among first-degree relatives but without type IIa or IIb present.

SYNONYMS: Fredrickson type IV hyperlipidemia; Endogenous hypertriglyceridemia.

DIFFERENTIAL DIAGNOSIS: Types I, IIb, III, V hyperlipidemia; Secondary causes of hypertriglyceridemia.

SYMPTOMS AND SIGNS: Type IV hyperlipidemia is an asymptomatic condition. Increased risk for premature coronary artery disease may exist, depending on family context and associated risk factors (low high-density lipoprotein [HDL], diabetes, hypertension).

ETIOLOGY/EPIDEMIOLOGY: A few causes are known, such as heterozygous lipoprotein lipase deficiency (at least 221 mutations currently known), but the etiology of most cases is unknown. Evidence exists for variants in apolipoprotein CIII leading to increased apo CIII levels and hypertriglyceridemia. Type IV hyperlipidemia is frequently associated with overweight and type 2 diabetes. Poorly controlled diabetes (either type 1 or 2) may produce severe elevations of plasma triglycerides and should be considered a secondary cause of hypertriglyceridemia. When due to heterozygous lipoprotein lipase deficiency, low HDL is commonly found, and obesity increases the likelihood of expression of hypertriglyceridemia.

DIAGNOSIS: A 12-hour fasting plasma lipid profile is sufficient for diagnosis. A chemistry profile including creatinine, blood urea nitrogen, and liver enzymes is helpful for ruling out secondary causes related to kidney and liver disease. A glucose level (and, if indicated, hemoglobin A_{1C}) is helpful to assess diabetes status. Thyroid-stimulating hormone determination is most useful for screening for hypothyroidism.

TREATMENT

Standard Therapies: Hygienic measures can be very important and include weight loss where indicated, increased exercise, and avoiding saturated fat, alcohol, or excess carbohydrate in the diet (especially sucrose). Oral estrogens can markedly increase plasma triglycerides (through increased VLDL production) and should be changed to a patch or other alternative. Fish (particularly oily fish such as salmon) and fish oil can be helpful (doses of 9–12 g of oil daily are usually required for substantial triglyceride lowering and are more typically used when fasting chylomicronemia is also present). Drug therapy includes fibrates and high-dose niacin. Statin drugs may also lower triglycerides, sometimes substantially.

REFERENCES

Austin MA, McKnight B, Edwards KL, et al. Cardiovascular disease mortality in familial forms of hypertriglyceridemia: a 20-year prospective study. *Circulation* 2000;101:2777–2782.

Gilbert B, Rouis M, Griglio S, de et al. Lipoprotein lipase (LPL) deficiency: a new patient homozygote for the preponderant mutation Gly188Glu in the human LPL gene and review of reported mutations: 75% are clustered in exons 5 and 6. *Ann Genet* 2001;44:25–32.

Hoffer MJ, Sijbrands EJ, De Man FH, et al. Increased risk for endogenous hypertriglyceridaemia is associated with an apolipoprotein C3 haplotype specified by the SstI polymorphism. *Eur J Clin Invest* 1998;28:807–812.

Nordestgaard BG, Abildgaard S, Wittrup HH, et al. Heterozygous lipoprotein lipase deficiency. Frequency in the general population, effect on plasma lipid levels, and risk of ischemic heart disease. *Circulation* 1997;96:1737–1744.

Samuels M, Forbey K, Reid J, et al. Identification of a common variant in the lipoprotein lipase gene in a large Utah kindred ascertained for coronary heart disease: the -93G/D9N variant predisposes to low HDL-C/high triglycerides. *Clin Genet* 2001;59:88–98.

RESOURCES

35, 357

---

42 The Primary Hyperoxalurias

Dawn S. Milliner, MD

DEFINITION: Primary hyperoxaluria is the metabolic overproduction of oxalate by the liver. Two types of primary hyperoxaluria (PH) have been well described: PH I and PH II.

SYMPTOMS AND SIGNS: Patients with PH I most often present clinically with urolithiasis during childhood, adolescence, or early adulthood, although the disease may remain unrecognized until the third or fourth decade of life. As long as renal function is well preserved, the excess oxalate is excreted by the kidney and the primary clinical problem is urolithiasis. With time, progressive damage to kidneys related to parenchymal deposition of calcium oxalate leads to end-stage renal disease. Some patients first come to medical attention due to end-stage renal failure and have no history of urolithiasis. Patients with PH II typically present in the first two decades of life with urolithiasis. Urine oxalate excretion tends to be lower in PH II patients than PH I. Considerable overlap exists between the two PH subtypes in both the amount of oxaluria and in the clinical features.

ETIOLOGY/EPIDEMIOLOGY: Both types of primary hyperoxaluria are autosomal-recessive inborn errors of metabolism. Type I PH is caused by a deficiency of the hepatic enzyme alanine:glyoxylate aminotransferase (AGT). The gene encoding human AGT maps to chromosome 2q36-37. A number of different mutations of the gene, as well as normal polymorphisms, have been recognized. Type II PH occurs much less frequently than PH I and is due to deficiency of hepatic hydroxypyruvate reductase (HPR). The gene encoding HPR has been localized to chromosome 9.

DIAGNOSIS: The diagnosis of PH I is strongly suggested by a urine oxalate excretion rate of greater than 1.2 mmol (105 mg)/1.73 m²/24 hours (normalized to body surface area in children) and an elevated urine glycolate. Oxalate excretion rates may be lower if renal function is significantly reduced. Liver biopsy for AGT enzyme analysis is often required to confirm the diagnosis. DNA analysis for known mutations or by linkage studies can also be diagnostic in PH I, although fewer than 50% of patients with PH I can currently be identified by DNA testing. The diagnosis of PH II is suggested by an elevated urine oxalate, elevated urine glycerate, and normal urine glycolate. The diagnosis can be confirmed by liver biopsy and analysis for HPR enzyme activity.

TREATMENT

Standard Therapies: Of patients with PH I, 20%–30% respond to pharmacologic doses of pyridoxine with a reduction in oxalate production to normal or near normal. High oral fluid intake to maintain a urine volume of 3–6 L daily in adolescents and adults is a mainstay of management in all patients other than those with end-stage renal failure. Neutral phosphate therapy should be considered in patients with adequately preserved renal function. Citrate and magnesium have also been advocated. Dialysis is inefficient for the removal of oxalate, and most dialysis regimens cannot keep pace with daily production. Renal transplantation can restore renal function, although the allograft remains vulnerable to oxalate injury due to persistent hyperoxaluria. Hepatic transplantation can correct the metabolic defect and is appropriate in patients with PH I with irreversible decline in renal function to a level associated with significant hyperoxalemia. Treatment of PH II consists of a high oral fluid intake and, in most patients, neutral phosphate therapy. Oral citrate and/or magnesium may be considered. Stone formation is easier to control, and there appears to be better preservation of renal function over time in patients with PH II when compared with PH I. However, end-stage renal disease can occur in PH II. Renal transplantation has been successful.

REFERENCES

Cochat P, Deloraine A, Rotily M, et al. Epidemiology of primary hyperoxaluria type 1. *Nephrol Dial Transplant* 1995;10:3–7.

Cramer SD, Ferree PM, Lin K, et al. The gene encoding hydroxypyruvate reductase (GRHPR) is mutated in patients with primary hyperoxaluria type II. *Hum Mol Genet* 1999;8:2063–2069.

Danpure CJ, Smith LH. The primary hyperoxalurias. In: Coe FL, Favus MJ, Pak CYC, et al., eds. *Kidney stones: medical and surgical management.* Philadelphia: Lippincott-Raven, 1996: 859–881.

Milliner DS, Eickholt JT, Bergstralh E, et al. Primary hyperoxaluria: results of long-term treatment with orthophosphate and pyridoxine. *N Engl J Med* 1994;331:1553–1558.

Milliner DS, Wilson DM, Smith LH. Phenotypic expression of primary hyperoxaluria: comparative features of types I and II. *Kidney Int* 2001;59:31–36.

RESOURCES

98, 354, 385

---

43 The Congenital Lactic Acidoses

Peter W. Stacpoole, MD, PhD

DEFINITION: The term CLA refers to a group of rare metabolic diseases variably characterized by episodic or persistent lactate accumulation in blood, urine and/or cerebrospinal fluid, invariably by progressive psychomotor deterioration, frequently by multiorgan system failure and, occasionally, by abnormalities of the head and face. (*See also,* Alpers disease; Barth syndrome; Cytochrome oxidase deficiency; Leber hereditary optic neuropathy; MELAS and MERFF syndromes.)

SYNONYMS: Mitochondrial myopathy; Pyruvate dehydrogenase (PDH) complex (PDC) deficiency; Respiratory (electron transport) chain deficiency; Oxidative-phosphorylation deficiency; Pyruvate carboxylase deficiency; Cytochrome oxidase (COX) deficiency: Leigh syndrome: MELAS; MERRF; NARP; Complex I-V deficiency; Kerns-Sayre syndrome; Chronic progressive external ophthalmoplegia: MNGIE; Pearson syndrome.

DIFFERENTIAL DIAGNOSIS: Fatty acid oxidation disorders; Glycogen storage disease; Hypoxic or other acquired causes of lactic acidosis; Other causes of neonatal or infantile psychomotor retardation.

SIGNS AND SYMPTOMS: In general, the major subtypes of CLA, such as those involving pyruvate dehydrogenase deficiency or defects in respiratory chain enzyme complexes, typically exhibit neurobehavioral, neurologic, and motor developmental delay within the first year of life. Some patients, however, particularly those with mutations in mitochondrial DNA, do not present with signs or symptoms until adulthood. Children born with a severe biochemical defect in one of the aforementioned enzymes often have fulminant lactic acidosis with acidemia in the neonatal period. Children born with less severe defects may have only mild to moderate (less than 5 mmol/L) hyperlactatemia or may exhibit normal basal venous lactate levels. Such patients, however, are vulnerable to environmental stresses, such as infection or an asthmatic attack, that may precipitate acute acid-base decompensation and life-threatening lactic acidosis. Patients may have microcephaly and cranial abnormalities due to hydrocephaly. *PDC deficiency* may give rise to a broad clinical spectrum, from overwhelming lactic acidosis in neonates to mild developmental delay or motor impairment that presents in childhood or adolescence. Circulating levels of lactate and pyruvate are increased proportionally and the blood lactate/pyruvate ratio is normal (# 20/1). The concentration of lactate in cerebrospinal fluid tends to be higher than in blood. Defects in *pyruvate carboxylase* may run the clinical gamut from mild lactic acidosis and cognitive defects to severe acidemia, mental retardation and early death. In this condition, the blood lactate/pyruvate ratio is also normal. *Fumarase deficiency*, a rare cause of CLA, has been associated with failure to thrive, developmental delay, hypotonia, lactic acidosis and increased urinary excretion of fumarate, a Krebs cycle intermediate. Other Krebs cycle defects include aconitase, the ketoglutarate dehydrogenase complex and succinate dehydrogenase. In *respiratory chain defects*, typically, lactate accumulation increases disproportionately compared to pyruvate, so that lactate/pyruvate ratio in blood usually exceeds 25/1. As in patients with PDC deficiency, those with respiratory chain defects tend to have cerebrospinal fluid lactate concentrations higher than corresponding blood levels. The onset of clinical manifestations in patients with *Leigh disease* is usually before the age of two years and may include optic atrophy, ophthalmoplegia, nystagmus, respiratory abnormalities, ataxia, hypotonia, spasticity and developmental delay. *Kearns-Sayre syndrome* (KSS) usually manifests before age 20 years with weakness of both extraoccular and limb muscles, atypical retinitis pigmentosa, and, sometimes, cardiac conduction defects. Patients whose symptoms begin after age 20 years are classified as having chronic *progressive external ophthalmoplegia* (CPEO). Both Kearns-Sayre and CPEO affected individuals may also exhibit signs and symptoms of multiple visceral organ dysfunction, including heart, nervous system, liver, lungs and gastrointestinal tract. *Pearson syndrome* often presents in infancy as failure to thrive, intestinal malabsorption, exocrine pancreatic insufficiency, diarrhea and sideroblastic anemia. Affected children may subsequently progress to manifest the Kearns-Sayre syndrome. Multiple organ systems can be affected in CLA, regardless of underlying biochemical defect, but their clinical expression is highly variable and unpredictable. Thus, patients may present with a remarkable array of signs and symptoms in addition to the more classic picture of hypo-

tonia, ataxia, and progressive neurodegeneration. Seizures, diabetes mellitus and other endocrine-deficient states, migraines, early hearing loss, vomiting, diarrhea, constipation, liver failure, blindness, renal tubular acidosis and other signs of renal insufficiency, heart failure, and peripheral neuropathy may be manifested to variable degrees and times in a given patient.

ETIOLOGY/EPIDEMIOLOGY: Limited data imply that CLA occurs in approximately 250–300 live births per year in the U.S., with a prevalence in the U.S. of at least 1,000 cases, but these are probably considerable underestimates. CLA is due to one or more inherited or sporadic mutations in DNA of the nucleus (nDNA) or mitochondria (mtDNA). With the exception of the few cases of CLA due to defects in gluconeogenic enzymes other than pyruvate carboxylase, all the enzyme defects leading to this disease reside in the mitochondria. Deficiency of the *pyruvate dehydrogenase complex* accounts for about 10%-15% of biochemically proven cases of CLA. All defects are due to mutations in nDNA, most frequently involving the E1α component of the complex. The E1α gene is X-linked. Because both males and females are affected clinically, this type of PDC deficiency is classified as X-linked co-dominant, and the effects in females can vary greatly. Most E1α mutations are sporadic. Defects in other components of the PDC are more rare. *Pyruvate carboxylase deficiency* is due to nDNA gene mutations and may also be secondary to defects in biotin metabolism. Deficiencies of enzymes of the tricarboxylic acid (Krebs cycle) may cause CLA, including *fumarase deficiency*. *Respiratory chain defects* are also known as oxidative-phosphorylation (OXPHOS) diseases or electron transport chain (ETC) diseases. They are due to mutations in genes encoding one or more of the five complexes involved in oxidative phosphorylation. As a group, respiratory chain defects constitute the largest collection of known causes of CLA. The defects may be due to nDNA or mtDNA gene mutations that may be inherited or sporadic. Maternal inheritance is the mode of transmission for mtDNA mutations, and these may give rise to deficiencies in complexes I, III, IV or V of the oxidative phosphorylation pathway. nDNA mutations may affect any of the five complexes and may be inherited as Mendelian traits or may occur sporadically. *MELAS* (mitochondrial encephalomyopathy, lactic acidosis and stroke-like episodes) and *MERRF* (myochronic epilepsy and ragged red fiber disease) occur as a result of mutations in mitochondrial transfer RNAs. NARP (neurogenic muscle weakness, ataxia and retinitis pigmentosa) is also due to mtDNA point mutations of a mtDNA encoded subunit of complex V (ATPase). *Leigh syndrome* (subacute necrotizing encephalomyopathy) refers to a set of specific neuropathologic or neuroradiographic findings that are associated with a variety of clinical manifestations and etiologies. Known causes of

Leigh syndrome include defects in pyruvate dehydrogenase, complexes I or IV of the respiratory chain, MERRF, NARP and mtDNA point mutations.

Pearson syndrome is also due to deletions of mtDNA and usually occurs sporadically. Other conditions caused by deletions of mtDNA are Leigh disease, Kearns-Sayre syndrome, and *Leber's hereditary optic neuropathy* (LHON). Other clinical conditions associated with one or more respiratory chain deficiencies include various forms of *mitochondrial myopathy*, *Barth syndrome*, which is an X-linked myopathy involving the cardiac and skeletal musculature, certain other *inherited cardiomyopathies*, and *Alpers disease*.

DIAGNOSIS: In the absence of hypoxia or other acquired causes (e.g., infection), patients who develop severe acidemia shortly after birth should be suspected of having CLA due to a profound deficiency in the activity of the affected enzyme. In patients with less severe defects, circulating lactate levels may be increased episodically or persistently. Cerebrospinal fluid lactate is more frequently elevated than blood lactate and is probably a more sensitive and specific marker of disease status in the central nervous system. The diagnosis is ultimately established on the basis of enzymologic or molecular genetic tests conducted in peripheral blood leukocytes or in biopsy material from skin, skeletal muscle or, occasionally, liver. Neuroimaging studies may be helpful in identifying clinical subsets of CLA and in following disease course, but are not a substitute for biochemical or molecular genetic investigations in establishing a diagnosis. Patients suspected of having CLA should be referred to a tertiary care health center for definitive diagnosis.

TREATMENT
Standard Therapies: There is no generally effective treatment of CLA beyond standard supportive care. Administration of large doses of biotin or thiamine have been successful, respectively, in cases of *biotinidase deficiency* or in extremely rare cases of *pyruvate dehydrogenase deficiency* due to mutations in the E1α gene. Carnitine, thiamine, biotin, lipoate, riboflavin, coenzyme Q or vitamin K plus ascorbate (vitamin C) and tocopherol (vitamin E) have been the most commonly used nutritional agents. Additional pharmacologic therapy is directed toward specific complications of CLA, such as seizures or cardiac failure.

Investigational Therapy: At present, dichloroacetate (DCA) is the only investigational drug that is considered to have the potential to treat a wide variety of causes of CLA.

REFERENCES
DiMauro S, Schon EA. Mitochondrial DNA mutations in human disease. *Am J Med Genetics.* 2001;106:18–26.
Kerr DS, Wexler ID, Zinn AB. Pyruvate metabolism and the tricarbocyclic acid cycle. In: Fernandes J, Saudubray J-M, van der Berghe GV, eds. *Inborn Metabolic Diseases.* 3rd ed. New York: Springer-Verlag; 2000:127–138.
Robinson BH. Lactic acidemia (disorders of pyruvate carboxylase, pyruvate dehydrogenase). In: Scriver CR, Beaudet AL, Sly WS, Valle D, eds. *The Metabolic and Molecular Bases of Inherited Disease.* 8th ed. New York: McGraw-Hill; 2001: 2275–2295.
Stacpoole PW, Barnes CL, Hurbanis MD, Cannon SL, Kerr DS. Treatment of congenital lactic acidosis with dichloroacetate. *Arch Dis Child.* 1997;77:535–541.

RESOURCES
58, 109, 228

44 Lesch-Nyhan Syndrome

Neil R.M. Buist, MB, ChB, DCH, and Susan C. Winter, MD, FAAP, FCMG

DEFINITION: Lesch-Nyhan syndrome is an X-linked disorder of purine metabolism caused by a severe deficiency of hypoxanthine-guanine phosphoribosyl transferase (HGPRT) activity. Severe choreoathetosis, with or without self-mutilating behavior, is associated with hyperuricemia.

SYNONYMS: Severe HGPRT deficiency with choreoathetosis; HPRT deficiency; HGPRT deficiency.

DIFFERENTIAL DIAGNOSIS: Severe choreoathetosis from any other hereditary or acquired cause including cerebral palsy and other self-mutilating conditions. These include, but are not limited to, athetoid cerebral palsy, postkernicterus, ischemic or toxic damage to the basal ganglia, and glutaric aciduria type I.

SYMPTOMS AND SIGNS: Infants may appear normal or irritable with delayed motor development. Urinary urates can cause faint orange staining of diapers. At approximately 1 year, choreoathetosis with concomitant motor delay becomes evident. Within 2–3 years, severe choreoathetosis with extreme difficulties of coordination and speech is established. More than 80% of patients exhibit uncontrollable self-abusive behavior, including biting lips, tongue, limbs, and digits; they may also exhibit similar behavior toward others. Most patients are believed to be mentally retarded because of their extraordinary difficulty with communication and movement; however, affected individuals can have normal intellect. Renal stones are frequent and recurrent because of massive excretion of purines.

ETIOLOGY/EPIDEMIOLOGY: Lesch-Nyhan syndrome is an X-linked, recessively inherited disorder caused by a severe mutation of the HGPRT gene (Xq26-q27.2). Less severe mutations of HGPRT are common and cause hyperuricemia in adults with its attendant complications.

DIAGNOSIS: The blood uric acid level is always elevated but may be scarcely above the upper limits of normal. Enzyme assay in red blood cell or cultured skin fibroblasts is confirmatory. Prenatal diagnosis by chorionic villus sampling or amniocentesis is routine, and DNA analysis for family and carrier testing is sometimes informative. The new mutation rate is believed to be approximately 30% of cases and there are many private mutations.

TREATMENT
Standard Therapies: Standard therapy includes allopurinol to normalize the blood uric acid levels. This drug has no effect on the neurologic manifestations, and xanthine/urate renal stones still develop. Fluid intake should be as high as possible to keep the urine dilute, and urine pH should be maintained above 7 with bicarbonate. Extra-ordinary efforts are required for education and home management. Special feeding devices and communication boards are helpful. Muscle relaxants such as baclofen or benzodiazepines and antidepressants can be helpful for older patients. Wheelchairs must be fitted with limb restraints for use only when requested or needed to prevent self-mutilation. Dental obturators or extraction of teeth may be needed to control self- mutilation. Later complications caused by uric acid accumulation include renal stones, renal failure, gouty arthritis, or arthropathy; the dystonia can lead to severe arthropathy.

Investigational Therapies: Controlling the dystonia by medications or stereotactic surgery is being explored.

REFERENCES
Gilbert-Barness E, Barness LA. *Metabolic diseases, foundations of clinical management, genetics, and pathology.* Natick, MA: Eaton Publishing, 2000.
McKusick VA, ed. Online Mendelian Inheritance in Man, OMIM [database online]. Bethesda, MD: National Center for Biotechnology Information, National Library of Medicine, 2000. MIM# 308000.
Scriver CR, Beaudet AL, Sly WS, et al., eds. *The metabolic and molecular bases of inherited disease,* 8th ed. New York: McGraw-Hill, 2001.

RESOURCES
58, 238, 239

45 Familial Lipoprotein Lipase Deficiency

Pierre N.M. Demacker, PhD, and Anton F.H. Stalenhoef, MD, PhD

DEFINITION: Lipoprotein lipase (LPL) deficiency is a disorder characterized by massive accumulation of chylomicrons in the plasma, resulting in a milky appearance.

SYNONYMS: Familial chylomicronemia syndrome; Type I hyperlipoproteinemia.

DIFFERENTIAL DIAGNOSIS: Type V hyperlipoproteinemia; Hyperchylomicronemia due to apolipoprotein C-II deficiency.

SYMPTOMS AND SIGNS: Milky plasma is a characteristic feature. Diagnosis is usually made when the patient is younger than 10, based on problems with breast-feeding while an infant, repeated episodes of abdominal pain, recurrent attacks of pancreatitis, eruptive cutaneous xanthomas over the elbows, knees, and buttocks, hepatosplenomegaly, and lipemia retinalis. Improvement is rapid on complete restriction of fat intake.

ETIOLOGY/EPIDEMIOLOGY: The LPL enzyme is bound to the endothelial surface along the capillary endothelium in muscle and adipose tissue. Absence of this enzyme or its cofactor causes disturbed clearance of triglycerides from circulation. Familial lipoprotein lipase deficiency is an autosomal-recessive disorder. Heterozygotes show a 50% reduction in normal lipoprotein lipase activity, although their triglyceride levels are normal or slightly elevated. Numerous mutations have been detected in the LPL gene. Untreated diabetes or excessive use of alcohol induces another form of hyperchylomicronemia (type V hyperlipidemia), particularly in the presence of a mutation in one of the alleles of the LPL gene. In type V, very-low-density lipoprotein concentrations are also increased.

DIAGNOSIS: Along with the clinical characteristics, milky plasma and sensitivity to the amount of fat in the diet are typical. Whole blood shows white layers of fat. Plasma after refrigeration for 24–48 hours, or after centrifugation of the hematocrit blood cells, shows a broad white layer at the meniscus, usually above clear plasma. Plasma triglycerides at first visit usually exceed 50 mM. The excess lipids in the plasma interfere in several clinical chemistry methods due to the volume or to the turbidity of the fat layer. Intraveneously injected heparin (50–100 IE/kg body weight) releases LPL from endothelial tissues. Blood taken at 15 minutes after injection is measured for lipase activity using a triglyceride-rich emulsion, after precipitation of hepatic lipase.

TREATMENT
Standard Therapies: The only method of treatment is limiting the total amount of fat in the patient's diet. Alcohol and drugs that increase triglyceride synthesis (oral contraceptives) should be avoided. Drugs are not effective in decreasing chylomicronemia. Patients usually learn to avoid food containing fat. To be pain free, however, they often need to restrict their dietary fat intake severely, to approximately 0.5 g/kg body weight. Many patients have been successfully treated by a diet rich in medium-chain fatty acids.

REFERENCE
Brunzell JD. Familial lipoprotein lipase deficiency and other causes of the chylomicronemia syndrome. In: Scriver CR, Beaudet AL, Sly WS, et al., eds. *The metabolic base of inherited disease.* Vol. 2. New York: McGraw-Hill, 1995:1913–1927.

RESOURCES
109, 354

46   Lowe Syndrome

Richard A. Lewis MD, MS

DEFINITION: Lowe syndrome is an X-linked disorder characterized by congenital cataract, muscular hypotonia, areflexia, severe psychomotor retardation, vitamin D–resistant rickets, and renal tubular acidosis and aminoaciduria.

SYNONYMS: Oculo-cerebro-renal syndrome of Lowe; OCRL1.

DIFFERENTIAL DIAGNOSIS: Renal tubular syndrome, Fanconi type; Zellweger cerebrohepatorenal syndrome.

SYMPTOMS AND SIGNS: Males with Lowe syndrome are born with bilateral dense congenital cataracts; half of them have at birth or develop (usually within the first year) infantile glaucoma, with or without buphthalmos and secondary corneal clouding. Patients manifest severe psychomotor retardation (mean IQ in the moderate to severe range), failure to thrive and growth retardation after the first year, a shrill high-pitched cry, muscular hypotonia, reduced deep tendon reflexes, and renal tubular aminoaciduria, although not necessarily present until age 2 years. Secondary features include frontal bossing and prominent forehead, thin hair, adiposity in the first year with wasting later, and cryptorchidism. Metabolic acidosis with hypophosphatemia and hyperphosphaturia, carnitine wast-

ing, and generalized aminoaciduria are seen usually after age 1 year. Bone fractures occur in one third and rickets in one half of patients, probably due to complications of weakened bone structure from the metabolic disease. Maladaptive behaviors may occur, ranging from temper tantrums, to stubbornness and irritability, to stereotypy and mannerisms, to negativism.

ETIOLOGY/EPIDEMIOLOGY: Lowe syndrome is an X-linked disorder mapped to Xq25-q26.1. The gene *OCRL1* spans 58 kb of genomic sequence and is composed of 24 exons and encodes an enzyme phosphatidylinositol 4,5 bisphosphate 5-phosphatase.

DIAGNOSIS: Males are diagnosed by the presence of congenital cataracts (and also infantile glaucoma) and the clinical appearance of distinctive facies, cryptorchidism, and aminoaciduria. Either the deficiency of the OCRL enzyme or direct DNA mutational analysis of *OCRL1* confirms the clinical impression. Female carriers for OCRL have a distinctive, characteristic appearance in the lens, typically present after puberty (although it may be present earlier).

TREATMENT
Standard Therapies: Cataract surgery as early in life as feasible will optimize visual function, but most children maintain nystagmus and reduced acuity. Patients should be

monitored for glaucoma and a 'keloidlike' corneal degeneration. Seizures occur in approximately one half of boys with Lowe syndrome. Behavior modification may moderate the stereotypy and negativism. Hypotonia may influence motor milestones and scoliosis and thus require physical therapy and bracing. Renal tubular acidosis requires replacement of bicarbonate, L-carnitine, potassium, and phosphate. Supplemental citrate and vitamin D metabolite may reduce the risk of kidney stones.

REFERENCES

Attree O, Olivos IM, Okabe I, et al. The Lowe oculocerebrorenal syndrome gene encodes a novel protein highly homologous to inositol polyphosphate-5-phosphatase. *Nature* 1992;358: 239–242.

Lin T, Lewis RA, Nussbaum RL. Molecular confirmation of carriers for Lowe syndrome. *Ophthalmology* 1999;106:119–122.

Lin T, Orrison BM, Suchy SF, et al. Mutations are not uniformly distributed throughout the *OCRL1* gene in Lowe syndrome patients. *Mol Genet Metab* 1998;64:58–61.

Lowe CU, Terry M, MacLachan EA. Organic aciduria, decreased renal ammonia production, hydrophthalmos, and mental retardation: a clinical entity. *Am J Dis Child* 1952;83:164–184.

Lowe Mutational Database. *www.nhgri.nih.gov/DIR/GDRB/Lowe.*

McKusick VA, ed. Online Mendelian Inheritance in Man, OMIM [database online]. Bethesda, MD: National Center for Biotechnology Information, National Library of Medicine, 2000. Entry no. 309000; last update March 5, 2001.

Suchy SF, Olivos-Glander IM, Nussbaum RL. Lowe syndrome, a deficiency of a phosphatidylinositol 4,5-bis-phosphate 5-phosphatase in the Golgi apparatus. *Hum Mol Genet* 1995; 4:2245–2250.

RESOURCES

249, 358, 462

---

47 Alpha-Mannosidosis

Dag Malm, MD, PhD

DEFINITION: Alpha-mannosidosis is an inborn disorder that results in mental retardation, skeletal changes, hearing loss, and recurrent infections.

DIFFERENTIAL DIAGNOSIS: Other lysosomal storage diseases, e.g., aspartylglucosaminuria; Beta-mannosidosis.

SYMPTOMS AND SIGNS: Mannosidosis belongs to the group of lysosomal storage diseases. It encompasses a continuum of clinical findings from an early lethal form to less symptomatic forms initially diagnosed in juveniles. The more severe types cause early death, mainly due to infections, whereas other types are characterized in juveniles by the presence of mild to moderate mental retardation, reduced hearing, characteristic coarse features, immunodeficiency, clinical or radiographic skeletal abnormalities, and the presence of primary central nervous system disease, mainly in the cerebellum, causing ataxia. The onset of mannosidosis is usually before age 2, probably even at birth. In some subjects, the course of alpha-mannosidosis is insidiously progressive, and patients live into the sixth decade. The condition is frequently associated with corneal opacities, aseptic destructive arthritis, and metabolic myopathy.

ETIOLOGY/EPIDEMIOLOGY: The condition is caused by mutation in or in the vicinity of the alpha-mannosidase gene. The human lysosomal alpha-mannosidase enzyme (MANB; LAMAN) has been biochemically characterized and the gene cloned and sequenced. Polymerase chain reaction–based strategies have been developed to detect known mutations. The incidence is approximately 1 in 250,000 live births. It is seen in both sexes.

DIAGNOSIS: Alpha-mannosidosis should be suspected in individuals with mental retardation, hearing deficiency, ataxia, skeletal abnormalities, and coarse features. Detection of vacuoles in lymphocytes and/or mannose-rich sugars in urine should heighten the suspicion, but the finding is not specific for the disease. The diagnosis of alpha-mannosidosis relies on demonstration of deficient MANB (LAMAN) enzyme activity in peripheral blood leukocytes or other nucleated cells such as fibroblasts. If the familial mutation is known, genetic testing can be performed.

TREATMENT

Standard Therapies: Medical measures include the following: treatment of infections with antibiotics if necessary; detection and treatment of infections/accumulation of fluid in the middle ear; treatment of hearing deficiency early with hearing devices; adaptation of glasses to improve vision; physiotherapy with muscle training avoiding stress upon the joints; and adaptation of wheelchair if necessary. Orthopedic surgery should be performed with caution because of osteoporosis and poor healing of bone. Educational/social measures include: learning sign languages when the reduced hearing cannot be compensated; kindergarten for development of social skills; speech therapy; specialist teachers to maximize learning; and planning for a possible future with a wheelchair.

Investigational Therapies: The effectiveness of bone marrow transplantation is being evaluated, but if performed, it is important that it be done as early as possible.

REFERENCES

Berg T, et al. Spectrum of mutations in alpha-mannosidosis. *Am J Hum Genet* 1999;64:77–88.

Nilssen O, et al. α-Mannosidosis: functional cloning of the lysosomal α-mannosidase cDNA and identification of a mutation in two affected siblings. *Hum Mol Genet* 1997; 6:717–726.

Riise HMF, et al. Genomic structure of the human lysosomal alpha-mannosidase gene (MANB). *Genomics* 1997;42:200–207.

Tollersrud OK, et al. Purification of bovine lysosomal alpha-mannosidase, characterization of its gene and determination of two mutations that cause alpha-mannosidosis. *Eur J Biochem* 1997;246:410–419.

Wall DA, et al. Bone marrow transplantation for the treatment of alpha-mannosidosis. *J Pediatr* 1998;133:282–285.

RESOURCES

255, 314, 354

---

48 Maple Syrup Urine Disease

Dean J. Danner, PhD

DEFINITION: Maple syrup urine disease (MSUD) is an inborn error of metabolism that results from the inability of the branched chain amino acids (BCAAs)—leucine, isoleucine, and valine—to undergo catabolism. The branched chain amino and the transaminated ketoacids accumulate in the cells and fluids of the body.

SYNONYM: Branched chain ketoacidemia.

DIFFERENTIAL DIAGNOSIS: Dihydrolipoamide dehydrogenase deficiency; Hypervalinemia; Hyperleucine; Isoleucinemia; Organic aciduria.

SYMPTOMS AND SIGNS: Newborns usually present with failure to thrive, lethargy, poor sucking response, and coma. A sweet odor in cerumen and body fluids, especially urine, akin to maple syrup or burnt coffee is present. Laboratory tests show elevated ketoacids in urine, and plasma BCAAs along with alloisoleucine are elevated. Abnormal neurologic responses may be found, but no characteristics specific to the disease are known. Brain edema can occur at different sites with each episode of metabolic decompensation. Infections that cause cellular protein degradation, or lapse in diet restrictions with increased protein intake, can cause the aforementioned complications.

ETIOLOGY/EPIDEMIOLOGY: The disorder is inherited as an autosomal-recessive trait. It is reported to occur in all racial and ethnic groups with an equal distribution among females and males. In the overall population, the frequency is 1 in 185,000 live births. In the Old World Mennonites in the United States, the incidence is 1 in 176. Inbreeding also has raised the incidence in regions of the Middle East. The catalytic activity of the branched chain α-ketoacid dehydrogenase complex is contained in the protein products of four genes each located on a different chromosome in the nucleus. Mutations in any of three of these genes can result in the clinical phenotype specific for MSUD.

DIAGNOSIS: Newborn screening programs have been used to identify individuals at risk for MSUD by assessment of plasma leucine concentrations. Many clinicians use the Guthrie test of bacterial growth rings; these need to be confirmed with high-performance liquid chromatography or ion exchange amino acid analysis. With the advent of tandem mass spectrometry in newborn screening, more accurate quantitation is possible on the initial sample. When newborn screening is not available or the screening process does not detect MSUD, suspicion is raised that the individual is affected by episodes of vomiting, lethargy, seizures, failure to thrive, or by the unusual odor. Diagnostic procedure should include urine analysis for ketoacidosis using dinitrophenyl hydrazine and a complete plasma amino acid profile. True confirmation is made by enzyme assay on peripheral lymphocytes or on cells cultured from the individual's skin.

TREATMENT

Standard Therapies: Treatment must be considered in two aspects: acute care in crisis and continued care throughout life. With acute care of the newborn or when metabolic decompensation occurs at any time, the main objective is to rapidly reduce the plasma leucine concentration. Several methods have been used, including various forms of dialysis. Most centers prefer a nasogastric or intravenous administration of a total parenteral nutrition solution devoid of BCAA. Lifetime treatment consists of a protein-modified diet used to maintain the plasma BCAA concentrations within normal limits.

Investigative Therapies: Gene therapy is being explored. Studies are being developed to better understand the neurologic consequences of the genetic mutations and the use of special diets.

REFERENCES

Chuang DT, Shih VE. Maple syrup urine disease. In: Scriver CR, Beaudet AL, Sly WS, et al., eds. *The metabolic and molecular bases of inherited disease*, 8th ed. New York: McGraw-Hill, 2001:1971–2005.

Danner DJ, Doering CB. Human mutations affecting branched chain α-ketoacid dehydrogenase. *Front Biosci* 1998;3:517–524.

Menkes JH, Hurst PL, Craig JM. A new syndrome: progressive familial infantile cerebral dysfunction associated with unusual urinary substance. *Pediatrics* 1954;14:462–467.

Nellis MM, Danner DJ. Gene preference in maple syrup urine disease. *Am J Hum Genet* 2001;68:232–237.

RESOURCES

58, 256, 354

---

49 MELAS and MERRF

*Petra Kaufmann, MD,
John M. Shoffner, MD,
Kris Engelstad, BS, and
Darryl C. De Vivo, MD*

DEFINITION: MELAS (mitochondrial encephalomyopathy, lactic acidosis, and strokelike episodes) and MERRF (myoclonus epilepsy and ragged red fibers) are clinical syndromes that have been associated with mitochondrial DNA point mutations. They are multisystem disorders that adversely affect many organs, particularly the nervous system and muscle.

SYNONYM: Mitochondrial encephalopathies.

DIFFERENTIAL DIAGNOSIS: For MELAS: Sickle cell anemia; Heart defects; Coagulopathies; Moyamoya disease; Lipoprotein disorders; Cancer; Venous thrombosis; Homocystinuria; CADASIL; Carotid or vertebral artery disease. For MERRF: Unverricht-Lundborg disease; Lafora body disease; Neuronal ceroid lipofuscinosis; Sialidosis; Ramsay Hunt syndrome; Dentatorubral-pallidolysian atrophy.

SYMPTOMS AND SIGNS: MELAS is a multisystem disorder defined by the following features: mitochondrial encephalopathy evident as dementia or seizures; lactic acidosis as manifestation of the respiratory chain defect; and strokelike episodes at a young age. Also, patients often experience migraine-like headaches, recurrent vomiting, gastrointestinal symptoms, exercise intolerance, muscle weakness, neuropathy, ataxia, short stature, and hearing loss. MERRF is a clinical syndrome characterized by myoclonus epilepsy and other seizure types and ragged red fibers as manifestation of the respiratory chain defect. Ataxia and neuropathy are common. Short stature, hearing loss, mild cognitive difficulties, and depression are also common. Occasionally, patients have multiple lipomas or hypoparathyroidism. Migraines are characteristic. Mild behavioral and cognitive deficits are present. Mean age of onset is 24 years.

ETIOLOGY/EPIDEMIOLOGY: MELAS and MERRF are maternally inherited. MELAS is commonly associated with an A-to-G transition at nucleotide 3243 within the mitochondrial DNA, less commonly with other mitochondrial DNA point mutations. MERRF is commonly associated with an A-to-G transition at nucleotide 8344, less commonly with a T-to-C transition at nucleotide 8356. The prevalence of MELAS and MERRF is difficult to estimate because of the clinical variability. The point prevalence of mitochondrial encephalomyopathies in children younger than 16 years was estimated as 1 in 21,000 in one study. The frequency of the 3243 mitochondrial point mutation was calculated to be greater than 16 in 100,000 in another study.

DIAGNOSIS: Diagnosis of MELAS or MERRF is made based on the clinical picture and, often, family history. Physical examination may show pigmentary changes of the retina or subtle signs of peripheral neuropathy. Laboratory tests include blood lactate and pyruvate. Neuroimaging in MELAS often shows fluctuating, predominantly occipital lesions. Basal ganglia calcification and diffuse cerebral atrophy are seen in MELAS and MERRF. Genetic testing of DNA extracted from blood leukocytes, fibroblasts, urine sediment, hair follicles, or muscle tissue can confirm the genetic diagnosis. Muscle biopsy specimens morphologically often show ragged red fibers, the histologic hallmark of mitochondrial dysfunction.

TREATMENT

Standard Therapies: There is no cure for either MELAS or MERRF. Symptomatic treatment of seizures with antiepileptic medications and of glucose and thyroid abnormalities with the appropriate medical measures is indicated. To attempt to improve the primary metabolic defect, a vitamin cocktail of coenzyme Q 10, L-carnitine, and alpha lipoic acid is recommended.

Investigational Therapies: Dichloroacetate is being investigated in patients with MELAS.

REFERENCES

De Vivo DC, Jackson AH, Wade C, et al. Dichloroacetate treatment of MELAS-associated lactic acidosis. *Ann Neurol* 1990;28:437.

Hirano M, Pavlakis SG. Mitochondrial myopathy, enecephalopathy, lactic acidosis, and strokelike episodes (MELAS): current concepts. *J Child Neurol* 1994;9:4–13.

Pavlakis SG, Phillips PC, DiMauro S, et al. Mitochondrial myopathy, encephalopathy, lactic acidosis, and stroke-like episodes: a distinctive clinical syndrome. *Ann Neurol* 1984;16:481–488.

Shoffner JM, Lott MT, Lezza A, et al. Myoclonic epilepsy and ragged-red fiber disease (MERRF) is associated with a mitochondrial DNA tRNALys mutation. *Cell* 1990;61:1213–1217.

RESOURCES

109, 265, 368, 478

---

50   Menkes Disease

John H. Menkes, MD

DEFINITION: Menkes disease is an X-linked multifocal degenerative disease of cerebral gray matter marked by reduced serum copper and ceruloplasmin, and caused by a defect in a copper-transporting P-type adenosine triphosphatase. The disease is characterized by developmental delay and deterioration, seizures, and colorless, friable hair. The severity of clinical expression of Menkes disease varies considerably.

SYNONYMS: Kinky hair disease; Trichopoliodystrophy.

DIFFERENTIAL DIAGNOSIS: Pollitt syndrome; Biotin deficiency; Argininosuccinic aciduria; Trichothiodystrophy; Battered child syndrome.

SYMPTOMS AND SIGNS: Menkes disease is considerably variable in the severity of its clinical expression. In the neonatal period, infants present with hypothermia, hypoglycemia, and impaired weight gain. When the disease becomes apparent later in life, the most common initial symptoms are seizures, delayed development, and hypotonia. The face has a cherubic appearance with a depressed nasal bridge, ptosis, and reduced facial movements. The hair is colorless and friable. The most common abnormality of hair (30%–50% of scalp hair) is pili torti, a hair shaft that is flattened and twisted on its own axis. The optic discs are pale; hydronephrosis and hydroureter, osteoporosis, metaphyseal spurring, and a diaphyseal periosteal reaction occur. Subdural effusions are common. Electroencephalography and visual evoked potentials are severely abnormal. Heterozygotes are mostly asymptomatic.

ETIOLOGY/EPIDEMIOLOGY: The frequency of occurrence is 0.8–2 per 100,000 live male births. The gene for Menkes disease is located on the long arm of the X chromosome (Xq13). It encodes for a copper-transporting ATPase. The gene product is a metal-binding protein with considerable structural similarity to the protein produced by the Wilson disease gene. Numerous mutations have been described, and nearly every family has its private mutation.

DIAGNOSIS: The clinical history of developmental arrest or regression, hypotonia and seizures, and the unusual hair should suggest the diagnosis. Reduced levels of serum ceruloplasmin and copper confirm the diagnosis. Copper levels in cord blood and during the neonatal period can be normal or higher than normal. The prenatal diagnosis is based on the increased copper content of cultured amniocytes and chorionic villus samples.

TREATMENT

Standard Therapies: Treatment with copper histidine has been used at several medical centers. Because of the clinical variability of the disease, its effectiveness has not been verified.

REFERENCES

Danks DM, Campbell PE, Stevens BJ, et al. Menkes' kinky hair syndrome: an inherited defect in copper absorption with widespread effects. *Pediatrics* 1972;50:188–201.

Kaler SG. Menkes disease. *Adv Pediatr* 1994;41:263–304.

McKusick VA, ed. Online Mendelian Inheritance in Man (OMIM) [database online]. Bethesda, MD: National Center for Biotechnology Information, National Library of Medicine, 2000. Entry no. 309400; last update April 29, 2002.

Menkes JH. Menkes disease and Wilson disease: two sides of the same copper coin. *Eur J Paediatr Neurol* 1999;3:147–158.

Menkes JH, Alter M, Weakley D, et al. A sex-linked recessive disorder with growth retardation, peculiar hair, and focal cerebral and cerebellar degeneration. *Pediatrics* 1962;29:764–779.

Vulpe C, Levinson B, Whitney S, et al. Isolation of a candidate gene for Menkes disease and evidence that it encodes a copper-transporting ATPase. *Nat Genet* 1993;3:7–13.

RESOURCES

262, 368

51 Methylmalonate Semialdehyde Dehydrogenase Deficiency

*K. Michael Gibson, PhD,
and Kenneth L. Chambliss, MD, PhD*

DEFINITION: Methylmalonate semialdehyde dehydrogenase (MMSDH) deficiency is an autosomal-recessive disorder affecting the catabolism of L-valine, one of the branched chain amino acids. The index and only confirmed patient was asymptomatic, except for persistent elevation of blood methionine and urine 3-hydroxyisobutyric acid.

SYNONYMS: 3-hydroxyisobutyric aciduria; Hypermethioninemia; Combined semialdehyde dehydrogenase deficiency.

DIFFERENTIAL DIAGNOSIS: 3-hydroxyisobutyric aciduria; Idiopathic hypermethioninemia.

SYMPTOMS AND SIGNS: No clinical symptoms may exist. The index patient was found to have isolated and persistent hypermethioninemia upon routine newborn screening. Follow-up analysis included urine organic acids, which showed a number of abnormalities, including elevation of urine 3-hydroxyisobutyric, 3-hydroxypropionic, 3-aminoisobutyric, and 2-(hydroxymethyl) butyric acids, as well as elevation of blood beta-alanine. A sibling of the patient also manifested persistent hypermethioninemia but none of the associated organic aciduria; thus, the hypermethioninemia was believed to be unrelated to the organic aciduria.

ETIOLOGY/EPIDEMIOLOGY: Only a single male patient with this urine organic aciduria pattern has been described. The pattern of metabolites strongly suggests a

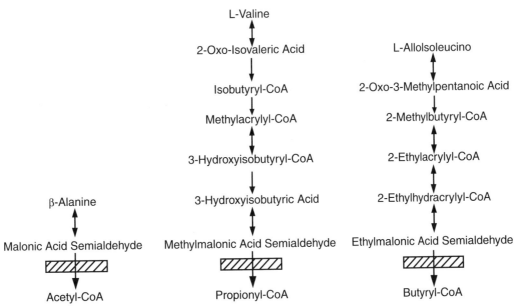

FIGURE 10.1 Catabolic pathways for B-alanine, L-valine, and t-alloisoleucine. Cross-hatched boxes indicate the site of potential combined enzyme deficiency in a patient with 3-hydroxyisobutyric and 2-ethylhydracrylic aciduria. *CoA*, coenzyme A. (Reprinted from *J Inherit Metab Dis* 1993;16:563–597; with permission.)

combined deficiency of the semialdehyde dehydrogenase enzymes acting on malonic, methylmalonic, and ethylmalonic semialdehyde (on the beta-alanine, L-valine, and L-alloisoleucine catabolic pathways, respectively).

DIAGNOSIS: The primary approach to clinical diagnosis is difficult, because the index patient did not manifest symptoms. Routine blood amino acid analysis and urine organic acid analyses should suffice to identify the abnormal metabolite patterns. Enzymatic diagnosis requires specific synthesis of highly unstable semialdehyde substrates. Instead, fibroblasts from suspected patients can be incubated with the appropriately radiolabeled precursors (beta-alanine and L-valine) and the evolution of radiolabeled carbon dioxide quantified. Confirmation has been achieved by identification of a disease-associated mutation in the MMSDH gene obtained from fibroblasts of the proband.

TREATMENT
Standard Therapies: Beyond the potential for L-carnitine intervention or mild protein restriction, no therapeutic intervention is required.

REFERENCES
Chambliss KL, Gray RGF, Rylance G, et al. Molecular characterization of methylmalonate semialdehyde dehydrogenase deficiency. *J Inherit Metab Dis* 2000;23:497–504.
Gibson KM, Lee CF, Bennett MJ, et al. Combined malonic, methylmalonic and ethylmalonic acid semialdehyde dehydrogenase deficiencies: an inborn error of beta-alanine, L-valine and L-alloisoleucine metabolism? *J Inherit Metab Dis* 1993;16:563–567.
Pollitt RJ, Green A, Smith R. Excessive excretion of beta-alanine and of 3-hydroxypropionic, *R*- and *S*-3-aminoisobutyric, *R*- and *S*-3-hydroxyisobutyric and *S*-2-(hydroxymethyl) butyric acids probably due to a defect in the metabolism of the corresponding malonic semialdehydes. *J Inherit Metab Dis* 1985;8:75–79.
Roe CR, Struys E, Kok RM, et al. Methylmalonic semialdehyde dehydrogenase deficiency: psychomotor delay and methylmalonic aciduria without metabolic decompensation. *Mol Genet Metab* 1998;65:35–43.

RESOURCES
354, 403

52 Mucolipidosis II and III

*Joseph Muenzer, MD, PhD,
and Barbara Wedehase, LCSW, CGC*

DEFINITION: Mucolipidosis II (I-cell disease; ML II) and mucolipidosis III (psuedo-Hurler polydystrophy; ML III) are genetic disorders caused by abnormal lysosomal enzyme trafficking. The enzyme UDP-N-acetylglucosamine-1-phosphotransferase, which is involved in the synthesis of the recognition marker mannose-6-phosphate, is defective, resulting in decreased intracellular lysosomal enzyme levels and increased levels in serum and body fluid.

DIFFERENTIAL DIAGNOSIS: Hurler syndrome; Hunter syndrome; Maroteaux-Lamy syndrome.

SYMPTOMS AND SIGNS: Infants with ML II usually have coarse facial features and restricted joint movement, and develop severe developmental delays. Gingival hyperplasia, skeletal abnormalities (kyphoscoliosis, lumbar gibbus), hepatomegaly, umbilical and inguinal hernias, deafness, and delayed growth are also seen. Linear growth slows during the first year, and optimal growth is generally obtained by age 2 years. Corneal clouding and cardiac

murmurs are commonly observed and respiratory infections frequently found. Noisy breathing with snoring and sleep apnea are also commonly reported. Death usually occurs in early childhood, although some patients survive into their teens. Children with ML III typically do not show features of the disorder until ages 2–4 years and may survive into adulthood. Stiffness of the hands and shoulders may be an early feature, with later development of carpal tunnel syndrome, deterioration of hip joints, scoliosis, and short stature. Corneal clouding and cardiac insufficiency are uncommon. Almost 50% of individuals with ML III have learning disabilities or mental retardation.

ETIOLOGY/EPIDEMIOLOGY: ML II and III are inherited in an autosomal-recessive manner. The disease is caused by a mutation in the UDP-N-acetylglucosamine-1-phosphotransferase gene that is located on chromosome 4q21-q23. The prevalence of ML II and III is unknown because both are often misdiagnosed. They occur in all ethnic groups and both males and females are affected. One estimate of prevalence is 1 in 1 million births, although in the French-Canadian population in a region of Quebec, the estimated prevalence of ML II is 1 in 6,000 births, most likely due to a founder effect.

DIAGNOSIS: Diagnosis of ML II and III is made on the basis of finding elevated lysosomal enzyme activity in serum or decreased enzyme levels in white blood cells or cultured fibroblasts. ML II and III cannot be differentiated by measurement of lysosomal enzymes because enzyme activity is similar in both disorders; thus, diagnosis is based on clinical presentation. Prenatal diagnosis can be made by measuring lysosomal enzyme activity in cultured amniotic cells or chorionic villus material.

TREATMENT

Standard Therapies: There is no definitive treatment. Treatment of respiratory infections with antibiotics and yearly flu shots is important. Physical therapy is encouraged to maintain joint function and mobility as long as possible. Total hip replacement has been most effective in post-pubertal individuals with ML III. Hearing aids tend to be underused, affecting the individual's ability to learn and communicate. Sleep studies can determine the degree of obstructive sleep apnea, and nighttime continuous positive airway pressure or bilevel positive airway pressure can open the airway. Intubation may be difficult because of a narrow trachea and may require placement with a flexible broncho-scope. Injury to the spinal cord can occur from repositioning of the neck during anesthesia, or intubation and difficulty with extubation may result in a tracheostomy.

Investigational Therapies: Bone marrow transplantation was tried in 2 patients with ML II, but the response was limited.

REFERENCES

Beck M, Barone R, Hoffmann R, et al. Inter- and intrafamilial variability in mucolipidosis II (I-cell disease). *Clin Genet* 1995; 47:191–200.

Kelly TE, Thomas GH, Taylor HA, et al. Mucolipidosis III (pseudo-Hurler polydystrophy): clinical and laboratory studies in series of 12 patients. *Johns Hopkins Med J* 1975;137: 156–175.

Kornfeld S, Sly WS. I-cell and pseudo-Hurler polydystrophy: disorders of lysosomal enzyme phosphorylation and localization. In: Scriver CR, Beaudet AL, Sly WS, et al., eds. *The metabolic and molecular bases of inherited disease*, 7th ed. New York: McGraw-Hill, 1995:2495–2508.

RESOURCES

109, 314, 354, 440

---

53 Mucolipidosis IV

Gregory M. Pastores, MD

DEFINITION: The term *mucolipidosis* is used to refer to a heterogeneous group of at least four disorders associated with distinct enzyme/protein deficiencies. Mucolipidosis IV (ML IV) is a neurodegenerative lysosomal storage disorder with onset in the first decade of life.

DIFFERENTIAL DIAGNOSIS: Other disorders associated with corneal clouding; Mucopolysaccharidoses; GM1 gangliosidoses; Sialidosis; I-cell disease; Pseudo-Hurler polydystrophy.

SYMPTOMS AND SIGNS: Characteristic clinical features include psychomotor retardation with minimal expressive language development. Although initially associated with hypotonia (evidenced by poor head control), affected children eventually develop spasticity (especially in the legs with scissoring and tight heel cords). Additional signs include ophthalmologic abnormalities, such as corneal clouding, retinal degeneration, strabismus, and nystagmus.

ETIOLOGY/EPIDEMIOLOGY: The disorder is inherited in an autosomal-recessive fashion. Individuals of Ashkenazi Jewish ancestry account for more than 80% of cases, which has been attributed to a founder effect. The disease gene has been mapped to the short arm of chromosome 19 (p13.2–13.3), and various causal mutations in a novel gene named mucolipin (*MCOL1*) have been described. Investigations of heterozygote frequency among the Ashkenazi Jewish population indicate an estimated 1 in 100–127 individuals are carriers.

DIAGNOSIS: Familiarity with the clinical features, and in certain cases the presence of a positive family history (particularly among individuals of Ashkenazi Jewish ancestry) should prompt consideration of the diagnosis. Mutation analysis enables confirmation of the clinical diagnosis, reliable carrier detection, appropriate genetic counseling, and rapid, accurate prenatal diagnosis in families at risk. Histologic studies show the presence of heterogeneous lysosomal storage of laminated membranous material and granular, amorphous vacuoles in neurons, axons, and other cell types. Normal enzyme activity for certain lysosomal storage disorders should exclude sialidosis, I-cell disease, and pseudo-Hurler polydystrophy, which are associated with other features not evident in patients with ML IV. Biochemical analyses show increased gangliosides, phospholipids, and acid mucopolysaccharides in cultured skin fibroblasts and brain tissue. These findings are associated with signs of neuronal loss and astrocytosis in cerebral cortex, basal ganglia, deep cerebellar nuclei, and brainstem nuclei. Involvement of the corneal epithelium with an intact Bowman membrane should enable distinction from the mucopolysaccharidoses and GM1 gangliosidoses. MRI brain scans show the presence of hypoplastic corpus callosum, white matter signal abnormalities (suggestive of delay or arrest of myelination), signs of increased iron deposition in the thalamus and basal ganglia, and cerebellar/ cerebral atrophy in older patients.

TREATMENT

Standard Therapies: Management is primarily supportive and includes the instillation of artificial tears into each conjunctival sac. Excessive salivation may be controlled with glycopyrrolate. Baclofen and regular physical therapy have been recommended for children with spasticity. Signing and communication board training have been encouraged to facilitate socialization.

REFERENCES

Acierno JS Jr, Kennedy JC, Falardeau JL, et al. A physical and transcript map of the *MCOLN1* gene region on human chromosome 19p13.3-p13.2. *Genomics* 2001;73:203–210.

Bargal R, Avidan N, Olender T, et al. Mucolipidosis type IV: novel *MCOLN1* mutations in Jewish and non-Jewish patients and the frequency of the disease in the Ashkenazi Jewish population. *Hum Mutat* 2001;17:397–402.

Bassi MT, Manzoni M, Monti E, et al. Cloning of the gene encoding a novel integral membrane protein, mucolipidin, and identification of the two major founder mutations causing mucolipidosis type IV. *Am J Hum Genet* 2000;67:1110–1120.

Edelmann L, Dong J, Desnick RJ, et al. Carrier screening for mucolipidosis type IV in the American Ashkenazi Jewish population. *Am J Hum Genet* 2002;65:773–778.

Sun M, Goldin E, Stahl S, et al. Mucolipidosis type IV is caused by mutations in a gene encoding a novel transient receptor potential channel. *Hum Mol Genet* 2000;9:2471–2478.

Wang ZH, Zeng B, Pastores GM, et al. Rapid detection of the two common mutations in Ashkenazi Jewish patients with mucolipidosis type IV. *Genet Test* 2001;5:87–92.

RESOURCES

109, 266, 314, 354

54   The Mucopolysaccharide Storage (MPS) Diseases

Joe T.R. Clarke, MD, PhD

DEFINITION: The mucopolysaccharide storage (MPS) diseases are a group of inherited metabolic disorders caused by disturbances in the normal breakdown of mucopolysaccharides. There are several different types, including Hurler disease and variants (MPS-IH, MPS-IH/S, MPS-IS), Hunter disease (MPS-II), Sanfilippo disease (MPS-III), Morquio disease (MPS-IV), Maroteaux-Lamy disease (MPS-VI), and Sly disease (MPS-VII). Classification is usually based on the specific enzyme defect causing the disease (Table 10.1). All the MPS storage diseases have certain characteristics in common. All occur with a frequency of 1 in 100,000 births or less, and all but one are in-

TABLE 10.1 Summary of the Specific Enzyme Defects in the Different MPS Storage Diseases		
Disease	**Enzyme**	**Enzyme Source**
Hurler disease and variants (MPS-IH, MPS-IH/S, MPS-IS)	■ α-L-iduronidase	■ L, F
Hunter disease (MPS-II	■ Iduronate-2-sulfatase	■ S, L, F
Sanfilippo disease, type A (MPS-IIIA)	■ Heparan-*N*-sulfatase	■ L, F
Sanfilippo disease, type B (MPS-IIIB)	■ α-*N*-Acetylglucosaminidase	■ L, F
Sanfilippo disease, type C (MPS-IIIC)	■ Acetyl-CoA:α-glucosaminide acetyltransferase	■ F
Sanfilippo disease, type D (MPS-IIID)	■ *N*-Acetylglucosamine-6-sulfatase	■ L, F
Morquio disease, type A (MPS-IVA)	■ *N*-Acetylgalactosamine-6-sulfatase	■ L, F
Morquio disease, type B (MPS-IVB)	■ β-Galactosidase	■ S, L, F
Maroteaux-Lamy disease (MPS-VI)	■ *N*-Acetylgalactosamine-4-sulfatase (arylsulfatases B)	■ L, F
Sly disease (MPS-VII)	■ β-Glucuronidase	■ S, L, F

L, peripheral blood leukocytes; F, cultured skin fibroblasts; S, serum.

herited as autosomal-recessive conditions (Hunter disease is inherited as an X-linked recessive disorder). All except for Sanfilippo disease interfere with growth, causing short stature. All cause deformities of the bones and joints that interfere with mobility and often cause osteoarthritis, especially of the large, weight-bearing joints.

SYMPTOMS AND SIGNS: In MPS-IH, affected children usually show signs of recurrent ear infections, persistent nasal congestion, snoring during sleep, and disproportionate enlargement of the head in the first few months of life. Almost all affected infants have an umbilical hernia, and many have inguinal hernias. Cloudiness of the corneas is present. Affected infants often grow abnormally rapidly in the first year of life, and the head grows faster. They also develop an unusual facial appearance caused by the large head, prominent brow with puffy-looking eyelids, small nose with forward-facing nostrils, thick lips and earlobes, and large tongue. Growth slows during the second year and ultimately stops by age 3–5 years. The abdomen of affected infants is protuberant, and the liver and spleen are enlarged. The fingers are short and stubby. Later in the course of the disease, they become stiff and immobilized in a bent position. The elbows, shoulders, hips, ankles, and knees also become stiff and fixed in flexion. The spine is often angulated, with a sharp bend just below the chest. Skeletal radiographs show severe deformities of the long bones, skull, spine, pelvis, hands, and feet. A few affected infants develop cardiomyopathy in the first few months of life and die within a few weeks or months. In most patients, the progression of the disease is slower, but death generally occurs before age 10–11 years, usually from pneumonia.

In MPS-IS (Scheie disease), affected individuals may not have many problems until late in childhood. Most patients come to medical attention as a result of short stature, joint pain, or the incidental discovery of clouding of the corneas. The facial appearance of affected patients is usually normal. Many show some stiffness of joints, but it is usually not severe enough to cause significant disability. Skeletal radiographs show deformities of the spine, long bones and joints, pelvis, hands, and skull, similar to those in Hurler disease, although milder.

Children with MPS-IH/S (Hurler-Scheie disease) generally come to medical attention in the middle of the first decade of life as a result of skeletal problems: short stature, joint deformities, and stiffness of joints. Umbilical and inguinal hernias are common, and most patients have clinically significant enlargement of the liver and spleen. Skeletal radiographs show moderately severe deformities of the long bones, skull, spine, pelvis, hands, and feet. The most serious complications involve the cardiovascular system and the lungs. Thickening and stiffness of the heart valves, along with progressive weakening of the heart muscle, causes major disability, usually by the mid-teens.

MPS-IIA is a severe form of Hunter disease. Affected boys begin having problems in the first year of life, usually with recurrent ear infections, persistent nasal congestion, and snoring during sleep. They also have disproportionate enlargement of the head. Many affected infant boys have an umbilical hernia, and many have inguinal hernias as well. Their growth is often abnormally rapid in the first year of life, and their heads grow faster. They also develop an unusual facial appearance. Growth slows during the second year and ultimately stops by age 3–5 years. The liver and spleen are enlarged. The fingers are short and stubby. Later in the course of the disease, they become stiff and immobilized in a bent position. The elbows, shoulders, hips, ankles, and knees also become stiff and fixed in flexion. The spine is often angulated, with a sharp bend just below the chest.

In MPS IIB, the most common complaints are short stature or joint pain. Early signs of the disease may include problems with the heart valves, and congestive heart failure may occur. The facial appearance is usually normal, at least for many years. Most show some progressive stiffening of joints. Skeletal radiographs show mild deformities of the spine, long bones and joints, pelvis, hands, and skull, similar to those in Scheie disease. The corneas of the eyes are almost always clear; however, affected individuals are at risk for glaucoma and of degeneration of the retina later in life. Osteoarthritis occurs in most patients. Most men with MPS-IIB develop high-frequency hearing impairment. Many patients develop difficulty breathing and tire quickly during exercise as a result of restriction of expansion of the chest.

Children with Sanfilippo disease usually come to medical attention in the third or fourth year of life because of developmental delay, especially affecting speech, and severe behavior abnormalities. The facial appearance, growth, bones, and joints of young children with Sanfilippo disease are generally normal. Only after age 6 years do they begin to develop subtle changes in facial appearance typical of MPS diseases. Growth is often normal for many years, although radiographs of the spine, skull, pelvis, and long bones generally show at least mild changes. Seizures are a common problem. They are often generalized tonic-clonic seizures, although complex partial seizures or atypical absence attacks may occur.

Morquio disease occurs in two forms: type A and type B. Type A is more common, but the two types are clinically indistinguishable. Children with Morquio disease typically come to attention late in the first year of life or even later as a result of deformities of the chest (flaring of the lower ribs or abnormal prominence of the breast bone), loose joints, abnormally short neck, or joint deformities, such as knock-knees. Affected children have a characteristic facial appearance, subtle clouding of the corneas of the eyes, and mild enlargement of the liver and spleen. Skeletal radiographs typically show flattening of the vertebrae. The long bones of the arms and legs are shorter and thicker than normal. The skull is large for the rest of the body. One of the most characteristic radiographic findings is poor development of the connection between the first and second vertebrae in the neck caused by near or complete absence of the odontoid process. The instability of this joint constitutes one of the more serious threats to the survival of affected individuals. A relatively trivial injury may cause the two vertebrae to slip on each other, pressing on, then cutting the spinal cord. Children show marked growth retardation from early in life. The elbows, wrists, hips, knees, and other large joints are abnormally flexible, causing overall instability. The deformity of the chest causes a strain on the heart and lungs, which may ultimately cause chronic respiratory failure. High-frequency hearing impairment is common.

Maroteaux-Lamy disease is clinically almost indistinguishable from Scheie disease. Affected individuals may not have many problems until middle childhood. Most patients come to medical attention as a result of short stature, complaints of joint pain, or the incidental discovery of clouding of the corneas. The facial appearance is usually normal. Many show some stiffness of joints, but this is usually not severe enough to cause significant disability until adulthood. Intelligence is generally unaffected, although some patients may have mild to moderate mental handicap. Skeletal radiographs show deformities of the spine, long bones and joints, pelvis, hands, and skull, similar to those in Scheie disease.

Involvement of joints causes some osteoarthritis in most patients. Accumulation of MPS and secondary scarring of the heart valves causes leakage and obstruction that may cause heart failure. High-frequency hearing loss is common in adults. Accumulation of MPS and secondary fibrosis of the membranes surrounding the spinal cord may cause pressure, resulting in generalized muscle weakness or quadriplegia, requiring surgical decompression and fusion of the spine in the neck area.

The clinical features of Sly disease vary markedly; however, all patients appear to have impaired growth and short stature, changes in the bones visible on routine radiography, and some degree of mental handicap, which may be severe. Sly disease is slowly progressive, and survival into adulthood is common. Osteoarthritis is a common complication.

ETIOLOGY/EPIDEMIOLOGY: Hurler disease occurs in approximately 1 in 75,000 births. It is caused by deficiency of the lysosomal enzyme, alpha-L-iduronidase, and is associated with excessive excretion of dermatan sulfate and heparan sulfate in the urine. Hunter disease is an X-linked recessive disorder caused by deficiency of lysosomal sulfoiduronate sulfatase. It affects approximately 1 in 75,000 boys born (approximately 1 in 150,000 babies born). Sanfilippo disease occurs in 1 in 100,000 births. It is caused by deficiency of one of four different lysosomal enzymes involved in the breakdown of heparan sulfate. Sanfilippo disease is therefore subclassified into four types, according to the specific enzyme defect shown in Table 10.2. All are inherited as autosomal-recessive disorders. Sly disease affects approximately 1 in 1 million babies born. It is caused by deficiency of lysosomal beta-glucuronidase.

DIAGNOSIS: Diagnosis of the MPS disorders is by appropriate specific enzyme analysis of peripheral blood leukocytes or cultured skin fibroblasts. Prenatal diagnosis is possible by enzymic (alpha-L-iduronidase) or molecular genetic analysis of fetal material obtained by chorionic villus sampling or by analysis of cultured amniotic fluid cells. Carrier detection is unreliable except by mutation analysis, when the specific mutation causing disease is known.

TREATMENT
Standard Therapies: Hurler disease responds well to treatment by bone marrow transplantation (BMT). If affected infants undergo BMT in the first year of life, they continue to develop normally. Growth and facial appearance are often normal, although skeletal problems often develop as the child approaches puberty, and many children treated early by BMT have to undergo orthopedic surgical treatment of skeletal complications, especially of the spine. Treatment by BMT after 18 months appears to stabilize the developmental handicap and results in some improvement in facial appearance and growth. Treatment of children for whom a suitable BMT donor cannot be found, or in whom the procedure fails, is supportive. Although Scheie disease is slowly progressive, life expectancy for patients who undergo successful treatment of various complications, such as problems with heart valves, is close to normal. Involvement of joints causes some osteoarthritis in most patients with the disease, and many undergo surgical replacement of large joints as young adults. Corneal transplantation may be necessary. Glaucoma is treatable by surgery or medications. Treatment of MPS-IIA and Sanfilippo disease is supportive, because BMT does not materially influence the course of either disease.

Investigational Therapies: Treatment of Hunter disease by enzyme replacement is being explored, as is enzyme replacement for some subtypes of MPS-IIA and Sanfilippo disease. Research suggests that BMT and enzyme replacement therapy might be beneficial in the treatment of Sly disease.

REFERENCES
Beighton P, McKusick VA. *Heritable disorders of connective tissue,* 5th ed. St. Louis: CV Mosby, 1993.
Froissant R, et al. Identification of iduronate sulfatase gene alterations in 70 unrelated Hunter patients. *Clin Genet* 1998;53: 362–368.
Kjellen L, Lindahl V. The proteoglycans structures and functions. *Ann Rev Biochem* 1991;60:443–475.
Peters C, Shapiro EG, Krivit W. Hurler syndrome: past, present and future. *J Pediatr* 1998;133:7–9.

54a   MPS-IH (Hurler Disease)

Joe T.R. Clarke, MD, PhD

DEFINITION: As in all mucopolysaccharide storage (MPS) diseases, Hurler disease is an inherited metabolic disorder caused by disturbances in the normal breakdown of mucopolysaccharides.

SYNONYMS: MPS-IH/S; MPS-IS.

DIFFERENTIAL DIAGNOSIS: Other MPS storage diseases.

SYMPTOMS AND SIGNS: Affected children usually show signs of recurrent ear infections, persistent nasal congestion, snoring during sleep, and disproportionate enlargement of the head in the first few months of life. Almost all affected infants have an umbilical hernia, and many have inguinal hernias. The corneas are cloudy. Affected infants often grow abnormally rapidly in the first year of life, and the head grows faster. They also develop an unusual facial appearance caused by the large head, prominent brow with puffy-looking eyelids, small nose with forward-facing nostrils, thick lips and earlobes, and large tongue. Growth slows during the second year and ultimately stops by age 3–5 years. The abdomen of affected infants is protuberant, and the liver and spleen are enlarged. The fingers are short and stubby. Later in the course of the disease, they become stiff and immobilized in a bent position. The elbows, shoulders, hips, ankles, and knees also become stiff and fixed in flexion. The spine is often angulated, with a sharp bend just below the chest. Skeletal radiographs show severe deformities of the long bones, skull, spine, pelvis, hands, and feet. A few affected infants develop cardiomyopathy in the first few months of life and die within a few weeks or months. In most patients, the progression of the disease is slower, but death generally occurs before age 10–11 years, usually from pneumonia.

ETIOLOGY/EPIDEMIOLOGY: Hurler disease affects approximately 1 of every 75,000 babies born. It is caused by deficiency of the lysosomal enzyme, alpha-L-iduronidase, and is associated with excessive excretion of dermatan sulfate and heparan sulfate in the urine.

DIAGNOSIS: Diagnosis is by enzyme analysis of peripheral blood leukocytes or cultured skin fibroblasts. Prenatal diagnosis is possible by enzymic (alpha-L-iduronidase) or molecular genetic analysis of fetal material obtained by chorionic villus sampling or by analysis of cultured amniotic fluid cells obtained by amniocentesis. Carrier detection is unreliable except by mutation analysis, when the specific mutation causing disease is known.

TREATMENT

Standard Therapies: Hurler disease responds well to treatment by bone marrow transplantation (BMT). If affected infants undergo BMT in the first year of life, they continue to develop normally. Growth and facial appearance are often normal, although skeletal problems often develop as the child approaches puberty, and many children treated early by BMT have to undergo orthopedic surgical treatment of skeletal complications of the disease, especially of the spine. Treatment by BMT after 18 months appears to stabilize the developmental handicap and results in some improvement in facial appearance and growth. Treatment of children for whom a suitable BMT donor cannot be found, or in whom the procedure fails, is supportive.

REFERENCES

Beighton P, McKusick VA. *Heritable disorders of connective tissue,* 5th ed. St. Louis: CV Mosby, 1993.

Kjellen L, Lindahl V. The proteoglycans structures and functions. *Ann Rev Biochem* 1991;60:443–475.

Peters C, Shapiro EG, Krivit W. Hurler syndrome: past, present and future. *J Pediatr* 1998;133:7–9.

RESOURCES

109, 314, 440

54b   MPS-IS (Scheie Disease)

Joe T.R. Clarke, MD, PhD

DEFINITION: As in all mucopolysaccharide storage (MPS) diseases, Scheie disease is an inherited metabolic disorder caused by disturbances in the normal breakdown of mucopolysaccharides.

DIFFERENTIAL DIAGNOSIS: Other MPS storage diseases.

SYMPTOMS AND SIGNS: Affected individuals may not have many problems until late in childhood. Most patients come to medical attention as a result of short stature, joint pain, or the incidental discovery of clouding of the corneas. The facial appearance of affected patients is usually normal. Many show some stiffness of joints, but it is usually not severe enough to cause significant disability. Skeletal radiographs show deformities of the spine, long bones and joints, pelvis, hands, and skull, similar to those in Hurler disease, although milder.

DIAGNOSIS: Test results of the urine for MPS are generally positive, and further analysis shows increased excretion of both dermatan and heparan sulfate. The diagnosis is confirmed by demonstrating profound deficiency of alpha-L-iduronidase in peripheral blood leukocytes or cultured skin fibroblasts.

TREATMENT
Standard Therapies: Although Scheie disease is slowly progressive, life expectancy for patients who undergo successful treatment of various complications, such as problems with heart valves, is close to normal. Involvement of joints causes some osteoarthritis in most patients with the disease, and many undergo surgical replacement of large joints as young adults. Corneal transplantation may be necessary. Glaucoma is treatable by surgery or by medications.

REFERENCES
Beighton P, McKusick VA. *Heritable disorders of connective tissue,* 5th ed. St. Louis: CV Mosby, 1993.
Kjellen L, Lindahl V. The proteoglycans structures and functions. *Ann Rev Biochem* 1991;60:443–475.

54c   MPS-II (Hunter Disease)

Joe T.R. Clarke, MD, PhD

DEFINITION: As in all mucopolysaccharide storage (MPS) diseases, Hunter disease is an inherited metabolic disorder caused by disturbances in the normal breakdown of mucopolysaccharides.

DIFFERENTIAL DIAGNOSIS: Other MPS storage diseases.

SYMPTOMS AND SIGNS: MPS-IIA is a severe form of Hunter disease. Affected boys begin having problems in the first year of life, usually with recurrent ear infections, persistent nasal congestion, and snoring during sleep. They also have disproportionate enlargement of the head. Many affected infant boys have an umbilical hernia, and many have inguinal hernias as well. Affected infants often grow abnormally rapidly in the first year of life, and the head grows faster. They also develop an unusual facial appearance. Growth slows during the second year and ultimately stops by age 3–5 years. The liver and spleen are enlarged. The fingers are short and stubby. Later in the course of the disease, they become stiff and immobilized in a bent position. The elbows, shoulders, hips, ankles, and knees also become stiff and fixed in flexion. The spine is often angulated, with a sharp bend just below the chest. In MPS-IIB, the most common complaints are short stature or joint pain. Early signs of the disease may include problems with

the heart valves, and congestive heart failure may occur. The facial appearance of affected patients is usually normal, at least for many years. Most show some progressive stiffening of joints. Skeletal radiographs show mild deformities of the spine, long bones and joints, pelvis, hands, and skull, similar to those in Scheie disease. The corneas of the eyes are almost always clear; however, affected individuals are at risk for glaucoma and of degeneration of the retina later in life. Osteoarthritis occurs in most patients with the disease. Most men with MPS-IIB develop high-frequency hearing impairment. Many patients develop difficulty breathing and tire quickly during exercise as a result of restriction of expansion of the chest.

ETIOLOGY/EPIDEMIOLOGY: Hunter disease is an X-linked recessive disorder caused by deficiency of lysosomal sulfoiduronate sulfatase. It affects approximately 1 in 75,000 boys born (approximately 1 in 150,000 babies born).

DIAGNOSIS: The diagnosis is confirmed by demonstrating profound deficiency of sulfoiduronate sulfatase in serum or in leukocytes isolated from peripheral blood samples. Prenatal diagnosis of Hunter disease in fetuses is possible. Female carriers can sometimes be identified by enzyme analysis of leukocytes isolated from blood samples. Mutation analysis is particularly helpful in the identification of carriers of Hunter disease, but it requires the identification of the specific mutation causing the disease in the family of the woman being tested. This is often not practical.

TREATMENT
Standard Therapies: Treatment of MPS-IIA is supportive.

Investigational Therapies: Treatment of Hunter disease by enzyme replacement is being explored, as is enzyme replacement for some subtypes of MPS-IIA.

REFERENCES
Beighton, P, McKusick VA. *Heritable disorders of connective tissue,* 5th ed. St. Louis: CV Mosby, 1993.
Froissant R, et al. Identification of idurontate sulfatase gene alterations in 70 unrelated Hunter patients. *Clin Genet* 1998;53: 362–368.
Kjellen L, Lindahl V. The proteoglycans structures and functions. *Ann Rev Biochem* 1991;60:443–475.

RESOURCES
109, 314, 440

54d   MPS-III (Sanfilippo Disease)

Joe T.R. Clarke, MD, PhD

DEFINITION: As in all mucopolysaccharide storage (MPS) diseases, Sanfilippo disease is an inherited metabolic disorder caused by disturbances in the normal breakdown of mucopolysaccharides.

DIFFERENTIAL DIAGNOSIS: Other MPS storage diseases.

SYMPTOMS AND SIGNS: Children with Sanfilippo disease usually come to medical attention in the third or fourth year of life because of developmental delay, especially affecting speech, and severe behavioral abnormalities. The facial appearance, growth, bones, and joints of young children with Sanfilippo disease are generally normal. Only later, after age 6 years, do they begin to develop subtle changes in facial appearance typical of MPS diseases. Growth is often normal for many years, although radiography of the spine, skull, pelvis, and long bones generally show at least mild changes typical of MPS disease. Seizures are a common problem. They are often generalized tonic-clonic seizures, although complex partial seizures or atypical absence attacks may occur. The behavioral problems are similar to those in boys with Hunter disease. Affected children generally do not develop skills beyond the 3- to 4-year-old age level. By age 8–10 years, most children with the disease begin to show some regression.

ETIOLOGY/EPIDEMIOLOGY: Sanfilippo disease affects up to 1 in 100,000 babies born. It is caused by deficiency of one of four different lysosomal enzymes involved in the breakdown of heparan sulfate. Sanfilippo disease is therefore subclassified into four types, according to the specific enzyme defect. All are inherited as autosomal-recessive disorders.

DIAGNOSIS: Tests for MPS in the urine are usually positive, but are negative often enough to be unreliable as a screening test for the disease. Detailed chemical analysis of the MPS in urine shows predominance of heparan sulfate. The definitive diagnosis of the disease requires specific enzyme analysis. Some of the enzymes can be measured on white blood cells isolated from a small blood sample, but cultured skin fibroblasts are required to measure all of them.

TREATMENT
Standard Therapies: Treatment is supportive.

Investigational Therapies: Enzyme replacement is being explored.

REFERENCES
Beighton P, McKusick VA. *Heritable disorders of connective tissue,* 5th ed. St. Louis: CV Mosby, 1993.
Kjellen L, Lindahl V. The proteoglycans structures and functions. *Ann Rev Biochem* 1991;60:443–475.

RESOURCES
109, 314, 354, 362

54e   MPS-IV (Morquio Disease)

Joe T.R. Clarke, MD, PhD

DEFINITION: Morquio disease is a mucopolysaccharide (MPS) storage disease that occurs in two forms: type A, caused by deficiency of lysosomal N-acetylgalactosamine-6-sulfatase, and type B, caused by deficiency of lysosomal beta-galactosidase. Type A is the more common, but the two types are clinically indistinguishable.

DIFFERENTIAL DIAGNOSIS: Other MPS storage diseases.

SYMPTOMS AND SIGNS: Children with Morquio disease typically come to attention late in the first year of life or even later as a result of deformities of the chest (flaring of the lower ribs or abnormal prominence of the breast bone), loose joints, abnormally short neck, or joint deformities, such as knock-knees. Affected children have a characteristic facial appearance, subtle clouding of the corneas of the eyes, and mild enlargement of the liver and spleen. Early development and overall intelligence are typically normal. Skeletal radiographs typically show marked flattening of the vertebrae. The long bones of the arms and legs are characteristically shorter and thicker than normal. The skull is large for the rest of the body. One of the most characteristic radiographic findings is poor development of the connection between the first and second vertebrae in the neck caused by near or complete absence of the odontoid process. Children with Morquio disease show marked growth retardation from early in life. The elbows, wrists, hips, knees, and other large joints are abnormally flexible, causing overall instability. This interferes with efficient muscle action, producing an impression of muscle weakness. Instability of the joint between the first and second cervical vertebrae, caused by absence of the odontoid process, constitutes one of the more serious threats to the life of persons with Morquio disease. A relatively trivial injury may cause the two vertebrae to slip on each other, pressing on, then cutting the spinal cord. Intelligence is normal. Life expectancy is decreased somewhat by the deformities of the spine, which sometimes causes pressure on the spinal cord despite surgery to stabilize the bones. The deformity of the chest causes a strain on the heart and lungs, which may eventually cause chronic respiratory failure. High-frequency hearing impairment is common.

ETIOLOGY/EPIDEMIOLOGY: Both types are inherited as autosomal-recessive conditions; the two types never occur together in the same family.

DIAGNOSIS: Tests for MPS in the urine are often positive, but the test reaction is often weak. More detailed analysis shows the presence of excessive amounts of keratan sulfate. The diagnosis is confirmed by demonstrating profound deficiency of N-acetylgalactosamine-6-sulfatase (type A) or beta-galactosidase (type B) in peripheral blood leukocytes or cultured skin fibroblasts.

TREATMENT
Standard Therapies: Surgical decompression and fusion of the bones of the upper neck to the base of the skull can prevent destabilization of the cervical vertebrae and potential damage to the spinal cord.

REFERENCES
Beighton P, McKusick VA. *Heritable disorders of connective tissue,* 5th ed. St. Louis: CV Mosby, 1993.
Kjellen L, Lindahl V. The proteoglycans structures and functions. *Ann Rev Biochem* 1991;60:443–475.

RESOURCES
109, 314, 354, 462

54f   MPS-VI (Maroteaux-Lamy Disease)

Joe T.R. Clarke, MD, PhD

DEFINITION: As in all mucopolysaccharide storage (MPS) diseases, Maroteaux-Lamy disease is an inherited metabolic disorder caused by disturbances in the normal breakdown of mucopolysaccharides.

DIFFERENTIAL DIAGNOSIS: Other MPS storage diseases.

SYMPTOMS AND SIGNS: Maroteaux-Lamy disease is clinically almost indistinguishable from Scheie disease. Affected individuals may not have many problems until middle childhood. Most patients come to medical attention as a result of short stature, complaints of joint pain, or the incidental discovery of clouding of the corneas. The facial appearance of affected patients is usually normal. Many show some stiffness of joints, but this is usually not severe enough to cause significant disability until adulthood. Intelligence is generally unaffected, although some patients may have mild to moderate mental handicap. Skeletal radiographs show deformities of the spine, long bones and joints, pelvis, hands, and skull, similar to those in Scheie disease. Involvement of joints causes some osteoarthritis in most patients. Accumulation of MPS and secondary scarring of the heart valves causes leakage and obstruction that may cause heart failure. High-frequency hearing loss is common in adult patients. Accumulation of MPS and secondary fibrosis of the membranes surrounding the spinal cord may cause pressure, resulting in generalized muscle weakness, or even quadriplegia.

ETIOLOGY/EPIDEMIOLOGY: All MPS syndromes are inherited as autosomal-recessive disorders.

DIAGNOSIS: Tests of the urine for MPS are generally positive, and further analysis shows increased excretion of both dermatan and heparan sulfate. The diagnosis is confirmed by demonstrating profound deficiency of N-acetyl-galactosamine-4-sulfatase in peripheral blood leukocytes or cultured skin fibroblasts.

TREATMENT
Standard Therapies: The treatment is supportive and symptomatic. Surgical decompression and fusion of the spine in the neck area may be required.

REFERENCES
Beighton, P, McKusick VA. *Heritable disorders of connective tissue,* 5th ed. St. Louis: CV Mosby, 1993.
Kjellen L, Lindahl V. The proteoglycans structures and functions. *Ann Rev Biochem* 1991;60:443–475.

RESOURCES
109, 314, 354, 462

54g   MPS-VII (Sly Disease)

Joe T.R. Clarke, MD, PhD

DEFINITION: As in all mucopolysaccharide storage (MPS) diseases, Sly disease is an inherited metabolic disorder caused by disturbances in the normal breakdown of mucopolysaccharides.

DIFFERENTIAL DIAGNOSIS: Other MPS storage diseases.

SYMPTOMS AND SIGNS: The clinical features of Sly disease vary from patient to patient; however, all appear to have impaired growth and short stature, changes in the bones visible on routine radiography, and some degree of mental handicap, which may be severe. Sly disease is slowly progressive, and survival into adulthood is common. Osteoarthritis is a common complication.

ETIOLOGY/EPIDEMIOLOGY: This MPS storage disease is extremely rare, affecting only about 1 in 1 million babies born. It is caused by deficiency of lysosomal beta-glucuronidase.

DIAGNOSIS: Diagnosis is by appropriate specific enzyme analysis of peripheral blood leukocytes or cultured skin fibroblasts. Prenatal diagnosis is possible by enzymic (alpha-L-iduronidase) or molecular genetic analysis of fetal material obtained by chorionic villus sampling or by analysis of cultured amniotic fluid cells obtained by amniocentesis. Carrier detection is unreliable except by mutation analysis, when the specific mutation causing disease is known.

TREATMENT
Investigational Therapies: Research experience with bone marrow transplantation and with enzyme replacement therapy of mice with experimental MPS-VII suggests that either might be beneficial in the treatment of the disease in humans, but so far neither has been tried.

REFERENCES
Beighton P, McKusick VA. *Heritable disorders of connective tissue,* 5th ed. St. Louis: CV Mosby, 1993.
Kjellen L, Lindahl V. The proteoglycans structures and functions. *Ann Rev Biochem* 1991;60:443–475.

RESOURCES
109, 314, 354, 462

55   Multiple Carboxylase Deficiency (Biotinidase Deficiency)

William M. Nyhan, MD, PhD

DEFINITION: Biotinidase deficiency causes multiple carboxylase deficiency in which biotin levels in blood and urine are low. Major manifestations may be neurologic or cutaneous.

SYNONYM: Late-onset multiple carboxylase deficiency.

DIFFERENTIAL DIAGNOSIS: Holocarboxylase synthetase deficiency.

SYMPTOMS AND SIGNS: Biotinidase deficiency usually presents after 3 months, so it is really a late infantile rather than late-onset multiple carboxylase deficiency. It may also appear earlier, or as late as 4 years. The classic infantile presentation is with episodic ketoacidosis typical of an organic acidemia. Some patients, however, present first with convulsions. With time, patients develop cutaneous manifestations. Alopecia is usually partial or patchy, as are skin eruptions. Periorificial cracking lesions are common. An initial diagnosis has been acrodermatitis enteropathica. Complicating monilial infection is regularly observed. Keratoconjunctivitis may lead to corneal ulceration. Development may be delayed. Ataxia may be intermittent or of such severity that the patient cannot walk. Cerebellar atrophy and gliosis have been noted histopathologically. Immunodeficiency has been documented in deficiency of both T and B cells. In the presence of extensive moniliasis, responses to *Candida* antigen both *in vitro* and *in vivo* have been absent. Neurosensory deficits in both optic and auditory nerves have been late developments. Retinal dysplasia as well as optic atrophy occurs. Spastic diplegia is an even later development in patients not diagnosed or treated until adolescence or adulthood.

ETIOLOGY/EPIDEMIOLOGY: Biotinidase deficiency is autosomal recessive. The gene has been mapped to chromosome 3p25, and it has been cloned. Several mutations have been identified. Deficiency of biotinidase leads to deficiency of the carboxylases, propionyl CoA carboxylase, 3-methylcrotonyl CoA carboxylase, and pyruvate carboxy-

lase. Prevalence is approximately 1 in 60,000 births in the United States, with no particular ethnic predominance.

DIAGNOSIS: The earliest diagnosis is made in neonatal screening programs in which assay for the enzyme in blood spots is carried out. Organic acid analysis can detect the characteristic multiple carboxylase pattern of marked elevation of 3-hydroxyisovaleric acid and usually of 3-methylcrotonylglycine and lactic acid, along with smaller elevations of 3-hydroxypropionic acid and 3-methylcitric acid. Some patients are diagnosed as part of a workup for chronic lactic acidemia. A rapid method for distinguishing this disease is to assay activity of the carboxylases in lymphocytes in the presence and absence of preincubation with biotin. Cultured fibroblasts from patients with this disease have normal carboxylase activity. The definitive assay of biotinidase is usually carried out in serum. It has also been demonstrated in liver and fibroblasts. Mutational analysis can be used in genetic diagnosis in a family in which the mutation is known.

TREATMENT

Standard Therapies: Treatment is with biotin. An oral dose of 10 mg daily is usually enough to eliminate or prevent all manifestations of the disease. Losses of optic or auditory nerve function are not recovered completely, although improvement may occur. Spastic paraparesis once developed does not remit.

REFERENCES

Lott IT, Lottenberg S, Nyhan WL, et al. Cerebral metabolic change after treatment in biotinidase deficiency. *J Inherit Metab Dis* 1993;16:399–407.

Norrgaard KJ, Pomponio RJ, Hymes J, et al. Mutations causing profound biotinidase deficiency in children ascertained by newborn screening in the United States occur at different frequencies than in symptomatic children. *Pediatr Res* 1999;46: 20–27.

Nyhan WL, Ozand PT. *Atlas of metabolic diseases.* London: Arnold, 1998:33–40.

RESOURCES

58, 109, 354

56 Multiple Carboxylase Deficiency (Holocarboxylase Synthetase Deficiency)

William M. Nyhan, MD, PhD

DEFINITION: Holocarboxylase synthetase is the cause of a form of multiple carboxylase deficiency that usually presents in the early days of life. Its major clinical manifestations are life-threatening ketoacidosis, dermatosis, and alopecia.

SYNONYM: Neonatal form (biotin responsive) multiple carboxylase deficiency.

DIFFERENTIAL DIAGNOSIS: Propionic acidemia; biotinidase deficiency.

SYMPTOMS AND SIGNS: Infants with holocarboxylase synthetase deficiency usually develop overwhelming illness in the first hours or days of life. Initial anorexia or vomiting is followed by lethargy, acidosis, and hyperpnea, leading to coma, dehydration, and, in the absence of intervention, death. Massive ketosis is accompanied by lactic acidemia and metabolic acidosis. Patients treated with effective parenteral fluid and electrolyte therapy recover, but then undergo repeated similar crises of ketoacidosis until diagnosis. With time, an erythematous dermatosis appears, usually as a bright red, total body eruption. It may be scaly or weeping and is commonly complicated by monilia. It resembles ichthyosis and seborrheic dermatitis, but it looks just like human biotin deficiency. It is accompanied by alopecia totalis. Immunologic deficiency may lead to infection, and patients have been shown to have a diminution in T-cell number and in their specific responses to *Candida*. A few patients have had neurologic abnormalities including seizures, athetosis, hypotonia, and hypertonia.

ETIOLOGY/EPIDEMIOLOGY: The disease is autosomal recessive. The fundamental defect in holocarboxylase synthetase has been documented in lymphocytes and cultured fibroblasts. This enzyme activates biotin by forming the adenylate and then attaching it to the lysine of the carboxylase proteins, conferring on them enzyme activity. The enzymes propionyl CoA carboxylase, 3-methylcrotonyl CoA carboxylase, and pyruvate carboxylase are all deficient, and this leads to the abnormal biochemistry that characterizes the disease. The gene is on chromosome 21q22.1. Prevalence data are not available.

DIAGNOSIS: The diagnosis is usually made by organic acid analysis. Quantification is important to distinguish this disorder from propionic acid. The abnormal multiple carboxylase pattern is of large amounts of 3-hydroxyisovaleric acid and usually of 3-methylcrotonylglycine along with lactic acid and smaller amounts of 3-hydroxypropionic acid and methylcitric acid. The diagnosis may be confirmed by assay of the carboxylases and by assay of holocarboxylase synthetase. Prenatal diagnosis has been carried out by means of both of these assays of cultured amniocytes and chorionic villus cells, as well as by gas chromatography mass spectrometry for 3-hydroxyisovaleric acid. The gene has been cloned and mutations identified, and this information can be used for genetic diagnosis in a family in which the mutation is known.

TREATMENT

Standard Therapies: Patients are extraordinarily sensitive to biotin. An oral dose of 10 mg per day is usually sufficient to reverse or prevent all manifestations of the disease. Prenatal treatment has been successful.

REFERENCES

Burri BJ, Sweetman L, Nyhan WL. Mutant holocarboxylase synthetase. Evidence for the enzyme defect in early infantile biotin-responsive multiple carboxylase deficiency. *J Clin Invest* 1981;68:1491–1495.

Nyhan WL, Ozand PT. *Atlas of metabolic diseases.* London: Arnold, 1998:27–32.

Thuy LP, Belmont J, Nyhan WL. Prenatal diagnosis and treatment of holocarboxylase synthetase deficiency. *Prenat Diagn* 1999; 19:108–112.

Yang X, Aoki Y, Li X, et al. Haplotype analysis suggest that the two predominant mutations in Japanese patients with holocarboxylase synthetase deficiency are founder mutations. *J Hum Genet* 2000;45:358–362.

RESOURCES

58, 109, 354

57 Multiple Sulfatase Deficiency

Grazia M.S. Mancini, MD, PhD,
and Otto P. van Diggelen, PhD

DEFINITION: Multiple sulfatase deficiency (MSD) is an autosomal-recessive disorder associated with the deficiency of at least seven different sulfatase enzymes. The disease belongs to the lysosomal storage diseases, as most of these sulfatases are lysosomal enzymes and the storage material is found inside the lysosomal compartment.

SYNONYM: Mucosulfatidosis.

DIFFERENTIAL DIAGNOSIS: Metachromatic leukodystrophy; X-linked ichthyosis with steroid sulfatase deficiency; Hunter disease; Mucopolysaccharidosis III (Sanfilippo disease); Mucolipidosis II.

SYMPTOMS AND SIGNS: Two main phenotypes can be distinguished: one similar to the mucopolysaccharidoses with neurologic symptoms, skeletal changes, and facial coarsening, and the other closely resembling metachromatic leukodystrophy, with ichthyosis and without facial and skeletal changes. The "Saudi variant" is a form of MSD with skeletal changes, mild white matter changes, and no ichthyosis. The main symptoms are late-infantile onset of psychomotor regression, loss of acquired skills and speech, deambulation and swallowing difficulties, pyramidal symptoms, Babinski sign and loss of deep tendon reflexes, epilepsy with generalized tonic-clonic and myoclonic seizures, and loss of eye contact (cerebral blindness and retinal degeneration). Brain MRI shows generalized white matter destruction, similar to that of metachromatic leukodystrophy. Skin signs include vulgar ichthyosis, which can be subtle and not apparent until toddler age, and mild to moderate hirsutism. The skeletal changes, typical of multiple dysostosis, can be mild or completely absent.

ETIOLOGY/EPIDEMIOLOGY: The disorder is one of the rarest lysosomal storage diseases; only approximately 50 cases have been described. The basic defect lies in a posttranslational modification essential to confer enzymatic activity to all sulfatases: the modification of a cysteine residue in the catalytic center into formyl-glycine. The gene for this disease and the chromosomal locus are unknown.

DIAGNOSIS: The disease is clinically suspected at the observation of a leukodystrophy associated with ichthyosis or with dysostosis multiplex and facial coarsening. Enzymatic confirmation is seen in peripheral blood leukocytes, therefore the tissue of choice for the diagnosis, which shows the deficiency of several sulfatases, particularly arylsulfatase A, arylsulfatase B, steroid-sulfatase, iduronate-sulfatase, heparan-sulfamidase, and N-acetylglucosamine-6-sulfatase. The degree of deficiency of each sulfatase can vary, hence the need to check several enzymes. Urine excretion of sulfatides is always elevated, but mucopolysaccharide levels can be moderately increased or normal. The deficiencies of sulfatases in cultured fibroblasts often are less pronounced, which may make it difficult to discriminate between metachromatic leukodystrophy and MSD, particularly in cases where mucopolysaccharide excretion is normal.

TREATMENT
Standard Therapies: No therapy exists except for supportive antiepileptic and muscle relaxant treatment.

REFERENCES
Basner R, et al. Multiple deficiency of mucopolysaccharide sulfatases in mucosulfatidosis. *Pediatr Res* 1979;13:1316–1318.
Hopwood JJ, Ballabio A. Multiple sulfatase deficiency and the nature of the sulfatase family. In: Scriver C, et al., eds. *The molecular and metabolic bases of inherited disease,* 8th ed. Vol. 3. New York: McGraw-Hill, 2001:3725–3732.
Mancini GMS, et al. Pitfalls in the diagnosis of multiple sulfatase deficiency. *Neuropediatrics* 2001;32:38–40.
Schmidt B, et al. A novel amino acid modification in sulfatases that is defective in multiple sulfatase deficiency. *Cell* 1995; 82:271–278.

RESOURCES
109, 335, 368

58 Niemann-Pick Disease, Type C

Marc C. Patterson, MD

DEFINITION: Niemann-Pick disease, type C (NPC) is an autosomal-recessive storage disorder characterized by progressive neurodegeneration, with or without organomegaly.

SYNONYMS: Juvenile Niemann-Pick disease; Niemann-Pick disease type II; Niemann-Pick disease, type D; Juvenile dystonic lipidosis; DAF syndrome (Downgaze paralysis, ataxia, foam cells); Neville-Lake disease; Lactosylceramidosis; Vertical supranuclear ophthalmoplegia with neurovisceral lipidosis; Sea-blue histiocytosis.

DIFFERENTIAL DIAGNOSIS: Biliary atresia; Congenital infections; Alpha-1-antitrypsin deficiency; Tyrosinemia; Leukemia; Lymphoma; Histiocytosis; Acquired infections; Malaria; Mitochondrial cytopathies; Glycine encephalopathy; Maple syrup urine disease; Absence seizures; Idiopathic torsion dystonia; Dopa-responsive dystonia; Wilson disease; Neuronal ceroid lipofuscinosis; Subacute sclerosing panencephalitis; HIV encephalopathy.

SYMPTOMS AND SIGNS: Presenting features vary with the patient's age at onset. Severely affected babies may have ascites *in utero*, detectable on ultrasonography, and most have severe liver disease with massive hepatosplenomegaly, jaundice, and failure to thrive. Many have extensive pulmonary infiltration with foam cells. Some children have early hypotonia and developmental delay; others may have a variable period of normal development before neurologic decline occurs. The classic form of the disease manifests in middle to late childhood with apparent clumsiness, subsequently evolving into overt ataxia. Impairment of vertical gaze (up or down) may be the initial neurologic finding. As the disease progresses, most children develop dystonia. Gelastic cataplexy, which may vary from head nods to complete collapse provoked by humorous stimuli, is characteristic, but occurs in only about 20% of patients. Some patients develop seizures that may be difficult to control. All eventually develop severe dysphagia that ultimately precludes oral feeding. Late-onset presentations with partial phenotypes are increasingly recognized. Adolescents and adults may present with subtle physical findings in the context of psychiatric illness, such as depression or schizophreniform illness.

ETIOLOGY/EPIDEMIOLOGY: Niemann-Pick disease, type C is a panethnic, autosomal-recessive disease resulting from mutations in NPC1 (in an estimated 95% of cases) or NPC2. Genetic isolates have been observed in Nova Scotia (French Acadians), Colorado, and New Mexico (Hispanics). The prevalence in Western Europe has been estimated at 1 in 150,000.

DIAGNOSIS: Invasive studies are now only rarely required, because a biochemical diagnosis can be made in most cases by studying lipid trafficking in cultured fibroblasts. Mutation analysis for the *NPC1* gene is available; more than 150 mutations have been described.

TREATMENT
Standard Therapies: Dystonia, epilepsy, and gelastic cataplexy respond in varying degrees to standard therapies. Supportive care with special attention to nutritional status and airway protection is critical; most patients eventually require gastrostomy feeding. Physical and speech therapy for patients and counseling support for family members is essential.

Investigational Therapies: Use of inhibitors of glycosphingolipid synthesis has shown promise.

REFERENCES

Chen C-S, Patterson MC, Wheatly CL, et al. Unexpected lysosomal accumulation of a fluorescent sphingolipid provides a general screening test for lipid storage diseases. *Lancet* 1999; 354;901–905.

Patterson M. Niemann-Pick disease, type C (September 2001). In: GeneClinics: Clinical Genetic Information Resource [database online]. Copyright, University of Washington, Seattle. Available at *www.geneclinics.org.*

Patterson MC, Di Bisceglie AM, Higgins JJ, et al. The effect of cholesterol-lowering agents on hepatic and plasma cholesterol in Niemann-Pick disease type C. *Neurology* 1993:43: 61–64.

Patterson MC, Vanier MT, Suzuki K, et al. Niemann-Pick disease, type C: a lipid trafficking disorder. In: Scriver CR, Beaudet AL, Sly WS, et al. *The metabolic and molecular bases of inherited disease,* 8th ed. New York: McGraw-Hill, 2001:3611–3633.

Vanier MT. Lipid changes in Niemann-Pick disease type C brain: personal experience and review of the literature. *Neurochem Res* 1999;24:481–489.

RESOURCES
109, 319, 335, 368

59   PEPCK Deficiency

Calum Sutherland, PhD

DEFINITION: Phosphoenolpyruvate carboxylase (GTP-oxaloacetate carboxylase, E.C. 4.1.1.32, PEPCK) deficiency is a disorder that results in neonatal hypoglycemia as a result of low, or absent neonatal gluconeogenesis. Phosphoenolpyruvate carboxylase is a rate-controlling enzyme of gluconeogenesis in the liver and kidney. The enzyme is encoded by two genes—*PCK1* (cytosolic form) and *PCK2* (mitochondrial form)—and expression is limited to a few tissues, mainly the liver, kidney, and adipose. The few reported cases of PEPCK deficiency were characterized by liver enlargement and impairment, with increased fasting alanine levels and fatty liver and kidney deposits. Patients have not survived longer than 36 months.

SYNONYMS: PCK1 or PCK2 deficiency.

DIFFERENTIAL DIAGNOSIS: Glucose-6-phosphatase deficiency; Fructose-1,6-diphosphatase deficiency; Pyruvate carboxylase deficiency.

SYMPTOMS AND SIGNS: At or shortly after birth, the neonate may have an enlarged liver, apnea, and a moderate delay in motor functions. Poor appetite, vomiting, coma, and seizures may be present. All four patients reported have exhibited convulsions. Liver impairment produces increased liver enzymes, alanine, glycine, and glutamine levels. Hypoglycemia is always present and may be accompanied by mild lacticacidemia after fasting. In 1 case where only *PCK1* was impaired, the myocardium and kidney tubules exhibited fatty infiltration and the optic nerve was atrophied.

ETIOLOGY/EPIDEMIOLOGY: The small number of cases of PEPCK deficiency tentatively diagnosed (N = 4) makes it impossible to accurately assess etiology. Both male and female patients have been reported. The diagnosis of PEPCK deficiency in these cases was achieved by biochemical measurement of PEPCK activity, with no genetic or hereditary evidence for an inborn defect. The parents and siblings of the patients were unaffected.

DIAGNOSIS: The diagnosis should be suspected after neonatal episodic hypoglycemia. Diagnosis should be confirmed by biochemical analysis of liver and/or kidney PEPCK expression and activity, along with liver enzyme, alanine, glycine, and glutamine levels. Other gluconeogenic enzyme activities/expression (e.g., glucose-6-phosphatase, pyruvate carboxylase) should be determined.

TREATMENT
Standard Therapies: In 1 case, coma was immediately reversed by glucose infusion; however, because of the rarity of this disorder, no treatment has been developed.

REFERENCES
Fiser RH, Melsher HL, Fisher DA. Hepatic PEPCK deficiency: a new cause of hypoglycemia in childhood [Abstract]. *Pediatr Res* 1974;8:432.

Hanson RW, Reshef L. Regulation of PEPCK gene expression. *Ann Rev Biochem* 1997;66:581–611.

Hommes FA, Bendien K, Elema JD, et al. Two cases of phosphoenolpyruvate carboxykinase deficiency. *Acta Paediatr Scand* 1976;65:233–240.

She P, Shiota M, Shelton KD, et al. PEPCK is necessary for the integration of hepatic energy metabolism. *Mol Cell Biol* 2000; 20:6508–6517.

Vidnes J, Sovik O. Gluconeogenesis in infancy and childhood. *Acta Paediatr Scand* 1976;65:307–312.

RESOURCES
109, 354, 478

60   Peroxisomal Biogenesis Disorders

Martina C. McGuinness, PhD, and Kirby D. Smith, PhD

DEFINITION: Peroxisome biogenesis disorders (PBDs) are a heterogeneous group of diseases characterized by alterations in the various proteins involved in peroxisome biogenesis and multiple defects in peroxisomal function. Clinically, PBDs are a group of lethal diseases with a continuum of severity of clinical symptoms ranging from the most severe form, Zellweger syndrome (ZS), to the milder forms, neonatal adrenoleukodystrophy (NALD), infantile Refsum disease (IRD), and Rhizomelic Chondrodysplasia Punctata (RCP).

SYNONYM: Cerebrohepatorenal syndrome.

DIFFERENTIAL DIAGNOSIS: X-linked adrenoleukodystrophy; "Adult" Refsum disease; Single enzyme defects in peroxisomal β-oxidation.

SYMPTOMS AND SIGNS: The disorders can often be recognized at birth due to a lack of muscle tone, an inability to suck and/or swallow, neonatal seizures, and dysmorphic features. Psychomotor delay, vision problems, liver enlargement, and renal cysts are also characteristic. Zellweger syndrome is the most severe form; patients have few, if any, functional peroxisomes in the liver and kidney and usually die during the first year of life. Patients have multiple congenital and metabolic abnormalities, including characteristic craniofacial abnormalities (high forehead, up-slanting palpebral fissures, hypoplastic supraorbital ridges, and epicanthal folds), ocular abnormalities (cataracts, glaucoma, corneal clouding, Brushfield spots, pigmentary retinopathy, and optic nerve dysplasia), severe hypotonia, seizures, chondrodysplasia punctata, and renal cysts. They also have neuronal migration defects and white matter abnormalities in the brain. Biochemical abnormalities include impaired degradation of peroxide, impaired very-long-chain fatty acid, pipecolic acid, and phytanic acid oxidation, and impaired plasmalogen, bile acid, cholesterol, and docosahexaenoic acid synthesis. Dysmorphic features are less striking in NALD and may be absent. The defects in plasmalogen synthesis and the degree of very-long-chain fatty acid accumulation are also less severe than in ZS. The neuronal and gray matter changes are less consistent and less severe than in ZS, but the white matter involvement is more striking. The clinical course of IRD is milder than that of NALD. Patients have an enlarged liver, mental retardation, sensorineural deafness, pigmentary degeneration of the retina, and moderately dysmorphic features including epicanthal folds, flat bridge of nose, and low-set ears. Patients often survive into the second decade of life. Rhizomelic chondrodysplasia (RCDP) is characterized clinically by severe growth failure, profound developmental delay, cataracts, rhizomelia, widespread epiphyseal calcifications, and ichthyosis. Patients have higher levels of phytanic acid and more severe deficiency of plasmalogens than patients with ZS, NALD, or IRD. Affected children usually die within the first two years of life, but may survive into their teens.

ETIOLOGY/EPIDEMIOLOGY: The PBDs are inherited in an autosomal-recessive manner with an incidence of approximately 1 in 50,000. All ethnic groups are affected. Some correlations between genotype and PBD have been found. Patients with classic RCDP are found in a single PBD complementation group, and the defective gene is *pex*7 encoding Pex7p, the PTS receptor. Mutations in pex7p result in abnormal import of peroxisomal matrix proteins carrying the PTS-2 import signal, including those involved in phytanic acid oxidation and plasmalogen synthesis.

DIAGNOSIS: Many of the biochemical pathways affected in PBDs can be assayed in the laboratory prenatally or postnatally. Ultrasonography can be used to detect renal cysts and enlarged livers.

TREATMENT
Standard Therapies: Treatment is usually symptomatic and supportive, such as special education programs, correction of auditory and vision deficits, steroid replacement therapy to correct adrenal insufficiency, and vitamin K to correct abnormal bleeding. Limited attempts to correct specific biochemical abnormalities by dietary supplementation and/or modification have had little or no effect on clinical outcome.

Investigational Therapies: Sodium-4-phenylbutyrate (4PBA) and other pharmacologic agents, including butyrate derivatives, are being explored.

REFERENCES
Gould SJ, Raymond GV, Valle D. The peroxisomal biogenesis disorders. In: Scriver CR, Beaudet AL, Valle D, eds. *The metabolic and molecular bases of inherited disease,* 8th ed. New York: McGraw-Hill, 2001:3181–3217.
McGuinness MC, Wei H, Smith KD. Therapeutic developments in peroxisome biogenesis disorders. *Exp Opin Invest Drugs* 2000; 9:1985–1992.
Moser HW. Genotype-phenotype correlations in disorders of peroxisome biogenesis. *Mol Genet Metab* 1999;68:316–327.
Wei HW, Kemp S, McGuinness MC, et al. Pharmacological induction of peroxisomes in peroxisome biogenesis disorders. *Ann Neurol* 2000;47:286–296.

RESOURCES
58, 335, 368, 477

61   Phenylketonuria

Juan Francisco Cabello, MD,
and Harvey L. Levy, MD

DEFINITION: Phenylketonuria (PKU) is an inherited metabolic disorder that can produce severe mental retardation. The biochemical genetic defect is a deficiency of the liver enzyme phenylalanine hydroxylase (PAH). This deficiency leads to elevated levels of the amino acid phenylalanine in the blood and other tissues.

SYNONYMS: PKU; Hyperphenylalaninemia.

DIFFERENTIAL DIAGNOSIS: Secondary hyperphenylalaninemia; Disorders of tetrahydrobiopterin (BH_4) deficiency (GTP cyclohydrolase I deficiency, 6-PTS deficiency, dihydropteridine reductase deficiency); Transient hyperphenylalaninemia; Tyrosinemia with secondary hyperphenylalaninemia; Galactosemia.

SYMPTOMS AND SIGNS: Untreated PKU is characterized by developmental delay leading to mental retardation, autism, microcephaly, delayed speech, seizures (particularly infantile spasms), eczema, and behavioral abnormalities.

ETIOLOGY/EPIDEMIOLOGY: Mutations in the *PAH* gene produce complete absence or profound deficiency of the enzyme PAH. The gene has been cloned and mapped to chromosome 12q24.1. More than 400 identified mutations have been associated with PKU and are inherited in an autosomal-recessive manner. The reported incidence of PKU from newborn screening programs ranges from 1 per 13,500 to 1 per 19,000 in the United States, with large variations among ethnic groups.

DIAGNOSIS: Diagnosis is usually made through neonatal screening. The infant should be referred to a metabolic specialist or center and for an evaluation that includes quantitative plasma amino acid levels, with particular attention to phenylalanine and tyrosine, and collection of additional blood and urine samples for pterin studies to evaluate the possibility of BH_4 deficiency with secondary hyperphenylalaninemia. Molecular genetic testing of the PAH gene may be used to specify the degree of PKU and for prenatal testing.

TREATMENT
Standard Therapies: Standard therapy includes a phenylalanine-restricted diet. Infants who have phenylalanine levels of >10 mg/dL should be started on treatment as soon as possible, ideally before 7–10 days of age. Those with levels between 7 and 10 mg/dL that persist more than a few days are usually started on dietary treatment. Those with phenylalanine levels of 3–6 mg/dL (non-PKU mild hyperphenylalaninemia) are not treated. Nutrition therapy involves the use of elemental amino acid medical products containing no phenylalanine, modified low-protein products, and a limited amount of natural food. The recommended blood phenylalanine levels on the diet are 2–6 mg/dL for individuals younger than 12 years, 2–10 mg/dL for adolescents, and 2–15 mg/dL for adults. The level should be monitored weekly during the first year of life and every other week thereafter. Lifelong dietary treatment is recommended. During episodes of intercurrent infections or stress protein, intake should be further restricted because of catabolism. Essential nutrients such as Ca, Fe, and Zn can be deficient and should be supplemented if necessary. Genetic counseling should be provided for the family. Measurement of the blood phenylalanine level in each parent should be obtained at the initial evaluation of the infant.

Investigational Therapies: Somatic gene therapy and enzymatic treatment as ancillary to the diet are being explored.

REFERENCES
Dougherty F, Levy H. Present newborn screening for phenylketonuria. *MRDD Res Rev* 1999;5:144–149.
Levy H. Phenylketonuria: old disease, new approach to treatment. *Proc Natl Acad Sci USA* 1999;96:1811–1813.
National Institutes of Health Consensus Statement, 2000. Phenylketonuria: screening and management. Available at *www.consensus.nih.gov.*
Scriver C, Kaufman Eisensmith R, Woo S. The hyperphenylalaninemias. In: Scriver CR, Beaudet AL, Sly WS, et al., eds. *The metabolic and molecular bases of inherited disease,* 7th ed. New York: McGraw-Hill, 1995:1015–1075.

RESOURCES
100, 324, 362, 391

62   Maternal Phenylketonuria

Juan Francisco Cabello, MD, and Harvey L. Levy, MD

DEFINITION: Maternal phenylketonuria is a disorder characterized by teratogenic effects in the offspring of a woman with phenylketonuria.

DIFFERENTIAL DIAGNOSIS: Fetal alcohol syndrome.

SYMPTOMS AND SIGNS: The most constant features are microcephaly and mental retardation in affected offspring. Congenital heart disease, facial dysmorphism, and low birth weight are also frequently observed (Insert Fig. 48). The effects are dose responsive, varying with the levels of phenylalanine during pregnancy and the duration of fetal exposure. Typically, there are no unusual complications of pregnancy, labor, and delivery.

ETIOLOGY/EPIDEMIOLOGY: The teratogenic effect is due to the maternal phenylketonuria and not related to whether the offspring has phenylketonuria. All offspring will be carriers of the mutation, but only occasionally (1 in 100) will have phenylketonuria. Phenylalanine readily crosses the placenta and is concentrated 1.2- to 1.9-fold in fetal blood. Phenylalanine is likely the toxic agent, but this is unproven. The maternal genotype does not have an independent influence over the frequency or severity of the teratogenic effects, but acts through the severity of the maternal hyperphenylalaninemia.

DIAGNOSIS: Pregnancies in phenylketonuric women are high risk. If a mother has one or more offspring with unexplained microcephaly and developmental delay, she should be tested for phenylalanine, because she may have undiagnosed phenylketonuria.

TREATMENT

Standard Therapies: A phenylalanine-restricted diet should be administered and monitored at a metabolic center. Pregnancies should be planned to achieve phenylalanine levels below 6 mg/dL 3 months before conception. The maternal phenylalanine level should be maintained at 2–6 mg/dL during the pregnancy with weekly or twice weekly monitoring. A comprehensive approach that provides psychosocial support for the family during the pregnancy and careful follow-up for the infant is essential.

REFERENCES

Lenke R, Levy H. Maternal phenylketonuria and hyperphenylalaninemia. An international survey of the outcome of untreated and treated pregnancies. *N Engl J Med* 1980;303: 1202–1208.

Levy H, Ghavami M. Maternal phenylketonuria: a metabolic teratogen. *Teratology* 1996;53:176–184.

Levy H, Waisbren S, Lobbregt D, et al. Maternal mild hyperphenylalaninemia: an international survey of offspring outcome. *Lancet* 1994;344:1589–1594.

National Institutes of Health, 2000. Consensus Development Conference Statement. Phenylketonuria: Screening and Management. Available at *www.consensus.nih.gov*.

Platt L, Koch R, Hanley W, et al. The international study of pregnancy outcome in women with maternal phenylketonuria: report of a 12-year study. *Am J Obstet Gynecol* 2000;182: 326–333.

RESOURCES

100, 324, 362, 391

63   Phosphoglycerate Kinase Deficiency

Jan Aasly, MD, PhD

DEFINITION: Phosphoglycerate kinase (PGK) deficiency is an X-linked disorder that causes jaundice, splenomegaly, hemolytic anemia, and mental retardation in infants and may cause exercise-induced pain, stiffness, and cramps with myoglobinuria in young males.

SYNONYM: Glycogenosis type X.

DIFFERENTIAL DIAGNOSIS: In newborns with jaundice: Sickle cell anemia; Thalassemia. In young males: Myophosphorylase deficiency (McArdle disease; glycogenosis type V); Muscle phosphofructokinase deficiency (Tarui disease; glycogenosis type VII).

SYMPTOMS AND SIGNS: The three main features are hemolytic anemia, mental retardation, and myopathy, which may coexist or manifest in combinations. Infants with PGK deficiency are born with nonimmune hydrops, jaundice, hepatomegaly and splenomegaly, hemolytic anemia, and mental retardation. All patients with childhood PGK deficiency have some degree of mental retardation with delayed language acquisition; some have epilepsy and strokes. Later in life, nonspherocytic hemolytic anemia is the most common clinical presentation. Most adult patients are moderately affected, and heterozygous females may show mild hemolytic anemia without crisis and have no myopathy or mental retardation. The third manifestation, myopathy with exercise-induced stiffness, cramps, myalgia, and rhabdomyolysis is seen in adolescents and young adult males. Myoglobinuria is a sign of extensive necrosis of muscle cells and typically triggered by a sudden start of vigorous exercise. The cramps are often severe and incapacitate the patient for hours. Splenomegaly is not seen in patients with pure myopathy; neither is hemolysis or anemia. Muscle biopsies have a normal appearance.

ETIOLOGY/EPIDEMIOLOGY: Phosphoglycerate kinase deficiency is inherited in an X-linked recessive manner. PGK catalyses the transfer of the acylphosphate group of 1,3-diphosphoglycerate to adenosine diphosphate with formation of 3-phosphoglycerate and adenosine triphosphate in the terminal stage of the glycolytic pathway. The ubiquitous PGK, which exits universally in various tissues, is encoded by a single structural gene on the X-chromosome q13. Several mutations are known to induce hemolytic anemia in different families. Mental retardation or myopathy, or the combination of both, is rare; probably fewer than 15 affected patients from different ethnic groups have been described.

DIAGNOSIS: PGK deficiency should be suspected in children with nonimmune hemolytic crisis and mental retardation and in children/young adults with exercise-induced

cramps and rhabdomyolysis. The ischemic forearm test is positive with no increase in lactate formation. Creatine kinase and myoglobin content in urine are usually normal between attacks. The PGK activity in muscle cells, erythrocytes, leukocytes, or fibroblasts is low, usually at or below 5% compared with normal controls. Electromyography and MRI of muscles are normal.

TREATMENT

Standard Therapies: In newborns with severe hemolytic crisis, splenectomy usually has a dramatic effect. After episodes of severe rhabdomyolysis, maintenance fluids and mannitol should be given to prevent acute renal failure due to myoglobin deposition, and alkalinizing agents to prevent acidosis and acute tubular necrosis. There is no other specific therapy. Patients with myopathy should be told to avoid sudden, vigorous exercise.

REFERENCES

Aasly J, van Diggelen OP, Boer AM, et al. Phosphoglycerate kinase deficiency in two brothers with McArdle-like clinical symptoms. *Eur J Neurol* 2000;7:111–113.

DiMauro S, Dalakas M, Miranda A. Phosphoglycerate kinase deficiency: a new cause of recurrent myoglobinuria. *Trans Am Neurol Soc* 1981;106:202–205.

Kraus A, Langston M, Lynch B. Red cell phosphoglycerate kinase deficiency: a new cause of non-spherocytic hemolytic anemia. *Biochem Biophys Res Commun* 1968;30:173–177.

Tarui S. Glycolytic defects in muscle: aspects of collaboration between basic science and clinical medicine. *Muscle Nerve* 1995;3(suppl):2–9.

Tsujino S, Shanske S, DiMauro S. Molecular genetic heterogeneity of phosphoglycerate kinase (PGK) deficiency. *Muscle Nerve* 1995;3(suppl):45–49.

RESOURCES
58, 109, 364

64   Acute Intermittent Porphyria

Karl E. Anderson, MD

DEFINITION: Acute intermittent porphyria (AIP) results from a deficiency of porphobilinogen (PBG) deaminase, the third enzyme in the heme biosynthetic pathway. The disease affects the nervous system and causes abdominal pain and potentially life-threatening muscle weakness.

SYNONYMS: Intermittent acute porphyria; Pyrroloporphyria; Swedish porphyria.

DIFFERENTIAL DIAGNOSIS: ALAD porphyria; Hereditary coproporphyria (HCP); Variegate porphyria (VP); Severe forms of functional bowel disease; Guillain-Barré syndrome.

SYMPTOMS AND SIGNS: Symptoms develop during adult life and are usually intermittent and in the form of attacks lasting for several days or longer. Pain in the abdomen, back, extremities, and elsewhere can be severe and accompanied by nausea, vomiting, abdominal distention, constipation, and bladder dysfunction. Other common findings are tachycardia, hypertension, restlessness, and fine tremors. Peripheral neuropathy is primarily motor, but may be accompanied by extremity pain that can be severe. Weakness usually begins in proximal muscles and more often in the arms than the legs. Cranial and sensory nerves can be affected. Progression to respiratory and bulbar paralysis and death may occur, especially if the disease is not recognized. Central nervous system involvement can lead to anxiety, insomnia, hallucinations, depression, and seizures. Hyponatremia can contribute to seizures. Attacks are more common in women. The disease may predispose to chronic hypertension and renal impairment. Some patients develop chronic pain. The disease is often associated with mild liver dysfunction. The risk for liver cancer is increased.

ETIOLOGY/EPIDEMIOLOGY: The disorder is inherited in an autosomal-dominant manner with highly variable penetrance. It is the result of mutations in the PBG deaminase gene. Up to 200 different mutations of this gene are known to cause the disease. The prevalence is estimated at 2–5 in 100,000. All ethnic groups are affected. Prevalence is considerably greater in northern Sweden, where one mutation is common, and may be somewhat greater in other populations of northern European origin. Most individuals who inherit a mutation causing AIP never develop symptoms. Known exacerbating influences include certain drugs, hormones, and nutritional alterations.

DIAGNOSIS: The diagnosis should be suspected in patients with unexplained abdominal pain, especially when accompanied by muscle weakness, other neurologic symptoms, or hyponatremia. Dark or reddish urine is sometimes a clue. The diagnosis of acute porphyria is readily established or excluded by measuring PBG in urine. If urinary PBG is substantially increased, further testing is needed to determine whether the patient has HCP or VP rather than AIP.

TREATMENT

Standard Therapies: Hospitalization for symptomatic and supportive treatment is often required during attacks. Narcotic analgesics are usually required for pain and small to moderate doses of a phenothiazine for nausea, vomiting, anxiety, and restlessness. Chloral hydrate can be used for insomnia. Diazepam in low doses is probably safe if a minor tranquilizer is required. Bladder distention may require catheterization. Specific therapies are intravenous glucose and heme. Carbohydrate loading may be adequate for mild attacks and can be given orally as sucrose, glucose polymers, or carbohydrate-rich foods. Intravenous glucose can be given if oral intake is not feasible. Heme therapy is most effective and should be initiated early in an attack. Management should include efforts to prevent future attacks and detect latent porphyria in relatives. Gonadotropin-releasing hormone analogues can prevent frequent cyclic attacks, as can periodic heme infusions.

Investigational Therapies: Tin mesoporphyrin and other inhibitors of heme breakdown are being studied to determine whether they may prolong or enhance the benefits of heme therapy.

REFERENCES
Anderson KE, Sassa S, Bishop D, et al. Disorders of heme biosynthesis: X-linked sideroblastic anemia and the porphyrias. In: Scriver CR, Beaudet AL, Sly WS, et al., eds. *The metabolic and molecular bases of inherited disease,* 8th ed. New York: McGraw-Hill, 2000:2991–3062.

Anderson KE, Spitz IM, Bardin CW, et al. A GnRH analogue prevents cyclical attacks of porphyria. *Arch Intern Med* 1990; 150:1469–1474.

Kauppinen R, Mustajoki P. Prognosis of acute porphyria: occurrence of acute attacks, precipitating factors, and associated diseases. *Medicine* 1992;71:1–13.

Tenhunen R, Mustajoki P. Acute porphyria: treatment with heme. *Semin Liver Dis* 1998;18:53–55.

RESOURCES
41, 109, 354

---

65   ALA-Dehydratase–Deficient Porphyria

Karl E. Anderson, MD

DEFINITION: ALA-dehydratase–deficient porphyria (ADP) is the result of a deficiency of delta-aminolevulinic acid (ALA) dehydratase (ALAD). Most symptoms resemble those that occur in other acute porphyrias, such as acute intermittent porphyria (AIP).

SYNONYM: Doss porphyria.

DIFFERENTIAL DIAGNOSIS: Acute intermittent porphyria; Hereditary tyrosinemia; Exposure to lead and other chemicals that can inhibit ALAD.

SYMPTOMS AND SIGNS: Attacks of abdominal pain, peripheral neuropathy, and other neurologic manifestations are identical to those that occur in AIP, but may begin in childhood. Drugs, steroids, and nutritional factors may provoke symptoms, as in other acute porphyrias. Hemolysis is sometimes present. Failure to thrive and developmental retardation during childhood may be a feature in severe cases. Cutaneous photosensitivity is not present.

ETIOLOGY/EPIDEMIOLOGY: Delta-aminolevulinic acid dehydratase is significantly reduced, often to 1%–2% of normal. The enzyme deficiency is inherited as an autosomal-recessive trait, and the parents have approximately half-normal enzyme activity. A variety of different mutations of the ALAD gene have been found in the few reported cases of ADP. Disease severity may depend in part on the severity of the inherited mutations and the degree of residual enzyme activity. The increased amount of coproporphyrin III found in this and other disorders in which ALA accumulates may originate from metabolism of excess ALA to coproporphyrin III in tissues other than the tissue of origin. The disease has been recognized mostly in Europe, but can occur in any population.

DIAGNOSIS: Urinary ALA and coproporphyrin III and erythrocyte zinc protoporphyrin are increased. These findings strongly suggest any condition associated with ALAD deficiency. It is important to document the deficiency by measuring the enzyme activity in erythrocytes, to exclude other causes of this enzyme deficiency, and to determine the underlying mutation of the ALAD gene.

TREATMENT
Standard Therapies: Acute attacks may be treated as in AIP. Drugs known to exacerbate other acute porphyrias should be avoided, although the efficacy of this approach in ADP is uncertain.

REFERENCES
Anderson KE, Sassa S, Bishop D, et al. Disorders of heme biosynthesis: X-linked sideroblastic anemia and the porphyrias. In: Scriver CR, Beaudet AL, Sly WS, et al., eds. *The metabolic and molecular bases of inherited disease,* 8th ed. New York: McGraw-Hill, 2000:2991–3062.
Sassa S. ALAD porphyria. *Semin Liver Dis* 1998;18:95–101.

66   Congenital Erythropoietic Porphyria

Herbert L. Bonkovsky, MD

DEFINITION: Congenital erythropoietic porphyria (CEP) is an autosomal-recessive disease caused by the inherited deficiency of the enzyme uroporphyrinogen-III synthase.

SYNONYM: Günther disease.

DIFFERENTIAL DIAGNOSIS: Hepatoerythropoietic porphyria; Hereditary coproporphyria; Variegate porphyria; Pseudoporphyria.

SYMPTOMS AND SIGNS: Typically, the disorder manifests shortly after birth. The major symptoms are due to marked overproduction and accumulation of uroporphyrin-I, which causes severe photosensitivity and fragility of the skin; erythrocytic fragility producing hemolytic anemia; red discoloration of the teeth, fingernails, and urine; and stunted growth. The disease is often associated with splenomegaly and the development of iron overload. The iron overload is related to the hemolytic anemia and sometimes also to transfusional or intravenous heme therapy, both of which supply extra iron to patients.

ETIOLOGY/EPIDEMIOLOGY: Many mutations of the gene for urogen-III cosynthase have been identified in patients and kindreds. The most common mutation reported in European and American countries has been the *C73R* mutation. Many patients are compound heterozygotes in whom the *C73R* mutation is found on one chromosome and some other mutation on the second chromosome. The gene encoding the urogen-III cosynthase protein contains 10 exons and is located on chromosome 10 in the chromosomal region 10q25.3. The disorder is seen equally in both sexes.

DIAGNOSIS: Diagnosis is established by the demonstration of increases in uroporphyrin in the urine and plasma of affected individuals. Special high-performance liquid chromatography or other separation techniques can distinguish the I isomer from the III isomer and lead to a firm diagnosis. Diagnosis may also be made by sequencing of the urogen-III cosynthase gene.

TREATMENT

Standard Therapies: Treatment involves the avoidance of sun or other strong light. Some modest additional benefit may accrue from the use of large doses of beta carotene. High doses of activated charcoal given orally several times a day may be capable of binding porphyrins within the gastrointestinal tract and enhancing their excretion, thereby preventing an enterohepatic circulation of the porphyrins, but the doses of charcoal required are sizable and unlikely to be tolerable over the long term. Another approach is to reduce the overproduction of porphyrins. Hypertransfusion of blood, particularly of young red blood cells, has been somewhat effective. Patients with splenomegaly and hypersplenism may benefit from splenectomy. In some patients, administration of intravenous heme can lead to some downregulation of the overproduction of porphyrins. Other patients have seemed to benefit from administration of hydroxyurea, to dampen red cell overproduction. Definitive therapy has been successfully delivered in a few patients who have undergone bone marrow or stem cell transplantation, with replacement or supplementation of their abnormal red blood cell precursors with normal precursors.

Investigational Therapies: Gene therapy may be tried.

REFERENCES
Bonkovsky HL, Barnard G. The porphyrias. In: Rakel RE, ed. *Conn's current therapy.* Philadelphia: WB Saunders, 2000:447–453.

Fontanellas A, Bensidhoum M, De Salamanca ER, et al. A systematic analysis of the mutations of the uroporphyrinogen III synthase gene in congenital erythropoietic porphyria. *Eur J Hum Genet* 1996;4:274–282.

Kieffer IZ, Langer B, Eyer D, et al. Successful cord blood stem cell transplantation for congenital erythropoietic porphyria (Günther's disease). *Bone Marrow Transplant* 1996;18:217–220.

Takamura N, Hombrados I, Tanigawa K, et al. Novel point mutation in the uroporphyrinogen III synthase gene causes congenital erythropoietic porphyria of a Japanese family. *Am J Med Genet* 1997;70:299–302.

Thomas C, Ged C, Nordmann Y, et al. Correction of congenital erythropoietic porphyria by bone marrow transplantation. *J Pediatr* 1996;129:453–456.

RESOURCES
41, 109, 354

---

67   Porphyria Cutanea Tarda

Karl E. Anderson, MD

DEFINITION: Porphyria cutanea tarda (PCT) causes blistering lesions on sun-exposed areas of the skin. It is the most common and readily treated form of porphyria, and is caused by a deficiency of uroporphyrinogen decarboxylase in the liver.

SYNONYM: Symptomatic porphyria.

DIFFERENTIAL DIAGNOSIS: Pseudoporphyria; Hereditary coproporphyria (HCP); Variegate porphyria (VP); Congenital erythropoietic porphyria; Erythropoietic protoporphyria.

SYMPTOMS AND SIGNS: Vesicles and bullae develop on sun-exposed areas, especially the backs of the hands, forearms, and face (Insert Fig. 49). The sun-exposed skin is friable, and minor trauma may lead to bullae or denudation of the skin. Small white plaques ("milia") may precede or follow vesicle formation. Other skin manifestations may include hypertrichosis, hyperpigmentation, scarring, thickening, and calcification. Liver dysfunction is common, and the risk of hepatocellular carcinoma is increased. Porphyria cutanea tarda associated with end-stage renal disease is often especially severe.

ETIOLOGY/EPIDEMIOLOGY: A normal or increased amount of hepatic iron is an essential finding in this disease. Iron may catalyze the formation of free radicals that inactivate or form an inhibitor of uroporphyrinogen decarboxylase. Hepatic uroporphyrinogen decarboxylase activity is decreased, whereas the amount of enzyme protein is normal. With treatment, the enzyme activity gradually increases. The disorder is most common in men. In women, estrogen use is almost always one of the contributing factors. Many other clinically identifiable factors contribute, including alcohol use, smoking, hepatitis C, HIV, and hemochromatosis. In addition, approximately 20% of patients have an inherited partial deficiency of uroporphyrinogen decarboxylase, which acts as a predisposing factor. Patients with this inherited enzyme deficiency are classified as having familial (type II), and those without it are classified as having sporadic (type I) PCT. The inherited enzyme deficiency in type II is an autosomal-dominant trait, and can result from many different mutations of the uroporphyrinogen decarboxylase gene.

DIAGNOSIS: Plasma porphyrins are increased in patients with skin lesions due to any type of porphyria, including PCT. A normal plasma porphyrin concentration, therefore, excludes PCT. If the plasma porphyrins are increased, the fluorescence spectrum of plasma can distinguish VP and EPP from PCT. Urine porphyrins are also increased, with a predominance of uroporphyrin and heptacarboxyl porphyrin. Isocoproporphyrins are increased in feces but are more difficult to measure. Urine porphobilinogen is normal, and delta-aminolevulinic acid is normal or only slightly increased. Familial (type II) PCT is distinguished from type I by an approximately 50% deficiency of the decarboxylase in nonhepatic tissues, such as erythrocytes.

TREATMENT

Standard Therapies: The preferred treatment is a course of phlebotomies at 1- to 2-week intervals. This virtually always leads to a remission of the disease, usually after about 5–6 units of blood are removed. Many more phlebotomies may be needed in patients who also have hemochromatosis. Patients are advised to discontinue alcohol, estrogens, iron supplements, or other contributing factors. Recurrences do not develop in most patients, but can be treated in the same manner. A course of low-dose chloroquine 125 mg twice weekly or hydroxychloroquine 100 mg twice weekly for several months is usually effective when repeated phlebotomies are contraindicated. Treatment of hepatitis C is generally addressed after the PCT has been treated.

REFERENCES

Anderson KE, Sassa S, Bishop D, et al. Disorders of heme biosynthesis: X-linked sideroblastic anemia and the porphyrias. In: Scriver CR, Beaudet AL, Sly WS, et al., eds. *The metabolic and molecular bases of inherited disease,* 8th ed. New York: McGraw-Hill, 2000:2991–3062.

Egger NE, Goeger DE, Payne DA, et al. Porphyria cutanea tarda: multiplicity of risk factors including *HFE* mutations, hepatitis C and inherited uroporphyrinogen decarboxylase deficiency. *Dig Dis Sci* 2002;47:419–426.

Elder GH. Porphyria cutanea tarda. *Semin Liver Dis* 1998;18:67–75.

Phillips JD, Jackson LK, Bunting M, et al. A mouse model of familial porphyria cutanea tarda. *Proc Natl Acad Sci USA* 2001;98:259–264.

RESOURCES

41, 109, 354

---

68 Variegate Porphyria and Hereditary Coproporphyria

Karl E. Anderson, MD

DEFINITION: Variegate porphyria (VP) and hereditary coproporphyria (HCP) are the result of inherited deficiencies of protoporphyrinogen oxidase and coproporphyrinogen oxidase, respectively. Affected individuals may present with neurologic attacks identical to those that occur in acute intermittent porphyria (AIP). Blistering skin lesions identical to those found with porphyria cutanea tarda (PCT) occur commonly in VP, and less commonly in HCP.

SYNONYMS: For VP: Porphyria variegata; South African genetic porphyria.

DIFFERENTIAL DIAGNOSIS: Acute intermittent porphyria; Porphyria cutanea tarda.

SYMPTOMS AND SIGNS: Attacks of abdominal pain, peripheral motor neuropathy, and other neurologic manifestations are identical to those that occur in AIP (see AIP entry). The cutaneous blistering lesions, which are much more common in VP than HCP, are identical to those of PCT. These may occur apart from the neurovisceral symptoms. Drugs, steroids, and nutritional factors that are detrimental in AIP provoke exacerbations of HCP and VP.

ETIOLOGY/EPIDEMIOLOGY: HCP and VP are a result of deficiencies of approximately 50% of coproporphyrinogen oxidase and protoporphyrinogen oxidase, respectively. These deficiencies are inherited as autosomal-dominant traits with variable penetrance. Most individuals who inherit these deficiencies remain asymptomatic for all or most of their lives. Many different mutations in the genes for these enzymes are described. VP is prevalent in

South Africa, where most affected persons are descendants of a couple who emigrated from Holland in the late 1600s. A few homozygous cases of HCP and VP have been described.

DIAGNOSIS: Urinary delta-aminolevulinic acid and porphobilinogen are commonly increased during acute attacks, but with clinical improvement these may normalize more readily than in AIP. Increases in urinary and fecal porphyrins are more persistent. A marked, isolated increase in fecal coproporphyrin (especially isomer III) is distinctive for HCP. Fecal coproporphyrin and protoporphyrin are about equally increased in VP. The fluorescence spectrum of plasma porphyrins (at neutral pH) is characteristic and useful for rapidly distinguishing VP from the other porphyrias. The plasma porphyrin concentration is usually normal and skin photosensitivity rare in HCP. The affected enzymes can be measured to detect latent cases, using cells other than erythrocytes; however, these assays are not widely available. If the specific mutation is known in a patient, latent disease can be reliably detected in relatives by DNA methods.

TREATMENT
Standard Therapies: Acute attacks are treated as in AIP. The skin manifestations of VP may be chronic and difficult to treat except by protection from sunlight. Phlebotomies

and chloroquine, which are effective in PCT, are not effective in VP and HCP. As with AIP, the overall prognosis has improved with better identification of latent cases, avoiding harmful drugs, and better treatment during acute attacks.

REFERENCES
Anderson KE, Sassa S, Bishop D, et al. Disorders of heme biosynthesis: X-linked sideroblastic anemia and the porphyrias. In: Scriver CR, Beaudet AL, Sly WS, et al., eds. *The metabolic and molecular bases of inherited disease,* 8th ed. New York: McGraw-Hill, 2000:2991–3062.

Kirsch RE, Meissner PN, Hift RJ. Variegate porphyria. *Semin Liver Dis* 1998;18:33–41.

Lamoril J, Puy H, Whatley SD, et al. Characterization of mutations in the CPO gene in British patients demonstrates absence of genotype-phenotype correlation and identifies relationship between hereditary coproporphyria and harderoporphyria. *Am J Hum Genet* 2001;68:1130–1138.

Martasek P. Hereditary coproporphyria. *Semin Liver Dis* 1998;18:25–32.

Whatley SD, Puy H, Morgan RR, et al. Variegate porphyria in Western Europe: identification of PPOX gene mutations in 104 families, extent of allelic heterogeneity, and absence of correlation between phenotype and type of mutation. *Am J Hum Genet* 1999;65:984–994.

RESOURCES
41, 109, 354

---

69   Erythropoietic Protoporphyria

Micheline M. Mathews-Roth, MD

DEFINITION: Erythropoietic protoporphyria (EPP) is an inherited deficiency of the enzyme ferrochelatase, resulting in the accumulation of excessive amounts of protoporphyrin in red blood cells and plasma. This accumulation causes the development of increased sensitivity of exposed skin to the visible light rays of the solar spectrum and, in some patients, to certain artificial light sources.

SYNONYMS: Protoporphyria; Erythrohepatic protoporphyria.

DIFFERENTIAL DIAGNOSIS: Polymorphous light eruption; Solar urticara; Variegate porphyria; Hereditary coproporphyria; Congenital erythropoietic porphyria; Hepatoerythropoietic porphyria; Porphyria cutanea tarda.

SYMPTOMS AND SIGNS: Patients with EPP experience pain, burning, or itching of light-exposed skin with some degree of redness or swelling. Usually, there are no prominent skin lesions, but some patients develop bullae or some areas of increased pigmentation and thickening of the skin. These symptoms usually start in childhood. Liver function is usually normal, but some patients with EPP develop protoporphyrin-containing gallstones and cholecystitis and bile duct obstruction, necessitating surgery. Rarely, a patient may develop severe liver damage that can progress to liver failure, requiring liver transplantation. Rapidly increasing protoporphyrin levels may signal onset of liver disease.

ETIOLOGY/EPIDEMIOLOGY: EPP is inherited as an autosomal-dominant trait, with poor penetrance; some people who carry the defective gene develop no symptoms. The disorder is due to mutations in the ferrochelatase gene, which is located on chromosome 18q.21.3. The prevalence of EPP has been estimated to be about 1 in 35,000. Males and females are affected equally, and EPP has been found in all races.

DIAGNOSIS: EPP should be suspected in any individual who reports skin discomfort on light exposure, especially if it occurs through window glass or from artificial light. The disorder is definitively diagnosed by finding elevated levels of protoporphyrin in erythrocytes and in plasma.

TREATMENT
Standard Therapies: Exposure to light should be decreased by the use of protective clothing. Opaque sunscreens may be helpful. An oral beta-carotene preparation, Lumitene (Tishcon Corp.), improves sunlight tolerance. This therapy has no effect on porphyrin levels. Patients should be monitored annually with liver function tests and protoporphyrin levels to watch for any signs of liver disease. Estrogen and drugs that impair bile flow should be avoided, as should consumption of alcohol. If surgery is required, the patient's skin, as well as internal organs, should be protected from the operating room lights.

Investigational Therapies: The orphan product L-cysteine is being tested for the prevention/reduction of photosensitivity.

REFERENCES
Desnick RJ. The porphyrias. In: Fauci AS, Braunwald E, Isselbacher KJ, et al, eds. *Harrison's principles of internal medicine,* 14th ed. New York: McGraw-Hill, 1998:2152–2158.

Mathews-Roth MM. Erythropoietic protoporphyria: beta-carotene and cysteine. *Dermatol Ther* 1997;4:81–85.

Pawliuk R, Bachelot T, Wise RJ, et al. Long-term cure of the photosensitivity of murine erythropoietic protoporphyria by preselective gene therapy. *Nat Med* 1999,5:768–773.

RESOURCES
41, 109, 147, 354

70   Pyruvate Kinase Deficiency

Ernest Beutler, MD

DEFINITION: Red cell pyruvate kinase deficiency is the most common hereditary nonspherocytic hemolytic anemia.

DIFFERENTIAL DIAGNOSIS: Hereditary nonspherocytic hemolytic anemia due to unstable hemoglobins and due to other enzyme defects—including glucose-6-phosphate dehydrogenase deficiency, glucose phosphate isomerase deficiency, triosephosphate isomerase deficiency, and glutathione synthetase deficiency.

SYMPTOMS AND SIGNS: The predominant symptoms are those of anemia. Splenomegaly is often present. The reticulocyte count is often greatly elevated, particularly in patients who have undergone splenectomy. The severity of the disease may vary from a mild, relatively well-compensated anemia to severe anemia requiring intravenous support through red cell transfusion.

ETIOLOGY/EPIDEMIOLOGY: Pyruvate kinase deficiency is inherited in an autosomal-recessive manner. It is caused by mutations of the *PKLR* gene, the gene that encodes the liver and red cell type of pyruvate kinase. The gene is located on chromosome 1 q21. The gene frequency for deficient alleles in the European population is approximately 7×10^{-3}.

DIAGNOSIS: The diagnosis depends on the results of a red cell enzyme assay or a screening test. Because the white cell pyruvate kinase is not encoded by *PKLR* but rather by a different gene, *PKM*, it is important that the red cells be freed of contaminating leukocytes. Prenatal diagnosis is best based on DNA sequence analysis.

TREATMENT
Standard Therapies: Mild cases require no treatment. Clinically severe disease is treated by blood transfusions and by splenectomy. The latter is delayed as long as possible in small children to allow the immune system to mature. Hematopoietic stem cell transplantation has rarely been performed and should be curative.

REFERENCES
Beutler E, Gelbart T. Estimating the prevalence of pyruvate kinase deficiency from the gene frequency in the general white population. *Blood* 2000;95:3585–3588.

Bianchi P, Zanella A. Hematologically important mutations: red cell pyruvate kinase (third update). *Blood Cells Mol Dis* 2000;26:47–53.

Demina A, Boas E, Beutler E. Structure and linkage relationships of the region containing the human L-type pyruvate kinase (*PKLR*) and glucocerebrosidase (*GBA*) genes. *Hematopathol Mol Hematol* 1998;11:63–71.

Hirono A, Kanno H, Miwa S, et al. Pyruvate kinase and related hemolytic anemias. In: Scriver CR, Beaudet AL, Sly WS, et al.,

eds. *The metabolic and molecular bases of inherited disease*, 8th ed. New York: McGraw-Hill, 2000.

Miwa S, Fujii H. Molecular basis of erythroenzymopathies associated with hereditary hemolytic anemia: tabulation of mutant enzymes. *Am J Hematol* 1996;51:122–132.

RESOURCES
228, 356

---

71   Sandhoff Disease

*Cynthia J. Tifft, MD, PhD,
and Richard L. Proia, PhD*

DESCRIPTION: Sandhoff disease is a neurodegenerative, inborn error of metabolism caused by a deficiency of the α subunit of enzymes α-hexosaminidase A (Hex A) and α-hexosaminidase B (Hex B).

SYNONYM: G_{M2} gangliosidosis variant O.

DIFFERENTIAL DIAGNOSIS: Tay-Sachs disease; G_{M2} activator deficiency.

SYMPTOMS AND SIGNS: Sandhoff disease is historically classified into infantile- (acute), juvenile- (subacute), or adult- (chronic) onset forms. The neurologic findings are clinically indistinguishable from Tay-Sachs disease. The early-onset form is generally recognized at 4–6 months of age with visual inattentiveness, mild motor weakness, and an exaggerated startle response. Ophthalmology evaluation shows a cherry-red spot, which although not pathognomonic, is strongly suggestive of G_{M2} gangliosidosis. Developmental skills plateau, and progressive loss of vision, hearing, and motor skills ensues. By 8–10 months, children develop seizures, and by 12 months feeding and swallowing become more difficult, leading to recurrent aspiration. Progressive macrocephaly develops and by 16–18 months the children become vegetative. Death by 2–5 years is common. In contrast to Tay-Sachs disease, patients with Sandhoff disease also develop hepatosplenomegaly and oligosacchariduria. Juvenile Sandhoff disease develops at 2–10 years with ataxia and incoordination followed by developmental regression and dementia. Affected children become spastic and develop seizures by the end of the first decade. Visual loss due to optic atrophy and retinitis pigmentosa is seen later in the course of the disease. Decerebrate rigidity and a vegetative state develop by 10–15 years, and death is usually by aspiration or intercurrent infection.

The adult or chronic form of Sandhoff is highly variable in its age of onset, presenting symptoms, and rate of progression. Patients are often misdiagnosed for several years after the onset of symptoms, which may include dystonia, ataxia, choreoathetoid movements, signs of spinocerebellar or motor neuron involvement, or psychosis. The disorder is slowly progressive over decades.

ETIOLOGY/EPIDEMIOLOGY: Sandhoff disease is an autosomal-recessive disorder caused by mutations in the *HEXB* gene on chromosome 5q13. More than 26 mutations have been described. In contrast to Tay-Sachs disease, there is no ethnic predilection in Sandhoff disease. The incidence, based on carrier screening, is estimated to be 1 in 309,000 or 15–20 births per year in North America.

DIAGNOSIS: The diagnosis should be suspected based on findings of developmental regression and a cherry red spot on ophthalmologic evaluation. Loss of developmental milestones in an older child as well as unexplained gait disturbance or movement disorder in an adult should also prompt investigation. The diagnosis is made by demonstrating markedly reduced α-hexosaminidase A and B activity in peripheral leukocytes. Prenatal diagnosis is available.

TREATMENT
Standard Therapies: These disorders are uniformly fatal, but supportive care can improve the quality of life for a limited time in some patients.

Investigational Therapies: Several approaches to therapy including bone marrow transplantation, substrate inhibitor drugs, and implantation of neuronal stem cells are being investigated.

REFERENCES
Gravel RA, Kaback MM, Proia RL, et al. The GM2 gangliosidoses. In: Scriver CR, Beaudet AL, Sly WS, et al., eds. *The metabolic*

and molecular bases of inherited disease, 7th ed. New York: McGraw-Hill, 1995:3827–3876.

Johnson WG. The clinical spectrum of hexosaminidase deficiency disease. *Neurology* 1981;31:1453.

Sandhoff K, Andreae U, Jatzkewitz H. Deficient hexosaminidase activity in an exceptional case of Tay-Sachs disease with additional storage of kidney globoside in visceral organs. *Pathol Eur* 1968;3:278.

Wada R, Tifft CJ, Proia RL. Microglial activation precedes acute neurodegeneration in Sandhoff disease and is suppressed by bone marrow transplantation. *Proc Natl Acad Sci USA* 2000; 97:10954–10959.

RESOURCES
288, 335, 368

---

72 Sialidosis

Peter J. Meikle, PhD

DEFINITION: Sialidosis is one of a group of more than 40 genetic disorders known as lysosomal storage disorders.

SYNONYMS: Cherry red spot and myoclonus syndrome; Glycoprotein neuraminidase deficiency; Lipomucopolysaccharidosis type I; Mucolipidosis type I; Neuraminidase deficiency; Sialidase deficiency; Sialidosis type I; Sialidosis type II.

DIFFERENTIAL DIAGNOSIS: Apartylglucosaminuria; α-Fucosidosis; Galactosialidosis; G_{M1} Gangliosidosis; G_{M2} Gangliosidosis; α-Mannosidosis; β-Mannosidosis; Mucolipidosis type II/III; Mucopolysaccharidoses.

SYMPTOMS AND SIGNS: As with most lysosomal storage disorders, sialidosis can manifest with a broad spectrum of clinical severity, although all phenotypes result from a deficiency of the α-sialidase enzyme. Sialidosis has been divided into two broad subtypes. Type I is the late-onset form of the disease and usually presents in the second to third decade of life with the development of gait abnormalities and/or problems with visual acuity. Ocular cherry red spots and generalized myoclonus are also noted at this stage. Additional symptoms in some patients include seizures, hyperreflexia, and ataxia. Sialidosis type II is the more severe form of the disease, presenting early in life with a severe mucopolysaccharidosis-like phenotype, including organomegaly, dystosis multiplex, and mental retardation. Additional clinical features may include coarse facial features, increased head size, and short stature. Cherry red spots and myoclonus are also observed in older children. Type II sialidosis has been subdivided into a congenital form, marked by severe clinical abnormalities at birth, and an infantile form, in which symptoms develop soon after birth. The congenital form is often associated with hydrops fetalis and neonatal ascities with stillbirth or death at an early age.

ETIOLOGY/EPIDEMIOLOGY: Sialidosis is inherited in an autosomal-recessive manner. No accurate figures are available for the incidence, but a figure of 1 in 4.2 million live births has been reported in the Australian population. The disease results from a deficiency of the lysosomal enzyme exo-α-sialidase (EC 3.2.1.18). The gene for this enzyme is located on chromosome 6p21.3. The cDNA has been cloned and a number of mutations identified.

DIAGNOSIS: Screening tests based on the identification of abnormal patterns and/or amounts of oligosaccharides in urine have been developed using thin-layer chromatography. These screens serve to identify an abnormality in glycoprotein degradation and can identify a range of glycoproteinoses/oligosaccharidoses. Sialic acid containing glycoconjugates can be specifically localized by resorcinol staining of the oligosaccharides. Positive diagnosis is made by direct measurement of the α-sialidase activity in a suitable tissue, usually cultured skin fibroblasts or white cells from a whole blood sample. Prenatal diagnosis is possible by enzyme determination in cultured amniotic cells or chorionic villi samples.

TREATMENT
Standard Therapies: No definitive treatment is available for this disorder.

REFERENCES
Holmes EW, O'Brien JS. Separation of glycoprotein derived oligosaccharides by thin-layer chromatography. *Anal Biochem* 1979;93:167–170.

Meikle PJ, Hopwood JJ, Clague AE, et al. Prevalence of lysosomal storage disorders. *JAMA* 1999;281:249–254.

Pshezhetsky AV, Richard C, Michaud L, et al. Cloning, expression and chromosomal mapping of human lysosomal sialidase and characterization of mutations in sialidosis. *Nat Genet* 1997;15:316–320.

RESOURCES
109, 314, 354, 440

73   Succinic Semialdehyde Dehydrogenase Deficiency

Phillip L. Pearl, MD,
and K. Michael Gibson, PhD

DEFINITION: Succinic semialdehyde deficiency (SSADH) is an autosomal-recessive disorder that affects the metabolism of GABA (gamma-amino-butyric acid), the major inhibitory neurotransmitter of the brain. It manifests as mental retardation, ataxia, and seizures.

SYNONYMS: 4-Hydroxybutyric aciduria; Gamma-hydroxybutyric aciduria.

DIFFERENTIAL DIAGNOSIS: Mental retardation-ataxia syndromes; Epileptic encephalopathy.

SYMPTOMS AND SIGNS: SSADH presents in childhood with psychomotor retardation with seizures, muscle hypotonia, and nonprogressive ataxia. Associated features include disproportionate language delay and behavioral abnormalities, including autistic traits, aggressiveness, anxiety, and hallucinations.

ETIOLOGY/EPIDEMIOLOGY: This is an autosomal-recessive disease caused by deficiency of the SSADH enzyme, which is involved in the metabolism of GABA. SSADH, in conjunction with GABA-transaminase, converts GABA to succinate. In the absence of SSADH, GABA converts to 4-hydroxybutyrate (gammahydroxybutyrate, GHB). The accumulation of GHB is believed to represent the toxic metabolite leading to the clinical syndrome. Mutations in the SSADH gene have been identified in some patients. The disorder has been identified in approximately 200 patients, with a fair proportion of consanguineous families.

DIAGNOSIS: The diagnosis should be suspected in mental retardation-ataxia syndromes of unknown etiology, particularly if accompanied by seizures or an epileptiform electroencephalogram. Electroencephalographic features are nonspecific and include generalized and focal spike-wave discharges, and background disorganization with slowing. MRI may show increased T2-weighted signal of the globus pallidus. The diagnosis will be primarily suspected, however, by abnormal urine organic acid testing, showing an accumulation of 4-hydroxybutyric acid. Urine organic acid testing may not specifically detect 4-hydroxybutyrate, in which case this accumulation will be masked in a larger urea peak and may be missed diagnostically. Confirmation of the diagnosis is readily achieved in peripheral blood cells.

TREATMENT

Standard Therapies: No standard therapies exist. Seizures are managed with antiepileptic drugs. Vigabatrin is a logical therapy, as its inhibition of GABA-transaminase leads to lack of formation of succinic semialdehyde, the substrate for SSADH. This agent has not produced consistent results. Valproate is not recommended.

Investigational Therapies: Benzodiazepines and opiate receptor antagonists are being investigated.

REFERENCES

Gibson KM, Hoffmann GF, Hodson AK, et al. 4-hydroxybutyric acid and the clinical phenotype of succinic semialdehyde dehydrogenase deficiency, an inborn error of GABA metabolism. *Neuropediatrics* 1998;29:14–22.

Gibson KM, Jakobs C. Disorders of beta- and gamma amino acids in free and peptide-linked forms. In: Scriver CR, Beaudet AL, Sly WS, et al., eds. *The metabolic and molecular bases of inherited disease,* 8th ed. New York: McGraw-Hill, 2001:2079–2105.

Gibson KM, Sweetman L, Nyhan WL, et al. Succinic semialdehyde dehydrogenase deficiency: an inborn error of gamma-aminobutyric acid metabolism. *Clin Chim Acta* 1983;133:33–42.

Matern D, Lehnert W, Gibson KM, et al. Seizures in a boy with succinic semialdehyde dehydrogenase deficiency treated with vigabatrin. *J Inherit Metab Dis* 1996;19:313–318.

RESOURCES

58, 361, 365, 368

74 Tangier Disease

Margaret E. Brousseau, PhD,
and Ernst J. Schaefer, MD

DEFINITION: Tangier disease (TD) is a genetic disorder characterized by severe deficiency of high-density lipoprotein cholesterol (HDL-C) concentrations in the plasma, as well as by the deposition of cholesteryl esters in tissues throughout the body. Sites of deposition include macrophages in the tonsils, liver, spleen, intestinal mucosa, lymph nodes, bone marrow, and Schwann cells.

SYNONYM: Familial high-density lipoprotein deficiency.

DIFFERENTIAL DIAGNOSIS: ApoA-I deficiency; ApoA-I/C-III deficiency; ApoA-I/C-III/A-IV deficiency; Familial lecithin:cholesteryl acyltransferase deficiency; Fish eye disease; Obstructive liver disease; Hepatic parenchymal diseases or tumors; Gaucher disease; Niemann-Pick, type C; Wolman disease; Acquired HDL deficiency states.

SYMPTOMS AND SIGNS: The classic clinical signs of TD are hyperplastic orange-yellow tonsils, splenomegaly, and relapsing peripheral neuropathy, each resulting from cholesteryl ester deposition. A severely reduced HDL-C level in combination with hyperplastic orange-yellow tonsils is virtually pathognomonic for TD. Aside from these findings, the clinical expression of TD is variable, with some patients presenting with hepatomegaly, abnormal rectal mucosa, corneal opacities, anemia, lymphadenopathy, thrombocytopenia, and/or premature coronary heart disease.

ETIOLOGY/EPIDEMIOLOGY: Tangier disease is caused by mutations in the gene encoding adenosine triphosphate-binding cassette 1, or *ABCA1*. Located on chromosome 9q31, *ABCA1* is a member of a large family of ATP-binding cassette transporters, which use ATP as a source of energy to transport one of the avidin-biotin complex transporters that transfer substrates to various cellular compartments. The clinical phenotype in TD is inherited in an autosomal-recessive mode, whereas the biochemical phenotype is autosomal codominant. Fewer than 100 cases of TD have been reported, with both genders and many different ethnic groups being affected.

DIAGNOSIS: In patients with unexplained hepatic or splenic enlargement, neuropathy, or corneal deposits, examination of the oropharynx and quantification of plasma total cholesterol, HDL-C, low-density lipoprotein cholesterol (LDL-C), and triglycerides are indicated. TD homozygotes have plasma levels of HDL-C and LDL-C that are typically <5% (<5 mg/dL) and <50% (<70 mg/dL) of normal, respectively. Although severely reduced, apolipoprotein A-I is detectable in the plasma. A definitive diagnosis can be made by identifying mutation(s) in the *ABCA1* gene through sequence analysis.

TREATMENT

Standard Therapies: No clear guidelines exist for treatment. Attempts to significantly raise plasma HDL-C levels have been unsuccessful. Other coronary disease risk factors should be treated, especially in patients with established coronary heart disease.

REFERENCES

Assmann G, von Eckardstein A, Brewer HB Jr. Familial high density lipoprotein deficiency: Tangier disease. In: Scriver CR, Beaudet AL, Sly WS, et al., eds. *The metabolic and molecular bases of inherited disease,* 7th ed. New York: McGraw-Hill, 1995:2053–2072.

Bodzioch M, Orso E, Klucken J, et al. The gene encoding ATP-binding cassette transporter 1 is mutated in Tangier disease. *Nat Genet* 1999;22:347–51.

Brooks-Wilson A, Marcil M, Clee SM, et al. Mutations in *ABC1* in Tangier disease and familial high-density lipoprotein deficiency. *Nat Genet* 1999;22:336–345.

Brousseau ME, Schaefer EJ, Dupuis J, et al. Novel mutations in the gene encoding ATP-binding cassette 1 in four Tangier disease kindreds. *J Lipid Res* 2000;41:433–441.

Fredrickson DS, Altrocchi PH, Avioli LV, et al. Tangier disease. *Ann Intern Med* 1961;55:1016–1031.

Remaley AT, Rust S, Rosier M, et al. Human ATP-binding cassette transporter 1 (ABC1): genomic organization and identification of the genetic defect in the original Tangier disease kindred. *Proc Natl Acad Sci USA* 1999;96:12685–12690.

Rust S, Rosier M, Funke H, et al. Tangier disease is caused by mutations in the gene encoding ATP-binding cassette transporter 1. *Nat Genet* 1999;22:352–355.

RESOURCES

335, 368

75 Tay-Sachs Disease

William G. Johnson, MD

DEFINITION: Tay-Sachs disease (TSD) is a progressive, neurodegenerative disorder that results from a genetically determined deficiency of the enzyme hexosaminidase that causes the accumulation of GM2-ganglioside and/or other complex lipids and/or mucopolysaccharides, especially in the neurons of cells.

SYNONYMS: GM2 gangliosidosis, type I; Cerebromacular degeneration; Hexosaminidase A deficiency; Juvenile Tay-Sachs disease.

DIFFERENTIAL DIAGNOSIS: Sandhoff disease; Alpers disease; Kufs disease; Leigh disease.

SYMPTOMS AND SIGNS: As a result of a successful program of carrier screening, later-onset variants of TSD are seen much more frequently than is progressive infantile encephalopathy, which in the past was far more prevalent. The infantile encephalopathy with cherry-red spots group includes three disorders: classic infantile Tay-Sachs disease (α locus), infantile Sandhoff disease (α locus), and the AB variant (activator-protein coenzyme locus). Infants with these conditions appear normal until 3–10 months. Listlessness and irritability are usually the first indications of the illness, and hyperacusis (myoclonic jerks in response to sound) is seen in approximately one half of infants. The macular cherry red spot is diagnostic. The weak and floppy infants present with hyperactive reflexes, clonus, and extensor plantar responses. Although seizures and myoclonus are obvious and frequent during the first year or more, the infants become decorticate, leading to a vegetative state, usually by 2 years. No significant enlargement occurs of liver or spleen. Progressive enlargement of the head is invariable if the disease has lasted more than 18 months. In the late infantile, juvenile, and adult GM2-gangliosidoses forms, dementia and ataxia with or without macular cherry red spots are almost invariable. These may be accompanied by muscle wasting and spasticity caused by anterior horn disease. Some patients with late-onset forms present with cerebellar ataxia or motor neuron disease. Lower motor neuron forms resemble Kugelberg-Welander or Aran-Duchenne syndrome. Patients with upper motor neuron forms present with symptoms and signs similar to those of amyotrophic lateral sclerosis.

ETIOLOGY/EPIDEMIOLOGY: The Tay-Sachs gene affects approximately 1 in 30 Ashkenazi Jews, and within this population the disease occurs in approximately 1 of 3,900 live births. In the general population, the disorder may be encountered in approximately 1 of 112,00 live births. The inheritance pattern is recessive and usually autosomal, but sometimes X-linked.

DIAGNOSIS: In infantile encephalopathy with cherry red spots, the brain, cerebellum, and spinal cord show grossly ballooned neurons throughout by light microscopy. Electron microscopy (rectal biopsy as tissue source) highlights membranous cytoplasmic bodies with regularly spaced concentric dark and pale lamellae. In classic Tay-Sachs, hexosaminidase A is absent and hexosaminidase B is increased. For late infantile, juvenile, and adult GM2-gangliosidoses forms, rectal biopsy for electron microscopy of autonomic neurons, natural substrate hexosaminidase assays, and DNA-based diagnosis are key tests.

TREATMENT
Standard Therapies: No specific treatment exists for TSD in any of its variants. Treatment is supportive and palliative.

REFERENCES
Johnson WG. Lysosomal and other storage diseases. In: Rowland LP, ed. *Merritt's neurology,* 10th ed. Philadelphia: Lippincott Williams & Wilkins, 2000:514–518.
Kaback MM, Desnick RJ. Tay-Sachs disease: from clinical description to molecular defect. *Adv Genet* 2001;44:1–9.
Platt FM, Jeyakumar M, Andersson U, et al. Inhibition of substrate synthesis as a strategy for glycolipid lysosomal storage disease therapy. *J Inherit Metab Dis* 2001;24:275–290.
Risch N. Molecular epidemiology of Tay-Sachs disease. *Adv Genet* 2001;44:233–252.

RESOURCES
231, 299, 335, 368

76   Tetrahydrobiopterin Deficiency

Beat Thöny, PhD, and Nenad Blau, PhD

DEFINITION: Tetrahydrobiopterin (BH4) deficiency is a genetic neurologic disorder present at birth. Impairment of the metabolism of the coenzyme BH4 due to autosomal-recessive or -dominant mutations (for autosomal-dominant mutations, see Dopa-responsive dystonia) leads to lowered levels of the monoamine neurotransmitters dopamine and serotonin. In many variants, BH4 deficiency is accompanied by an abnormally high blood level of the amino acid phenylalanine.

SYNONYMS: BH4 deficiency; Atypical phenylketonuria; Malignant hyperphenylalaninemia.

DIFFERENTIAL DIAGNOSIS: Classic phenylketonuria (PKU).

SYMPTOMS AND SIGNS: Symptoms of BH4 deficiency usually include neurologic disturbances, muscle tone and coordination abnormalities, seizures, microcephaly, hypersalivation, hypotonia of the trunk, hypertonia of the limbs, and delayed motor development. The classical forms of BH4 deficiency, i.e., autosomal-recessive deficiency of GTP cyclohydrolase I, 6-pyruvoyl tetrahydropterin synthase, and dihydropteridine reductase, present with hyperphenylalaninemia. Patients do not respond to a low-phenylalanine diet. Patients with sepiapterin reductase deficiency present with normal plasma phenylalanine levels but with symptoms and signs related to monoamine neurotransmitter deficiency, including dystonia.

ETIOLOGY/EPIDEMIOLOGY: BH4 deficiencies are inherited as autosomal-recessive or -dominant traits. Cofactor deficiencies are due to mutations in the genes encoding the BH4 metabolic enzymes, including GTP cyclohydrolase I, 6-pyruvoyl-tetrahydropterin synthase, sepiapterin reductase, and dihydropteridine reductase (mutations in the carbinolamine dehydratase lead only to transient hyperphenylalaninemia without neurologic problems).

DIAGNOSIS: BH4 deficiencies are often found in newborn screening for hyperphenylalaninemia (Guthrie card). Further differentiation requires measurements of urinary biopterin and neopterin and a BH4 loading test, as well as enzymatic measurements in red blood cells, and determination of monoamine neurotransmitter and biopterin metabolites in cerebrospinal fluids. In case of sepiapterin reductase deficiency, the blood phenylalanine levels are normal, although symptoms and signs related to monoamine neurotransmitter deficiency are present. Determination of neurotransmitter metabolites in cerebrospinal fluids and biopterin-metabolite production in *in vitro*–cultivated and cytokine-stimulated primary skin fibroblasts is recommended.

TREATMENT

Standard Therapies: Treatment should be started as early as possible to prevent potentially severe and irreversible neurologic damage. To control high plasma phenylalanine levels, oral daily doses of synthetic BH4 are mandatory to restore liver phenylalanine hydroxylase activity. To treat the neurologic disturbances, a combined and lifelong therapy with the neurotransmitter precursors L-dopa/carbidopa and 5-hydroxytryptophan is required.

Investigational Therapies: Some patients with low compliance are treated with the monoamine A inhibitor Deprenyl (selegiline) or with the catechol-O-methyl transferase inhibitors.

REFERENCES

Blau N, Blaskovics M. Hyperphenylalaninemia. In: Blau N, Duran M, Scriver CR, eds. *Physician's guide to the laboratory diagnosis of metabolic diseases.* New York: Chapman & Hall, 1996:65–78.

Blau N, Thöny B, Cotton RGH, et al. Disorders of tetrahydrobiopterin and related biogenic amines. In: Scriver CR, Beaudet AL, Sly WS, et al., eds. *The metabolic and molecular bases of inherited disease.* New York: McGraw-Hill, 2001: 1275–1776.

Bonafé L, Thöny B, Penzien JM, et al. Mutations in the sepiapterin reductase gene cause a novel tetrahydrobiopterin-dependent monoamine neurotransmitter deficiency without hyperphenylalaninemia. *Am J Hum Genet* 2001;69:269–277.

Thöny B, Auerbach G, Blau N. Tetrahydrobiopterin biosynthesis, regeneration and functions. *Biochem J* 2000;3471–3516.

RESOURCES

58, 109, 368

77   Trimethylaminuria

Eileen P. Treacy, MD,
and Deborah M. Lambert, MSc

DEFINITION: Trimethylaminuria (TMAuria) is a condition associated with a decreased ability to oxidize dietary-derived odorous trimethylamine (TMA) to the non-odorous metabolite trimethylamine N-oxide (TMANO) caused by an inherited or acquired deficiency in N-oxidation of trimethylamine. This results in an excretion of free trimethylamine in urine, sweat, and bodily secretions and a fishlike odor.

SYNONYMS: Fish-odor syndrome; FMO, adult liver form.

DIFFERENTIAL DIAGNOSIS: Odor due to organic aciduria (e.g., isovaleric aciduria); Fishlike odor due to dimethylglycinuria or consumption of high doses of carnitine (TMA precursor).

SYMPTOMS AND SIGNS: The condition presents with an unpleasant, rotten fish odor. Onset of symptoms may be in the newborn period or in adulthood, but generally is first noted in the early (school-age) childhood period. Symptoms are exacerbated by the consumption of foods rich in choline or TMA precursors, hot weather, emotional stress, or exercise. In females, symptoms may be exacerbated perimenstrually. The odor may be quite severe and offensive, leading to social isolation of those affected. Individuals with severe TMAuria possibly have decreased clearance of biogenic amines and altered metabolism of some medications.

ETIOLOGY/EPIDEMIOLOGY: TMAuria occurs in both sexes but is more common in females. The incidence varies in different populations: many reported patients are of British Isles or Australian-British origin, with others reported from Germany and Asia. The liver flavin-containing monooxygenase enzyme FMO3 mediates oxidation of TMA. Rare mutations (abolished enzyme activity) and common polymorphisms (decreased enzyme activity) encoded by the *FMO3* gene on chromosome 1q21-23 have been described. The phenotype results from overloading a deficient TMA N-oxidation system.

DIAGNOSIS: The diagnosis should be suspected with the characteristic fishlike odor. Diagnostic testing of trimethylamine and trimethylamine N-oxide is available at only a few referral centers. Diagnosis is made by an excess of TMA either alone or in combination with increased TMANO. Confirmation may be provided by molecular analysis of the *FMO3* gene.

TREATMENT

Standard Therapies: Standard therapy includes supportive, counseling, and dietary intervention. The dietary treatment consists of a decrease in foods containing choline and lecithin. Professional dietary advice is recommended to maintain a well-balanced diet with adequate mineral and vitamin supplementation. The diet may resolve milder cases and improve the symptoms in severe cases. In unresponsive severe cases, intermittent use of a gut-sterilizing antibiotic such as metronidazole may help.

Investigational Therapies: Riboflavin may be useful in milder cases. Local agents such as gut absorbents, charcoal, and local skin adsorbents are being investigated.

REFERENCES

Dolphin CT, Janmohamed A, Smith RL, et al. Missense mutation in flavin-containing mono-oxygenase 3 gene, *FMO3* underlies fish-odour syndrome. *Nat Genet* 1997;17:491–494.

Lambert DM, Mamer OA, Akerman BR, et al. *In vivo* variability of TMA oxidation is partially mediated by polymorphisms of the *FMO3* gene. *Mol Genet Metab* 2001;73 (in press).

Mitchell SC, Smith RL. Trimethylaminuria: the fish malodor syndrome. *Drug Metab Disposition* 2001;29:517–521.

Treacy EP, Akerman B, Chow LML, et al. Mutations of the flavin-containing monooxygenase gene *(FMO3)* cause trimethylaminuria, a defect in detoxication. *Hum Mol Genet* 1998;7:839–845.

Zchoscke J, Kohlmueller D, Quak E, et al. Mild trimethylaminuria caused by common variants in *FMO3* gene. *Lancet* 1999;354:834–835.

RESOURCES

58, 109, 416

78   Tyrosinemia Type I

Elizabeth Holme, MD

DEFINITION: Tyrosinemia type I is an inborn error of metabolism caused by a deficiency of fumarylactoacetase, which is the last enzyme in the tyrosine degradation pathway. Accumulation of fumarylacetoacetate, maleylacetoacetate, and succinylacetone causes liver and kidney damage. Succinylacetone is a potent inhibitor of 5-aminolevulinic acid dehydratase and porfyrin synthesis.

SYNONYMS: Hepatorenal tyrosinemia; Fumarylacetoacetase deficiency.

DIFFERENTIAL DIAGNOSIS: Liver disease of other causes (hypertyrosinemia and liver failure); Hypophosphatemic rickets of other causes; Neonatal transient hypertyrosinemia; Tyrosinemia type II; Tyrosinemia type III; Tyrosinemia of prematurity; Hawkensinosis.

SYMPTOMS AND SIGNS: The age at onset of symptoms varies from the neonatal period to adolescence. Most patients present during infancy with signs of liver failure preceded by failure to thrive. Often, a marked coagulopathy exists, although other signs of liver disease are subtle. Even in the infant with liver failure, the jaundice is modest and the level of liver transaminases is not exceedingly high. The α-fetoprotein concentration is often highly increased. Sepsis is common. Signs of hypophosphatemic bone disease may exist, secondary to renal tubular dysfunction, which is often more pronounced when the onset of symptoms is during childhood. Rarely, the presenting symptom is a porphyria-like neurologic crisis. If untreated, the mortality rate during infancy is high. Children who survive past 2 years of age have progressive liver disease with an exceptionally high risk for development of hepatocellular carcinoma (HCC). Survival beyond adolescence is rare.

ETIOLOGY/EPIDEMIOLOGY: Tyrosinemia type I is inherited in an autosomal-recessive manner. The disease is due to mutations in the fumarylacetoacetase gene, located on chromosome 15q 23–25. The incidence is estimated to be 1 in 100,000 to 1 in 200,000, but is variable in different ethnic groups. The incidence is high in Quebec province in Canada.

DIAGNOSIS: The diagnosis should be suspected in any child with signs of liver disease and/or rickets and renal tubular dysfunction and in children with hypertyrosinemia. The diagnosis is made by identification of succinylacetone and related substances in urine or plasma. Other laboratory findings are high plasma tyrosine level, and in acutely ill patients, an increase in methionine. Erythrocyte 5-aminolevulinate dehydratase (porphobilinogen synthase) activity is low and there is a large urinary excretion of 5-aminolevilinate (5-ALA).

TREATMENT

Standard Therapies: For many years, treatment with a diet restricted in phenylalanine and tyrosine was the only available treatment. Dietary treatment may alleviate acute symptoms but does not stop progression of the liver disease and development of HCC. Since 1992, NTBC [2-(2-nitro-4-trifluoromethylbenzoyl)-1,3-cyclohexanedione] has been available for treatment of tyrosinemia type I. The drug blocks tyrosine degradation and production of toxic metabolites, but gives an increased tyrosine concentration, which has to be controlled by diet.

REFERENCES

Holme E, Lindstedt S. Tyrosinaemia type I and NTBC (2-(2-nitro-4-trifluoromethylbenzoyl)-1,3-cyclohexanedione. *J Inherit Metab Dis* 1998;21:507–517.

Holme E, Lindstedt S. Nontransplant treatment of tyrosinemia. *Clin Liver Dis* 2000;4;805–814.

Lindstedt S, Holme E, Lock EA, et al. Treatment of hereditary tyrosinemia, type I by inhibition of 4-hydroxyphenylpyruvate dioxygenase. *Lancet* 1992;2:813–817.

Mitchell GA, Grompe M, Lambert M, et al. Hypertyrosinemia. In: Scriver CR, Beaudet AL, Sly WS, et al., eds. *The metabolic and molecular bases of inherited disease*, 8th ed. New York: McGraw-Hill, 2001:1777–1805.

RESOURCES

58, 98, 109, 416

79   Urea Cycle Disorders

Asad I. Mian, MB, BS,
and Brendan Lee, MD, PhD

DEFINITION: The urea cycle is a metabolic pathway that converts excess nitrogen into urea. Deficiency of any enzyme in the pathway causes a urea cycle disorder (UCD). The triad of hyperammonemia, encephalopathy, and respiratory alkalosis is characteristic of the UCDs.

SYNONYMS: Carbamyl phosphate synthetase I deficiency; Ornithine transcarbamylase (OTC) deficiency; Argininosuccinate synthetase deficiency (citrullinemia); Argininosuccinate lyase deficiency (argininosuccinic aciduria); Arginase deficiency; N-acetyl glutamate synthetase deficiency.

DIFFERENTIAL DIAGNOSIS: Severe dehydration; Organic acidemias; Fatty acid oxidation defects; Disorders of pyruvate metabolism; Lysinuric protein intolerance; Hyperornithinemia, hyperammonemia, homocitrullinuria syndrome; Transient hyperammonemia of the newborn; Portosystemic circulatory shunt, e.g., patent ductus venosus.

SYMPTOMS AND SIGNS: A UCD typically manifests in a full-term newborn who appears well for the first 24–48 hours after birth. The infant becomes symptomatic once feeding has been initiated secondary to the protein load of human milk or formula. Initial signs include somnolence and poor feeding, usually followed by vomiting, lethargy, and coma. A common early sign in newborns with hyperammonemia is central hyperventilation leading to respiratory alkalosis, which may be a result of cerebral edema. Increasing edema may also cause abnormal posturing and progressive encephalopathy with hypoventilation and respiratory arrest. Approximately 50% of infants with severe hyperammonemia have seizures. Atypical presentations after the newborn period are seen in patients with partial urea cycle enzyme deficiencies. This delayed presentation is most common with partial OTC deficiency, but it may occur with other UCDs. Children may present atypically with chronic vomiting, developmental delay, seizure disorder, and psychiatric illness.

ETIOLOGY/EPIDEMIOLOGY: The overall incidence of the UCDs is approximately 1 per 8,200 live births. The diseases are due to mutations in genes encoding enzymes of the urea cycle. The inheritance pattern is autosomal recessive, except for OTC deficiency. Since OTC is X-linked, hemizygous males are usually more severely affected than females. The clinical severity in affected females depends on the pattern of X-inactivation in the liver and ranges from asymptomatic to almost as severe as in an affected male.

DIAGNOSIS: The laboratory hallmark of a UCD is an elevated ammonia concentration. Initial diagnostic tests should include arterial pH and CO_2 tension, serum lactate, serum glucose, serum electrolytes to calculate the anion gap, plasma amino acids, urine organic acids, urine orotic acid, and acylcarnitine profile. An elevated plasma ammonia concentration combined with normal blood glucose and anion gap strongly suggests a UCD. Additional testing is required to identify the specific enzyme deficiency; quantifying plasma levels of different metabolites of the urea cycle is helpful.

TREATMENT
Standard Therapies: Neurologic abnormalities and impaired cognitive function are significantly correlated with the duration of hyperammonemia and encephalopathy; thus, treatment should be started as soon as a UCD is suspected. Symptomatic newborns with hyperammonemia should be cared for in a center experienced in the diagnosis and treatment of metabolic disorders. The initial approach should include rehydration and maintenance of good urinary output, curtailment of protein intake, and removal of excess ammonia using medications and dialysis. Pharmacologic therapy of hyperammonemia consists of administration of sodium phenylacetate and sodium benzoate. Arginine and citrulline may need to be supplemented depending on the specific UCD. In the presentation of massive hyperammonemia, hemodialysis is indicated, since pharmacotherapy and other forms of dialysis will be inadequate to rapidly decrease ammonia levels. In centers that are not equipped to perform neonatal hemodialysis, immediate transfer should be considered.

Investigational Therapies: A combined preparation of sodium phenylacetate and sodium benzoate (Ammonul) is available as an investigational drug for intravenous use in the acute setting. Some patients with UCDs may be candi-

dates for liver transplantation. Gene therapy may become available. For maintenance therapy, oral sodium phenylbutyrate (Buphenyl) is FDA approved for chronic treatment.

REFERENCES

Brusilow SW, Horwich AL. Urea cycle enzymes. In: Scriver CR, Beaudet AL, Sly WS, et al., eds. *The metabolic and molecular bases of inherited disease,* 8th ed. New York: McGraw-Hill, 2001:1909–1963.

Brusilow SW, Maestri NE. Urea cycle disorders: diagnosis, pathophysiology, and therapy. *Adv Pediatr* 1996;43:127.

Lee B, Goss J. Long-term correction of urea cycle disorders. *J Pediatr* 2001;138(suppl):62–71.

Summar M. Current strategies for the management of neonatal urea cycle disorders. *J Pediatr* 2001;138(suppl):30–39.

RESOURCES

37, 58, 109, 336, 354, 383

80 Wilson Disease

George J. Brewer, MD

DEFINITION: Wilson disease is an autosomal-recessive inherited disease of copper toxicity causing liver disease and often a neurologic movement disorder and behavioral disturbance, usually presenting in teenagers or young adults.

SYNONYM: Hepatolenticular degeneration.

DIFFERENTIAL DIAGNOSIS: Hepatitis; Cirrhosis; Liver failure; Parkinsonism; Essential tremor; Mood disorder; Depression; Substance abuse.

SYMPTOMS AND SIGNS: Patients with Wilson disease can present initially with a liver disease, a movement disorder, or a behavioral disturbance. The liver disease may mimic viral hepatitis, chronic active hepatitis, or cirrhosis. The patient may present with hepatic failure, which may be mild, moderate, or severe. The predominant signs and symptoms of the movement disorder include dysarthria, tremor, incoordination, and dystonia. Behavioral disturbances may antedate obvious liver or neurologic disease by several years and include loss of ability to focus on tasks, loss of control of emotions, depression, suicidal thoughts, sexual exhibitionism, and, occasionally, delusions or hallucinations.

ETIOLOGY/EPIDEMIOLOGY: The disease is the result of a mutation in gene *ATP7B,* which plays an important role in liver excretion of excess copper into the bile for loss in the stool. In most populations, the disease occurs at a rate of approximately 1 in 40,000 people. It affects both sexes equally.

DIAGNOSIS: Initial workup should include a thorough history, physical examination, blood counts (including platelets), and liver function tests. The presence of concomitant liver and brain disease is strongly suggestive of Wilson disease. Relative youth is a strong clue. Useful tests include 24-hour urine copper, an ophthalmologic slit-lamp examination for Kayser-Fleischer rings, and a serum ceruloplasmin. The gold standard for diagnosis is quantitative liver copper, measured from a needle biopsy sample.

TREATMENT
Standard Therapies: All patients require lifelong anticopper therapy. Zinc acetate (Galzin) is recommended for maintenance therapy, treatment of presymptomatic patients, and for pregnant patients. A combination of trientine (Syprine) and zinc is recommended for the initial 4 months of treatment for hepatic patients. In patients with severe hepatic failure, hepatic transplantation is indicated. Penicillamine (Cuprimine), which has many toxic side effects, should be avoided in the initial treatment of neurologic symptoms, because it worsens the neurologic condition of approximately 50% of patients.

Investigational Therapies: An experimental drug, tetrathiomolybdate, is being developed.

REFERENCES
Brewer GJ. Recognition, diagnosis, and management of Wilson's disease. *Proc Soc Exp Biol Med* 2000;223:39–49.

Brewer GJ. *Wilson's disease: a clinician's guide to recognition, diagnosis, and treatment.* Hingham, MA: Kluwer, 2001 (in press).

Brewer GJ, Dick RD, Johnson VD, et al. Treatment of Wilson's disease with zinc: XV long-term follow-up studies. *J Lab Clin Med* 1998;132:264–278.

Brewer GJ, Johnson V, Dick RD, et al. Treatment of Wilson disease with ammonium tetrathiomolybdate. II. Initial therapy in 33 neurologically affected patients and follow-up with zinc therapy. *Arch Neurol* 1996;53:1017–1025.

Thomas GR, et al. The Wilson disease gene: spectrum of mutations and their consequence. *Nat Genet* 1995;9:210–217.

RESOURCES
39, 368, 494

Neurologic Disorders

1   Agenesis of the Corpus Callosum

Richard Bittar, MBBS, PhD

DEFINITION: Agenesis of the corpus callosum is a disorder of neuronal migration resulting in partial or complete absence of the corpus callosum.

SYNONYMS: Cerebral dysgenesis; Callosal agenesis.

DIFFERENTIAL DIAGNOSIS: Chiari malformations; Encephaloceles; Dandy-Walker cysts; Other neuronal migration disorders.

SYMPTOMS AND SIGNS: Type I callosal agenesis is either asymptomatic or is associated with mild neurologic manifestations such as mild mental retardation, epilepsy, or impaired bimanual coordination. It is not associated with other disorders. Type II callosal agenesis is associated with more severe neurologic problems, including failure to thrive, seizures, spasticity, hemi/diplegia, and moderate to severe mental retardation. It is associated with other chromosomal syndromes or neuronal migration disorders, and patients may have hydrocephalus or microcephaly.

ETIOLOGY/EPIDEMIOLOGY: Incidence is unknown. Etiology is usually either genetic (sporadic, autosomal dominant, and X-linked inheritance patterns) or metabolic (e.g., neonatal adrenoleukodystrophy), with the causative insult occurring *in utero*.

DIAGNOSIS: The investigative algorithm for developmental delay or seizures should include cerebral CT and MRI. These will demonstrate the partial or complete absence of the corpus callosum and may also show a high-riding (upwardly displaced and enlarged) third ventricle, widely spaced frontal horns, dilatation of the occipital horns, and evidence of other neuronal migration disorders.

TREATMENT
Standard Therapies: Management requires a multidisciplinary approach involving pediatricians, neurologists, orthopedic surgeons, and occupational and physical therapists. Seizures are treated with anticonvulsants. Genetic counseling is important. Some patients may be suitable for surgery to treat intractable epilepsy.

REFERENCES
Barkovich AJ, Simon EM, Walsh CA. Callosal agenesis with cyst: a better understanding and a new classification. *Neurology* 2001;56:220–227.
Finlay DC, Peto T, Payling J, et al. A study of three cases of familial related agenesis of the corpus callosum. *J Clin Exp Neuropsychol* 2000;22:731–742.
Goodyear PW, Bannister CM, Russell S, et al. Outcome in prenatally diagnosed agenesis of the corpus callosum. *Fetal Diagn Ther* 2001;16:139–145.
Zannolli R, Mostardini R, Pucci L, et al. Corpus callosum agenesis, multiple cysts, skin defects, and subtle ocular abnormalities with a *de novo* mutation [45,XX,der(5), t(514)(pter; q11.2)]. *Am J Med Genet* 2001;102:29–35.

RESOURCES
12, 79, 190, 368

2   Primary Visual Agnosia

Glyn W. Humphreys, PhD

DEFINITION: Primary visual agnosia is a neurologic disorder consequent on lesions to the posterior ventral cortex (particularly regions of the occipital and temporal lobes supplied by the posterior cerebral artery). It is characterized by a deficit in recognizing and naming common objects from vision; tactile recognition and naming of the object to a verbal definition can be intact. Face and word recognition can also be affected. It is found in its most profound form after bilateral damage, but can occur in milder forms after unilateral lesions. Unilateral lesions to the right hemisphere are associated with poor face recognition, and unilateral lesions to the left hemisphere with poor word recognition.

DIFFERENTIAL DIAGNOSIS: Optic aphasia; Semantic dementia.

SYMPTOMS AND SIGNS: Patients are unable not only to name visually presented objects, but also to provide accurate descriptions about the nature of the object and what it might be used for, confirming a diagnosis of impaired recognition as well as impaired naming. Patients may be able to copy objects even when they cannot recognize them. However, even when copying is impaired, aspects of visual perception can be shown to be intact, because patients may remain able to perform simple visual matching tasks, and they may often reach and grasp objects appropriately. A distinction can be drawn between apperceptive and associative agnosia. In apperceptive agnosia, basic visual perception may be disrupted although visually directed actions can be spared. In associative agnosia, basic visual perception can be spared, but patients are unable to match their percepts with their stored memories, and so fail to recognize the objects. Long-term memory for objects can be intact, as shown by asking the patient to draw from memory. A variety of psychophysical tests can be conducted to pinpoint the nature of the visual process that is disrupted in a given patient. Tests of reading (particularly varying the lengths of the words) and face recognition should be performed, because these abilities are also likely to be affected. In addition, color perception can be disrupted, although stereo-depth perception may be spared.

ETIOLOGY/EPIDEMIOLOGY: This syndrome occurs as a result of damage to posterior regions of the cortex (typically bilateral), and can be found after stroke, tumor, or head injury.

DIAGNOSIS: As indicated by the symptoms, diagnosis should include tests of the following: naming visually presented objects, recognition of visually presented objects (e.g., describing their use), copying objects, drawing from memory, tactile recognition and naming (using the same objects as tested for vision), and naming to auditory definitions (for the same objects as tested for vision). Additional psychophysical tests can include perceptual matching, object decision (judging whether an object is real), associative matching, and recognition from unusual viewpoints.

TREATMENT
Standard Therapies: Retraining procedures have focused on having patients pay detailed attention to critical features of objects and to restoring any loss of stored memories. Patients typically improve at recognizing real objects compared with line drawings, reflecting the use of information about surfaces and three-dimensional depth.

REFERENCES
Humphreys GW. *Case studies in the neuropsychology of vision.* London: Psychology Press, 1999.
Riddoch MJ, Humphreys GW. *The Birmingham Object Recognition Battery.* London: Psychology Press, 1993.
Riddoch MJ, Humphreys GW, Gannon T, et al. Memories are made of this: the effects of time on stored visual knowledge in a case of visual agnosia. *Brain* 1999;122:537–559.

RESOURCES
197, 368

3 Aicardi Syndrome

Adele Schneider, MD

DEFINITION: Aicardi syndrome is a neurodevelopmental disorder characterized by agenesis of the corpus callosum, chorioretinal lacunae, infantile spasms, and mental retardation.

SYNONYMS: Agenesis of corpus callosum-chorioretinal abnormality; Agenesis of corpus callosum-infantile spasms-ocular anomalies.

DIFFERENTIAL DIAGNOSIS: Congenital toxoplasmosis; Microphthalmia-linear skin defects (MLS) syndrome; Goltz syndrome.

SYMPTOMS AND SIGNS: Microcephaly is common in this condition. Variable brain abnormalities include partial or complete agenesis of the corpus callosum, abnormal cerebral ventricles, choroid plexus cysts and papillomas, and cortical migration defects. The Dandy-Walker variant with midline cerebellar hypoplasia, gray matter heterotopias, and cortical malformations such as lissencephaly, pachygyria, or polymicrogyria is frequently reported. Hemispheric and ventricular asymmetries and absence of the pineal gland have been reported. Mental retardation and seizure disorder occur. Seizures develop in early infancy. Typical electroencephalographic (EEG) findings consist of multifocal epileptiform activity occurring in a burst suppression pattern, showing complete asynchrony between the two hemispheres. Chorioretinal lacunae may be seen in association with microphthalmia, colobomas of optic nerve and choroid, persistent pupillary membrane, scleral ectasia, and glial tissue extending from the disc (Insert Fig. 50). Hypoplastic optic nerves and chiasm have been described and, rarely, anophthalmia. Visual impairment is common. Other findings may include vertebral and rib anomalies, scoliosis, oral clefts, and hypotonia. Hepatoblastoma, embryonal carcinoma, lipoma, and metastatic angiosarcoma have also been described.

ETIOLOGY/EPIDEMIOLOGY: All patients described were female or had Klinefelter syndrome with karyotype 47,XXY. The syndrome is believed to be an X-linked dominant, male lethal mutation on the short arm of the X chromosome. All cases appear to represent new mutations. Some overlap of findings is noted in Aicardi, Goltz, and MLS syndrome. All are considered to be male lethal conditions. These three conditions may be caused by a defect in the same gene or genes at Xp22, or they may be caused by different but contiguous genes.

DIAGNOSIS: Clinical diagnosis is based on eye, brain, and EEG findings. Seizures usually present in the first year of life, possibly as infantile spasms. Studies should include imaging of the brain (MRI or CT), ophthalmologic evaluation, EEG, and skeletal films for vertebral and rib anomalies. A significant EEG finding is the independent activity of each hemisphere. Other studies may be indicated based on results of the clinical examination, such as chromosome study with G-banding. Prenatal diagnosis by high-resolution ultrasonography would detect cerebral malformations and microphthalmia.

TREATMENT

Standard Therapies: Standard therapy is anticonvulsants, although seizures may be difficult to control. Frequent pneumonias should be treated with antibiotics. Early intervention for developmental delay and vision therapy for low vision or blindness is indicated in some individuals. Feeding tube or gastrostomy should be used if indicated.

REFERENCES

Bromley B, Krishnamoorthy KS, Benacerraf BR. Aicardi syndrome: prenatal sonographic findings. A report of two cases. *Prenat Diagn* 2000;20:344–346.

Costa T, Greer W, Rysiecki G, et al. Monozygotic twins discordant for Aicardi syndrome. *J Med Genet* 1997;34:688–691.

Jones KL. *Smith's recognizable patterns of human malformation,* 5th ed. Philadelphia: WB Saunders, 1997.

Neidich JA, Nussbaum RL, Packer RJ, et al. Heterogeneity of clinical severity and molecular lesions in Aicardi syndrome. *J Pediatr* 1990;116:911–917.

Smith CD, Ryan SJ, Hoover SL, et al. Magnetic resonance imaging of the brain in Aicardi syndrome: report of 20 patients. *J Neuroimaging* 1996;6:214–221.

RESOURCES

13, 77, 197, 368

---

4   Alexander Disease

Michael Brenner, PhD,
Anne B. Johnson, MD,
James E. Goldman, MD, PhD,
and Albee Messing, VMD, PhD

DEFINITION: Alexander disease is an often fatal neurologic disorder, characterized by the widespread presence in astrocytes of protein aggregates, termed Rosenthal fibers.

SYNONYMS: Fibrinoid leukodystrophy; Dysmyelinogenic leukodystrophy with megalobarencephaly.

DIFFERENTIAL DIAGNOSIS: Canavan disease; Vacuolating leukoencephalopathy; Leigh encephalopathy; Adrenoleukodystrophy; Metachromic leukodystrophy; Krabbe leukodystrophy; Tay-Sachs disease; Glutaric aciduria type 1; Multiple sclerosis; Merosin-deficient congenital muscular dystrophy; Cerebral palsy and tumor (especially brain stem tumors in juvenile and adult forms).

SYMPTOMS AND SIGNS: The most common is the infantile form, which manifests between birth and 2 years. Patients show an enlarged head and extensive myelin deficiency, most marked in the frontal cerebrum. This is accompanied by progressive and severe developmental and motor deficits. Clinical signs include loss of mental and physical developmental milestones, megalencephaly, seizures, hydrocephalus, spasticity, vomiting, hyperreflexia, and eventual paralysis of the limbs. This form is progressive and usually fatal by age 10 years. The juvenile and adult forms progress more slowly. The juvenile form typically manifests between 2 and 10 years, and the adult form after 10 years. Primary clinical signs for both juvenile and adult forms are speech problems, difficulty swallowing and/or breathing, ataxia, spasticity, and vomiting. Mental decline often develops slowly, but may not occur.

ETIOLOGY/EPIDEMIOLOGY: Fewer than 100 cases of Alexander disease have been described, but no precise estimates of incidence or prevalence are available. No racial, ethnic, geographic, or sex preference has been observed. Most cases of Alexander disease are sporadic, but a few families have more than one affected member. Heterozygous mutations in the coding region of GFAP, an astrocyte-specific intermediate filament protein, are associated with most cases of the sporadic infantile form and some of the later onset forms. The GFAP mutations are dominant, and except for a reported family of adult-onset cases, arise *de novo*. The exact mechanism by which the mutations cause disease is not known, however. The failure to find GFAP mutations for several patients indicates that other causes of the disease exist.

DIAGNOSIS: The conditions in the differential diagnosis should be excluded if tests are available to do so. MRI, in conjunction with clinical signs, is helpful and can usually differentiate Alexander disease from other leukodystrophies and from vacuolating leukoencephalopathy, tumor, and merosin-deficient congenital muscular dystrophy.

Identification of one of the known GFAP mutations in patient DNA probably provides a definitive diagnosis; however, a negative result does not preclude the disease. Finding a mutation in an affected child opens the possibility of fetal testing for subsequent pregnancies. The definitive diagnosis remains demonstration of disseminated Rosenthal fibers in a biopsy or autopsy sample.

TREATMENT
Standard Therapies: There is no treatment other than supportive therapy.

REFERENCES
Brenner M, Johnson AB, Boespflug-Tanguy O, et al. Mutations in *GFAP*, encoding glial fibrillary acidic protein, are associated with Alexander disease. *Nat Genet* 2001;27:117–120.
Messing A, Goldman JE, Johnson AB, et al. Alexander disease: new insights from genetics. *J Neuropathol Exp Neurol* 2001; 60:563–573.
Van der Knaap MS, Naidu S, Breiter SN, et al. Alexander disease: diagnosis with MR imaging. *Am J Neuroradiol* 2001;22: 541–552.

RESOURCES
58, 368, 462, 477

5   Alexander Syndrome

Alpers Syndrome

*Sanjiv Sahoo, MD,
Tena Rosser, MD,
and Phillip L. Pearl, MD*

DEFINITION: Alpers syndrome is a rapidly progressive encephalopathy of infancy and early childhood caused by degeneration of cerebral gray matter. When associated with hepatic failure, the disease is called Alpers-Huttenlocher syndrome.

SYNONYMS: For Alpers syndrome: Alpers disease; Diffuse progressive degeneration of the gray matter; Progressive infantile poliodystrophy; Poliodystrophia cerebri progressiva; Spongy glioneuronal dystrophy; Spongy degeneration of the gray matter; Diffuse cerebral degeneration of infancy. For Alpers-Huttenlocher syndrome: Progressive neuronal degeneration with liver disease; Diffuse degeneration of cerebral gray matter with hepatic cirrhosis; Early childhood hepatocerebral degeneration.

DIFFERENTIAL DIAGNOSIS: Leigh disease and other mitochondrial disorders; Progressive myoclonic epilepsies; Neuronal ceroid lipofuscinosis; Tay-Sachs disease.

SYMPTOMS AND SIGNS: Most patients develop symptoms between ages 2 and 13 months, but onset may occur in early or late childhood. Late presentation with visual symptoms, subacute encephalopathy, and seizures in previously healthy teenagers has been reported. Typically, patients have an insidious onset of progressive developmental delay, profound hypotonia, bouts of vomiting, and failure to thrive. An antecedent event such as a viral infection, dehydration, vaccination, or status epilepticus is sometimes identified. Seizures are the presenting symptom in approximately 25% of patients, whereas in others epilepsy occurs after a period of neurologic deterioration. Epilepsia partialis continua, status epilepticus, and myoclonus are prominent. Visual symptoms are common, initially manifesting as migraine-like illness with flashing aura and pain behind the eyes, and nausea and vomiting. Homonymous hemianopia and cortical blindness ensue. Other features may include chorea, ataxia, and deafness. Signs of hepatic dysfunction may be apparent before onset of seizures. Late-stage disease is characterized by severe spastic quadriplegia, intractable epilepsy, cortical blindness, and hepatic failure. Most patients do not survive beyond age 3 years or more than 2–3 years after onset of symptoms.

ETIOLOGY/ EPIDEMIOLOGY: Autosomal-recessive inheritance is presumed. Males and females are affected equally. Multiple enzymatic abnormalities have been identified in this disorder.

DIAGNOSIS: Definitive diagnosis can only be made post-mortem, based on brain and liver pathology, but use of biochemical, electrophysiologic, and radiologic testing can support the diagnosis during a patient's lifetime. Routine workup to exclude other metabolic neurodegenerative diseases is warranted, including plasma amino acids, urine organic acids, serum lactate/pyruvate, ammonia, and liver function tests. Muscle and skin biopsy may be required to rule out mitochondrial disorders and neuronal ceroid lipofuscinosis, respectively.

TREATMENT
Standard Therapies: Management is supportive. Traditional anticonvulsants are used to treat epilepsy; however, valproic acid has been associated with hepatic failure in these patients.

Investigational Therapies: Potential treatment strategies are based on supplying electron transport chain cofactors and substrates, L-carnitine, and antioxidants. Sodium succinate, lipoic acid, ascorbic acid, niacin, riboflavin, and coenzyme Q10 have all been recommended. When lactic acidosis is prominent, the experimental agent dichloro-acetate has been used.

REFERENCES
Gauthier-Villers M, Landrieu P. Respiratory chain deficiency in Alpers syndrome. *Neuropediatrics* 2001;32:150–152.
Harding BN. Progressive neuronal degeneration of childhood with liver disease (Alpers-Huttenlocher syndrome): a personal review. *J Child Neurol* 1990;5:273–287.
Harding BN, Alsanjari N, Smith SJM, et al. Progressive neuronal degeneration of childhood with liver disease (Alpers' disease) presenting in young adults. *J Neurol Neurosurg Psychiatry* 1995;58:320–325.
Lyon G, Adams RD, Kolodny EH. Alpers syndrome. In: Lyon G, Adams RD, Kolodny EH, eds. *Neurology of hereditary metabolic diseases in children,* 2nd ed. New York: McGraw-Hill, 1996:81–84.
Naviaux KN, Nyhan WL, Barshop BA. Mitochondrial DNA polymerase gamma deficiency and mt DNA depletion in a child with Alpers syndrome. *Ann Neurol* 1999;45:54–58.

RESOURCES
58, 145, 288, 478

---

6   Alternating Hemiplegia of Childhood

Fernando Dangond, MD

DEFINITION: Alternating hemiplegia of childhood (AHC) is characterized by paroxysmal attacks of limb weakness and tonic "fits," usually manifesting in childhood. A familial syndrome of AHC has also been described.

SYNONYMS: Familial alternating hemiplegia (FAH); Familial alternating hemiplegia of childhood (FAHC).

DIFFERENTIAL DIAGNOSIS: Moyamoya disease; Seizures; Postictal paralysis; Hemiplegic migraine.

SYMPTOMS AND SIGNS: Infants with AHC present with episodes of one-sided limb weakness (hemiparesis or hemiplegia), sometimes associated with facial weakness.

Rarely, patients may also present with attacks of quadriplegia or monoparesis. The episodes may last minutes to hours, and subside spontaneously. Patients remain alert and are able to communicate verbally. Some patients also present with "tonic fits"; it is uncertain whether these represent tonic seizures or paroxysmal dystonic postures. A subset of patients may experience true epilepsy. Patients have preserved ability to track objects with a conjugate gaze and seemingly remain alert during episodes of bilateral tonic fits. The episodes of hemiplegia or tonic fits alternate and may occur daily, weekly, or once every few months. Baseline clinical examinations may show dystonia, choreoathetosis, or abnormal eye movements including nystagmus. It is widely believed that with age, patients with AHC develop psychomotor retardation or cognitive impairment. Children with early onset and increased frequency of attacks have a greater risk of developmental delay.

ETIOLOGY/EPIDEMIOLOGY: Alternating hemiplegia of childhood is primarily a sporadic disease. The familial syndrome is believed to be autosomal dominant. It is possible that genes located within the affected chromosomal regions may be involved in triggering the syndrome. Because of its paroxysmal nature and exclusivity to the central nervous system, the familial syndrome may be caused by mutations/rearrangements of a gene involved in the structure of neuronal membrane channels, such as a calcium channel, or involved in other neuronal membrane function but using calcium for its proper activity. No association has been shown of AHC with mutations of the calcium channel gene responsible for hemiplegic migraine, *CACNA1A*. Other calcium channel or energy pathway/calcium-dependent genes could be responsible, or alternatively, mitochondrial dysfunction or dysregulated neuronal metabolism could play a role in this disease.

DIAGNOSIS: No peripheral blood marker or imaging tests exist for AHC. Single-photon emission CT scanning shows asymmetric metabolism in brain regions during the attacks in some patients, but this technique is only used for investigational purposes. The diagnosis must be made based on the clinical findings.

TREATMENT
Standard Therapies: Flunarizine is the only medication that reliably has helped treat AHC by reducing the duration, frequency, and severity of the episodes. Chloral hydrate and niaprazine have also been used.

Investigational Therapies: Other calcium channel blockers are being investigated, especially in countries where flunarizine is not available.

REFERENCES
Dangond F, Garada B, Murawski BJ, et al. Focal brain dysfunction in a 41-year old man with familial alternating hemiplegia. *Eur Arch Psychiatry Clin Neurosci* 1997;247:35–41.
Kramer U, Nevo Y, Margalit D, et al. Alternating hemiplegia of childhood in half-sisters. *J Child Neurol* 2000;15:128–130.
Mikati M. Alternating hemiplegia of childhood. *Pediatr Neurol* 1999;21:764.
Mikati MA, Maguire H, Barlow CF, Ozelius L, et al. A syndrome of autosomal dominant alternating hemiplegia: clinical presentation mimicking intractable epilepsy; chromosomal studies; and physiologic investigations. *Neurology* 1992;42:2251–2257.
Siemes H, Cordes M. Single-photon emission computed tomography investigations of alternating hemiplegia of childhood. *Dev Med Child Neurol* 1993;35:346–350.
Silver K, Andermann F. Alternating hemiplegia of childhood: a study of 10 patients and results of flunarizine treatment. *Neurology* 1993;43:36–41.
Veneselli E, Biancheri R. Alternating hemiplegia of childhood: treatment of attacks with chloral hydrate and niaprazine. *Eur J Pediatr* 1997;156:157–158.

RESOURCES
20, 368

---

7 Amyotrophic Lateral Sclerosis

Rup Tandan, MD, FRCP

DEFINITION: Amyotrophic lateral sclerosis (ALS) is an age-dependent fatal paralytic disorder caused by degeneration of motor neurons in the motor cortex, brainstem, and spinal cord. It is a syndrome of both upper and lower motor neuron dysfunction at several levels of the neuraxis (such as bulbar, cervical, thoracic, or lumbosacral region) without involvement of other neurologic systems.

SYNONYMS: Lou Gehrig disease; Charcot disease; Motor neuron disease.

DIFFERENTIAL DIAGNOSES: Cervical spondylotic myeloradiculopathy; Spinal muscular atrophies; Hereditary spastic paraparesis; Kennedy disease; Inclusion body myositis; Multisystem atrophy.

SYMPTOMS AND SIGNS: Most commonly, patients present with symptomatic weakness, although they may have a history of muscle cramping and atrophy before weakness is apparent. Frequently, hyperreflexia occurs in limbs in which muscles are starting to atrophy due to denervation, with an absence of sensory disturbance in the same distribution. At onset, limb involvement occurs about 3 times more often than bulbar involvement, and upper limbs are slightly more often affected than lower limbs. The pattern of involvement is frequently asymmetric or focal. If more upper motor neurons are predominantly affected, the symptoms are primarily clumsiness and stiffness, whereas lower motor neuron degeneration manifests as weakness. Bulbar symptoms include hoarseness, slurring of speech, choking on liquids, and difficulty initiating swallowing. Paresthesias and sensory symptoms may affect up to 25% of patients. Disease progression and duration vary widely. Bowel, bladder, and sexual functioning and cognition are usually spared.

ETIOLOGY/EPIDEMIOLOGY: Broadly, the three types of ALS usually considered in epidemiologic studies are classic sporadic ALS, classic familial ALS (FALS), and a variant of ALS, sometimes called Guamanian ALS, found in the Western Pacific, that is characterized by the cooccurrence of parkinsonism and/or dementia in some patients. Sporadic ALS has an incidence of 1–2 in 100,000 with fairly uniform distribution worldwide and equal representation among racial groups. The incidence is greatest in persons aged 50–70 years. The male:female ratio is approximately 1.5:1. Genetic studies have identified several missense mutations in the gene encoding Cu/Zn superoxide dismutase (*SOD1*) on the long arm of chromosome 21 as the cause of the disease in approximately one fifth of autosomal-dominant cases. In sporadic ALS, abnormalities in a specific transporter protein that removes glutamate from the spinal fluid into the brain are implicated in the potential role of glutamatergic toxicity in the disease. The only consistent epidemiologic associations in sporadic ALS thus far have been with long-term exposure to heavy metals, particularly lead, and a family history of parkinsonism and dementia.

DIAGNOSIS: No definitive diagnostic test exists. According to the revised El Escorial criteria formulated at the Airlie House Conference in 1999, the diagnosis requires signs of upper or lower motor neuron degeneration by clinical, electrophysiologic, or neuropathologic examination, and progressive spread of signs from one region to other regions, together with the absence of the following: electrophysiologic evidence of other disease processes that might explain the signs of upper and/or lower motor neuron degeneration; and neuroimaging evidence of other disease processes that might explain the observed clinical and electrophysiologic signs.

TREATMENT
Standard Therapies: No treatment is available that stops the progression of the disease. The glutamate antagonist and benzothiazole compound, riluzole, is the only disease-modifying agent approved by the U.S. Food and Drug Administration for the treatment of ALS. Riluzole has a modest effect in extending the life span of patients by an average of approximately 3 months, and allows patients to stay in milder stages of the disease for longer as compared with placebo. Drugs such as baclofen, quinine, and diazepam can be used to reduce cramping, and anticholinergic agents such as amitriptyline or scopolamine can be

used to control sialorrhea. Amitriptyline or lithium may be used to control pseudobulbar symptoms. Physical therapy can help control spasticity and maintain strength and function. Occupational therapists can provide splints and aids that can extend the patient's ability to function independently. A speech therapy evaluation can provide instructions that help to prolong the patient's ability to communicate and swallow, and assist in procuring needed augmentative communication devices. Bilevel positive airway pressure not only provides short-term symptomatic relief of respiratory muscle fatigue and sleep apnea, but also improves quality of life and prolongs survival. Percutaneous endoscopic gastrostomy can provide nutritional support, prevent malnutrition and dehydration, and may improve quality of life and survival.

REFERENCES
Aboussan LS, Khan SU, Banerjee M, et al. Objective measures of the efficacy of non-invasive positive-pressure ventilation in amyotrophic lateral sclerosis. *Muscle Nerve* 2001;127:403–409.
Bradley WG, Anderson F, Bromberg M, et al., and the ALS CARE Study Group. Current management of ALS. Comparison of the ALS CARE Database and the AAN Practice Parameter. *Neurology* 2001;57:500–504.
Chio A, Finocchiaro E, Meineri P, et al., and the ALS Percutaneous Endoscopic Gastrostomy Study Group. Safety and factors related to survival after percutaneous endoscopic gastrostomy in ALS. *Neurology* 1999;53:1123–1125.
Kasarskis EJ, Scarlatta D, Hill R, et al., and the BDNF Phase III and the ALS CNTF Treatment Study (ACTS) Groups. A retrospective study of percutaneous endoscopic gastrostomy in ALS patients during the BDNF and CNTF trials. *J Neurol Sci* 1999;169:118–125.
Kleopa KA, Sherman M, Neal B, et al. BiPAP improves survival and rate of pulmonary function decline in patients with ALS. *J Neurol Sci* 1999;164:82–88.
Lacomblez L, Bensimon G, Leigh PN, et al. Dose-ranging study of riluzole in amyotrophic lateral sclerosis. *Lancet* 1996;347:1425–1431.
Miller RG, Rosenberg JA, Gelinas DF, et al., and the ALS Practice Parameters Task Force. Practice parameter: the care of the patient with amyotrophic lateral sclerosis (an evidence-based review). Report of the Quality Standards Subcommittee of the American Academy of Neurology. *Neurology* 1999;52:1311–1323.
Mitsumoto H. Diagnosis and progression of ALS. *Neurology* 1997;48(suppl 4):2–8.
Ringel SP, Murphy JR, Alderson MK, et al. The natural history of amyotrophic lateral sclerosis. *Neurology* 1993;43:1316–1322.
Riviere M, Meininger V, Zeisser P, et al. An analysis of extended survival in patients with amyotrophic lateral sclerosis treated with riluzole. *Arch Neurol* 1998;55:526–528.

RESOURCES
43, 237, 368

8 Apraxia

John C.M. Brust, MD

DEFINITION: The term *apraxia* refers not to a disease but to a variety of syndromes involving motor performance. Broadly, apraxia is a disturbance of skilled movement not explained by weakness, cerebellar ataxia, abnormal tone or posture, bradykinesia, deafferentation, movement disorder (such as tremor, chorea, or athetosis), dementia, aphasia, or poor cooperation.

SYMPTOMS AND SIGNS: Failure to perform an act at all is not apractic; it must be performed incorrectly. Parts of the act might be omitted, abnormally sequenced, or incorrectly oriented in space. Four types of testing detect apraxia: (a) gesture ("Show me how you would . . ."); (b) imitation ("Watch how I . . ., then you do it"); (c) use of an actual object ("Here is a . . . Show me how you would use it"); and (d) imitation of examiner using the object. Tests include limb gestures (waving goodbye, hitchhiking), limb manipulation (opening a door with a key, flipping a coin), buccofacial gesture (sticking out tongue), buccofacial manipulation (blowing out a match), and serial acts (folding a letter, putting it in an envelope, sealing the envelope, and placing a stamp on it).

In ideomotor apraxia, the patient is unable to perform learned or complex motor acts even though both primary executive skills and the "idea" of the act (its time-space-form program or "engram") are preserved. Affected patients accurately describe what they are supposed to do and correctly perform individual components of the act. Moreover, when the mode of input is switched (e.g., by being handed real objects, such as a match or scissors, or, less often, watching the examiner perform the act), the act is performed correctly. Ideomotor apraxia can be viewed as a functional disconnection between engram and execution. In ideational apraxia, the lesion appears to involve the engram itself; the patient cannot accurately describe the act, and presentation of the real object produces no improvement. In limb-kinetic apraxia, the act is understood, but neither the act nor its individual components can be performed, with or without the objects. The lesion appears to affect the executive apparatus but not enough to cause frank weakness.

ETIOLOGY/EPIDEMIOLOGY: Depending on the type of apraxia, the lesion can be in one or both cerebral hemispheres (including the thalamus) or the corpus callosum. Gait apraxia suggests frontal lobe pathology. Such lesions can be cerebrovascular, traumatic, neoplastic, infective, demyelinating, or degenerative.

DIAGNOSIS: The presence of apraxia is established by neurologic examination. The causal lesion is then determined by standard neurodiagnostic tests, especially imaging.

TREATMENT
Standard Therapies: Therapy depends on cause, e.g., stroke versus neoplasm. Little information exists on the efficacy of rehabilitation medicine strategies in the treatment of apraxia.

REFERENCES
Geschwind N. The apraxias: neural mechanisms of disorders of learned movement. *Am Sci* 1975;63:188–195.

Heilman KM, Rothi LJG. Apraxia. In: Heilman KM, Valenstein E, eds. *Clinical neuropsychology,* 3rd ed. New York: Oxford University Press, 1993:141–163.

Watson RT, Heilman KM. Callosal apraxia. *Brain* 1983;106: 391–403.

RESOURCES
284, 368

9 Arnold-Chiari Syndrome

Sanjiv Sahoo, MD,
and Phillip L. Pearl, MD

DEFINITION: The Chiari malformation is a congenital anomaly of the hindbrain characterized by downward elongation of the brainstem and cerebellum into the cervical portion of the spinal cord. There are four types (I–IV). Although Chiari type II is the Arnold-Chiari malformation, all types are commonly called Arnold-Chiari syndrome.

SYNONYMS: Chiari malformations; Congenital tonsillar ectopia (type I); Cerebellar hypoplasia (type IV).

DIFFERENTIAL DIAGNOSIS: Low intracranial pressure; Tonsillar herniation; Dandy-Walker syndrome; Basilar impression; Posterior fossa tumors; Multiple sclerosis, Syringomyelia.

SYMPTOMS AND SIGNS: Patients with Chiari type I present in childhood or adulthood. Increased intracranial pressure, hydrocephalus, headache, vertigo, ataxia, Ménière-type hearing loss, or upper limb weakness may be present. Lower bulbar dysfunction (dysphagia, dysphonia, vocal cord paralysis, diminished gag) may be present. If syringomyelia is associated, symptoms may include headache, neck pain, or back pain. Many other symptoms have been reported including cough syncope, oculomotor disturbances, sleep apnea, torticollis, persistent crying, progressive leg weakness, and incontinence. Chiari II is more severe than Chiari I and manifests at birth in infants with meningomyelocele and hydrocephalus.

ETIOLOGY/EPIDEMIOLOGY: Arnold-Chiari malformation is possibly secondary to a developmental arrest of the posterior fossa and overgrowth of the neural tube in embryonic life. Some cases of acquired Chiari I malformations have occurred after lumboperitoneal shunting in children and are believed to be due to a "craniospinal pressure gradient." Types III and IV are rare. Type III is represented by an occipitocervical meningocele including brainstem and cerebellar tissue components. Familial aggregates suggest a genetic component. Type IV denotes cerebellar and brainstem hypoplasia.

DIAGNOSIS: Neuroimaging, specifically MRI, is the hallmark of diagnosis. In Type I, abnormal extension of the cerebellar tonsils at least 3–5 mm below the foramen magnum with or without hydrocephalus, syringomyelia, or syringobulbia. Patients may have basilar impression, occipitalization of the atlas, a kinked cervical cord, or C1 spina bifida. Type II Chiari describes additional caudal displacement of the medulla and fourth ventricle with brainstem distortion (S-shaped kink) at the foramen magnum and beaking of the midbrain tectum. There may be additional skull base and cervical spine defects and occasionally agenesis of the corpus callosum. In Type III Chiari malformation, displaced cerebellar tonsils and brainstem extend into a meningoencephalocele or occipitocervical encephalocele. Type IV Chiari malformation describes cerebellar and brainstem hypoplasia rather than displacement.

TREATMENT
Standard Therapies: The surgical management for the Chiari malformation ranges from suboccipital decompression and duroplasty to additional steps that may be necessary for an associated syrinx, such as myelotomy or shunting. Asymptomatic children should be monitored for symptoms and advised to avoid contact sports because minor trauma can often result in significant symptoms. Type II patients born with spina bifida and hydrocephalus require a combination of surgical procedures after birth, including repair of the meningomyelocele and ventriculperitoneal shunting for hydrocephalus. Later, development of bulbar dysfunction or central sleep apnea may require a more specific surgical approach. Prevention of Arnold-Chiari malformation is directly linked to the screening and prevention of neural tube defects, e.g., spina bifida.

REFERENCES

Feldstein NA. Management of Chiari I malformations with holocord syringohydromyelia. *Pediatr Neurosurg* 1999;3:143–149.

Milhorat TH. Chiari I malformation redefined: clinical and radiographic findings for 364 symptomatic patients. *Neurosurgery* 1999;44:1005–1017.

Sakamoto H. Expansive suboccipital cranioplasty for the treatment of syringomyelia associated with Chiari malformation. *Acta Neurochir* 1999;141:949–960.

Shuman RM. The Chiari malformations: a constellation of anomalies. *Semin Pediatr Neurol* 1995;2:220–226.

Wu YW. Pediatric Chiari I malformations: do clinical and radiologic features correlate? *Neurology* 1999;53:1271–1276.

RESOURCES
42, 190, 368

---

10   Batten Disease

Paul Richard Dyken, MD

DEFINITION: Batten disease is a neurologic degenerative disease. It is the chronic juvenile form of the neuronal ceroid-lipofuscinoses, which are characterized by the accumulation of autofluorescing ceroid-lipofuscin within neurons and other supporting cells of the central nervous system (CNS).

SYNONYMS: Neuronal ceroid-lipofuscinosis (NCL); Chronic juvenile NCL; NCL-1; CLN-3; Juvenile amaurotic familial idiocy; Autofluorescing lipidosis; Juvenile lipidosis with macular degeneration; Retinitis pigmentosa with neurodegeneration.

SYMPTOMS AND SIGNS: Clinically, behavioral and visual symptoms slowly progress over several years after onset, which is usually between ages 5 and 15 years. Frequently, the first sign is the onset and progression of epileptic seizures and motor symptoms. Both pyramidal and extrapyramidal dysfunction are present in the form of paresis, paralysis, and hyperreflexia, leading ultimately to dementia and complete immobility. The three phases in the clinical presentation are as follows. Phase I, to age 5 years, is characterized by moderate behavioral and visual symptoms; phase II, lasting from 5 to 10 years, is an ambulatory degenerative phase, characterized by dementia, blindness, seizures, and motor deterioration; phase III, lasting from 10 to 20 years, is the nonambulatory vegetative phase when spasticity, quadriparesis, myoclonus, seizure resolution, and loss of vegetative functions occur. In almost all instances of NCL, but in Batten disease particularly, the visual problem is a centrally originating lesion in the pigment epithelium of the outer boundary of the retina. This macular lesion, and the corresponding loss of central vision, is the most obvious feature of the disease. As the disease progresses, the process extends peripherally, sometimes with the deposit of streaks of pigment that resemble the lesion of true retinitis pigmentosa.

ETIOLOGY/EPIDEMIOLOGY: The clinical features are caused by the progressive accumulation of waxy, autofluorescent pigments identified as ceroid-lipofuscin within neurons and supporting elements of the brain, especially the cerebral cortex. The pathogenic basis is genetic and may be an enzymatically controlled inborn error of metabolism. Batten disease is found in all parts of the world and affects all races and genders equally. The genetic defect has been mapped to chormosome 16p12.1.

DIAGNOSIS: The disease should be suspected in young patients presenting with retinitis pigmentosa, ataxia, and/or myoclonic seizures. Particularly important is the characteristic appearance in the retina, which is invariably present. A family history of the disorder is also helpful for diagnosis. It has been suggested that the criteria for diagnosis should be (a) typical clinical history and findings, and (b) histologic confirmation by examination of skin, conjunctiva, lymphocytes, and/or brain.

TREATMENT

Standard Therapies: Aggressive palliative treatment is indicated, particularly in the early years of the disorder when neurologic and ophthalmologic disabilities are often mild. In phase I, cerebral stimulants or tranquilizers to control disturbances in behavior and schoolwork are indicated. Training in Braille can be useful for patients whose psychologic and neurologic disabilities are minimal. Aggressive anticonvulsant therapy is helpful for epileptic seizures. Phenytoin, however, may have disadvantages because some side effects mimic some of the features of Batten disease.

Investigational Therapies: Treatment with antioxidants is being investigated, as is the drug phosphocysteamine.

REFERENCES
Dyken PR. Reconsideration of the classification of the neuronal ceroid-linofuscinoses. *Am J Med Genet* 1988;5(suppl):69–84.

Dyken PR. The neuronal ceroid-lipofuscinoses. In: Berg BO, ed. *Principles of child neurology.* New York: McGraw-Hill, 1996: 1495–1512.

Gardner M, Mole S, Mitchison H. The 8th International Congress on Neuronal Ceroid Lipofuscinoses (Batten Disease) [Abstract]. *Eur J Paediatr Neurol* 2001;106:A1.

Luiro K, Kopra O, Lehtovirta M, et al. CLN3 protein is targeted to neuronal synapses but excluded from synaptic vesicles: new clues to Batten disease. *Hum Mol Genet* 2001;10:2123–2131.

Zhang Z, Butler JD, Levin SW, et al. Lysosomal ceroid depletion by drugs: therapeutic implications for a hereditary neurodegenerative disease of childhood. *Nat Med* 2001;7:478–484.

RESOURCES
68, 109, 368

11   Beckwith-Wiedemann Syndrome

Adeline Vanderver, MD,
and Phillip L. Pearl, MD

DEFINITION: Beckwith-Wiedemann syndrome (BWS) is a somatic overgrowth syndrome characterized by neonatal hyperinsulinemic hypoglycemia, hemihypertrophy, macrosomia, macroglossia, omphalocele, organomegaly, and predisposition to intraabdominal embryonal tumors.

SYNONYMS: Wiedemann-Beckwith syndrome; Exomphalos-macroglossia-gigantism syndrome.

DIFFERENTIAL DIAGNOSIS: Prematurity; Infant of diabetic mother; Maternal isoimmune disease; Hypoxia or shock and ensuing global ischemia; Seizures; Hepatic dysfunction; Congenital adrenal insufficiency; Inborn errors of metabolism; Perlman nephroblastosis syndrome; Simpson-Golabi-Behmel syndrome; Sotos syndrome; Weaver syndrome.

SYMPTOMS AND SIGNS: The syndrome is characterized by macroglossia, neonatal hyperinsulinemic hypoglycemia, and macrosomia. Patients often have hemihypertrophy and organomegaly, as well as anterior abdominal wall defects and a predisposition to intraabdominal embryonal tumors. Patients have a higher incidence of problems related to gestation, including prematurity, as well as polyhydramnios and, less frequently, preeclampsia. Craniofacial dysmorphism is a constant finding and includes microcephaly, capillary hemangioma or naevus flammeus of the forehead, a characteristic earlobe crease, posterior helical ear pits, exophthalmos, and a flattened nasal dorsum. Cardiac malformations occur in 6%–16% of patients and include obstructive subaortic stenosis and secundum atrial septal defect. Other congenital malformations such as renal abnormalities and intestinal malrotation may occur. Patients have an increased risk of embryonal tumors, including Wilm tumor, hepatoblastoma, neuroblastoma, rhabdomyosarcoma, and adrenocortical carcinoma. Wilm tumor represents approximately 60% of tumors in these children.

ETIOLOGY/EPIDEMIOLOGY: Prevalence is approximately 1 in 17,000 births. Most cases are sporadic, although some familial cases (approximately 15%) have been described with an uncertain mode of inheritance. The syndrome is associated with a defect of genomic imprinting at chromosomal locus 11p15.

DIAGNOSIS: Diagnosis is made chiefly on clinical findings. Abnormal findings on renal imaging include nephromegaly, cortical and medullary cysts, and medullary dysplasia, although most affected children have normal kidneys on ultrasonographic imaging. Cytogenetic analysis looking for abnormalities of chromosome 11p15.5 and genomic transmission is also often done.

TREATMENT
Standard Therapies: Neonatal hypoglycemia is usually managed with extra feedings or a brief period of intravenous dextrose in the immediate neonatal period. The increased frequency of intraabdominal embryonal tumors has led to efforts at early diagnosis with screening techniques. Studies support the use of serial abdominal ultrasonography every 3 months until the age of 7–8 years for early diagnosis of Wilm tumor. Serial α-fetoprotein measurements in infancy and early childhood for the diagnosis of occult hepatoblastoma have also been suggested. Macroglossia is treated if it causes dentoskeletal problems, psychosocial consequences, or functional deficits such as difficulty swallowing or feeding, drooling, altered or delayed speech, or upper airway obstruction. Surgical reduction and oral regulation therapies have been used. The macroglossia may occasionally self correct during development.

REFERENCES
Choyke PL, Siegel MJ, Craft AW, et al. Screening for Wilms tumor in children with Beckwith-Wiedmann syndrome or idiopathic hemihypertrophy. *Med Pediatr Oncol* 1999;32:196–200.
DeBaun MR, Tucker MA. Risk of cancer during the first four years of life in children from the Beckwith-Wiedemann Syndrome Registry. *J Pediatr* 1998;132:398–400.
Elliot M, Bayly R, Cole T, et al. Clinical features and natural history of Beckwith-Wiedemann syndrome: presentation of 74 new cases. *Clin Genet* 1994;46:168–174.
Everman DB, Shuman C, Dzolganovski B, et al. Serum α-fetoprotein levels in Beckwith-Wiedemann syndrome. *J Pediatr* 2000;137:123–127.
Porteus MH, Narkool P, Neuberg D, et al. Characteristics and outcome of children with Beckwith-Wiedeman syndrome and Wilm's tumor: a report from the National Wilms Tumor Study Group. *J Clin Oncol* 2000;18:2026–2031.

RESOURCES
69, 293, 352, 379

12   Binswanger Disease

Rodger J. Elble, MD, PhD

DEFINITION: Binswanger disease is a dementing disorder in which large blotchy areas of subcortical white matter degeneration occur with varying numbers of lacunar infarcts in, but not limited to, the subcortical white matter, basal ganglia, and thalamus.

SYNONYM: Subcortical arteriosclerotic encephalopathy.

DIFFERENTIAL DIAGNOSIS: Alzheimer disease; Chronic subdural hematoma; Frontotemporal dementia; Late-onset leukodystrophies; Multiple sclerosis; Multiple system atrophy; Normal pressure hydrocephalus; Parkinson disease and dementia with Lewy bodies; Progressive supranuclear palsy.

SYMPTOMS AND SIGNS: Binswanger pathology may be an asymptomatic incidental finding on CT or MRI head scans, or it may cause varying degrees of dementia with focal neurologic deficits, impaired gait, urinary urgency, and incontinence. The disease is usually gradually progressive, punctuated by acute episodes of neurologic deterioration. The gait disturbance is initially no more than a mild impairment of balance with reduced velocity, shortened steps, and slightly widened base. Arm swing is typically preserved. In more advanced cases, there is hesitation, freezing, inappropriate foot placement, inappropriate postural synergies, and absent or greatly limited rescue reactions when balance is lost. The abnormalities of gait are strongly influenced by the patient's emotion and environment, and because of this, performance can be bafflingly variable. Furthermore, these abnormalities are most noticeable when the patient makes transitional movements such a rising from a chair or bed.

ETIOLOGY/EPIDEMIOLOGY: Advanced age seems to be the most consistent predictor of extensive white matter degeneration. Men and women are both affected. Patchy subcortical white matter degeneration in the elderly probably has multiple causes and can occur independently of microinfarction in the white matter, basal ganglia, and thalamus. Arteriosclerosis plays an important role in many but not all cases. Younger patients (age <60–70 years) almost invariably have long-standing hypertension, often in combination with diabetes mellitus. In the absence of these risk factors, the radiologic and clinical picture of Binswanger disease in a young or middle-aged adult may be caused by a rare autosomal-dominant arteriopathy called CADASIL (cerebral autosomal-dominant arteriopathy with subcortical infarcts and leukoencephalopathy).

DIAGNOSIS: Diagnosis is made by CT and MRI. CADASIL DNA testing is indicated when symptoms begin before age 60, there is a family history of early dementia and cerebrovascular symptoms, and a strong personal and family history of atherosclerotic risk factors is absent.

TREATMENT
Standard Therapies: Treatment of vascular risk factors such as antiplatelet medication for stroke prophylaxis is recommended. Concomitant neurologic disease may be treatable (e.g., Parkinson disease, depression, sleep disorders). Cholinesterase inhibitors (donepezil, rivastigmine, or galantamine) might be tried if coexistent Alzheimer disease is suspected. Supportive care from physical therapists and occupational therapists is useful. Speech therapists can assist in the evaluation of dysphagia, which can cause life-threatening aspiration pneumonia. Caregivers must be informed about the nature of the gait disturbance, because a patient's gait may seem bizarre to the uneducated, and the variable performance is often baffling.

REFERENCES
Blass JP, Hoyer S, Nitsch R. A translation of Otto Binswanger's article, "The delineation of the generalized progressive paralyses." *Arch Neurol* 1991;48:961–972.
Brilliant M, Hughes L, Anderson D, et al. Rarefied white matter in patients with Alzheimer disease. *Alzheimer Dis Assoc Disord* 1995;9:39–46.
Caronti B, Calandriello L, Francia A, et al. Cerebral autosomal dominant arteriopathy with subcortical infarcts and leukoencephalopathy (CADASIL). *Acta Neurol Scand* 1988;98:259–267.
Huang K, Wu L, Luo Y. Binswanger's disease: progressive subcortical encephalopathy or multi-infarct dementia? *Can J Neurol Sci* 1985;12:88–94.
Román GC. Senile dementia of the Binswanger type. A vascular form of dementia in the elderly. *JAMA* 1987;258:1782–1788.

RESOURCES
23, 368, 369

13   Brown-Séquard Syndrome

Patricia Winchester, PT, PhD

DEFINITION: The Brown-Séquard syndrome is classically defined as a spinal hemiplegia resulting from the effect of a disease of, or an injury to, the lateral half of the spinal cord. This syndrome results in contralateral absent or diminished sensation to pinprick and temperature due to interruption of the spinothalamic tract and ipsilateral proprioceptive and motor loss below the level of spinal cord lesion due to interruption of the dorsal columns and corticospinal tract.

SYNONYM: Brown-Séquard plus syndrome.

DIFFERENTIAL DIAGNOSIS: Central cord syndrome; Anterior cord syndrome.

SYMPTOMS AND SIGNS: The neurologic signs include ipsilateral spastic motor loss; ipsilateral loss or impaired position sense, light touch, and vibration sense; and contralateral loss of sensation to pinprick and temperature, all below the neurologic level of injury; and ipsilateral loss of all sensation at the neurologic level of injury.

ETIOLOGY/EPIDEMIOLOGY: The incidence of Brown-Séquard syndrome has been reported to be approximately 2% of all traumatic spinal cord injuries. Brown-Séquard syndrome can be associated with trauma, tumors, degenerative diseases, inflammation, hemorrhage, and other medical causes.

DIAGNOSIS: The classification of Brown-Séquard syndrome is primarily based on the clinical neurologic examination. The neurologic signs caudal to the hemisected region of the spinal cord are used to clinically diagnose the Brown-Séquard syndrome. In some instances, evidence from MRI or surgical observations can support the diagnosis.

TREATMENT
Standard Therapies: There are no specific surgical therapies, other than stabilization of the unstable spine in the event of a fracture dislocation.

REFERENCES
Bohlman HH. Acute fractures and dislocations of the cervical spine. An analysis of three hundred hospitalized patients and review of the literature. *J Bone Joint Surg [Am]* 1979;61: 1119–1142.

Bosch A, Stauffer ES, Nickel VL. Incomplete traumatic quadriplegia: a ten year review. *JAMA* 1971;216:473–478.

Maynard FM, Bracken MB, Creasey G, et al. International standards for neurological and functional classification of spinal cord injury patients (revised 1996). *Spinal Cord* 1997;35: 266–274.

Roth EJ, Park T, Pang T, et al. Traumatic cervical Brown Sequard and BS Plus syndromes: the spectrum of presentations and outcomes. *Paraplegia* 1991;29:582–589.

RESOURCES
152, 368

14   Cerebro-Oculo-Facio-Skeletal Syndrome

Tena Rosser, MD,
and Phillip L. Pearl, MD

DEFINITION: Cerebro-oculo-facio-skeletal syndrome is a neurodegenerative disorder of the brain and spinal cord associated with craniofacial and skeletal abnormalities.

SYNONYMS: Neurogenic arthrogyposis; Pena-Shokeir II syndrome.

DIFFERENTIAL DIAGNOSIS: Cockayne syndrome; Neu-Laxova syndrome; Seckel syndrome.

SYMPTOMS AND SIGNS: The neurodegenerative process is suspected to begin *in utero,* but infants are usually born at term with normal birth weights. Most infants can be diagnosed at birth; however, some develop the phenotype over the first weeks or months of life. Patients show generalized hypotonia with hyporeflexia or areflexia. Neuroimaging studies show reduced white matter with gray matter mottling. Associated abnormalities include agenesis of the corpus callosum, calcifications of hemispheric white matter and basal ganglia, hypoplasia of the optic tracts and chiasm, hypoplasia of temporal lobes and hippocampus, focal microgyria, and focal subependymal gliosis at the third ventricle. Infantile spasms can occur. Patients are severely mentally retarded. Multiple craniofacial anomalies occur. Microcephaly is a uniform feature. Evaluation of the face shows a prominent root of the nose, large ear pinnae, micrognathia, and an upper lip overhanging the lower lip. Ophthalmologic findings include microphthalmia, nystagmus, cataracts, and blepharophimosis with deep-set eyes. Skeletal anomalies include camptodactyly, rocker-bottom feet, and flexure contractures at the elbows and knees. The second metatarsal may be displaced posteriorly or there may be a longitudinal groove in the soles along the second metatarsal. Additional dysmorphic features may include widely spaced nipples, renal defects, hirsutism, osteoporosis, and kyphoscoliosis. Patients show progressive deterioration, and rarely survive beyond 5 years.

ETIOLOGY/EPIDEMIOLOGY: The syndrome is transmitted by autosomal-recessive inheritance. It affects males and females and occurs in many ethnic groups.

DIAGNOSIS: Diagnosis is based on clinical presentation in addition to imaging and pathologic studies. Radiographs show characteristic proximal displacement of second metatarsals. Neuroimaging studies show gray and white matter changes as well as areas of dysgenesis. Pathologic examination of the iliac crest shows extensive cell necrosis.

TREATMENT
Standard Therapies: Treatment is supportive and symptomatic.

REFERENCES
Del Bigio MR, Greenberg CR, Rorke LB, et al. Neuropathologic findings in eight patients with cerebro-oculo-facio-skeletal (COFS) syndrome. *J Neuropathol* 1997;56:1147–1157.
Harden CL, Tuchman AJ, Daras M. Infantile spasms in COFS syndrome. *Pediatr Neurol* 1991;7:302–304.
Hwang WS, Trevenen CL, Greenberg C, et al. Chondro-osseus changes in cerebro-oculo-facial-skeletal syndrome. *J Pathol* 1982;138:33–40.
Jones KL. *Smith's recognizable patterns of human malformation,* 4th ed. Philadelphia: WB Saunders, 1998.

RESOURCES
96, 149, 368

15   Charcot-Marie-Tooth Polyneuropathy Syndrome

Carlos A. Garcia, MD

DEFINITION: Charcot-Marie-Tooth (CMT) polyneuropathy syndrome represents a clinically and genetically heterogeneous group of disorders that produce progressive deterioration of the peripheral nerves manifested by distal leg and hand weakness.

SYNONYMS: Peroneal muscular atrophy; Hereditary motor and sensory neuropathy I and II; Hypertrophic neuropathy; Roussy-Levy syndrome; Dejerine-Sottas syndrome; Congenital hypomyelination neuropathy; Hereditary neuropathy with liability to pressure palsies (HNPP).

DIFFERENTIAL DIAGNOSIS: Acquired chronic neuropathies including chronic inflammatory demyelinating polyneuropathy; Multifocal motor neuropathy; Distal muscular dystrophy of Welander; Distal myopathy of Miyoshi; Autosomal-dominant spinal muscular atrophy.

SYMPTOMS AND SIGNS: Clinical symptoms appear in the first or second decade with gait disturbances, foot deformities (Insert Fig. 51), or loss of balance. Infants and children manifest the disease by walking on their toes. Later, the foot drops with each step, forcing the patient to flex the hip, giving the steppage or equine gait. Pes cavus deformity and hammer toes develop with age. Atrophy of the legs may be a prominent feature. Cold intolerance in the legs is common. Weakness of the intrinsic hand muscles occurs late. The thumb lies flat in the plane of the hand instead of opposing the other fingers, giving the appearance of claw hand. Hand tremors are a frequent complaint. Enlargement of the nerves can be seen in slender, predominantly male patients. Muscle stretch reflexes disappear early and plantar responses are frequently flexor or show no response. Mild sensory loss to pricking pain in the legs in a stocking distribution and decreased vibratory sense are often seen. Hip dysplasia is usually asymptomatic until adolescence.

ETIOLOGY/EPIDEMIOLOGY: The syndrome is a hereditary disorder that can occur sporadically or as an autosomal-dominant, autosomal-recessive, or X-linked trait. Two major types are distinguished by physiologic and pathologic findings, CMT1 or demyelinating type, and CMT2 or neuronal form. Genetic linkage studies have identified several loci for CMT1 and some for CMT2. CMT1A is an autosomal-dominant neuropathy that accounts for 70% of all CMT cases. It is due to a submicroscopic duplication on chromosome 17 (17p12) that encodes the peripheral myelin protein 22 (PMP22). CMT1B accounts for less than 10% of CMT1 cases and is due to point mutations in the *MPZ* gene that encodes for the myelin protein zero in chromosome 1. Autosomal-recessive forms are rare and at least in some patients are due to mutations in the periaxin gene on chromosome 19.

DIAGNOSIS: The diagnosis is suspected when a patient shows signs of chronic peripheral neuropathy. Because of the extremely variable clinical picture, molecular diagnostic testing makes the definitive diagnosis.

TREATMENT
Standard Therapies: No medical treatment is available to stop the progression of the disease. Symptomatic treatment is important. The tremor is aggravated by coffee and nicotine and responds to β-blockers. Nonsteroidal antiinflammatory medication and analgesics relieve low back and leg pains. Avoidance of alcohol and some medications that can worsen the neuropathy is important. Diet in obese patients to achieve an appropriate weight for the patient's size and frame will make ambulation easier and less painful in the legs and back. Physical and occupational therapy are helpful. Stretching of the heel cord by daily therapy is important. Early in the course of the disease, high-top shoes or boots that fit properly are important. Shoe inserts that

are molded to the patient's feet are the next step. Ankle-foot-orthosis (AFO) braces are required in most patients. Surgery is indicated in hip dysplasia. Surgery of the feet is directed toward correcting the pes cavus, the heel varus, and the hammer toes. Tendon transplants in the hand can restore strength to the thumb.

REFERENCES
Garcia CA. Familial neuropathies. In: Johnson RT, Griffin JW, eds. *Current therapy in neurologic disease,* 5th ed. St. Louis: Mosby–Year Book, 1997:386.
Garcia CA. A clinical review of Charcot-Marie-Tooth. *Ann N Y Acad Sci* 1999;883:69–76.
Lupski JR, Garcia CA. Charcot-Marie-Tooth peripheral neuropathies and related disorders. In: Scriver CR, Beaudet AL, Sly WS, et al., eds. *The metabolic and molecular bases of inherited diseases,* 8th ed. New York: McGraw-Hill, 2001:5759–5788.
Mersiyanova IV, Perepelov AV, Polyakov AV, et al. A new variant of Charcot-Marie-Tooth disease type 2 is probably the result of a mutation in the neurofilament-light gene. *Am J Hum Genet* 2000;67:37.

RESOURCES
90, 368

---

16 Sydenham Chorea

Michael S. Okun, MD

DEFINITION: Sydenham chorea is a disease characterized by involuntary, purposeless, rapid movements of the limbs; muscular weakness; and emotional lability. It may occur in isolation or as a major manifestation in 10%–25% of cases of rheumatic fever.

SYNONYMS: Acute chorea; Chorea minor; Juvenile chorea; Rheumatic chorea; Sydenham disease; St. Vitus dance; Lupus.

DIFFERENTIAL DIAGNOSIS: PANDAS (postinfectious autoimmune neuropsychiatric disorders associated with streptococcal infection); Tourette syndrome; Secondary chorea.

SYMPTOMS AND SIGNS: Patients may present with emotionality, a hyperkinetic movement disorder, a gait disorder, or a combination of these features. The child may exhibit facial grimacing and have motor impersistence when asked to keep the tongue protruded. Initially, the child may complain of difficulty with handwriting. The movement disorder is characterized by chorea that may in-

volve the face, bucco-oral-lingual region, trunk, and all extremities. The child may make a clucking sound when trying to speak as the tongue is thrust toward the bottom of the mouth. The movements are purposeless and exacerbated by emotional stress. As with other movement disorders, the chorea of Sydenham disappears in sleep. Intentional movements such as grabbing or drinking exacerbate the movement abnormalities. Subtle chorea may be observed during activating movements, walking, or holding the hands outstretched in front of the body. It usually resolves within 3 weeks to 3 months but may last longer. Movements may recur during the first year, and occasionally they have been known to recur later in life, particularly during times of stress, including pregnancy and intercurrent illnesses. Chorea that is not self-limiting should prompt a more complete search for an underlying cause, including metabolic and systemic illnesses, proprionic acidemia, glutaric aciduria, methylmalonic acidemia, antiphospholipid and anticardiolipin antibody, underlying cerebral palsy, polycythemia vera, pregnancy, and lupus and other connective tissue diseases.

ETIOLOGY/EPIDEMIOLOGY: The syndrome usually follows streptococcal infection. Sydenham chorea may appear in isolation or as a major manifestation of rheumatic fever, although chorea occurs in only 10%–25% of cases of rheumatic fever. It occurs most commonly between the ages of 7 and 14 and more frequently in girls. It is rare after adolescence.

DIAGNOSIS: The evaluation for potential Sydenham chorea should include serologic testing for antistreptolysin titer, anti-DNAse, and streptozyme levels. All or none of these titers may be positive. Children should be checked for active carditis, and clinicians should note that if rheumatic fever is present, arthritis does not accompany chorea.

TREATMENT

Standard Therapies: Treatment should include prophylaxis with a penicillin or penicillin equivalent drug with coverage of a broad range of streptococcal species. A Dobhoff tube may need to be temporarily placed for feeding, and the child should be put on aspiration precautions. The movement disorder is usually self-limiting within weeks, but may be cautiously treated (and only if absolutely necessary) with low doses of benzodiazepines such as clonazepam or an atypical dopamine blocker such as olanzapine. Severe cases may warrant nonselective dopamine blockers such as haloperidol or pimozide, but when using these drugs the clinicians should be aware of potential long-term consequences including tardive dyskinesia and tardive dystonia. The medication history should be obtained carefully because many drugs including oral contraceptive pills can cause chorea. Sydenham chorea usually resolves within 3 weeks to 3 months, but has been reported to

last longer. Movements may recur during the first year, and occasionally have been known to recur later in life, particularly during times of stress, including pregnancy and intercurrent illnesses. Chorea that is not self-limiting should prompt a more complete search for an underlying cause, including metabolic and systemic illnesses, proprionic acidemia, glutaric aciduria, methylmalonic academia, antiphospholipid and anticardiolipin antibody, underlying cerebral palsy, polycythemia vera, pregnancy, lupus, and other connective tissue diseases. Another recently described disorder, PANDAS (postinfectious autoimmune neuropsychiatric disorders associated with streptococcal infection), can also manifest with a movement disorder as well as neuropsychiatric manifestations, and may belong to the same spectrum of diseases as Sydenham.

REFERENCES

Aron AM, Freeman JM, Carter S. The natural history of sydenham's chorea. *Am J Med* 1965;38:83–95.

Cardoso F, Vargas AP, Oliveira LD, et al. Persistent Sydenham's chorea. *Mov Disord* 1999;14:805–807.

Markowitz M, Kuttner A. *Rheumatic fever: diagnosis, management, and prevention.* Philadelphia: WB Saunders, 1969.

Shannon K, Fenichel G. Pimozide treatment of Sydenham's chorea. *Neurology* 1990;50:186.

Swedo SE, Leonard HL. Childhood movement disorders and obsessive compulsive disorder. *J Clin Psychiatry* 1994;55 (suppl):32–37.

RESOURCES
177, 368, 487

---

17   Complex Regional Pain Syndrome Type I

Sanjiv Sahoo, MD,
and Phillip L. Pearl, MD

DEFINITION: Complex regional pain syndrome (CRPS) is a diagnostic term applied to patients with pain associated with various combinations of sensory, motor, and circulatory manifestations. Complex regional pain syndrome I is diagnosed when, in the absence of overt or sufficient neuropathy, there is ongoing pain, allodynia, or hyperalgesia disproportionate to any inciting event or underlying condition.

SYNONYMS: Reflex sympathetic dystrophy; Minor causalgia; Posttraumatic pain syndrome; Sympathetically mediated pain; Shoulder hand syndrome; Sudeck atrophy.

DIFFERENTIAL DIAGNOSIS: Postherpetic neuralgia; Painful neuropathies including diabetic neuropathy, compression neuropathies, and causalgia; Pain dysfunction syndrome; Cumulative trauma disorder; Repetitive strain injury; Overuse syndrome; Tennis elbow; Nonspecific thoracic outlet syndrome; Fibromyalgia; Posttraumatic vasoconstriction; Undetected fracture; Peripheral vascular disease; Conversion disorder.

SYMPTOMS AND SIGNS: Symptoms include pain and sensory changes, autonomic dysfunction, trophic changes in the skin and subcutaneous tissues, motor impairment, and psychological abnormalities. The pain is disproportionate to the inciting event and is usually described as spontaneous burning or stinging. The pain distribution is usually distal but is sometimes proximal, including truncal or facial. There is hyperesthesia to minor mechanical stimuli such as a draft. There may be an extreme sensitivity to temperature changes in the environment. Patients frequently experience an asymmetry of color, temperature, or sweating of the affected limb. The affected limb may be perceived as swollen and stiff, with a decreased range of movement, and with "jumping" movements, myoclonus, dystonia, or tremor. Trophic changes include thin, shiny skin; coarse hair; thick nails; and muscle wasting. When symptoms are present for less than a year, the affected limb is more likely to be warm, dilated, and responsive to sympatholytic intervention. When present for more than a year, the affected area is more likely to be cold, pale, and less responsive to sympatholytic therapy.

ETIOLOGY/EPIDEMIOLOGY: Controversy persists regarding the role of the sympathetic nervous system. Investigations are ongoing as to the likely mechanisms at the nerve fiber (C-fiber unmyelinated polymodal nociceptive axons), spinal, and supraspinal levels.

DIAGNOSIS: The diagnosis is clinical and there are no specific laboratory tests.

TREATMENT
Standard Therapies: Management requires a coordinated interdisciplinary approach. Functional restoration, starting with desensitization using reactivation techniques and contrast baths, is followed by gradual joint mobilization, concomitant pain control, muscle strengthening, and vocational rehabilitation. The medications most commonly used include tricyclic antidepressant agents and the antiepileptics: gabapentin, phenytoin, carbamazepine, and lamotrigine. Agents for abortive management include ketoprofen, steroids, opioids, cutaneous lidocaine, clonidine, intravenous regional blockade with bretylium, intravenous phentolamine, and paravertebral/epidural blocks. Capsaicin, nifedipine, and calcitonin have mixed efficacy. Sympathectomy has not shown long-term benefits.

REFERENCES
Harden RN. A clinical approach to complex regional pain syndrome. *Clin J Pain* 2000;16(suppl):26–32.
Sandroni P, Low PA. Complex regional pain syndrome I (CRPS I): prospective study and laboratory evaluation. *Clin J Pain* 1998; 14:282–289.
Stanton Hicks M. Complex regional pain syndrome (type I, RSD; type II, causalgia): controversies. *Clin J Pain* 2000;16(suppl): 33–40.
Tahmoush AJ. Quantitative sensory studies in complex regional pain syndrome type 1/RSD. *Clin J Pain* 2000;16:340–344.
Verdugo RJ. Abnormal movements in complex regional pain syndrome: assessment of their nature. *Muscle Nerve* 2000;23: 198–205.

RESOURCES
368, 414, 415, 422

18 | Corticobasal Degeneration

Irene Litvan, MD

DEFINITION: Corticobasal degeneration (CBD) is a neurodegenerative disease that manifests clinically with two main forms: lateralized, in which motor problems develop over one extremity and then spread to the others; and dementia, in which changes in personality, difficulty planning events, inattention, and language disturbances are observed.

SYNONYMS: Corticodentatonigral degeneration with neuronal achromasia; Corticonigral degeneration with neuronal achromasia; Cortical-basal ganglionic degeneration.

DIFFERENTIAL DIAGNOSIS: Parkinson disease; Focal form of Alzheimer disease; Pick disease; Progressive supranuclear palsy.

SYMPTOMS AND SIGNS: It is believed that 50% of patients present with the lateralized CBD form. Typically, patients present with a clumsy (loss of purposeful movement), jerky (myoclonus), and stiff (rigid) arm that may eventually develop a fixed posture (dystonia, contractures) and may be felt as "alien." Infrequently, patients present with leg rather than arm/hands problems, and trouble walking may be an early problem. Symptoms progressively spread to the other extremities and, eventually, all four extremities are affected. Patients who present with a dementia form may lose the ability to plan events, become disinhibited, have a shortened attention span, and later may develop bilateral motor (parkinsonism) and urinary (incontinence) problems. The symptoms tend to progress steadily for an average of 7 years, but the disease duration varies.

ETIOLOGY/EPIDEMIOLOGY: Men and women are affected equally. The disease has not been reported in a person younger than 40; typically, patients present in their early 60s. It is estimated that 5 patients per 100,000 subjects have this disease, with approximately 0.62–0.92 new patients per 100,000 subjects per year; however, frequently CBD is not diagnosed during the patient's life. Although some families with FTDP-17 may present with either form of the disease, the role of genetics in the most common, sporadic, form is not clear. Pathologically, the clinical problems correspond to lesions affecting the frontal, parietal, and basal ganglia brain areas. The lesions observed in the affected areas are characterized by the abnormal aggregation of the tau protein in various types of brain cells: neurons, astrocytes, and oligodendroglia. These lesions are observed in both the white and gray matter. Most patients seem to have polymorphism in the tau chromosome, tau H1 haplotype, but this is also found in more than half of the normal population.

DIAGNOSIS: Distinguishing CBD from similar neurodegenerative diseases is often difficult at early stages of the disease. No laboratory markers exist. The diagnosis involves a careful neurologic examination. Autopsy confirmation remains the only definitive diagnostic tool. Eye movement recording and MRI may help rule out other disorders as well as detect abnormalities that may support the diagnosis.

TREATMENT

Standard Therapies: No medications can slow the progression of CBD, and few offer relief of symptoms. Levodopa and other dopaminergic drugs used in Parkinson disease are rarely beneficial, but may help the slowness and stiffness some patients experience. Jerking may be controlled with drugs such as clonazepam. Physical therapy may be useful to maintain mobility and range of motion of stiff joints, which in turn, may prevent pain and contractures. Botox injections may alleviate the contractures and pain; however, they do not restore the ability to control movements. Weighted walkers may help maintain independence. Botox injections may also be used to treat the difficulty in opening or closing eyelids some patients develop. Occupational therapy is useful to evaluate home safety and to provide adaptive equipment that could lead to increased functional independence. A speech therapist may help the patient improve articulation and volume and advise on communication aids, as well as assess and treat any swallowing disturbances that may develop, preventing aspiration pneumonias.

REFERENCES

Kompoliti K, Goetz CG, Boeve BF, et al. Clinical presentation and pharmacological therapy in corticobasal degeneration. *Arch Neurol* 1998;55:957–961.

Togasaki DM, Tanner CM. Epidemiologic aspects. *Adv Neurol* 2000;82:53–59.

Wenning GK, Litvan I, Jankovic J, et al. Natural history and survival of 14 patients with corticobasal degeneration confirmed at postmortem examination. *J Neurol Neurosurg Psychiatry* 1998;64:184–189.

RESOURCES

368, 487

---

19   Cyclic Vomiting Syndrome

*Jennifer Howard, RN,
Kathleen Adams, RN,
and B.U.K. Li, MD*

DEFINITION: Cyclic vomiting syndrome (CVS) is a disorder characterized by recurrent, discrete, stereotypical spells of rapid-fire vomiting, between which the child is completely well.

SYNONYMS: Abdominal migraine; Periodic syndrome.

DIFFERENTIAL DIAGNOSIS: Malrotation with intermittent volvulus and other partial obstructions; Peptic disorders; Chronic sinusitis; Brainstem neoplasms, Chiari malformation; Acute hydronephrosis; Mitochondrial encephalopathies; Fatty acid oxidation disorders; Urea cycle defects; Acute intermittent porphyria.

SYMPTOMS AND SIGNS: Children with CVS vomit at a peak pace of every 5–15 minutes, an intensity unmatched by any other known vomiting disorder. Other major symptoms include pallor, lethargy, anorexia, nausea, retching, abdominal pain, and dehydration. These episodes tend to be stereotypical within individuals as to the time of onset (usually early morning hours), major symptoms, and episode duration (24–36 hours). The patient returns to completely normal health for a period of days or weeks. An acute episode is commonly mistaken for a bout of gastroenteritis because of the concomitant vomiting, low-grade fever, and diarrhea. Children with CVS are substantially more ill than those with the "stomach flu," because of the shocklike pallor and profound listlessness.

ETIOLOGY/EPIDEMIOLOGY: Cyclic vomiting syndrome has been observed to occur in all races, with a ratio of girls:boys of 55:45. The median age of onset is 6 years, but the correct diagnosis is usually not made for an average of 2.6 years. It appears to be primarily a disorder of children; however, more adults are being diagnosed with CVS. The cause is unknown. It may be a migraine variant, a hypothalmic surge of corticotropin-releasing factor, mitochondropathy, or a form of dysautonomia.

DIAGNOSIS: Because CVS remains a diagnosis of exclusion, potential testing includes small bowel radiography, endoscopy, abdominal ultrasonography, intracranial imaging, and metabolic screening (including glucose, electrolytes, lactate, NH_3, amino acids and urine organic acids, δ-ALA, and porphobilinogen).

TREATMENT

Standard Therapies: The treatment remains empiric. The goals are to prevent or reduce the frequency of vomiting episodes, and if unsuccessful, to abort or attenuate episodes once they begin. To prevent episodes, first-line therapy for those with more frequent episodes includes daily use of antimigraine agents (propranolol, cyproheptadine, amitriptyline), especially in those patients with a family history of migraine, or prokinetic medications. To abort episodes, especially in those with less frequent episodes, antiemetics (ondansetron, granisetron) or antimigraine agents (triptans) may be tried at the onset of attacks. During episodes, intravenously administered glucose-containing (D_{10}) fluids plus ondansetron and lorazepam are often helpful. Attempts at various preventative or abortive therapies may be necessary before an effective regimen is found. In some instances, specific triggering substances (cheese, chocolate, and monosodium glutamate) or positive or negative psychological stressors can be identified and either avoided or attenuated. Family support and a nurturing patient-physician relationship are critical to improvement.

Investigational Therapies: Medications being investigated include new antimigraine triptans, antiepileptics (e.g., gabapentin and topamirate), tackykinin receptor antagonists (potent antiemetics), and CRF antagonists (to truncate the stress response).

REFERENCES

Li BUK, ed. Proceedings of the International Symposium on Cyclic Vomiting Syndrome. *J Pediatr Gastroenterol Nutr* 1995;21(suppl):1–62.

Li BUK, Balint JP. Cyclic vomiting syndrome: evolution in understanding of a brain-gut disorder. *Adv Pediatr* 2000;47:117–160.

Li BUK, Issenman R, Sarna SK, eds. Proceedings of the 2nd International Symposium on Cyclic Vomiting Syndrome. *Dig Dis Sci* 1999;44(suppl):1–120.

RESOURCES

127, 301, 354

---

20   Dandy-Walker Syndrome

*Raj Kumar, MD,
and Jaideep Chandra, MS*

DEFINITION: Dandy-Walker syndrome (DWS) is an uncommon cranial anomaly characterized by vermian aplasia with varying degrees of cerebellar hypoplasia, enlarged fourth ventricle, and atresia of the outlet foramina of the fourth ventricle resulting in a large posterior fossa.

DIFFERENTIAL DIAGNOSIS: Dandy-Walker variants; Posterior fossa arachnoid cyst; Blake pouch; Mega cisterna magna.

SYMPTOMS AND SIGNS: The mean age of presentation is 3–4 years, and the age range is 9 months to 12 years. The most common symptom is macrocrania, and signs of raised pressure or hydrocephalus predominate the findings. Cerebellar dysfunction, in the form of truncal ataxia, is seen in older children. Signs of brainstem dysfunction such as hemiparesis or respiratory difficulties are less common. Gait disturbance is another symptom. Cranial nerve palsies are rare. Associated intracranial anomalies include agenesis of corpus callosum, corpus callosum cysts, gyral anomalies, occipital encephalocele, heterotopias of cerebrum and cerebellum, malformation of brainstem, and aqueductal stenosis. A few patients have associated extracranial anomalies such as cardiovascular malformations and renal, facial, or limb abnormalities.

ETIOLOGY/EPIDEMIOLOGY: Some researchers have theorized that DWS occurs as a result of the atresia of foramina of Luschka and Magendie, which causes enlargement of the fourth ventricle and aplasia of the vermis. Other researchers believe that this occurs as a result of the failure of regressive changes in posterior medullary velum leading to cyst formation along with aplasia of vermis. The basic defect occurs between the 4th and 7th weeks of gestation. The etiology is probably multifactorial, and not only teratogenic influences but also single gene deletions and chromosomal aberrations may be involved. The disorder also forms a part of certain autosomal-recessive syndromes. The sex incidence is approximately 60% males to 40% females.

DIAGNOSIS: Clinically, the disorder should be suspected in a patient with macrocrania who has a widened lambdoid suture and a prominent occiput. Transillumination of the posterior fossa shows a cyst and a high torcula. The fontanels may be bulging and other signs of hydrocephalus such as limited upward gaze, enlarged head size, and crackpot sign may be elicited. In older children, cerebellar dysfunction and mental and developmental retardation may be found. Antenatal diagnosis is possible with high-resolution ultrasonagraphy or an MRI study. MRI with cerebrospinal fluid flow dynamic study is the modality of choice for the diagnosis and detection of associated anomalies, as well as for management decisions.

TREATMENT
Standard Therapies: Three options are available: excision of the cyst, cystoperitoneal shunt (CP), or a combined ventriculo-cystoperitoneal shunt (VCP). CP is the primary modality of treatment, and may be combined with drainage of the lateral ventricle if aqueductal stenosis coexists.

REFERENCES
Kumar R, Jain MK, Chhabra DK. Dandy Walker syndrome: different modalities of treatment and outcome in 42 cases. *Child Nervous System* 2001;17:348–352.

Mapstone TB. *Pediatric neurosurgery,* 3rd ed. Philadelphia: WB Saunders, 1994:234–241.

McLaurin R, Crone KR. Dandy Walker syndrome. In: Wilkins RH, Rengachary SS, eds. *Neurosurgery,* 2nd ed. New York: McGraw-Hill, 1996:3669–3672.

Osenbach RK, Menezes AH. Diagnosis and management of the Dandy Walker malformation: 30 years of experience. *Pediatr Neurosurg* 1992;18:179–189.

Zayne D, Jonathan P. Midline developmental abnormalities of the posterior fossa: correlation of classification and outcome. *Pediatr Neurosurg* 1996;24:111–118.

RESOURCES
190, 303, 368

21   Dejerine-Sottas Syndrome

*Tena Rosser, MD,
and Phillip L. Pearl, MD*

DEFINITION: Dejerine-Sottas syndrome (DSS) is a hereditary demyelinating sensorimotor polyneuropathy of infancy and childhood. Clinically, patients show progressive hypotonia, generalized weakness, motor delay, and areflexia with slow nerve conduction velocities (NCV).

SYNONYMS: Hereditary motor and sensory neuropathy (HMSN) type III; Charcot-Marie-Tooth disease type III; Hypertrophic neuropathy of infancy; Hypertrophic interstitial neuropathy of infancy.

DIFFERENTIAL DIAGNOSIS: HMSN type IA or IB; HMSN type II; HMSN type IV; Congenital hypomyelination neuropathy; Giant axonal neuropathy; Infantile neuroaxonal dystrophy; Childhood chronic inflammatory demyelinating polyneuropathy.

SYMPTOMS AND SIGNS: Age of onset and clinical course are variable. In the classic form, children present with hypotonia, weakness, and delayed motor milestones at birth or in early infancy. In most patients, disease is evident before age 1 year. Older children may present with hand weakness or ataxia. A progressive and debilitating sensorimotor peripheral polyneuropathy then ensues. Weakness initially affects the distal lower extremities and gradually involves proximal and upper extremity musculature, eventually resulting in generalized muscle wasting and weakness. Walking is delayed until after 2 years. Hand and foot deformities develop in late childhood. Areflexia is invariably present. Hypertrophic nerves are often palpable within the first decade. Sensory loss is profound and involves all modalities. A severe sensory ataxia results. Progressive sensorineural hearing loss often occurs. Pupillary abnormalities, nystagmus, cranial neuropathies with facial and bulbar weakness, and phrenic nerve involvement with diaphragmatic weakness are found less frequently. A characteristic facial appearance with thick, prominent lips (*levre de tapir*) has been noted in some patients. Common orthopedic complications include scoliosis, short stature, pes cavus, and claw hand deformities. Severe disability is inevitable but symptoms appear to plateau in early adulthood.

ETIOLOGY/EPIDEMIOLOGY: The syndrome is a genetically heterogeneous condition and there is considerable genetic overlap with the other hereditary motor and sensory neuropathies. Inheritance is generally by autosomal-dominant or autosomal-recessive transmission. *De novo* mutations also occur and are responsible for sporadic cases. Dejerine-Sottas syndrome phenotypes have been associated with abnormalities in the peripheral myelin protein (*PMP-22*), myelin protein zero (*MPZ/Po*), and early growth response-2 (*EGR-2*) genes. How mutations in these myelin genes cause demyelinating polyneuropathy is still being determined.

DIAGNOSIS: The diagnosis is made by testing nerve conduction velocities and by sural nerve biopsy in light of a history and physical examination consistent with the condition. NCVs are extremely slow, typically less than 6–12 m/s. Sural nerve biopsy shows hypomyelination with evidence of ongoing demyelination-remyelination. Classic hypertrophic onion bulbs, myelin breakdown products, and inflammation are present. An elevated cerebrospinal fluid protein supports the diagnosis. Genetic testing for a duplication of chromosome 17p11.2, which is responsible for approximately 70%–90% of HSMN type IA, should be performed.

TREATMENT
Standard Therapies: No specific treatment exists; management is primarily supportive. Early intervention services such as physical, occupational, and speech therapy can improve long-term function. Orthopedic and assistive devices such as splints, braces, crutches, and wheelchairs prolong mobilization.

REFERENCES
Harding AE. From the syndrome of Charcot, Marie and Tooth to disorders of peripheral myelin proteins. *Brain* 1995;118: 809–818.
Ouvrier RA. Correlation between the histopathologic, genotypic, and phenotypic features of hereditary peripheral neuropathies in childhood. *J Child Neurol* 1996;11:133–146.
Ouvrier RA, McLeod JG, Conchin TE. The hypertrophic forms of hereditary motor and sensory neuropathy: a study of hypertrophic Charcot-Marie-Tooth disease (HMSN type I) and Dejerine-Sottas disease (HMSN type III) in childhood. *Brain* 1987;110:121–148.
Schaumburg HH, Berger AR, Thomas PK. *Disorders of peripheral nerves,* 2nd ed. Philadelphia: FA Davis, 1992.
Tyson J, Ellis D, Fairbrother U, et al. Hereditary demyelinating neuropathy of infancy: a genetically complex syndrome. *Brain* 1997;120:47–63.

RESOURCES
270, 368

22 Diencephalic Syndrome

Roger J. Packer, MD

DEFINITION: Diencephalic syndrome is a disorder of infancy characterized by profound emaciation with failure to thrive, despite apparently normal caloric intake.

SYNONYM: Russell syndrome.

DIFFERENTIAL DIAGNOSIS: Failure to thrive; Infantile anorexia; Gastrointestinal disease; Neurodegenerative diseases.

SYMPTOMS AND SIGNS: Diencephalic syndrome usually affects young children between 18 months and 3 years of age. Patients most commonly present with a history of normal development and weight gain, followed by either a prolonged period of failure to gain weight or of weight loss. The individual may have anorexia or even apparently excessive appetite. Over time, usually significant loss of subcutaneous tissue occurs with an associated emaciated appearance. The child may have a relatively large head, as compared with body weight. Overall development is often slowed, despite a paucity of abnormal neurologic findings. Affected children may have nystagmus and tremor, and on careful examination they may have unilateral or bilateral visual loss and optic pallor.

ETIOLOGY/EPIDEMIOLOGY: There is no known genetic predisposition to the syndrome. Patients most commonly have a low-grade glial tumor of the hypothalamic region that may anteriorly infiltrate the optic chiasm region or extend posteriorly and inferiorly to the intrapeduncular fossa or basal cisterns. The cause of the weight loss associated with the tumors is unknown, but it may be due to diminished appetite and/or increased energy expenditure due to a hypermetabolic state. Other possibilities are excessive growth hormone secretion, activation of pituitary peptides that contain lipolytic activity, or the secretion of a yet-to-be defined lipid-mobilizing compound. Childhood brain tumors arise in 2.5–3.5 per 100,000 children at risk per year.

DIAGNOSIS: The diagnosis is suspected in a child who has failed to thrive despite apparently normal caloric intake. A history of relatively normal development prior to the onset of weight loss and lack of clear-cut gastrointestinal difficulties is suggestive of the diencephalic syndrome. Careful assessment may demonstrate relative macrocephaly, unsteadiness, nystagmus, and/or visual impairment. The diagnosis is usually readily confirmed by either CT or MRI. Features of CT usually include a hypodense or isodense tumor, often relatively poorly demarcated with little associated edema. Enhancement is variable and tends to be more prominent with pilocytic astrocytomas than with other types of low-grade tumors. On MRI, the hypothalamic tumor is usually either hypointense or isointense on T1-weighted images and shows an increased signal on T2-weighted images. Enhancement is often minimal, especially in nonpilocytic infiltrating lesions.

TREATMENT

Standard Therapies: Treatment options are limited. Supplemental feeding without other types of intervention usually is insufficient, as the tumor will continue to grow and cause increasing emaciation. Extensive surgical resections have been reported to result in transient tumor control; however, total removal of the tumor is usually impossible given its location and infiltrating nature. The most common form of treatment has been biopsy or partial resection followed by radiation therapy. More recently, chemotherapy has been reported to be effective in some children with the diencephalic syndrome secondary to low-grade gliomas.

REFERENCES

Danoff BF, Kramer S, Thompson N. The radiotherapeutic management of optic gliomas of children. *Int J Radiat Oncol Biol Phys* 1980;6:45–50.

Gropman AL, Packer RJ, Nicholson HS, et al. Treatment of diencephalic syndrome with chemotherapy. *Cancer* 1998;83:166–172.

Markesbery WR, McDonald JV. Diencephalic syndrome. A long-term survival. *Am J Dis Child* 1973;125:123–125.

Menezes AH, Bell WE, Perret GC. Hypothalamic tumors in children: their diagnosis and management. *Child Brain* 1977;3:265–280.

Scott EW, Mickle JP. Pediatric diencephalic gliomas: a review of 18 cases. *Pediatr Neurosci* 1987;13:225–232.

RESOURCES

30, 190, 303

---

23 Familial Dysautonomia

Felicia B. Axelrod, MD

DEFINITION: Familial dysautonomia (FD) is an autosomal-recessive disease that primarily affects individuals of Ashkenazi Jewish extraction. It affects development and survival of unmyelinated sensory and autonomic neurons and is characterized by widespread sensory dysfunction and variable autonomic dysfunction.

SYNONYMS: Riley-Day syndrome; Hereditary sensory and autonomic neuropathy type III (HSAN 3).

DIFFERENTIAL DIAGNOSIS: Congenital autonomic dysfunction with universal pain loss; Hereditary sensory and autonomic neuropathy type II (HSAN 2).

SIGNS AND SYMPTOMS: Signs of the disorder are present from birth and neurologic function slowly deteriorates with age so that symptoms and problems will vary with time. Clinical symptoms are related to complications of sensory and autonomic dysfunction. Lack of overflow tears with emotional crying is consistent, but can be considered normal until after age 9 months. In the neonatal period, difficulty feeding and low tone are common. Deep tendon reflexes are decreased. Developmental delay and failure to thrive may be noted. Motor skills and expressive language are usually more affected than receptive language and cognitive skills. The gait may be clumsy and the speech nasal. Many of the symptoms are related to dysphagia and gastroesophageal reflux resulting in aspiration and frequent pneumonia. Decreased response to pain and temperature, scoliosis, labile blood pressures, periodic erythematous blotching of the skin, and increased sweating may also be present.

ETIOLOGY/EPIDEMIOLOGY: FD appears confined to individuals of Ashkenazi Jewish extraction. The carrier rate has been estimated to be 1 in 30, with a disease frequency of 1 in 3,600 live births. The gene is *IKBKAP* and two mutations have been found responsible for FD. The gene is located on the distal long arm of chromosome 9 (q31). Males and females are affected in equal numbers.

DIAGNOSIS: Definitive diagnosis can be made by DNA diagnostic testing for the two mutations in the *IKBKAP* gene. However, a *de novo* diagnosis is based on "cardinal" clinical criteria, i.e., alacrima, absent fungiform papillae, depressed patellar reflexes, lack of an axon flare after intradermal histamine, and both parents being of Ashkenazi Jewish extraction. Further supportive evidence is provided by findings of decreased response to pain and temperature, orthostatic hypotension, periodic erythematous blotching of the skin, and increased sweating. In addition, cinesopha-grams may show delay in cricopharyngeal closure, tertiary contractions of the esophagus, gastroesophageal reflux, and delayed gastric emptying.

TREATMENT
Standard Therapies: The disease process cannot be arrested. Treatment is preventative, symptomatic, and supportive. It must be directed toward specific problems, which can vary considerably among patients and at different ages. In the early years, the major goal is to prevent aspiration and maintain good nutrition while promoting normal development. When medical management is not sufficient, fundoplication with gastrostomy is advised. In the later years, spine fusion may be required for correction of severe spine curvature. Diazepam and clonidine are frequently used as treatment for vomiting. To promote more blood pressure stability, fludrocortisone and midodrine are suggested.

REFERENCES
Axelrod FB. Familial dysautonomia. In: Mathias CJ, Bannister R. *Autonomic failure,* 4th ed. New York: Oxford University Press, 1999:402–418.
Axelrod FB, Maayan CH. Familial dysautonomia. In: Burg FD, Ingelfinger JR, Walk ER, et al., eds. *Gellis and Kagen's current pediatric therapy,* 16th ed. Philadelphia: WB Saunders, 1999: 466–469.
Blumenfeld A, Slaugenhaupt SA, Liebert CB, et al. Precise genetic mapping and haplotype analysis of the familial dysautonomia gene on human chromosome 9q31. *Am J Hum Genet* 1997;64: 1110–1118.
Laplaza J, Turajane T, Axelrod FB, et al. Non-spinal orthopaedic problems in familial dysautonomia. *J Pediatr Orthop* 2001; 21:229–232.
Slaugenhaupt SA, Blumenfeld A, Gill SP, et al. Tissue-specific expression of a splicing mutation in the *IKBKAP* gene causes familial dysautonomia. *Am J Hum Genet* 2001;68:598–604.

RESOURCES
137, 138, 294, 368

24 Primary Empty Sella Syndrome

Kathleen Colleran, MD

DEFINITION: Primary empty sella (PES) is a defect of the diaphragma sellae. The PES syndrome consists of the anatomic finding in association with headache, visual disturbances, and benign intracranial pressure.

SYNONYMS: Empty sella; Empty sella tursica.

DIFFERENTIAL DIAGNOSIS: Prior pituitary surgery; Radiation; Sheehan syndrome; Hemorrhage of a pituitary tumor.

SYMPTOMS AND SIGNS: PES is an anatomic finding rarely associated with clinical symptoms. Headache is the most common symptom, but it is unclear whether the two are related. Rarely, PES may be associated with benign intracranial hypertension, visual disturbances, pseudotumor cerebri, or cerebrospinal fluid (CSF) rhinnorhea. Pituitary hypofunction is uncommon but may occur. Usually this consists of decreased hormone reserve, without clinical manifestations, and is seen only on dynamic endocrine testing. Mild hyperprolactinemia is more common, occurring in approximately 15% of individuals with PES. In children, growth hormone deficiency may be seen rarely.

ETIOLOGY/EPIDEMIOLOGY: Primary empty sella results from a congenital defect in the diaphragma sellae

lining the sella tursica, which allows the subarachnoid membrane to herniate through it. The CSF within the subarachnoid space exerts pressure on the sella tursica, enlarging and flattening it. The pituitary gland, normally located in this space, is compressed during this process, thus giving the appearance of an empty sella tursica. Autopsy studies suggest the prevalence of PES is 5%–23%. The PES syndrome is less common, occurring in less than 1% of cases of primary empty sella. It is more common in middle-aged, obese, multiparous women.

DIAGNOSIS: PES is diagnosed by MRI or CT. Causes of secondary empty sella including pituitary tumor, resection, Sheehan syndrome, or radiation should be excluded.

TREATMENT
Standard Therapies: Treatment is supportive. If endocrine dysfunction occurs, the affected hormones should be replaced.

REFERENCES
Braatvedt CD, Corrall RM. The empty sella syndrome: much ado about nothing. *Br J Hosp Med* 1992;47:523–525.
Cacciari E, Zucchini S, Ambrosetto P, et al. Empty sella in children and adolescents with possible hypothamamic-pituitary disorders. *J Clin Endocrinol Metab* 1994;78:767–771.

Gallardo E, Schachter D, Caceres E, et al. The empty sella: results of treatment in 76 successive cases and high frequency of endocrine and neurological disturbances. *Clin Endocrinol* 1992;37:529–533.

Valensi P, Combes M, Perret G, et al. TSH and prolactin responses to thyrotropin releasing hormone (TRH) and domperidone in patients with empty sella syndrome. *J Endocrinol Invest* 1996;19:293–297.

RESOURCE

368

---

25   Progressive Myoclonus Epilepsy

Michael R. Pranzatelli, MD

DEFINITION: Progressive myoclonus epilepsy (PME) is a syndrome of more than a dozen different diseases that share worsening of symptoms over time and the presence of both myoclonus and epilepsy. Patients may have more than one type of seizure, and the rate of progression may be slow or fast, depending on the underlying disease.

DIFFERENTIAL DIAGNOSIS: Myoclonic epilepsy; Juvenile myoclonus epilepsy.

SYMPTOMS AND SIGNS: Myoclonus (rapid muscle jerks) is usually the worst problem because it is not helped as much by anticonvulsants, which control the epilepsy. Abundant in the morning, it increases with stress and illness. A buildup of myoclonic jerks typically leads to a convulsion. Myoclonus often interferes with coordination, and ataxia can be a problem. Mental function may be impaired in PME, leading especially to problems with memory and depression. Some individuals have a neurogenic bladder, gastrointestinal or thyroid problems, lipomas, and visual or hearing impairment. Due to inactivity, obesity is common and further restricts activity.

ETIOLOGY/EPIDEMIOLOGY: The most common causes of PME are mitochondrial encephalomyopathy (MERRF, MELAS, others), EPM1 (also called Unverricht-Lündborg disease or Baltic myoclonus), Lafora disease (EPM2A), Batten disease (neuronal ceroid lipofuscinosis), cerebral storage disorders, other neurodegenerative disorders, and biotin-responsive encephalopathy. Mitochondrial myopathy refers to disorders in which the function of mitochondria is abnormal owing to gene mutations. EPM1 is caused by a repeat expansion mutation in the cystatin B gene on chromosome 21. Lafora disease, one of the most severe types of PME, results from a gene mutation on chromosome 6. Most types of Batten disease are associated with blindness; for two of the forms, gene mutations have been discovered. Cerebral storage disorders include many rare diseases in which abnormal deposits form in the brain, such as GM2 gangliosidosis, sialidosis, Tay-Sachs disease, and Gaucher disease. In degenerative disorders, such as neuroaxonal dystrophy and dentatorubro-pallidoluysian atrophy, other neurologic abnormalities (ataxia, neuropathy) are present besides those associated with PME. Biotin-responsive disorders are a rare but reversible cause of PME.

DIAGNOSIS: The following tests are usually necessary to determine the diagnosis: molecular genetic studies on blood samples, back-averaging (electroencephalography/electromyography), 24-hour video-telemetry, sleep study, neuropsychological testing, SPECT or positron emission tomographic scan, magnetic resonance spectroscopy, spinal fluid tests, skin or muscle biopsy, and tests of vision, hearing, and bladder function.

TREATMENT

Standard Therapies: The treatment of myoclonus always begins with a thorough search for reversible causes. Genetic counseling is recommended. Clonazepam, divalproex sodium, and primidone or phenobarbital are the standard anticonvulsants for myoclonus. The following anticonvulsants help treat both myoclonus and seizures: levetiracetam, topiramate, and zonisamide. For patients who experience exacerbations of myoclonus or seizures during their menstrual periods, low-dose oral contraceptives or acetazolamide may also help. Chloral hydrate helps patients whose sleep is disrupted by myoclonus, and it is also excellent for myoclonic emergencies during the day. Treatment with a serotonin synaptic reuptake inhibitor, in conjunction with counseling, is effective for patients who experience depression.

Investigational Therapies: Treatments being investigated include piracetam, 5-hydroxy-L-tryptophan, vigabatrin, and N-acetylcysteine.

REFERENCES

Bespalova IN, et al. Novel cystatin B mutation and diagnostic PCR assay in Unverricht-Lündborg (Baltic) progressive

myoclonus epilepsy patient. *Am J Med Genet* 1997;74:467–471.
Pranzatelli MR, Nadi NS. Mechanism of action of antiepileptic and antimyoclonic drugs. In Fahn S, et al., eds. *Negative motor phenomena.* Vol. 67. Advances in neurology. Philadelphia: Lippincott-Raven, 1995.

Roger J. Progressive myoclonus epilepsies. In: Dam M, Gram L, eds. *Comprehensive epileptology.* New York: Raven, 1981:215–231.

RESOURCES
145, 322, 368

26 Fahr Disease

Bala V. Manyam, MD

DEFINITION: All cases of bilateral striopallidodentate calcinosis are included under the term *Fahr disease,* although the proper name should be bilateral striopallidodentate calcinosis (BSPDC), a descriptive term.

SYNONYMS: Symmetric cerebral calcification; Idiopathic calcification of cerebral capillaries; Symmetric calcification of the basal ganglia; Idiopathic nonarteriosclerotic calcification of cerebral vessels; Idiopathic familial cerebrovascular ferrocalcinosis; Symmetrical intracranial advanced pseudocalcium; Pallido-dentate calcifications; Idiopathic basal ganglia calcification.

DIFFERENTIAL DIAGNOSIS: Hypoparathyroidism.

SYMPTOMS AND SIGNS: No specific symptoms and signs exist for Fahr disease. Movement disorders may account for 55% of all symptomatic patients; of these, parkinsonism is the most common. Less common are chorea, tremor, dystonia, athetosis, and orofacial dyskinesia. Other neurologic manifestations include cognitive impairment, speech disorder, cerebellar signs, psychiatric features, pyramidal signs, and gait disorder. Occasional symptoms include sensory changes, pain sizers, and urinary incontinence.

ETIOLOGY/EPIDEMIOLOGY: Autosomal-dominant, familial, and sporadic cases have been described. The locus of autosomal-dominant BSPDC in one large family is reported on chromosome 14q. In one family with autosomal-dominant inheritance, cerebrospinal fluid homocarnosine was increased compared with the sporadic form. Calcium is the major element present, and it accounts for the radiologic appearance of the disease. Mucopolysaccharides, traces of aluminum, arsenic, cobalt, copper, molybdenum, iron, lead, manganese, magnesium, silver, phosphorus, and zinc are also present. Calcium and other mineral deposits were found in the perivascular spaces, walls of capillaries, arterioles, and small veins. Of the 99 patients who have been identified, two thirds were symptomatic. The disease is slightly more common in men.

DIAGNOSIS: The diagnosis is established by CT or MRI evidence of bilateral, almost symmetric, calcifications of one or more of the following areas: basal ganglia, dentate nuclei, thalamus, and cerebral white matter (Insert Fig. 52). Diagnosis is further based on normal childhood growth and development and the absence of parathyroid and other known neurologic disorders. Symptoms, if they occur, usually manifest in the fourth decade of life, whereas calcification may be found in the second decade of life.

TREATMENT
Standard Therapies: No specific treatment is known. In 1 patient, disodium etidronate showed symptomatic benefit without reduction in calcification.

REFERENCES
Geschwind DH, Loginov M, Stern JM. Identification of a locus on chromosome 14q for idiopathic basal ganglia calcification (Fahr disease). *Am J Hum Genet* 1999;65:764–772.
Loeb JA. Functional improvement in a patient with cerebral calcinosis using a bisphosphonate. *Mov Disord* 1998;13:345–349.
Manyam BV, Bhatt MH, Moore WD, et al. Bilateral strio-pallidodentate calcinosis: CSF, imaging, and electrophysiological studies. *Ann Neurol* 1992;31:379–384.
Manyam BV, Walters AS, Keller IA, et al. Parkinsonism associated with autosomal dominant bilateral striopallidodentate calcinosis. *Parkinsonism Rel Disord* 2001;7:269–295.
Manyam BV, Walters AS, Narla KR. Bilateral striopallidodentate calcinosis: clinical characteristics of patients seen in a registry. *Mov Disord* 2001;16:258–264.

RESOURCES
151, 368

27   Frey Syndrome

Jens-Jörg von Lindern, MD, DMD

DEFINITION: Frey syndrome is a sequela of operative procedures in the region of the parotid gland. It occurs frequently after conservative and radical parotidectomies and sometimes after purulent parotitis, tumors, trauma, typhoid fever, and irritation of the auriculotemporal nerve by dislocated temporomandibular fractures.

SYNONYMS: Frey-Baillarger syndrome; Gustatory sweating; Auriculotemporal syndrome; Sudation parotidienne.

DIFFERENTIAL DIAGNOSIS: General hyperhidrosis.

SYMPTOMS AND SIGNS: Frey syndrome becomes symptomatic when undesirable sweating occurs in the cheek, retroauricular, and temporal regions after eating. Symptoms can also occur in the distribution of the greater auricular nerve. There can be flushing and warmness with overheating of the affected areas of the skin, which in some cases is associated with pain. Pain can also occur initially as a preliminary sign or be the only symptom. Typically, the symptoms occur several weeks or months after surgery.

ETIOLOGY/EPIDEMIOLOGY: The precise pathophysiology of Frey syndrome is unclear. Hypothetical explanations are based on the dense parasympathetic innervation in the region of the parotid. Parasympathetic secretory fibers from the glossopharyngeal nerve to the parotid gland pass by means of the tympanic nerve, superficial petrosal nerve, and otic ganglion (Jacobson anastomosis) to the auriculotemporal nerve, which branches off the trunk of the mandibular nerve. Frey syndrome can be explained by local terminal inhibition of the physiologic reflex or by malinnervation due to misdirection of the parasympathetic fibers of the auriculotemporal nerve for the parotid gland in the process of postoperative regeneration. The incidence depends on the size of the glandular compartment re-

moved and on the intensity of the diagnostic procedures used to verify the presence of the syndrome. Follow-up examinations show that approximately 30%–50% of postparotidectomy patients experience the symptoms described, and approximately 15% rate their symptoms as severe.

DIAGNOSIS: In response to targeted questioning, 30%–50% of postparotidectomy patients report having the typical symptoms. The Minor Iodine-Starch Test provides reliable verification of hyperhidrosis.

TREATMENT
Standard Therapies: Treatment of Frey syndrome has been unsatisfactory. In addition to surgical measures such as excision of the affected skin or the interposition of fascia lata, muscle flaps, or Silastic sheeting, there are also drug treatments involving the systemic or topical application of anticholinergics or antihidrotics. An innovative method of treatment consists of the local intracutaneous injection of type A botulinum toxin in the affected areas.

REFERENCES
Brin MF. Interventional neurology: treatment of neurological conditions with local injection of botulinum toxin. *Arch Neurobiol* 1991;54:7–23.
Drobik C, Laskawi, R. Frey's syndrome: treatment with botulinum toxin. *Acta Otolaryngol (Stockh)* 1995;115:459–461.
Frey L. Le syndrome du nerf auriculo-temporal. *Rev Neurol (Paris)* 1923;40:97–104.
Gardner WJ, McCubbin JW. Auriculotemporal syndrome: gustatory sweating due to misdirection of regenerated nerve fibers. *JAMA* 1956;160:272–277.
von Lindern J-J, Niederhagen B, Bergé S, et al. Frey's syndrome: treatment with type A botulinum toxin. *Cancer* 2000;89: 1659–1663.

RESOURCE
368

28   Frontotemporal Dementia (Pick Disease)

John H. Growdon, MD

DEFINITION: Frontotemporal dementia (FTD) is a diagnostic term that encompasses a spectrum of chronic progressive neurodegenerative disorders associated with lobar atrophy. The two characteristic clinical patterns are gradual and progressive changes in personality and behavior, and progressive language dysfunction.

SYNONYMS: Pick disease; Semantic dementia; Primary progressive aphasia; Frontal lobe dementia; Frontotemporal lobar degeneration with and without motor neuron disease.

DIFFERENTIAL DIAGNOSIS: Alzheimer disease; Parkinson disease; Diffuse Lewy body disease; Huntington disease; HIV encephalopathy; Schizophrenia; Sequelae of multiple strokes.

SYMPTOMS AND SIGNS: In the most common form of FTD, patients present with early and prominent changes in personality and social conduct. They have difficulty modulating behavior in social situations and are often uninhibited. They are impulsive, lack judgment, and may display frank antisocial behavior. Throughout the illness, they show little insight or personal concern for their actions. The other clinical phenotype of FTD is characterized by early and progressive language dysfunction. The most common problem is with expressive language. The patient has difficulty selecting and using the correct words; comprehension is usually preserved. Many patients become mute. Although memory loss occurs in both forms of FTD, it is relatively mild early in the illness and is often overshadowed by the behavioral and language difficulties.

ETIOLOGY/EPIDEMIOLOGY: Frontotemporal dementia usually begins between ages 35 and 75 years, and affects men and women equally. Some patients have a history of another affected family member. A few cases are caused by mutations in the tau gene on chromosome 17.

DIAGNOSIS: Clinical criteria for the diagnosis of FTD specify that (a) there are early and progressive changes in personality, behavior, and/or language function; (b) these changes are sufficiently severe to impair social and occupational functioning; and (c) the course of illness has a gradual onset and steady continuous decline. No diagnostic tests are 100% sensitive and specific. Anatomic brain images with CT or MRI typically show asymmetric or symmetric atrophy of the anterior temporal and frontal lobes. Functional neuroimaging with SPECT or positron emission tomography may detect decreased cerebral perfusion and glucose metabolism in the anterior temporal and frontal lobe regions, even when atrophy is not pronounced.

TREATMENT
Standard Therapies: No treatments reverse the signs of FTD, nor even retard the course of illness. Anxiolytic, antipsychotic, and mood-stabilizing drugs may be prescribed for treating specific symptoms.

REFERENCES
Binetti G, Locascio J, Corkin S, et al. Differences between Pick disease and Alzheimer disease in clinical appearance and rate of cognitive decline. *Arch Neurol* 2000;57:225–232.
Brun A, England B, Gustafson L, et al. Clinical and neuropathological criteria for frontotemporal dementia: the Lund criteria. *J Neurol Neurosurg Psychiatry* 1994;57:416–418.
McKhann GM, Albert MS, Grossman M, et al. Clinical and pathological diagnosis of frontotemporal dementia. *Arch Neurol* 2001;58:1803–1809.
Neary D, Snowden JS, Gustafson L, et al. Frontotemporal lobar degeneration: a consensus on clinical diagnostic criteria. *Neurology* 1998;51:1546–1554.
Snowden JS, Neary D, Mann DM. *Fronto-temporal lobar degeneration.* London: Churchill-Livingston, 1996.
Spillantine MG, Bird TD, Ghetti B. Frontotemporal dementia and Parkinsonism linked to chromosome 17: a new group of tauopathies. *Brain Pathol* 1998;8:387–402.

RESOURCES
22, 368, 369

29 Gerstmann Syndrome

*Steven W. Anderson, PhD,
and Arthur Benton, PhD*

DEFINITION: The Gerstmann syndrome is a combination of specific cognitive deficits (right-left disorientation, finger agnosia, agraphia, and acalculia) that, when it occurs in pure form, is strongly indicative of a focal lesion in the posterior parietal region of the brain, usually of the left hemisphere.

DIFFERENTIAL DIAGNOSIS: Alzheimer disease; Other conditions causing diffuse brain dysfunction.

SYMPTOMS AND SIGNS: The cardinal symptoms of the syndrome, i.e., difficulty in identifying the fingers of both hands, difficulty in discriminating between the right and left sides of one's body, and loss of the ability to write and to calculate, are rarely encountered in the precise form first described by the Viennese neurologist Josef Gerstmann. Instead, far more frequent are combinations of two or three Gerstmann symptoms with other specific indications of posterior parietal lobe disease, e.g., acalculia, agraphia, and constructional apraxia (sometimes labeled Leonhard syndrome) or acalculia, agraphia, and defective recognition of faces (sometimes labeled Zeh syndrome). Gerstmann symptoms, whether occurring in isolation or in combination with "non-Gerstmann" symptoms, are best regarded as manifestations of a broader parietal symptom complex which is sufficiently limited to have localizing implications.

ETIOLOGY/EPIDEMIOLOGY: Gerstmann syndrome and similar posterior parietal symptom combinations are usually the result of focal cerebrovascular disease in a posterior branch of the left middle cerebral artery or a border zone infarct, usually involving the angular gyrus or subjacent white matter (Brodmann area 39). In rare cases, traumatic brain injury or an expanding neoplasm in this same region can cause all or elements of the symptoms of this syndrome.

DIAGNOSIS: Provided that general mental impairment and significant aphasic disorder can be excluded as primary factors, the presentation of deficits such as agraphia, acalculia, and right-left confusion should alert the clinician to the possibility of focal posterior parietal lobe disease. Neuropsychologic evaluation can be useful in determining the presence of less obvious deficits such as finger agnosia and constructional apraxia, and for evaluating other relevant spheres of cognition. Structural and functional neu-

roimaging may be of further value in determining whether evidence exists of underlying neurologic abnormality.

TREATMENT
Standard Therapies: Gerstmann syndrome and similar symptom combinations are outcomes, not diseases. Primary treatment is directed to the underlying neurologic abnormality. Cognitive rehabilitation may be useful for those aspects of the syndrome that interfere with performance of daily activities, such as agraphia and acalculia.

REFERENCES
Benton AL. Gerstmann's syndrome. *Arch Neurol* 1992;49:445–447.
Critchley M. The enigma of Gerstmann's syndrome. *Brain* 1966; 89:183–198.
Mayer E, Martory M-D, Pegna AJ, et al. A pure case of Gerstmann syndrome with a subangular lesion. *Brain* 1999;122:1107–1120.
Morris HH, Luders H, Lesser RP, et al. Transient neuropsychological abnormalities (including Gerstmann's syndrome) during cortical stimulation. *Neurology* 1984;34:877–883.

RESOURCE
233

---

30   Guillain-Barré Syndrome

Jane Pritchard, BM, BCh

DEFINITION: Guillain-Barré syndrome (GBS) is an acute-onset neuropathy. It is usually demyelinating but can be axonal in type. Subtypes include acute inflammatory demyelinating polyradiculoneuropathy (AIDP), acute motor axonal neuropathy (AMAN), acute motor and sensory axonal neuropathy (AMSAN), and Miller-Fisher syndrome (MFS; external ophthalmoplegia, ataxia, and areflexia).

SYNONYMS: Acute febrile polyneuritis; Acute infective polyneuritis; Landry-Guillain-Barré syndrome; Landry-Guillain-Barré-Strohl syndrome; Idiopathic polyneuritis.

DIFFERENTIAL DIAGNOSIS: Toxin (e.g., arsenic, solvents) and drug exposure (e.g., nitrofurantoin); Acute intermittent porphyria; Vasculitic neuropathy; Infection (e.g., borreliosis, diphtheria); Lymphomatous infiltration.

SYMPTOMS AND SIGNS: Approximately two thirds of patients have a history of an antecedent infection in the

weeks before the onset of neurologic symptoms, most frequently *Campylobacter jejuni* affecting the gastrointestinal tract or *Mycoplasma pneumoniae*, Epstein-Barr virus, or cytomegalovirus affecting the respiratory tract. Patients typically first develop ascending distal numbness and paresthesia, then progressive weakness of all four limbs. The patient soon becomes areflexic. The weakness is symmetric and in one third of patients is predominantly proximal, in one third predominantly distal, and in the rest both proximal and distal strength is affected. Cranial nerve involvement may occur with bilateral facial weakness, external ophthalmoplegia, and progressive bulbar dysfunction. Most patients reach a nadir within 2 weeks, but always in less than 4 weeks, then their condition plateaus for approximately 1 week before beginning to improve. Approximately 25% of patients require ventilatory support. In the long term, 80% of patients have good recovery, 10% are not fit to return to work, and 10% die, usually from the complications of immobility.

ETIOLOGY/EPIDEMIOLOGY: Two cases of GBS occur per 100,000 population per year. The syndrome occurs at any age, becoming more common with advancing age, with an additional peak in young adults. It is more common in men (ratio 1.25:1). It is believed to be an autoimmune disease, the immune-mediated attack directed against the myelin sheath and axon triggered by an antecedent infection in a susceptible individual.

DIAGNOSIS: The diagnosis is clinical, supported by laboratory investigations. A patient suspected to have GBS should always be admitted to the hospital (in case deterioration in respiratory function or cardiac arrhythmia occur) where nerve conduction studies should be performed to characterize the disease as axonal or demyelinating. A lumbar puncture should show acellular cerebrospinal fluid but with a mildly elevated protein level. Results of both of these investigations can be normal in the first week of the illness. Serum can be assayed for antibodies against gangliosides, which are found in many patients with GBS.

TREATMENT
Standard Therapies: Plasma exchange and intravenous immunoglobulin are equally efficacious in improving outcome in bed-bound patients when administered within the first 2 weeks of onset of symptoms. It is essential to monitor vital capacity and cardiac rhythm in the early stages of the illness. Analgesia and drugs to treat neuropathic pain (e.g., carbamazepine and gabapentin) may be needed together with subcutaneous heparin to prevent the formation of deep vein thromboses.

REFERENCES
Hughes RA. *Guillain-Barré syndrome.* Heidelberg: Springer-Verlag, 1990.
Hughes RAC, Raphael JC, Swan AV, et al. Intravenous immunoglubulin for Guillain-Barré syndrome (Cochrane Review). In: *The Cochrane Library,* Issue 2, 2002. Oxford: Update Software.
Hughes RAC, van der Meché FGA. Corticosteroids for Guillain-Barré syndrome (Cochrane Review). In: *The Cochrane Library,* Issue 2, 2002. Oxford: Update Software.
Raphael JC, Chevret S, Hughes RAC, et al. Plasma exchange for Guillain-Barré syndrome (Cochrane Review). In: *The Cochrane Library,* Issue 2, 2002. Oxford: Update Software.

RESOURCES
27, 171, 368

---

31   Holoprosencephaly

Jeffrey E. Ming, MD, PhD

DEFINITION: Holoprosencephaly (HPE) is a structural anomaly in which the forebrain fails to completely separate into distinct right and left halves.

SYNONYMS: Holotelencephaly; Middle interhemispheric fusion.

DIFFERENTIAL DIAGNOSIS: Smith-Lemli-Opitz syndrome; Chromosomal abnormalities (including trisomy 13).

SYMPTOMS AND SIGNS: A wide spectrum of clinical findings exists in HPE. In the most severe form, there is complete continuity across the midline of the forebrain with a single ventricle (alobar HPE). In the lobar form, the lateral ventricles are separated but the forebrain is still partially continuous across the midline. The clinical range occurs in a continuum from alobar HPE to continuity only across the most ventral basal portion of the cerebral cortex.

Hydrocephalus may occur. Pituitary anomalies may be present and may be associated with hypernatremia (due to diabetes insipidus), adrenal hypoplasia, hypothyroidism, and hypogonadism. Craniofacial anomalies are commonly present, although some affected children have relatively normal facies. Affected individuals often have hypotelorism, cleft lip/palate (often midline), a flat hypoplastic nose, and microcephaly. More severe defects of the eyes (e.g., cyclopia) and face may also occur. Developmental delay and mental retardation are almost invariably present in all patients with brain malformations. Seizures may also occur.

ETIOLOGY/EPIDEMIOLOGY: The disorder occurs in approximately 1 in 16,000 live births. Males and females are affected in a large number of ethnic groups. The etiology is heterogeneous, and both environmental (e.g., maternal diabetes) and genetic causes have been noted. Approximately one half of patients have a cytogenetic abnormality, most frequently trisomy 13. Although most cases occur sporadically, autosomal-dominant transmission has been noted. Pedigrees consistent with autosomal-recessive and X-linked inheritance have also been described. Mutations in each of several genes have been noted in affected individuals, and genes identified causing HPE in humans include *sonic hedgehog*, *ZIC2*, *TGIF*, and *SIX3*.

DIAGNOSIS: Facial features characteristic for HPE may suggest the diagnosis in the newborn period. CT or MRI of the brain can confirm the diagnosis. Severe cases of HPE can often be detected on prenatal ultrasonography at approximately 16 weeks' gestation, although less severe forms may not be reliably detected. A prenatal history should be obtained to determine if any teratogen exposure occurred. A karyotype for chromosome analysis should be obtained.

TREATMENT

Standard Therapies: Treatment is based on the specific organ system involved and is symptomatic and supportive. Appropriate interventions for seizures, hydrocephalus, cleft lip/palate, feeding difficulties, and developmental delay should be instituted as indicated. The physician should be alert for signs of pituitary dysfunction. Referral to a clinical geneticist is indicated to obtain a karyotype and for evaluation for associated syndromes and recurrence risk estimation. Features consistent with familial transmission of the disease (e.g., a single central maxillary incisor) should be carefully assessed in parents and family members.

REFERENCES

Ming JE, Muenke M. Holoprosencephaly: from Homer to Hedgehog. *Clin Genet* 1998;53:155–163.

Muenke M, Beachy PA. Holoprosencephaly. In: Scriver CR, Beaudet AL, Valle D, et al., eds. *The metabolic and molecular bases of inherited disease,* 8th ed. New York: McGraw-Hill, 2001:6203–6230.

RESOURCES

75, 156, 195

32 Huntington Disease

Adam Rosenblatt, MD

DEFINITION: Huntington disease is a hereditary, progressive, neurodegenerative disorder characterized by a movement disorder, cognitive decline, and various psychiatric disturbances.

SYNONYM: Huntington chorea.

DIFFERENTIAL DIAGNOSIS: Sydenham chorea; Benign familial chorea; Chorea-acanthocytosis; Wilson disease; Friedrich ataxia; Spinocerebellar ataxia; Dentatorubro-pallidoluysian atrophy.

SYMPTOMS AND SIGNS: Symptoms begin insidiously and progress slowly over many years, until the death of the affected individual. Onset is typically in the fourth or fifth decade of life, but may take place any time from childhood to old age. Affected individuals may have a motor, cognitive, or psychiatric onset, but motor symptoms seem to be most common and are the only unequivocal signs. The movement disorder consists of the presence of irregular involuntary jerking or writhing movements (chorea or choreoathetosis) and impairment of voluntary movements. Chorea usually begins in the distal extremities, becomes more extravagant over time, involving the limbs, head, face, and trunk, and usually recedes later in the course of the illness. Voluntary movement impairments generally become significant somewhat later and involve abnormal eye movements, slow and uncoordinated fine movements, dysarthria, dysphagia, and gait disturbance. In the final stages, victims tend to become rigid. Weight loss is a common problem, and death usually occurs as a result of immobility and inanition. The typical life expectancy is 15–20 years from onset. The cognitive disorder is characterized by loss of cognitive speed and flexibility, seen first in complex or multiple cognitive tasks. As the condition progresses, cognitive impairments become more extensive and result in a global dementia. Psychiatric disorders in Huntington disease are more variable and are not always seen, but common problems include depression and personality changes consisting of irritability, apathy, explosiveness, disinhibition, and perseveration.

ETIOLOGY/EPIDEMIOLOGY: Huntington disease is caused by an expansion in the normal number of CAG triplets in the huntington gene of chromosome 4. Several genetic diseases exist in which such triplets, coding for the amino acid glutamine, are expanded, leading to cell death. In Huntington disease, the basal ganglia, particularly the head of the caudate nucleus, are affected first, but atrophy and brain cell loss are more global late in the course. The number of CAG triplets is inversely correlated with the age of onset. Particularly when passed in the paternal line, the expanded sequence is vulnerable to further expansion, causing anticipation in the age of onset of 6–8 years on average when passed from father to child. Males and females are affected in equal numbers. The prevalence is between 1 in 10,000 and 1 in 20,000 individuals.

DIAGNOSIS: Diagnosis is made on the basis of family history, neurologic examination showing the characteristic movement disorder, and confirmatory genetic testing. A direct genetic assay makes presymptomatic and prenatal testing possible as well. Because of the typically late onset of symptoms, the absence of a family history does not preclude diagnosis.

TREATMENT
Standard Therapies: There are no standard therapies, nor any therapies known to influence the rate of progression. Medications such as neuroleptics, benzodiazepines, and dopamine-depleting agents such as reserpine and tetra-

benazine may be used to suppress chorea. Psychiatric treatment can be effective for depression and behavioral disturbances associated with Huntington disease. Cognitive decline and motor impairments are usually treated with environmental changes and conservative management. Patients may require a high caloric intake to maintain weight and may need a special diet because of dysphagia.

REFERENCES
Folstein SF. *Huntington's disease. A disorder of families.* Baltimore: Johns Hopkins Press, 1989.
Harper PS. *Huntington's disease.* London: WB Saunders, 1996.
Rosenblatt A, Ranen NG, Nance MA, et al. *A physician's guide to the management of Huntington's disease,* 2nd ed. New York: Huntington's Disease Society of America, 1999.

RESOURCES
177, 189, 368, 487

---

33 Hydranencephaly

Gary N. McAbee, DO, JD

DEFINITION: Hydranencephaly is a congenital disorder that results from the failure of normal brain development or a secondary destructive process and manifests within several weeks of birth. The hallmark of the disorder is the severe destruction of cerebral hemispheres with only remnants of nonfunctioning cortex. The intracranial space is filled with cerebrospinal fluid. The brainstem remains partially or completely intact.

DIFFERENTIAL DIAGNOSIS: Severe congenital hydrocephalus; Massive subdural effusions; Holoprosencephaly.

SYMPTOMS AND SIGNS: Typically, infants appear healthy at birth. Facial features are normal, which distinguishes hydranencephaly from other major central nervous system malformations. The head circumference is normal or large, or progressively enlarges within the first few weeks of life. It is the enlarged head circumference that often alerts the physician that a neurologic problem exists. Other neurologic signs, including hypotonia or spasticity, motor weakness, irritability, or depressed mental status, also become evident within several weeks of life. "Stiffening" episodes, which mimic seizures, as well as "normal" infant behaviors such as yawning, crying, and smiling anomalies occur, although rarely. Death typically occurs within weeks or months. Prolonged survival to the age of 19 years has been reported.

ETIOLOGY/EPIDEMIOLOGY: Almost all patients have prenatal onset. The pathogenesis is variable, but has been attributed to either a developmental or severely destructive process of the cortex, such as an infection or toxin that affects the major blood vessels supplying the brain. Genetics may play a role in a small number of cases.

DIAGNOSIS: Diagnosis is suspected by the absence of the cortex on either fetal or postnatal ultrasonography; CT or MRI is needed to confirm. Ventricular shunting may be needed to exclude other causes such as massive hydrocephalus.

TREATMENT
Standard Therapies: No treatment is available other than appropriate nursing care and shunting, if required.

REFERENCES
Gershoni-Baruch R, Zekaria D. Deletion (13)(q22) with multiple congenital anomalies, hydranencephaly and penoscrotal transposition. *Clin Dysmorphol* 1996;5:289–294.
Halsey J. Hydranencephaly. In: Vinken P, Bruyn G, Klawans H, eds. *Handbook of clinical neurology.* Amsterdam: Elsevier Science, 1987:337–353.
McAbee G, Chan A, Erde E. Prolonged survival with hydranencephaly: report of two cases and literature review. *Pediatr Neurol* 2000:23;80–84.

RESOURCES
190, 368, 462

34   Hydrocephalus

Sanjiv Sahoo, MD,
and Phillip L. Pearl, MD

DEFINITION: Hydrocephalus is defined as enlargement of the ventricles of the brain with an abnormal increase in the amount of cerebrospinal fluid (CSF) relative to the brain tissue.

SYNONYM: Internal hydrocephalus.

DIFFERENTIAL DIAGNOSIS: In children: Aqueductal stenosis; Chiari II malformation; Choroid plexus papilloma; Dandy-Walker malformation; Hydranencephaly; Intrauterine infections; Intraventricular hemorrhage; Meningitis; Mucopolysaccharidoses; Nonketotic hyperglycinemia; Tumors, X-linked genetic type. In adults: Arachnoid villi seeding by ependymomas; Binswanger disease; Cerebellar infarcts or hemorrhages; Chronic meningitis; Mass lesions; Hemorrhage; High CSF protein content; Parkinson disease; Vein of Galen malformation; Venous sinus thrombosis.

SYMPTOMS AND SIGNS: In neonates and young children, irritability, lethargy, poor feeding, headaches, vomiting, diplopia, blurring of vision, ataxic gait, spasticity, seizures, and failure to thrive are characteristic. The child may have a bulging fontanelle, thinning of the skull, separation of the sutures, engorged scalp veins, an enlarged head circumference, ocular movement abnormalities, sluggish pupillary reaction and decreased response to visual threat, downward orbital displacement, cracked pot sound on skull percussion, optic atrophy, papilledema, spasticity, and increased reflexes. Children with otic hydrocephalus may have fever and purulent ear discharge. After the sutures are closed, affected children present with symptoms of raised intracranial tension. If hydrocephalus is long-standing and untreated, there may be associated endocrine dysfunction with short stature, diabetes insipidus, and menstrual irregularities. In adults, acute hydrocephalus presents with headaches, vomiting, blurred vision, diplopia, seizures, mutism, mental status changes, gait disturbance, and hyperreflexia along with focal signs from focal lesions. The triad of dementia, gait apraxia, and urinary incontinence characterize normal pressure hydrocephalus (NPH).

ETIOLOGY/EPIDEMIOLOGY: Hydrocephalus results from ventricular obstruction, overproduction or defective absorption of CSF, and *ex vacuo* dilatation of the ventricles.

The various types include communicating (nonobstructive), noncommunicating (obstructive), NPH, and *ex vacuo* hydrocephalus. Normal pressure hydrocephalus is a disorder of the elderly, whereas the other types occur in children and adults.

DIAGNOSIS: Hydrocephalus can be diagnosed by the following investigations. Fundoscopic examination may show papilledema in acute hydrocephalus. In chronic hydrocephalus, it may manifest as either papilledema or optic atrophy. If NPH is suspected, a therapeutic high-volume lumbar tap may be performed after baseline gait evaluation and neuropsychological testing. Chronic meningitis may be ruled out in a subacute presentation. CT or MRI of the brain may show hydrocephalus. Venous ophthalmodynamometry may be used in the differential diagnosis of malfunction of ventricular shunts, gastrointestinal disorders, hypertensive hydrocephalus, and brain atrophy in children. Transcranial Doppler ultrasonography is a noninvasive method of evaluating hydrocephalus.

TREATMENT

Standard Therapies: Emergent neurosurgical consultation is warranted. If elevated intracranial pressure and impending herniation secondary to obstruction of flow of CSF from edema are present, hyperventilation, mannitol, and dexamethasone may be used to lower the edema in the interim. Shunting can be of the following types: ventriculostomy, ventriculocisternal, ventriculoperitoneal, ventriculopleural, and ventriculoatrial. Permanent shunts are not necessary if the hydrocephalus is treated therapeutically.

REFERENCES

Davson H, Welch K, Segal MB. *Physiology and pathophysiology of the cerebrospinal fluid.* New York: Churchill Livingstone, 1987.

Fishman RA. *Cerebrospinal fluid in diseases of the nervous system,* 2nd ed. Philadelphia: WB Saunders, 1992.

Hamid RA. Pediatric neuroanesthesia, hydrocephalus. *Anesthesiol Clin North Am* 2001;19:207–218.

Malm J. Three-year survival and functional outcome of patients with idiopathic adult hydrocephalus syndrome. *Neurology* 2000;55:576–578.

Van Hove JL. Acute hydrocephalus in nonketotic hyperglycinemia. *Neurology* 2000;54:754–756.

RESOURCES

190, 303, 368

35 Hyperekplexia

Maria T. Acosta, MD,
William M. McClintock, MD,
and Phillip L. Pearl, MD

DEFINITION: Hyperekplexia is characterized by an excessive startle response elicited by auditory, visual, or tactile stimulation that would fail to produce a response in unaffected individuals.

SYNONYMS: Startle disease; Stiff baby syndrome; Congenital stiff man syndrome.

DIFFERENTIAL DIAGNOSIS: Startle epilepsy; Cryptogenic focal epilepsy with exclusively reflex seizures; Epilepsy; Cerebral palsy; Jumping Frenchmen of Maine; Myriachit; Latah.

SYMPTOMS AND SIGNS: The disorder occurs in two forms: a major form and a minor form. The major form is characterized by hypertonia that disappears spontaneously by the end of the first year of life, excessive startle response, falling attacks without unconsciousness, episodic generalized shaking, generalized hyperreflexia, and unsteady gait. The minor form is characterized by an isolated, inconstant excessive startle response. Hyperekplexia usually presents during the neonatal period as stiff baby syndrome. The onset of stiffness becomes evident a few hours after birth, and the shoulder girdle muscles are hypertonic. The child may have difficulty swallowing and frequent choking. The hypertonia usually disappears during sleep, although repetitive and violent movements may be seen during the hypnagogic stage. The neonatal form improves spontaneously during the first year of life, although developmental delay in the gross motor sphere may be present. Umbilical and inguinal hernias are frequently associated.

ETIOLOGY/EPIDEMIOLOGY: Most cases are dominantly inherited, but recessive inheritance has been observed. The major form of hyperekplexia is typically familial. Linkage analyses demonstrate genetic homogeneity in typical cases linked to DNA markers in the long arm of chromosome 5q. Familial cases demonstrate point mutations in the alpha-1 subunit of the inhibitory glycine receptor. Glycine is an important inhibitory neurotransmitter in the brainstem and spinal cord, and binds to a ligand-gated channel conducting chloride ions. The pri-

mary physiologic abnormality seems to be related to the reticular activating neurons in the brainstem. One possibility is that mutations causing hyperekplexia might enable the glycine receptor to respond to GABA as an agonist, leading ultimately to paradoxic excitation.

DIAGNOSIS: Clinical identification of familial carriers has been suggested by the presence of an exaggerated non-habituating startle response to the glabellar tap in the absence of other neurologic signs. A careful family history is important. The attacks are different from epileptic seizures because ictal electroencephalography does not show paroxysmal activity. Results of neuroimaging are normal. Spectroscopic imaging in four patients showed a reduction of the relative resonance intensity of N-acetylaspartate in frontal, central, and parietal areas.

TREATMENT

Standard Therapies: Hyperekplexia responds to drugs that can act as GABA agonists, such as clonazepam, phenobarbital, sodium valproate, and perhaps vigabatrin. Clonazepam, a GABA-A receptor agonist, is the usual treatment of choice, but may not completely suppress symptoms. Clobazam has also been effective. The attacks can be prevented by sudden flexion of the head and limbs. Genetic counseling is necessary for affected families, because early identification is important to prevent neonatal complications.

REFERENCES

Bernasconi A, Cendes F, Shoubridge EA, et al. Spectroscopic imaging of frontal neuronal dysfunction in hyperekplexia. *Brain* 1998;21:1507–1512.

Cokar O, Gelisse P, Livet MO, et al. Startle response: epileptic or nonepileptic? The case for "flash" SMA reflex seizures. *Epilepsia Disord* 2001;3:7–11.

Gherpelli JLD, Nogueira AR, Troster EJ, et al. Hyperekplexia, a cause of neonatal apnea: a case report. *Brain Dev* 1995; 17:114–116.

Stevens H. Jumping Frenchmen of Maine (myriachit). *Trans Am Neurol Assoc* 1964;89:65–67.

Surtees R. Inborn error of neurotransmitter receptors. *J Inherit Metab Dis* 1999;22:374–380.

RESOURCE

368

36 Infantile Spasms

Susan Koh, MD

DEFINITION: Infantile spasms (IS) are age-dependent myoclonic seizures consisting of brief head nods or truncal flexion or extension occurring in clusters.

SYNONYMS: West syndrome; Saalam seizures; Infantile myoclonic seizures.

DIFFERENTIAL DIAGNOSIS: Myoclonic seizures; Tonic seizures; Benign myoclonus of infancy; Neonatal sleep myoclonus.

SIGNS AND SYMPTOMS: Infantile spasms look like clusters of brief truncal flexion or extension occurring on awakening or falling asleep. Jerks of the trunk, arms, legs, or head are faster than tonic seizures and slower than myoclonic seizures (approximately 1–2 seconds). Spasms can be asymmetric with crying between each spasm and can be associated with eye movements/nystagmus or autonomic features. The spasms may be either extensor type (with back arching and arms and legs extended), flexion (trunk flexion with flexion of the arms and legs), or mixed type (trunk flexion and arms and legs extended). Infantile spasms are usually associated with developmental delay. Often, if the IS ends, development stops declining, and therefore the spasms should be treated as soon as possible. Children may continue to have spasms into adolescence and adulthood called juvenile or tonic spasms.

ETIOLOGY/EPIDEMIOLOGY: Infantile spasms occur in children younger than 2 years, with a peak age of onset at 4–7 months. Incidence has been 0.24–0.60 per 1,000 live births, and there is no gender preference. Causes include tuberous sclerosis, Aicardi syndrome, hypoxic ischemic encephalopathy, aminoacidopathies, pyridoxine dependency, nonketotic hyperglycinemia, mitochondrial disease, meningoencephalitis, trauma, strokes, congenital infection (TORCH), Down syndrome, incontinentia pigmenti, Sturge-Weber syndrome, and congenital malformations.

DIAGNOSIS: Evaluation includes a physical examination, especially for skin lesions, and an eye examination. Other important tests include electroencephalography (EEG), MRI, and metabolic workup, including serum amino acids, urine organic acids, serum ammonia, liver function tests, serum pyruvate, serum and cerebrospinal fluid (CSF) lactate, CSF glycine, and a pyridoxine test. EEG usually shows a characteristic background pattern called hypsarrhythmia, with high amplitude; asynchronous, disorganized, slow waves; and multifocal independent spike discharges. Ictal EEG may show an electrodecremental response, slow waves, or paroxysmal fast activity.

TREATMENT

Standard Therapies: ACTH, a type of intramuscular steroid, is most often used. Oral steroids at 2 mg/kg/day are less efficacious with more recurrences. Side effects for ACTH include increased appetite, cushingoid appearance, growth retardation, acne, irritability, infections and immunosuppression, hypertension, osteoporosis, hypokalemic alkalosis, cardiac hypertrophy, and hyperglycemia. Patients must be monitored weekly for blood pressure, glucose, and electrolytes. If side effects occur, ACTH can be reduced, changed to methylprednisolone, or antihypertensive medications and salt-restricted diets can be added. Other medications that have been used include high-dose vitamin B6/pyridoxine, benzodiazepines, and valproic acid, which have not been as effective as ACTH. Topiramate, lamotrigine, zonisamide, and tiagabine have also been suggested as possible treatments. Epilepsy surgery is a possibility if all anticonvulsant therapy has failed and an epileptogenic origin can be found through videotelemetry, positron emission tomographic scans, ictal SPECT, and MRI scans.

Investigational Therapies: Experimental drugs include vigabatrin, which is excellent for children who have tuberous sclerosis and infantile spasms.

REFERENCES

Cossette P, Rivello JJ, Carmant L. ACTH versus vigabatrin therapy in infantile spasms: a retrospective study. *Neurology* 1999;52: 1691–1694.

Dulac O, Plouin P, Jambaque I. Predicting favorable outcome in idiopathic West syndrome. *Epilepsia* 1993;34:747–756.

Holmes GL, Vigevano F. Infantile spasms. In: Engel J, Pedley TA, eds. *Epilepsy: a comprehensive textbook.* Philadelphia: Lippincott-Raven, 1997:627–642.

Snead OC III, Benton JW, Myers GL. ACTH and prednisone in childhood seizure disorders. *Neurology* 1983;33:966–970.

Wong M, Trevathan E. Infantile spasms. *Pediatr Neurol* 2001;24: 89–98.

RESOURCES

145, 219, 368, 491

37   Joubert Syndrome

Maria T. Acosta, MD, and Phillip L. Pearl, MD

DEFINITION: Joubert syndrome is an autosomal-recessive form of agenesis of the cerebellar vermis. Clinical manifestations include hypotonia, developmental delay, mental retardation, ataxia, abnormal respiratory patterns, abnormal eye movements, and retinal dystrophy.

SYNONYMS: Joubert-Boltshauser syndrome; Cerebellar vermis agenesis; CPD IV; Cerebello-parenchymal disorder IV.

DIFFERENTIAL DIAGNOSIS: Rett syndrome; Mohr syndrome; Dandy-Walker malformation; COACH syndrome; Ritscher-Schinzel syndrome; 3C (cranio-cerebello-cardiac) syndrome; CHARGE association; Occipital encephalocele; Arima syndrome; Senior-Loken syndrome; Cerebellar vermian hypoplasia; Oligophrenia; Congenital ataxia; Coloboma; Hepatic fibrosis syndrome; Juvenile nephrophthisis due to *NPH1* mutations.

SYMPTOMS AND SIGNS: Affected children present with nonspecific features such as hypotonia, ataxia, and developmental delay. Careful examination of the face shows a characteristic appearance: large head, prominent forehead, high rounded eyebrows, epicanthal folds, ptosis (occasionally), upturned nose with evident nostrils, open mouth, tongue protrusion and rhythmic tongue motions, and, occasionally, low-set and tilted ears. Oculomotor alterations are common and include decreased smooth pursuit and vestibuloocular reflex cancellation, partial to complete oculomotor apraxia both in the horizontal and vertical directions, and hypometric saccades if oculomotor apraxia is not complete. A classification into two groups has been proposed on the basis of the presence or absence of retinal dystrophy. The group with retinal dystrophy has a high prevalence of multicystic renal disease. Respiratory alterations are prominent. In the neonatal period, most children have hyperpnea intermixed with central apnea. Congenital hepatic fibrosis has also been reported, usually in association with congenital medullary cystic renal disease. The renal cysts are multiple, small, and cortical, and affected kidneys also have interstitial chronic inflammation and fibrosis. Polydactyly and soft tissue tumors of the tongue occur less frequently.

ETIOLOGY/EPIDEMIOLOGY: The biochemical and genetic basis of Joubert syndrome is unknown, and a specific chromosomal locus for this disorder has not been identified. Recent studies suggest that Joubert syndrome may result from a specific gene defect. *PAX* (*PAX2, PAX5, PAX8*) and *EN* family genes contribute to midhindbrain formation and cerebellar development. Other investigations have identified the nephrophthisis (*NPH*) gene complex as potentially causing Joubert syndrome. In the autosomal-recessive form (type A), homozygous deletions have been described as causative in more than 80% of patients. In type B Joubert syndrome, different combinations of the extrarenal symptoms with the *NPH* gene occur. Joubert syndrome with retinal dystrophy and renal cysts may represent a variant of the carbohydrate-deficient glycoprotein syndrome.

DIAGNOSIS: The diagnosis is established by clinical and neuroimaging findings. The typical presentation includes developmental delay, abnormal eye movements, and episodes of abnormal breathing. Neuroimaging on axial sections demonstrates the "molar tooth sign"—deep posterior interpeduncular fossa, thick and elongated superior cerebellar peduncles, and hypoplastic or aplastic superior cerebellar vermis.

TREATMENT
Standard Therapies: There is no specific treatment. Symptomatic therapy and genetic counseling are recommended.

REFERENCES
Chance PF, Cavalier L, Satran D, et al. Clinical nosologic and genetic aspects of Joubert and related syndromes. *J Child Neurol* 1999;14:660–666.

Fennell EB, Gitten JC, Dede DE, et al. Cognition, behavior, and development in Joubert syndrome. *J Child Neurol* 1999;14:592–596.

Maria BL, Boltshauser E, Palmer SC, et al. Clinical features and revised diagnostic criteria in Joubert syndrome. *J Child Neurol* 1999;14:583–590.

van Beek EJR, Majoie CBLM. Case 25: Joubert syndrome. *Radiology* 2000;216:379–382.

Yachnis AT, Rorke LB. Neuropathology of Joubert syndrome. *J Child Neurol* 1999;14:655–659.

RESOURCES
136, 219, 368

38 | Kernicterus

Sanjiv Sahoo, MD,
and Phillip L. Pearl, MD

DEFINITION: Kernicterus (yellow nuclei) is a condition caused by bilirubin toxicity to the basal ganglia and various brainstem nuclei in neonates.

SYNONYMS: Bilirubin encephalopathy; Neonatal hyperbilirubinemia.

DIFFERENTIAL DIAGNOSIS: Icterus neonatorum or neonatal jaundice secondary to hemolytic diseases; Intrauterine infections; Concealed hemorrhage; Hypothyroidism; Gilbert syndrome; Crigler-Najjar syndrome; Breast milk jaundice.

SYMPTOMS AND SIGNS: No neurologic symptoms are obvious in 15% of affected infants. Kernicterus can occur in an acute or chronic form. Jaundice usually begins in the first 24 hours after birth. In the acute form, in phase I (first 1–2 days), the neonate has a poor suck, shrill cry, stupor, hypotonia, and seizures. In phase II (middle of first week), the neonate presents with opisthotonous, retrocollis, hypertonia of extensor muscles, and fever. In phase III (after the first week), the neonate presents with hypertonia. In the chronic form, the affected infant presents in the first year with delayed motor skills, hypertonia, obligatory tonic neck reflexes, and active deep tendon reflexes. After the first year, movement disorders (choreoathetosis, ballismus, and tremor), paralysis of upward gaze, and sensorineural hearing loss are prominent features. Lower IQ, especially in males, is noted. The mortality rate approaches 4% in infants.

ETIOLOGY/EPIDEMIOLOGY: In neonates unconjugated bilirubin is not readily excreted, and the ability to conjugate bilirubin is limited. These factors lead to physiologic jaundice starting on day 2. When an aggravating factor is present, hyperbilirubinemia progresses to levels over 17 mg/dL, which are no longer considered physiologic. Bilirubin has a neurotoxic effect and can inhibit mitochondrial enzymes, interfere with DNA synthesis, induce DNA strand breakage, inhibit protein synthesis and phosphorylation, inhibit the uptake of tyrosine, and interfere with the function of NMDA receptor ion channels. It also has an affinity for membrane phospholipids, and inhibits ion exchange, leading to neuronal swelling, which occurs in bilirubin encephalopathy.

DIAGNOSIS: The diagnosis is based on clinical and laboratory evaluation of a neonate who presents with jaundice. The current American Academy of Pediatrics (AAP) guidelines recommend that any infant who is jaundiced before 24 hours should undergo laboratory testing (including serum or transcutaneous bilirubin levels) to assess the level of hyperbilirubinemia and be followed up in 2–3 days. Testing should be performed to rule out sepsis, hemolytic diseases, metabolic/genetic diseases, and for assessment of hypoxemia, acidosis, and hypoalbuminemia. Measurement of end-tidal carbon monoxide in exhaled air is used as an index of bilirubin production. MRI may show increased T2-weighted signal intensity in the globus pallidus, correlating with the level of bilirubin deposited in the basal ganglia.

TREATMENT
Standard Therapies: Phototherapy is the standard treatment. It is usually discontinued once the bilirubin levels decrease by 4–5 mg/dL. Exchange transfusion is used successfully to rapidly eliminate circulating bilirubin as well as antibodies against targeted erythrocytes. Exchange transfusion is an invasive procedure with potential complications, and is reserved for patients in whom intensive phototherapy has failed. Phenobarbital has been used to induce hepatic enzymes in neonates and has also been given to at-risk mothers in the last week of pregnancy with beneficial effects. Once bilirubin has accumulated, raising brain pH by alkalinization may be attempted either by bicarbonate infusion or by ventilator strategies to lower the partial pressure of CO_2 and thus raise blood pH.

REFERENCES
Cook RW. New approach to prevention of kernicterus. *Lancet* 1999;353:1814–1815.

Dennery PA, Seidman DS, Stevenson DK. Neonatal hyperbilirubinemia. *N Engl J Med* 2001;344:581–590.

Hansen TW, Tommarello S. Effect of phenobarbital on bilirubin metabolism in rat brain. *Biol Neonate* 1998;73:106–111.

Maisels JM. Neonatal jaundice and kernicterus. *Pediatrics* 2001; 108:763–765.

RESOURCES
39, 365, 388

39   Kleine-Levin Syndrome

Daniel G. Glaze, MD

DEFINITION: Kleine-Levin syndrome (KLS) is a sleep disorder characterized by episodes of hypersomnia lasting up to several weeks that typically occur weeks or months apart with normal functioning between episodes. The episodes are associated with compulsive hyperphagia and behavioral/psychiatric disturbances. Between attacks, affected individuals have no symptoms.

SYNONYMS: Periodic hypersomnia; Recurrent hypersomnia.

DIFFERENTIAL DIAGNOSIS: Obstructive sleep apnea syndrome; Narcolepsy; Periodic limb movement disorder; Menstrual-associated sleep disorders; Seizures; Atypical depression.

SYMPTOMS AND SIGNS: Episodes typically begin in early adolescence, but onset may occur in adulthood. Episodes generally last several days to several weeks, and recur 2–12 times a year. Patients may sleep as long as 18–20 hours of the 24-hour day during somnolent episodes. They wake to eat and void; urinary incontinence does not occur. Patients may demonstrate binge eating and weight gains of 2–5 kg during an episode. The monosymptomatic type (episodic hypersomnia only) may be associated with weight loss. Episodes of hypersomnia may be precipitated by acute febrile illnesses, sleep deprivation, alcohol use, and severe somatic stress. During an episode patients may experience behavior changes that include disorientation, forgetfulness, depression, depersonalization, and hallucinations. Irritability, aggression, and impulsive behaviors can also occur. Patients may show disinhibited behaviors or depression during an episode. Transient dysphoria, insomnia, elation, restlessness, or sexual hyperactivity has been reported to follow the period of somnolence. Social, school, and occupational impairment during attacks is severe. Between hypersomnia episodes, patients appear to have no increased occurrence of medical or psychiatric problems in comparison with the general population, and appear to function and sleep normally.

ETIOLOGY/EPIDEMIOLOGY: The constellation of symptoms suggests a disorder of hypothalamic and limbic function. Although several single case studies report neuroendocrine abnormalities, a study of 5 patients failed to find evidence of hypothalamic, endocrine, or circadian dysfunction during symptomatic periods. The HLA haplotype DR1, DQ1 has been reported in several cases of KLS. Prevalence is unknown. The disorder is more frequently described in males, but the true sex ratio is unknown. Rarely, KLS can reoccur in families.

DIAGNOSIS: The diagnosis is based on the clinical symptoms. Delay in diagnosis occurs frequently. The diagnosis should be suspected in individuals with a complaint of excessive sleepiness and episodes of somnolence lasting for at least 18 hours a day, recurring at least once or twice a year, and lasting a minimum of 3 days. There should be no associated medical or mental disorder such as epilepsy or depression, or other sleep disorders such as narcolepsy, sleep apnea syndrome, or periodic limb movement disorder. If the disorder is solely one of recurrent episodes of hypersomnia, it is diagnosed as hypersomnia monosymptomatic type. If it is associated with voracious eating or hypersexuality, it is diagnosed as the KLS type of hypersomnia.

TREATMENT
Standard Therapies: Therapy is supportive with consideration to protect the individual from injury during an episode and to the psychosocial, educational, and job-related impact of KLS. There are no curative therapies. Anecdoctal reports suggest that amantadine, sodium valproate, carbamazepine, and melatonin may have benefit. Patients may continue to have recurrent episodes of hypersomnia despite treatment with these agents. Stimulants to lessen the severity of an attack have been used with minimal effect.

REFERENCES
American Sleep Disorders Association. *The international classification of sleep disorders,* revised ed. Rochester, MN: Davies, 1997:43–46.

Kelser A, Gadoth N, Vainstein G, et al. Klein Levin syndrome (KLS) in young females. *Sleep* 2000;23:563–567.

Malhotra S, Das MK, Gupta N, Muralidharan R. A clinical study of Kleine-Levin syndrome with evidence for hypothalamic-pituitary axis dysfunction. *Biol Psychiatry* 1997;42:299–301.

Mayer G, Leonhard E, Krieg J, et al. Endocrinological and polysomnographic findings in Kleine-Levin syndrome: no evidence for hypothalamic and circadian dysfunction. *Sleep* 1998;21:278–284.

Papacostas SS, Hadjivasihs V. The Kleine-Levin syndrome. Report of a case and review of the literature. *Eur Psychiatry* 2000;15:231–235.

RESOURCES
330, 367, 368

40   Kluver-Bucy Syndrome

L. Anne Hayman, MD,
and Emese Nagy, MD, PhD

DEFINITION: Kluver-Bucy syndrome is usually a result of damage in both anterior temporal lobes, including the deep gray matter of the amygdala. Symptoms include three or more of the following: visual agnosia, hypermetamorphosis (increased exploration), hyperorality with dietary changes, placidity, and increased sexual behavior.

DIFFERENTIAL DIAGNOSIS: Temporolimbic disorders; Schizophrenia; Affective disorders.

SYMPTOMS AND SIGNS: Because of individual variations in the degree of anatomic structural damage and patients' ability to compensate, a broad spectrum of behavioral abnormalities exists. There are six core symptom groups for both children and adults: (a) visual agnosia (sometimes auditory agnosia and very rarely tactile agnosia occur); (b) emotional disturbances (placidity, loss of fear/anxiety or diminished aggression, apathy, blunted affection, and petlike compliance); (c) hypermetamorphosis (a strong tendency to attend to and touch visual stimuli); (d) hyperorality (patients tend to place objects to their mouth; some have even died as a result); (e) dietary change (usually weight gain, which can lead to bulimia); and (f) indiscriminate hypersexuality.

ETIOLOGY/EPIDEMIOLOGY: Bilateral damage to the temporal lobes or amygdala occurs in a variety of clinical settings. Surgical irradiation and chemotherapeutic injuries have been reported. Herpes simplex encephalitis is a relatively common cause. Bilateral damage to the temporal lobes or amygdala has also been described in association with Alzheimer disease, Pick disease, adrenoleukodystrophy, toxoplasmosis and hypoglycemia, Huntington disease, vascular lesions, anoxia, subarachnoid hemorrhage, transtentorial herniation, systemic lupus erythemathosus, and neuroleptic medication. It has been reported in children after traumatic brain injury, tubercular meningitis, heat stroke, and in association with shigellosis. Kluver-Bucy syndrome can also occur after unilateral anterior left temporal lobectomy and bilateral thalamic infarctions.

DIAGNOSIS: All six symptoms are rarely present in a single case, and only three are needed to make the diagnosis. Brain imaging can help by showing characteristic sites of damage.

TREATMENT
Standard Therapies: Kluver-Bucy syndrome occurs transiently in patients with traumatic brain injury, and its presence is correlated with a better global outcome. Behavioral therapy may be beneficial. Dietary restrictions are necessary in patients with appropriate symptoms. Carbamazepine may help reduce rage attacks. Propranolol may reduce restlessness, promote sleep, and reduce verbal and physical aggression. Leuprolide may control hypersexuality and sexual aggression. Selective serotonergic reuptake inhibitors (fluoxetine, sertraline) may help control aggression, aggressive impulses, hyperorality, and hypersexuality.

REFERENCES
Clarke DJ, Brown NS. Kluver-Bucy syndrome and psychiatric illness. *Br J Psychiatry* 1990;157:439–441.
Hoshmand H, Sepdbam T, Vries JK. Kluver-Bucy syndrome: successful treatment with carbamazepine. *JAMA* 1974;229:1782.
Ott BR. Leuprolide treatment of sexual aggression in a patient with dementia and the Kluver-Bucy syndrome. *Clin Neuropharmacol* 1995;18:443–447.
Slaughter J, Bobo W, Childers MK. Selective serotonin reuptake inhibitor treatment of post-traumatic Kluver-Bucy syndrome. *Brain Injury* 1999;13:59–62.
Stewart JT. Carbamazepine treatment of a patient with Kluver-Bucy syndrome. *J Clin Psychiatry* 1985;46:496–497.
Varga E, Haher EJ, Simpson GM. Neuroleptic induced Kluver-Bucy syndrome. *Biol Psychiatry* 1975;10:65–68.

RESOURCES
22, 368, 370

41   Korsakoff Syndrome

Sanjiv Sahoo, MD,
and Phillip L. Pearl, MD

DEFINITION: Korsakoff syndrome is disproportionate impairment in memory relative to other aspects of cognitive function. Occasionally, patients have confabulations. When associated with Wernicke syndrome (triad of confusion, ataxia, and ophthalmoplegia), it is known as Wernicke-Korsakoff syndrome (WKS).

SYNONYM: Psychosis polyneurotica.

DIFFERENTIAL DIAGNOSIS: Alcoholic pellagra encephalopathy; Alcoholic psychosis; Delirium tremens; Alcoholic dementia; Wernicke encephalopathy; Transient global amnesia; Herpes encephalitis; Temporal lobe infarctions; Bilateral posterior cerebral artery infarctions; Ruptured anterior communicating artery aneurysm; Head trauma; Third ventricle or thalamic tumor; Multiple sclerosis; Temporal lobe epilepsy; Alzheimer disease.

SYMPTOMS AND SIGNS: Korsakoff syndrome occurs in the setting of chronic alcoholism, malnourishment, or chronic illness such as AIDS, dialysis, hyperemesis gravidarum, gastroplasty, or gastric carcinoma. Patients may present with Wernicke triad of ataxia, confusion, and ophthalmoplegia or nystagmus, and a prodromal agitation, and then develop profound amnesia associated with confabulation. Peripheral neuropathy is usually present. The disease may have an acute onset of less than 8 weeks, or a more insidious onset. The amnesia is disproportionate to cognitive impairment. Typically, the working/immediate memory and the procedural memory are intact along with the less affected semantic memory. The short-term/explicit memory is severely affected, with greater defects in the consolidation than the encoding phase. This results in poor anterograde memory. Retrograde memory is also affected over several decades of the patient's past. The often quoted statement that confabulation is a patient's compensatory device to diminish embarrassment caused by a memory gap is unproven.

ETIOLOGY/EPIDEMIOLOGY: The prevalence of WKS in the United States is 1%–2%. The syndrome occurs because of a deficiency of dietary thiamine. Alcohol further reduces thiamine absorption, diminishes hepatic stores, and inhibits the activity of the enzyme required to convert thiamine to its active form. Anterograde amnesia correlates with third ventricle volume, suggesting that atrophic lesions in the nuclei in the midline of the thalamus may be responsible.

DIAGNOSIS: Studies, including routine laboratory screens, liver function tests, and ammonia level, are recommended to rule out entities with potentially similar presentations. Thiamine and erythrocyte transketolase activity may be reduced. Serum and cerebral spinal fluid pyruvate may be mildly elevated. CT and MRI are recommended to rule out tumors, infarcts, and hemorrhages, and in Korsakoff syndrome may identify cortical atrophy with widening of the interhemispheric fissure, third ventricle, and lateral ventricles. Shrunken mammillary bodies may be noted on MRI. Rarely, hypodensity of the thalamus may be seen on CT. Single-photon emission CT (SPECT) has shown reduced tracer uptake throughout the cortex, except the posterior temporal cortex. Fluorodeoxyglucose positron emission tomography shows bilateral reduction in metabolism in interconnected limbic-hippocampal regions, including the thalamic nuclei, as well as the frontal basal cortex. Neuropsychologic testing may also help in diagnosis.

TREATMENT

Standard Therapies: Parenteral thiamine 50–100 mg intravenously (divided 2–3 times daily) should be given for several days, because intestinal absorption is impaired in alcoholics. Hypomagnesemia can compromise the treatment response, and replacement therapy should be considered. Maintenance treatment with oral thiamine 50–100 mg 3 or 4 times daily for several months should be instituted. An over-the-counter food supplement, thiamine propyl disulphide, although not FDA-approved, is also available. A balanced diet should be resumed. Abstinence from alcohol and institution of psychotherapy are important.

REFERENCES

Cook CC. Prevention and treatment of Wernicke-Korsakoff syndrome. *Alcohol Alcohol* 2000;35(suppl 1):19–20.

Cook CC, Hallwood PM, Thomson AD. B vitamin deficiency and neuropsychiatric syndromes in alcohol misuse. *Alcohol Alcohol* 1998;33:317–336.

Kopelman MD. The Korsakoff syndrome. *Br J Psychiatry* 1995; 166:154–173.

Zubaran C, Fernandes JG, Rodnight R. Wernicke-Korsakoff syndrome. *Postgrad Med J* 1997;73:27–31.

RESOURCES

154, 354

42   Kuf Disease

Paul Richard Dyken, MD

DEFINITION: The adult form of neuronal ceroid-lipofuscinosis (NCL), Kuf disease, is characterized by distention of the cytoplasm of neurons with accumulation of lipoprotein pigments. Kuf disease is distinguished by (a) adult onset, (b) autosomal-recessive or sporadic inheritance, (c) accumulation of ceroid-lipofuscin within neurons, and (d) a characteristic clinical picture consisting of progressive motor symptoms (either cerebellar, extrapyramidal, or pyramidal), seizures, and dementia.

SYNONYMS: Adult-onset NCL; Late-onset amaurotic familial idiocy; CLN-4; NCL-4; Spatform der amauroischen idiote.

DIFFERENTIAL DIAGNOSIS: Boehme disease; Batten disease; Gaucher disease; Jansky-Bielschowsky disease; Niemann-Pick disease.

SYMPTOMS AND SIGNS: The clinical symptoms of Kuf disease suggest two types. The largest group consists of patients who have epileptic seizures along with involuntary movement and myoclonia. The smaller group consists of patients with either a motor problem or pure dementia. Because patients present such clinical diversity without distinct pathology, Kuf disease may not represent a single disease sui generis.

ETIOLOGY/EPIDEMIOLOGY: The etiology has not been determined. The pathogenesis, however, is most probably related to the accumulation of ceroid-lipofuscin within selective neurons and supporting elements of the central nervous system. The seizures are probably reflec- tions of neuronal membrane instability that allow a progressively worsening hyperexcitability and a propensity toward the "electrical discharge" of epilepsy. Although there is some suggestion of autosomal-recessive inheritance, it is possible the disease is simply sporadic without genetic basis. Average age of onset is approximately 30 years, and duration of illness is 15–20 years.

DIAGNOSIS: Commonly, mild but steadily progressive dementia occurs, usually associated with adult-onset seizures that ultimately become refractive. Visual or retinal abnormalities are rare if they occur at all. Family history is usually negative. Occasionally, patients die undiagnosed, and the condition is discovered during postmortem examination.

TREATMENT
Standard Therapies: No curative therapies are known. Palliative therapies depend on the symptoms expressed.

REFERENCES
Boehme DH, Cottrell JC, Leonberg SC, et al. A dominant form of neuronal ceroid-lipofuscinosis. *Brain* 1971;94:745–756.
Dyken PR. Reconsideration of the classification of the neuronal ceroid-lipofuscinoses. *Am J Med Genet* 1988;5(suppl):69–84.
Dyken PR. The neuronal ceroid-lipofuscinoses. In: Berg BO, ed. *Principles of child neurology.* New York: McGraw-Hill, 1996: 1495–1512.
Wisniewski KE. Pheno/genotypic correlations of neuronal ceroid lipofuscinoses. *Neurology* 2001;57:576–581.

RESOURCES
94, 368, 462

43   Landau-Kleffner Syndrome

John F. Mantovani, MD

DEFINITION: Landau-Kleffner syndrome (LKS) is a neurologic disorder of childhood characterized by the loss of comprehension and expression of verbal language in association with severely abnormal electroencephalographic (EEG) findings.

SYNONYMS: Acquired epileptiform aphasia; Acquired aphasia with convulsive disorder.

DIFFERENTIAL DIAGNOSIS: Acquired deafness; Structural lesions of the posterior frontal and/or superior temporal lobes such as tumor, abscess, or vascular malformation; Regressive form of autism; Childhood disintegrative disorder; Neurodegenerative disorders affecting cortical/gray matter function; Rett syndrome.

SYMPTOMS AND SIGNS: The disorder typically begins between the ages of 4 and 7 years. Affected children often appear to have acquired deafness since they fail to respond to verbal language and in some cases to nonverbal sounds. A significant minority of children develop serious behavioral dysfunction, including hyperactivity, temper outbursts, or withdrawn behaviors, but rarely the severe social impairments seen in autism.

ETIOLOGY/EPIDEMIOLOGY: Although it is generally believed that the epileptiform discharge disrupts the brain's auditory and linguistic processing connections and leads to the aphasia, the cause of the epileptiform activity itself is unknown. Many possible causes have been suggested, including genetic tendencies, autoimmune disorders, and other inflammatory processes. The syndrome occurs in both sexes with a male preponderance and has occurred in siblings on rare occasion.

DIAGNOSIS: In addition to linguistic regression, the diagnosis requires the presence of severely epileptiform activity on EEG, particularly during sleep. Approximately 70% of affected children also have obvious seizures, most often simple or complex partial seizures and/or atypical absence in type. In addition to EEG, a newer technique, magnetoencephalography (MEG), is being used in some centers. Brain imaging with MRI is recommended to exclude structural lesions. Additional testing includes behavioral and/or brainstem evoked audiometry and standardized psychometric and speech/language testing.

TREATMENT
Standard Therapies: The standard therapeutic approach begins with antiepileptic drugs, particularly "spike-suppressing" medications such as divalproex, ethosuximide, and benzodiazepines. Other antiepileptic drugs that may be beneficial are lamotrigine and felbamate.

Investigational Therapies: When antiepileptic drugs are ineffective, other approaches include the ketogenic diet or immunosuppression with intravenous or oral corticosteroids. Treatment with intravenous immunoglobulin and calcium-channel blocking drugs may also be beneficial. A neurosurgical procedure, multiple subpial transection (MST), is being used in several centers for selected children who fail to improve linguistically within 2 years and those who develop steroid dependency or toxicity.

REFERENCES
DaSilva EA, Chugani D, Muzik O, et al. Landau-Kleffner syndrome: metabolic abnormalities in temporal lobe are a common feature. *J Child Neurol* 1997;12:489–495.
Grete CL, VanSlyke P, Hoeppner JAB. Language outcome following multiple subpial transactions for Landau-Kleffner syndrome. *Brain* 1999;122:561–566.
Lewine JD, Andrews R, Chez M, et al. Magnetoencephalopgraphic patterns of epileptiform activity in children with regressive autistic spectrum disorders. *Pediatrics* 1999;104:405–418.
Mantovani JF. Autistic regression and Landau-Kleffner syndrome: progress or confusion? *Dev Med Child Neurol* 2000;42:349–353.
Robinson RO, Baird G, Robinson G, et al. Landau-Kleffner Syndrome: course and correlates with outcome. *Dev Med Child Neurol* 2001;43:243–247.

RESOURCES
145, 284, 368, 370

44   Primary Lateral Sclerosis

*Sanjiv Sahoo, MD,
and Phillip L. Pearl, MD*

DEFINITION: Primary lateral sclerosis (PLS) is a nonhereditary disorder characterized by progressive spinobulbar spasticity, related to the exclusive loss of precentral pyramidal neurons, with secondary pyramidal tract degeneration and preservation of anterior horn motor neurons. It is uncertain if it is an independent disease or a variant of amyotrophic lateral sclerosis (ALS).

SYNONYMS: Spastic spinal paralysis; Upper motor neuron disease.

DIFFERENTIAL DIAGNOSIS: ALS; Cervical and compressive myelopathies; Multiple sclerosis; Spinal cord tumors; Leukodystrophy; Chiari malformations; Lathyrism; Vitamin B_{12} deficiency; Hereditary spastic paraparesis; Neurosyphilis; Lyme disease; HIV; Human T-cell leukemia virus-1.

SYMPTOMS AND SIGNS: Patients with PLS usually present in the fifth decade of life with slowly progressive upper motor neuron signs and symptoms of progressive symmetric weakness, initially involving the lower extremities and then the upper extremities. Other manifestations include spasticity, loss of dexterity, pseudobulbar palsy, dysphagia, dysarthria, hyperreflexia, and presence of Babinski responses. Rarely, detrusor hyperreflexia with neurogenic incontinence may appear late in the course of the disease, unlike ALS, in which bladder involvement is absent. Sensory, autonomic, cognitive, visual, and extrapyramidal involvement is conspicuously absent. Occasionally, patients with apparent PLS develop lower motor neuron signs very late in the course and are then diagnosed with ALS, but they appear to have a slower clinical course than typical ALS. Overall the prognosis for PLS is better than that for ALS, with slower progression, often spanning several decades.

ETIOLOGY/EPIDEMIOLOGY: PLS is a rare nonhereditary disease. There appears to be atrophy of the precentral gyrus with loss of Betz cells in layer 5 of the cortex, gliosis in layers 3 and 5, and demyelination of the corticospinal tracts. The etiology is unknown.

DIAGNOSIS: The diagnosis is one of exclusion. ALS, which combines both upper and lower motor neuron dysfunction, cannot be excluded within 3 years of onset because lower motor neuron features may develop late. Various diagnostic tests may be helpful, including electromyography and nerve conduction studies. MRI and CT of the spine and brain may help to exclude other neurologic diseases. Newer experimental techniques include cortical motor magnetic stimulation showing prolonged evoked latencies, FDG-PET demonstrating decreased glucose uptake in precentral cortex, and magnetic resonance spectroscopy of the motor cortex showing decreased levels of N-acetyl-aspartate (NAA), creatine, and glutamate, normal choline levels, decreased NAA/choline ratio, and elevated choline/creatine ratios. Muscle or nerve biopsy is not always performed, although either can be used to confirm denervation in ALS.

TREATMENT

Standard Therapies: No therapy is curative. Symptomatic treatment consists of antispasticity drugs such as baclofen, used orally or intrathecally, or tizanidine. Phenol injections may be tried. Botulinum-A injection may be helpful in focal spasticity. Physical and occupational therapy are indicated.

REFERENCES

Donaghy M. Classification and clinical features of motor neuron diseases and motor neuropathies in adults. *J Neurol* 1999;246: 331–333.

Le Forestier N. What's new in primary lateral sclerosis? *Rev Neurol* 2000;156:364–371.

Le Forestier N. Primary lateral sclerosis: further clarification. *J Neurol Sci* 2001;185:95–100.

Rowland LP. Primary lateral sclerosis: disease, syndrome, both or neither. *J Neurol Sci* 1999;170:1–4.

Swash M. What is primary lateral sclerosis? *J Neurol Sci* 1999;170: 5–10.

RESOURCES

43, 237, 269, 368

---

45   Lennox-Gastaut Syndrome

*Maria T. Acosta, MD,
and Phillip L. Pearl, MD*

DEFINITION: Lennox-Gastaut syndrome (LGS) is an epileptic syndrome occurring in children ages 1–8 years.

SYNONYM: Childhood epileptic encephalopathy with diffuse slow spike waves.

DIFFERENTIAL DIAGNOSIS: Myoclonic variant of LGS; Myoclonic astatic epilepsy.

SYMPTOMS AND SIGNS: The syndrome begins in childhood and is accompanied by mental retardation, which may become apparent only with time. Multiple seizure types occurring frequently on a daily basis characterize LGS. The most frequently occurring are tonic, tonic-clonic, myoclonic, atypical absences, and "head drops," which represent a form of atonic, tonic, or myoclonic seizures. It is not unusual for some children with LGS to have hundreds of seizures per day, with the highest frequency during drowsiness and inactivity. Tonic seizures, typically associated with "ballet posturing" with the arms extended over the head, are the hallmark. They are typically brief, lasting seconds to a minute. Atypical absences and generalized tonic-clonic seizures are seen in more than half of patients. Myoclonic seizures can occur either in isolation or as a part of atypical absence seizures. Mental retardation is present before onset of the seizures in 20%–60% of patients. Some patients with idiopathic or cryptogenic etiologies have normal IQ and development before seizure onset. Fluctuations in cognitive abilities may occur and to some degree correlate with the intensity of electroencephalographic (EEG) abnormalities. Behavior problems are also common, ranging from hyperactivity to frankly psychotic and autistic behavior.

ETIOLOGY/EPIDEMIOLOGY: The etiology of LGS is divided into primary/cryptogenic and secondary/symptomatic causes, including cerebral dysgenesis, tuberous sclerosis, congenital infections, stroke, perinatal hypoxia, central nervous system infections, and metabolic disorders. The pathophysiology is unknown. The syndrome accounts for 1%–4% of childhood epilepsy, but 10% of cases that begin in the first 5 years. Epidemiologic studies in the Western, industrialized world demonstrate a consistent proportion across populations. The annual incidence is 2 in 100,000 children. Prevalence ranges from 0.1 to 0.28 per 1,000. There is a male predominance. The mean age at epilepsy onset is 26–28 months.

DIAGNOSIS: The triad of diagnostic elements is as follows: (a) multiple seizure types, including tonic, atypical absence, and atonic; (b) EEG with 1.5- to 2.5-Hz slow spike-wave background; and (c) mental retardation.

TREATMENT
Standard Therapies: No treatment provides a satisfactory response for patients with LGS. The response to antiepileptic drugs (AEDs) is variable. Polypharmacy is generally needed to achieve maximal seizure control. Valproate is generally considered the first-line treatment based on its wide spectrum of action. Benzodiazepines are also a first-line AED option, but are associated with side effects of tachyphylaxis. Newer pharmacologic agents such as vigabatrin, topiramate, lamotrigine, felbamate, and zonesamide are also being used. The ketogenic diet produces seizure control comparable with the AEDs. Surgical therapies include corpus callosotomy and the vagus nerve stimulator. Therapeutic options tend to need revisions throughout the life cycle of these patients.

REFERENCES
Espinosa E, Acosta MT, Nunez LC. Refractory epilepsy. In: Espinosa E, Dunoyer C, eds. *Neuropediatrics,* 2nd ed. Bogota, Colombia: Editora Guadalupe, 2001:392–396.
Farrell K. Secondary generalized epilepsy and Lennox-Gastaut syndrome. In: Wyllie E, ed. *The treatment of epilepsy. Principles and practice.* Malvern, PA: Lea & Febiger, 1993:604–611.
Glauser TA, Morita DA. Encephalopathic epilepsy after infancy. In: Pellock JM, Dodson WE, Bourgeois BFD, eds. *Pediatric Epilepsy diagnosis and therapy,* 2nd ed. New York: Demos Medical, 2001:201–208.
Holmes G. Generalized seizures. In: Swaiman KF, Ashwal S, eds. *Pediatric neurology: principles and practice,* 3rd ed. St. Louis: CV Mosby, 1999:642–645.

RESOURCES
145, 235, 236, 368

46   Leukodystrophy (Canavan Disease)

Leonie van Passel-Clark, MD, and Phillip L. Pearl, MD

DEFINITION: Canavan disease (CD) is a neurodegenerative disorder characterized by degeneration of the white matter in the central nervous system during infancy due to a defect in the enzymatic breakdown of N-acetylaspartic acid.

SYNONYMS: Canavan-Van Bogaert-Bertrand disease; Spongy degeneration of the central nervous system; Aspartoacylase (ASPA) deficiency.

DIFFERENTIAL DIAGNOSIS: Alexander disease; G_{M2} gangliosidosis; Other childhood leukodystrophies; Hydrocephalus.

SYMPTOMS AND SIGNS: In the infantile form, the most common one, the onset of symptoms occurs between ages 3 and 6 months. In addition to macrocephaly, it is characterized by rapid psychomotor regression, optic atrophy, feeding difficulties, and hypotonia transforming into spasticity, with death usually occurring in the second decade. Seizures can occur, particularly of the myoclonic type. There is no peripheral nervous system or other organ involvement. The congenital form presents with lethargy, irritability, and dysphagia; marked hypotonia; and Cheyne-Stokes breathing, and survival rarely lasts more than a few weeks. A juvenile form has also been recognized, with onset usually after 5 years or later in the form of progressive cerebellar dysfunction and cognitive decline. This form is characterized by the absence of macrocephaly and sporadic occurrence.

ETIOLOGY/EPIDEMIOLOGY: The disease occurs at a higher frequency in individuals of Ashkenazi Jewish ancestry, the estimated carrier frequency being 1 in 40 persons. The disease is autosomal recessive, with the affected gene for aspartoacylase located on chromosome 17. In Ashkenazi Jewish people, three mutations have been found that are responsible for 99% of cases. In patients not of

Ashkenazi background, there is no clear uniformity in the causative mutations. Due to the reduced ability to hydrolyze N-acetylaspartic acid (NAA), this substance accumulates in the brain, urine, and serum, where it can be measured. N-acetyl-aspartyl-glutamate, a presumed product of NAA, has been shown to disrupt the N-methyl-D-aspartate receptor in brain, and may have pathophysiologic relevance to the lesions in CD.

DIAGNOSIS: The disease should be suspected when the clinical presentation described is encountered, but it is difficult to distinguish from other leukodystrophies; therefore, the following additional tests can be used. Abnormal amounts of NAA can be found in urine, blood, and cerebrospinal fluid. Deficiency of aspartoacylase can be shown in cultured skin fibroblasts; less than 40% of normal is diagnostic. MRI will show low signal intensity on T1-weighting and high signal intensity on T2-weighting, indicative of markedly increased water content. Prenatal testing is possible through the measurement of NAA or enzyme activity in the amniotic fluid and chorionic villus sampling for DNA testing, the latter being the method of choice. Carriers can be identified through DNA testing as well, although testing is more accurate in the Ashkenazi Jewish population due to the uniformity of the mutations.

Magnetic resonance spectroscopy can show an increase of the NAA:choline ratio.

TREATMENT

Standard Therapies: No established treatment is available.

Investigational Therapies: Experimental treatment protocols involving transfer of the gene encoding ASPA, in conjunction with adeno-associated virus-based plasmids containing recombinant ASPA, have yielded encouraging results.

REFERENCES

Brismar J, Brismar G, Gascon G, et al. Canavan disease: CT and MRI imaging of the brain. *AJNR* 1990;11:805–810.

Gordon N. Canavan disease: a review of recent developments. *Eur J Paediatr Neurol* 2001;5:65–69.

Leone P, Janson CG, Bilaniuk L, et al. Aspartoacylase gene transfer to the mammalian central nervous system with therapeutic implications for Canavan disease. *Ann Neurol* 2000;48:9–10.

Traeger EC, Rapin I. The clinical course of Canavan disease. *Pediatr Neurol* 1998;18:207–212.

RESOURCES

58, 335, 368, 477

---

47 Leukodystrophy (Krabbe Disease)

Leonie van Passel-Clark, MD, and Phillip L. Pearl, MD

DEFINITION: Krabbe disease is a dysmyelinating disorder of the central and peripheral nervous system caused by a genetic deficiency of the lysosomal enzyme galactocerebrosidase (GALC), a key component in metabolic pathways of myelin turnover and breakdown.

SYNONYMS: Globoid cell leukodystrophy; Galactosylceramide lipidosis; Krabbe leukodystrophy.

DIFFERENTIAL DIAGNOSIS: Metachromatic leukodystrophy; Adrenoleukodystrophy; Canavan disease; Alexander disease; Pelizaeus-Merzbacher disease; Nonprogressive encephalopathies of prenatal origin and fetal encephalitis; Aminoacidopathies in neonates; Leigh disease, G_{M2} gangliosidosis; Chronic gastrointestinal disease.

SYMPTOMS AND SIGNS: In the infantile form, the median age of onset is 4 months, with a range of 1–7 months.

Initial symptoms are irritability and hypersensitivity to stimuli, which are then followed by progressive hypertonicity in the skeletal muscles. Within 2–4 months after onset, the child has lost all previously achieved milestones and is in a permanent position of opisthotonus. Blindness occurs, and before 1 year, 90% of affected infants either die or are in a chronic persistent vegetative state. Peripheral neuropathy can accompany especially the infantile presentation. The cerebrospinal fluid protein content is elevated. In the juvenile or adult forms, the onset may manifest as a spastic paraparesis with progressive visual failure. Evidence of a polyneuropathy tends to become more obvious with advancing age. Low nerve conduction velocities and a high cerebrospinal fluid protein content, constant findings in the early form of the disease, are lacking in 50% of the cases of juvenile/adult onset.

ETIOLOGY/EPIDEMIOLOGY: The *GALC* gene maps to chromosome 14q24.3 to 14q32.1, and various Krabbe disease–causing mutations have been identified. The disease displays autosomal-recessive inheritance. Galactocerebrosidase deficiency results in the accumulation of galactosylsphingosine, which is considered to be neurotoxic to both the central and peripheral nervous systems.

DIAGNOSIS: MRI shows diffuse demyelination of the cerebral hemispheres, but this may be difficult to distinguish from a normal myelination pattern in a very young patient. At that time, CT may be more helpful because it may show hyperdense areas in the thalami, in the bodies of the caudate nuclei, or in the posterior periventricular regions. Cerebral calcifications and density abnormalities in the cerebral and cerebellar white matter can be seen and, in a child that has not received cranial radiation, are fairly specific for Krabbe disease. Motor nerve conduction velocity of peripheral nerves is usually prolonged, and the cerebrospinal fluid shows increased protein content, usually in a range between 70 and 450 mg /100 mL. Deficient activity of GALC in leukocytes or cultured fibroblasts is diagnostic. Enzymatic assays on chorionic villus or cultured amniotic fluid cells provide the possibility of prenatal diagnosis.

TREATMENT

Standard Therapies: No curative treatment is available. Care is supportive, with nutritional assistance. Allogeneic hematopoietic stem cell transplantation is helpful in slowing the progression of disease, but mainly in the later onset form with slower progression.

Investigational Therapies: Researchers are exploring options to supply GALC activity by transplanted cells or viral vectors to still functional endogenous oligodendrocytes.

REFERENCES

Berger J, Moser HW, Forss-Petter S. Leukodystrophies: recent developments in genetics, molecular biology, pathogenesis and treatment. *Curr Opin Neurol* 2001;14:305–312.

Demaerel P, Wilms G, Vendru P, et al. MRI findings in globoid cell leukodystrophy. *Neuroradiology* 1990;32:520–522.

Randell E, Connolly-Wilson M, Duff A, et al. Evaluation of the accuracy of enzymatically determined carrier status for Krabbe disease by DNA based testing. *Clin Biochem* 2000;33:217–220.

Sasaki M, Sakuragawa N, Takashima S, et al. MRI and CT findings in Krabbe disease. *Pediatr Neurol* 1991;7:283–288.

Wenger DA, Rafi MA, Luzi P, et al. Krabbe disease: genetic aspects and progress towards therapy. *Mol Genet Metab* 2000;70:1–9.

RESOURCES

58, 109, 368, 477

---

48   Metachromatic Leukodystrophy

*Tena Rossser, MD,
and Phillip L. Pearl, MD*

DEFINITION: Metachromatic leukodystrophy (MLD) is a lysosomal storage disease that results in accumulation of cerebroside sulfate (sulfatide) in the central and peripheral nervous systems as well as in non-neural tissues. Clinically, MLD is characterized by cognitive decline, behavioral changes, spasticity, weakness, ataxia, and optic atrophy.

SYNONYMS: Sulfatidosis; Sulfatide lipidosis; Arylsulfatase A (ASA) deficiency; Leukoencephalopathy.

DIFFERENTIAL DIAGNOSIS: Adrenoleukodystrophy; Alexander disease; Canavan disease; Krabbe disease; Pelizaeus-Merzbacher disease.

SYMPTOMS AND SIGNS: Three variants have been described: late infantile, late childhood (juvenile), and adult. In the late infantile form, children have normal development until approximately 10–25 months, when irritability, hypotonia, and gait disturbance develop. Lower extremity spasticity appears and evolves to spastic quadriplegia with decerebrate posturing in late stages. Bulbar weakness with loss of speech occurs. Peripheral neuropathy develops, causing hyporeflexia and sensory ataxia. Cognitive decline occurs relatively late but progresses rapidly. Seizures are infrequent. Ophthalmologic complications include strabismus and optic atrophy with cortical blindness. Cherry red spots may occur. Most affected children die by age 8–10 years. The juvenile form is more variable, with onset ranging from 4–10 years. Typically, behavioral disturbances, learning disabilities, and a spastic, ataxic gait mark the onset of disease. Dementia and spasticity are progressive and disabling. Seizures and movement disorders occur more frequently than in the late infantile form. Children generally survive 5–10 years after the onset of symptoms. Onset of the adult form commonly presents in the third or fourth decade with dementia or psychiatric disturbances, such as personality change, aggressiveness, disinhibition, hallucinations, and poor memory. Slow progression with further mental deterioration, severe ataxia, and spastic paraplegia occur. Peripheral neuropathy may also be apparent. Seizures are occasionally noted. Patients survive 10–20 years after the onset of symptoms.

ETIOLOGY/EPIDEMIOLOGY: The prevalence of the late infantile form is 1 in 40,000 and of the juvenile form is 1 in 150,000. The adult form is believed to be rare. All forms are transmitted as an autosomal-recessive trait. Many ethnic groups are affected. Two lysosomal enzyme defects are responsible for MLD phenotypes: ASA deficiency and deficiency of saposin B, a cerebroside sulfate activator protein.

DIAGNOSIS: The disorder is diagnosed by demonstrating decreased or absent ASA activity in leukocytes or fibroblasts in addition to the presence of sulfatides in urine or body tissues. A nonpathologic ASA pseudodeficiency (ASA-PD) exists in approximately 1% of the general population; ASA-PD can be ruled out by DNA analysis. Multiple additional studies help confirm the diagnosis, including sural nerve biopsy, brainstem evoked potentials, visual evoked potentials, somatosensory evoked potentials, and brain MRI.

TREATMENT
Standard Therapies: Management is primarily supportive and symptomatic.

Investigational Therapies: Bone marrow transplantation has been attempted in all three forms with variable results. Adenoviral and retroviral gene transfer are also being explored.

REFERENCES
Hageman ATM, Gabreels FJM, De Jong JGN, et al. Clinical symptoms of adult metachromatic leukodystrophy and arylsulfatase A pseudodeficiency. *Arch Neurol* 1995;52:408–413.

Kaye EM. Update on genetic disorders affecting white matter. *Pediatr Neurol* 2001;24:11–24.

Kim TS, Kim IO, Kim WS, et al. MR of childhood metachromatic leukiodystrophy. *AJNR* 1997;18:733–738.

Krivit W, Aubourg P, Shapiro E, et al. Bone marrow transplantation for globoid cell leukodystrophy, adrenoleukodystrophy, metachromatic leukodystrophy, and Hurler syndrome. *Curr Opin Hematol* 1999;6:377–382.

RESOURCES
58, 309, 368, 477

---

49 | Classic Lissencephaly

Joseph O. Gleeson, MD

DEFINITION: Classic lissencephaly is an inborn error of brain development owing to a defect in the migration of neurons from their place of origin along the lining of the lateral ventricle to the developing cerebral cortical gray matter. The result is a smooth cerebral cortex that either has simplified broadened gyral pattern (pachygyria) or lacks gyri and sulci altogether (agyria).

SYNONYMS: Pachygryia; Agyria.

DIFFERENTIAL DIAGNOSIS: Polymicrogyria; Cobblestone lissencephaly; Congenital hydrocephalus.

SYMPTOMS AND SIGNS: Head circumference is usually small to normal at birth, but head growth stalls in the first few months of life. Typically, profound developmental delay and mental retardation occur, and seizures begin in the first 3 years of life. Spasticity is not a feature of classic lissencephaly, but is a feature of polymicrogyria, which can help distinguish between these two disorders. Medical complications include feeding difficulties, aspiration pneumonia, gut motility defects, and infections. Lifespan is much shorter than normal.

ETIOLOGY/EPIDEMIOLOGY: Classic lissencephaly occurs either sporadically or as an X-linked dominant trait. Approximately 60%–70% of patients with the sporadic form display *de novo* heterozygous mutations or deletions in the lissencephaly-1 (*LIS1*) gene on 17p13.3. In rare instances in which an unaffected parent carries a chromosomal translocation, the parent is at risk for having a second child with lissencephaly. Approximately 20% of patients display mutations in the doublecortin gene on Xq23.3. A significant risk of recurrence for lissencephaly exists in this setting, and genetic counseling is advised. Mutations in the doublecortin (*DCX*) gene are also seen in some patients with the related disorder subcortical band heterotopia (double cortex). Often, individuals with double cortex and lissencephaly occur in the same family. The prevalence is estimated at 1 in 100,000. All ethnic groups are affected.

DIAGNOSIS: Because of failure of gyri to form, lissencephaly may be identified during pregnancy at midgestation with ultrasonography, and confirmed with MRI.

However, the diagnosis is not typically made until after birth. Lissencephaly should be suspected in a child with developmental delay or seizures who has an abnormal gyral pattern on brain imaging. Molecular diagnosis can be made in most patients with typical physical findings and abnormalities seen on imaging, which can be helpful in genetic counseling,

TREATMENT

Standard Therapies: Treatment is generally aimed at maximizing the child's development and in preventing the medical complications that are associated with lissencephaly. Specific therapy awaits improved understanding of the molecular mechanisms of neuronal migration.

REFERENCES

Barkovich AJ, Hevner R, Guerrini R. Syndromes of bilateral symmetrical polymicrogyria. *AJNR* 1999;20:1814–1821.

de Rijk-van Andel JF, van der Knaap MS, Valk J, et al. Neuroimaging in lissencephaly type I. *Neuroradiology* 1991;33:230–233.

Gleeson JO. Classical lissencephaly and double cortex (subcortical band heterotopia): LIS1 and doublecortin. *Curr Opin Neurol* 2000;13:121–125.

Golden JA. Cell migration and cerebral cortical development. *Neuropathol Appl Neurobiol* 2001;27:22–28.

Okamura K, Murotsuki J, Sakai T, et al. Prenatal diagnosis of lissencephaly by magnetic resonance image. *Fetal Diagn Ther* 1993;8:56–59.

RESOURCES

243, 244, 368, 453

---

50 Locked-in Syndrome

Sanjiv Sahoo, MD,
and Phillip L. Pearl, MD

DEFINITION: Locked-in syndrome is a neuromuscular syndrome composed of quadriplegia, aphonia, occasional absent horizontal eye movements with intact vertical eye movements, and a state of wakefulness.

SYNONYMS: Deefferented state; Cerebromedullospinal disconnection; Pseudocoma.

DIFFERENTIAL DIAGNOSIS: Akinetic mutism; Catatonia; Guillain-Barré syndrome; Bilateral lacunar infarcts; Tentorial herniation; Myasthenia gravis; Poliomyelitis; Polyneuritis; Bilateral brainstem tumors.

SYMPTOMS AND SIGNS: Patients with locked-in syndrome are quadriplegic, aphonic, and occasionally lack horizontal eye movements secondary to the involvement of the ventral pons, its corticospinal tracts, and bilateral sixth nerve fascicles. In the early stages of a basilar artery thrombosis, a "herald hemiparesis" may result from partial infarction of the brainstem before progressing to bilateral involvement. The patient is fully awake due to the sparing of the reticular formation. Vertical eye movements and blinking are spared and the patient may be able to convey his wishes through eye blinking.

ETIOLOGY/EPIDEMIOLOGY: Males and females are equally affected. The syndrome results from bilateral ventral pontine lesions such as infarction, basilar artery thrombosis, tumors, hemorrhage, trauma, and central pontine myelinolysis.

DIAGNOSIS: The diagnosis is usually made clinically. MRI and MR angiography can be used to rule out tumors, infarcts, hemorrhages, and herniation. The scans may show brainstem infarcts, basilar artery thrombosis, and tumors. Brainstem auditory evoked responses may be helpful in localizing brainstem involvement. Electromyography and nerve conduction study may be used to rule out a peripheral cause for deefferentation.

TREATMENT

Standard Therapies: Reversal of basilar artery thrombosis with intraarterial thrombolytic therapy may be attempted up to 6 hours after symptom onset. Tumors may be managed with intravenous steroids and radiation. Hemorrhage may be managed conservatively. Rehabilitation and supportive care are helpful in patients who show some recovery. Devices to help in communication may be used.

REFERENCES

Cabezudo JM, Olabe J, Lopez-Anguera A. Recovery from locked in syndrome after posttraumatic bilateral distal vertebral artery occlusion. *Surg Neurol* 1986;25:185–190.

Hawkes CH. "Locked-in" syndrome: report of seven cases. *BMJ* 1974;4:379.

Phan TG. Intra-arterial thrombolysis for vertebrobasilar artery circulation ischemia. *Crit Care Clin* 1999;15:719–742.

Plum F, Posner JB. *The diagnosis of stupor and coma,* 3rd ed. Philadelphia: FA Davis, 1980.

RESOURCES

79, 368

51   Machado-Joseph Disease

Taeun Chang, MD,
and Phillip L. Pearl, MD

DEFINITION: Machado-Joseph disease (MJD) is a central nervous system disorder involving cerebellar ataxia and ophthalmoplegia. There are three phenotypes.

SYNONYMS: Joseph disease; Spinocerebellar ataxia 3; Spinocerebellar atrophy III; Azorean neurologic disease; Spinopontine atrophy; Nigrospinodentatal degeneration; Ataxin 3.

DIFFERENTIAL DIAGNOSIS: Other spinocerebellar ataxias (particularly SCA1); Friedreich ataxia; Marie ataxia; Hallervorden-Spatz disease; Olivopontocerebellar atrophy; Parenchymatous cortical degeneration of the cerebellum; Progressive supranuclear palsy.

SYMPTOMS AND SIGNS: Cerebellar ataxia and ophthalmoplegia are common symptoms of all three types of MJD. Other minor findings include facial and lingual fasciculations, bulging eyes due to lid retractions, extrapyramidal (parkinsonian) symptoms such as rigidity and bradykinesia, bulbar symptoms (dysarthria, dysphagia), distal motor weakness with hyperreflexia, and dystonia. Type 1 is characterized by early onset of symptoms, usually at approximately 25 years, and prominent pyramidal signs and dystonic postures. Type 2 is the most common, with a mean onset of approximately age 40 years. Pyramidal signs may or may not be present. Type 3 has a late onset (mean, approximately 47 years) and slow progression with prominent amyotrophy.

ETIOLGY/EPIDEMIOLOGY: The disease is an autosomal-dominant neurologic disorder caused by a (CAG)n trinucleotide expansion in a gene located on chromosome 14q. The gene has been mapped to chromosome 14q24.3-q31. The normal allele has 13–36 CAG repeats, whereas the expanded allele has anywhere between 67 and 200 repeats. The disorder was originally described in the Machado family on the Azorean island of San Miguel, in the Thomas family, who migrated from San Miguel to Massachusetts, and in the Joseph family, who migrated from the Azorean island of Flores to California. The disorder has also occurred in other families of diverse non-Azorean descent. Pathology shows sparing of the inferior olivary nuclei and Purkinje cells unlike other hereditary ataxias. Instead, there is significant involvement of the dentate nuclei and substantia nigra.

DIAGNOSIS: Genetic testing, clinical presentation, and positive family history establish the diagnosis.

TREATMENT
Standard Therapies: Treatment is symptomatic and supportive. Genetic testing is recommended for families in which at least one member has been diagnosed with the disease.

REFERENCES
Higgins JJ, Nee LE, et al. Mutations in American families with spinocerebellar ataxia (SCA) type 3: SCA3 is allelic to Machado-Joseph disease. *Neurology* 1996;46:208–213.
Junck L, Fink JK. Machado-Joseph disease and SCA3: the genotype meets the phenotypes. *Neurology* 1996;46:4–8.
Kawaguchi Y, Okamoto T, et al. CAG expansions in a novel gene for Machado-Joseph disease at chromosome 14q32.1. *Nat Genet* 1994;8:221–228.
Silveira I, Lopes-Cendes I, et al. Frequency of spinocerebellar ataxia type 1, dentatorubropallidoluysian atrophy, and Machado-Joseph disease mutations in a large group of spinocerebellar ataxia patients. *Neurology* 1996;46:214–218.
Twist EC, Casaubon LK, et al. Machado-Joseph disease maps to the same region of chromosome 14 as the spinocerebellar ataxia type 3 locus. *J Med Genet* 1995;32:25–31.

RESOURCES
205, 368

52   Megalocornea and Mental Retardation

*Ania Porazinski, MD,
and Shachar Tauber, MD*

DEFINITION: Megalocornea (MC) is characterized by a nonprogressive and symmetric corneal enlargement in the absence of congenital glaucoma. The cornea may measure 13.0–16.5 mm in diameter and in most cases is histologically normal. Megalocornea may appear in association with other abnormalities of the anterior segment, including iris hypoplasia, iridocorneal dysgenesis, cataract, mosaic corneal dystrophy, refractive errors, and glaucoma. A subset of MC associated with mental retardation (MR) and other craniofacial, neurologic, and osteoarticular anomalies is referred to as megalocornea-mental retardation syndrome (MMR).

SYNONYM: Neuhauser syndrome.

DIFFERENTIAL DIAGNOSIS: Congenital glaucoma; Dwarfism; Down syndrome; Marfan syndrome; Weil-Marchesani syndrome; Rothmund-Thompson syndrome; Alport syndrome; Osteogenesis imperfecta; Mucolipidosis type II; Oculocerebrorenal syndrome; Walker-Warburg syndrome.

SYMPTOMS AND SIGNS: All patients present with delayed psychomotor development, megalocornea, and variable expressivity of other anomalies. Craniofacial deformity may include microcephalia, round facies, macrocephaly, frontal bossing, broad nasal base, hypertelorism, epicanthus, abnormal auricles, prominent globes, long upper lip, high/narrow palate, and small chin. Neurologic abnormalities may include hypotony, seizures, ataxia, abnormal movements, and hyperactivity. Osteoarticular clinically abnormal findings may include distal flexion fingers, kyphosis-scoliosis, plano/valgus and club feet, and joint hyperlaxity.

ETIOLOGY/EPIDEMIOLOGY: At least 20 case reports have been published of MMR since Neuhauser first de-scribed the association of MC with MR. The etiology may be related to abnormal embryologic development. Most cases are X-linked recessive and have been mapped to the Xq21.3-q22 region. Sporadic, AR, and AD cases have also been reported. The inheritance pattern and genetic mutations are unknown. A classification of MMR syndrome into four distinct types addresses the heterogeneity of this syndrome suggested by the discrepancies and broad variations in its clinical presentation. More males are affected than females.

TREATMENT

Standard Therapies: A team approach involving medical and subspecialty physicians is indicated in the care and management of these patients. Congenital glaucoma must be ruled out by intraocular pressure, gonioscopy, and optic nerve evaluation. Refractive error should be managed either by spectacles or contact lenses. Evaluation of the anterior segment including lens iris and cornea should be made to rule out any associated disorders of the eye. The patient should be evaluated for signs of strabismus. The family should be offered genetic counseling.

REFERENCES
Antinola G, et al. Megalocornea-mental retardation syndrome. *Am J Med Genet* 1994;52:196–197.
Del Guiudice E, et al. Megalocornea and mental retardation syndrome: two new cases. *Am J Med Genet* 1987;26:417–420.
Grenbech-Jensen M. Megalocornea and mental retardation syndrome: a new case. *Am J Med Genet* 1989;32:468–469.
Santolaya JM. Additional case of Neuhauser megalocornea and mental retardation syndrome with congenital hypotonia. *Am J Med Genet* 1992;43:609–611.
Verloes A, et al. Heterogeneity versus variability in megalocornea-mental retardation syndromes. *Am J Med Genet* 1993;46:132–137.

RESOURCES
96, 288, 355, 368

53   Melkersson-Rosenthal Syndrome

Sunil N. Dutt, MS, FRCS Ed,
and Richard M. Irving, MD, FRCS

DEFINITION: Melkersson-Rosenthal syndrome (MRS) is a neuromucocutaneous disorder causing localized edema and inflammation in the face and oral cavity. In the complete form of the syndrome, the classic triad of recurrent facial paralysis, faciolabial edema, and fissured tongue is characteristic.

DIFFERENTIAL DIAGNOSIS: Recurrent (alternating) facial paralysis of unknown origin; Angioneurotic edema; Hereditary angioneurotic edema.

SYMPTOMS AND SIGNS: Patients with MRS present with a recurrent episodic condition with intermittent periods of remission. The initial orofacial features include edema of the face, lips, gingivae, buccal mucosa, and tongue; gingival erosions, burning sensation of the tongue; and facial palsy. During the course of an attack that may last from several days to months, these symptoms and signs may be exaggerated. Three clinical forms have been described: complete, monosymptomatic, and oligosymptomatic. Patients can present with localized cheilitis only and this variant is probably a fairly common cause of constant lip swelling. The facial nerve is involved in 19%–31% of cases. The palsy may initially be a mild paresis but may become complete with progression of the disease. Over several years, the episodes become more frequent and prolonged, resulting in distorting and disfiguring sequelae such as facial myokimia, synkinesis, and increasing residual paralysis.

ETIOLOGY/EPIDEMIOLOGY: Nearly 300 cases of the disease have been reported. The prevalence may be higher, because the facial nerve is affected in only about a third of cases. The disease exhibits a slight female preponderance. The condition is an autosomal-dominant disorder with variable expression. Families with two, three, and four generations of affected individuals have been reported. The "Melkersson-Rosenthal gene" may be situated at 9p11.

DIAGNOSIS: The diagnosis is clinical based on recurrent oral and faciolabial features and facial paralysis, often with a positive family history. Demonstrating a noncaseating epithelioid granuloma by a labial biopsy may be mandatory for diagnosis. Imaging techniques including high-resolution CT and MRI are useful in excluding other causes of facial paralysis such as tumors. Genetic studies may be useful in screening families affected by the disease.

TREATMENT

Standard Therapies: Most of the symptoms and signs seem to resolve spontaneously, but symptoms occur with increasing frequency and persist for longer durations if the condition is untreated. Non-neurologic manifestations may be treated by corticosteroids (topical, intralesional, or systemic). Medications such as dapsone, clofazimine, sulfasalazine, and antihistamines have been found useful. Limited success has been reported with radiotherapy, sulfazopyridine, and reduction cheiloplasty. Systemic and intralesional steroids are perhaps the most effective forms of therapy in controlling progression and reducing some of the orofacial granulomatous edema. Surgical management of facial paralysis is controversial. Results of surgical decompression of the nerve in its entire intratemporal course have been encouraging. A total decompression is recommended for a significant increase in frequency, duration, and severity of facial paralysis leading to disabling sequelae such as synkinesis and persistent residual paresis. Patients should be made aware that the procedure is not curative and that the other orofacial manifestations need to be addressed and managed with oral or intralesional steroids.

REFERENCES

Dutt SN, Mirza S, Irving RM, et al. Total decompression of facial nerve for Melkersson-Rosenthal syndrome. *J Laryngol Otol* 2000;114:870–873.

House JW, Brackmann DE. Facial nerve grading system. *Otolaryngol Head Neck Surg* 1985;93:146–147.

Smeets E, Fryns JP, Van den Berghe H. Melkersson-Rosenthal syndrome and de novo t(9;21)(p11;p11) translocation. *Clin Genet* 1994;45:323–324.

Zimmer WM, Rogers III RS, Reeve CM, et al. Orofacial manifestations of Melkersson-Rosenthal syndrome. *Oral Surg Oral Med Oral Pathol* 1992;74:610–619.

RESOURCES

27, 368

54   Ménière Disease

*Hoda Hachicho, MD,
and Phillip L. Pearl, MD*

DEFINITION: Ménière disease is an idiopathic disease involving the membranous inner ear characterized by vertigo, hearing loss, and tinnitus. The hearing loss is fluctuating, usually low frequency, and sensorineural. Over time, hearing loss and tinnitus may become permanent.

SYNONYMS: Hydrops labyrinthi; Endolymphatic hydrops.

DIFFERENTIAL DIAGNOSIS: Acoustic neuroma; Multiple sclerosis; Cerebellar or brainstem tumors; Benign paroxysmal positional vertigo; Labyrinthitis; Autoimmune inner ear disease; Diabetes mellitus; Thyroid disease; Syphilis; Anemia.

SYMPTOMS AND SIGNS: In typical Ménière disease, the attacks of vertigo are abrupt and last several minutes to an hour or longer. The vertigo is rotational and usually severe, interfering with standing and walking. Varying degrees of nausea and vomiting, low-pitched tinnitus, feeling of fullness in the ear, and diminution in hearing are present. Nystagmus is present in the acute attack. It is horizontal in type, usually with a rotatory component. As the attack subsides, hearing improves, as does the sensation of fullness in the ear. With further attacks, deafness may develop. Patients with frequent attacks may report a mild state of disequilibrium and reluctance to move the head or turn quickly. A few patients experience sudden, violent falling attacks that they describe as a sensation of being pushed or knocked to the ground without warning. Early in the disease, deafness affects mainly low tones and fluctuates in severity. Later, fluctuation is less, and high tones are affected.

ETIOLOGY/EPIDEMIOLOGY: No gender difference exists. Onset is usually in the fifth decade. Although cases are mostly sporadic, rare hereditary forms have been described. The main pathologic change consists of an increase in the volume of endolymph and distention of the endolymphatic system. Sustained or frequent pressure/volume changes can cause irreversible damage to the delicate inner ear sensory systems.

DIAGNOSIS: The diagnosis should be suspected by the presence of episodic vertigo, fluctuating-ascending hearing loss, aural fullness, and tinnitus. Routine audiometric studies typically show a low-frequency fluctuating sensorineural hearing loss early in the course, with gradual progression to a flat, more severe loss.

TREATMENT
Standard Therapies: The therapeutic goal is significant, sustained hearing improvement and freedom from reccurent attacks of vertigo. Once an affected individual loses the reversibility component, chances for improved hearing are diminished. There is no known cure, but 80% of patients appear to respond to conservative treatment with a variety of systemic medical and dietary regimens. Acute medical treatment includes vestibular suppressants and antiemetic drugs. Maintenance therapy usually includes diet modification with reduced sodium intake combined with other pharmacologic interventions. Diuretics including thiazides and carbonic anhydrase inhibitors have been used. Vasodilators, calcium channel blockers, aminoglycosides, and steroids may be considered in patients refractory to diuretics. Many nondestructive and destructive surgical approaches to inner ear endolymphatic hydrops problems are routinely performed in attempts to alter, improve, or selectively ablate inner ear functions. There is no consensus regarding the best surgical approach. The most common destructive procedures are vestibular nerve section and labyrinthectomy. The most common nondestructive procedure is endolymphatic sac surgery.

REFERENCES
Arenberg IK, Graham MD, eds. *Treatment options for Ménière's disease. Endolymphatic sac surgery: do it or don't do it.* San Diego: Singular Publishing Group, 1998:1–6.
Brookes GB. Medical management of Ménière's disease. *Ear Nose Throat J* 1997;76:634–640.
Hoffer ME, Balough B, Henderson J, et al. Use of sustained release vehicles in the treatment of Ménière's disease. *Otolaryngol Clin North Am* 1997;30:1159–1166.
Van De Heyning PH. Definition, classification and reporting of Ménière's disease and its symptoms. *Acta Otolaryngol* 1997; 526(suppl):5–9.
Weber PC, Adkins WY Jr. The differential diagnosis of Ménière's disease. *Otolaryngol Clin North Am* 1997;30:1061–1074.

RESOURCES
124, 261, 370, 485

55   Moyamoya Syndrome

R. Michael Scott, MD

DEFINITION: Moyamoya syndrome is a cerebral blood vessel disease that causes progressive narrowing of the arteries at the base of the brain, accompanied by a progressive dilation of small perforating arteries in the same area, which then supply the brain distal to the area of stenosis.

DIFFERENTIAL DIAGNOSIS: Fibromuscular dysplasia; Cerebral artery dissection; Cerebral arteritis; Hemiplegic migraine.

SYMPTOMS AND SIGNS: In children, symptoms range from transient ischemic attacks (~40%) to complete strokes (~40%). Alternating hemiplegia may occur in some patients. Seizures, involuntary choreiform movements, or headaches may also occur in the pediatric group. Intracranial or subarachnoid hemorrhage due to rupture of collateral vessels at the base of the brain or in the ventricular system occurs relatively infrequently in this population. In the adult population, approximately 40%–65% of patients present with hemorrhage, most commonly in the basal ganglia, thalamus, or within the ventricular system.

ETIOLOGY/EPIDEMIOLOGY: The cause of the syndrome is unknown. The major symptoms are caused by (a) progressive reduction in blood supply to the brain, leading to stroke, transient ischemic attacks, headache, and seizures; (b) thrombi forming at the sites of stenoses, with similar symptoms resulting from thrombosis of the involved vessel or distal embolism; and (c) brain hemorrhage within the basal ganglia or within the ventricles resulting from rupture of the thin-walled, dilated collateral vessels. A 7%–12% familial incidence has been reported in Japan, but a multifactorial etiology seems to be operant in many cases diagnosed in the Western hemisphere, including associations of the syndrome with a variety of congenital disorders including neurofibromatosis, Down syndrome, previous history of congenital cardiac surgery, and prior cranial X-irradiation. In Japan, the syndrome is believed to occur at approximately 1 case per million population per year with an overall male:female ratio of 1:1.6. A recent report from Japan suggests that a specific gene locus for the familial form of the disease has been identified.

DIAGNOSIS: Results of MRI and magnetic resonance angiography demonstrate reduced caliber of vessels in the circle of Willis, dilated "moyamoya" vessels passing through the basal ganglia, and often, evidence of previous ischemic injury to the brain. Electroencephalographic studies may also show a characteristic pattern of "rebuildup." Cerebral blood flow studies such as SPECT, positron emission tomography, and xenon-CT may show areas of reduced brain perfusion and instability of blood flow. Cerebral angiography is diagnostic, demonstrating the severe constrictions of the intracranial internal carotid, middle cerebral, and anterior cerebral arteries, along with the characteristic moyamoya vessels passing through the basal ganglia.

TREATMENT

Standard Therapies: Numerous surgical procedures have been use to increase cerebral blood flow, including so-called indirect procedures, which provide an avenue to the brain surface through which new collateral blood flow can develop, or direct anastomotic procedures, such as the superficial temporal to middle cerebral anastomosis. Antiplatelet medication likely also plays an important role, reducing the formation of microthrombi at areas of major vessel stenosis and reducing the likelihood of subsequent cerebral embolization. Headache may be helped by antimigraine medications, including calcium channel blockers and antiserotonin agents.

REFERENCES

Adelson P, Scott R. Pial synangiosis for moyamoya syndrome in children. *Pediatr Neurosurg* 1995;23:26–33.

Ohaegbulam C, Magge S, Scott RM. Moyamoya syndrome. In: McLone DG, ed. *Pediatric neurosurgery: surgery of the developing nervous system.* Philadelphia: WB Saunders, 2001:1077–1092.

Scott R. Surgical treatment of moyamoya syndrome in children. In: Chapman P, ed. *Concepts in pediatric neurosurgery.* New York: S Karger, 1985:198–212.

Suzuki J, Takaku A. Cerebrovascular "moyamoya" disease. A disease showing abnormal net-like vessels in base of brain. *Arch Neurol* 1969;20:288–299.

RESOURCES

153, 368

56   Rare Variants of Multiple Sclerosis

Barbara S. Giesser, MD

DEFINITION: Although multiple sclerosis (MS) is the most common demyelinating disorder of the central nervous system, there are rare clinical variants. These include Balo concentric sclerosis, Devic syndrome, Marburg variant, Schilder disease, and MS with onset in childhood.

SYNONYMS: Neuromyelitis optica q.v. (Devic); Myelinoclastic diffuse sclerosis (Schilder).

DIFFERENTIAL DIAGNOSIS: Adrenoleukodystrophy; Subacute sclerosing panencephalitis; Metabolic leukodystrophies.

SYMPTOMS AND SIGNS: Balo concentric sclerosis usually presents in adults, but cases in children have been reported. Typical features may include headache, seizures, alteration of consciousness, or cognitive loss. The course is generally monophasic and rapidly progressive, in contrast to MS, which most commonly waxes and wanes. Devic syndrome is characterized by concurrent or temporally associated optic neuritis and myelopathy. In contrast to MS, brainstem, cerebellar, and cognitive deficits tend not to occur. Only about 10% of patients with Devic syndrome go on to develop typical MS. Marburg variant is a rapidly progressive monophasic demyelinating illness that tends to present in otherwise healthy young adults, and the time course to death is generally months to a year. Schilder disease is usually a disorder of children or young adults. Common presenting features may be similar to those of a mass lesion, e.g., headache, hemiparesis, or hemianopsia. The course tends to be progressive, and may have periods of superimposed acute worsening. Multiple sclerosis in childhood, i.e., before age 15, only accounts for 3%–5% of cases, with onset before age 10 accounting for less than 1%. Although the symptoms may be similar to those of adult MS (weakness, incoordination, tremor, sensory deficits), atypical presentations such as seizures or encephalopathy may occur.

ETIOLOGY/EPIDEMIOLOGY: The cause of MS and its variants remains unknown. Devic disease occurs in multiple ethnic groups, but more commonly in Asians. Childhood MS affects more equal numbers of males and females than does adult MS.

DIAGNOSIS: The variants of MS have important pathologic as well as clinical differences. Balo concentric sclerosis gets its name from the characteristic alternating rings of demyelination and preserved myelin. Cerebrospinal fluid (CSF) tends to resemble that of MS, with frequent occurrence of oligoclonal bands and increased intrathecal IgG. Schilder disease tends to present radiographically as a large single hemispheric or bilaterally symmetric hemispheric lesions, suggesting tumor, but without pronounced mass effect or edema. In addition to demyelination, axonal destruction and diffuse inflammatory changes are seen. Patients with Devic syndrome tend to have normal results on MRI of the brain and swelling and cavitation of the spinal cord. The oligoclonal bands and increased intrathecal immunoglobulin synthesis that are seen in approximately 90% of patients with MS tend not to occur in Devic syndrome. MS with onset in childhood has been reported to have more normal CSF, with the number of oligoclonal bands increasing with disease progression.

TREATMENT

Standard Therapies: Corticosteroids are usually useful in decreasing severity of acute presentations through their antiinflammatory actions. Other strategies may include intravenous immunoglobulin, immunosuppressive therapy, or plasmapheresis. Treatment to ameliorate symptoms such as spasticity, weakness, pain, ataxia, or genitourinary dysfunction includes pharmacologic and rehabilitative modalities.

REFERENCES

Garell PC, Menezes AH, Baumbach G, et al. Presentation, management and follow up of Schilder's disease. *Pediatr Neurosurg* 1998;29:86–91.

Mandler RN, Davis LE, Jeffery DR, et al. Devic's neuromyelitis optica: a clinicopathologic study of 8 patients. *Ann Neurol* 1993;34:162–168.

Mendez MF, Pogacar S. Malignant monophasic MS or "Marburg's disease." *Neurology* 1998;38:1153–1155.

Miller A, Bourdette D, Cohen JA, et al. Multiple sclerosis. *Continuum* 1999;5:50–56.

Selcen D, Anlar B, Renda Y. MS in childhood: report of 16 cases. *Eur Neurol* 1996;36:79–84.

RESOURCES

116, 315, 368, 487

57   Multiple System Atrophy

Niall P. Quinn, FRCP

DEFINITION: Multiple system atrophy (MSA) is a degenerative disease of the nervous system characterized by varying combinations of parkinsonism, cerebellar symptoms, and autonomic failure.

SYNONYMS: Shy-Drager syndrome; Sporadic olivopontocerebellar atrophy or degeneration; Striatonigral degeneration.

DIFFERENTIAL DIAGNOSIS: Parkinson disease; Progressive supranuclear palsy; Corticobasal degeneration; Other forms of (spino) cerebellar degeneration or hereditary olivopontocerebellar atrophy; Pure autonomic failure.

SYMPTOMS AND SIGNS: Autonomic signs include erectile dysfunction in males, bladder disturbance (having to pass water at night; daytime frequency, urgency, or incontinence; incomplete bladder emptying; or retention of urine), and often faintness on standing or after meals, sometimes with a loss of consciousness. Signs of parkinsonism include slowness, stiffness, and often tremor, usually responding poorly to levodopa preparations used to treat Parkinson disease, although up to 30% of patients show an initially good response. Signs of cerebellar dysfunction include incoordination, slurred speech, and unsteadiness, often leading to falls. Other symptoms include rapid eye movement (REM) sleep behavior disorder, snoring, sleep apnea, inspiratory sighs and stridor, neurologic weepiness, myoclonic twitches of the fingers, cold extremities, and Raynaud phenomenon. Half of patients develop pyramidal signs but not weakness or a spastic gait.

ETIOLOGY/EPIDEMIOLOGY: The cause of MSA is unknown. No genetic risk factors have been identified, and no familial cases have been proven. Males and females are about equally affected. Peak incidence is in the early 50s. Prognosis varies widely, but median survival from the first symptom is 9–10 years. Population prevalence has been estimated at 4.4 per 100,000.

DIAGNOSIS: Diagnosis is clinical. Ancillary investigations may assist in diagnosis, or exclude other conditions. These include cardiovascular autonomic function tests, external anal or urethral sphincter electromyography, and MRI brain scan.

TREATMENT
Standard Therapies: Levodopa preparations, dopamine agonists, and amantadine are used to treat parkinsonism. High-salt diet; elastic tights; head-up tilt of the bed at night; postural "tricks;" and fludrocortisone, midodrine, and/or L-threo-DOPS are used to treat postural faintness. Sildenafil is used for impotence, although it may worsen faintness. Anticholinergic drugs (e.g., oxybutynin) and intermittent self-catheterization are used to treat urinary symptoms. Continuous positive pressure ventilation is the standard treatment for sleep apnea, and clonazepam is used for REM sleep behavior disorder. Tricyclics or selective serotonin reuptake inhibitors are used to treat neurologic weepiness.

REFERENCES
Gilman S, Low PA, Quinn N, et al. Consensus statement on the diagnosis of multiple system atrophy. *J Neurol Sci* 1999;163: 94–98.

Quinn N. Multiple system atrophy—the nature of the beast. *J Neurol Neurosurg Psychiatry* 1989;(suppl):78–89.

Quinn N. Multiple system atrophy. In: Marsden CD, Fahn S, eds. *Movement disorders*, 3rd ed. London: Butterworth-Heinemann, 1987:262–281.

Wenning GK, Ben-Shlomo Y, Magalhães M, et al. Clinical features and natural history of multiple system atrophy. *Brain* 1994; 117:835–845.

RESOURCES
368, 487

58   Narcolepsy

Meeta Goswami, MD, MPH, PhD

DEFINITION: Narcolepsy is a sleep disorder of neurologic origin characterized by excessive daytime sleep (EDS) episodes. It is typically associated with cataplexy and other rapid eye movement (REM) features such as sleep paralysis, and with hypnagogic hallucinations. Associated features include disrupted nocturnal sleep and automatic behavior.

SYNONYMS: Excessive daytime sleepiness; Cataplexy; Abnormal REM sleep; Gelineau syndrome; Narcoleptic syndrome.

DIFFERENTIAL DIAGNOSIS: Idiopathic hypersomnolence; Sleep apnea; Upper airway resistance syndrome; Hypothyroidism; Hypoglycemia; Depression; Drug withdrawal; Fugue states; Hysteria; Akinetic seizures; Epilepsy; Muscular disorders; Vestibular disorders; Drop attacks; Psychological or psychiatric disorders.

SYMPTOMS AND SIGNS: People with narcolepsy have repeated episodes of EDS that generally last from a few minutes to an hour. Characteristically, patients report feeling refreshed after a brief nap. Cataplexy, which occurs in 60%–70% of cases, is a unique feature of narcolepsy and is characterized by a sudden loss of bilateral muscle tone precipitated by deep emotion or a stressful situation. The person does not lose consciousness. Sleep paralysis is the inability to move or speak during the transition between sleep and wakefulness. Hypnagogic hallucinations are extremely vivid dreams or images occurring at sleep onset and include visual, tactile, kinetic, and auditory experiences. All four symptoms occur in approximately 20% of patients. Other common complaints are disturbed nocturnal sleep, memory problems, and fatigue.

ETIOLOGY/EPIDEMIOLOGY: The disorder is linked to brain chemicals called hypocretins/orexin, which play an important role in regulating sleep and appetite. Nongenetic factors are also involved in the pathophysiology of narcolepsy. Narcolepsy is estimated to occur in 0.03%–0.16% of the general population. The first symptoms of narcolepsy generally appear between the ages of 13 and 30. Men and women are equally affected.

DIAGNOSIS: The diagnosis is established by multiple all-night polysomnography testing, showing short sleep latencies of less than 10 minutes and two or more sleep-onset REM periods, i.e., REM appearing within 20 minutes after sleep onset. Genetic testing for HLA-DQB1*0602 may indicate a predisposition to this disorder.

TREATMENT
Standard Therapies: The central nervous system stimulants currently prescribed for EDS are amphetamine, methamphetamine, methylphenidate, pemoline, and dextroamphetamine, which is most commonly prescribed. Modafinil is accepted by many clinicians as the first-line treatment for narcolepsy. Tricylic antidepressants are prescribed for cataplexy, hypnagogic hallucinations, and sleep paralysis. Protriptyline is the drug of choice in the United States. Other medications prescribed are impramine, desmethylimipramine, and clomipramine. Fluoxitene, a serotonin-uptake blocker, is also effective in reducing cataplexy. Counseling and support services are recommended to cope with the profound psychosocial impact of narcolepsy, which includes depression, social isolation, job loss, and marital discord.

Investigational Therapies: Investigational medications include gamma-hydroxybuterate, monamine oxidase inhibitors (e.g., nardil and deprenyl), viloxazine hydrochloride, fluvoxamine, zimeldine, and femoxitine. Research is being done on abnormalities of dopamine receptors, genetic studies, and the use of histamine H3 antagonists.

REFERENCES
Aldrich MS. Narcolepsy. *Neurology* 1992;42:34–43.
Chemelli RM, et al. Narcolepsy in orexin knockout mice: molecular genetics of sleep regulation. *Cell* 1999;98:437–451.
Beusterien KM, et al. Health-related quality of life effects of modafinil for treatment of narcolepsy. *Sleep* 1999;22:757–765.
Lin L, et al. The sleep disorder canine narcolepsy is caused by a mutation in the hypocretin (orexin) receptor 2 gene. *Cell* 1999;98:365–376.
Mignot E. Genetic and familial aspects of narcolepsy. In: Fry J, ed. Current issues in the diagnosis and management of narcolepsy. *Neurology* 1998;50(suppl 1):16–22.

RESOURCES
278, 279, 316, 368

59 Neu-Laxova Syndrome

Renata Laxova, MD, PhD

DEFINITION: Neu-Laxova syndrome is a lethal autosomal-recessive multiple malformation syndrome, characterized by severe intrauterine growth retardation (IUGR), microcephaly, typically recognizable facial appearance, flexion deformities, ichthyosis, and edema.

DIFFERENTIAL DIAGNOSIS: Cerebro-oculo-facial and other fetal akinesia syndromes; Multiple pterygia syndromes; Other syndromes associated with severe IUGR; Dysmorphism; Microcephaly; Edema; Other arthrogryposis syndromes.

SYMPTOMS AND SIGNS: The pregnancy is usually associated with oligohydramnios, reported weak or absent fetal movements, early delivery (average 32 weeks), small placenta, and an infant who is invariably severely intrauterine-growth retarded in all parameters, microcephalic, and edematous. Facial characteristics of affected infants include a sloping forehead, small cranium, little or no scalp hair, round, protruding eyes with occasional cataracts, absent eyelids and lashes, flat short nose, depressed nasal bridge, vertical nares, unusually configured small ears, and open mouth circumvented by thick everted lips. The neck is short, sometimes hyperextended. Limbs are short, frequently edematous, with severe flexion contractures and pterygia. Syndactyly and overlapping of digits are frequently observed, as is edema of hands and feet, resulting in an appearance sometimes reminiscent of inflated rubber gloves with short digits. Skeletal anomalies, such as radioulnar synostosis and bowing have been described, as have joint dislocations. The skin is thin, scaly, frequently ichthyotic, and edematous. The subcutaneum is thick and yellow, resulting in a "shiny tight" appearance of the skin. Genitalia are hypoplastic. Occasional organic malformations include kidneys and cardiovascular system. Open neural tube defects as well as facial clefting malformations have sometimes been observed.

ETIOLOGY/EPIDEMIOLOGY: The underlying cause is unknown. The syndrome has occurred in both sexes and has resulted from several consanguineous (first cousins included) unions. It is assumed to be inherited as an autosomal-recessive trait. Fewer than 100 instances have been reported, from several ethnic groups. Most infants are stillborn or die neonatally.

DIAGNOSIS: The diagnosis is usually clinical, based on the phenotypic appearance, premature delivery, and the specific constellation of characteristic features. Imaging of the central nervous system invariably shows lissencephaly, pachygyria, agenesis of the corpus callosum, and cerebral and cerebellar hypoplasia. Histologic evaluation of the skin shows keratotic epidermis and infiltration of the dermis by fat lobules.

TREATMENT

Standard Therapies: No curative or specific treatments exist. Until the cause is clarified, patients should receive symptomatic management in the form of cardiac, ophthalmologic, audiologic, and psychologic support as applicable. Most important is physical therapy (movement of joints) in the surviving infant. Support must be available for the parents, siblings, and extended family in helping them to understand the nature and course of the infant's disorder. Supportive genetics counseling and explanation of potential recurrence risks is strongly recommended. Prenatal diagnosis should be offered to those who wish to have information during a potential subsequent pregnancy.

REFERENCES

Curry CJR. Letter to the editor: further comments on the Neu-Laxova syndrome. *Am J Med Genet* 1982;13:441.

Laxova R, Ohdra PT, Timothy JAD. A further example of a lethal autosomal recessive condition in siblings. *J Ment Def Res* 1972;16:139.

Lyons-Jones K. Neu-Laxova syndrome. In: *Smith's recognizable patterns of human malformation*, 5th ed. Philadelphia: WB Saunders, 1997:180–181.

Neu RL, et al. A lethal syndrome of microcephaly with multiple congenital anomalies in three siblings. *Pediatrics* 1971;47:610.

Pivnick EK, Gilbert-Barness E, Laxova RL, et al. Long term survival and trisomy 8 mosaicism in a patient with Neu-Laxova syndrome. 2001.

Shapiro I, et al. Neu-Laxova syndrome: prenatal ultrasonographic diagnosis, clinical and pathological studies, and new manifestations. *Am J Med Genet* 1992;43:602.

RESOURCE

368

---

60 Neurofibromatosis Type 1

M. Priscilla Short, MD

DEFINITION: Neurofibromatosis type 1 (NF1) is characterized by benign tumors involving peripheral nerves (neurofibromas), café-au-lait skin macules, and axillary and inguinal freckling. Other findings may include bony lesions, learning disabilities, short stature, and optic glioma.

SYNONYMS: Von Recklinghausen disease; Peripheral neurofibromatosis.

DIFFERENTIAL DIAGNOSIS: Neurofibromatosis type 2; Multiple café-au-lait spots; McCune-Albright syndrome; Tuberous sclerosis.

SYMPTOMS AND SIGNS: Various aspects of the disease emerge with age. At birth, the most common finding is multiple café-au-lait spots. Features that occur in early childhood include axillary and inguinal freckling, Lisch nodules, and large head and short stature. Congenital bony lesions are also seen, particularly pseudoarthrosis and sphenoid wing hypoplasia. Learning disabilities including hyperactivity are common. Optic gliomas sometimes occur. Rarely, hypertension may be noted related to renal artery stenosis or pheochromocytoma of the adrenal gland. As children enter adolescence, most will have the characteristic Lisch nodules on the irises, and cutaneous neurofibromas begin to appear and continue into early adulthood. Scoliosis may become apparent. Malignant nerve sheath tumors may occur in early to mid-adulthood and typically arise in plexiform neurofibromas. Typically, neurologic function is maintained, although pain may be associated with size and location. Rare occurrence of stroke has been reported. Other rare complications include late or early onset of puberty, astrocytomas of the brain and spinal cord, cerebrovascular malformation, and seizure disorders.

ETIOLOGY/EPIDEMIOLOGY: NF1 is inherited as an autosomal-dominant disorder in nearly half of patients and as a new mutation in the remaining patients. The disease is due to a mutation in the neurofibromin gene on chromosome 17. The incidence of NF1 is reported to be 1 in 3,500, and the prevalence has been estimated to be 1 in 4,400. It occurs equally in both sexes and it is not associated with a specific ethnic or racial group.

DIAGNOSIS: Two of the following features are necessary to make a clinical diagnosis of NF1: six or more café-au-lait spots more than 5 mm in diameter in prepubertal children and larger than 15 mm after puberty; two or more neurofibromas of any type or one plexiform neurofibroma; freckling in the axillary or inguinal region; an optic glioma; two or more Lisch nodules; a distinctive, bony lesion, such as sphenoid wing dysplasia or thinning of a long bone with or without pseudoarthrosis; or a first-degree relative with NF1 by these criteria.

TREATMENT

Standard Therapies: Routine pediatric ophthalmologic evaluation is recommended, as is MRI for any children with detected visual changes or neurologic changes. Neurofibromas can be surgically removed. For learning disabilities, early attention and intervention such as special education is recommended. For patients with progression of optic glioma, chemotherapy and, less often, radiation therapy are recommended. Plexiform neurofibromas can grow and produce problems related to location and size and surgical removal is a consideration. Because the tumor is integral to a functional nerve, excision can produce neurologic deficits. In some cases, surgical debulking may preserve essential function with minor sensory loss. Malignant degeneration of a plexiform neurofibroma occurs in less than 10% of patients. Current therapy includes strategic timing of radiation, surgery, and chemotherapy. If renal artery stenosis or a pheochromocytoma is present, surgical treatment is effective.

Investigational Therapies: Aspects of NF1 under investigation include plexiform neurofibromas, optic gliomas, pheochromocytomas, and malignant nerve sheath tumors.

REFERENCES
Friedman JM, Gutmann DH, MacCollin M, et al., eds. *Neurofibromatosis: phenotype, natural history and pathogenesis,* 3rd ed. Baltimore: John Hopkins University Press, 1999.
Friedman JM. Neurofibromatosis 1. Available at *www.geneclinics.org.*
Gutmann DH, Aylsworth A, Carey JC, et al. The diagnostic evaluation and multidisciplinary management of neurofibromatosis 1 and neurofibromatosis 2. *JAMA* 1997;278:51–57.
Huson SM, Hughes RAC, eds. *The neurofibromatoses: a pathogenetic and clinical overview.* London: Chapman & Hall Medical, 1994.

RESOURCES
317, 341, 346, 368

61 Neurofibromatosis Type 2

M. Priscilla Short, MD

DEFINITION: Neurofibromatosis type 2 (NF2) is a distinctly different disease from neurofibromatosis type 1 (NF1) and is characterized by bilateral vestibular schwannomas (benign nerve sheath tumors) that cause symptoms of hearing loss, balance problems, and, in cases of large tumors, palsies of other cranial nerves and cerebellar dysfunction.

SYNONYMS: Neurofibromatosis, central type; Bilateral acoustic neuromas; Bilateral vestibular schwannomas.

DIFFERENTIAL DIAGNOSIS: Neurofibromatosis type 1; Multiple schwannomatosis.

SYMPTOMS AND SIGNS: Loss of hearing is the most common presenting symptom of patients with NF2 secondary to compression of the acoustic branch of the 8th cranial nerve by schwannomas developing on the vestibular branch. Hearing loss can be gradual or occur more suddenly. Mild tinnitus or ringing in the ear is common, as is disturbance of balance. Less commonly, individuals present with visual disturbance related to lenticular opacities or with skin bumps. Meningiomas arise in NF2, but generally do not precede the appearance of schwannomas. More serious neurologic problems such as weakness in the arms or legs can arise when tumors are large or glial tumors arise involving the brainstem or spinal cord. In a few patients, symptoms and signs of a peripheral neuropathy that resembles Charcot-Marie-Tooth disease have been present. Malignant degeneration of schwannomas is rare.

ETIOLOGY/EPIDEMIOLOGY: The disorder is inherited in an autosomal-dominant manner in nearly 50% of cases. It is due to a mutation in a gene encoding for merlin, a cytoskeletal protein on chromosome 22. The prevalence is estimated at 1 in 37,000 individuals. No apparent gender or racial predilection exists. There is some suggestion of genotype/phenotype correlation, with some types of mutations associated with more mild disease manifestations.

DIAGNOSIS: The diagnostic criteria include individuals with bilateral vestibular schwannomas as visualized by MRI, a parent or child with bilateral vestibular schwannomas, NF2, plus either a unilateral vestibular schwannoma detected before the age of 30 or two of any of the following findings: meningiomas, glioma, schwannoma, or juvenile posterior subcapsular lenticular opacity. Given the availability of mutational analysis for further confirmation, NF2 should also be considered in anyone who presents with a unilateral vestibular schwannoma before the age of 30 and one of the following: meningioma, glioma, schwannoma, juvenile posterior subcapsular lenticular opacities/juvenile cortical cataracts. Likewise, the diagnosis should be considered for an individual who has multiple meningiomas and one of the following: glioma, schwannoma, or the previously described lenticular abnormality.

TREATMENT

Standard Therapies: Routine audiology tests to assess pure tone acuity and speech threshold are important in assessing treatment options for patients. Given the typical slow growth of NF2-associated tumors, repeat studies should be done before consideration of surgery unless the size of the tumor is endangering the patient's life. Timing of surgery should take into consideration the bilateral nature of disease and the goal of maintaining usable hearing for as long as possible. Surgical approach likewise is informed by the same goal, with preservation of the 8th nerve if possible. For some patients, particularly those who are poor surgical candidates, noninvasive gamma knife therapy may be used for tumor reduction. For patients who have minimal hearing left, auditory brainstem implants provide some hearing. Brainstem implants along with lip reading instruction provide some patients with serviceable hearing.

Investigational Therapies: The effectiveness of fractionated radiotherapy on vestibular schwannomas is being explored. The use of the tyrosine kinase inhibitor STI571 for NF2-associated meningiomas is also being investigated.

REFERENCES

Friedman JM. Neurofibromatosis 1. Available at *www.geneclinics. org.*

Friedman JM, Gutmann DH, MacCollin M, et al., eds. *Neurofibromatosis: phenotype, natural history and pathogenesis,* 3rd ed. Baltimore: John Hopkins University Press, 1999.

Gutmann DH, Aylsworth A, Carey JC, et al. The diagnostic evaluation and multidisciplinary management of neurofibromatosis 1 and neurofibromatosis 2. *JAMA* 1997;278:51–57.

Huson SM, Hughes RAC, eds. *The neurofibromatoses: a pathogenetic and clinical overview.* London: Chapman & Hall Medical, 1994.

RESOURCES

74, 317, 341, 370

62 Neuroleptic Malignant Syndrome

Adelaide S. Robb, MD

DEFINITION: Neuroleptic malignant syndrome (NMS) is a constellation of symptoms characterized by severe muscle rigidity and elevated temperature in individuals taking neuroleptic medications.

SYNONYM: Malignant catatonia.

DIFFERENTIAL DIAGNOSIS: Malignant hyperthermia; Drug reactions and interactions including monoamine oxidase inhibitors with or without tricyclics, serotonergic agents, meperidine, lithium toxicity, amphetamines, fenfluramine, cocaine, and phencyclidine; Anticholinergic syndromes; Serotonin syndrome; Central nervous system (CNS) or systemic infections; Neurologic conditions; Abrupt discontinuation of antiparkinsonian medications in a patient with Parkinson disease; Treatment with dopamine depleting agents; Heat stroke; Lethal catatonia in patients with untreated schizophrenia or mania.

SYMPTOMS AND SIGNS: NMS presents as a constellation of major and minor symptoms in patients who are being treated with neuroleptics. The three major symptoms are high fever, muscle rigidity, and elevated creatine phosphokinase (CPK). Minor manifestations include tachycardia, tachypnea, diaphoresis, altered consciousness, abnormal blood pressure, leukocytosis, and myoglobinuria.

ETIOLOGY/EPIDEMIOLOGY: The incidence of the disorder is 0.4%–1.4% of all patients treated with neuroleptics. The symptoms are more likely to occur in patients taking high-potency neuroleptics. Males and females are both affected, and it occurs in all ethnic groups. Increased risks include prior history of NMS, use of high-potency neuroleptics, male gender, being elderly, nonpsychiatric CNS pathology (Alzheimer disease, mental retardation), and extreme agitation.

DIAGNOSIS: The diagnosis is confirmed after examining the patient, obtaining the history, and ruling out other causes of high fever, agitation, and autonomic instability. Physical tests may include vital signs, electrocardiography, spinal tap, and blood and urine cultures. Laboratory examination should include complete blood count with differential count, CPK with MB bands, urinalysis and urine myoglobin, liver function tests, electrolytes, serum urea nitrogen, creatinine, and glucose. Urine and blood toxicology screens are also helpful to rule out use of illicit drugs associated with hyperthermia.

TREATMENT

Standard Therapies: Standard therapy is supportive with vigorous intravenous hydration, antipyretics, and immediate cessation of the neuroleptic medication. Evaluation for sepsis is always medically indicated. Benzodiazepines may be used if sedation is needed for an underlying psychiatric illness. Disease-specific therapies include muscle relaxants and dopaminergic agents, including bromocriptine, levodopa-carbidopa, and amantadine. Dantrolene is a skeletal muscle relaxant used to treat malignant hyperthermia and NMS. It can be used with or without dopaminergic agents. When patients are restarted on neuroleptics, a different class of drug and preferably a lower potency agent should be used.

Investigational Therapies: Electroconvulsive therapy is used as an alternate/investigational treatment. If muscle necrosis is severe, hemodialysis may be needed to prevent renal failure due to extensive myoglobinuria.

REFERENCES

Addonizio G, Susman V, Roth S. Neuroleptic malignant syndrome: review and analysis of 115 cases. *Biol Psychiatry* 1987; 22:1004–1020.

American Psychiatric Association. *Diagnostic and statistical manual of mental disorders,* 4th ed. Washington, DC: American Psychiatric Association, 1994.

Delay J, Pichot P, Lemperiere T. Un neroleptique majeur non phenothiazin et non resepenique, l'haloperidol, dans le traitement des psychoses. *Ann Med Psychol* 1960;118:145–152.

Robb AS, Chang WL, Lee HK, et al. Risperidone-induced neuroleptic malignant syndrome in an adolescent. *J Child Adolesc Psycopharmacol* 2000;10:327–330.

Silva R, Munoz D, Alpert M, et al. Neuroleptic malignant syndrome in children and adolescents. *J Am Acad Child Adolesc Psychiatry* 1999;38:187–194.

RESOURCES

254, 367, 376

63 Neuromyelitis Optica

Brian G. Weinshenker, MD

DEFINITION: Neuromyelitis optica (NMO) is an inflammatory demyelinating disease of the central nervous system that selectively targets the optic nerves and spinal cord.

SYNONYMS: Devic disease/syndrome; Opticospinal variant of multiple sclerosis (MS).

DIFFERENTIAL DIAGNOSIS: MS; Sarcoidosis; MS-like presentation associated with Leber mutations in mitochondrial DNA (Harding disease); Glioma; Dural arteriovenous fistula; Optic nerve glioma.

SYMPTOMS AND SIGNS: NMO manifests as acute or subacute attacks of visual loss or blindness, motor weakness, sensory impairment, and bladder and bowel dysfunction. Although the attacks range widely in severity, compared with those of MS, they are more severe. Attacks are followed by some degree of recovery, but ultimately disability accumulates in most cases, which can lead to severe neurologic impairment and/or death. Neuromyelitis optica may be monophasic with nearly simultaneous bilateral optic neuritis and myelitis. More commonly, it is a relapsing disease with repeated attacks of unilateral optic neuritis and myelitis separated by periods of remission. Attacks often occur in clusters separated by weeks or months. If the upper cervical spinal cord is involved, fatal respiratory failure may occur. Lesions in the cord may extend into the lower brainstem and result in nausea or bulbar symptoms. Patients with NMO may experience systemic symptoms, including fever or malaise at onset. Radicular pain, which is infrequent in MS, is common. Paroxysmal tonic spasms are common. Although tonic spasms also occur in MS, they are more frequent and severe in NMO.

ETIOLOGY/EPIDEMIOLOGY: NMO occurs in individuals of all races; however, there is a predilection for Asians and possibly Africans. Individuals of any age may be affected, but typically NMO occurs in late middle-aged women. Equal numbers of men and women have monophasic NMO, but women are fourfold to fivefold more commonly affected by the relapsing form. NMO is likely an autoimmune disease.

DIAGNOSIS: The diagnosis is primarily clinical, but paraclinical investigations are helpful. Spinal cord lesions are longitudinally extensive on MRI and extend over three or more vertebral segments, which is unusual in MS. MRI scans of the brain are usually normal or do not show the typical lesions of MS, except in patients who exhibit enhancement and/or swelling of the optic nerve and chiasm during an acute attack of optic neuritis. Spinal fluid analyses typically do not show the oligoclonal bands that are found in MS. During an attack, pleocytosis may be prominent with more than 50 white blood cells/mm^3, and occasionally neutrophilic pleocytosis may occur. Serologic evidence for autoimmunity is common. Various autoantibodies may be detected, the most common of which are antibodies to extractable nuclear antigens and in particular to SS-A antigen.

TREATMENT

Standard Therapies: For acute attacks, the standard treatment is high-dose intravenous corticosteroids, typically methylprednisolone. Plasma exchange may be effective in patients with inflammatory demyelinating disease, including neuromyelitis optica, who experience acute severe attacks that do not respond to intravenous corticosteroids. For long-term suppression of the disease, no specific treatment has been proven, but azathioprine is regarded by many clinicians as first-line therapy. For treatment of paroxysmal tonic spasms, low doses of carbamazepine or other anticonvulsants are highly effective. Complications such as spasticity are managed with baclofen or other antispasticity agents.

REFERENCES

Mandler RN, Ahmed W, Dencoff JE. Devic's neuromyelitis optica: a prospective study of seven patients treated with prednisone and azathioprine. *Neurology* 1998;51:1219–1220.

Mandler RN, Davis LE, Jeffery DR, et al. Devic's neuromyelitis optica: a clinicopathological study of 8 patients. *Ann Neurol* 1993;34:162–168.

O'Riordan J, Gallagher H, Thompson A, et al. Clinical, CSF, and MRI findings in Devic's neuromyelitis optica. *J Neurol Neurosurg Psychiatry* 1996;60:382–387.

Weinshenker BG, O'Brien PC, Petterson TM, et al. A randomized trial of plasma exchange in patients with acute CNS inflammatory demyelinating disease. *Ann Neurol* 1999;46:878–886.

Wingerchuck DM, Hogancamp WF, O'Brien PC, et al. The clinical course of neuromyelitis optica (Devic's syndrome). *Neurology* 1999;53:1107–1114.

RESOURCES

27, 355, 368

64   Congenital Hypomyelination Neuropathy

*Tena Rosser, MD,
and Phillip L. Pearl, MD*

DEFINITION: Congenital hypomyelination neuropathy (CHN) is a hereditary congenital polyneuropathy with onset in infancy characterized clinically by hypotonia, nonprogressive muscle weakness, areflexia, and slow nerve conduction velocities. It lies within the emerging spectrum of hereditary myelinopathies.

SYNONYMS: Congenital hypomyelinating neuropathy; Congenital amyelinating neuropathy.

DIFFERENTIAL DIAGNOSIS: Hereditary motor and sensory neuropathy (HMSN) type III or Dejerine-Sottas syndrome (DSS); Giant axonal neuropathy; Infantile neuroaxonal dystrophy.

SYMPTOMS AND SIGNS: Neonatal and infantile forms of CHN have been described. The neonatal form generally presents as severe hypotonia at birth, often with respiratory failure. Prolonged ventilatory support may be necessary into early childhood. Arthrogryposis multiplex has been documented in some patients. Children who survive beyond the neonatal period are occasionally able to crawl or walk with assistance. Infantile CHN manifests between ages 3 and 8 months with hypotonia, poor head control, delayed motor development, and poor feeding. The neurologic examination often shows muscle atrophy with wasting and areflexia. Several patients are able to stand and walk with assistance by age 2–3 years. Thus, strength may improve with time. Sensory ataxia is evident in older children. Associated orthopedic complications include scoliosis, pes planus, and pes cavus. Cognitive development may be normal. Seizures have been reported. The long-term prognosis is not well documented and is highly variable.

ETIOLOGY/EPIDEMIOLOGY: The disorder occurs sporadically and most likely results from impaired myelin formation. Mutations in the peripheral myelin protein-22 (PMP-22), myelin protein zero (MPZ/Po), and early growth response 2 (*EGR2*) genes have all been reported. These genetic defects have considerable overlap with the various hereditary motor and sensory neuropathies.

DIAGNOSIS: Nerve conduction velocities (NCVs) and sural nerve biopsy in conjunction with clinical history and physical examination establish the diagnosis. Traditionally considered a severe form of DSS, CHN is increasingly believed to be a distinct entity within the spectrum of congenital myelinopathies. These two disorders can be differentiated on a clinical as well as a pathophysiologic basis. In CHN, NCVs are severely delayed. In many patients they are undetectable but when present are typically less than 5–10 m/s. Sural nerve biopsy shows two possible patterns: absent myelin with no onion bulb formation or severe hypomyelination with atypical onion bulbs, described as concentric whirls of redundant basement membrane. In contrast to DSS, there is no evidence of demyelination, inflammation, or myelin breakdown products in CHN. Axons are normal. Central nervous system myelination is not affected.

TREATMENT

Standard Therapies: Management is primarily supportive. Ventilatory support may be required through the neonatal period and occasionally into early childhood. Thorough developmental evaluation with early interventional services such as physical, occupational, and speech therapy can help maximize each patient's individual abilities. Lower extremity braces, crutches, wheelchairs, and other assistive devices aid in mobilization and in performing activities of daily living. Aggressive management of the complications of hypotonia, such as recurrent infections and feeding problems, may also improve quality of life.

REFERENCES

Boylan KB, Ferriero DM, Greco CM, et al. Congenital hypomyelination neuropathy with arthrogryposis multiplex congenita. *Ann Neurol* 1992;31:337–340.

Fabrizi GM, Simonati A, Taioli F, et al. PMP22 related congenital hypomyelination neuropathy. *J Neurol Neurosurg Psychiatry* 2001;70:123–126.

Harding AE. From the syndrome of Charcot, Marie, and Tooth to disorders of peripheral myelin proteins. *Brain* 1995;118:809–818.

Mandich P, Mancardi GL, Varese A, et al. Congenital hypomyelination due to myelin protein zero Q215X mutation. *Ann Neurol* 1999;45:676–678.

Phillips JP, Warner LE, Lupski JR, et al. Congenital hypomyelinating neuropathy: two patients with long-term follow-up. *Pediatr Neurol* 1999;20:226–232.

RESOURCES

27, 368

65　Giant Axonal Neuropathy

Adeline Vanderver, MD,
and Phillip L. Pearl, MD

DEFINITION: Giant axonal neuropathy is a progressive mixed peripheral neuropathy with central nervous system (CNS) involvement associated with abnormal cytoskeletal proteins.

SYNONYM: Giant axonal disease.

DIFFERENTIAL DIAGNOSIS: Infantile neuroaxonal dystrophy; Early-onset Friederich ataxia; Vitamin B_{12} deficiency; Neurotoxins; Renal tubular acidosis.

SYMPTOMS AND SIGNS: Children with giant axonal neuropathy present in early infancy and childhood, usually by age 3 years but occasionally later. Patients have progressive gait disturbance, pale kinky hair, long curly eyelashes, and a prominently high forehead. Findings on examination may include both peripheral and CNS findings such as hypotonia, distal weakness, diminished tendon reflexes, and gait disturbance, or, conversely, more prominent seizures, cerebellar signs, mental retardation, and spasticity. Cranial nerves may also be affected, with optic atrophy or external opthalmoplegia. The generalized hypotonia is not accompanied by fasciculations. Some case reports have suggested a peculiar posture of the lower extremities consisting of eversion of the feet with thigh adduction and splaying of the legs. Skeletal abnormalities have been described but are likely secondary to motor disease and include scoliosis and foot deformities among others. Patients presenting in infancy may have a history of neonatal respiratory or feeding problems. Motor milestones may be delayed if onset of symptoms occurs before the acquisition of independent walking. Different systems may be variably involved. Rapid progression leads to early death, often by adolescence and nearly always by the third decade.

ETIOLOGY/EPIDEMIOLOGY: Early reports of parental consanguinity and affected siblings suggested an autosomal-recessive pattern of inheritance. Recent gene mapping led to the identification of a locus on 16q24 (*GAN*).

This locus was subsequently found to encode the expression of a novel, ubiquitous protein named gigaxonin. A possible genetic heterogeneity suggested by a difference in clinical course in Tunisian patients led to linkage of a locus also on 16q24 named *GAN1*. No exact incidence of this disorder has been reported.

DIAGNOSIS: When performed, results of electroencephalography and visual, auditory, and somatosensory evoked potentials have been abnormal. Electromyography shows axonal neuropathy. Peripheral nerve biopsies are notable for axonal loss with striking abnormalities of remaining fibers. Segmental distention occurs of distal axons with bundles of neurofilaments, or giant axonal swellings. Central nervous system findings show similar axonal swellings filled with neurofilaments. Pathologic findings with accumulation of other intermediate filaments have also been described in Schwann, endothelial, perineurial, and endoneurial cells, in melanocytes, and in fibroblasts, suggesting a generalized disorganization of cytoskeletal intermediate filaments.

TREATMENT
Standard Therapies: The only treatment is supportive care.

REFERENCES
Berg BO, Rosenberg SH, Asbury AK. Giant axonal neuropathy. *Pediatrics* 1972;49:894–899.
Bomont P, Cavalier L, Blondeau F, et al. The gene encoding gigaxonin, a new member of the BTB/kelch repeat family, is mutated in giant axonal neuropathy. *Nat Genet* 2000;26:370–374.
Flanigan KM, Crawford TO, Griffin JW, et al. Localization of the giant axonal neuropathy gene to chromosome 16q24. *Ann Neurol* 1998;43:143–148.
Igisu H, Ohta M, Tabira T, et al. Giant axonal neuropathy, a clinical entity affecting the central as well as the peripheral nervous system. *Neurology* 1975;25:717–721.
Swaiman KE, Ashwal S, eds. *Pediatric neurology: principles and practice*, 3rd ed. St. Louis: CV Mosby, 1999:1189–1190.

RESOURCE
368

66   Hereditary Sensory Neuropathy Type I

Sylvia Mandler, MD, and Phillip L. Pearl, MD

DEFINITION: The hereditary sensory neuropathies are a clinically and genetically heterogeneous group of degenerative disorders affecting sensory neurons. Classification into several subtypes is based on clinical symptoms, age at onset, and mode of inheritance. Clinically, they variably combine severe sensory symptoms, trophic skin alterations, and dysautonomia. Hereditary sensory neuropathy type I (HSN-I) is an autosomal-dominant progressive degeneration of dorsal root ganglia and motor neurons. It is the most common hereditary disorder of peripheral sensory neurons.

SYNONYMS: Hereditary sensory and autonomic neuropathy type I (HSAN-I); Thevenard disease.

DIFFERENTIAL DIAGNOSIS: Charcot-Marie-Tooth 2B; Roussy-Levy syndrome; Dejerine-Sottas syndrome; Hereditary neuropathy with liability to pressure palsies (tomaculous neuropathy); Pure neuritic leprosy; Morvan disease; Acroosteolysis.

SYMPTOMS AND SIGNS: Onset is usually during the second or third decade of life. Initial symptoms are typically sensory loss in the feet, which may be followed by distal muscle wasting and weakness. "Burning feet" may be the only manifestation, which is characteristically improved by cold and exacerbated by heat. Loss of pain sensation may lead to chronic skin ulcers and distal amputations. In severe cases, patients have recurrent perforating ulcers of the feet and somatic shooting pains, similar to the lightning pains of tabes dorsalis. Skin lesions may lead to chronic skin ulcers, osteomyelitis, and extrusion of bone fragments. Restless legs and lancinating pain also may occur. Patients may develop progressive deafness over several years. Neurologic examination shows disappearance of ankle and knee reflexes. Loss of pain, touch, and temperature sensation occurs, primarily affecting the feet and sometimes the hands. Cranial nerves are normal except for the auditory nerve.

ETIOLOGY/EPIDEMIOLOGY: The disorder is an autosomal-dominant condition and the locus has been mapped to chromosome 9q22.1-22.3. This corresponds to the gene *SPTLC1*, encoding serine palmitoyltransferase and expressed in the dorsal root ganglia. In one study, mutation screening showed three different missense mutations resulting in changes to two amino acids in all affected members of 11 HSN-I families. Other mutations are described, some associated with increased *de novo* glucosyl ceramide synthesis in lymphoblast cell lines of affected individuals. Increased ceramide synthesis triggers apoptosis and is associated with massive cell death during neural tube closure, raising the possibility that neural degeneration in HSN-I is due to ceramide-induced apoptotic cell death.

DIAGNOSIS: The diagnosis is based on clinical findings of a distal sensory neuropathy, distal muscle wasting, and sometimes hearing loss. Nerve conduction velocities show evidence of an axonal neuropathy. Sural nerve biopsies show marked loss of myelinated fibers and comparable loss of unmyelinated fibers. No biochemical marker is known for these conditions.

TREATMENT
Standard Therapies: Treatment is palliative and symptomatic. Daily visual inspection and early treatment of ulcers and infections are indicated. Somatic shooting pains may be treated with medications commonly used for peripheral neuropathy, such as amitryptiline, carbamazepine, and gabapentin.

REFERENCES
Bejaoui K, McKenna-Yasek D, Hosler BA, et al. Confirmation of linkage of type 1 hereditary sensory neuropathy to human chromosome 9q22. *Neurology* 1999;52:510–515.

Campbell AM, Hofman HL. Sensory radicular neuropathy associated with muscle wasting in two cases. *Brain* 1964;87:67–74.

Danon MJ, Carpenter S. Hereditary sensory neuropathy: biopsy study of an autosomal dominant variety. *Neurology* 1985;35: 1226–1229.

Dawkins JL, Hulme DJ, Brahmbhatt SB, et al. Mutations in *SPTLC1*, encoding serine palmitoyltransferase, long chain base subunit-1, cause hereditary sensory neuropathy type 1. *Nat Genet* 2001;27:309–312.

Denny-Brown D. Hereditary sensory radicular neuropathy. *J Neurol Neurosurg Psychiatry* 1952;14:237–252.

RESOURCE
368

67   Hereditary Sensory Neuropathy Type II

Sylvia Mandler, MD,
and Phillip L. Pearl, MD

DEFINITION: The hereditary sensory neuropathies are still in the process of being classified. Hereditary sensory neuropathy type II (HSN II) is a progressive disorder of peripheral sensory nerves in which impairment of sweating is a cardinal sign. The mode of transmission may be recessive. A dominantly inherited form has also been described.

SYNONYM: Hereditary sensory autonomic neuropathy type II.

DIFFERENTIAL DIAGNOSIS: Charcot-Marie-Tooth 2B; Hereditary neuropathy with liability to pressure palsies (tomaculous neuropathy); Acroosteolysis; Dejerine-Sottas syndrome.

SYMPTOMS AND SIGNS: In general, all patients have insensitivity to pain and anhidrosis. Onset of symptoms usually occurs in the second decade of life, with decreased sensation involving the feet and legs. Mutilating acropathy is not as common as in HSN-I, but patients may present with penetrating foot ulcers and acral sensory impairment. Some patients may have muscle hypertrophy caused by sustained muscle contractions. Some children with this condition have presented with slowly progressive gait spasticity, and others with temperature elevation due to impairment of sweating. They may also be cognitively impaired for unclear reasons.

DIAGNOSIS: Absence of sensory nerve action potentials with normal motor nerve conduction velocities are typical. Sural nerve biopsy shows total loss of myelinated fibers with relative preservation of unmyelinated fibers. Sweating induced by iontophoretic pilocarpine is decreased on the dorsum of the feet. Histamine testing evokes no axonal flare. Morphometric analysis of sudomotor nerves around sweat glands shows a decreased number of nerve terminals. Sweat glands appear normal on skin biopsy.

TREATMENT
Standard Therapies: Treatment is palliative and symptomatic. The sweating impairment may cause a body temperature increase unrelated to infection.

REFERENCES

Bye AM, Baker WD, Pollard J, et al. Hereditary sensory neuropathy type II without trophic changes. *Dev Med Child Neurol* 1990;32:164–171.
Cavanagh NP, Eames RA, Galvin RJ, et al. Hereditary sensory neuropathy with spastic paraplegia. *Brain* 1979;102:79–94.
Dyck PJ, Ohta M. Neuronal atrophy and degeneration predominantly affecting peripheral sensory neurons. In: *Peripheral neuropathy*. Toronto: WB Saunders, 1975:791–824.
Nukada H, Pollock M, Haas LF. The clinical spectrum and morphology of type II hereditary sensory neuropathy. *Brain* 1982;105:647–665.
Robinson GC, Jan JE, Miller JR. A new variety of hereditary sensory neuropathy. *Hum Genet* 1977;35:153–161.

RESOURCE
368

68   Obstetric Brachial Plexus Palsy

Christina Strömbeck, MD,
and Hans Forssberg, MD, PhD

DEFINITION: An obstetric brachial plexus (OBP) injury is caused by a traction injury of two or more nerves in the brachial plexus (C5 to Th1) during delivery. Injury involving C5–6 nerves causes a palsy of the arm but not the hand (Erb-Duchennes paralysis). Injury of C8 to Th1 causes a palsy of the hand (Klumpke paralysis). If all the nerves in the plexus are involved, the entire arm and hand will be affected.

SYNONYMS: OBP lesion; Erb-Duchenne paralysis; Klumpke paralysis.

DIFFERENTIAL DIAGNOSIS: Fracture of the clavicle and humerus; Artrogryphosis; Hemiplegic or monoplegic form of cerebral palsy.

SYMPTOMS AND SIGNS: In newborns, upper plexus injury including C5–6 results in a flaccid arm without movement in the shoulder joint and elbow joint. The arm is often in adduction and internal rotation of the shoulder joint and the forearm are in pronation. The Moro reflex is absent but the grasp reflex is normal. These injuries usually lead to the milder form of nerve injury, which has a favorable prognosis with spontaneous recovery in approximately 75% of all infants who have symptoms at birth. If C7 also is injured, the wrist is in volar flexion with ulnar deviation and the fingers are flexed. In rare cases, the phrenic nerve is affected, but usually it recovers within 1–3 months. In the complete OBP lesion (C5 to Th1), the entire arm-hand is flaccid. There is often a Horner sign (mios-, ptos-, or enophthalmus). Upper OBP may lead to a decreased abduction, flexion, and external rotation in the shoulder joint, often with humeroscapular contractures. In the forearm, the strength is reduced in all directions. Flexion contractures are common in the elbow joint. Even if the child has good hand and forearm function, he or she often uses the arm in a position of extreme internal rotation. Affected children with complete lesions often gain some function in the shoulder joint and elbow joint but no or only minor activity in the hand. The sensibility of the arm and hand is also influenced.

ETIOLOGY/EPIDEMIOLOGY: An OBP injury is caused by a traction injury during delivery. The incidence is approximately 1–2 per 1,000 births in countries with well-developed obstetric services. The injury is more common in children with birth weight exceeding +2 SD. Nerve fibers sustain different types of damage. The mildest form is an edema in the peripheral nerve (neurapraxia) where the function of the nerve fibers returns within a couple of weeks. In a more severe form, the nerve fibers are disrupted while the myelin sheath remains intact (axonotmesis). In these cases, the function usually returns within months. In the most severe injuries, the nerve fiber is totally disrupted (neurotmesis), or the roots are pulled out of the spinal cord (root avulsion). Patients with OBP lesions often have all types of nerve fiber damage.

DIAGNOSIS: The newborn has a typical birth history; the affected arm is flaccid and the Moro reflex is asymmetric. If the disorder is suspected after the infant period, diagnosis is based on the typical clinical presentation.

TREATMENT
Standard Therapies: Physiotherapy with gentle range of motion exercises should start as soon as possible to avoid contractures, particularly the internal rotation contracture of the shoulder and the flexion contracture of the elbow. Surgery often has to be performed to correct subluxation or luxation of the shoulder joint. In severe OBP lesions, reconstructive microsurgery of the damaged nerves can regain connectivity between motor neurons and muscles. This operation should be performed during the first year of life. If the paralysis persists without improvement in a complete plexus injury after 2 months and in an upper plexus injury after 3–6 months, the child should be seen by a surgeon. Electromyography can be used to explore whether there is a regeneration process of the nerve fibers (reinnervation potentials) or if the damage is permanent (denervation potentials). Before microsurgery, CT or MRI myelography of the spinal cord can be performed to discover root avulsions of the nerve.

REFERENCES
Eng GD, Koch B, Smokvina MD. Brachial plexus palsy in neonates an children. *Arch Phys Med Rehabil* 1978;59:458–464.
Gilbert A, Tassin JL. Surgical repair of the brachial plexus in obstetric paralysis. *Chirurgie* 1984;110:70–75.
Narakas AO. Obstetrical brachial plexus injuries. In: Lamb DW, ed. *The paralyzed hand.* Edinburgh: Churchill Livingstone, 1986:116–135.
Strömbeck C, Krumlinde-Sundholm L, Forssberg H. Functional outcome at 5 years in children with obstetrical brachial plexus palsy with and without microsurgical reconstruction. *Dev Med Child Neurol* 2000;42:148–157.

RESOURCES
70, 71, 368

---

69   Opsoclonus-Myoclonus Syndrome

Michael R. Pranzatelli, MD

DEFINITION: Opsoclonus-myoclonus syndrome (OMS) is a disorder of opsoclonus, myoclonus, ataxia, and encephalopathy. Opsoclonus is an unusual disorder of eye movement in which both eyes dart involuntarily. *Myoclonus* means brief, involuntary muscle jerks.

SYNONYMS: Kinsbourne syndrome; Dancing eyes–dancing feet.

DIFFERENTIAL DIAGNOSIS: Acute cerebellar ataxia.

SYMPTOMS AND SIGNS: Myoclonus occurs with movement, worsens with agitation or stimulation, and may be present at rest. The patient may appear tremulous or have gross jerking. Face, eyelids, limbs, fingers, head, and trunk are involved. During the peak of the illness, sitting or standing is difficult or impossible. Patients also have trouble speaking, eating, or sleeping, and exhibit drooling, rage attacks, head tilt, or other abnormalities. Children appear to be nervous, irritable, or lethargic, whereas adults may have mental clouding.

ETIOLOGY/EPIDEMIOLOGY: The syndrome often follows an apparent viral infection, such as the flu. Most children are younger than 2 years when diagnosed. Males and females are nearly equally affected. Viral infections account for almost half of the cases of OMS. Because some patients who present with flulike symptoms later turn out to have a tumor, the presence of a viral infection should not preclude the search for a tumor. Tumors are found in approximately half of patients with OMS. The most common ones in children with OMS are neuroblastoma and ganglioneuroblastoma, which occur in the chest or abdomen. These tumors derive from neural crest cells, the same embryonic forerunners of brain cells. The most widely accepted theory is that the syndrome is autoimmune.

DIAGNOSIS: The search for neuroblastoma includes chest and abdominal CT scans, MIBG scan, and measurement of urinary catecholamines. Screening for serum antibodies is now a routine clinical laboratory test. Other tests are available only as research tools. IgG and IgM antibodies to neurofilament, a structural protein in the cerebellum and peripheral nerve, have been reported. Screening blood and spinal fluid for abnormal leukocytes is also important.

TREATMENT
Standard Therapies: If possible, the treatment is to remove the tumor. This may alleviate the OMS, but tumor removal often does not help and may worsen symptoms. Adrenocorticotrophic hormone (ACTH) is the gold standard for treatment. It must be given by intramuscular injection over a 20-week period. Initially, high-dose injections are given twice daily; subsequently, injections are given on alternate days during maintenance and tapering. Human intravenous immune globulins (IVIGs) are commercial preparations of antibodies that have been purified from plasma pools of healthy blood donors. Improvement may take a few weeks, and monthly doses are required to maintain remission. Azathioprine is one of the easiest immunosuppressive agents to use. It should be started at a low dose and slowly advanced over weeks. Blood tests to monitor peripheral leukocyte count, platelet count, and liver function are necessary. The delay to onset of therapeutic effect is 6–12 months, and maximum benefit may not be seen for 2 years.

Investigational Therapies: Cyclophosphamide, methotrexate, and other forms of chemotherapy are sometimes given to children with neuroblastoma. Drugs under evaluation include inhibitors of activated lymphocytes.

REFERENCES
Brodeur GM, Castelberry RP. Neuroblastoma. In: Pizzo PA, Poplack DG, eds. *Principles and practice of pediatric oncology,* 3rd ed. Philadelphia: Lippincott-Raven, 1997:761–797.
Pranzatelli MR. The neurobiology of opsoclonus-myoclonus. *Clin Neuropharmacol* 1992;15:186–228.
Pranzatelli MR. The immunopharmacology of the opsoclonus-myoclonus syndrome. *Clin Neuropharmacol* 1996;19:1–47.
Pranzatelli MR. Friendly fire. *Discover* 2000;April:35–36.
Pranzatelli MR. Paraneoplastic syndromes: an unsolved murder. *Semin Pediatr Neurol* 2000;7:188–130.

RESOURCES
322, 368, 381

70   Progressive Supranuclear Palsy

Rodger J. Elble, MD, PhD

DEFINITION: Progressive supranuclear palsy (PSP) is a degenerative disease with the classic presentation of supranuclear vertical gaze palsy, parkinsonism, postural instability, axial dystonia, pseudobulbar palsy, and dementia.

SYNONYM: Steele-Richardson-Olszewski syndrome.

DIFFERENTIAL DIAGNOSIS: Parkinson disease; Diffuse Lewy body disease; Multiple system atrophy; Corticobasal degeneration; Frontotemporal dementia; Creutzfeldt-Jakob disease.

SYMPTOMS AND SIGNS: The clinical presentation is variable. The hallmark of the disease is the progressive supranuclear impairment of eye movement, particularly in the downward direction. This abnormality, however, may not develop until late in the illness, if at all, and may not be detected except in the examination of saccadic eye movements from one target to another. Patients exhibit various combinations and degrees of poor balance, akinesia with freezing, parkinsonism without rest tremor, ataxia, dysarthria, dysphagia, axial dystonia, and dementia. The dysarthria is usually a mixture of hypophonia and pseudobulbar dysarthria, with variable degrees of festination and ataxia. Labile laughter or crying and palilalia are not uncommon. Cognitive and personality changes consist mainly of reduced motivation, initiative, concentration, impulse control, memory, and organizational skills, reflecting pathology in the frontal lobes and basal ganglia. Falls are common, and in contrast to Parkinson disease, typically begin early in the course of the illness, resulting in the early use of a wheelchair and other assistive devices. The facial expression is often fixed, but (unlike in Parkinson disease) the eyebrows and eyelids are often raised, creating a startled or wild-eyed look. In addition, the head may be tilted backward, instead of forward.

ETIOLOGY/EPIDEMIOLOGY: The prevalence is believed to be at least 6 per 100,000 people. Men and women are both affected. The illness typically begins insidiously in the fifth decade of life or later and is relentlessly progressive with severe disability or death developing in 5 years. The etiology is unknown, but this disease belongs to a large group of diseases in which intracytoplasmic neurofibrillary tangles are found in the affected areas of the brain. These tangles consist of abnormally phosphorylated tau protein, which is a normal component of the neuronal cytoskeleton. Neuronal loss, gliosis, and tangle formation are variably found in the frontal cortex, nucleus basalis of Meynert, basal ganglia, brainstem, cerebellar dentate nucleus, and spinal cord.

DIAGNOSIS: No diagnostic test exists. The condition is frequently confused with Parkinson disease and multiple system atrophy, and misdiagnosis by movement disorder specialists is common. The key features favoring the diagnosis of PSP are early disturbance of gait and balance, impaired downward gaze, and absence of rest tremor.

TREATMENT
Standard Therapies: Treatment is symptomatic and supportive. Prevention of injurious falls and aspiration quickly becomes the main concern. Speech therapists can assist in the evaluation of swallowing, and occupational and physical therapists are helpful in maximizing the safety of ambulation. Antiparkinson medications are usually tried but provide little or no benefit. Cholinesterase inhibitors (donepezil, rivastigmine, and galantamine) are occasionally helpful in the treatment of cognitive impairment. As in Parkinson disease, depression and sleep disturbances are common and usually respond to pharmacotherapy.

REFERENCES
Litvan I, Agid Y, Jankovic J, et al. Accuracy of clinical criteria for the diagnosis of progressive supranuclear palsy (Steele-Richardson-Olszewski syndrome). *Neurology* 1996;46:922–930.
Litvan I, Campbell G, Mangone CA, et al. Which clinical features differentiate progressive supranuclear palsy (Steele-Richardson-Olszewski syndrome) from related disorders? A clinicopathological study. *Brain* 1997;120:65–74.
Schrag A, Ben-Shlomo Y, Quinn NP. Prevalence of progressive supranuclear palsy and multiple system atrophy: a cross-sectional study. *Lancet* 1999;354:1771–1775.
Steele JC, Richardson JC, Olszewski J. Progressive supranuclear palsy: a heterogeneous degeneration involving brainstem, basal ganglia and cerebellum with vertical gaze and pseudobulbar palsy, nuchal dystonia and dementia. *Arch Neurol* 1964; 10:333–358.

RESOURCES
368, 442, 487

---

71   Subacute Sclerosing Panencephalitis

Paul R. Dyken, MD

DEFINITION: Subacute sclerosing panencephalitis (SSPE) is a progressive neurologic disease resulting from an altered rubeola virus attacking the nervous system.

SYNONYMS: Subacute sclerosing leukoencephalitis; Slow measles encephalitis or encephalopathy; Persistent measles infection; Diffuse sclerosis; Dawson disease; Van Bogaert-Dawson disease; Pette-Doring panencephalomyelitis.

DIFFERENTIAL DIAGNOSIS: Slow virus diseases; Neurodegenerative diseases.

SYMPTOMS AND SIGNS: After apparent full recovery from an episode of rubeola infection, there may be an asymptomatic period of 7–8 years. Early symptoms of stage I consist of disturbances in behavior and mentation such as irritability, distraction, shortened attention, impulsiveness, and forgetfulness. These evolve into temper tantrums, outbreaks of abberant behavior, failing intellectual abilities, and frank dementia. Occasional epileptic seizures occur. Neurologic impairment at this stage varies between 0 and 30% and may last for 6 months. Stage II, during which neurologic disability progresses from 33% to 55%, is characterized by involuntary movements known as massive myoclonus, consisting of sudden and repetitive movements involving more than one muscle group and both appendicular and axial musculature. Fully developed, these involuntary movements are severe, frequent, and disabling. In stage III, the involuntary movements disappear as encephalitic lesions give way to encephalopathic lesions in the basal ganglion. Immobility, rigidity, tremor (but not myoclonus), and increasing spasticity occur, and dementia worsens. Disability ranges between 55% and 80%, and the patient is completely bedridden. Stage IV is the terminal phase of the disease and may include stabilization at a plateau of severe disability that may last for years.

ETIOLOGY/EPIDEMIOLOGY: The disorder is due to the latent effects of rubeola virus as altered by the host's immune response. It is hypothesized that the matrix or M-protein of the virus becomes defective or damaged at the time the virus makes first contact with the host, usually in infancy when the immune system is immature. This condition allows a viable but altered portion of the virus (a virion) to escape to the nervous system, where the altered measles virus harbors in neurons and glia cells. Virion transmission from one cell to the next is slow and the virus is relatively dormant for years. Ultimately, the virus breaks out and thereafter does serious and rapid damage to the nervous system. The disorder is seen throughout the world, but has been decreasing in countries with effective national immunization programs for measles.

DIAGNOSIS: The rate at which symptoms develop distinguishes the classic forms of SSPE. The diagnosis rests on two essentials: (a) the presence of a typical or atypical clinical picture, and (b) elevated measles antibody titers in the spinal fluid or demonstration of measles antigen or typical viral cellular inclusions within the brain. Neuroimaging, electroencephalography, cerebral spinal fluid analysis for nonspecific gammaglobulin, and antibodies and tests for specific IgG synthesis are helpful for diagnosis.

TREATMENT

Standard Therapies: Many palliative therapies are available. In the early phases, behavioral management and/or anticonvulsants may be prescribed. Carbamazepine seems to be useful as both an anticonvulsant and as an anti–abnormal movement agent. Cerebral stimulants or tranquilizers have occasionally been helpful for hyperkinetic patients in stage I. In the severely disabled state, vigorous care of infection, sphincter function, feeding, and other life essentials are mandatory. None of these therapies are curative, however, and the best therapy is prevention.

Investigational Therapies: Oral inosiplex (Isoprinsine) alone, intrathecal synthetic interferon-α alone, and a combination of inosiplex and interferon are being investigated.

REFERENCES
Anlar B, Kose G, Gurer Y, et al. Changing epidemiological features of subacute sclerosing panencephalitis. *Infection* 2001;29: 192–195.

Dyken PR. Subacute sclerosing panencephalitis. Current status. *Neurol Clin* 1985;3:179–196.

Dyken PR. Neuroprogressive diseases of post-infectious origin: a review of a resurging subacute sclerosing panencephalitis (SSPE). *Ment Retard Dev Disabil Res Rev* 2001;7:217–225.

Dyken PR, Swift A, DuRant RH. Long-term follow-up of patients with subacute sclerosing panencephalitis treated with Inosiplex. *Ann Neurol* 1982;11:359–364.

RESOURCES
334, 359

---

72 | Hereditary Spastic Paraplegia

Jonathan K. Fink, MD

DEFINITION: Hereditary spastic paraplegia (HSP) refers to a group of clinically similar inherited disorders in which the primary symptom is bilateral lower extremity weakness and spasticity. It is classified as "uncomplicated" (pure) if neurologic abnormalities are limited to weakness and spasticity in the legs, often accompanied by mild impairment of vibration sensation in the toes, and urinary urgency. It is classified as "complicated" if, in addition, the inherited syndrome includes other abnormalities such as mental retardation, distal amyotrophy, peripheral neuropathy, extrapyramidal disturbance, optic atrophy, retinitis pigmentosa, cataracts, or gastroesophageal reflux.

SYNONYMS: Familial spastic paraplegia; Familial spastic paraparesis; Strumpell-Lorrain syndrome.

DIFFERENTIAL DIAGNOSIS: Multiple sclerosis; Vitamin B_{12} deficiency; Adrenomyeloneuropathy or other leukodystrophy; Structural disorder affecting the brain or spinal cord; Dopa-responsive dystonia.

SYMPTOMS AND SIGNS: Gait disturbance in uncomplicated HSP may begin at any age and usually progresses insidiously. Many individuals with early childhood onset of symptoms, however, have little worsening even over several decades. Neurologic examination of patients with uncomplicated HSP shows bilateral lower extremity spasticity and weakness, hyperreflexia, extensor plantar response, and often, mildly impaired vibration sensation in the toes. Although upper extremity deep tendon reflexes may be mildly brisk, subjects with uncomplicated HSP maintain normal upper extremity strength, tone, and dexterity. Pes cavus is often present. Significant variation occurs in the age at which gait disturbance begins and the degree of functional impairment within a given family, among families with the same genetic type of HSP, and among different genetic types of HSP.

ETIOLOGY/EPIDEMIOLOGY: Hereditary spastic paraplegia may be inherited as an autosomal-dominant, autosomal-recessive, or X-linked disorder. Genetic loci for HSP are designated SPG (spastic gait loci) 1–16. The most common type of dominantly inherited HSP is that due to the *SPG4* gene on chromosome 2p. Mutations in this gene (which encode the protein spastin) account for approximately 45% of dominantly inherited HSP. The only other dominantly inherited HSP gene identified is *SPG3A,* which encodes the protein atlastin. *SPG3A* mutations cause approximately 25% of childhood-onset, dominantly inherited HSP. The functions of spastin and atlastin are not known. *SPG7* gene mutations cause a rare form of autosomal-recessive HSP. The *SPG7* gene encodes paraplegin, a mitochondrial metalloprotease. *Proteolipid protein* gene mutations cause the childhood-onset, slowly progressive form of X-linked HSP. L1 cell adhesion molecule (*L1CAM*) gene mutations cause several X-linked congenital neurologic disorders, including X-linked spastic paraplegia.

DIAGNOSIS: Hereditary spastic paraplegia is diagnosed on the basis of (a) lower extremity spasticity, weakness, hyperreflexia, extensor plantar response, often accompanied by mildly impaired distal vibratory sense impairment, and urinary urgency that usually progresses insidiously; (b) family history of similarly affected relatives; and (c) exclusion of alternate disorders. Laboratory, neuroimaging, and neurophysiologic studies are helpful to exclude other disorders. Routine laboratory tests, cerebrospinal fluid analysis, electromyography, and nerve conduction studies are normal in uncomplicated HSP. Prenatal testing for the most common form of dominantly inherited HSP and X-linked HSP due to PLP gene mutation is available.

TREATMENT
Standard Therapies: No treatment will reverse or retard the underlying axonal degeneration in HSP. Treatment is directed toward maintaining and improving muscle tone and strength through physical therapy. Antispasticity medications (such as Baclofen) are often helpful to reduce muscle spasticity. Ankle-foot orthotic devices may be useful to improve gait. Oxybutinin is useful to reduce urinary urgency.

REFERENCES
Fink JK. Hereditary spastic paraplegia. In: Rimoin DL, Pyeritz RE, Connor JM, et al., eds. Emery and Rimoin's principles and practice of medical genetics, 4th ed. London: Churchill Livingston, 2001:3124–3145.

Fink JK. Progressive spastic paraparesis: hereditary spastic paraplegia and its relation to primary and amyotrophic lateral sclerosis. *Semin Neurol* 2001;21:199–208.

Fink JK, Hedera P. Hereditary spastic paraplegia: genetic heterogeneity and genotype-phenotype correlation. *Semin Neurol* 1999;19:301–309.

RESOURCES
187, 368, 487

---

73   Parkinson Disease

Abraham N. Lieberman, MD

DEFINITION: Idiopathic Parkinson disease (PD) is a slowly progressive disease of the nervous system marked by rigidity, tremor, bradykinesia, and postural instability. Degenerative processes are especially noticeable in the substantia nigra and are accompanied by a decrease in dopamine levels in the striatum.

SYNONYMS: Paralysis agitans; Shaking palsy.

DIFFERENTIAL DIAGNOSIS: Essential tremor; Multiple system atrophy; Progressive supranuclear palsy; Parkinson plus; Corticobasilar degeneration.

SYMPTOMS AND SIGNS: The principal symptoms are limb rigidity and tremor. The tremor is usually present at rest, with the limbs relaxed, and absent with the limbs innervated or moving, and it is usually asymmetric in the beginning stages. Tremor is absent in 30% of patients. Bradykinesia, slowness, or paucity of movement is the most prominent and disabling symptom. Postural instability is also a principal symptom. Secondary symptoms include difficulty in walking with festination, anteropulsion or retropulsion, and freezing; seborrhea; dementia (30% of patients, especially the elderly, may develop dementia); autonomic nervous system impairment; hypomimia or masked facies; sialorrhea; dysphagia; and kyphoscoliosis. Secondary symptoms, alone or in combination, are neither sufficient nor essential for the diagnosis of PD.

ETIOLOGY/EPIDEMIOLOGY: In the United States, the prevalence is approximately 3,500 patients per million population, with an incidence of approximately 500 patients per million population. Although PD is mainly a disorder of old age with a peak incidence at age 60 years, 5% of patients develop PD younger than age 40 years and 15% of patients develop PD younger than age 50 years. The juvenile form affects teenagers. The sex ratio is 55% male to 45% female, and whites are affected more often than blacks. The cause is unknown. Several genes may be related to PD. One is found at 4q21-q23 that codes for *alpha-synnuclein*; another at 4q21 that codes for *PARKIN 1*; another at 2p13 that codes for *PARKIN 3*; another at 4p13 that codes for *PARKIN 4*; and another at 6q25.2-q27.

DIAGNOSIS: If a patient has two or more of the primary symptoms, one of which is either resting tremor or bradykinesia, the diagnosis of PD is virtually certain. Positron emission tomographic scans or SPECT scans may, in some instances, be used to confirm difficult diagnoses. MRI may be useful in the differential diagnosis.

TREATMENT
Standard Therapies: Levodopa combined with carbidopa in a single tablet (Sinemet) is the most effective anti-PD drug and works by restoring dopamine levels in the striatum. Dopamine agonists such as pergolide, pramipexole, and ropinerole act directly without the need for dopamine. Because the long-term use of Sinemet may be associated with dyskinesias, there is an increased tendency to start newly diagnosed PD patients with an agonist and, at a later date, add Sinemet. Other agents sustain the effect of levodopa, including the COMT-inhibitor entacopone, and, to a lesser extent, the MAO-B inhibitors selegiline or deprenyl. Other useful anti-PD drugs include amantadine and several anticholinergic drugs. Thalamotomy has been used to control a disabling tremor that could not be controlled by drugs. Pallidotomy has been used to control disabling dyskinesias. Deep brain stimulation may be effective in some patients.

Investigational Therapies: Many new drugs are being tested worldwide for their potential ability to halt or retard the progression of PD. Newer techniques of transplanting neural and other cells and tissues in treating PD are also being explored.

REFERENCES
Aminoff MJ. Parkinson's disease. *Neurol Clin* 2001;19:119–128.
Bhatia K, et al., for the Parkinson's Disease Consensus Working Group. Updated guidelines for the management of Parkinson's disease. *Hosp Med* 2001;62:456–470.
Melton L. Neural transplantation: new cells for old brains. *Lancet* 2000;355:2142.
Widner H. Neural tissue xerografting in neurogenrative disorders: countdown to a clinical trial. *Transplant Proc* 2000;32:1174.

RESOURCES
65, 359, 368, 389

---

74 Parsonage-Turner Syndrome

Sanjiv Sahoo, MD,
and Phillip L. Pearl, MD

DEFINITION: Parsonage-Turner syndrome is characterized by sudden onset of shoulder and upper arm pain followed by marked upper arm weakness or atrophy.

SYNONYMS: Acute brachial neuropathy; Brachial neuritis; Acute brachial radiculitis; Acute brachial plexitis; Acute shoulder neuritis; Paralytic neuritis; Multiple or localized neuritis of the shoulder girdle.

DIFFERENTIAL DIAGNOSIS: Cervical disc disease; Rotator cuff tear; Impingement syndromes; Adhesive capsulitis; Calcific tendonitis; Poliomyelitis; Amyotrophic lateral sclerosis; Herpes zoster; Tumors of the spinal cord or brachial plexus; Chronic inflammatory demyelinating polyneuropathy; Vasculitis; Traumatic compressive nerve injuries.

SYMPTOMS AND SIGNS: Patients may present with the disorder several weeks after an infection or immunization or in the absence of an obvious inciting event. The disorder is usually heralded by the sudden onset of burning, lancinating, boring, throbbing, or aching severe pain in the shoulder girdle and upper arm. Patients have been awakened at night with the sudden onset of pain, which can radiate up the neck or down the lateral arm to the elbow. The symptoms may remain intense for hours to weeks. Patients find comfort in keeping the shoulder and arm adducted and elbow flexed, the so-called "flexion-adductor sign." As pain subsides, weakness appears in a lower motor neuron fashion with flaccidity and atrophic wasting. The distribution of weakness may involve a single nerve to several trunks and often presents as a mononeuritis multiplex pattern. The suprascapular, axillary, long thoracic, and musculocutaneous nerves are most commonly involved. Less commonly affected are the radial, anterior interosseous, median, and phrenic nerves. Rarely, the posterior interosseous and lateral antebrachial cutaneous nerves and cranial nerves IX–XII are involved. Dyspnea has been noted with phrenic nerve involvement. Sensory loss is minimal to absent and usually mirrors the affected nerves. Tendon reflexes are often diminished, and fasciculations are occasionally seen. When the contralateral side is also affected, the presentation is usually asymmetric or subclinical. The weakness usually resolves over months, with complete spontaneous recovery anticipated by 3 years, although phrenic nerve involvement may have a more prolonged recovery.

ETIOLOGY/EPIDEMIOLOGY: The exact cause is unknown. Factors believed to incite brachial neuritis include trauma, infection, viral diseases, heavy exercise, surgery, hepatitis B vaccination, influenza vaccination, tetanus toxoid administration and other immunizations, and childbirth. These suggest an autoimmune basis. A hereditary form has been described. Coxsackie virus type II or B was found in many patients in an outbreak in Czechoslovakia, but no single pathogen could explain the occurrence of brachial neuritis. The annual incidence is estimated at 1.64 cases per 100,000 persons with a male predominance of 2.1–11.5:1. Most cases occur in individuals aged 20–60 years, although the syndrome has been reported in all age groups.

DIAGNOSIS: The diagnosis is made clinically, aided by electrodiagnostic studies.

TREATMENT
Standard Therapies: The syndrome is a self-limiting entity, and the overall treatment is supportive. Rest is recommended because movement aggravates the pain. Analgesics including narcotics may be indicated at onset for a few weeks because of severe debilitating pain. Immobilization of the affected upper extremity or use of a sling may be helpful in preventing stretching of the affected muscles. Steroids are frequently used, although without proven benefit. As the pain subsides, passive range of motion exercises and rehabilitation of all affected muscle groups are recommended. Surgical intervention with stabilization of the scapula or tendon transfers is reserved for the rare patient with poor recovery.

REFERENCES
England JD. The variations of neuralgic amyotrophy. *Muscle Nerve* 1999;22:435–436.
McCarty EC, Tsairis P, Warren RF. Brachial neuritis. *Clin Orthop* 1999;368:37–43.
Miller JD, Pruitt S, McDonald TJ. Acute brachial plexus neuritis: an uncommon cause of shoulder pain. *Am Fam Physician* 2000;62:2067–2072.

RESOURCES
27, 351

---

75 Pelizaeus-Merzbacher Disease

Leonie van Passel-Clark, MD, and Phillip L. Pearl, MD

DEFINITION: Pelizaeus-Merzbacher disease (PMD) is an X-linked disorder characterized by dysmyelination of the central nervous system (CNS) caused by mutations involving the proteolipid protein (*PLP*) gene.

SYNONYMS: Sudanophilic leukodystrophy; Tigroid leukoencephalopathy.

DIFFERENTIAL DIAGNOSIS: Metachromatic leukodystrophy; Krabbe disease; Adrenoleukodystrophy; Canavan disease; Alexander disease; Genetic disorders of the mitochondrial respiratory chain; Mitochondrial encephalomyelopathy with lactic acidosis and stroke-like episodes (MELAS); Aicardie-Goutières syndrome; Congenital muscular dystrophies; Cerebral autosomal-dominant arteriopathy with subcortical infarcts and leukencephalopathy (CADISIL); Cockayne syndrome; Zellweger disease; Multiple sclerosis; Leigh disease; Sjögren-Larsson disease.

SYMPTOMS AND SIGNS: In classic PMD, the symptoms begin before age 1 year, ambulation with assistance is possible, and speech is usually present. Symptoms are restricted to the central nervous system and the disease does not affect other organ systems. The disorder most commonly occurs in boys, with nystagmus, spastic quadriparesis, ataxia, and delay in cognitive development. A severe connatal form of PMD can be distinguished, with symptoms becoming apparent during the neonatal period. Seizures may be present, and speech and ambulation are never achieved. Clinical signs include dysarthria, optic atrophy, nystagmus, head nodding, delayed developmental milestones, ataxia, choreoathetosis, and spasticity in all four limbs.

ETIOLOGY/EPIDEMIOLOGY: Pelizaeus described in 1885 a family with five male infants having a peculiar form of spastic paraplegia in combination with other CNS abnormalities. Merzbacher reexamined the family in 1910 and concluded the disease was X-linked. The disease was linked to the *PLP* gene in 1985, when the gene was mapped to the X-chromosome and an animal model was developed (the jumpy mouse). Proteolipid protein functions as an integral component of myelin and a trophic factor in the genesis of oligodendrocytes, without which myelogenesis is impaired.

DIAGNOSIS: The diagnosis is suspected when a male infant develops nystagmus and abnormal head movements, and family history is suggestive for X-linked transmission. Symptoms should be restricted to the CNS. Supportive diagnostic studies include the following: a symmetric pattern of delayed myelination may be visualized on MRI, with low signal intensity from the lentiform nuclei or thalamus, suggesting iron deposition. Brainstem auditory and somatosensory evoked potentials are consistently abnormal. Visual evoked potentials may show prolonged latencies. Cerebrospinal fluid studies are normal. A definite diagnosis can be established by demonstration of a defect in the *PLP* gene. Carrier detection and prenatal diagnosis are possible using chorionic villi. Different mutations in the same codon of the *PLP* gene may help in correlating genotype with phenotype.

TREATMENT

Standard Therapies: Supportive care includes occupational therapy, optimizing nutrition, and treatment of spasticity. There is no specific therapy.

REFERENCES

Garbern J, Cambi F, Shy M, et al. The molecular pathogenesis of Pelizaeus-Merzbacher disease. *Arch Neurol* 1999;56:1210–1214.

Hodes ME. Different mutations in the same codon of the proteolipid protein gene may help in correlating genotype with phenotype in PMD/X-linked spastic paraplegia. *Am J Med Genet* 1999;15:132–139.

Merzbacher L. Eine eigenartige familiär-hereditäre Erkrankungsform. *Z Ges Neurol Psychiatry* 1910;3:1–138.

Pelizaeus F. Ueber eine eigentümliche form spastischer Lähmung mit Cerebralerscheinlungen auf hereditären Grundlage. *Arch Psychiatr Nerven* 1885;16:698–710.

RESOURCES

109, 368, 477

---

76 Congenital Bilateral Perisylvian Syndrome

Ruben I. Kuzniecky, MD

DEFINITION: Congenital bilateral perisylvian syndrome (CBPS) is a malformation of cortical development caused by polymicrogyria. Bilateral perisylvian lesions result in a typical pseudobulbar paresis, mental retardation, and seizures.

SYNONYM: Bilateral perisylvian polymicrogyria.

SYMPTOMS AND SIGNS: Infants with CBPS may have hypotonia at birth and difficulty feeding. In less affected patients, other symptoms begin to appear more noticeably at the time of speech development with dysarthria and drooling. Severely affected individuals may also be mute, based on oromotor disturbance. By contrast, comprehension is relatively preserved. Seizures occur in infancy and childhood in 60%–85% of patients. Pyramidal signs may be present and may be bilateral or asymmetric. Cognitive function ranges from normal to severe mental retardation. Seizures are usually of multiple type, including generalized tonic-clonic seizures, atonic attacks, partial onset seizures, or atypical absence. Perioral seizures characterized by clonic bucal activity are rare, but specific milder forms of the disorder have been described with mild dysarthria and dysphasia. In mildly affected patients, seizures are less common.

ETIOLOGY/EPIDEMIOLOGY: The cause of the syndrome is unknown. Pedigrees in the familial forms are consistent with X-linked inheritance although some are compatible with autosomal-dominant or autosomal-recessive inheritance. Perisylvian polymicrogyria has been found in several chromosomal syndromes, most prominently in the deletion of the chromosome 22q11.2. Prevalence and relative incidence are unknown. All ethnic groups are affected. A slight male predominance has been reported.

DIAGNOSIS: The diagnosis should be suspected based on the clinical findings of prominent oromotor dysfunction characterized by dysarthria, limitation of tongue movements, and relatively preserved comprehension. Results of electroencephalography usually demonstrate generalized spike and wave discharges or multifocal epileptiform activity. Typical findings of bilateral perisylvian polymicrogyria on MRI studies make the diagnosis.

TREATMENT
Standard Therapies: Treatment is directed at seizure control. Monotherapy or polytherapy have been used. Speech and physical therapy are helpful. If seizures become intractable, surgical procedures such as corpus callosum section may be useful in the treatment of drop attacks. No antiepileptic drug appears to be more effective than others.

REFERENCES
Kuzniecky R, and the CBPS Group. The congenital bilateral perisylvian syndrome: a study of 31 patients. *Lancet* 1993;341: 608–612.
Kuzniecky R, Andermann F, and the CBPS Group. The congenital bilateral perisylvian syndrome: imaging features. *Am J Neuroradiol* 1994;15:139–144.
Kuzniecky R, Andermann F, Guerrini R, and the CBPS Multicenter Collaborative Study. The epileptic spectrum in the congenital bilateral perisylvian syndrome. *Neurology* 1994;44: 379–385.

RESOURCES
156, 368, 453, 465

77 Adult Polyglucosan Body Disease

Caroline M. Klein, MD, PhD

DEFINITION: Adult polyglucosan body disease is a metabolic disorder caused by abnormal accumulation of polyglucosan bodies, which are spheroids composed of branched polysaccharides, in multiple systemic tissues, including nerve, muscle, liver, kidney, and lung. Clinical manifestations are typically related to neurologic involvement and include upper and lower motor neuron dysfunction, distal sensory loss in the lower extremities, loss of sphincter control, and dementia.

SYNONYM: Polyglucosan disease.

DIFFERENTIAL DIAGNOSIS: Adrenomyeloneuropathy; Metachromatic leukodystrophy; Pelizaeus-Merzbacher disease; Hereditary spastic paraplegia.

SYMPTOMS AND SIGNS: Onset of symptoms occurs in mid to late adulthood (fifth to seventh decade of life). Symptoms are insidious in onset and progressive in nature, with a variable time course until death. Patients may present with progressive gait problems due to weakness and spasticity. Brisk reflexes, fasciculations, extensor plantar responses, and occasionally extrapyramidal signs, such as slowed, low-volume speech, poor balance, and unilateral tremor, may be found. Symmetric sensory loss occurs in the distal lower limbs. Sphincter dysfunction manifests as neurogenic bladder and fecal incontinence. Features of dementia may include impaired short-term memory, verbal comprehension, naming, attention, and visuospatial processing. CT or MRI scans typically reveal atrophy of the cerebral cortex and spinal cord, along with diffuse hyperintense subcortical white matter signal abnormalities.

ETIOLOGY/EPIDEMIOLOGY: Adult polyglucosan body disease has an unknown prevalence; fewer than 50 cases have been reported. No gender predominance is known. Polyglucosan bodies are composed of glucose polymers with 1,4 α-D-glucoside linkages configured as branched polysaccharides. Biochemically, these bodies are similar to corpora amylacea and Lafora bodies, but they have a wider distribution in the nervous system and other organs in this disease. A subgroup of Ashkenazi Jewish patients diagnosed with adult polyglucosan body disease has been found to have a mutation in the glycogen-branching enzyme gene, and an autosomal-recessive pattern of inheritance has been proposed. In view of this mutation, adult polyglucosan body disease may represent an adult variant of glycogen storage disease type IV, which is an early childhood metabolic disorder.

DIAGNOSIS: Clinical evaluation should include a careful neurologic examination, including mental status testing. Electrodiagnostic testing to confirm the presence of peripheral neuropathy and CT or MRI studies of the brain and cervical spinal cord are helpful to document atrophy and white matter changes. Demonstration of multiple, large polyglucosan bodies in sural nerve or axillary skin biopsy strongly supports the diagnosis in the typical clinical setting. Postmortem examination of brain, spinal cord, peripheral nerve, and other systemic tissues is necessary for pathologic confirmation of this diagnosis. Glycogen branching enzyme activity, measured in blood leukocytes, may be helpful for patients with a positive family history, particularly if they are of Ashkenazi Jewish heritage.

TREATMENT

Standard Treatment: There are no known treatments for adult polyglucosan body disease. The clinical course is progressive until death, which occurs within 3–20 years from onset. Treatment is supportive, addressing symptoms such as impaired mobility and gait dysfunction, incontinence, and dementia. No current investigational therapies are known.

REFERENCES

Busard HLSM, Gabreels-Festen AAWM, Renier WO, et al. Adult polyglucosan body disease: the diagnostic value of axilla skin biopsy. *Ann Neurol* 1991;29:448–451.

Gray F, Gherardi R, Marshall A, et al. Adult polyglucosan body disease (APBD). *J Neuropathol Exp Neurol* 1988;47:459–474.

Klein CM, Bosch EP, Dyck PJ. Probable adult polyglucosan body disease. *Mayo Clin Proc* 2000;75:1327–1331.

Lossos A, Meiner Z, Barash V, et al. Adult polyglucosan body disease in Ashkenazi Jewish patients carrying the Tyr^{329}Ser mutation in the glycogen-branching enzyme gene. *Ann Neurol* 1998;44:867–872.

Rifai Z, Klitzke M, Tawil R, et al. Dementia of adult polyglucosan body disease. *Arch Neurol* 1994;51:90–94.

RESOURCES

43, 58, 368

78 Chronic Inflammatory Demyelinating Polyneuropathy

Richard A. Lewis, MD

DEFINITION: Chronic inflammatory demyelinating polyneuropathy (CIDP) is an acquired disorder of peripheral nerves and nerve roots. Typically, patients present with progressive symmetric numbness and weakness of arms and legs over at least 12 weeks. In many ways, CIDP is the chronic equivalent of acute inflammatory demyelinating polyneuropathy, the most common form of Guillain-Barré syndrome. The many variants of CIDP include polyneuropathy associated with monoclonal gammopathies of undetermined significance (particularly IgM kappa), multifocal motor neuropathy (MMN), multifocal sensorimotor demyelinating neuropathy with persistent conduction block (Lewis-Sumner syndrome), CIDP associated with diabetes mellitus, and chronic inflammatory sensory polyneuropathy.

SYNONYM: Chronic inflammatory demyelinating polyradiculoneuropathy.

DIFFERENTIAL DIAGNOSIS: Central nervous system disorders; Spinal cord disorders; Multiple sclerosis; Myopathies; Diabetes mellitus; Charcot-Marie-Tooth disease; Vitamin deficiences, particularly B vitamins; Systemic lupus erythematosus; Rheumatoid arthritis; Sjögren syndrome; Sarcoidosis; HIV; Hepatitis B and C.

SYMPTOMS AND SIGNS: Most patients present with slowly progressive symmetric weakness of arms and legs. The length of time that one has progressive symptoms be-fore being considered to have CIDP is somewhat arbitrary; however, patients with symptoms that progress for more than 12 weeks are considered by most experts to have CIDP. Accompanying paresthesias, burning pain, and numbness are frequently present, but motor symptoms and distal weakness tend to predominate. Some patients have double vision, swallowing problems, and facial weakness. The variants of CIDP may manifest with multifocal abnormalities, consistent with a mononeuritis multiplex. When sensory and motor symptoms occur in the distribution of individual nerves, the Lewis-Sumner variant should be considered. If pure motor symptoms occur, MMN should be considered. Some patients have a purely sensory disorder and present with numbness and ataxia. Neurologic examination usually shows symmetric weakness and atrophy with reduction or loss of deep tendon reflexes. The sensory abnormalities tend to involve vibration, light touch, and position sense with pain.

ETIOLOGY/EPIDEMIOLOGY: The disorder can occur at any age. Males and females are equally affected. The specific cause is unknown, but evidence suggests that most of the disorders considered part of the CIDP syndrome may be caused by antibodies directed against antigens present on peripheral nerves.

DIAGNOSIS: The critical tests required for diagnosis are nerve conduction studies and electromyography. Laboratory evaluations should include serum glucose and Hgb-A1C, serum immunofixation electrophoresis, hepatitis profile, HIV testing, antinuclear antibody, and rheumatoid factor. In some cases, genetic testing for inherited neuropathies including CMT-1A, CMT-1B, CMT-X, and hereditary neuropathy with liability to pressure palsies may be indicated.

TREATMENT

Standard Therapies: Most of the many therapeutic options are of significant benefit in approximately 70% of patients. Some of the variants of CIDP are not as responsive to treatment as others. Intravenous immunoglobulin (IVIG) and plasmapheresis are equally effective in CIDP, whereas IVIG, but not plasmapheresis, has been effective in MMN. Oral prednisone has been beneficial in many forms of CIDP. Azathioprine has been used along with prednisone in an attempt to reduce the steroid dosage and avoid the side effects, but azathioprine, by itself, may not be effective. Mycophenolate, which has a similar effect on the immune system as azathioprine but without the potential liver toxicity, may be useful. Cyclosporine may be of benefit. Cyclophosphamide may be a potent agent against many forms of CIDP. Rituxan, a monoclonal antibody directed against B cells, has been reported to be effective in MMN and in the neuropathy associated with IgM kappa monoclonal gammopathy.

REFERENCES

Dyck PJ, Prineas J, Pollard JD. Chronic inflammatory demyelinating polyneuropathy. In: Dyck PJ and Thomas PK, eds. *Peripheral neuropathy*, 3rd ed. Philadelphia: WB Saunders, 1993.

Gorson KC, Chaudhry VV. Chronic inflammatory demyelinating polyneuropathy. *Curr Treat Options Neurol* 1999;1:251–262.

Rotta FT, Sussman AT, Bradley WG, et al. The spectrum of chronic inflammatory demyelinating polyneuropathy. *J Neurol Sci* 2000;173:129–139.

Saperstein DS, Katz JS, Amato AA, et al. Clinical spectrum of chronic acquired demyelinating polyneuropathies. *Muscle Nerve* 2001;24:311–324.

RESOURCES

27, 171, 368

79 Pseudotumor Cerebri

Bradley K. Farris, MD

DEFINITION: Pseudotumor cerebri (PTC) is characterized by papilledema and elevated intracranial pressure in the presence of normal results of neuroimaging and cerebral spinal fluid studies.

SYNONYMS: Benign or idiopathic intracranial hypertension.

DIFFERENTIAL DIAGNOSIS: Cerebral venous thrombosis; Meningitis (septic/aseptic); Leptomeningeal carcinomatosis; Pseudopapilledema with migraine headache; Structural abnormality (Chiari type I malformation, arachnoid cyst).

SYMPTOMS AND SIGNS: PTC typically occurs in relatively obese females in their second to fourth decades of life. It is unusual in men. Chronic, progressive global headache with or without nausea is common, associated with transient obscurations of vision. The visual loss can occur with head position (orthostatic amaurosis) or eye position (gaze evoked amaurosis). Ophthalmologic examination usually shows bilateral papilledema (may be asymmetric), with decreased visual acuity and loss of peripheral visual field in late stages.

ETIOLOGY/EPIDEMIOLOGY: PTC typically has no known cause. Pathophysiologically, either cerebrospinal fluid (CSF) production is too great for normal absorption mechanisms, or CSF production is normal and the absorption rate is decreased. Obstruction of cerebral venous outflow, endocrine and metabolic dysfunction, exposure to exogenous drugs, and systemic illness can be associated with the development of the disease.

DIAGNOSIS: Normal results from MRI scan secure the diagnosis. Magnetic resonance venography of the brain, with a lumbar puncture showing elevated opening pressure and otherwise normal studies, may be diagnostic. An empty sella is a common finding on MRI scan.

TREATMENT

Standard Therapies: Once the diagnosis is established and the cause is believed to be idiopathic (i.e., not venous obstruction), vision needs to be formally assessed with fundoscopy, visual acuity, and visual field analysis. If immediate visual loss is not a threat, acetazolamide is often beneficial in reducing intracranial pressure and associated papilledema. Too rapid tapering of the diuretic can result in rebound papilledema. In medication-resistant patients, or when rapid visual loss is present, surgical optic nerve decompression or lumbar/ventricular-peritoneal shunting should be considered. Optic nerve decompression can also be considered in patients with chronic papilledema and minimal headache.

REFERENCES

Banta JT, Farris BK. Pseudotumor cerebri and optic nerve sheath decompression. *Ophthalmology* 2000;107:1907–1912.

Johnston I, Paterson A. Benign intracranial hypertension. I. Diagnosis and prognosis. *Brain* 1974;97:289–300.

Miller NR. Papilledema. In: Miller NR, Newman NJ, eds. *Walsh & Hoyt's clinical neuro-ophthalmology,* 5th ed. Vol. 1. Baltimore: Williams & Wilkins, 1998:523–538.

Wall M, George D. Idiopathic intracranial hypertension. A prospective study of 50 patients. *Brain* 1991;114:155–180.

RESOURCES

79, 368, 407

---

80   Restless Legs Syndrome

Michael H. Silber, MB, ChB

DEFINITION: Restless legs syndrome (RLS) is a neurologic disorder characterized by discomfort in the legs precipitated by rest, relieved by activity, and associated with an irresistible need to move.

SYNONYM: Ekbom syndrome.

DIFFERENTIAL DIAGNOSIS: Arthritis; Peripheral neuropathy; Claudication.

SYMPTOMS AND SIGNS: Patients describe the discomfort in many ways, including creeping, crawling, bugs under the skin, tingling, aching, and burning. Some patients have the desire to move without a definite abnormal sensation. RLS is usually felt in both legs, although one may predominate. It may sometimes be felt in the arms. Stretching and walking can relieve the sensations. Sitting down, especially in the evening or on long journeys, and lying in bed at night precipitate the problem, which leads to insomnia. Eighty percent of patients have involuntary periodic limb movements during sleep.

ETIOLOGY/EPIDEMIOLOGY: The syndrome is familial in approximately 50% of patients. Associated disorders include chronic renal failure, iron deficiency, and peripheral neuropathy. Males and females are equally affected, although the symptoms may become worse during pregnancy. Most patients are undiagnosed or untreated, but studies suggest a prevalence of 2%–10%. The disorder may start at any age, including during childhood, but the prevalence increases with age. Remissions and exacerbations may occur.

DIAGNOSIS: The diagnosis is based on the history. Hematocrit and serum ferritin concentration should be measured if a history exists of menorrhagia or gastrointestinal blood loss, if RLS is of recent onset or unexpectedly worsening, or if the patient does not respond to first-line medications. Serum creatinine and glucose concentrations may also be relevant.

TREATMENT

Standard Therapies: Oral iron replacement should be considered if serum ferritin concentration is less than 50 µg/L. Dopaminergic agents are usually the first line of therapy. These include carbidopa/levodopa for mild RLS and pramipexole for moderate or severe symptoms. Levodopa, especially in doses greater than 200 mg daily, may cause augmentation (the development of RLS earlier in the day when the drug is administered before sleep). Other agents for mild RLS include low-potency opioids (such as codeine) or benzodiazepines (such as temazepam). For severe RLS, combination therapy (such as pramipexole with gabapentin or a benzodiazepine) or high-potency opioids (such as oxycodone) may be tried.

REFERENCES

Hening W, Allen R, Earley C, et al. The treatment of restless legs syndrome and periodic limb movement disorder. *Sleep* 1999;22:970–999.

Montplaisir J, Boucher S, Poirier G, et al. Clinical, polysomnographic and genetic characteristics of restless legs syndrome: a study of 133 patients diagnosed with new standard criteria. *Mov Disord* 1997;12:61–65.

Montplaisir J, Nicolas A, Denesle R, et al. Restless legs syndrome improved by pramipexole: a double-blind randomized trial. *Neurology* 1999;52:938–943.

Sun ER, Chen CA, Ho G, et al. Iron and the restless legs syndrome. *Sleep* 1998;371–377.

RESOURCES

368, 417, 487

81   Rett Syndrome

Ignatia B. Van den Veyver, MD,
and Daniel G. Glaze, MD

DEFINITION: Rett syndrome (RTT) is an X-linked dominant neurodevelopmental disorder (Insert Fig. 53).

DIFFERENTIAL DIAGNOSIS: Autism; Angelman syndrome; Infantile or juvenile neuronal ceroid lipofuscinosis.

SYMPTOMS AND SIGNS: Girls with classic Rett syndrome have apparently normal early development, but subtle nonspecific signs, including early deceleration of head growth. At 6–18 months, they enter a short developmental stagnation phase after which they regress. They lose purposeful hand skills and language skills. They acquire stereotyped hand movements (wringing, washing, clapping), seizures, gait apraxia, and ataxia. Girls with Rett syndrome often have autonomic dysfunction with episodes of blue discoloration and temperature instability of the extremities. Many have episodes of alternating apnea and hyperapnea while awake. Somatic growth failure frequently manifests between ages 3 and 5 years. Oral motor dysfunction can occur, and gastrointestinal dysmotility may lead to constipation and gastroesophageal reflux. Scoliosis can develop. Kyphosis may develop in older females with Rett. After this regression period, there is a stabilization phase with some recovery, including acquisition of nonverbal communication skills, some hand use, and decreased severity of seizures, breathing abnormalities, and nutrition problems. There is no further cognitive decline. Although Rett syndrome is primarily seen in females, a few males who have a severe neonatal encephalopathy leading to early death (before age 2 years) have been born in RTT families.

ETIOLOGY/EPIDEMIOLOGY: Rett syndrome affects about 1 in 10,000 to 1 in 23,000 girls and is seen in all ethnic groups. It is caused by mutations in the X-linked *MECP2* gene, which encodes methyl-CpG-binding protein 2.

DIAGNOSIS: Mutation analysis can be offered to all patients with a suggestive phenotype. Mutations may not be found in up to 10%–20% of patients who fit all the criteria of classic Rett syndrome and in a higher percentage in variant forms. In individuals with no mutations, a fuller diagnostic evaluation should be done, including molecular genetic screening for Angelman syndrome, imaging studies of the brain, and screening for metabolic disorders.

TREATMENT
Standard Therapies: There is no cure for Rett syndrome, but several therapies may improve the quality and length of life. These include physical therapy (promote and maintain ambulation), occupational therapy (promote hand use and oral motor skills), hydrotherapy, hippotherapy (horseback riding), music therapy, and therapies directed to the development of nonverbal communication skills. Hand or elbow splints may improve hand use. Supplemental oral feeding or feeding by means of gastrostomy may be necessary to ensure adequate caloric intake and somatic growth. Symptomatic treatment is directed to management of seizures, constipation, and gastroesophageal reflux.

Investigational Therapies: L-carnitine is being investigated. Also, some researchers are investigating treatments aimed at supporting the function of the defective gene.

REFERENCES
Amir RE, Van den Veyver IB, Schultz R, et al. Influence of mutation type and X chromosome inactivation on Rett syndrome phenotypes. *Ann Neurol* 2000;47:670–679.

Amir RE, Van den Veyver IB, Wan M, et al. Rett syndrome is caused by mutations in X-linked MECP2, encoding methyl-CpG-binding protein 2. *Nat Genet* 1999;23:185–188.

Shahbazian M, Zoghbi HY. Molecular genetics of Rett syndrome and clinical spectrum of *MECP2* mutations. *Curr Opin Neurol* 2001;14:171–176.

Trevathan E, et al. Diagnostic criteria for Rett syndrome. The Rett Syndrome Diagnostic Criteria Work Group. *Ann Neurol* 1988;23:425–428.

Zoghbi HY, Francke U. Rett syndrome. In: Scriver CR, Beaudet AL, Sly WS, et al., eds. *The metabolic and molecular bases of inherited disease,* 8th ed. New York: McGraw-Hill, 2000: 6329–6338.

RESOURCES
211, 368, 462

82   Rosenberg-Chutorian Syndrome

William J. Kimberling, PhD

DEFINITION: Rosenberg-Chutorian syndrome is a disorder involving vision loss due to atrophy of the optic nerve, hearing loss, and muscle weakness of the distal arms and legs.

SYNONYMS: Motor and sensory neuropathy; Optic atrophy; Sensorineural hearing loss.

DIFFERENTIAL DIAGNOSIS: Charcot-Marie-Tooth syndrome; Hagemoser syndrome; Iwashita syndrome.

SYMPTOMS AND SIGNS: The neurosensory hearing loss occurs in infancy and progresses to severe to profound. Night blindness is the first manifestation of the visual impairment, occurring at approximately age 20 years; this is followed by a severe loss of visual acuity. Results of electroretinography are normal, and patients do not have retinitis pigmentosa. The muscles of the lower legs become weak by age 5 years, after which the ability to walk deteriorates. Later, the distal arms and hands become involved. Sensation is decreased below the knees and elbows in adults. Biopsies of the muscles demonstrate severe neurogenic atrophy, and motor conduction studies show decreased nerve conduction.

ETIOLOGY/EPIDEMIOLOGY: This is an X-linked genetic disorder, but there is some phenotypic manifestation in the carrier female. Only 3 cases have been reported.

DIAGNOSIS: Diagnosis requires a careful evaluation by a team of clinicians including a geneticist, ophthalmologist, otolaryngologist, and neurologist. Laboratory test results are normal. The gene has not been identified.

TREATMENT
Standard Therapies: A cochlear implant may help the hearing loss. Braces and other assistive devices may be needed for movement.

REFERENCES
Iwashita H, Inoue N, Araki S, et al. Optic atrophy, neural deafness, and distal neurogenic myotrophy. *Arch Neurol* 1970;22:357–364.
Pauli RM. Sensorineural deafness and peripheral neuropathy [Letter]. *Clin Genet* 1984;26:383–384.
Rosenberg RN, Chutorian A. Familial opticoacoustic nerve degeneration and polyneuropathy. *Neurology* 1967;17:827–832.

RESOURCES
288, 368

83   Santavuori Disease

Susan Sklower-Brooks, MD

DEFINITION: Santavuori disease is a neurodegenerative disorder of infancy caused by mutations in *CLN1* leading to deficiency of palmitoyl protein thioesterase (PPT). The disorder is characterized by hypotonia, loss of vision, psychomotor regression, and partial complex seizures. There is intralysosomal storage of ceroid lipofuscin in characteristic granular omiophilic deposits (GRODs). Deficiency of PPT may also lead to later onset disease with accumulation of GRODs.

SYNONYMS: Neuronal ceroid lipofuscinosis, infantile Finnish type; Infantile neuronal ceroid lipofuscinosis; Santavuori-Haltia disease.

DIFFERENTIAL DIAGNOSIS: Other forms of neuronal ceroid lipofuscinosis.

SYMPTOMS AND SIGNS: Infants with Santavuori disease generally have onset of symptoms between 10 and 18 months. There is decline in head growth, hypotonia, psychomotor regression, and visual loss. Irritability is a prominent finding. By age 2 years, severe visual impairment is present. Optic atrophy and macular and retinal changes occur with early extinction of the electroretinograms and visual evoked potentials. Hypointensity of the thalami on T-weighted images and high-signal rims in the periventricular white matter are seen on MRI before 1 year. The electroencephalogram becomes flat at approximately 3 years. Later onset forms of PPT deficiency, termed variant late-infantile and variant juvenile neuronal ceroid lipofuscinosis, account for half of the cases seen in the United States. In the former, the onset is between 18 months and 3 years, whereas in the latter onset is between 6 and 14 years. Symptoms include visual loss, psychomotor regression, and seizures.

ETIOLOGY/EPIDEMIOLOGY: Santavuori disease results from mutations within the *CLN1* gene mapped to chromosome 1p32. *CLN1* encodes PPT. The disorder is inherited in an autosomal-recessive pattern and is most prevalent in Finland, where the carrier frequency is 1 in 70.

DIAGNOSIS: The ERG is extinguished early. Ultrastructural examination of various tissues shows GRODs. Analysis of PPT in peripheral blood leukocytes or cultured cells confirms the diagnosis. Identification of mutation within *CLN1* is also diagnostic. Prenatal diagnosis can be offered for subsequent pregnancies.

TREATMENT
Standard Therapies: Treatment is symptomatic and palliative. It may include anticonvulsants and GABA agonists. Genetic counseling is recommended for families.

Investigational Therapies: Bone marrow transplantation is being investigated.

REFERENCES
Brooks SS. Genetic counseling in the neuronal ceroid lipofuscinosis. In: Wisniewski KE, Zhong N, eds. *Batten disease: diagnosis, treatment, and research.* San Diego: Academic, 2001:159–167.
McKusick VA, ed. Online Mendelian Inheritance in Man (OMIM) [database online]. Bethesda, MD: National Center for Biotechnology Information, National Library of Medicine, 1999. Entry no. 256730; last update October 28, 1999.
Santavuori P, Gottlob I, Haltia M, et al. CLN1 infantile and other types of NCL with GROD. In: Goebel HH, Mole SE, Lake BD, eds. *The neuronal ceroid lipofuscinoses (Batten disease).* Amsterdam: IOS Press, 1999.
Wisniewski KE, Kida E, Golabek AA, et al. Neuronal ceroid lipofuscinosis: classification and diagnosis. In: Wisniewski KE, Zhong N, eds. *Batten disease: diagnosis, treatment, and research.* San Diego: Academic, 2001:12–15.

RESOURCES
58, 68, 355, 368

84   Schwartz-Jampel Syndrome

Riley J. Snook, MD, and Robert M. Pascuzzi, MD

DEFINITION: Schwartz-Jampel syndrome (SJS) is a progressive hereditary disorder characterized by short stature, myopathy, myotonia, continuous muscle fiber activity, joint contractures, bony deformities, distinctive facies, and ocular abnormalities.

SYNONYMS: Schwartz-Jampel-Aberfeld syndrome; Chondrodystrophic myotonia.

DIFFERENTIAL DIAGNOSIS: Thomsen disease (myotonia congenita); Marden-Walker syndrome; Stuve-Wiedemann syndrome; Morquio disease (osteochondrodystrophy).

SYMPTOMS AND SIGNS: In the classic form of SJS, affected patients at birth generally show only evidence of bony abnormalities and muscle hypertrophy. Most of the symptoms and signs are usually noted in the first 2–3 years of life. Bony deformities are varied, including hip dysplasia, kyphoscoliosis, talipes-equinovarus, pectus carinatum, high arched palate, irregularities of articular surfaces, flat-tening of the femoral head, platybasia, and small flattened vertebral bodies. The typical facial appearance includes small, narrow palpebral fissures, small mouth with pursed lips, receded chin, low lying ears, and a fixed facial expression. Ocular abnormalities include myopia and, possibly, varying degrees of external ophthalmoparesis. Skeletal muscles tend to be hypertrophic, especially in proximal distribution in males. Muscles are stiff and resistant to passive or active range of motion. Joint contractures usually involve the elbows and wrists. Power is reduced, especially in distal muscles where progressive atrophy may develop. Action and percussion myotonia are prominent findings in nearly all patients. Continuous muscle activity in the form of quivering, rippling movements in limb and facial muscles is often present. Gait is usually stiff and wide based, and posture is often stooped or hunchbacked. Intelligence and higher cortical function are normal.

ETIOLOGY/EPIDEMIOLOGY: The inheritance of SJS is unclear. Most reported cases are isolated or in siblings, suggesting an autosomal-recessive pattern of inheritance. The few reported occurrences in successive generations suggest an autosomal-dominant inheritance with complete or variable penetrance of the phenotype. Genetic studies in a few cases have localized the SJS locus to 1p36.1-p34, which maps to a gene encoding perlecan (*HSPG2*), a heparin sulfate proteoglycan highly expressed in basement membranes and cartilage; however, studies in other patients affected with SJS have shown evidence against linkage to 1p36.1-p34.

DIAGNOSIS: Diagnosis is usually by history and clinical examination. Radiography may show varying levels of bony deformity. Electromyography needle examination may show continuous low-voltage, high-frequency discharges at rest increasing with needle insertion, percussion of muscle, or volitional muscle activation, as well as myokymic discharges. Muscle enzymes including creatine kinase and lactate dehydrogenase have been reported as mildly elevated or normal. Muscle biopsy typically shows nonspecific dystrophic changes.

TREATMENT
Standard Therapies: Treatment is generally symptomatic. Physical and occupational therapy and orthopedic management may be required for bony deformities and contractures. Phenytoin and carbamazepine have been used to treat the myotonia and continuous muscle fiber activity in some patients with modest symptomatic improvement. Chest wall deformity resulting in restrictive lung disease may require noninvasive ventilation (bilevel positive airway pressure).

REFERENCES
McKusick VA, ed. Online Mendelian Inheritance in Man (OMIM) [database online]. Bethesda, MD: National Center for Biotechnology Information, National Library of Medicine, 2000. Entry no. 2558800; last update March 12, 2001.
Pascuzzi RM. Schwartz-Jampel syndrome. *Semin Neurol* 1991;11: 267–273.
Schwartz O, Jampel RS. Congenital blepharophimosis associated with a unique generalized myopathy. *Arch Ophthalmol* 1962; 68:52–57.

RESOURCES
351, 368

85   Lumbar Spinal Stenosis

Michael Cornefjord, MD, PhD

DEFINITION: Lumbar spinal stenosis is a spinal disorder induced by narrowing of the central spinal canal and/or the nerve root canals. The narrowing of the spinal canal leads to mechanical compression of the dural sac and/or individual spinal nerve roots, which may lead to motor and/or sensory neural deficits and radiating pain in the legs.

SYNONYMS: Pseudoclaudication; Neurogenic claudication.

DIFFERENTIAL DIAGNOSIS: Claudicatio intermittens; Osteoarthritis of the hips.

SYMPTOMS AND SIGNS: The most common type of spinal stenosis is the acquired degenerative type, induced by degenerative changes in the facet joints, intervertebral discs, and ligamentous structures in the lumbar spine. Symptoms typically begin in middle-aged or older adults and usually have a slow progression. The most typical symptoms are lumbar pain and/or radicular leg pain relieved by rest, but increased by activity. Many patients also describe decreased walking capacity, due to radiating pain, weakness, and numbness in the legs while walking longer distances. Typically, patients walk with short steps and with a reduced lumbar lordosis or flexed lumbar spine. Symptoms are increased if the lumbar spine is in hyperextension, for example, while walking downhill, but relieved by flexion.

ETIOLOGY/EPIDEMIOLOGY: Lumbar spinal stenosis is found in both males and females. The annual incidence is estimated to be 40–60 per million population. Central lumbar spinal stenosis can be classified as congenital/developmental or acquired. The congenital/developmental type can be subdivided into dwarfism, such as achondroplasia, and idiopathic types. Acquired stenosis can have many causes, for example, developmental/degenerative spinal stenosis, posttraumatic stenosis, iatrogenically induced stenosis, and miscellaneous conditions such as acromegaly, cysts of ligamentum flavum, and Paget disease.

DIAGNOSIS: The diagnosis should be suspected based on the clinical picture described. Findings often include a typical gait pattern, with short steps and a flexed lumbar spine. The straight leg raising test may be positive, the knee and/or ankle reflexes may be reduced, and sensory as well as some degree of motor paresis, involving one or more nerve roots, may be found. The investigation should include a test of the cauda equina function; however, clinical findings often vary and can be absent or sparse. Plain radiography can give an indication of spinal stenosis, showing decreased disc height, spondylosis, short pedicles, and osteoarthritis in the facet joints. The diagnosis is confirmed radiologically with MRI scan or myelography, the latter with or without a preceding CT scan.

TREATMENT
Standard Therapies: Conservative treatment is often recommended for patients with mild or moderate symptoms. This includes nonsteroidal antiinflammatory drugs or nonopioid analgesics when needed, recommendations to be physically active, and sometimes physical exercises supervised by a physiotherapist. Long-term improvement occurs in the natural course in approximately 30% of patients. Surgical treatment may be needed in patients with moderate or severe symptoms who do not improve following a conservative regimen. This includes decompression of the compressed nerve roots with or without a concomitant fusion. Patients who have signs of instability, for example, a degenerative spondylolisthesis, are generally treated with a posterolateral fusion in the same surgical session.

REFERENCES
Cornefjord M, Byrod G, Brisby H, et al. A long-term (4- to 12-year) follow-up study of surgical treatment of lumbar spinal stenosis. *Eur Spine J* 2000;9:563–570.
Johnson KE, Udén A, Rosén I. The natural course of lumbar spinal stenosis. *Clin Orthop* 1992;279:82–86.
Katz JN, Lipson SJ, Lew RA, et al. Lumbar laminectomy alone or with instrumented or noninstrumented arthrodesis in degenerative lumbar spinal stenosis. Patient, selection, costs, and surgical outcomes. *Spine* 1997;22:1123–1131.
Schonstrom N, Willen J. Imaging lumbar spinal stenosis. *Radiol Clin North Am* 2001;39:31–53.

86   Stiff Person Syndrome

Mary Kay Floeter, MD, PhD

DEFINITION: Stiff person syndrome is an acquired disorder characterized by progressive muscle stiffness and superimposed spasms. It usually begins insidiously in young adults, first involving axial muscles and progressing to affect proximal leg muscles. Patients have a characteristic stiff-legged gait, lordotic posture, and stimulus-induced spasms.

SYNONYMS: Stiff man syndrome; Moersch-Woltman syndrome.

DIFFERENTIAL DIAGNOSIS: Progressive encephalomyelitis with rigidity and myoclonus; Neuromyotonia; Myelopathy with spasticity; Dystonia; Rheumatologic disorders producing muscle stiffness; Muscle spasms secondary to injury.

SYMPTOMS AND SIGNS: Muscle stiffness generally starts in the back or neck muscles. Early on, stiffness may be present only intermittently, but it gradually becomes fixed. Both the agonist and antagonist muscle groups are affected, causing abdominal wall rigidity, hyperlordosis, and difficulty bending. As the disease progresses, stiffness of proximal leg muscles develops, often asymmetrically, leading to a slow, stiff gait. In some patients, stiffness may progress to involve the arms or face. Except for the stiffness, the neurologic examination is normal. Deep tendon reflexes are often brisk, but Babinski signs are not present. The most disabling problem is episodic spasms, which are often painful. They may involve the entire body or only a localized region, and often lead to falls. Spasms are precipitated by unexpected noises or tactile stimuli as well as by anxiety-producing situations. In some cases, no precipitant is evident. Spasms involving the chest and respiratory muscles can be serious and lead to ventilatory compromise. Spasms may last several minutes, but occasionally last for hours, requiring emergency medical treatment with ventilatory support.

ETIOLOGY/EPIDEMIOLOGY: Stiff person syndrome may be an autoimmune disorder. Two thirds of patients have antibodies to GAD-65, a protein in inhibitory nerve cells. Rarely, stiff person syndrome is associated with cancers such as breast cancer or small cell lung cancer. Both men and women are affected. The incidence and prevalence of the disorder are unknown.

DIAGNOSIS: The diagnosis must be made clinically. Electromyography can be helpful to rule out neuromyotonia and to demonstrate the continuous motor unit firing in the stiff muscles. A response to benzodiazepines provides support for the diagnosis. Thyroid function tests, vitamin B_{12}, and serum glucose should be assessed to seek associated conditions, and in newly diagnosed patients, a search for underlying malignancies is recommended.

TREATMENT
Standard Therapies: Benzodiazepines, such as diazepam or clonazepam, are the primary symptomatic treatment for muscle stiffness and episodic spasms. Many patients also

benefit from baclofen, usually given in addition to benzodiazepines. Other medications reported to have benefit in a small number of patients include vigabatrin, valproate, and gabapentin. Some patients had symptomatic improvement with plasmapheresis or intravenous immunoglobulin. Steroid treatment also occasionally has been effective.

Investigational Therapies: Controlled trials are needed to determine which patients are most suitable for immunomodulatory treatment, and which treatments are most effective.

REFERENCES

Barker RA, Revesz T, Thom M, et al. Review of 23 patients affected by the stiff man syndrome: clinical subdivision into stiff trunk (man) syndrome, stiff limb syndrome, and progressive encephalomyelitis with rigidity. *J Neurol Neurosurg Psychiatry* 1998;65:633–640.

Dalakas MC, Fujii M, Li M, et al. High-dose intravenous immune globulin for stiff-person syndrome. *N Engl J Med* 2001;345: 1870–1876.

Dalakas MC, Fujii M, Li M, et al. The clinical spectrum of anti-GAD antibody-positive patients with stiff-person syndrome. *Neurology* 2000;55:1531–1535.

Khanlou H, Eiger G. Long-term remission of refractory stiff-man syndrome after treatment with intravenous immunoglobulin. *Mayo Clin Proc* 1999;74:1231–1232.

Levy LM, Dalakas MC, Floeter MK. The stiff-person syndrome: an autoimmune disorder affecting neurotransmission of gamma-aminobutyric acid. *Ann Intern Med* 1999;131:522–530.

RESOURCES

27, 368

---

87   Syringobulbia

Sanjiv Sahoo, MD,
and Phillip L. Pearl, MD

DEFINITION: Syringobulbia denotes the presence of a fluid-filled cavity within the brainstem. The term is clinically applied to brainstem symptoms in patients with syringomyelia (see also Syringomyelia entry).

SYNONYM: Brainstem syrinx.

DIFFERENTIAL DIAGNOSIS: Posttraumatic syrinx; Neoplasm-related syrinx; Congenital syrinx; Postinflammatory syrinx from arachnoiditis due to syphilis, tuberculosis, early childhood meningitis, subarachnoid hemorrhage, epidural infection, or spinal surgery; Reactions to radiographic oil-based dyes; Transverse myelitis; Radiation necrosis; Spinal cord infarction.

SYMPTOMS AND SIGNS: Usually, syringobulbia presents after syringomyelia, although isolated cases of syringobulbia have been documented. Patients with syringobulbia have bulbar symptoms involving the cranial nerves and present with diplopia, dysphonia, dysphagia, perioral paresthesias, vertigo, nystagmus, tinnitus, hearing loss, ptosis, Horner syndrome, facial palsy, palatal palsy, accessory nerve palsy, and hypoglossal palsy. Syncope and respiratory arrest may occur. Periodic limb movements have been described in a few patients, especially during sleep. Rarely, nausea, vomiting, and feeding difficulties may be early symptoms. Death has been reported within 6–27 years of onset of brainstem symptoms in patients with syringobulbia. Rapid and sometimes fatal deterioration can occur from bleeding into syringobulbia clefts.

ETIOLOGY/EPIDEMIOLOGY: No consensus exists as to the pathophysiology of syrinx formation. Most believe that a syrinx forms because of alterations in flow dynamics of the cerebrospinal fluid (CSF). Various views exist as to the origin of bulbar symptoms.

DIAGNOSIS: Diagnosis is made by means of neuroimaging. MRI can detect a syrinx less than 1 cm in diameter and any underlying lesion causing the syrinx. CT myelography may be used if there is a contraindication to MRI. Lateral radiographs of the skull may show basilar invagination, or flattening of the basal, small posterior fossa, or evidence of preexisting hydrocephalus or bone disease. Plain radiographs of the spine may show spina bifida and kyphoscoliosis. Electromyography can investigate abnormal movements and shows spontaneous bursts of grouped action potentials in muscles innervated by the same spinal segment.

TREATMENT

Standard Therapies: The various surgical approaches to syringobulbia usually must be combined with treatment for syringomyelia. Syringomyelia is approached with options including simple myelotomy, shunting procedures, craniovertebral decompression (CVD), upper cervical laminectomy, duroplasty, and terminal ventriculostomy. Syringobulbia is approached with CVD and shunting procedures. Although no clear-cut guidelines exist as to the procedure of choice, CVD, with or without duroplasty or shunting, is efficacious in congenital syringobulbia. Cord shunting procedures are sometimes reserved only for patients in whom other modalities fail.

REFERENCES

Morgan D, Williams B. Syringobulbia: a surgical appraisal. *J Neurol Neurosurg Psychiatry* 1992;55:1132–1141.

Nogues M. Gastrointestinal symptoms in syringomyelia and syringobulbia. *Neurology* 1999;52:432–433.

Williams B. Surgical treatment of syringobulbia. *Neurosurg Clin North Am* 1993;4:553–571.

Williams B. Syringobulbia: a surgical review. *Acta Neurochir (Wien)* 1993;123:190–194.

Winkelmann J, Wetter TC, Trenkwalder C, et al. Periodic limb movements in syringomyelia and syringobulbia. *Mov Disord* 2000;15:752–753.

RESOURCES

42, 333, 368

---

88 Syringomyelia

Sanjiv Sahoo, MD, and Phillip L. Pearl, MD

DEFINITION: Syringomyelia is the occurrence of a longitudinally disposed fluid-containing cavity within the spinal cord.

SYNONYM: Syrinx.

DIFFERENTIAL DIAGNOSIS: Posttraumatic syrinx; Neoplasm-related syrinx (intramedullary and extramedullary tumors of the cord); Congenital syrinx (Chiari related); Myelocystocele; Postinflammatory syrinx from arachnoiditis due to syphilis; Tuberculosis; Early childhood meningitis; Subarachnoid hemorrhage; Epidural infection; Spinal surgery and possible reactions to radiographic oil-based dyes; Transverse myelitis; Radiation necrosis; Spinal cord infarction.

SYMPTOMS AND SIGNS: Occurrence is usually insidious, with the exception of abrupt occurrence after a precipitating event such as a bout of coughing or the Valsalva maneuver. Usually, patients present with lower motor neuron signs at the level of the lesion and upper motor neuron signs below the level of the lesion. Patients may present with atrophic weakness and claw deformity of the hands and worsening gait spasticity suggestive of a progressive myelopathy. Numbness and paresthesias are associated in a capelike distribution. A dissociated sensory loss affects only the spinothalamic modalities (pain and temperature) and spares light touch, proprioception, and vibratory sensation. Abnormal flushing and sweating are frequently associated with syringomyelia. Patients may have occipital headaches, neck or back pain, radicular pain, and areas of segmental dysesthesia. Joints may be affected due to loss of sensation, causing a neuropathic monoarthritic disease or Charcot joint, primarily affecting the shoulder.

The neurologic deficits may be symmetric. Reflexes are brisk below the level of the lesion, and extensor Babinski responses are present on neurologic examination. Kyphoscoliosis is commonly seen in children and may be the earliest feature. Periodic limb movements have been described in a few patients, especially during sleep. Rarely, nausea, vomiting, abdominal pain, and feeding difficulties may be early symptoms. Patients may have bulbar symptoms involving the cranial nerves if the syrinx extends superiorly into the brainstem.

ETIOLOGY/EPIDEMIOLOGY: No consensus exists as to the pathophysiology of syrinx formation. A syrinx likely forms because of alterations in cerebrospinal fluid flow dynamics. The subarachnoid space may be occluded at the foramen magnum, causing enlarged pulsatile cervical pressure waves that compress the spinal cord from outside and propagate syrinx fluid caudally with each heartbeat. A transmission of pressure waves from the fourth ventricle may occur, producing syrinx progression. It is also possible that raised intraabdominal or intrathoracic pressure causes epidural vein engorgement and subsequent transmission of dural pressure to the interstitial spaces or the central canal of the spinal cord.

DIAGNOSIS: Diagnosis is established by neuroimaging. MRI is the procedure of choice, and can detect a syrinx less than 1 cm in diameter and any underlying primary lesion that may be present. CT-myelography may be used in the presence of a metallic implant or pacemaker, which poses a contraindication to MRI. Electromyography may show spontaneous synchronous bursts of grouped action potentials in muscles innervated by the same spinal segment.

TREATMENT

Standard Therapies: The various surgical approaches to syringomyelia include simple myelotomy, shunting procedures, craniovertebral decompression, upper cervical laminectomy, duroplasty, terminal ventriculostomy, and resection of tumors or other causative lesions.

REFERENCES

Goel A, Desai K. Surgery for syringomyelia: an analysis based on 163 surgical cases. *Acta Neurochir (Wien)* 2000;142:293–301.
Heiss JD, Patronas N. Elucidating the pathophysiology of syringomyelia. *J Neurosurg* 1999;91:553–562.
Oldfield EH. Syringomyelia. *J Neurosurg* 2001;95(suppl):153–155.
Palma L. Pathophysiology of syringomyelia. *J Neurosurg* 2000;92:1071–1073.
Siver JR. History of post-traumatic syringomyelia: post-traumatic syringomyelia prior to 1920. *Spinal Cord* 2001;39:176–183.

RESOURCES

42, 368

---

89   Tardive Dyskinesia

Daniel Tarsy, MD

DEFINITION: Tardive dyskinesia (TD) is a movement disorder that appears in delayed fashion after treatment with antipsychotic drugs (APD). Several variants or subtypes have been described such as tardive dystonia, tardive akathisia, tardive tics, tardive myoclonus, tardive stereotypy, and tardive tremor.

DIFFERENTIAL DIAGNOSIS: Wilson disease; Huntington disease; Other APD-induced extrapyramidal syndromes; Meige syndrome; Idiopathic torsion dystonia.

SYMPTOMS AND SIGNS: A mixture of orofacial dyskinesia, athetosis, dystonia, chorea, tics, and facial grimacing that may involve the oral region, face, trunk, and extremities is characteristic. Rhythmic tremor occurs rarely. In older patients, oral, facial, and lingual dyskinesias are conspicuous, including involuntary eyelid, tongue, lip, and jaw movements. Extremity dyskinesia may include twisting, spreading, and "piano-playing" finger movements; tapping foot movements; and extensor postures of the toes. Axial dystonia may include retrocollis, torticollis, shoulder shrugging, rocking and swaying, and rotatory or thrusting hip movements. Severe orofacial dyskinesia is disfiguring and may interfere with speech, eating, or breathing, whereas truncal dystonia interferes with gait and mobility. Tardive dyskinesia may appear as early as several months after APD exposure, although it usually occurs after 2 or more years of treatment.

ETIOLOGY/EPIDEMIOLOGY: The prolonged course of TD suggests structural alterations in the brain. Blockade of postsynaptic dopamine receptors may be a likely mechanism for all APD-induced extrapyramidal syndromes. Evidence also exists for dopamine receptor supersensitivity after repeated APD treatment. The disorder could also result from loss of striatal interneurons, which exert a feedback influence on dopamine neurons. An excitotoxic mechanism may cause selective destruction of a localized population of basal ganglia neurons. The prevalence of TD over and above background prevalence of spontaneous dyskinesia is approximately 15%. In prospective studies, incidence of new TD cases is 5% per year with a cumulative incidence of 20% at 4 years and 40% after 8 years of APD exposure. Patients older than 50 years are at increased risk for TD and have a poorer prognosis for remission.

DIAGNOSIS: Diagnosis is based on the presence of dyskinesia, a history of APD exposure, and exclusion of other causes of involuntary movements.

TREATMENT
Standard Therapies: Emphasis should be on prevention, early detection, and management of early and potentially reversible cases. The use of APDs for longer than 3 months requires careful evaluation of indications and risks and should be limited to situations where there is no alternative therapy. Because prompt APD withdrawal results in a better prognosis for recovery, patients taking APDs should be regularly examined for signs of TD. Botulinum toxin injections can be of value in management of localized forms of tardive dystonia such as retrocollis, blepharospasm, or jaw dystonia. Tetrabenazine and reserpine are presynaptic dopamine depletors with efficacy in TD but often limited by hypotension, sedation, and fatigue. Vitamin E has been widely used for treatment of TD with unproven benefit. In some patients with persistent TD that has failed to remit off APD, it may be necessary to resume APD treatment to suppress TD.

REFERENCES

Casey DE. "Seroquel" (quetiapine): preclinical and clinical findings of a new atypical antipsychotic. *Exp Opin Invest Drugs* 1996;5:939–957.
Jankovic J. Tardive syndromes and other drug-induced movement disorders. *Clin Neuropharmacol* 1995;18:197–214.

Tarsy D. Akathisia. In: Joseph AB, Young RR, eds. *Movement disorders in neurology and neuropsychiatry.* Boston: Blackwell, 1992: 88–99.

Tarsy D, Baldessarini RJ. Behavioral supersensitivity to apomorphine following chronic treatment with drugs which interfere with the synaptic function of catecholamines. *Neuropharmacology* 1974;13:927–940.

Tarsy D, Kaufman D, Sethi KD, et al. An open-label study of botulinum toxin A for treatment of tardive dystonia. *Clin Neuropharmacol* 1997;20:90–93.

RESOURCES

367, 368, 460

90 Tarsal Tunnel Syndrome

Ruth A. Cook, MSN, ANP, and Martin J. O'Malley, MD

DEFINITION: Tarsal tunnel syndrome is a symptom complex associated with entrapment neuropathy of the posterior tibial nerve or one of its terminal branches.

SYNONYM: Entrapment neuropathy–posterior tibial nerve.

DIFFERENTIAL DIAGNOSIS: Diabetic neuropathy; Reflex sympathetic dystrophy; Plantar fasciitis; Subtalar DJD; Posterior tibial tendonitis; Sciatica (L5 to dorsum of foot, S1 to heel).

SYMPTOMS AND SIGNS: Clinical symptoms are often difficult to delineate clearly. Pain is poorly localized. Patients may describe radiating pain from the medial malleolus to the heel and sole of the foot that occasionally radiates up the calf. They may also describe pain of the foot that is global. Paresthesias, "burning" pain, and numbness on the plantar surface of the foot or toes are common. Pain is usually not found at the insertion of the plantar fascia. The symptoms are often exacerbated by activity and relieved when shoes are removed and the feet elevated, but some patients experience pain at night. Percussion (Tinel sign) over the posterior tibial nerve will recreate symptoms, but results of the gross sensory examination are usually normal.

ETIOLOGY/EPIDEMIOLOGY: Causes of tarsal tunnel syndrome include space-occupying lesions, which may increase pressure in the fibroosseus tunnel. These include ganglion, lipoma, or neurilemoma. Other factors that may lead to nerve compression are varicosities, proliferative synovitis, subtalar coalition, enlarged or displaced os trigonum, and nonunion of the sustentaculum tali after calcaneal fracture.

DIAGNOSIS: A positive Tinel sign is often the first diagnostic finding. Radiographs of the foot and ankle are necessary and may show a significant bony abnormality. Electro-diagnostic studies (electromyography) are nearly 90% accurate in identifying posterior tibial nerve entrapment and differentiating other sources of pain such as radiculopathy or neuropathy. MRI may be useful if a space-occupying lesion is strongly suspected. Pain relief after injection of xylocaine into the tarsal tunnel may help make the diagnosis.

TREATMENT

Standard Therapies: Conservative treatment should be tried initially and consists of rest, contrast baths, nonsteroidal antiinflammatory drugs, change of shoe wear to avoid tightness, and nonrigid orthotics. In patients with a flexible flat foot and significant pronation, an orthotic with a medial longitudinal arch support may decrease stretch on the nerve. Some believe that arch support in patients who do not exhibit abnormal foot biomechanics should be avoided to minimize compression over the abductor hallucis. A corticosteroid injection and immobilization may be helpful. Surgery is recommended for severe symptoms that do not respond to conservative measures in several weeks to months. The most favorable outcomes are in cases where a space-occupying lesion exists. Release should include incision of the flexor retinaculum overlying the nerve. No role is established for internal neurolysis. Extensive dissection around the nerve should be avoided to minimize scarring and protect vascularity. Inadequate distal release of either the medial or lateral terminal nerve branch may be a reason for surgical failure.

Investigational Therapies: Nerve wrapping with autologous vein grafts and peripheral nerve stimulation are being investigated. Intractable pain is treated with an implanted nerve stimulator.

REFERENCES

Kaplan PE, Kernahan WT. Tarsal tunnel syndrome. *J Bone Joint Surg [Am]* 1981;63:96.

Schon LC, Glennon TP, Baxter DE. Heel pain syndrome: electrodiagnostic support for nerve entrapment. *Foot Ankle* 1993;14:129.

RESOURCE

351

91   Thalamic Pain Syndrome

Sanjiv Sahoo, MD,
and Phillip L. Pearl, MD

DEFINITION: Thalamic pain syndrome is a clinical syndrome characterized by hemihypesthesia, allodynia, hyperpathia, transient hemiparesis, hemichoreoathetosis, and aching burning pain and paresthesias in the affected hemibody, caused by a thalamic lesion on the opposite side.

SYNONYM: Dejerine-Roussy syndrome.

DIFFERENTIAL DIAGNOSIS: Thalamic tumor; Thalamic stroke; Lesions in the spinothalamocortical afferent sensory pathways including the parietal cortex, subcortical white matter, medial lemniscus, and dorsolateral medulla.

SYMPTOMS AND SIGNS: The rate of onset of symptoms depends on the underlying cause. The syndrome tends to manifest abruptly in the event of a stroke, and insidiously with gradual progression in the presence of a tumor. There is a predilection for right-sided diencephalic lesions, although either side can be involved, leading to contralateral mild hemiparesis that rapidly improves over days. This is accompanied by spontaneous severe burning, aching, paroxysmal pain, and paresthesias, which may develop immediately to several months later. There is associated allodynia to even nonnoxious stimuli and hyperpathia. Patients experience pain and numbness over the entire distribution of face, arm, leg, and trunk, more prominently distally than proximally. The pain may disturb sleep and may be incessant or paroxysmal. Chorea is mild and usually restricted to the hand. Some patients have mild hemiataxia, visual field defects, and a distorted sense of taste. The syndrome manifests somewhat laterally, with left-sided lesions having slightly greater vibratory sensory loss. Proprioception and stereognosis appear to be densely affected. Reflexes on the affected side may be slightly increased, and plantar responses may be normal.

ETIOLOGY/EPIDEMIOLOGY: The usual age of presentation is approximately 60 years, but a range of 18–85 years has been reported. The geniculothalamic artery is often affected in thalamic strokes. The ventroposterolateral thalamic nuclei along with the intralaminar, reticular, and central thalamic nuclei appear to be involved in the relay and generation of nociceptive stimuli.

DIAGNOSIS: The diagnosis is made clinically. Other causes of pain, whether localized or referred, must be ruled out. CT and MRI are used to rule out tumors, infarct, or cerebral hemorrhage. Hyperdensity or hypodensity of the thalamus may be seen on CT depending on whether the stroke is hemorrhagic or nonhemorrhagic, respectively. Increased T2-weighted signal or diffusion-weighted imaging (DWI) by means of MRI may show acute stroke in the thalamus or elsewhere. Somatosensory evoked potentials may be useful in the identification and localization of sensory deficits, and are usually absent on the affected side in central thalamic pain syndrome.

TREATMENT
Standard Therapies: The immediate management depends on the underlying cause. Strokes should be managed accordingly and tumors addressed by neurosurgery, oncologic therapies, and the use of steroids as required. Further stroke prophylaxis is warranted. Various analgesics for pain management may be tried, including narcotics, although success is limited. Pain prophylaxis with tricyclic antidepressants and anticonvulsants, including agents such as gabapentin, have met with variable success. Supportive care, rehabilitation, and psychotherapy are indicated.

REFERENCES
Mauguiere F, Desmids JE. Thalamic pain syndrome of Dejerine-Roussy. Differentiation of four subtypes assisted by somatosensory evoked potentials data. *Arch Neurol* 1988;45:1312–1320.
Nasreddine ZS, Saver JL. Pain after thalamic stroke: right diencephalic predominance and clinical features in 180 patients. *Neurology* 1997;48:1196–1199.
Pearce JM. The thalamic syndrome of Dejerine and Roussy. *J Neurol Neurosurg Psychiatry* 1988;51:676.
Sanchez-Valiente S. Treatment of neuropathic pain with gabapentin. *Rev Neurol* 1998;26:618–620.

RESOURCE
368

92   Tourette Syndrome

Gerald Erenberg, MD

DEFINITION: Tourette syndrome is a neuropsychological disorder characterized by a changing pattern of motor and vocal tics that wax and wane in intensity and change form over time. Onset is in childhood, and many persons find that their tics disappear or become significantly reduced as they enter adulthood.

SYNONYM: Chronic motor and vocal tic disorder.

DIFFERENTIAL DIAGNOSIS: Myoclonus; Dystonia; Sydenham chorea; Stereotypies; Wilson disease; Athetotic cerebral palsy.

SYMPTOMS AND SIGNS: Tics are sudden, rapid, purposeless, recurrent, nonrhythmic, stereotypic motor movements or vocalizations. The onset of tics is in childhood, usually between the ages of 5 and 10 years. Onset can be gradual or explosive. Persons with Tourette syndrome often have comorbid psychological conditions. The two most common are attention-deficit/hyperactivity disorder and obsessive-compulsive disorder. Other comorbid conditions found commonly in persons with Tourette syndrome include higher than expected incidences of anxiety and autistic spectrum disorder. The pattern to the tics is highly unpredictable. They may disappear and reappear or may continue at different levels from the time of onset. The associated comorbid behavioral conditions can occur before or coincident with the onset of tics, or after the tics have started. The intensity of the tics varies widely. In some individuals, the tics are relatively infrequent and usually inconspicuous. In others, the tics are frequent and highly visible. No physical degeneration is associated with tics, but repetitive motions may lead to some pain. The involuntary utterance of obscenities was once believed to be a universal part of Tourette syndrome, but it is now known that this phenomenon only occurs in a minority of persons with this disorder.

DIAGNOSIS: The diagnosis is clinical, based on the history and confirmed by the presence of tics during a physical examination. Tourette syndrome does not cause an abnormality on any of the available clinical diagnostic tests. The specific diagnostic criteria used are those listed in the American Psychiatric Association's *Diagnostic and Statistical Manual* (DSM).

TREATMENT

Standard Therapies: Medication is the standard treatment where it is necessary. In persons with mild tics, no treatment is necessary. For those whose symptoms are more pervasive and bothersome, medications are available that diminish either the tics or the various associated behavioral patterns. Medications that block the effect of dopamine, such as haloperidol, pimozide, and risperidone, are the mainstay of therapy. Clonidine, although an antihypertensive, can be beneficial and is commonly used. Medications for the associated conditions include the usual treatments for attention deficit disorder and obsessive-compulsive disorder.

Investigational Therapies: New medications are being investigated, including nicotine, baclofen, and medications that actually activate the dopamine rather than block it. Nonpharmaceutical treatments such as habit-reversal therapy are also being investigated. Some interest is also being shown in deep brain stimulation as a potential treatment for very severe cases.

REFERENCES

Cohen DJ, Bruun RD, Leckman JF. *Tourette's syndrome and tic disorders: clinical understanding and treatment.* New York: John Wiley & Sons, 1988.

Kurlan R. *Handbook of Tourette's syndrome and related tic and behavioral disorders.* New York: Marcel Decker, 1993.

Jankovic J. Tourette's syndrome. *N Engl J Med* 2001;345:1184–1192.

Shapiro AK, Shapiro ES, Young JG, et al. *Gilles de la Tourette syndrome,* 2nd ed. New York: Raven, 1988.

RESOURCES

368, 467, 487

93 Trigeminal Neuralgia

Peter J. Jannetta, MD

DEFINITION: Trigeminal neuralgia is a symptom of sharp, lancinating, often repetitive, shocklike facial pain.

SYNONYMS: Tic doloureux; Trifacial neuralgia.

DIFFERENTIAL DIAGNOSIS: Dental caries; Gum disease; Atypical trigeminal neuralgia; Thalamic syndrome of Dejerine-Rossea.

SYMPTOMS AND SIGNS: The primary symptom is facial pain, usually starting in the V2 distribution, V2 cheek, or V3 jaw distribution, which may spread over the rest of the face in time. Pain starts and stops suddenly. After prolonged pain, repetitive very severe pains, many years of pain, or after some medications, sharp jabbing pain can be accompanied, or even superceded, by a more constant burning pain. Describing the pain, the patient will not touch the affected area. They have so-called trigger points where a light touch precipitates an attack. Most patients have a positional component to their pain, i.e., they find a position that precipitates the pain or relieves it. Up to 30% of patients have mild sensory loss in the distribution of the pain.

ETIOLOGY/EPIDEMIOLOGY: The incidence and prevalence are unknown. At least 10,000 to 15,000 new cases occur each year. Women are more prone to developing the condition than are men by a ratio of 3:2. The cause in almost all cases is compression by a blood vessel of the trigeminal nerve in the cerebellopontine angle. Occasionally, a benign tumor causes trigeminal neuralgia. In a small percentage of patients, multiple sclerosis is the cause.

DIAGNOSIS: History is the most important feature for diagnosis. Patients believe they have a dental problem and see a dentist. Unfortunately they receive dental treatment, which is not helpful. MRI with and without contrast should be performed to look for tumors, abnormal blood vessels, and multiple sclerosis.

TREATMENT
Standard Therapies: The treatment of trigeminal neuralgia has historically been to replace the pain with numbness. Current techniques of doing this include percutaneous radiofrequency rhizotomy, where a needle is placed into the ganglion of the nerve through the cheek and the nerve is burned, and percutaneous glycerol rhizotomy, where a chemical is placed around the nerve through a needle in the cheek. Some neurosurgeons have treated trigeminal neuralgia with percutaneous balloon compression, placing a small balloon in the area of the ganglion of the nerve, again through the cheek, and blowing it up. The definitive procedure is microvascular decompression (the Jannetta procedure), where the blood vessel is carefully moved and held away from the nerve using microsurgical techniques by means of a small thumbnail-sized opening behind the mastoid bone. This is the benchmark of treatment because it has the best long-term results and the fewest side effects in experienced hands.

Investigational Therapies: Investigational therapies include high-energy focused radiation, using gamma rays.

REFERENCES
Barker FG II, Jannetta PJ, Bissonette DJ, et al. The long-term outcome of microvascular decompression for trigeminal neuralgia. *N Engl J Med* 1996;334:1077–1083.
Weigel G, Casey KF. *Striking back: a trigeminal neuralgia handbook.* Trigeminal Neuralgia Association, 2000.

RESOURCES
320, 368, 469

94 Tuberous Sclerosis

David J. Kwiatkowski, MD, PhD

DEFINITION: Tuberous sclerosis is a familial tumor syndrome in which patients develop hamartomas in the brain, skin, heart, kidneys, and lungs. Involvement of the brain causes the greatest morbidity in most patients, but the disease is highly variable.

SYNONYM: Tuberous sclerosis complex (TSC).

DIFFERENTIAL DIAGNOSIS: Idiopathic epilepsy; Mental retardation; Acne; Multiple endocrine neoplasia type I.

SYMPTOMS AND SIGNS: Tuberous sclerosis most often presents in early childhood as a seizure disorder. Infantile spasms, partial motor, and complex partial seizures are all common, and are due to the hallmark cortical tubers. Cortical tubers also cause autism, other forms of development delay, and mental retardation, which varies from mild to profound. A second brain lesion, the subependymal nodule, is usually clinically silent but can grow, causing cerebrospinal fluid obstruction. Skin lesions include facial angiofibromas, red papules, or nodules in a centrofacial distribution; hypomelanotic macules, also known as white spots; forehead plaque; Shagreen patch; and ungual fibromas. Facial angiofibromas develop during middle childhood, whereas ungual fibromas appear later. Cardiac rhabdomyomas develop antenatally and typically spontaneously resolve over a period of years. Hemodynamic compromise at birth occurs in a few patients (<5%). Subclinical lung involvement by lymphangiomyomatosis is common in adult women with TSC and causes clinical symptoms in approximately 5%. Kidney lesions include both cysts and angiomyolipomas. The latter tumors can grow, causing renal dysfunction by mass effect and distortion, and are prone to bleeding. Rarely, angiomyolipomas become malignant.

ETIOLOGY/EPIDEMIOLOGY: Tuberous sclerosis is inherited in an autosomal-dominant manner. It is caused by mutations in either the *TSC1* or *TSC2* genes. Birth incidence is approximately 1 in 6,000–10,000, and all ethnic groups are affected. Two thirds of cases are sporadic, due to new mutations.

DIAGNOSIS: Any of the hallmark features described should suggest the diagnosis. When multiple systems are involved, the diagnosis is clear. Diagnosis of patients who lack brain manifestations can be challenging. Imaging studies of the brain (CT or MRI), heart (ultrasonography), and kidneys (ultrasonography or CT), and careful dermatologic and ophthalmologic examinations are part of a full diagnostic evaluation.

TREATMENT

Standard Therapies: In most patients, initial treatment is directed at control of seizures. Educational and developmental monitoring should be performed at regular intervals, and special needs addressed. Serial monitoring of brain and kidney lesions by radiographic imaging is recommended. Brain subependymal lesions may require surgical removal. Renal angiomyolipomas may require removal or vascular interruption. Cosmetic procedures are valuable for control of facial angiofibromas.

REFERENCES
Cheadle JP, Reeve MP, Sampson JR, et al. Molecular genetic advances in tuberous sclerosis. *Hum Genet* 2000;107:97–114.

Gomez M, Sampson J, Whittemore V. *The tuberous sclerosis complex,* 3rd ed. Oxford, UK: Oxford University Press, 1999.

Roach ES, DiMario FJ, Kandt RS, et al. Tuberous Sclerosis Consensus Conference: recommendations for diagnostic evaluation. *J Child Neurol* 1999;14:401–407.

Roach ES, Gomez MR, Northrup H. Tuberous Sclerosis Complex Consensus Conference: revised clinical diagnostic criteria. *J Child Neurol* 1998;13:624–628.

RESOURCES
145, 368, 471

---

95 Vascular Malformation of the Brain/ Brain Arteriovenous Malformation

Donna Golakovich, RN, and Karel G. terBrugge, MD

DEFINITION: A congenital disorder of unknown etiology, brain arterial venous malformations (BAVMs) are characterized by a network of abnormal "channels" (nidus) between the arterial feeders and the draining veins. Arterial venous malformations may be small (micro-AVMs) with normally sized arteries and draining veins and a nidus smaller than 1 cm in diameter. Macro-AVMs have arteries and veins that are usually larger than normal. The nidus creates a shortened arteriovenous blood transit time.

SYNONYM: Brain arterial venous fistula (BAVF).

DIFFERENTIAL DIAGNOSIS: Brain aneurysm; Brain hemorrhagic stroke; Brain tumor.

SYMPTOMS AND SIGNS: A person with a BAVM can remain asymptomatic throughout life. Patients present mainly with hemorrhage, seizures, progressive neurologic deficit, or headache. Hemorrhage in a patient represents a change in the compliance of the vascular system. There is a 3%–4% risk of hemorrhage per year; of these, 10% are fatal, and there is a 40%–50% incidence of permanent neurologic disability. Patients with AVMs in the temporal region have the highest incidence of seizures. Neurologic deficit and seizures could be caused by ischemia or mechanical compression of brain tissue.

ETIOLOGY/EPIDEMIOLOGY: Between 0.14% and 0.8% of the population per year may present with BAVMs. There is an equal distribution between sexes and among races. The disorder is believed to be a congenital defect or dysfunction of the embryonic capillary maturation process, which exhibits change with aging.

DIAGNOSIS: The topographic location of a malformation is best assessed by MRI or CT. Angiography permits the anatomic identification of the arterial feeders and the draining veins.

TREATMENT

Standard Therapies: Treatment should be performed only if it will result in an improvement over the expected natural history of the disorder. The main objective of any treatment is to completely and permanently exclude the lesion from the circulation. Three main methods exist: embolization, surgery, and stereotactic radiosurgery. Each method can be performed alone or in combination. With curative embolization, a permanent nonbiodegradable agent must be used to form a cast of the pathologic an-

gioarchitecture. Complete obliteration by embolization has been reported in 10%–40% of AVMs. The goal of presurgical and preradiosurgical embolization is the elimination of deep-feeding arterial supply and overall size and flow reduction through the nidus. The Spetzler-Martin scale is used to assess surgical risk. This classification considers the size, location (eloquence), and venous drainage pattern of the lesion. A Spetzler-Martin grade 5 AVM is considered inoperable. Surgery alone should be performed only when complete excision can be accomplished. With BAVMs smaller than 3 cm, stereotactic radiosurgery is an option. Focal targeted irradiation may thrombose the nidus, obtaining occlusion after a period of 14–24 months.

REFERENCES
Al-Yamany M, terBrugge K, Willinsky R, et al. Palliative embolisation of brain arteriovenous malformations presenting with progressive neurological deficit. *Int Neuroradiol* 2000;6:177–183.

Redekop G, terBrugge K, Montanera W, et al. Arterial aneurysms associated with cerebral arteriovenous malformations: classifications, incidence and risk of hemorrhage. *J Neurosurg* 1998;89:539–546.

RESOURCE
368

96 Walker-Warburg Syndrome

Christopher A. Walsh, MD, PhD

DEFINITION: Walker-Warburg syndrome is a condition associated with hydrocephalus, with lissencephaly, eye abnormalities, and muscular dystrophy.

SYNONYMS: HARD ± E syndrome; Warburg syndrome; Cerebrooculomuscular syndrome.

DIFFERENTIAL DIAGNOSIS: Muscle-eye-brain disease; Fukuyama muscular dystrophy; Lissencephaly with cerebellar hypoplasia.

SIGNS AND SYMPTOMS: The primary features in the brain are type II "cobblestone" lissencephaly and cerebellar malformations, or cerebellar hypoplasia. Many children also present with encephalocele. Hydrocephalus is generally present because of the cerebellar malformations such as Dandy-Walker. Clinically, patients usually have neonatal seizures and profound developmental delay. The many possible eye abnormalities include microphthalmia,

macrophthalmia, cataracts, glaucoma, and abnormal retinas. Most children with Walker-Warburg syndrome also have muscular dystrophy that presents as significantly low muscle tone with poor reflexes. Less common features include cleft lip, cleft palate, intrauterine growth retardation, microtia, absent auditory canals, and renal cysts. Life expectancy of children with Walker-Warburg syndrome depends on the severity of the disease.

ETIOLOGY/EPIDEMIOLOGY: Walker-Warburg syndrome is inherited as an autosomal-recessive disorder. It has been reported throughout the world.

DIAGNOSIS: Walker-Warburg syndrome is typically diagnosed in the period shortly after birth, although some diagnoses have been made prenatally on the basis of ultrasonography and fetal MRI findings. The diagnosis is made clinically. MRI can be used to detect type II lissencephaly and hydrocephalus. Serum creatinine kinase levels help in diagnosing myopathy. Diagnoses made prenatally are made on the basis of brain and eye abnormalities in conjunction with family history. An ophthalmologic examination is indicated to look for any of the eye abnormalities that may go along with this syndrome.

TREATMENT
Standard Therapies: Treatment is generally palliative.

REFERENCES
Chemke J, Czernobilsky B, Mundel G, et al. A familial syndrome of central nervous system and ocular malformations. *Clin Genet* 1975;7:1–7.

Dobyns WB, Kirkpatrick JB, Hittner HM, et al. Syndromes with lissencephaly II. *Am J Med Genet* 1985;22:157–195.

Dobyns WB, Pagon RA, Armstrong D, et al. Diagnostic criteria for Walker-Warburg syndrome. *Am J Med Genet* 1989;32:195–210.

Donnai D, Farndon PA. Walker-Warburg syndrome (Warburg syndrome, HAD ± E syndrome). *J Med Genet* 1986;23:200–203.

RESOURCES
190, 368

12

Neuromuscular Disorders

1 Ataxia, Baltic/Mediterranean/ Unverrich-Lundborg Myoclonic Epilepsy

R. Stanley Burns, MD

DEFINITION: Baltic/Mediterranean/Unverrich-Lundborg myoclonic epilepsy is an autosomal-recessive disorder with an onset during childhood or adolescence (age 6–15 years) characterized by progressive and disabling myoclonus associated with generalized seizures, mild cognitive impairment, and progressive ataxia.

SYNONYMS: Progressive myoclonic epilepsy (PME); Ramsay-Hunt syndrome.

DIFFERENTIAL DIAGNOSIS: Lafora body disease; Myoclonic epilepsy with ragged red fibers; Neuronal ceroid lipofuscinosis; Sialidosis type I; Dentatorubropallidoluysian atrophy.

SYMPTOMS AND SIGNS: Either generalized seizures or myoclonus can be the initial symptom. The disorder is characterized by stimulus-sensitive myoclonus triggered by touch, noise, light, or voluntary movement. The myoclonus worsens over time and eventually becomes incapacitating. Generalized tonic-clonic seizures, absence, and drop attacks can occur. The frequency of the seizures is low, and they can be controlled with medications. The rate of progression is variable, and the phenotype is relatively broad. In addition to the core features of myoclonus, seizures, dementia, and ataxia, other neurologic signs include pyramidal signs, hyporeflexia, distal muscle wasting, and autonomic dysfunction. Scoliosis also may occur.

ETIOLOGY/EPIDEMIOLOGY: Baltic myoclonus, Mediterranean myoclonus, and Unverrich-Lundborg disease are now known to be the same disease. This disease is due to a mutation (minisatellite expansion in the promotor region) in the *EPM1* gene (locus 21q22.3) that codes for the protease inhibitor cystatin B. The mechanism is not yet understood. The disease is more common in Finland (estimated incidence of 1 in 20,000), Estonia, and the Mediterranean countries.

DIAGNOSIS: Patients present with progressive myoclonic epilepsy. The clinical picture as described is suggestive of the diagnosis. Electroencephalography typically shows background slowing with paroxysmal bursts. Somatosensory evoked potentials show giant potentials. A skin biopsy with examination by electron microscopy can show membrane-bound inclusions in sweat glands. Diagnosis is made by DNA analysis demonstrating a mutation in the *EPM1* gene.

TREATMENT
Standard Therapies: Treatment with antiepileptic drugs (clonazepam, valproic acid, piracetam) can reduce myoclonus and, as a result, significantly improve motor function. Treatment with phenytoin can worsen the condition and should be avoided.

REFERENCES
Buchhalter JR. Inherited epilepsies. In: Pulst SM, ed. *Neurogenetics.* New York: Oxford University Press, 2000:345.
Dicter MA, Buchhalter JR. The genetic epilepsies In: Rosenberg RN, Prusiner SB, DiMauro S, et al., eds. *The molecular and genetic basis of neurological disease,* 2nd ed. Boston: Butterworth-Heinemann, 1997:769.
McKusick VA, ed. Online Mendelian Inheritance in Man (OMIM) [database online]. Bethesda, MD: National Center for Biotechnology Information, National Library of Medicine, 2000. Entry no. 254800.

RESOURCES
145, 322, 368

2 Episodic Ataxia Type I

R. Stanley Burns, MD

DEFINITION: Episodic ataxia type I is an autosomal-dominant, childhood-onset (age 2–15 years), nonprogressive disorder characterized by short-duration (seconds to minutes) attacks of ataxia and rhythmic movements associated with persistent myokymia of the hands and face.

SYNONYMS: Hereditary myokymia and periodic ataxia; Kinesigenic paroxysmal ataxia; Episodic ataxia and neuromyotonia; Familial paroxysmal kinesigenic ataxia.

DIFFERENTIAL DIAGNOSIS: Partial epilepsy; Paroxysmal kinesigenic choreoathetosis; Intermittent metabolic ataxias; Lesions of brainstem; Other disorders producing myokymia.

SYMPTOMS AND SIGNS: Sudden, rapid movements trigger the attacks of ataxia; onset is marked by paresthesias. Attacks occur up to 15 times per day with a refractory period of approximately 1 hour. The attacks are most frequent during the first and second decades of life. Associated signs include rhythmic movements (tremor of mandible, head nodding, shaking, or rocking of body) and dystonia in some patients. Other neurologic signs include persistent myokymia of face and hand muscles, the occurrence of carpopedal spasms ("priest hand"), and, in some patients, epilepsy.

ETIOLOGY/EPIDEMIOLOGY: Episodic ataxia type 1 is due to a mutation in the *KCNA1* gene (locus 12p13) that encodes a δ-subunit of a voltage-dependent potassium channel that is concentrated in synaptic terminals and parnodal regions and expressed in the cerebellum and peripheral nerves. The paresthesias and myokymia are believed to be due to hyperexcitability of peripheral nerve axons. The central nervous system manifestations are likely caused by increased transmitter release. Disease prevalence is estimated at 1 in 500,000, and it occurs in both sexes.

DIAGNOSIS: Clinically, sudden, short-lived attacks of ataxia provoked by movement and associated with muscle activity at rest in the absence of vertigto and nystagmus is highly characteristic of episodic ataxia type 1. Results of CT and MRI brain scans are normal. Electromyography (EMG) shows spontaneous motor unit activity of myokymia in hand muscles with ischemic provocation and reactivity of the myokymia discharges. Muscle biopsy with histology shows small, intensely staining fibers of both types. A definitive diagnosis can be made based on EMG evidence of myokymia and DNA analysis demonstrating a mutation in the *KCNA1* gene.

TREATMENT

Standard Therapies: Carbonic anhydrase inhibitors (acetozolamide 125–375mg/day; sulthiame 100–300 mg/day) or antiepilepitic drugs (carbamazepine; phenytoin) may be used for treatment.

REFERENCES
Brunt ER. Episodic ataxia type 1. In: Klockgether T, ed. *Handbook of ataxia disorders*. New York: Marcel Dekker, 2000:487–515.

Jen J, Ptacek L. Channelopathies: episodic disorders of the nervous system. In: Scriver CR, Beaudet AL, Sly WS, et al., eds. *The metabolic and molecular bases of inherited disease,* 8th ed. New York: McGraw-Hill, 2001:5228–5230.

McKusick VA, ed. Online Mendelian Inheritance in Man (OMIM) [database online]. Bethesda, MD: National Center for Biotechnology Information, National Library of Medicine, 2000. Entry no. 150120.

Moon SL, Koller WC. Hereditary periodic ataxias. In: Vinken PJ, Bruyn GW, Klawans HL, eds. *Handbook of clinical neurology*, Vol. 60. New York: Elsevier Science, 1991:433–443.

RESOURCES
289, 368, 487

---

3 Episodic Ataxia Type II

R. Stanley Burns, MD

DEFINITION: Episodic ataxia type II is an autosomal-dominant disorder with an onset during childhood or adulthood (7th week to 5th decade) characterized by episodes of ataxia and vertigo lasting hours to a day and associated with interictal nystagmus. It is associated with a slowly progressive ataxia and cerebellar atrophy late in life.

SYNONYM: Familial periodic ataxia.

DIFFERENTIAL DIAGNOSIS: Episodic ataxia type I; Intermittent metabolic ataxias.

SYMPTOMS AND SIGNS: Episodes of ataxia can occur spontaneously or be triggered by stress, exercise, fatigue, alcohol, or caffeine. Prodromal symptoms include sweating, flushing, a feeling of heaviness of the head, light-headedness, and sensory symptoms. The episodes are frequently associated with vertigo, nausea, vomiting, or headache. One episode per month to five per week may occur, and they last hours or up to a day. Persistent gaze-evoked and/or spontaneous downbeat nystagmus is found between episodes. Migraine headaches are frequently present at the same time.

ETIOLOGY/EPIDEMIOLOGY: Episodic ataxia type II is due to a mutation in the *CACNA1A4* gene (locus) that codes for a δ_{1A}-subunit of a brain-specific, voltage-dependent calcium channel. Episodes of ataxia are believed to be due to a transient impairment in the activation or de-activation of these calcium channels. Persistent or progressive neurologic deficits are believed to be due to chronic and excessive entry of calcium into cells or release of intercellular calcium-activating signaling pathways. Episodic ataxia type II affects both sexes.

DIAGNOSIS: Episodic ataxia and vertigo associated with persistent gaze-evoked and spontaneous downbeat nystagmus is characteristic of episodic ataxia type II in children and young adults. A slowly progressive cerebellar ataxia with a history of episodes of ataxia or vertigo earlier in life and a family history of migraine headaches is a characteristic presentation of episodic ataxia type II in older adults. The MRI brain scan is found to be normal or to show atrophy of the cerebellar vermis. A variety of abnormalities of the electroencephalogram have been reported. Auditory evoked potentials are abnormal in some cases. Diagnosis is made by DNA analysis demonstrating a mutation in the *CACNA1A4* gene.

TREATMENT
Standard Therapies: Treatment with carbonic anhydrase inhibitors (acetozolamide 500–750 mg/day) can significantly reduce the symptoms. Other treatment agents include valproic acid. Treatment with phenytoin should be avoided because it can worsen the attacks in some cases.

REFERENCES
Baloh RW, Jen JC. Episodic ataxia type 2 and spinocerebellar ataxia type 6. In: Klockgether T, ed. *Handbook of ataxia disorders.* New York: Marcel Dekker, 2000:447–467.
Jen J, Ptacek L. Channelopathies: episodic disorders of the nervous system. In: Scriver CR, Beaudet AL, Sly WS, et al., eds. *The metabolic and molecular bases of inherited disease,* 8th ed. New York: McGraw-Hill, 2001:5228–5230.
Kramer PL, Smith E, Carrero-Valenzuela R, et al. Autosomal dominant episodic ataxia represents at least two genetic disorders. *Ann Neurol* 1994;36:279.
Vighetto A, Froment JC, Trillet M, et al. Magnetic resonance imaging in familial paroxysmal ataxia. *Arch Neurol* 1988;45:547–549.

RESOURCES
289, 368, 487

---

4 Friedreich Ataxia

R. Stanley Burns, MD

DEFINITION: Friedreich ataxia is an autosomal-recessive disorder with an onset during childhood or adolescence (age 4–17 years; mean, 9 years) characterized by progressive gait and limb ataxia (first in lower extremities, later in all limbs), dysarthria, a reduction or absence in position sense and areflexia in the lower extremities, the presence of Babinski signs (extensor toe signs), pes cavus, scoliosis, and hypertrophic cardiomyopathy.

SYNONYMS: Classic or typical Friedreich ataxia; Arcadian form of Friedreich ataxia; Friedreich ataxia with retained reflexes; Late-onset Friedreich ataxia.

DIFFERENTIAL DIAGNOSIS: Charcot-Marie-Tooth disease, type 1; Ataxia with isolated vitamin E deficiency; Abetalipoproteinemia; Familial hypobetalipoproteinemia; Refsum disease.

SYMPTOMS AND SIGNS: Although most patients develop symptoms before the end of puberty, some patients have presented as late as the seventh decade of life. The usual presenting symptoms include gait ataxia, generalized clumsiness, or scoliosis. In rare cases, cardiac symptoms or tremor are the presenting symptoms. The most prominent clinical findings are gait and limb ataxia. These are associated with optic atrophy, dysarthria, a loss of vibration and position sense and areflexia in the lower extremities, Babinski signs, and muscle atrophy and weakness (upper motor neuron syndrome; neurogenic and disuse atrophy). Friedreich ataxia is a multisystem disorder that can affect the heart and endocrine and skeletal systems. A hypertrophic cardiomyopathy with concentric left ventricular and septal hypertrophy occurs. The cardiac pathology includes hypertrophied or necrotic muscle fibers, interstitial fibrosis, and granular iron deposits in muscle fibers. Diabetes mellitus occurs in up to 40% of patients. Scoliosis and pes cavus are highly characteristic of this disorder.

ETIOLOGY/EPIDEMIOLOGY: Friedreich ataxia is due to a GAA repeat expansion mutation in the *frataxin* gene (locus) that codes for the protein frataxin, a transport protein that plays a role in the export of reduced iron (Fe^{2+}) out of mitochondria. The normal repeat length varies between 7 and 22 repeats. In patients with Friedreich ataxia, the repeat length is in the range of 120–1,700 repeats. The repeat expansion mutation reduces but does not completely suppress expression of frataxin and leads to a deficiency of frataxin with a loss of function. As a result, iron accumulates within mitochondria and is believed to produce oxidative damage, particularly to iron-sulfur proteins, including components of the respiratory chain enzyme complexes (I, II, and III). The damage to mitochondria and energy metabolism is believed to be responsible for cell death.

DIAGNOSIS: Findings considered to be essential to the diagnosis of classic Friedreich ataxia are vibration and position sense loss in the lower extremities, areflexia in the lower extremities, abnormal sensory nerve action potentials on nerve conduction velocity studies, and the presence of scoliosis. Diagnosis is established by DNA analysis demonstrating that the patient is homozygous for the GAA repeat expansion mutation (in both alleles) of the *frataxin* gene.

TREATMENT

Standard Therapies: Patients should be chronically treated with coenzyme Q10 (300 mg/day) and vitamin E (2,000 mg/day) until the results of experimental drug trials are completed.

Investigational Therapies: Desferrioxamine (an iron chelating agent), idebenone (a coenzyme Q10 analogue), and the combination of coenzyme Q10/vitamin E are being investigated.

REFERENCES

Koenig M. Friedreich ataxia and AVED. In: Scriver CR, Beaudet AL, Sly WS, et al., eds. *The metabolic and molecular bases of inherited disease,* 8th ed. New York: McGraw-Hill, 2001:5852–5853.

Koenig M, Durr A. Friedreich ataxia In: Klockgether T, ed. *Handbook of ataxia disorders.* New York: Marcel Dekker, 2000:151–161.

Manyam BV. Friedreich disease. In: Vinken PJ, Bruyn GW, Klawans HL, eds. *Handbook of clinical neurology.* Vol. 60. New York: Elsevier Science, 1991:299–333.

McKusick VA, ed. Online Mendelian Inheritance in Man (OMIM) [database online]. Bethesda, MD: National Center for Biotechnology Information, National Library of Medicine, 2000. Entry no. 229300.

RESOURCES

165, 270, 289, 368

---

5 Ataxia, Kearns-Sayre Syndrome/Chronic Progressive External Ophthalmoplegia

R. Stanley Burns, MD

DEFINITION: The central feature of Kearns-Sayre syndrome (KSS) and chronic progressive external ophthalmoplegia (CPEO) plus is progressive external ophthalmoplegia with ptosis and gaze palsies.

DIFFERENTIAL DIAGNOSIS: Maternally inherited progressive external ophthalmoplegia; Pearson syndrome; NARP syndrome.

SYMPTOMS AND SIGNS: The term *Kearns-Sayre syndrome* refers to individuals who develop external ophthalmoplegia before age 20 years that is associated with pigmentary retinal degeneration and myopathy and variably with cerebellar ataxia, an increased cerebrospinal fluid (CSF) protein level (>100 mg/dL), and cardiac conduction defects. The term *chronic progressive external ophthalmo-plegia* is used to refer to individuals who develop a "pure" progressive external ophthalmoplegia with an onset after age 20 years. The term *CPEO plus* refers to individuals who develop progressive external ophthalmoplegia after age 20 years that is associated with other clinical manifestations. The neurologic features of KSS and CPEO plus include optic atrophy, sensorineural hearing loss, cerebellar ataxia, spasticity, dementia, seizures, and peripheral neuropathy. Clinical features of other organ system involvement include pigmentary retinal degeneration, proximal myopathy, cardiomyopathy, cardiac conduction defects and arrhythmias, proximal renal tubule dysfunction, diabetes mellitus, hypoparathyroidism, and growth hormone deficiency.

ETIOLOGY/EPIDEMIOLOGY: In most cases, KSS and CPEO plus are due to spontaneous deletions of the mitochondrial DNA (mtDNA) of up to 50% of the genome, which is believed to occur in the oocyte or during embryogenesis. The disorders can also be caused by mtDNA duplications that are maternally inherited. The clinical phenotype associated with mtDNA duplications are indistinguishable from those related to deletions. These types of molecular rearrangements lead to defects in mitochondrial respiratory chain enzymes (complexes I, II, and IV) and energy metabolism. The mtDNA with deletions is found in all tissues of the body. The percentage of deleted mtDNA molecules increases with age, possibly explaining the progressive nature of the condition.

DIAGNOSIS: The clinical criteria for the diagnosis of KSS include an onset before age 20 years, the findings of external ophthalmoplegia and pigmentary retinopathy, and the presence of at least one of the following: cerebellar ataxia, a cardiac conduction defect, or a CSF protein level greater than 100 mg/dL. The cardinal features of CPEO plus are external ophthalmoplegia and a proximal myopathy. Bood lactate and pyruvic acid can be elevated. Lumbar puncture with CSF analysis can show elevated levels of lactate and of total protein (>100 mg/dL). The electrocardiogram can show heart block. MRI brain scan abnormalities include white matter changes and basal ganglia calcification. Magnetic resonance spectroscopy can demonstrate an increase in the brain levels of lactic acid. Histochemical studies of muscle tissue obtained by biopsy can show ragged red fibers representing an increased number and peripheral location of mitochondria in muscle fibers. Diagnosis is made by mtDNA analysis of muscle tissue.

TREATMENT
Standard Therapies: Chronic treatment of KSS and CPEO plus with coenzyme Q10 and L-carnitine has been recommended. A cardiac pacemaker can prevent sudden death from heart block.

REFERENCES
Lyon G, Adams RD, Kolodny EH. *Neurology of hereditary metabolic diseases of children.* New York: McGraw-Hill, 1996.
McKusick VA, ed. Online Mendelian Inheritance in Man (OMIM) [database online]. Bethesda, MD: National Center for Biotechnology Information, National Library of Medicine, 2000. Entry no. 530000.
Pulst SM. *Neurogenetics.* New York: Oxford University Press, 2000.
Reichmann H. Ataxia in mitochondrial disorders. In: Klockgether T, ed. *Handbook of ataxia disorders.* New York: Marcel Dekker, 2000:325–341.
Wallace DC, Lott MT, Brown MD, et al. Mitochondria and neuro-ophthalmologic diseases. In: Scriver CR, Beaudet AL, Sly WS, et al., eds. *The metabolic and molecular bases of inherited disease,* 8th ed. New York: McGraw-Hill, 2001:2481–2484.

RESOURCES
288, 351, 355, 368

6   Ataxia, Refsum Disease

R. Stanley Burns, MD

DEFINITION: Refsum disease is an autosomal-recessive disorder characterized by the development of night blindness and loss of peripheral vision during late childhood or adolescence associated with the loss of smell and hearing, peripheral neuropathy, and ataxia. It is a multiple organ system disease affecting the eye, heart, skin, and skeleton in addition to the nervous system. The disease state results from the accumulation of phytanic acid in the body from dietary sources due to a reduced capacity to metabolize this compound.

SYNONYMS: Heredipathia atactica polyneuritiformis; Phytanic acid oxidose deficiency; Hereditary motor and sensory neuropathy, group IV.

DIFFERENTIAL DIAGNOSIS: Friedreich ataxia; Tangier disease; Dejerine-Sottas hypertrophic peripheral neuropathy; Charcot-Marie Tooth disease; Speilmeyer-Vogt disease; Tay-Sachs disease.

SYMPTOMS AND SIGNS: The characteristic symptoms include night blindness, loss of peripheral vision, loss of the sense of smell, limb weakness, and incoordination. In addition to ataxia and a peripheral neuropathy, the neurologic signs include retinitis pigmentosa, miosis with a poor pupillary response, anosmia, impairment of deep (vibration and position sense) and superficial (touch and pain) sensation, areflexia in the lower extremities, and distal muscle atrophy and weakness. Signs of involvement of other organ systems include posterior subcapsular cataracts, acute angle closure glaucoma, ichthyosis, cardiac arrhythmias, cardiomyopathy with rhabdomyolysis, and shortened terminal phalanges of the thumb and fourth metatarsal of the foot.

ETIOLOGY/EPIDEMIOLOGY: The disease is due to a mutation in the gene that codes for the enzyme protein phytanoyl-CoA hydrolase (PAHX) (locus 10pter-p11.2). This enzyme is involved in the oxidation (alpha-oxidation) of phytanic acid to pristanic acid within peroxisomes. A defect in this enzyme results in a reduced capacity to eliminate phytanic acid and ultimately to high fat stores and intoxication with phytanic acid. Refsum disease has been reported most often in individuals from Scandinavia and Western Europe. The prevalence in the United Kingdom is estimated to be 1 in 1 million.

DIAGNOSIS: The combination of retinitis pigmentosa, anosmia, and shortened terminal phalanges of the thumb and fourth metatarsal of the foot is highly characteristic. Electroretinography shows an absence of response. Lumbar puncture with cerebrospinal fluid analysis shows an elevated total protein level. The blood level of creatine kinase can be increased. Studies show low nerve conduction velocities. Electrocardiography characteristically shows an atrioventricular conduction or bundle block. Diagnosis is made by demonstration of elevated plasma levels of phytanic acid and reduced activity of phytanoyl-CoA hydrolase in cultured fibroblasts obtained by skin biopsy.

TREATMENT

Standard Therapies: Refsum disease is treated with a low phytanic acid diet (<10 mg/day). Patients are advised to avoid rapid weight loss because this can release phytanic acid from body fat. Plasma exchange is used to eliminate phytanic acid from the body in acutely ill patients.

REFERENCES

Gibberd FB, Wierzbicki AS. Heredopathia atactica polyneuritiformis, Refsum disease. In: Klockgether T, ed. *Handbook of ataxia disorders.* New York: Marcel Dekker, 2000:235–256.

McKusick VA, ed. Online Mendelian Inheritance in Man (OMIM) [database online]. Bethesda, MD: National Center for Biotechnology Information, National Library of Medicine, 2000. Entry no. 266500.

Skjeldal AH, Stokke O, Refsum S. Heredopathia atactica polyneuritiformis (phytanic acid storage disease; Refsum's disease; HMSN type IV). In: Vinken PJ, Bruyn GW, Klawans HL, eds. *Handbook of clinical neurology.* Vol. 60. New York: Elsevier Science, 1991:225–242.

Wanders RJA, Jakobs C, Skjeldal OH. Refsum disease. In: Scriver CR, Beaudet AL, Sly WS, et al., eds. *The metabolic and molecular bases of inherited disease,* 8th ed. New York: McGraw-Hill, 2001:3303–3321.

RESOURCES

58, 325, 368, 419

---

7 Ataxia-Telangiectasia

Richard A. Gatti, MD

DEFINITION: Ataxia-telangiectasia (A-T) is a progressive neurologic disease of childhood, with onset of truncal ataxia typically between ages 1 and 3 years. One in three patients develops cancer, usually lymphoma or leukemia, during their lifetime.

SYNONYM: Louis-Bar syndrome.

DIFFERENTIAL DIAGNOSIS: Friedreich ataxia; Spinocerebellar ataxias; Mre11 deficiency; Episodic ataxia; Brain tumor; Inner ear infection; Hexaminadase deficiency; Vitamin E deficiency; Beta-lipoprotein abnormalities; Urea cycle defects; Maple syrup disease; Isovaleric acidosis; 2-Hydroxyglutaric aciduria; Hartnup disease; Pyruvate dysmetabolism; Multiple sulfatase deficiency; Mitochondrial disease; Niemann-Pick syndrome; Late-onset globoid cell leukodystrophy; Adrenoleukodystrophy; Sialidosis type I; Ceroid lipofuscinosis; Metachromatic leukodystrophy.

SYMPTOMS AND SIGNS: Symptoms and signs include progressive cerebellar ataxia, ocular apraxia, dysarthria, drooling, severe twitching, choreoathetosis, decreased deep tendon reflexes, motor retardation, nystagmus, recurrent infections, and flat facies. Telangiectasias over the bulbar conjunctiva and other places also may occur, usually several years after the onset of ataxia.

ETIOLOGY/EPIDEMIOLOGY: The primary neurologic lesion is in the cerebellum, which appears grossly atrophied by age 5 in most patients. Immunohistochemistry of the cerebellum shows significant loss of Purkinje cells and granule cells and disrupted axonal fibers in the white matter. The primary cause of these lesions is unclear. On a molecular level, most patients are lacking the protein encoded by a mutated *ATM* (ataxia-telangiectasia mutated) gene. The prevalence varies with ethnicity, according to the frequency of inbreeding. In the United States, A-T occurs in approximately 1 in 100,000 live births. American parents are frequently unrelated to one another. Both sexes are affected equally, and A-T is found in all races.

DIAGNOSIS: The diagnosis is made clinically, based on a wide-based gait, with progressive cerebellar ataxia. Serum α-fetoprotein (AFP) is elevated in 85% of patients; however, AFP levels sometimes remain elevated until age 2 years in unaffected children and, thus, can be misleading. Liver enzymes are often elevated. An MRI scan is often useful, showing cerebellar atrophy. T-cell and B-cell functions are usually abnormal, sometimes severely. IgA and

IgG2 levels are decreased in 60%–80% of patients. IgG responses to challenge with polysaccharide antigens is poor in most patients. Karyotyping often shows characteristic translocations between chromosome 14q11-12 and other sites, such as 7p11, 7q32, and 14q32. Western blotting can be used to detect the ATM protein intracellularly; this is absent in 85% of patients. In certain families, genetic studies can also be performed to establish whether linkage of the suspected diagnosis exists to chromosome 11q23, the site of the *ATM* gene.

TREATMENT

Standard Therapies: There is no known therapy for reversing or preventing the progression of the cerebellar ataxia. Some symptoms, however, such as uncontrollable twitching movements and drooling are amenable to therapy. Steroids sometimes decrease the severity of the ataxia; however, this effect is transient and does not warrant long-term use. Physical therapy on a regular basis helps to prevent contractures of hands and feet and scoliosis secondary to extended time in a wheelchair. Antioxidants, such as vitamin E, vitamin C, and alpha-lipoic acid, and free-radical scavengers are recommended to counteract the inadequate responses of A-T cells *in vitro* to DNA damage from oxidative free radicals produced by the normal metabolism of food. These agents are also believed to reduce the risk of cancer. Chemotherapy is complicated in patients with A-T because of hypersensitivity not only to ionizing radiation but also to some radiomimetic and alkylating agents.

REFERENCES

Becker-Catania SG, Chen G, Hwang MJ, et al. Ataxia-telangiectasia: phenotype/genotype studies of ATM protein expression, mutations, and radiosensitivity. *Mol Genet Metab* 2000;70: 122–133.

Boder E. Ataxia-telangiectasia: an overview. In: Gatti RA, Swift M, eds. *Ataxia-telangiectasia: genetics, neuropathology, and immunology of a degenerative disease of childhood.* New York: Alan R. Liss, 1985:1–63.

Gatti RA. Ataxia-telangiectasia. In: Scriver CR, Beaudet AL, Sly WS, et al., eds. *Metabolic and molecular bases of inherited disease,* 8th ed. New York: McGraw-Hill, 2001:705–732.

Huo YK, Wang Z, Hong J-H, et al. Radiosensitivity of ataxia-telangiectasia, X-linked agammaglobulinemia and related syndromes. *Cancer Res* 1994;54:2544–2547.

RESOURCES

62, 63, 289, 368

---

8 | Ataxia with Isolated Vitamin E Deficiency

R. Stanley Burns, MD

DEFINITION: Ataxia with isolated vitamin E deficiency (AVED) is an autosomal-recessive disorder with an onset during childhood or adulthood (age 2–52 years) characterized by the development of ataxia and a peripheral neuropathy and associated with retinitis pigmentosa, cardiomyopathy, scoliosis, and pes cavus. The course of illness is chronic and progressive. The clinical picture resembles that found in Friedreich ataxia. If untreated, patients become wheelchair bound after an average disease duration of 13 years.

DIFFERENTIAL DIAGNOSIS: Friedreich ataxia; Abetalipoproteinemia; Familial hypobetalipoproteinemia; Refsum disease.

SYMPTOMS AND SIGNS: Ataxia with isolated vitamin E deficiency is a multisystem disorder that involves the central and peripheral nervous system and other organ systems, including the eye, heart, and skeletal system. The neurologic signs include a sensory and cerebellar ataxia, loss of vibration and position sense and areflexia in the lower extremities, the presence of Babinski reflexes (extensor toe signs), and dystonia. Signs of involvement of other organs include retinitis pigmentosa, retinal deposits (white-yellow spots in peripheral retina), cardiomyopathy, scoliosis, and pes cavus.

ETIOLOGY/EPIDEMIOLOGY: Ataxia with isolated vitamin E deficiency is due to a mutation in the α-*TTP* gene (locus 8q13) that codes for the α-tocopherol transfer protein. The α-tocopherol transfer protein specifically transfers the RRR stereoisomer of α-tocopherol (RRR α-tocopherol) from chylomicron reminants into very-low-density lipoproteins in the liver. The deficiency of the α-tocopherol transfer protein leads to rapid elimination (approximately 1 day) and absent recycling of vitamin E. The absorption of vitamin E from the intestine and secretion into plasma in chylomicrons is normal. Vitamin E is a free radical scavenger and its absence is believed to lead to oxidative damage to cells in the body. The prevalence of this disorder is estimated to be less than 1 in 1 million, except in Tunisia, where it might be as high as 1 in 100,000. Consanguinity is a factor in most cases.

DIAGNOSIS: The diagnosis is based on the findings of a very low level of vitamin E in blood with normal levels of lipoproteins and lipids and no evidence of fat malabsorption. Somatosensory evoked potentials show delays in conduction at the cervical and cortical levels. The MRI brain scan in some cases shows signal hyperintensity in the periventricular white matter on T2-weighted images, dilatation of the cisterna magna, or generalized cerebral atrophy. Morphologic changes found on light and electron microscopy examination of nerve biopsy tissue samples include a reduction in large myelinated fibers, evidence of nerve regeneration, and the presence of dense bodies in Schwann cells. Increased peroxidation sensitivity of red blood cells on hemolysis by acidified glycerol, H_2O_2, or NaN_3 and lipid peroxidation by the thiobarbituric acid method can be demonstrated.

TREATMENT

Standard Therapies: Treatment consists of the administration of 800 mg of RRR α-tocopherol (vitamin E) twice daily with meals containing fat. Treatment with α-tocopherol produces an arrest of progression and, in some cases, an improvement in existing neurologic deficits.

REFERENCES

Cavalier L, Ouahchi K, Kayden HJ, et al. Ataxia with isolated vitamin E deficiency: heretogeneity of mutations and phenotypic variability in a large number of families. *Am J Hum Genet* 1998;62:301–310.

Koenig M. Ataxia with isolated vitamin E deficiency. In: Klockgether T, ed. *Handbook of ataxia disorders.* New York: Marcel Dekker, 2000:223–234.

Koenig M. Friedreich's ataxia and AVED. In: Scriver CR, Beaudet AL, Sly WS, et al., eds. *The metabolic and molecular bases of inherited disease,* 8th ed. New York: McGraw-Hill, 2001:5852–5853.

McKusick VA, ed. Online Mendelian Inheritance in Man (OMIM) [database online]. Bethesda, MD: National Center for Biotechnology Information, National Library of Medicine, 2000. Entry no. 600415, 277460.

RESOURCES

145, 368

---

9 Central Core Disease

Gloria D. Eng, MD

DEFINITION: Central core disease is a neuromuscular disorder of infancy and childhood manifested by hypotonia and some delay in the acquisition of motor milestones. It is frequently diagnosed later in adolescence and adulthood because of associated skeletal problems requiring surgery. It is of particular significance because of its association with malignant hyperthermia.

DIFFERENTIAL DIAGNOSIS: Multicore (minicore) myopathy; Congenital fiber-type disproportion.

SYMPTOMS AND SIGNS: Breech presentation has been frequently reported in the birth process of affected individuals. Hypotonia, delay in walking and running, evidence of negligible facial weakness, and greater weakness of shoulder and hip girdle muscles rather than distal limb muscles have been described. Skeletal problems may include congenital dislocation of the hips, dislocating patellae, kyphoscoliosis, and, rarely, pes cavus or planus. Finger contractures also occur. Cardiac abnormalities are rare. Intelligence of affected individuals is normal to superior.

ETIOLOGY/EPIDEMIOLOGY: The candidate gene is localized on chromosome 19q.13.1 and is allelic with *RYR1* (ryanodine receptor gene responsible for susceptibility to malignant hyperthermia). Transmission is autosomal dominant.

DIAGNOSIS: Creatine phosphokinase levels are usually normal or slightly increased. Electrodiagnostic studies show normal nerve conduction velocity determinations. The electromyogram may be almost normal, especially in younger children, but may show short-duration, low-amplitude motor unit action potentials with some increase in polyphasic potentials. Fibrillation potentials are rare. When performing biopsy of muscle, cores are best delineated by succinate dehydrogenase or NADH-dehydrogenase reacted sections. Confusion arises if muscle biopsy is obtained too soon after a malignant hyperthermic crisis; rhabdomyolysis may obscure the finding of cores.

TREATMENT

Standard Therapies: Attention must be directed to alignment and posture in infants. Adaptive seating with careful head and trunk support is necessary. Very weak infants may require tube feeding. Physical and occupational therapists should provide hands-on therapies, but, more importantly, they should instruct the parents on handling, exercising, and stretching the limbs; help provide seating and mobility devices; and check fit of braces to back or limbs as prescribed by a pediatric orthopedist or physiatrist. Any operative event, including dental care, should be done in a setting well-monitored by an anesthesiologist with the necessary precautions to handle a possible malignant hyperthermic event.

REFERENCES
Dubowitz V. *Muscle disorders in childhood,* 2nd ed. Philadelphia: WB Saunders, 1995:135–142.
Griggs RC, Mendell JR, Miller RG. *Evaluation and treatment of myopathies.* Philadelphia: FA Davis, 1995:213–215.

McCarthy TV, Quane KA, Lynch PJ. Ryanodine receptor mutations in malignant hyperthermia and central core disease. *Hum Mutat* 2000;15:410–417.
Rowe PW, Eagle M, Pallitt C, et al. Multicore myopathy: respiratory failure and paraspinal muscle contractures are important complications. *Dev Med Child Neurol* 2000;42:340–343.

RESOURCES
254, 368, 376

10 Creutzfeldt-Jakob Disease

Stephen J. DeArmond, MD, PhD

DEFINITION: Creutzfeldt-Jakob disease (CJD) is a rapidly progressive, invariably fatal, neurodegenerative disease caused by abnormalities of the prion protein (PrP) that result in nerve cell death and the formation of prions.

SYNONYMS: Transmissible spongiform encephalopathy; Prion disease.

DIFFERENTIAL DIAGNOSIS: Atypical Alzheimer disease; Pick disease; Huntington disease; Cerebellar disorders and amyotrophic lateral sclerosis with dementia.

SYMPTOMS AND SIGNS: Patients with prion diseases present with a broad spectrum of clinical symptoms and signs, including dementia, ataxia, insomnia, paraplegia, paresthesias, and deviant behavior. Clinical features suggestive of CJD are often preceded by a prodromal period in which nonspecific clinical signs occur, including fatigue, sleep disturbances, memory disturbances, behavioral changes, vertigo, and ataxia. The most characteristic clinical presentation is a rapidly progressive mental deterioration with dementia; a broad spectrum of motor disturbances including myoclonus and other extrapyramidal, cerebellar, pyramidal, and/or anterior horn cell signs; and an electroencephalogram (EEG) showing periodic short-wave activity. Usually, CJD runs a relatively rapid course, leading to death within 4–12 months from the start of symptoms and signs.

ETIOLOGY/EPIDEMIOLOGY: The disorder occurs sporadically approximately 90% of the time (sporadic CJD), is dominantly inherited approximately 10% of the time (familial CJD), and rarely is acquired by infection with prions. Of sporadic CJD cases, 95% occur in patients older than 50 years and are believed to be caused either by an acquired mutation of the prion protein gene (*PRNP*) or by rare spontaneous conversion of the normal PrP isoform, PrP^C, to the protease-resistant isoform, designated PrP^{Sc}. All familial CJD cases are genetically linked to point mutations or insertions of the *PRNP* gene. Two main categories of CJD cases are acquired by infection: iatrogenic CJD acquired through medical procedures, and a variant of CJD in the United Kingdom and Europe acquired by ingestion of bovine spongiform encephalopathy (mad cow disease)–contaminated food. The incidence of all forms of CJD is equal between the sexes.

DIAGNOSIS: When the quartet of dementia, myoclonus, periodic EEG activity, and rapid progression is seen in a patient, the diagnosis is relatively certain. Definitive diagnosis requires identification of protease-resistant PrP^{Sc}. This can be done in life by brain biopsy or, in variant CJD, by biopsy of the pharyngeal tonsils. Definitive diagnosis often is made at autopsy.

TREATMENT
Standard Therapies: There is no known therapy; however, a small number of promising pharmacologic agents is being tested.

REFERENCES
Brown P, Will RG, Bradley R, et al. Bovine spongiform encephalopathy and variant Creutzfeldt-Jakob disease: background, evolution, and current concerns. Bethesda, MD: Centers for Disease Control and Prevention, 2001:1–13. Available at *www.cdc.gov/ncidod/EID/vol7no1/brown.htm.*
DeArmond SJ, Ironside JW. Neuropathology of prion diseases. In: Prusiner SB, ed. *Prion biology and diseases.* Cold Spring Harbor, NY: Cold Spring Harbor Laboratory Press, 1999:585–652.
DeArmond SJ, Prusiner SB. Prion diseases. In: Graham DI, Lantos PL, eds. *Greenfield's neuropathology,* 6th ed. London: Arnold (Oxford University Press), 1997:235–280.
Prusiner SB. Shattuck Lecture: neurodegenerative diseases and prions. *N Engl J Med* 2001;344:1516–1526.
Prusiner SB, Scott MR, DeArmond SJ, et al. Prion protein biology. *Cell* 1998;93:337–348.

RESOURCES
22, 122, 359, 368

11 Dystonia

Mahlon R. DeLong, MD

DEFINITION: Dystonia is a neurologic movement disorder characterized by involuntary muscle contractions that force the body into abnormal, sometimes painful, movements or postures. It can affect any part of the body, including the arms and legs, trunk, neck, eyelids, face, or vocal cords. It is classified in three ways: age of onset, body distribution of symptoms, and etiology.

SYNONYMS: Generalized dystonia; Focal dystonia.

DIFFERENTIAL DIAGNOSIS: Chronic motor tics; Cerebral palsy; Clubfoot; Scoliosis.

SYMPTOMS AND SIGNS: The symptoms may begin during childhood (early-onset), in adolescence, or during adulthood. Cases of childhood-onset and adolescent-onset (<28 years) dystonia typically begin in early childhood after a period of normal physical development. Dystonia may initially present in the limbs, particularly the foot and leg, and spread to other body areas. The appearance of symptoms in adult-onset dystonia (>28 years) typically occurs between ages 30 and 50 years after decades of normal physical function. Symptoms tend to remain focal, affecting one part of the body. When dystonia manifests, the symptoms may change significantly with different tasks. For example, dystonia of the foot may occur when walking forward but disappear completely when walking backward or while sitting in a chair. Classification is done by the number and specific areas of the body that are affected. Focal dystonia, the most frequent type of dystonia, affects one single area of the body; segmental dystonia affects at least two or more adjacent areas of the body; multifocal dystonia appears in two or more areas of the body that are not adjacent; generalized dystonia involves several body areas on both sides of the body; and hemidystonia affects either the left or the right side of the body exclusively.

ETIOLOGY/EPIDEMIOLOGY: Two broad categories exist to classify dystonia by the basic cause of symptoms: primary and secondary. Primary dystonia is defined by the existence of dystonia alone without any underlying disorder. It may be caused by abnormal functioning of the basal ganglia. An imbalance of dopamine may underlie several forms of dystonia, but more research is required for a better understanding of the brain mechanisms involved. Secondary forms of dystonia may be attributed to birth injury, exposure to certain medications (including neuroleptics), trauma, toxins, or stroke. Secondary dystonia may be symptomatic and occur in association with other disorders such as Wilson disease. Variant forms of dystonia are marked by atypical clinical features and may be etiologically distinct from the classic form. Dopa-responsive, paroxysmal, X-linked dystonia-parkinsonism, myoclonic, and rapid-onset dystonia-parkinsonism are all considered variant forms (see also separate entries).

DIAGNOSIS: The diagnosis rests on physical and neurologic examination and family history. Genetic tests are available for DYT1 childhood-onset dystonia and dopa-responsive dystonia. Specific biochemical tests may assist in the diagnosis of dopa-responsive dystonia.

TREATMENT
Standard Therapies: Treatment is intended to help lessen the symptoms of spasms, pain, and disturbed postures and functions. The three treatment options are oral medications, botulinum toxin injections, and surgery. These therapies may be used alone or in combination. Physical therapy and speech therapy may also play a role. Oral medications may lessen the symptoms of pain, spasm, and abnormal posturing and function. The categories of medications used include anticholinergics and benzodiazepines. Some patients with primary dystonia respond to drugs that increase dopamine such as levodopa or bromocriptine; however, many patients respond to agents that block or deplete dopamine, such as standard antipsychotics. Botulinum toxin is injected into specific muscles to reduce involuntary contractions. Surgery may be considered when symptoms fail to respond to other treatments. Surgery is undertaken to interrupt, at various levels of the nervous system, the pathways responsible for the abnormal movements. Some operations intentionally damage small regions of the thalamus (thalamotomy), globus pallidus (pallidotomy), or other deep centers in the brain. Deep brain stimulation has been tried with some success.

Investigational Therapies: Research into more effective treatments and ultimately a cure for dystonia is being pursued primarily in the field of genetics and animal models. Investigations into drug therapeutics and surgical procedures are also under way.

REFERENCES
Fahn S, Marsden CD, DeLong MR. *Dystonia 3.* Vol. 78. Advances in neurology. Philadelphia: Lippincott-Raven, 1998.
King J, Tsui C, Calne DB. *Handbook of dystonia.* New York: Marcel Dekker; 1995.

11a   Blepharospasm

Mahlon R. DeLong, MD

DEFINITION: Blepharospasm is a focal dystonia characterized by increased blinking and involuntary closing of the eyes. Vision is normal; visual disturbance is due solely to the forced closure of the eyelids.

SYNONYM: Benign essential blepharospasm.

DIFFERENTIAL DIAGNOSIS: Ptosis; Blepharitis; Hemifacial spasm; Chronic motor tic.

SYMPTOMS AND SIGNS: Blepharospasm affects the eye muscles and usually begins gradually with excessive blinking and/or eye irritation. In the early stages, it may occur with only specific precipitating stressors, such as bright lights, fatigue, and emotional tension. It occurs in both eyes almost exclusively. As the condition progresses, symptoms may occur frequently during the day. The spasms disappear in sleep, and some people find that after a good night's sleep, spasms do not appear for several hours after waking. In some cases, the spasms may intensify so that the eyelids remain forcefully closed for several hours at a time. Blepharospasm may occur in conjunction with dystonia of the mouth and/or jaw. In such cases, spasms of the eyelids are accompanied by jaw clenching or mouth opening, grimacing, and tongue protrusion.

ETIOLOGY/EPIDEMIOLOGY: Blepharospasm is likely caused by abnormal functioning of the basal ganglia. The cause is unknown. An imbalance of dopamine, a neurotransmitter in the basal ganglia, may underlie several different forms of dystonia. Although some patients may have a history of eye trauma, a relationship between trauma and blepharospasm has not been established. In most people it develops spontaneously with no known precipitating factor. Cases of inherited blepharospasm have been reported, usually in conjunction with early-onset generalized dystonia, which is associated with the *DYT1* gene. Blepharospasm may be secondary or symptomatic, occurring in association with other disorders such as tardive dystonia, parkinsonian syndromes, and Wilson disease.

DIAGNOSIS: Diagnosis of blepharospasm is based on information from the affected individual and the physical and neurologic examination. There is no test to confirm the diagnosis.

TREATMENT
Standard Therapies: The three options for treatment are oral medications, botulinum toxin injections, and surgery, used alone or in combination. Approximately one third of patients improved when treated with oral medications such as clonazepam, trihexyphenidyl, and baclofen, but the degree of improvement is usually unsatisfactory and at the expense of side effects. Botulinum toxin injections are the primary and most effective form of treatment. Minute doses of the toxin are injected intramuscularly into several sites above and below the eyes. Benefits can begin in 1–14 days after the treatment and last for an average of 3–4 months. Side effects are infrequent and transient. Surgery is recommended only after other therapies are tried. Protractor myectomy (removal of some or all of the muscles responsible for eyelid closure) has proven to be the most effective surgical treatment for blepharospasm. Complementary therapies may supplement medical treatment. Dark glasses are a common aid; the glasses perform two functions by reducing the intensity of sunlight, which may aggravate the blepharospasm, and by hiding the patient's eyes from curious onlookers. The use of sensory tricks may also be effective in relieving spasms. Some of the most common are pulling on the upper eyelid, pinching the neck, talking, humming, yawning, singing, sleeping, reading, looking down, or concentrating.

REFERENCES
Fahn S, Marsden CD, DeLong MR. *Dystonia 3.* Vol. 78. Advances in neurology. Philadelphia: Lippincott-Raven, 1998.
King J, Tsui C, Calne DB. *Handbook of dystonia.* New York: Marcel Dekker, 1995.

RESOURCES
72, 140, 368

11b   Cervical Dystonia (Spasmodic Torticollis)

Mahlon R. DeLong, MD

DEFINITION: Cervical dystonia is a focal dystonia characterized by neck muscles contracting involuntarily, causing abnormal movements and posture of the head and neck. This term is used generally to describe spasms in any direction: forward (anterocollis), backward (retrocollis), and sideways (torticollis). The movements may be sustained or jerky. Spasms in the muscles or pinching nerves in the neck can result in considerable pain and discomfort.

SYNONYM: Spasmodic torticollis.

DIFFERENTIAL DIAGNOSIS: Wry neck; Stiff neck; Arthritis; Local orthopedic or congenital problems.

SYMPTOMS AND SIGNS: In cervical dystonia, the neck muscles contract involuntarily in various combinations. Sustained contractions cause abnormal posture of the head and neck, whereas periodic spasms produce jerky head movements. The severity may vary from mild to severe. Movements are often partially relieved by a gentle touch on the chin or other parts of the face. Features such as cognition, strength, and the senses, including vision and hearing, are normal.

ETIOLOGY/EPIDEMIOLOGY: Cervical dystonia is believed to be due to abnormal functioning of the basal ganglia. An imbalance of dopamine may underlie several forms of dystonia, but more research is required. A history of head or neck injury may be obtained, but the exact relationship between trauma and dystonia is still unclear. The interval from trauma to the onset of dystonia can be years. Cases of inherited cervical dystonia have been reported, usually in conjunction with early-onset generalized dystonia, which is associated with the *DYT1* gene.

DIAGNOSIS: Diagnosis is based on information from the affected individual and the physical and neurologic examination. There is no test to confirm the diagnosis.

TREATMENT

Standard Therapies: Treatment for dystonia is intended to lessen the symptoms of spasms, pain, and disturbed postures and functions. Most therapies are symptomatic, attempting to cover up or relieve the muscle spasms. No single strategy is appropriate for every case. Three options exist for treating cervical dystonia: oral medications, botulinum toxin injections, and surgery. These may be used alone or in combination. No drugs appear to be uniformly effective. The categories of drugs that may help to relieve symptoms include anticholinergic, dopaminergic, and GABAergic drugs. Botulinum toxin injections are the primary and most effective form of treatment. Surgery may be considered when patients are no longer receptive to other treatments. Surgery may lose its effects over the years, but it may provide some relief. Surgical approaches include muscle resection, anterior cervical rhizotomy, and selective peripheral denervation (the Bertrand Procedure). Complementary care, such as physical therapy and speech therapy, may also have a role, depending on the form of dystonia. A soft cervical collar is sometimes helpful. The use of sensory tricks may also be effective in dealing with cervical dystonia. These may include lightly touching the chin or back of the head. Different sensory tricks work for different people, and if a person finds a sensory trick that works, it usually works consistently.

Investigational Therapies: Research into more effective treatments and ultimately a cure for dystonia is being pursued primarily in the field of genetics and animal models. Investigations into drug therapeutics and surgical procedures are also under way.

REFERENCES

Fahn S, Marsden CD, DeLong MR. *Dystonia 3*. Vol. 78. Advances in neurology. Philadelphia: Lippincott-Raven, 1998.
King J, Tsui C, Calne DB. *Handbook of dystonia*. New York: Marcel Dekker, 1995.

RESOURCES

139, 332, 368, 487

11c   Dopa-Responsive Dystonia

Mahlon R. DeLong, MD

DEFINITION: Dopa-responsive dystonia (DRD) is an umbrella term used to describe dystonia that responds to levodopa. DRD is characterized by progressive difficulty walking. Symptoms may be similar to early-onset generalized dystonia.

SYNONYMS: Segawa disease; Hereditary progressive dystonia with marked diurnal variation.

DIFFERENTIAL DIAGNOSIS: Cerebral palsy; DYT1 childhood-onset dystonia; Spastic paraplegia; Disorders that cause childhood-onset parkinsonism.

SYMPTOMS AND SIGNS: Dopa-responsive dystonia classically manifests as a dystonic gait disorder in early childhood. Although patients usually present with symptoms at approximately age 7 years, manifestations of DRD may appear at any age. The most common complaint of people with DRD is having problems walking. Symptoms may appear minor (such as muscle cramps after exercise) or present later in life in a form that more closely resembles Parkinson disease. Features of parkinsonism that may occur include slowness of movements, instability or lack of balance, and, less commonly, tremor of the hands at rest. Symptoms of DRD are often worse later in the day and may increase with exertion. They are almost always better in the morning after sleep.

ETIOLOGY/EPIDEMIOLOGY: DRD is believed to be caused by abnormal functioning of the basal ganglia. An imbalance of dopamine may underlie several different forms of dystonia, but more research is required for a better understanding of the brain mechanisms involved. Two genes responsible for DRD have been identified: one gene codes for the production of an enzyme called GTP cyclohydrolase and another codes for an enzyme called tyrosine hydroxylase; both of these enzymes contribute to the production of dopamine. These defective genes disrupt the normal production of dopamine, which reduces the levels of dopamine in the body, thereby causing motor problems. The most commonly identified form of DRD is a dominantly inherited condition caused by mutations in the GTP cyclohydrolase 1 gene (*GTP-CH1*). Another common form of DRD is caused by a mutation in the recessively inherited tyrosine hydroxylase gene (*hTH*). Approximately 40% of patients with DRD do not have a mutation in the *GTP-CH1* or the *hTH* gene. Other known inherited metabolic conditions may cause DRD (including autosomal-recessive deficiencies of GTP-CH1 and aromatic L-amino acid decarboxylase and other defects of tetrahydrobiopterin metabolism). These recessively inherited conditions often affect cognitive function, which is not associated with the dominantly inherited DRD.

DIAGNOSIS: The diagnosis is not made by one definitive test, but by a series of clinical observations and specific biochemical assessments. Defining the exact etiology may not be possible. A therapeutic trial with levodopa remains the most practical initial approach to diagnosis; however, dystonia that responds to levodopa may result from multiple conditions.

Not all patients respond immediately to levodopa, and not all individuals who are carriers exhibit symptoms. A detailed family history is an important element of diagnosis. Obtaining a cerebrospinal fluid sample (by means of lumbar puncture) is another important component. Specific metabolic defects may be detected by an oral phenylalanine loading test, but the test is not 100% sensitive and the scope is limited.

TREATMENT

Standard Therapies: Treatment for dystonia is designed to help lessen the symptoms of spasms, pain, and disturbed postures and functions. Most therapies are symptomatic, attempting to cover up or release the dystonic spasms. No single strategy is appropriate for every case. Symptoms can usually be treated effectively with levodopa. In many cases, full physical functionality is restored. Levodopa responsiveness has been reported to be effective in people who have been symptomatic for as long as 50 years before treatment. Stable response after years of continuous treatment has also been reported.

Investigational Therapies: Research into more effective treatments and ultimately a cure for dystonia is being pursued primarily in the field of genetics. Investigations into drug therapeutics and surgery are also under way.

REFERENCES
Fahn S, Marsden CD, DeLong MR. *Dystonia 3*. Vol. 78. Advances in neurology. Philadelphia: Lippincott-Raven, 1998.

King J, Tsui C, Calne DB. *Handbook of dystonia*. New York: Marcel Dekker, 1995.

RESOURCES
139, 332, 368, 487

11d   Embouchure Dystonia

Mahlon R. DeLong, MD

DEFINITION: Embouchure dystonia is a term used to describe a type of dystonia that affects musicians who play brass and woodwind instruments. The term *embouchure* refers to the adjustment of the mouth to fit the mouthpiece of a brass or wind instrument. The anatomy of this form of dystonia includes muscles of the mouth, face, jaw, and tongue.

SYNONYMS: Task-specific mouth, lip, tongue, and/or face dystonia.

DIFFERENTIAL DIAGNOSIS: Lack of preparation or concentration with regard to rehearsing music; Psychiatric condition.

SYMPTOMS AND SIGNS: The abnormal movements that characterize embouchure dystonia are often subtle and occur only while the musician is playing or buzzing into the mouthpiece of an instrument. Symptoms may occur as involuntary, abnormal contractions of the muscles in the face, including involuntary puckering, excessive elevation of the corners of the mouth, and involuntary closing of the mouth. Symptoms may also include air leaks at the corners of the mouth. This may be more noticeable at higher registers and may be accompanied by a noticeable tremor. Some musicians' difficulties are limited to sustained notes in particular registers or to certain passages of music at specific speeds. The dystonia is typically painless but may elicit intense psychological stress.

ETIOLOGY/EPIDEMIOLOGY: Embouchure dystonia is believed to be caused by abnormal functioning of the basal ganglia. An imbalance of dopamine may underlie forms of dystonia, but more research is required for a better understanding of the brain mechanisms involved.

DIAGNOSIS: Musicians may perceive the early symptoms of dystonia as the result of faulty technique or lack of sufficient preparation. Therefore, many musicians do not seek medical help until the condition is pronounced. Diagnosis is based on information from the affected individual and the physical and neurologic examination. There is no test to confirm the diagnosis and, in most cases, laboratory tests are normal.

TREATMENT
Standard Therapies: Oral medications, including trihexyphenidyl, clonazepam, and baclofen, are often used to treat segmental and generalized dystonias and may offer some relief for focal dystonias. Botulinum toxin is an option, but the anatomy of the area must be carefully considered to avoid unacceptable oral weakness. Stress can aggravate dystonia symptoms, and often, stress management and treating depression can result in an improvement of dystonia.

Investigational Therapies: Research into more effective treatments and ultimately a cure for dystonia is being pursued primarily in the field of genetics and animal models. Investigations into drug therapeutics are also under way.

REFERENCES
Fahn S, Marsden CD, DeLong MR. *Dystonia 3*. Vol. 78. Advances in neurology. Philadelphia: Lippincott-Raven, 1998.
King J, Tsui C, Calne DB. *Handbook of dystonia*. New York: Marcel Dekker, 1995.

RESOURCES
139, 332, 368, 487

11e   Laryngeal Dystonia (Spasmodic Dysphonia)

Mahlon R. DeLong, MD

DEFINITION: Spasmodic dysphonia (SD), a focal form of dystonia, involves involuntary spasms of the vocal cord muscles, causing interruptions of speech and affecting voice quality.

DIFFERENTIAL DIAGNOSIS: Muscle tension dysphonia; Voice strain; Essential tremor; Vocal effects of Parkinson disease; Stuttering; Psychogenic voice symptoms.

SYMPTOMS AND SIGNS: Two types of SD have been identified. In the more common adductor type, speaking causes abnormal involuntary excessive contraction of the muscles that bring the vocal cords together. This causes a tight voice quality, often with abrupt initiation and termination of voicing, resulting in a broken speech pattern and short breaks in speech. In the abductor type, there is excessive contraction of the muscles that separate the vocal cords, resulting in a breathy, whispering voice pattern. Clinicians have identified three subtypes of SD. One is a combination of adductor and abductor symptoms in which an individual may demonstrate both types of spasms as he speaks. In a second subtype, SD symptoms are accompanied by a voice tremor. A third subtype involves a primary voice tremor so severe the patient experiences adductor voice disruptions during the tremor. Symptoms may improve or disappear when whispering, laughing, or singing. Symptoms may vary during the day, become aggravated by certain types of speaking (especially talking on the phone), or increase during stressful situations. It may manifest at any age, but frequently begins between ages 40 and 50 years.

ETIOLOGY/EPIDEMIOLOGY: In most cases, the cause is unknown. SD is probably a central nervous system disorder and a focal form of dystonia. Dystonia disorders are believed to be due to abnormal functioning in the basal ganglia. Possible mechanisms involved in the triggering of SD are being researched, including familial factors, inflammation, and/or injury that may lead to central nervous system changes in laryngeal motor control. Onset is usually gradual. The disorder may co-occur with other dystonias such as blepharospasm, oromandibular dystonia, or cervical dystonia.

DIAGNOSIS: SD is one of the most frequently misdiagnosed conditions in speech-language pathology. Because there is no definitive test for SD, the diagnosis rests on the presence of characteristic clinical symptoms in the absence of other conditions that may mimic SD. It is important that an interdisciplinary team of professionals evaluate and provide accurate differential diagnosis. This team usually includes a speech-language pathologist to evaluate voice production and voice quality, a neurologist to carefully search for other signs of dystonia or other neurologic conditions, and an otolaryngologist to examine the vocal cords.

TREATMENT
Standard Therapies: Treatment is designed to help lessen the symptoms of the vocal spasms and improve the quality of the patient's voice. Most therapies are symptomatic, attempting to cover up or release the dystonic spasms. Oral medications provide little relief of the symptoms. Local injections of botulinum toxin into the vocal cord muscles are the most effective treatment. Persons with the more common adductor form of SD typically respond better to botulinum toxin injections than those with the abductor form. Surgery for SD is being reexamined for individuals in whom botulinum toxin injections no longer provide relief. Selective laryngeal adductor denervation-reinnervation surgery involves cutting the nerve to the affected vocal cord and reinnervating the muscle to prevent atrophy. General voice relaxation techniques and speech therapy may play an adjunct role in treatment. These include reducing vocal effort, loudness, intonation, and rate of utterance while increasing pause time between phrases. Some patients benefit from the use of a voice amplifier for the phone or of a self-contained microphone used in conjunction with any FM radio.

Investigational Therapies: Research into effective treatments and ultimately a cure for dystonia is being pursued primarily in the field of genetics. Investigations into drug therapeutics and surgical procedures are also under way.

REFERENCES
Fahn S, Marsden CD, DeLong MR. *Dystonia 3*. Vol. 78. Advances in neurology. Philadelphia: Lippincott-Raven, 1998.
King J, Tsui C, Calne DB. *Handbook of dystonia*. New York: Marcel Dekker, 1995.

RESOURCES
139, 140, 331, 370

11f   Myoclonic Dystonia

Mahlon R. DeLong, MD

DEFINITION: Myoclonic dystonia is characterized by rapid jerks alone or in combination with the sustained muscular contractions and postures of dystonia.

SYNONYMS: Hereditary dystonia with lightning jerks responsive to alcohol; Hereditary essential myoclonus.

SYMPTOMS AND SIGNS: Myoclonic movements are the most prominent clinical feature in most patients. The distribution of these rapid jerks is variable but most frequently affects the central part of the body, including the shoulders, arms, neck, and trunk. The face and legs are rarely affected. The jerks may occur synchronously or asynchronously in different muscle groups. The dystonic symptoms of prolonged muscle spasms or abnormal posture may also be present. The symptom distribution of myoclonic dystonia more often affects the upper body, whereas typical childhood-onset dystonia usually affects the legs. The age of onset is in the first or second decade of life, although some cases of adult onset have been reported. The course is benign in most cases. Most frequently, the disorder appears to be slowly progressive for a few years after onset, stabilizes, then fluctuates slightly over the years, or shows a mild, spontaneous improvement. As with all forms of dystonia, features such as cognition, strength, and the senses, including vision and hearing, are normal.

ETIOLOGY/EPIDEMIOLOGY: Myoclonic dystonia is often a familial disorder seen in successive generations. The mode of inheritance is autosomal dominant, with a high but incomplete penetrance and variable severity. Research to map and identify the gene or genes responsible for the disorder is ongoing. Sporadic cases may arise, but these instances may actually be genetic cases in which the family history is "masked" by reduced penetrance.

DIAGNOSIS: Diagnosis is based on family history and results of the physical and neurologic examinations. If the condition occurs with both myoclonus and dystonia, it may be classified as myoclonic dystonia or hereditary dystonia with lightning jerks responsive to alcohol. If dystonia is not present or is only a minor component, it may be classified as hereditary essential myoclonus. Whether all classifications are an expression of a single genetic disorder is not known.

TREATMENT
Standard Therapies: Treatment should be directed toward lessening the symptoms of spasms, pain, and disturbed postures and functions. Most therapies are symptomatic. No single strategy is appropriate for every case. Medications that have been tried include benztropine, clonazepam, neuroleptics, and dopamine agonists, but response to drugs for the treatment of myoclonic dystonia is poor. A striking feature in some people with myoclonus is the alleviation of symptoms upon ingestion of alcohol, but response varies greatly even within individual families.

Investigational Therapies: Research into more effective treatments and ultimately a cure for dystonia is being pursued primarily in the field of genetics and animal models. Investigations into drug therapeutics are also under way.

REFERENCES
Fahn S, Marsden CD, DeLong MR. *Dystonia 3*. Vol. 78. Advances in neurology. Philadelphia: Lippincott-Raven, 1998.
King J, Tsui C, Calne DB. *Handbook of dystonia*. New York: Marcel Dekker, 1995.

RESOURCES
139, 331, 368, 487

11g   Oromandibular Dystonia and Meige Syndrome

Mahlon R. DeLong, MD

DEFINITION: Oromandibular dystonia is a focal dystonia characterized by forceful contractions of the jaw and tongue, causing difficulty in opening and closing the mouth and often affecting chewing and speech. When oromandibular dystonia is combined with blepharospasm, it may be referred to as Meige syndrome.

SYNONYM: Jaw dystonia.

DIFFERENTIAL DIAGNOSIS: Temporomandibular joint disease (TMJ).

SYMPTOMS AND SIGNS: Oromandibular dystonia is often associated with dystonia of the cervical muscles (cervical dystonia/spasmodic torticollis), eyelids (blepharospasm), or larynx (spasmodic dysphonia). The combination of upper and lower dystonias is sometimes called cranial-cervical dystonia. The symptoms typically begin between the ages of 40 and 70 years and appear to be more common in women than in men. Oromandibular dystonia may be a continuous disorder that persists even during sleep, or it may be task specific, occurring only during activities such as speaking or chewing. Difficulty in swallowing is common if the jaw is affected, and spasms in the tongue can also make swallowing difficult. Cognition and the senses are normal. Although dystonia is not fatal, it is chronic and prognosis is difficult to predict.

ETIOLOGY/EPIDEMIOLOGY: Oromandibular dystonia may be attributed to abnormal functioning of the basal ganglia. An imbalance of dopamine may underlie several forms of dystonia, but more research is required for a better understanding of the brain mechanisms involved. Cases of inherited cranial dystonia have been reported, usually in conjunction with early-onset generalized dystonia, which is associated with the *DYT1* gene. Oromandibular dystonia may be secondary, or symptomatic, occurring in association with other disorders such as tardive dystonia, Wilson disease, Parkinson disease, and X-linked dystonia-parkinsonism.

DIAGNOSIS: Diagnosis is based on information from the affected individual and the physical and neurologic examination. There is no test to confirm the diagnosis.

TREATMENT
Standard Therapies: The two treatment options are oral medications and botulinum toxin injections, either used alone or in combination. The structure of the jaw is too complex for denervation surgery. No drugs appear to be uniformly effective. Approximately one third of patients' symptoms improve when treated with oral medications such as clonazepam, trihexyphenidyl, diazepam, tetrabenazine, and baclofen, but the degree of improvement is usually unsatisfactory and there are side effects. Approximately 70% of patients experience some reduction of spasm and improvement of chewing and speech after an injection of botulinum toxin into the masseter, temporalis, and lateral pterygoid muscles. Side effects such as swallowing difficulties, slurred speech, and excess weakness in injected muscles may occur, but these are usually transient and well tolerated. The use of sensory tricks may also be effective in reducing spasms. Some of the most common tricks for dystonia affecting the face include lightly touching the lips or chin, chewing gum, talking, biting on a toothpick, or putting a finger near an eye or underneath the chin to keep the jaw closed. Speech and swallowing therapy may lessen spasms, improve range of motion, and strengthen unaffected muscles.

Investigational Therapies: Research into more effective treatments and ultimately a cure for dystonia is being pursued primarily in the field of genetics and animal models. Investigations into drug therapeutics are also under way.

REFERENCES
Fahn S, Marsden CD, DeLong MR. *Dystonia 3.* Vol. 78. Advances in neurology. Philadelphia: Lippincott-Raven, 1998.
King J, Tsui C, Calne DB. *Handbook of dystonia.* New York: Marcel Dekker, 1995.

RESOURCES
72, 139, 368, 487

11h   Paroxysmal Dystonias and Dyskinesias

Mahlon R. DeLong, MD

DEFINITION: Paroxysmal dystonia is a form of paroxysmal dyskinesia (PD) characterized by relatively brief attacks of dystonic movements and postures with a return to normal posture between episodes. PDs are movement disorders in which the abnormal movements are present only during the attacks. Between attacks, the person is neurologically normal. PDs are currently classified into four types: paroxysmal kinesigenic (action-induced) dyskinesia (PKD), paroxysmal nonkinesigenic dyskinesia (PNKD), paroxysmal exertion-induced dyskinesia (PED), and paroxysmal hynogenic (nocturnal) dyskinesia (PHD).

SYNONYMS: Paroxysmal kinesigenic choreoathetosis; Paroxysmal dystonic nonkinesigenic choreoathetosis.

DIFFERENTIAL DIAGNOSIS: Seizure disorder; Psychiatric disorder.

SYMPTOMS AND SIGNS: PKD may be characterized by attacks which may occur up to 100 times per day, are often precipitated by a startle, a sudden movement, a particular movement, or other factors. The attacks are usually short, lasting seconds or minutes. The symptoms may be preceded by an unusual sensation in the limbs and may be limited to one side of the body or to a single limb. Most people with PKD have dystonia, and some have a combination of chorea and dystonia or ballism. The frequency of attacks in PNKD is less than that of PKD, ranging from two per year to three per day. Fatigue, alcohol, caffeine, excitement, and other factors may trigger symptoms. The attacks generally last a few seconds to 4 hours or longer. The attacks may begin in one limb and spread throughout the body, including the face. A person affected by PNKD may not be able to communicate during an attack but remains conscious and continues to breathe normally. Attacks of PED are triggered by prolonged exercise and may last 5–30 minutes. The attacks may occur once a day to twice a month. PHD is characterized by attacks of dystonia, chorea, or ballism during non-REM sleep. These attacks may occur 5 times a year to 5 times a night and usually last 30–45 seconds. The attacks may also sometimes occur during the day. PHD is probably a broad condition consisting of several different types of attacks and clinical manifestations.

ETIOLOGY/EPIDEMIOLOGY: PDs are generally attributed to dysfunction in the basal ganglia, but much has yet to be learned about how and why PD occurs. Some regard PKD as a form of epilepsy involving specific parts of the brain (i.e., the basal ganglia and thalamus). A growing resource of evidence suggests that PKD may belong to a group of disorders similar to the inherited episodic ataxias, which are known to be associated with disorders of ion channels.

Although the exact origin may not be known, most cases of PD are inherited or sporadic. A gene for PNKD has been located on chromosome 2q, and a gene for PKD on chromosome 16. Cases of PD that are not considered inherited or sporadic and are associated with specific factors and conditions are classified as "secondary." These include multiple sclerosis, cerebral palsy, metabolic disorders, physical trauma, cerebrovascular disease, and miscellaneous conditions, including supranuclear palsy and AIDS. Most conditions associated with PKD may also be associated with PNKD. A few cases of secondary PED and PHD have been reported. PDs have also been associated with encephalitis and injury to the brain due to stroke and tumors. Drugs such as cocaine and dopamine-blocking agents may also induce dyskinesias. In extremely rare cases, PD may be a manifestation of a psychiatric disorder, but legitimate cases of PD have often been inappropriately dismissed as "psychogenic." An inaccurate psychiatric diagnosis not only causes unnecessary suffering to the person affected by PD, but it may also preclude appropriate treatment options.

DIAGNOSIS: History and (ideally) video documentation of the attacks are important tools in diagnosing PD. The workup may also include electroencephalography, brain MRI or CT, blood chemistries, and calcium tests.

TREATMENT
Standard Therapies: The current poor understanding of the pathophysiology and biochemistry of PD often makes establishing a satisfactory treatment plan difficult. Treatment needs to be tailored to the individual, and it may be necessary to try several options before symptoms are diminished or alleviated. Patience on the part of both physician and patient may be needed. Anticonvulsant and/or anticholinergic and medications may be appropriate. The intermittent and transient nature of PD generally precludes the use of therapies such as botulinum toxin injections and surgery.

Investigational Therapies: Research into more effective treatments and ultimately a cure for dystonia is being pursued primarily in the field of genetics and animal models. Investigations into improved drug therapeutics are also under way.

REFERENCES
Fahn S, Marsden CD, DeLong MR. *Dystonia 3*. Vol. 78. Advances in neurology. Philadelphia: Lippincott-Raven, 1998.
Jankovic J, Tolosa E. *Parkinson's disease and movement disorders.* Baltimore: Williams & Wilkins, 1998
King J, Tsui C, Calne DB. *Handbook of dystonia.* New York: Marcel Dekker, 1995.

RESOURCES
139, 368

11i　Rapid-Onset Dystonia-Parkinsonism

Mahlon R. DeLong, MD

DEFINITION: Rapid-onset dystonia-parkinsonism (RDP), a rare hereditary form of dystonia, is characterized by the abrupt onset of slowness of movement (parkinsonism) and dystonic symptoms.

DIFFERENTIAL DIAGNOSIS: Parkinson disease.

SYMPTOMS AND SIGNS: The classic features of RDP include involuntary dystonic spasms in the limbs, promi-

nent involvement of the speech and swallowing muscles, slowness of movement, and poor balance. Onset of the combined dystonic and parkinsonian symptoms can be sudden, occurring over hours to days. Symptoms usually stabilize in less then 4 weeks, after which little progress is reported. The disorder usually occurs in adolescence or young adulthood (age range 15–45 years), but onset of mild dystonia-parkinsonism has been reported in individuals up to the age of 58 years.

ETIOLOGY/EPIDEMIOLOGY: The cause is not known, although the mode of inheritance is autosomal dominant.

Genetic linkage studies have excluded RDP from the genomic region encoding for *DYT1*, the gene responsible for early-onset dystonia, as well as *DYT5*, the gene responsible for dopa-responsive dystonia. Low levels of the dopamine metabolite homovanillic acid in cerebrospinal fluid indicate a deficit in the dopaminergic system. Additional research must be conducted to determine whether another internal trigger exists other than low dopamine metabolite levels that may initiate the cascade of biochemical changes leading to the abrupt onset of dystonia and parkinsonian symptoms. Understanding this possible "trigger" may provide further insights into the mechanism of both dystonia and Parkinson disease.

DIAGNOSIS: Diagnosis is based on neurologic examination. Results of tests such as CT or MRI are normal. A family history is required to distinguish the mild limb dystonia of RDP from early-onset dystonia.

TREATMENT
Standard Therapies: Treatment is limited. Levodopa/carbidopa or dopamine agonists may provide some mild improvement in select individuals.

Investigational Therapies: Research into more effective treatments and ultimately a cure for dystonia is being pursued primarily in the field of genetics and animal models. Investigations into drug therapeutics are also under way.

REFERENCES
Fahn S, Marsden CD, DeLong MR. *Dystonia 3*. Vol. 78. Advances in neurology. Philadelphia: Lippincott-Raven, 1998.
King J, Tsui C, Calne DB. *Handbook of dystonia.* New York: Marcel Dekker, 1995.

RESOURCES
139, 368, 389, 487

11j   Writer's Cramp

Mahlon R. DeLong, MD

DEFINITION: Writer's cramp is a task-specific focal dystonia of the hand. Symptoms usually appear when a person attempts a task that requires fine motor movements; they may initially appear only during a particular type of movement, such as writing or playing the piano, but the dystonia may spread to affect many tasks. Two types have been described: simple and dystonic. People with simple writer's cramp have difficulty with one specific task. For example, if writing activates the dystonia, as soon as the person picks up a pen or within writing a few words, dystonic postures of the hand begin to impede speed and accuracy. In dystonic writer's cramp, symptoms are present not only when the person is writing, but also when performing other task-specific activities, such as shaving, using eating utensils, or applying makeup.

SYNONYM: Focal hand dystonia.

DIFFERENTIAL DIAGNOSIS: Carpal tunnel syndrome; Overuse conditions; Lack of preparation or practice in musicians.

SYMPTOMS AND SIGNS: Common manifestations of simple writer's cramp include excessive gripping of the pen, flexion, and sometimes deviation of the wrist, elevation of the elbow, and occasional extension of a finger or fingers causing the pen to fall from the hand. Sometimes the disorder progresses to include elevation of the shoulders or retraction of the arm while writing. Tremor is usually not a symptom. The symptoms usually begin between ages 30 and 50 years. Cramping or aching of the hand is not typical. Mild discomfort may occur in the fingers, wrist, or forearm. A similar cramp may be seen in musicians, in certain athletes such as golfers, and in typists.

ETIOLOGY/EDPIDEMIOLOGY: Writer's cramp is believed to be due to abnormal functioning of the basal ganglia. Cases of inherited writer's cramp have been reported, usually in conjunction with early-onset generalized dystonia, which is associated with the *DYT1* gene. Both men and women are affected.

DIAGNOSIS: Diagnosis is based on information from the affected individual and the physical and neurologic examination. No test exists to confirm the diagnosis, and in most cases, laboratory tests are normal. Sometimes electromyography is helpful to identify which muscles are overactive and to what degree. Focal hand dystonia is responsible for only approximately 5% of all conditions affecting the hand.

TREATMENT
Standard Therapies: The two options to treat focal hand dystonia are oral medications and botulinum toxin injections, which may be used alone or in combination. Approximately 5% of those affected have symptoms improve

with the use of anticholinergic drugs, such as trihexyphenidyl and benztropine, but the degree of improvement is usually unsatisfactory, and side effects occur. Botulinum toxin injections into selected muscles are helpful, especially when significant deviation of the wrist or finger joints is present. Significant improvement in writing and reduction of pain is seen in at least two thirds of persons treated. A conservative approach to treatment may include avoiding writing with the affected hand and using other methods of communication such as typing or dictating into a tape recorder. Physical methods to help hand dystonia include learning to hold a pencil differently or using a special wax mold to change the alignment of the hand and arm while holding a pen or pencil. In some cases, attempting to use the shoulder and arm rather than the wrists and fingers to write may lessen symptoms. Sometimes a minimal change in writing style can make a difference. Approximately 60% of people with writer's cramp reduce their symptoms by writing vertically on a board rather than horizontally on a desk. Learning to write with the opposite hand may be helpful; however, in approximately 50% of affected individuals, the dystonia will eventually "jump" to the opposite hand. In some cases, writing with the left hand will trigger symptoms in the right hand, or vice versa. Physical therapy may help to improve local arm flexibility.

Investigational Therapies: Research into more effective treatments and ultimately a cure for dystonia is being pursued primarily in the field of genetics and animal models. Investigations into drug therapeutics are also under way.

REFERENCES

Fahn S, Marsden CD, DeLong MR. *Dystonia 3*. Vol. 78. Advances in neurology. Philadelphia: Lippincott-Raven, 1998.

King J, Tsui C, Calne DB. *Handbook of dystonia*. New York: Marcel Dekker, 1995.

11k   X-Linked Dystonia-Parkinsonism

Mahlon R. DeLong, MD

DEFINITION: X-linked dystonia-parkinsonism is a genetic form of dystonia found almost entirely among men from the Philippine island of Panay.

SYNONYM: Lubag.

SYMPTOMS AND SIGNS: Affecting mainly men, symptoms can appear as early as age 14 years. Young-onset patients tend to have focal dystonia that generalizes. In these patients, parkinsonism may replace dystonia symptoms or may develop with persistent dystonia. Patients with late-onset disease may present with parkinsonian features but without dystonia. The parkinsonian features of X-linked dystonia-parkinsonism are similar to those seen in idiopathic Parkinson disease with the exception that resting tremor is rarely seen.

ETIOLOGY/EPIDEMIOLOGY: X-linked dystonia-parkinsonism was first recognized in the Philippines among Panay Island families. Genetic analysis of large Filipino families indicates that the gene locus maps to chromosome Xq13. Pathologic and physiologic studies indicate that this disorder is caused by primary degeneration of the striatum with mosaic gliosis. Molecular genetic analysis indicates that the mutation responsible for X-linked dystonia-parkinsonism was introduced into the Olongo ethnic group of Panay more than 2,000 years ago.

DIAGNOSIS: X-linked dystonia-parkinsonism or Lubag is found almost exclusively among men from the Philippine Island of Panay. The diagnosis rests solely on information from the affected individual and the physical and neurologic examination.

TREATMENT

Standard Therapies: Dopaminergic agonists may cause a slight improvement in parkinsonian symptoms or induce dyskinesias. Anticholinergic drugs and benzodiazepines may have a slight effect on dystonia symptoms. The best hope for development of therapy may be based on an understanding of the etiology of the disease.

Investigational Therapies: Research into more effective treatments and ultimately a cure for dystonia is being pursued primarily in the field of genetics and animal models.

REFERENCES

Fahn S, Marsden CD, DeLong MR. *Dystonia 3*. Vol. 78. Advances in neurology. Philadelphia: Lippincott-Raven, 1998.

King J, Tsui C, Calne DB. *Handbook of dystonia*. New York: Marcel Dekker, 1995.

RESOURCES

139, 368, 389, 487

12   Hallervorden-Spatz Syndrome

Simon J. Hickman, MD, MRCP,
and Simon F. Farmer, PhD, FRCP

DEFINITION: Hallervorden-Spatz syndrome (HSS) is an incurable disorder that causes progressive extrapyramidal dysfunction and dementia. The pathologic features are iron deposition in the globus pallidus and substantia nigra, and widespread spheroid bodies.

SYNONYMS: Neurodegeneration with brain iron accumulation type 1; Pantothenate kinase–associated neurodegeneration.

DIFFERENTIAL DIAGNOSIS: Wilson disease; Huntington disease; Neuronal ceroid-lipofuscinosis; Early-onset Parkinson disease; GM_1 and GM_2 gangliosidoses.

SYMPTOMS AND SIGNS: Patients usually present in early childhood with dystonic posturing, rigidity, tremor, or choreoathetosis. Seizures, corticospinal tract involvement, dysarthria, dysphagia, retinitis pigmentosa, and optic atrophy are other possible features. Dementia and progressive motor decline usually follow, with death in early adulthood. A more aggressive course sometimes occurs with severe dystonia and opisthotonus. Patients may present in late childhood or adulthood. Their course is usually more indolent, with disease resembling atypical Parkinson disease with more prominent extrapyramidal features and less evidence of dementia.

ETIOLOGY/EPIDEMIOLOGY: Inheritance in most cases is autosomal recessive, although sporadic cases have also been described. Mutations from some, but not all patients, have been found on chromosome 20p13 in a gene encoding pantothenate kinase (*PANK2*). Dysfunction of *PANK2* may lead to the accumulation of cysteine, which can promote iron-induced lipid peroxidation and the formation of cell-damaging free radicals. This causes neuronal death and iron deposition, particularly in the globus pallidus and substantia nigra because of the naturally high local iron concentrations. Another candidate gene has been discovered, encoding a glial-derived neurotrophic receptor. Cases have been reported from the Americas, Europe, and Asia.

DIAGNOSIS: Diagnostic criteria have been proposed. All of the obligate features, at least two of the corroborative features, and no exclusionary features should be present. The obligate features include onset during the first two decades of life; progression of signs and symptoms; evi-

dence of extrapyramidal dysfunction; hypointense areas on MRI involving the basal ganglia, particularly the globus pallidus and the substantia nigra. The corroborative features include corticospinal tract involvement manifested by spasticity and/or a positive Babinski sign; progressive intellectual impairment; retinitis pigmentosa and/or optic atrophy; positive family history consistent with autosomal-recessive inheritance; and abnormal cytosomes in circulating lymphocytes and/or sea-blue histiocytes in bone marrow. The exclusionary features are abnormal ceruloplasmin levels and/or abnormalities in copper concentration or metabolism; the presence of overt neuronal ceroid-lipofuscinosis with severe visual impairment and/or difficult-to-control seizures; presence or family history of Huntington disease or other autosomal-dominant movement disorder; presence of caudate atrophy on imaging; a deficiency of hexosaminidase A or of GM_1-galactosidase; nonprogressive course; and absence of extrapyramidal signs.

TREATMENT

Standard Therapies: No treatment has been shown to alter the prognosis. Levodopa, bromocriptine, or trihexyphenidyl can often improve the dystonia. Focal dystonic spasms may be relieved by botulinum toxin injections. Baclofen can be used to treat spasticity and seizures may respond to either carbamazepine or phenytoin. Physiotherapy can help to maintain mobility. Speech therapy may be useful if dysarthria and dysphagia are present, although ultimately communication aids and gastrostomy feeding may be needed.

Investigational Therapies: Stereotactic pallidotomy is being investigated.

REFERENCES

First scientific workshop on Hallervorden-Spatz syndrome. *Pediatr Neurol* 2001;25:99–174.

Justesen CR, Penn RD, Kroin JS, et al. Stereotactic pallidotomy in a child with Hallervorden-Spatz disease. *J Neurosurg* 1999;90: 551–554.

Sethi KD, Adams RJ, Loring DW, et al. Hallervorden-Spatz syndrome: clinical and magnetic resonance imaging correlations. *Ann Neurol* 1988;24:692–694.

Zhou B, Westaway SK, Levinson B, et al. A novel pantothenate kinase gene (PANK2) is defective in Hallervorden-Spatz syndrome. *Nat Genet* 2001;28:345–349.

RESOURCES

109, 139, 357, 462

13 Lambert-Eaton Myasthenic Syndrome

Kevin T. Parsons, MD

DEFINITION: Lambert-Eaton myasthenic syndrome (LEMS) is an autoimmune disorder of the neuromuscular junction characterized by the gradual onset of symmetric proximal muscular weakness especially affecting the thigh and pelvic muscles. Of all LEMS cases, 60% are associated with a small cell lung cancer, and the onset of LEMS symptoms often begins prior to the detection of the cancer.

SYNONYMS: Eaton-Lambert syndrome; Myasthenic syndrome.

DIFFERENTIAL DIAGNOSIS: Myasthenia gravis; Botulism; Myopathies; Muscular dystrophy; Polyneuropathies.

SYMPTOMS AND SIGNS: Nearly all patients present with symmetric muscular weakness and easy fatigability of the thigh, pelvic, and especially the iliopsoas muscles. Onset is usually gradual, over several weeks to many months, affecting the patient's ability to engage in strenuous exercise and making climbing stairs and steep walkways difficult. Some patients also exhibit mild to moderate autonomic dysfunction, including dry mouth, difficulty swallowing, difficulty in articulation of speech, constipation, impotence, decreased sweating, postural hypotension, and drooping of the upper eyelids. Patients with or without cancer may also present with significant weight loss. Patients complain primarily of painless muscular weakness, and the physical examination can show signs of symmetric leg weakness and atrophy or be grossly normal and require active exercise for the weakness to be displayed. Muscle fasciculations are generally absent, and the deep tendon reflexes can be normal but are generally hypoactive or absent in advanced disease.

ETIOLOGY/EPIDEMIOLOGY: An estimated 400 cases are known worldwide. The syndrome is caused by autoantibodies against the P/Q voltage-gated calcium channel located on the nerve cell membrane at the neuromuscular junction. Affected patients with cancer are often older and nearly always have a long smoking history. In the 40% of LEMS cases where there is no associated cancer, disease onset can be at any age and the pathogenesis of the generation of the autoantibodies is unknown. Males and females are affected equally.

DIAGNOSIS: In patients presenting with symmetric muscular weakness, the diagnosis of LEMS should be considered and can be confirmed by a specialized electromyogram (EMG) and/or by the measurement of the blood level of calcium channel antibodies. The EMG may show initially decreased or normal amplitude, but after tetanic contraction, it usually shows a significant increase in amplitude over baseline (>100% in nearly half of LEMS patients).

TREATMENT

Standard Therapies: In LEMS patients with cancer, effective treatment of the cancer is the most beneficial treatment for LEMS. The most effective LEMS-specific treatment is 3,4-diaminopyradine (DAP), an orphan drug. More than 75% of LEMS patients will show significant improvement in muscular strength and endurance from treatment with DAP. DAP is often combined with mestinon to prolong its effectiveness. Other useful treatments include prednisone, chemotherapeutic agents such as imuran, intravenous gamma-globulin, and occasionally plasmapharesis.

REFERENCES

Deneviratne U, de Silva R. Lambert-Eaton myasthenic syndrome. *Postgrad Med J* 1999;75:516–520.

Takamori M, Komai K, Iwasa K. Antibodies to calcium channel and synaptotagmin in Lambert-Eaton myasthenic syndrome. *J Med Sci* 2000;319:204–208.

Tim RW, Massey JM, Sanders DB. Lambert-Eaton myasthenic syndrome: electrodiagnostic findings and response to treatment. *Neurology* 2000;54:2176–2178.

RESOURCES

27, 270, 368

14   Becker Muscular Dystrophy

Gyula Acsadi, MD, PhD

DEFINITION: Becker muscular dystrophy (BMD) is the allelic variant of Duchenne muscular dystrophy (DMD). Muscle dystrophy is a pathologic terminology, which entails the necrosis, atrophy, and fibroadipous displacement of skeletal muscle.

SYNONYMS: Pseudohypertrophic myopathy; Muscular dystrophy; Dystrophinopathy.

DIFFERENTIAL DIAGNOSIS: Duchenne muscular dystrophy; Congenital muscular dystrophy; Myotonic dystrophy; Limb-girdle muscular dystrophy; Metabolic myopathy.

SYMPTOMS AND SIGNS: Presentation and progression are strikingly variable. Some severely affected patients show delayed motor milestones similar to DMD, but experience a slower progression. The prominent hypertrophy of muscles in the early-onset form makes these children appear "muscular," but usually they have some clumsiness. Severely affected patients may become wheelchair bound later than is typical for DMD patients. These patients represent less than 10% of all BMD patients; the remaining 90% may show a milder and variable clinical phenotype with onset as late as age 65. The presentation of late-onset BMD includes proximal limb girdle weakness, episodic myoglobinuria, muscle cramps, muscle pain, cardiomyopathy, elevated creatine kinase level, muscle hypertrophy, or muscle atrophy. Most patients show slow deterioration of muscle strength, which may lead to loss of ambulation in their twenties or thirties, but others show milder progression and some remain asymptomatic.

ETIOLOGY/EPIDEMIOLOGY: BMD is caused by in-frame mutations of a 2.5 million base pairs gene located on the X-chromosome (Xp21). The protein product of the gene, dystrophin, is decreased in either quantity or size. Dystrophin is closely associated with the membrane cytoskeleton and likely takes part in plasma membrane stability during muscle contraction or stretching. The loss of dystrophin may lead to plasma membrane injury and a subsequent cascade of events leading to muscle cell necrosis. BMD affects approximately 1 in 7,000 males in all world populations.

DIAGNOSIS: Where a family history of the disease exists, diagnosis and prognosis can usually be based on the disease of older male relatives. Genetic testing can be done for diagnosis and counseling. For patients with no family history, multiplex polymerase chain reaction analysis of DNA for deletion mutations can confirm the diagnosis of a dystrophinopathy in approximately 65% of patients, and may often differentiate between DMD and milder BMD; however, not all BMD or DMD patients have deletion mutations large enough to detect. The gene is too large for routine gene sequencing, but a high proportion (70%–90%) of BMD patients show deletion of the gene. If a positive DNA test does not distinguish between severe DMD and milder BMD, or if the DNA test is negative, the dystrophin protein in a muscle biopsy should be analyzed by immuno-histochemistry of cryostat sections or immunoblotting (Western blots).

TREATMENT

Standard Therapies: The severity and clinical course of BMD are variable, and management is mostly symptomatic. Mildly affected patients may not require therapeutic intervention. More severely affected patients will likely need to be managed for contractures, and may require braces or wheelchairs. Corticosteroids may slow the progression of weakness and can prolong ambulation of DMD patients but no similar data are available for BMD. In patients with severe cardiomyopathy, heart transplantation should be considered.

Investigational Therapies: Therapies being explored include drugs to upregulate compensatory proteins (e.g., utrophin) and replacement of the defective dystrophin by gene therapy.

REFERENCES

Engel AG, Yamamoto M, Fischbeck KH. Dystrophinopathies. In: Engel AG, Franzini-Armstrong C, eds. *Myology,* 2nd ed. New York: McGraw-Hill, 1994:1130–1187.

Hartigan-O'Connor D, Chamberlain JS. Developments in gene therapy for muscular dystrophy. *Microsc Res Tech* 2000;48: 223–238.

Sandri M, El Meslemani AH, Sandri C, et al. Caspase 3 expression correlates with skeletal muscle apoptosis in Duchenne and facioscapulo human muscular dystrophy. A potential target for pharmacological treatment? *J Neuropathol Exp Neurol* 2001;60:302–312.

Saotome M, Yoshitomi Y, Kojima S, et al. Dilated cardiomyopathy of Becker-type muscular dystrophy with exon 4 deletion—a case report. *Angiology* 2001;52:343–347.

RESOURCES

270, 368, 441

15 | Duchenne Muscular Dystrophy

Gyula Acsadi, MD, PhD

DEFINITION: Duchenne muscular dystrophy (DMD) is the most common inherited muscle disease in children, characterized by progressive weakness, initial hypertrophy then atrophy of skeletal muscle, premature death, and X-linked inheritance.

SYNONYMS: Pseudohypertrophic myopathy; Muscular dystrophy; Dystrophinopathy.

DIFFERENTIAL DIAGNOSIS: Becker muscular dystrophy; Congenital muscular dystrophy; Myotonic dystrophy; Limb-girdle muscular dystrophy.

SYMPTOMS AND SIGNS: The main presentations include proximal muscle weakness, hypertrophy of the calf muscles, "waddling" gait, and elevated serum levels of creatine kinase. Other presenting symptoms are delayed walking, frequent falling, and tiptoe walking. Muscle hypertrophia is an early, characteristic sign. Deep tendon reflexes are absent in the upper extremities and knees even in the early stages, whereas ankle reflexes can be present until the terminal stages. The rate of deterioration is variable; however, most patients stop walking between age 9 and 13 years, and progressive scoliosis occurs after that. Most patients die around age 20 from respiratory insufficiency. Of affected boys, 30%–40% have a nonprogressive cognitive deficit.

ETIOLOGY/EPIDEMIOLOGY: The disease is caused by mutations of a 2.5 million base pairs gene located on the X chromosome (Xp21). The protein product of the gene, dystrophin, is missing in DMD. Dystrophin is closely associated with the membrane cytoskeleton and likely takes part in plasma membrane stability during muscle contraction or stretching. The loss of dystrophin may lead to plasma membrane injury and a subsequent cascade of events leading to muscle cell necrosis. The prevalence of DMD is approximately 1 in 3,500 male births worldwide.

DIAGNOSIS: Multiplex polymerase chain reaction analysis of DNA for deletion mutations can confirm the diagnosis in approximately 65% of patients. In patients testing negative for a gene deletion mutation, the next step is to analyze the dystrophin protein in a muscle biopsy, by either immunohistochemistry of cryostat sections or im-munoblotting. Dystrophin deficiency is generally considered specific for DMD.

TREATMENT

Standard Therapies: Corticosteroids may slow the progression of weakness and can prolong ambulation to some extent. Prednisone increases strength if administered relatively early in the disease. Deflazacort (not available in the United States) is equally effective in slowing the progression and has fewer side effects. The anabolic steroid oxandrolone, or creatin, may increase and maintain muscle strength. Tendon contractures are a major complication of DMD; physical therapy, with frequent stretching of the involved tendons, may alleviate or mitigate this problem. Achilles tendon contractures generally begin to limit mobility by the end of the first decade, and surgical tendon lengthenings are done frequently. Knee-foot orthosis is often used to prolong mobility and provide stability during ambulation. Bracing may also prevent contracture, and night splints are recommended in patients 4–5 years old and at the earliest sign of contractures. Later in the course of progression, patients generally require electric wheelchairs, because the hands and arms also lose strength as the ability to walk is lost. Wheelchair design and fitting are important for slowing of scoliosis. If scoliosis begins to limit vital capacity, spinal fusion may be considered.

Investigational Therapies: Drugs to upregulate compensatory proteins (e.g., utrophin) and the replacement of the defective dystrophin by gene therapy are being explored.

REFERENCES

Carpenter S, Karpati G. *Pathology of skeletal muscle.* New York: Oxford University Press; 2001.

Davies JE, Winokur TS, Aaron MF, et al. Cardiomyopathy in a carrier of duchenne's muscular dystrophy. *J Heart Lung Transplant* 2001;20:781–784.

Fenichel GM, Griggs RC, Kissel J, et al. A randomized efficacy and safety trial of oxandrolone in the treatment of Duchenne dystrophy. *Neurology* 2001;56:1075–1079.

Hartigan-O'Connor D, Chamberlain JS. Developments in gene therapy for muscular dystrophy. *Microsc Res Tech* 2000;48:223–238.

Sandri M, El Meslemani AH, Sandri C, et al. Caspase 3 expression correlates with skeletal muscle apoptosis in Duchenne and facioscapulo human muscular dystrophy. A potential target for pharmacological treatment? *J Neuropathol Exp Neurol* 2001;60:302–312.

RESOURCES

270, 368, 441

16   Emery-Dreifuss Muscular Dystrophy

Brenda Banwell, MD

DEFINITION: Emery-Dreifuss muscular dystrophy (EDMD) is a slowly progressive condition associated with early-onset contractures of the elbows and Achilles tendons, weakness and wasting of the proximal and distal muscles, and life-threatening cardiomyopathy with conduction block.

DIFFERENTIAL DIAGNOSIS: Limb-girdle muscular dystrophies; Duchenne and Becker muscular dystrophies; Rigid spine syndrome.

SYMPTOMS AND SIGNS: Contractures of the elbows and neck appear in childhood. Muscle weakness is usually noticed in late childhood or adolescence. Muscle wasting and weakness selectively affect biceps and triceps more than scapular muscles in the upper limbs. In the lower limbs, distal muscles are affected earlier than proximal muscles, although proximal weakness eventually develops and progresses slowly. Mild facial weakness is present in some patients. Tendon reflexes are reduced or absent in most patients. All patients have cardiac conduction disturbance. Atrial arrest develops over time, and may cause sudden death.

ETIOLOGY/EPIDEMIOLOGY: The disease exists in two forms: a more common X-linked form and an autosomal-dominant form (AD-EDMD). X-linked EDMD is caused by mutations in the *STA* gene at Xq28, encoding the protein emerin, and AD-EDMD is due to mutations in the *LMNA* gene at 1q11–21, which encodes the lamin A/C protein. Both emerin and lamin A/C localize to the nuclear envelope. How deficiency in nuclear membrane–associated proteins results in muscular dystrophy is unknown.

DIAGNOSIS: Clinical diagnosis is based on the unique combination of early-onset contractures, myopathy, and cardiac conduction block. Confirmation of the diagnosis of X-linked EDMD can be made by immunolocalization studies using antibodies directed against emerin. Diagnostic confirmation of AD-EDMD can be made by genetic studies in selected laboratories.

TREATMENT
Standard Therapies: The most critical aspect of care is careful cardiac assessment and timely insertion of a cardiac pacemaker. Patients should undergo regular electrocardiography (ECG) and Holter assessments; ECG alone is insufficient to detect early conduction and rhythm changes. General care of patients with muscular dystrophy includes stretching exercises to maintain as much range of motion at individual joints as possible and careful monitoring of scoliosis, especially during peak pubertal growth. Avoidance of smoking or exposure to second-hand smoke and prompt care of any intercurrent respiratory infection are also important health measures.

REFERENCES
Bione S, Maestrini E, Rivella S, et al. Identification of a novel X-linked gene responsible for Emery-Dreifuss muscular dystrophy. *Nat Genet* 1994;8:323–327.
Bonne G, Di Barletta MR, Varnous S, et al. Mutations in the gene encoding lamin A/C cause autosomal dominant Emery-Dreifuss muscular dystrophy. *Nat Genet* 1999;21:285–288.
Merlini L, Granata C, Dominici P, et al. Emery-Dreifuss muscular dystrophy: report of five cases in a family and review of the literature. *Muscle Nerve* 1986;9:481–485.
Mora M, Cartegni L, Di Blasi C, et al. X-linked Emery-Dreifuss muscular dystrophy can be diagnosed from skin biopsy or blood sample. *Ann Neurol* 1997;42:249–253.
Rowland LP, Fetell M, Olarte M, et al. Emery-Dreifuss muscular dystrophy. *Ann Neurol* 1979;5:111–117.

RESOURCES
270, 368, 441

17   Facioscapulohumeral Muscular Dystrophy

Rossella Tupler, MD, PhD

DEFINITION: Facioscapulohumeral muscular dystrophy (FSHD) is a hereditary disease characterized by progressive muscle weakness and wasting. Onset is usually in the second decade of life, but weakness can appear from infancy to late life. The disease initially involves facial muscles, followed by the scapula fixators and the scapular girdle muscles. Subsequently, the foot dorsiflexors and the pelvic girdle muscles become involved.

SYNONYM: Landouzy-Dejerine muscular dystrophy.

DIFFERENTIAL DIAGNOSIS: Scapuloperoneal muscular dystrophy; Limb girdle muscular dystrophies; Polymyositis; Spinal muscle atrophies; Coat syndrome; Moebius syndrome.

SYMPTOMS AND SIGNS: At onset, weakness affects facial muscles, especially the orbicularis oculi, orbicularis ori, and zigomaticus. Extraocular, masseter, temporalis, and pharyngeal muscles are spared. Patients are not able to close their eyelids, whistle, or drink through a straw. When smiling, the mouth moves transversely, and often asymmetrically. Later the disease spreads to the shoulder girdle muscles, primarily to the scapula fixators. Patients experience difficulty lifting or rotating their arms, and scapular winging is visible. The scapula is positioned more laterally, and rides upward and forward, giving the shoulders a forward-sloped appearance. The proximal part of the deltoid is affected, whereas the rest is spared. The pectoralis major is almost always weak and atrophic, resulting in a characteristic upward slope of axillary folds. Pectum excavatum can be observed. Respiratory capacity is reduced. Later, the weakness extends to the abdominal muscles. Involvement of pelvic girdle muscles appears in advanced stages of the disease in approximately half of patients. The tibialis anterior is affected early and the patient is unable to walk on tiptoes. The posterior leg muscles are spared. Sensorineural deafness and retinal vasculopathy may occur.

ETIOLOGY/EPIDEMIOLOGY: The incidence is 1 in 20,000. New mutation frequency is 1 in 320,000 newborns. The FSHD genetic locus has been assigned to the very distal part of the long arm of chromosome 4.

DIAGNOSIS: Diagnosis depends on a combination of clinical presentation, family history, and molecular genetic analysis. Electromyography detects nonspecific myopathic signs. Muscle biopsy shows increased variation of fiber size with sporadic small, angulated fibers and necrotic fibers. Inflammatory infiltration is frequently observed. Molecular diagnosis is possible using the probe p13E-11.

TREATMENT

Standard Therapies: Treatment is physical therapy to prevent the development of contractures and skeletal deformities.

Investigational Therapies: Albuterol and carnitine are being investigated.

REFERENCES

Deidda G, Cacurri S, Piazzo N, et al. Direct detection of 4q35 rearrangements implicated in facioscapulohumeral muscular dystrophy (FSHD). *J Med Genet* 1996;33:361–365.

Lunt PW. Facioscapulohumeral muscular dystrophy: diagnostic and molecular aspects. In: Demeer F, ed. *Neuromuscular diseases: from basic mechanisms to clinical management*. Vol. 18. Monographs in clinical neuroscience. Basel, Switzerland: Karger, 2000:44–60.

Padberg GW, Lunt PW, Koch M, et al. Facioscapulohumeral muscular dystrophy. In: Emery AEH, ed. *Diagnostic criteria for neuromuscular disorders*, 2nd ed. London: Royal Society Medicine Press, 1997:9–15.

Upadhyaya M, Maynard J, Rogers MT, et al. Improved molecular diagnosis of facioscapulohumeral muscular dystrophy (FSHD): validation of the differential double digestion for FSHD. *J Med Genet* 1997;34:476–479.

van der Maarel SM, Deidda G, Lemmers RJ, et al. *De novo* facioscapulohumeral muscular dystrophy: frequent somatic mosaicism, sex-dependent phenotype, and the role of mitotic transchromosomal repeat interaction between chromosomes 4 and 10. *Am J Hum Genet* 2000;66:26–35.

RESOURCES
150, 270, 368

18 Limb Girdle Muscular Dystrophy

Gyula Acsadi, MD, PhD

DEFINITION: Limb girdle muscular dystrophy (LGMD) is a heterogeneous group of muscle diseases in children and adults characterized by progressive weakness of proximal muscles.

SYNONYMS: Pelvifemoral muscular dystrophy; Pelviscapular muscular dystrophy; Proximal muscular dystrophy; Scapulohumeral muscular dystrophy; Scapuloperoneal syndrome; Erb muscular dystrophy; Leyden-Möbius muscular dystrophy; Sarcoglycanopathies.

DIFFERENTIAL DIAGNOSIS: Becker muscular dystrophy; Duchenne muscular dystrophy; Congenital muscular dystrophy; Myotonic dystrophy; Centronuclear myopathy; Nemaline rod myopathy; Central core disease; Multicore disease; Congenital fiber-type disproportion; Desmin myopathy; Myopathy with tubular aggregates;

Dermatomyositis; Inclusion body myositis; Endocrine myopathy; Toxic myopathy; Myopathy due to chronic corticosteroid therapy; Emery-Dreifuss muscular dystrophy; Facioscapulohumeral muscular dystrophy; Neurogenic scapuloperoneal syndrome; Glycogeneses; Lipid myopathies; Mitochondrial myopathy; Spinal muscular atrophy; Amyotrophic lateral sclerosis.

SYMPTOMS AND SIGNS: The main presentation is proximal muscle weakness of the pelvic and shoulder girdle. Age at onset, severity, and progression of symptoms vary. In approximately half of cases, weakness begins in the pelvic girdle muscles (Leyden and Möbius type), and then continues to involve the pectoral muscles. In the rest, the pectoral muscles are affected first. The trapezius, serratus anterior, sternal head of pectoralis major, spinati, biceps, and brachioradialis muscles are involved early in the pectoral form. The appearance is often characteristic: drooped shoulders, scapular winging, and anterior axillary fold. In the pelvic form, sacrospinalis, quadriceps, hamstrings, and hip muscles are especially involved, causing excessive lumbar lordosis and waddling gait.

ETIOLOGY/EPIDEMIOLOGY: Most cases are inherited as autosomal-recessive traits; the dominant form is less common. Approximately 15% of recessive cases are due to abnormalities in the plasma membrane–associated glycoprotein complex that is part of the dystrophin-glycoprotein-laminin complex. The estimated prevalence is approximately 65 per million population, and the incidence is 20 per million population per year, which is likely underestimated due to the heterogeneity of this disease. There is an increased incidence of some forms in genetically homogeneous populations.

DIAGNOSIS: The clinical diagnosis is based on the distribution of weakness and muscle atrophy. Electromyography helps differentiate the primary muscle involvement from peripheral neuropathy and motor neuron diseases. Creatine kinase is typically elevated in all forms. Muscle biopsy can confirm typical findings suggestive of primary muscle

disease. Usually, features similar to other muscular dystrophies are seen. The best approach for molecular diagnosis is from muscle biopsy. Specific deficiencies of the various proteins involved in LGMD can be investigated with a panel of antibodies using immunohistochemical techniques.

TREATMENT
Standard Therapies: The severity and clinical course are variable, and management is mostly symptomatic. Mildly affected patients may not require therapeutic intervention, but more severely affected patients will likely need to be managed for contractures, and may require braces or wheelchairs. Physical therapy to improve residual muscle strength and to help preserve optimum function must be used. The principal goals are to prevent contractures and deformities and to maintain upright posture and ambulation.

Investigational Therapies: Novel therapeutics for muscular dystrophies are being developed, including screenings of drugs to upregulate compensatory proteins and efforts to replace the defective relevant mutated gene using gene therapy.

REFERENCES
Bushby KM, Beckmann JS. The limb-girdle muscular dystrophies-proposal for a new nomenclature. *Neuromusc Disord* 1995;5:337–343.

Gordon ES, Hoffman EP. The ABC's of limb-girdle muscular dystrophy: alpha-sarcoglycanopathy, Bethlem myopathy, calpainopathy and more. *Curr Opin Neurol* 2001;14:567–573.

Richard I, Broux O, Allamand V, et al. Mutations in the proteolytic enzyme calpain3 cause limb-girdle muscular dystrophy type 2A. *Cell* 1995;81:27–40.

Verma A. Limb girdle muscular dystrophy. In: Gilman S, ed. *Neurobase.* Arbor, 2001.

RESOURCES
270, 368, 441

19   Myasthenia Gravis

Henry J. Kaminski, MD

DEFINITION: Myasthenia gravis is an autoimmune neuromuscular transmission disorder, which causes characteristic fatiguing muscle weakness, producing respiratory,

swallowing, and speech difficulties; limb weakness; drooping eyelids; and double vision.

DIFFERENTIAL DIAGNOSIS: Lambert-Eaton myasthenic syndrome; Congenital myasthenia; Amyotrophic lateral sclerosis; Myopathies. For ocular myasthenia: Chronic progressive ophthalmoplegia; Orbital mass lesions; Brainstem tumors.

SYMPTOMS AND SIGNS: The hallmark of myasthenia gravis is weakness that fatigues. Approximately half of patients present with double vision or ptosis, so-called ocular myasthenia, and a minority experience manifestations limited to the extraocular muscles. Of affected patients, 85% develop dysarthria, dysphagia, respiratory insufficiency, and limb weakness, all of which may occur in combination or in isolation. The weakness may be so severe as to require mechanical ventilation (myasthenic crisis). The severity of manifestations may fluctuate over time. Spontaneous remissions may occur.

ETIOLOGY/EPIDEMIOLOGY: Myasthenia gravis is caused by antibody-mediated attack of the skeletal muscle's neuromuscular junction, leading to the loss of acetylcholine receptors. The functional consequence is an impairment of neuromuscular transmission. A few patients are likely to have antibodies to other muscle proteins, which produce the same transmission defect. In 10%–15% of patients, the autoimmune attack is triggered by a thymoma. In the rest, there is no established etiology. The incidence of myasthenia gravis is estimated to be 3–9 per million population, with prevalence estimates ranging from 1–17 per 100,000. The disorder occurs more commonly in young woman, and the frequency of the disease increases with age in both sexes, with a male predominance at older ages.

DIAGNOSIS: The edrophonium (Tensilon) test, serum levels of acetylcholine receptor antibodies, and electrodiagnostic studies are used to confirm the diagnosis. The edrophonium test involves intravenous infusion of the drug followed by observation for improved strength (usually of an extraocular muscle), which occurs and resolves within minutes. Antibodies to the acetylcholine receptor are identified in 50% of ocular myasthenics and 90% of generalized myasthenics. A decremental response to repetitive stimulation by electromyography is observed in 80% of patients. Results of a single-fiber examination, a specialized electro-diagnostic test, may be abnormal in up to 95% of patients. Patients suspected of having myasthenia gravis should undergo CT or MRI of the chest to search for a thymoma.

TREATMENT

Standard Therapies: The choice of therapy depends on the severity of weakness. First-line treatment is with oral anticholinesterase medications, most commonly pyridostigmine bromide (Mestinon). Corticosteroids at doses of 60–80 mg/day of prednisone as initial therapy followed by gradual tapers, which include transfer to an every other day regimen, over several months are typically used. Immediate institution of high doses of corticosteroids often leads to greater weakness, and a gradual increase in dose over 2–3 weeks may be necessary. Improvement begins within 1–4 weeks. For patients intolerant of, or poorly responsive to, corticosteroids, azathioprine, cyclosporine, or mycophenolate, mofetil is used in combination with corticosteroids, or alone. The onset of action of azathioprine occurs in 6–9 months, whereas improvement with cyclosporine and mycophenolate mofetil occurs in 3–6 months. For severe weakness, plasma exchange or intravenous immunoglobulin may produce rapid improvement, but strength is maintained only for a few weeks, if no other therapy is initiated. Thymectomy is typically recommended for patients younger than 60 and without contraindications to surgery. The surgery is believed to improve the chance of remission. All patients with a thymoma should have the tumor removed. Medications including several antibiotics, β-blockers, penicillamine, and quinidine may exacerbate myasthenia gravis.

REFERENCES

Drachman DB. Myasthenia gravis. *N Engl J Med* 1994;330: 1797–1810.

Engel AG. *The myasthenic syndromes.* New York: Oxford University Press, 1999.

Kaminski HJ. Myasthenia gravis. In: Katirji B, Kaminski HJ, Preston DC, et al. *Neuromuscular disease in clinical practice.* Boston: Butterworth-Heinemann, 2002.

RESOURCES

270, 271, 272, 368

---

20 Myoclonus

John N. Caviness, MD

DEFINITION: Myoclonus is defined as sudden, brief, shocklike, involuntary movements caused by muscular contractions (positive myoclonus) or inhibitions (negative myoclonus or asterixis).

SYNONYM: Myoclonic jerk.

DIFFERENTIAL DIAGNOSIS: Tic disorder; Chorea; Dyskinesia.

SYMPTOMS AND SIGNS: The basic clinical manifestation of myoclonus is that of jerking, which interferes with movement control and balance, and results in disability. The particular clinical circumstances and associations can be classified as follows. Physiologic myoclonus occurs in neurologically normal people. The occurrence of myoclonus during sleep and sleep transitions is the most common example. Essential myoclonus is clinically significant and is usually the most prominent or only clinical finding. It usually progresses slowly or not at all. Hereditary (autosomal-dominant) and sporadic forms exist. Epileptic myoclonus refers to the presence of myoclonus in the setting of epilepsy. It can occur as one component of a seizure, as the only seizure manifestation, or as one of multiple seizure types within an epileptic syndrome. Symptomatic (secondary) myoclonus is the most common category and manifests usually in the setting of an identifiable underlying disorder. Myoclonus is often not the most prominent clinical symptom. Ataxia, dementia, and parkinsonism are common coexisting problems. Symptomatic causes of myoclonus comprise a widely diverse group of disease processes and include storage diseases, degenerative conditions, toxic-metabolic states, physical processes, infections, focal nervous system damage, paraneoplastic syndrome, and non-neurologic medical illnesses.

ETIOLOGY/EPIDEMIOLOGY: Myoclonus is caused by an abrupt and brief discharge of motor neurons to affected muscles. This excessive motor excitation may arise from the cortex, subcortical regions, segmental levels of the central nervous system, and, rarely, the peripheral nervous system. In the primary generalized epilepsies, facilitation between cortical and subcortical circuits plays a role (myoclonus with absence seizures). The incidence of myoclonus is 1.3 cases per 100,000 person-years, and the prevalence is 8.6 cases per 100,000 population.

DIAGNOSIS: The following minimal testing should be done in all unexplained cases of myoclonus: electrolytes, glucose, renal function tests, hepatic function tests, drug and toxin screen (if prompted by history), brain imaging, and electroencephalography. If results are negative, other imaging (cancer search, spinal cord imaging), paraneoplastic antibodies, tests for storage diseases and other metabolic derangements, cerebrospinal fluid examination, genetic testing, and clinical neurophysiologic testing may be indicated.

TREATMENT

Standard Therapies: Treatment is generally medical, symptomatic, and only mildly to moderately effective. Clonazepam and valproic acid are the most useful treatments. Side effects are common and often problematic.

Investigational Therapies: Tetrabenazine can be useful for subcortical or segmental myoclonus. Piracetam is being investigated for the symptomatic treatment of cortical-origin myoclonus.

REFERENCES

Brown P. Myoclonus: a practical guide to drug therapy. *CNS Drugs* 1995;3:22–29.

Caviness JN. Myoclonus. *Mayo Clin Proc* 1996;71:679–688.

Caviness JN, Alving LI, Maraganore DM, et al. The incidence and prevalence of myoclonus in Olmsted County, Minnesota. *Mayo Clin Proc* 1999;74:565–569.

Shibasaki H. Electrophysiologic studies of myoclonus. AAEE Minimonograph #30. *Muscle Nerve* 2000;23:321–335.

RESOURCES

145, 368, 381

---

21   Centronuclear and Myotubular Myopathy

Anne M. Connolly, MD

DEFINITION: Centronuclear and myotubular myopathies have centrally placed nuclei in muscle as their pathologic hallmark. Although no definite agreement exists between the two descriptive terms, *myotubular myopathy* is generally reserved for the X-linked form of the disease caused by mutations in the myotubularin gene (*MTM1*), whereas *centronuclear myopathy* is reserved to indicate autosomal-dominant or -recessive inheritance.

SYNONYMS: Centronuclear myopathy; Pericentronuclear myopathy; Type 1 fiber hypotrophy with central nuclei.

DIFFERENTIAL DIAGNOSIS: For the infantile form: Other congenital myopathies; Infantile facioscapulohumoral dystrophy. For children with later onset: Limb girdle muscular dystrophy; Mitochondrial myopathy; Facioscapulohumoral dystrophy.

SYMPTOMS AND SIGNS: In X-linked myotubular myopathy, infant boys are generally very weak, with presentation in the first days to weeks of life. Children with autosomal-recessive centronuclear myopathy may also present in infancy but tend to be more mildly affected. Patients with the autosomal-dominant form may present in the first year, early childhood, or young adulthood. Boys with the X-linked, severe form are hypotonic and weak. Respiratory failure may be present at birth. Distinctive facial features include long, thin face and high arched palate. Facial and extraocular weakness are often striking. Ptosis and limitation of extraocular movement may be partial or complete. Patients with the autosomal-dominant form present later and have less severe weakness. The pattern of weakness is scapuloperoneal, and leg cramps may develop. Ophthalmoplegia and facial weakness are common. The autosomal-recessive form tends to be intermediate in manifestation compared with the X-linked and dominant forms. Again, proximal more than distal weakness and ophthalmoplegia are common.

ETIOLOGY/EPIDEMIOLOGY: The gene responsible for the severe, X-linked disease, *MTM1,* encodes a phosphatase, myotubularin, which is highly conserved. The incidence for this form is 1 in 50,000 newborn males.

DIAGNOSIS: The diagnosis is usually suspected clinically in a hypotonic weak infant or young child. Older patients may complain of muscle cramps; physical examination will show facial weakness, ophthalmoplegia, and proximal weakness. Creatine kinase is usually normal; electromyography may show small, narrow, polyphasic motor unit potentials consistent with a myopathy. Diagnosis is established by muscle biopsy showing characteristic centrally placed nuclei.

TREATMENT

Standard Therapies: There are no medical therapies. Surgical treatment of contractures and scoliosis is helpful in patients who have milder courses.

REFERENCES

Appel S, Reichwald K, Zimmermann W, et al. Identification and localization of a new human myotubularin-related protein gene, *mtmr8,* on 8p22-p23. *Genomics* 2001;75:6–8.

Hammans SR, Robinson DO, Moutou C, et al. A clinical and genetic study of a manifesting heterozygote with X- linked myotubular myopathy. *Neuromuscular Disord* 2000;10:133–137.

Herman GE, Finegold M, Zhao W, et al. Medical complications in long-term survivors with X-linked myotubular myopathy. *J Pediatr* 1999;134:206–214.

Laporte J, Biancalana V, Tanner SM, et al. *MTM1* mutations in X-linked myotubular myopathy. *Hum Mutat* 2000;15:393–409.

Laporte J, Kress W, Mandel JL. Diagnosis of X-linked myotubular myopathy by detection of myotubularin. *Ann Neurol* 2001;50: 42–46.

Tanner SM, Schneider V, Thomas NS, et al. Characterization of 34 novel and 6 known *MTM1* gene mutations in 47 unrelated X-linked myotubular myopathy patients. *Neuromusc Disord* 1999;9:41–49.

RESOURCES

270, 275, 368

---

22 Congenital Myopathy with Fiber-Type Disproportion

Anne M. Connolly, MD

DEFINITION: Congenital myopathies with fiber-type variation can affect the ratio of type I to type II muscle fibers or the size of a specific fiber type. These nonspecific fiber-type changes can be present in a variety of congenital myopathies; however, congenital fiber-type disproportion with type I fiber hypotrophy has been recognized as a specific clinical entity. Affected children are hypotonic and weak, and muscle biopsies show type I predominance and hypotrophy.

SYNONYMS: Fiber-type atrophy; Fiber-type disproportion.

DIFFERENTIAL DIAGNOSIS: Other congenital myopathies including central core myopathy, central nuclear myopathy, and myotonic dystrophy; Spinal muscular atrophy; Facioscapulohumeral dystrophy.

SYMPTOMS AND SIGNS: Affected children are hypotonic at birth. Weakness varies, but a few children have had respiratory compromise in the first year of life. Although most children have had a nonprogressive course, five infants had rapidly progressive weakness and a dilated cardiomyopathy, with death occurring at 4–6 months. Congenital hip dislocation may occur in as many as 50% of patients. Contractures are common and involve both feet and hands. Although gross motor delay generally occurs, affected children do attain the ability to walk. Intellect is normal. Facial weakness is usually mild and, if present, should suggest possible facioscapulohumeral dystrophy. Motor examination shows proximal greater than distal weakness and decreased muscle stretch reflexes. Sensation is normal.

ETIOLOGY/EPIDEMIOLOGY: Fiber-type disproportion is described in both sexes. Although a few families have had apparent autosomal-dominant transmission, most children present in a sporadic fashion. Incidence is unknown.

DIAGNOSIS: Congenital fiber-type disproportion should be considered in the hypotonic, weak child. Creatine kinase is usually normal. Genetic testing should be done to exclude the more common spinal muscular atrophy. Electromyography may be helpful, showing a myopathic pattern with small, polyphasic, narrow duration motor unit potentials. The diagnosis is established with muscle biopsy that shows small type I fibers and often type I predominance.

TREATMENT
Standard Therapies: No medical therapies are known. Physical therapy and orthopedic treatment of contractures improve ambulation.

REFERENCES
Argov Z, Gardner-Medwin D, Johnson MA, et al. Congenital myotonic dystrophy: fiber type abnormalities in two cases. *Arch Neurol* 1980;37:693–696.
Barth PG, Wanders RJ, Ruitenbeek W, et al. Infantile fibre type disproportion, myofibrillar lysis and cardiomyopathy: a disorder in three unrelated Dutch families. *Neuromusc Disord* 1998;8:296–304.
Bartholomeus MG, Gabreels FJ, ter Laak HJ, et al. Congenital fibre type disproportion a time-locked diagnosis: a clinical and morphological follow-up study. *Clin Neurol Neurosurg* 2000;102:97–101.
Imoto C, Nonaka I. The significance of type 1 fiber atrophy (hypotrophy) in childhood neuromuscular disorders. *Brain Dev* 2001;23:298–302.
Marjanovic B, Cvetkovic D, Dozic S, et al. Association of Krabbe leukodystrophy and congenital fiber type disproportion. *Pediatr Neurol* 1996;15:79–82.
Unal I, Erdem S, Elibol B, et al. Rigid spine syndrome with fiber type disproportion. *Muscle Nerve* 1999;22:542–543.

RESOURCES
270, 368

---

23 Myofibrillar (Desmin and Desmin-Related) Myopathy

Anne M. Connolly, MD

DEFINITION: Myofibrillar myopathies are pathologically defined by accumulation of intermediate-filament protein in muscle. Clinically, they make up a heterogeneous group of patients who have distal weakness at presentation and frequently develop cardiomyopathy. Desmin is a muscle-specific intermediate-filament protein responsible for the structural integrity of the myofibrils, and is the most common intermediate-filament protein found to accumulate in muscle fibers. Mutations in the desmin gene (*DES*) have been identified in many but not all patients with pathologically defined desmin myopathy.

SYNONYMS: Myofibrillar myopathy; Distal myopathy; Desmin-related myopathy.

DIFFERENTIAL DIAGNOSIS: Nonaka distal myopathy; Miyoshi distal myopathy; Myotonic dystrophy; Myosin loss myopathy.

SYMPTOMS AND SIGNS: Patients with desmin myopathy usually present at age 20–30 years with weakness distally greater than proximally, with legs more affected than arms. The anterior compartment (tibialis anterior and toe extensor) muscles are preferentially affected. As weakness progresses, proximal limb, neck, and pharyngeal muscles are affected. Cardiac involvement occurs in more than 50% of patients. Cardiac symptoms include syncope and sometimes right bundle branch block. In some patients, cardiomyopathy alone may be the first manifestation of desmin myopathy. The phenotype for desmin-related myopathy is broader and includes younger children. The distinctive clinical feature remains distal more than proximal weakness.

ETIOLOGY/EPIDEMIOLOGY: Desmin, the most common myofibrillar myopathy, is inherited in an autosomal-dominant fashion, with onset at age 14–64 years. Compound heterozygotes and sporadic cases associated with chemotherapy have also been reported. The incidence is unknown.

DIAGNOSIS: Serum creatine kinase may be mildly elevated. Electromyographic changes include myopathic features (polyphasic, narrow, small motor unit potentials), and may also show fibrillation potential consistent with an irritable myopathy. These changes may be more striking in distal muscles. The diagnosis is established by muscle biopsy, which shows variability of muscle fiber size and increase in internal nuclei. The characteristic intermediate filament inclusions will immunostain positively for desmin, vimentin, and nestin.

TREATMENT

Standard Therapies: There are no medical therapies. The most important preventative treatment is to recognize the risk for underlying cardiomyopathy or arrhythmias, which may be treated medically. Orthotic use may be helpful if foot drop develops.

REFERENCES

Banwell BL. Intermediate filament-related myopathies. *Pediatr Neurol* 2001;24:257–263.

Barohn RJ, Amato AA. Distal myopathies. *Semin Neurol* 1999;19:45–58.

Bornemann A, Goebel HH. Congenital myopathies. *Brain Pathol* 2001;11:206–217.

Dalakas MC, Park KY, Semino-Mora C, et al. Desmin myopathy, a skeletal myopathy with cardiomyopathy caused by mutations in the desmin gene. *N Engl J Med* 2000;342:770–780.

Melberg A, Oldfors A, Blomstrom-Lundqvist C, et al. Autosomal dominant myofibrillar myopathy with arrhythmogenic right ventricular cardiomyopathy linked to chromosome 10q. *Ann Neurol* 1999;46:684–692.

Zhang J, Kumar A, Stalker HJ, et al. Clinical and molecular studies of a large family with desmin-associated restrictive cardiomyopathy. *Clin Genet* 2001;59:248–256.

RESOURCES

35, 357

---

24 Inclusion Body Myositis

Imelda Cabalar, MD,
and Paul H. Plotz, MD

DEFINITION: Inclusion body myositis (IBM) is an inflammatory disease of muscle that occurs mainly in older men, develops insidiously over several years, and manifests as weakness and a tendency to fall. It is characterized by the presence of rimmed vacuoles and either intracytoplasmic or intranuclear tubular or filamentous inclusions. A rare inherited form that may begin in childhood also exists.

SYNONYM: Inclusion body myopathy.

DIFFERENTIAL DIAGNOSIS: Polymyositis; Limb girdle muscular dystrophy; Facioscapulohumeral dystrophy; Metabolic myopathies; Toxic myopathies.

SYMPTOMS AND SIGNS: Patients with IBM typically present with muscle weakness and atrophy that develop insidiously over several years. Both proximal and distal muscles may be affected, and the involvement may be symmetric or asymmetric. Patients often have a history of falling and report lower extremity weakness, mainly of the quadriceps muscles. Dysphagia is present in 40% of patients, and facial weakness may be seen in some. Unlike polymyositis and dermatomyositis, it is not typically associated with skin changes, myocarditis, or interstitial lung disease. There is no increased risk of malignancy. Although the disease progresses slowly, it can be severely disabling.

ETIOLOGY/EPIDEMIOLOGY: The pathogenesis of IBM is unknown. It may be part of a spectrum of diseases that include polymyositis and dermatomyositis, but there is increasing belief that it is a distinct entity and that inflammation may not be present or play a role in some cases. The true incidence of IBM is unknown, but it is increasingly recognized as the most common form of myositis in older individuals.

DIAGNOSIS: Serum creatine kinase is often only mildly elevated or normal. Electromyography usually shows myopathic changes, and MRI may show atrophy and signal abnormalities in the affected muscles. Definitive diagnosis rests on the muscle biopsy, which may show endomysial inflammation and atrophy, but more importantly, muscle fibers with rimmed vacuoles lined with granular material. Hypertrophy of unaffected fibers is commonly present.

TREATMENT

Standard Therapies: Inclusion body myositis, unlike polymyositis and dermatomyositis, is relatively resistant to corticosteroids and other immunosuppressive agents. Mild or transient improvement has occurred with prednisone as well as a slowing of disease progression. If prednisone alone does not produce any improvement, a second-line agent such as azathioprine and/or methotrexate may be added. If no objective clinical improvement is seen after a trial of prednisone alone or in combination, pharmacologic therapy should be discontinued. Physical therapy is important to prevent further loss of function, avoid contractures, and preserve muscle strength in the remaining muscles.

REFERENCES

Amato A, Barohn R. Acquired neuromuscular diseases: idiopathic inflammatory myopathies. *Neurol Clin* 1997;15:615–648.

Barohn RJ, Amato A. Inclusion body myositis. *Curr Treat Options Neurol* 2000;2:7–12.

Miller FW. Inflammatory myopathies: polymyositis, dermatomyositis and related conditions. In: Koopman WJ, ed. *Arthritis and allied conditions: a textbook of rheumatology,* 13th ed. Baltimore: Williams & Wilkins, 1997.

Rose M, McDermott M, Thornton C, et al. A prospective natural history study of inclusion body myositis: implications for clinical trials. *Neurology* 2001;57:548–550.

RESOURCES

270, 274, 351

---

25 Myotonia Congenita

*Sudeep Shivakumar, BS,
and Edward C. Cooper, MD, PhD*

DEFINITION: Myotonia congenita is an inherited disorder of skeletal muscle. The muscles of affected individuals have normal strength but exhibit transient, uncontrolled stiffness following a voluntary contraction. Myotonia congenita is due to mutations in muscle chloride ion channels that are necessary for proper muscle relaxation.

SYNONYMS: Becker disease; Thomsen disease.

DIFFERENTIAL DIAGNOSIS: Myotonic dystrophy; Hyperkalemic periodic paralysis; Paramyotonia congenita; Neuromyotonia; Myokymia; Dystonia; Muscle cramps.

SYMPTOMS AND SIGNS: The main symptom is myotonia, which the patient experiences as muscle stiffness. Myotonia becomes noticeable within the first two decades of life, with the Thomsen form usually appearing from birth to early childhood, and the Becker form usually appearing later in the first decade. The myotonia is generalized, usually painless, and exhibits a "warm-up" phenomenon, in that it lessens during exercise. Muscle strength is normal, although transient weakness after muscle contraction is sometimes seen in Becker disease. This weakness is usually not disabling, and can be reversed fully by exercise. Muscle hypertrophy often occurs, especially in the lower limbs and buttocks. Hyperlordosis sometimes develops in Becker disease. Patients can grasp an object or close their eyes with normal strength and speed, but subsequent relaxation may be delayed briefly or for several seconds. Myotonia can sometimes be elicited with direct muscle percussion.

ETIOLOGY/EPIDEMIOLOGY: Patients with myotonia congenita have inherited mutations in the chloride channel gene *ClC-1* located on chromosome 7. These mutations reduce the number of functional chloride channels, causing muscle excitation to continue excessively and the symptom of sustained muscle contraction. Different specific mutations cause forms of myotonia congenita that are inherited in an autosomal-dominant (Thomsen disease) or autosomal-recessive (Becker disease) manner. The disorder has an incidence of between 0.3 and 0.6 per 100,000 population.

DIAGNOSIS: Diagnosis is based on the clinical picture and family history and supported by electromyography. The history should demonstrate muscle stiffness (distinguished from muscle weakness and muscle pain) that improves with activity, but worsens following rest. Hypertrophy may or may not be present. The pattern of inheritance is established by history and examination of relatives. Clinically apparent myotonia is accompanied by myotonic discharges, which are visible by needle electromyography testing (EMG). Serum creatine kinase may be mildly elevated (2–5 times normal), but this is a less specific finding than the EMG.

TREATMENT

Standard Therapies: For most patients, treatment is not necessary. Drugs that block muscle sodium channels (sometimes called "membrane-stabilizing" agents) are effective for reducing symptoms of muscle stiffness and weakness. Mexilitine, developed originally as an antiarrhythmic agent, usually reduces myotonic symptoms, although monitoring is required due to potential cardiac side effects. Phenytoin and carbamazepine may also be of benefit. In pregnancy, the benefits of these agents must be weighed against the potential teratogenic risks. Some patients with recessive myotonia congenita respond to treatment with acetazolamide, a carbonic anhydrase inhibitor.

REFERENCES

Cooper E, Jan LY. Ion channel genes and human neurological disease: Recent progress, prospects, and challenges. *Proc Natl Acad Sci USA* 1999;96:4759–4766.

Jentsch TJ, Friedrich T, Schriever A, et al. The CLC chloride channel family. *Eur J Physiol* 1999;437:783–795.

Ptacek L. The familial periodic paralyses and nondystrophic myotonias. *Am J Med* 1998;104:58–70.

Rudel R, Lehmann-Horn F, Ricker K. The nondystrophic myotonias. In: Engel AG, Franzini-Armstrong C, eds. *Myology: basic and clinical.* New York: McGraw-Hill, 1994.

RESOURCES
254, 270, 351, 368

---

26 Neuroacanthocytosis

Anne L. Foundas, MD,
and Jeffrey S. Kutcher, MD

DEFINITION: Neuroacanthocytosis (NA) is a degenerative, inherited disorder of the central nervous system, typically presenting in the third or fourth decade with orofacial dyskinesias and often involving chorea, tics, dystonia, parkinsonism, amyotrophy, and other symptoms. Acanthocytes are seen in abundance in the peripheral blood, accounting for at least 10% of all red blood cells.

SYNONYM: Choreoacanthocytosis.

DIFFERENTIAL DIAGNOSIS: Bassen-Kornzweig disease; HARP syndrome; Huntington disease.

SYMPTOMS AND SIGNS: Although clinical presentation varies, most patients begin to experience symptoms in the third or fourth decade of life. The most distinguishing feature is a severe eating dysfunction caused by progressive orofacial dyskinesias, resulting in expulsion of food by a protruding tongue. Patients often present with involuntary vocalizations, generalized chorea, cognitive impairment, and dystonic features. Peripheral neuropathies, amyotrophy, and seizures also occur. The rate of progression is variable. Death may follow within a few years of symptom onset, although some patients have been reported to live decades with the disease.

ETIOLOGY/EPIDEMIOLOGY: The exact cause is unknown but is presumed to be related to an abundance of acanthocytes in the blood and degeneration of at least the caudate nucleus but possibly the striatum and even the frontal lobes as well. Genetic linkage was established on chromosome 9q21. Neither the prevalence nor incidence of NA has been estimated. Inheritance is presumed to be recessive but may also be autosomal dominant or X-linked. Cases have been reported in both males and females.

DIAGNOSIS: The typical clinical presentation described earlier, with or without a significant family history, should lead to evaluation of a fresh (wet preparation) peripheral blood smear. Acanthocytes should account for at least 10% of the red blood cells. Serum creatine kinase is usually elevated. Electromyography may document a predominantly motor peripheral neuropathy. MRI of the brain may demonstrate caudate atrophy or T2-weighted hyperintensities in the striatum, whereas a positron emission tomographic scan may show decreased striatal glucose metabolism.

TREATMENT

Standard Therapies: Treatment is symptomatic and typically involves management of the abnormal movements, parkinsonism, and seizures. Dopamine-blocking agents such as haloperidol and dopamine-depleting agents such as reserpine have both been used with moderate symptomatic benefit. Patients with severe orofacial dyskinesias should be evaluated for swallowing function and nutritional status. Genetic counseling may be warranted.

REFERENCES

Brooks DJ, Ibanez V, Playford ED, et al. Presynaptic and postsynaptic striatal dopaminergic function in neuroacanthocytosis: A positron emission tomographic study. *Ann Neurol* 1991;30: 166–171.

Hardie RJ, Pullon HWH, Harding AE, et al. Neuroacanthocytosis. A clinical, hematological and pathological study of 19 cases. *Brain* 1991;114:13–49.

Kutcher JS, Kahn MJ, Andersson HC, et al. Neuroacanthocytosis masquerading as Huntington's disease: CT/MRI findings. *J Neuroimag* 1999;9:187–189.

Rinne JO, Daniel SE, Scaravilli F, et al. The neuropathological features of neuroacanthocytosis. *Mov Disord* 1994;9:297–304.

Stacy M, Jankovic J. Rare movement disorders associated with metabolic and neurodegenerative diseases. In: Robertson MM, Eapen V, eds. *Movement and allied disorders of childhood.* Chichester: Wiley, 1995:177–198.

RESOURCES
368, 487

27 Infantile Neuroaxonal Dystrophy

Robert E. Schmidt, MD, PhD

DEFINITION: Infantile neuroaxonal dystrophy (INAD) is an autosomal-recessive disorder in which presynaptic nerve terminals in the central and peripheral nervous systems accumulate a variety of subcellular organelles, resulting in axonal swellings (spheroids) that interfere with normal synaptic function.

SYNONYM: Seitelberger disease.

DIFFERENTIAL DIAGNOSIS: Metachromatic leukodystrophy; Infantile neuronal ceroid lipofuscinosis; Spinal muscular atrophy; Dejerine-Sottas disease; Rett syndrome; Leigh disease.

SYMPTOMS AND SIGNS: Infants with INAD typically exhibit developmental slowing and arrest, either failing to develop altogether or losing milestones within the first 6–24 months of life. Early symptoms may include weakness, loss of muscle tone, toe-walking, pendular nystagmus, squinting, and failing vision. Reflexes may be variably exaggerated or, more typically, lost, reflecting upper and lower motor neuron involvement. This often presents first in the lower extremities. Acquired skills, such as walking and speech, are lost. Affected children progressively lose motor and intellectual skills and eventually become bedridden, with global loss of neurologic function resulting in profound weakness, peripheral sensory deficits, cerebellar ataxia, blindness, optic atrophy, deafness, rigidity, and eventually complete mental deterioration with dementia and death, usually within the first 10 years of life. Autonomic involvement may result in urinary retention, loss of temperature regulation, decreased tearing, or chronic constipation. Although seizures are seen in occasional patients, they are not typical.

ETIOLOGY/EPIDEMIOLOGY: Infantile neuroaxonal dystrophy is inherited in an autosomal-recessive manner, although in some studies females are more often affected than males. The prevalence is undetermined. Genetic studies have mapped the chromosomal defect to 22q13, but the gene has not yet been identified. No predilection exists for any specific ethnic group. A subset of patients has a defect in the function of alpha-N-acetylgalactosaminidase, a lysosomal enzyme, but most patients do not. Dystrophic swelling of axon terminals may be the result of failure to balance orthograde (cell body-to-terminal) and retrograde (terminal-to-cell body) axonal transport or an abnormality in the process resulting in reversal of transport polarity (turnaround transport), delivering an excess of subcellular organelles to the nerve terminal.

DIAGNOSIS: The diagnosis may be made by biopsy examination of nerves in the skin (especially around sweat glands), conjunctiva, muscle, peripheral nerve, or rectum, or by brain biopsy. The diagnosis rests on the immunohistochemical or ultrastructural demonstration of 10–100 μm swollen dystrophic axons containing distinctive aggregates of tubulovesicular elements, often with a lucent cleft, normal and degenerating mitochondria, dense bodies, and amorphous granular material. A negative peripheral nerve biopsy does not exclude the diagnosis.

TREATMENT
Standard Therapies: There are no medical therapies.

REFERENCES

Aicardi J, Castelein P. Infantile neuroaxonal dystrophy. *Brain* 1979;102:727–748.

Ozmen M, Caliskan M, Goebel HH, et al. Infantile neuroaxonal dystrophy: diagnosis by skin biopsy. *Brain Dev* 1991;13:256–259.

Schindler D, Bishop DE, Wolfe DE, et al. Neuroaxonal dystrophy due to alpha-N-acetylgalactosaminidase deficiency. *N Engl J Med* 1989;320:1735–1740.

Yoshikawa S, Itoh Y, Nakano T, et al. Diminished retrograde transport causes axonal dystrophy in the nucleus gracilis: electron and light microscopic study. *Acta Neuropathol* 1985;68:93–100.

RESOURCES
355, 368, 477

28   Neuromyotonia

Angela Vincent, MB, BS, MSc

DEFINITION: Acquired neuromyotonia is an autoimmune condition that results in spontaneous muscle hyperactivity.

SYNONYMS: Undulating myokymia; Continuous muscle fiber activity; Quantal squander; Armadillo syndrome; Isaacs syndrome, neuromyotonia; Isaacs syndrome, neurotonia; Mertens syndrome; Continuous motor nerve discharges; Generalized myokymia; Idiopathic generalized myokymia.

DIFFERENTIAL DIAGNOSIS: Hereditary myotonias; Stiff person syndrome; Guillain-Barré syndrome; Some forms of neuroenvenomation; Episodic ataxia type 1.

SYMPTOMS AND SIGNS: The patient usually complains of excess muscle activity with fasciculations and cramps. There may be stiffness, pseudomyotonia, and, paradoxically, weakness in some muscle groups. Excessive sweating is frequent. The disease can occur at any age, but is most frequent in adults, with a slight male preponderance. In a proportion of cases, a thymic tumor is found; the disease can also be associated with myasthenia gravis. Autonomic and central nervous system symptoms, such as cardiac arrhythmias, excessive salivation, constipation, memory loss, confusion, hallucinations, change of personality, or sleep disorders, are found in fewer than 20% of patients, in whom the condition may be referred to as Morvan syndrome.

ETIOLOGY/EPIDEMIOLOGY: Acquired neuromyotonia is an acquired autoimmune disease. Autoantibodies directed against voltage-gated potassium channels have been identified in some patients. The antibodies to potassium channels are believed to reduce the number of functional potassium channels, thus leading to the neuronal hyperactivity responsible for muscle activity. The clinical benefits of plasma exchange, intravenous immunoglobulin therapy, or immunosuppressive treatments in these and the remaining patients suggests that all cases are likely to have an autoimmune etiology. The occurrence of thymic tumors in approximately 20% of cases, and coexisting myasthenia gravis in a similar proportion, also suggest an autoimmune etiology.

DIAGNOSIS: The diagnosis should be based on the presence of myokymia (muscle contractions), pseudomyokymia, and muscle cramps. The presence of spontaneous and repetitive motor unit potentials on electromyography confirms the diagnosis. These potentials, and visible muscle hyperactivity, continue during sleep (unlike stiff person syndrome) but should disappear if neuromuscular transmission is inhibited by local curare infusion. Potassium channel antibodies in 40% of cases confirm the autoimmune basis, and acetylcholine receptor antibodies should be sought if thymoma is suspected or predominant muscle weakness exists.

TREATMENT
Standard Therapies: Most patients do well on low doses of antiepileptic drugs such as carbamezipine or phenytoin. Steroids or steroids and azathioprine can be given, but they are seldom required. Plasma exchange and intravenous immune globulin treatment have been successful in individual cases, but their clinical benefits are not easy to predict. Thymoma should be treated by thymectomy.

REFERENCES
Hart IK. Acquired neuromyotonia: a new autoantibody-mediated neuronal potassium channelopathy. *Am J Med Sci* 2000;319:209–216.

Isaacs H. A syndrome of continuous muscle-fibre activity. *J Neurol Neurosurg Psychiatry* 1961;24:319–325.

Newsom-Davis J, Mills KR. Immunological associations of acquired neuromyotonia (Isaacs' syndrome). Report of five cases and literature review. *Brain* 1993;116:453–469.

Shillito P, Molenaar PC, Vincent A, et al. Acquired neuromyotonia: evidence for autoantibodies directed against K+ channels of peripheral nerves. *Ann Neurol* 1995;38:714–722.

Vincent A. Understanding neuromyotonia. *Muscle Nerve* 2000; 23:655–657.

RESOURCE

351

29 Spinal Bulbar Muscular Atrophy

Barry S. Russman, MD

DEFINITION: Spinal bulbar muscular atrophy (SBMA) is a gradually progressive neuromuscular disorder in which degeneration of lower motor neurons results in proximal muscle weakness, muscle atrophy, and fasciculations. It occurs only in males. Patients often show gynecomastia, testicular atrophy, and reduced fertility due to androgen insensitivity.

SYNONYMS: Kennedy syndrome; Spinal muscular atrophy; Spinal muscular atrophy with gynecomastia.

DIFFERENTIAL DIAGNOSIS: Spinal muscular atrophy type III; Adult onset spinal muscular atrophy; Limb girdle muscular dystrophy; Oral-pharyngeal muscular dystrophy; Amyotrophic lateral sclerosis.

SYMPTOMS AND SIGNS: The clinical diagnosis is suspected in males with the following characteristics: postadolescent onset of spinal lower motor neuron disease with proximal muscle weakness of the limbs or muscle cramps (which are sometimes accompanied by bulbar lower motor neuron disease with dysarthria and difficulty swallowing); fasciculations of the tongue, lips, or perioral region of the face; no signs of upper motor neuron disease such as hyperreflexia or spasticity; adolescent-onset signs of androgen insensitivity, including gynecomastia and/or small testes with oligospermia or azoospermia; and positive family history consistent with X-linked inheritance.

ETIOLOGY/EPIDEMIOLOGY: The disorder occurs in fewer than 1 in 50,000 live male births. It occurs in individuals of caucasian or Asian racial background. It appears to be much more common in the Japanese population than in any other ethnic group, as the result of a founder effect.

The etiology of SBMA relates to an expansion of the CAG trinucleotide repeat in the androgen receptor (*AR*) gene (chromosomal locus Xq11-q12).

DIAGNOSIS: The diagnosis is based on the presence of lower motor neuron disease and "mild" androgen insensitivity in a male. Polymerase chain reaction amplification can determine the CAG repeat number of the CAG repeat region within the *AR* gene.

TREATMENT

Standard Therapies: No specific treatment is available. Physical medicine and rehabilitation approaches, including the use of braces and walkers, offer the best prospect of keeping patients ambulatory. Neither antiandrogen therapies nor testosterone or its analogues are effective. Some patients have breast reduction surgery because of gynecomastia.

REFERENCES

Doyu M, Sobue G, Mukai E, et al. Severity of X-linked recessive bulbospinal neuronopathy correlates with size of the tandem CAG repeat in androgen receptor gene. *Ann Neurol* 1992;32: 707–710.

Harding AE, Thomas PK, Baraitser M, et al. X-linked recessive bulbospinal neuronopathy: a report of ten cases. *J Neurol Neurosurg Psychiatry* 1982;45:1012–1019.

La Spada AR, Wilson EM, Lubahn DB, et al. Androgen receptor gene mutations in X-linked spinal and bulbar muscular atrophy. *Nature* 1991;352:77–79.

Tanaka F, Doyu M, Ito Y, et al. Founder effect in spinal and bulbar muscular atrophy (SBMA). *Hum Mol Genet* 1996;5:1253–1257.

Warner CL, Griffin JE, Wilson JD, et al. X-linked spinomuscular atrophy: a kindred with associated abnormal androgen receptor binding. *Neurology* 1992;42:2181–2184.

RESOURCES

152, 224, 289, 368

30   Spinal Muscular Atrophy

Barry S. Russman, MD

DEFINITION: Spinal muscular atrophy (SMA) is manifested by slowly progressive loss of muscle strength. Classification of the form of SMA that has been mapped to chromosome 5q13 is based on clinical criteria. Approximately 80% of SMA falls into the severe category (SMA I). The other categories are SMA II (chronic SMA) and SMA III. Some forms of adult-onset motor neuron disease have been labeled SMA IV.

SYNONYMS: Werdnig-Hoffman Disease (SMA I); Intermediate or juvenile SMA (SMA II); Kugelberg-Welander disease (SMA III).

DIFFERENTIAL DIAGNOSIS: Prader-Willi syndrome; Adrenoleukodystrophy; Pompe disease; Spinal cord disorder; Congenital myasthenia gravis; Centronuclear myopathy; Nemaline myopathy; Central core disease; Myotonic muscular dystrophy; Congenital muscular dystrophy; Guillain-Barré syndrome; Duchenne muscular dystrophy; Becker muscular dystrophy; Glycogen storage diseases; Lipid myopathies.

SYMPTOMS AND SIGNS: Muscle weakness, lack of motor development, and poor muscle tone are the major clinical manifestations of SMA I. Infants with the gravest prognosis have problems sucking or swallowing. Some show abdominal breathing in the first few months of life. Muscle weakness is symmetric, and the ocular muscles are spared. Fasciculation of the tongue is often seen. A postural tremor of the fingers is generally seen in SMA II but only occasionally in SMA I. The onset of muscle weakness in SMA II patients is usually noted after 6 months of age. Consultation is sought when the child does not sit independently by age 9–12 months or is not standing by 1 year. Approximately 70% lack tendon reflexes. Patients with SMA III develop walking skills but may fall frequently or have trouble walking up and down stairs at age 2–3 years. Examination shows proximal limb weakness; the legs are more severely affected than the arms. As with SMA I and II, a normal sensory examination and absence of tendon reflexes in most affected individuals completes the clinical picture.

ETIOLOGY/EPIDEMIOLOGY: The disease occurs in both sexes. The incidence of SMA is 4–7.8 per 100,000 live births, giving a carrier frequency of 1 in 40 or 1 in 57. All cases of SMA linked to chromosome 5 are genetic. Many of the variants are also genetic, but linked to other chromosomes. A first gene for SMA, survival motor neuron gene (*SMN*), was isolated in 1995. A second gene, neuronal apoptosis inhibitory protein (*NAIP*) gene, was found to be deleted in 68% of cases of SMA I, but in only 2% of cases of SMA II and III. A third gene, *BTF2p44,* has been shown to be missing in 15% of SMA patients.

DIAGNOSIS: Finger trembling and flaccidity in a child who is alert and cognitively normal suggests the diagnosis. Blood chemistry values should be normal, but serum creatine kinase activity may be 1 to 2 times normal; if it is more than 10 times normal, another diagnosis such as muscular dystrophy or polymyositis should be considered. If the history and physical examination suggest SMA, a positive DNA test for deletion of the survival motor neuron gene negates the need for electrophysiologic testing and muscle biopsy. Electromyography shows regular spontaneous motor unit activity. Muscle biopsy shows group atrophy of type 1 and type 2 muscle fibers as opposed to the normal checkerboard pattern. Rare angulated and large type 1 fibers are scattered throughout.

TREATMENT

Standard Therapies: No specific treatment exists. Care is symptomatic, including use of orthotics, adaptive equipment, and respiratory care.

Investigational Therapies: The use of gabapentin in patients with SMA II and III and the use of riluzole in patients with SMA I are being explored.

REFERENCES

Iannaccone ST, Browne RH, Samaha FJ, et al. DCN/SMA group: a prospective study of SMA before age six years. *Pediatr Neurol* 1993;9:187–193.

Russman BS, Iannaccone ST, Buncher CR, et al. New observations on the natural history of SMA. *J Child Neurol* 1992;7:347–353.

Thomas NH, Dubowitz V. The natural history of type I (severe) SMA. *Neuromuscular Disord* 1994;4:497–502.

Zerres K, Rudnick-Schoneborn S, Forrest E, et al. A collaborative study on the natural history of childhood and juvenile onset proximal SMA (type II and III SMA): 569 patients. *J Neurol Sci* 1997;146:67–72.

31   Wieacker-Wolff Syndrome

Peter F. Wieacker, Dr Med

DEFINITION: Wieacker-Wolff syndrome is characterized by X-linked mental retardation, muscle atrophy, contractures, and oculomotor apraxia.

DIFFERENTIAL DIAGNOSIS: Allan-Herndon-Dudley syndrome; Arena syndrome; Apak ataxia–spastic diplegia; Goldblatt spastic paraplegia; Baar-Gabriel syndrome.

SYMPTOMS AND SIGNS: At birth, affected males show multiple contractures of the feet resulting in a pes calcaneovalgus. Further development is characterized by a slowly progressive, predominantly distal muscle atrophy, dyspraxia of the eyes, dysarthria, kyphoskoliosis, and mental retardation. Associated findings are ptosis, paresis of the nervus facialis with lagophthalmus, strabismus, and hyperopia.

ETIOLOGY/EPIDEMIOLOGY: Seven male patients in three generations of one family have been described.

DIAGNOSIS: The diagnosis is made by clinical examination. Muscle biopsy shows muscle cell atrophy suggestive of a neuropathy. Sensation and nerve conduction appear normal.

TREATMENT
Standard Therapies: Standard therapies include physical therapy to prevent progression of contractures, surgical correction of contractures, early support to minimize mental handicap, and speech therapy.

REFERENCES

Kloos DU, Jakubiczka S, Wienker T, et al. Localization of the gene for the Wieacker-Wolff syndrome in the pericentromeric region of the X-chromosome. *Hum Genet* 1997;100: 426–430.

Wieacker P, Wolff G, Wienker T. Close linkage of the Wieacker-Wolff syndrome to the DNA segment DXYS1 in proximal Xq. *Am J Med Genet* 1987;28:245–253.

Wieacker P, Wolff G, Wienker T, et al. A new X-linked syndrome with muscle atrophy, congenital contractures, and oculomotor apraxia. *Am J Med Genet* 1985;20:597–606.

RESOURCES

360, 368

13

Ophthalmologic Disorders

1 Aniridia

James D. Lauderdale, PhD

DEFINITION: Aniridia is a congenital inherited panocular eye disease characterized by bilateral partial agenesis of the iris, macular hypoplasia, and risk for acquired corneal opacification, cataracts, and glaucoma (see also WAGR syndrome and Gillespie syndrome).

SYNONYMS: AN1; AN2; Irideremia.

DIFFERENTIAL DIAGNOSIS: Rieger syndrome; Iridogoniodysgenesis; Peter anomaly with cataract; Peter anomaly.

SYMPTOMS AND SIGNS: Signs vary greatly. Photophobia, poor vision, and nystagmus are usually noted in infancy. Iris hypoplasia can range from an almost complete absence of the iris, through enlargement and irregularity of the pupil mimicking a coloboma, to small slitlike defects in the anterior iris layer that become visible only on slit-lamp examination. Associated defects may include nystagmus, strabismus, corneal clouding, cataract of various locations and degrees, foveal dysplasia, and optic nerve hypoplasia. All patients are at risk for developing glaucoma, which may be congenital. Aniridia accompanied by genitourinary abnormalities, mental retardation, and Wilms tumor is known as the WAGR syndrome (Wilms tumor, aniridia, genitourinary anomalies, and mental retardation). Aniridia accompanied by cerebellar ataxia and mental retardation is known as Gillespie syndrome. The lens and cornea in Gillespie syndrome are clear, whereas congenital cataract and corneal opacities (including epithelial haze and pannus formations) are relatively common among individuals with isolated autosomal-dominant aniridia.

ETIOLOGY/EPIDEMIOLOGY: Aniridia (AN2) is inherited as an autosomal-dominant trait. Approximately two thirds of cases are familial and one third are sporadic. The disease is associated with heterozygous null mutations within *PAX6*, a paired-box transcription factor, or with cytogenetic deletions of chromosome 11p13 that encompass *PAX6*. The prevalence is estimated at 1 in 60,000 to 1 in 100,000 live births. Males and females are affected in equal numbers. Evidence suggests that both AN1 and AN2 are linked to 11p. Therefore, it is likely that the only autosomal-dominant aniridia that maps to 11p13 remains and is designated AN2.

TREATMENT

Standard Therapies: Treatment is directed toward improvement and preservation of vision. If there is a refractive error, a patient may benefit from corrective lenses. Drugs may initially be helpful to control glaucoma, but surgery may be needed. Prophylactic surgery in early childhood is helpful to decrease the risk for glaucoma. Surgery is frequently necessary for visually significant cataracts in adults with aniridia. Genetic counseling is recommended for all patients. Those with WAGR syndrome should be evaluated with karyotype or fluorescence *in situ* hybridization for the deletion that raises the risk of associated Wilms tumor; abdominal sonography, CT, or laparotomy with renal biopsy may be necessary. Other treatment is symptomatic and supportive.

REFERENCES

Chen TC, Walton DS. Goniosurgery for prevention of Aniridic glaucoma. *Arch Ophthalmol* 1999;117:1144–1148.

Fantes J, Redeker B, Breen M, et al. Aniridia-associated cytogenetic rearrangements suggest that a position effect may cause the mutant phenotype. *Hum Mol Genet* 1995;4:415–422.

Glaser T, Ton CC, Mueller R, et al. Absence of *PAX6* gene mutations in Gillespie syndrome (partial aniridia, cerebellar ataxia, and mental retardation). *Genomics* 1994;19:145–148.

Hanson I, Jordan T, Van Heyningen V. Aniridia. In: Wright AF, Jay B, eds. *Molecular genetics of inherited eye disorders.* Switzerland: Harwood Academic, 1994:445–467.

Lauderdale JD, Wilensky JS, Oliver ER, et al. 3' deletions cause aniridia by preventing *PAX6* gene expression. *Proc Natl Acad Sci USA* 2000;97:13755–13759.

McKusick VA. *Mendelian inheritance in man,* 12th ed. Catalogs of human genes and genetic disorders. Baltimore: Johns Hopkins University Press, 1998.

RESOURCES

288, 355, 462

2   Blepharophimosis-Ptosis-Epicanthus Inversus Syndrome

Ludwine Messiaen, PhD, and Elfride De Baere, MD, PhD

DEFINITION: The blepharophimosis-ptosis-epicanthus inversus syndrome (BPES) is a genetic disorder subdivided into two types: in BPES type I a complex eyelid malformation is associated with premature ovarian failure (POF), whereas in BPES type II the eyelid defect is an isolated occurrence.

DIFFERENTIAL DIAGNOSIS: Congenital simple ptosis; Ptosis with external ophthalmoplegia; Ohdo blepharophimosis syndrome; Noonan syndrome; Marden-Walker syndrome; Schwartz-Jampel syndrome; Dubowitz syndrome; Smith-Lemli-Opitz syndrome; Michels syndrome.

SYMPTOMS AND SIGNS: Blepharophimosis is a narrowing of the horizontal aperture of the eyelids. In normal adults, the horizontal palpebral fissure measures 25–30 mm, whereas in patients with BPES it generally measures 20–22 mm. Ptosis is a drooping of the upper eyelid causing a narrowing of the vertical palpebral fissure. In this syndrome, ptosis is secondary to dysplasia of the musculus levator palpebrae superioris. An epicanthus inversus is a skinfold arising from the lower eyelid and running inward and upward. Telecanthus is a lateral displacement of the inner canthi, while the interpupillary distance is normal. Other features such as psychomotor and growth retardation, microcephaly, joint contractures, syndactyly, and cardiac defects may be associated with BPES. The female infertility seen in BPES type I is caused by POF and is characterized by primary or secondary amenorrhea, normal secondary sex characteristics, and hypergonadotropic hypogonadism, including elevated follicle-stimulating hormone and luteinizing hormone levels, and decreased estradiol and progesterone levels.

ETIOLOGY/EPIDEMIOLOGY: Most cases are sporadic, but autosomal-dominant inheritance has been observed in numerous families. The disease is caused by a mutation in the forkhead transcription factor gene *FOXL2*, which is located on chromosome 3q23. The disorder is rare and the prevalence is not known. In BPES type I there is complete penetrance; only affected males transmit the disease, because affected females are infertile. In BPES type II there is slightly reduced penetrance (96.5%), and both affected males and females transmit the disease.

DIAGNOSIS: The diagnosis should be suspected based on the findings of the complex eyelid malformation with or without ovarian failure. Mutation analysis in the *FOXL2* gene allows for the identification of an underlying germline mutation in approximately 65% of patients.

TREATMENT

Standard Therapies: The eyelid defect can be treated by ophthalmic plastic surgery: medial canthoplasty for the blepharophimosis, epicanthus inversus, and telecanthus, and a frontalis sling operation for correction of the ptosis. Surgery is hampered by the dysplastic structure of the eyelids. If the ptosis is not severe, surgery is generally performed when the child is 3–5 years of age. When the ptosis interferes with the child's vision, surgery is performed at an earlier age to allow proper visual development. Ovum donation is the only possible therapy for the female infertility at present, because normally differentiated follicles are lacking.

REFERENCES

Crisponi L, Deiana M, Loi A, et al. The putative forkhead transcription factor FOXL2 is mutated in blepharophimosis/ptosis/epicanthus inversus syndrome. *Nat Genet* 2001;27:159–166.

De Baere E, Dixon MJ, Small KW, et al. Spectrum of *FOXL2* gene mutations in blepharophimosis-ptosis-epicanthus inversus (BPES) families demonstrates a genotype-phenotype correlation. *Hum Mol Genet* 2001;10:1591–1600.

Hovav Y, Almagor M, Kafka I. Ovum donation for blepharophimosis-related infertility. *Hum Reprod* 1995;10:1555–1556.

Oley C, Baraitser M. *Congenital malformation syndromes.* New York: Chapman & Hall, 1995.

Steinkogler FJ, Kuchar A, Huber E, et al. Gore-Tex soft-tissue patch frontalis suspension technique in congenital ptosis and in blepharophimosis-ptosis syndrome. *Plast Reconstr Surg* 1993;92:1057–1060.

Zlotogora J, Sagi M, Cohen T. The blepharophimosis, ptosis, and epicanthus inversus syndrome: delineation of two types. *Am J Hum Genet* 1983;35:1020–1027.

RESOURCES

76, 96, 149, 295

3   Choroideremia

Richard A. Lewis, MD, MS

DEFINITION: Choroideremia is an X-linked progressive retinal dystrophy of the retinal pigment epithelium, choroid, and secondarily, the retina, characterized by night blindness, progressive loss of peripheral visual field in males, and a distinctive appearance of the retinal fundus. Classically, asymptomatic female carriers show a mosaic of reticular hyperpigmentation and hypopigmentation in the retinal pigment epithelium, accentuated in the peripheral retina.

SYNONYMS: Choroidal sclerosis; Tapetochoroidal dystrophy; Choroidoretinal degeneration; Rab geranylgeranyl transferase, component A deficiency; Rab escort protein 1 (REP1) deficiency.

DIFFERENTIAL DIAGNOSIS: Retinitis pigmentosa; Hyperornithinemia-gyrate atrophy of the retina and choroid (HOGA).

SYMPTOMS AND SIGNS: In the early stages, hypopigmentation of the peripheral pigment epithelium evolves to enlarging nummular zones of atrophy of the RPE and choriocapillaris, leaving bare the larger choroidal vessels against the bared sclera. Some islands of reactive hyperpigmented RPE may remain between these encroaching lacunae. Gradual encroachment on the macula occurs by the third or fourth decade of life, so that hemizygous males retain reasonable central acuity until late and a unique appearance of the posterior fundus. The inner retina is relatively well preserved so that retinal vascular attenuation and optic disc pallor do not occur until later in life. Female carriers are usually asymptomatic until age 60 or 70, but may have mild night blindness and difficulty with the rate of adaptation from light to dark or the reverse. With occasional lyonization, coarsening of the peripheral reticular pigmentation and even islands of RPE atrophy may be associated with a mild loss of peripheral field.

ETIOLOGY/EPIDEMIOLOGY: The disease is X-linked; the CHM gene maps to Xq21.2. The frequency is estimated at 1 in 50,000 population.

DIAGNOSIS: Clinical diagnosis is directed at diligent ophthalmoscopy of affected males. At-risk females (including the mothers and sisters of affected males) should also have dilated ophthalmoscopic examinations. A contiguous deletion syndrome also includes this locus and manifests choroideremia, mental retardation, and profound conductive deafness with stapes fixation resulting from mutations of the *POU3F4* gene, and a submicroscopic chromosomal deletion. Carriers manifest only the classic retinal carrier state. High-resolution karyotype (or appropriate molecular studies) will confirm the deletion.

TREATMENT

Standard Therapies: Standard therapies include conventional refraction and age-appropriate low vision aids. No dietary or pharmacologic intervention has been shown to be of benefit.

REFERENCES

Hodgson SV, Robertson ME, Fear CN, et al. Prenatal diagnosis of X-linked choroideremia with mental retardation, associated with a cytologically detectable X-chromosomal deletion. *Hum Genet* 1987;75:286–290.

Lewis RA, Nussbaum RL, Ferrell R. Mapping X-linked ophthalmic diseases. Provisional assignment of the locus for choroideremia to Xq13-q24. *Ophthalmology* 1985;92:800–806.

MacDonald IM, Mah DY, Ho YK, et al. A practical diagnostic test for choroideremia. *Ophthalmology* 1998;105:1637–1640.

Merry DE, Janne PA, Landers JE, et al. Isolation of a candidate gene for choroideremia. *Proc Natl Acad Sci USA* 1992;89:2135–2139.

Merry DE, Lesko JG, Sosnoski DM, et al. Choroideremia and deafness with stapes fixation: a contiguous gene deletion syndrome in Xq21. *Am J Hum Genet* 1989;45:530–540.

Seabra MC, Brown MS, Goldstein JL. Retinal degeneration in choroideremia: deficiency of Rab geranylgeranyl transferase. *Science* 1993;259:377–381.

RESOURCES

77, 295, 355

4   Coats Disease

Randall L. Goodman, MD,
and J. Michael Jumper, MD

DEFINITION: Coats disease is a nonhereditary developmental vascular disorder of the retina characterized by lipid leakage from telangiectatic retinal blood vessels, often with exudative retinal detachment.

SYNONYMS: Congenital retinal telangiectasias; Leber miliary aneurysms; Exudative retinopathy.

DIFFERENTIAL DIAGNOSIS: Retinoblastoma; Toxoplasmosis; Granuloma of *Toxocara*; Retinal detachment.

SYMPTOMS AND SIGNS: Patients usually present with decreased vision, strabismus, or leukocoria. The anterior segment eye examination is usually normal, although mild anterior uveitis may occur, especially with proteinaceous flare in the aqueous. On dilated retinal examination, telangiectatic blood vessels are invariably present, usually in the temporal or inferior retina. The exudation, however, affects areas remote from the vascular abnormalities, particularly the macula. White or yellow intraretinal and subretinal lipid accumulates along or around the abnormal blood vessels in a circumferential pattern, and two thirds of patients may have massive lipid exudation with exudative retinal detachment.

ETIOLOGY/EPIDEMIOLOGY: Coats disease is a sporadic condition of unknown etiology. Ninety-five percent of cases are unilateral, and 75% of affected persons are male. Most patients present in childhood (18 months to 10 years of age). The disease is not associated with other syndromes or systemic abnormalities, except for a similar and usually symmetric vasculopathy with facioscapulohumeral muscular dystrophy.

DIAGNOSIS: Upon suspicion of the diagnosis, the patient should be referred to an ophthalmologist for a dilated retinal examination. The best diagnostic method to differentiate Coats disease from similar conditions is indirect ophthalmoscopy. Results of slit-lamp biomicroscopy are usually normal. A fluorescein angiogram will show vascular nonperfusion, enlarged intercapillary spacing, variable capillary branching, and unusually large vessels with exceptional configurations in the areas of the telangiectatic vessels. B-scan ophthalmic echography may help differentiate Coats disease from rhegmatogenous retinal detachment or exophytic retinoblastoma. TORCH serum titers and a CT scan (for lack of intrinsic calcification) may distinguish Coats disease from other leukocorias.

TREATMENT: If untreated, Coats disease can lead to total retinal detachment and/or secondary glaucoma, sometimes requiring enucleation. Early treatment is aimed at destruction of the peripheral areas of abnormal blood vessels to stabilize vision and to prevent progression to retinal detachment. This is usually accomplished with retinal laser photocoagulation or trans-scleral cryotherapy to obliterate the leaking vessels. Once an exudative retinal detachment has occurred, a scleral buckling procedure or vitrectomy is often necessary. If the patient does not have macular exudation or extensive retinal detachment, a favorable visual outcome can be expected; however, approximately 25% of cases will become worse even with intervention.

REFERENCES

Coats G. Forms of retinal diseases with massive exudation. *R Lond Ophthalmol Hosp Rep* 1908;17:440–525.

Shields JA, Shields CL, HonaSG, et al. Clinical variations and complications of Coats' disease in 150 cases: the 2000 Sanford Gifford Memorial Lecture. *Am J Ophthalmol* 2001;131:561–571.

Shields JA, Shields CL, HonaSG, et al. Classification and management of Coats' disease: the 2000 Proctor Lecture. *Am J Ophthalmol* 2001;131:572–583.

RESOURCES

33, 77, 355

5 Cogan-Reese Syndrome

F. Jane Durcan, MD

DEFINITION: Cogan-Reese syndrome is a rare ophthalmic disorder that typically presents with unilateral glaucoma or decreased vision associated with corneal edema.

SYNONYMS: Iris nevus syndrome; Iridocorneal-endothelial (ICE) syndrome.

DIFFERENTIAL DIAGNOSIS: Benign nevi of the iris; Malignant melanoma; Lisch nodules; Essential iris atrophy; Chandler syndrome.

SYMPTOMS AND SIGNS: Patients with Cogan-Reese syndrome typically present in middle age with unilateral changes in the appearance of the iris. The classic presentation has fine pedunculated, pigmented lesions of the iris separated by areas of smooth atrophic flattened iris stroma with loss of stromal crypts (Insert Figs. 54 and 55). Features may also include corectopia (pupil out of its usual central position), atrophic areas of iris, peripheral anterior synechiae (PAS) (areas of peripheral iris adhesion to the cornea), and ectropion uveae (dragging of the posterior pigment epithelium around the border of the pupil onto the anterior surface of the iris). The growth of an endothelium-like cell layer across the structures of anterior chamber angle of the eye can lead to PAS and then obstruction of the drainage system of the eye. This can cause elevated intraocular pressure, which usually develops slowly enough that pain is not a symptom. The elevated intraocular pressure can evolve to glaucomatous optic nerve damage with loss of tissue (cupping) from the optic nerve and visual field loss. The increase in intraocular pressure may stress the corneal endothelium that is already compromised, and thus corneal edema, blurred vision, halos around lights, and discomfort from corneal epithelial breakdown may later occur.

ETIOLOGY/EPIDEMIOLOGY: Cogan-Reese syndrome is part of a spectrum of disorders known as the ICE syndromes. The term encompasses three entities: essential iris atrophy, Chandler syndrome, and Cogan-Reese syndrome. When corectopia, polycoria (multiple pupils), and PAS predominate, the syndrome is termed *essential iris atrophy*. When the beaten-metal appearance of the corneal endothelium and corneal edema predominate, the condition is called Chandler syndrome. The cause of the corneal endothelial abnormality is unknown. A male:female ratio ranges from 1:2 to 1:5. Most patients are middle aged, but the condition has been reported in children, and most are white. A family history usually shows no other cases. The disease is usually unilateral, but bilateral cases have been reported.

DIAGNOSIS: Diagnosis is made by clinical examination where a slit lamp shows the typical corneal and iris findings. Gonioscopy may show angle closure by PAS. Fundus examination may show optic nerve cupping if the intraocular pressure has been elevated for a long time.

TREATMENT
Standard Therapies: The major goal of therapy is protection of the optic nerve from permanent damage from elevated intraocular pressure. In the early stages of the disease, this may be accomplished using topical medications for glaucoma. Later, surgery to control pressure may include trabeculectomy, a glaucoma-filtering procedure that may fail when the membrane grows over and occludes the filter opening. The placement of an artificial tube may supplant the filter after it fails, but this, too, may become occluded by the progressive growth of the surface membrane. In its early stages, corneal edema may be treated with hypertonic saline eyedrops and ointments. When vision becomes severely affected, a corneal transplant may be necessary.

REFERENCES
Campbell DG, Shields MB, Smith TR. The corneal endothelium and the spectrum of essential iris atrophy. *Am J Ophthalmol* 1978;86:317–324.
Radius RL, Herschler J. Histopathology in the iris-nevus (Cogan-Reese) syndrome. *Am J Ophthalmol* 1980;89:780–786.
Shields MB. Progressive essential iris atrophy, Chandler's syndrome, and the iris nevus (Cogan-Reese) syndrome: a spectrum of disease. *Surv Ophthalmol* 1979;24:3–20.
Tester RA, Durcan FJ, Mamalis N, et al. Cogan-Reese syndrome. Progressive growth of endothelium over iris. *Arch Ophthalmol* 1998;116:1126–1127.
Wilson MC, Shields MB. A comparison of the clinical variations of the iridocorneal endothelial syndrome. *Arch Ophthalmol* 1989;107:1465–1468.

RESOURCES
168, 288, 355

6 Duane Syndrome

Nick J. Gutowski, MD

DEFINITION: Duane syndrome is a congenital form of strabismus characterized by horizontal eye movement limitation, specifically by globe retraction with palpebral fissure narrowing on attempted adduction.

SYNONYMS: Duane retraction syndrome; Retraction syndrome; Duane anomaly with radial ray defects and deafness; DR syndrome.

DIFFERENTIAL DIAGNOSIS: Sixth nerve palsy; Möbius syndrome; Congenital oculomotor apraxia; Infantile esotropia; Acquired orbital lesions that cause mechanical restriction of the globe.

SYMPTOMS AND SIGNS: Palpebral fissure narrowing and retraction of the affected eyeball on adduction tend to be constant findings. Three types of Duane syndrome are recognized. Type I, the most common, includes marked to moderate limitation of abduction and moderate to mild limitation of adduction. The palpebral fissure widens on attempted abduction, and a small angle esotropia is often present in primary position. In type II, the palpebral fissure narrows on adduction, but no limitation of abduction occurs. Both adduction and abduction are limited in type III. All three types frequently produce vertical eye movement anomalies with changes in the ocular axes. Strabismus, usually an esotropia in primary position, may occur. Cases are bilateral, but typically asymmetric; anisometropia and thus amblyopia occur uncommonly. Rarely, patients experience diplopia. Nystagmus, pupillary inequality, ptosis, midline cleft palate, or epibulbar dermoid also occasionally occur.

ETIOLOGY/EPIDEMIOLOGY: The prevalence of Duane syndrome is approximately 1 in 10,000 population worldwide; it accounts for 1%–4% of strabismus cases. The pathogenetic principle is paradoxic anomalous lateral rectus enervation of the affected eye by the inferior division of the third nerve, based on electromyographic and pathologic evidence (a hypoplastic or absent sixth nerve nucleus has been found). Duane syndrome is isolated in most cases, but approximately 10% are familial, most commonly autosomal dominant without associated abnormalities. Chromosomal loci for genes contributing to Duane syndrome with associated anomalies have been reported at 4q27–31, 8q12.2-q21.2, and 22pter→22q11.2. An autosomal-dominant form of Duane syndrome without associated abnormalities is linked to chromosome 2q31. There is a female gender and left eye preponderance.

DIAGNOSIS: The diagnosis is made readily with a history of congenital strabismus by testing horizontal eye movement limitations with the addition of globe retraction and palpebral fissure narrowing on attempted adduction. Assessment in an ophthalmology/orthoptic clinic is recommended.

TREATMENT

Standard Therapies: Anisometropic amblyopia should be recognized and treated promptly. Indications for surgery are a noticeable horizontal ocular deviation and an abnormal head position. Secondary indications for surgery are marked globe retraction on attempted adduction and a cosmetically unacceptable down-shoot and/or up-shoot of the eye in adduction. In some cases, regression of clinical features may occur in adulthood without therapy or with orthoptic treatments.

REFERENCES

Appukuttan B, Gillanders E, Juo S-H, et al. Localization of a gene for Duane retraction syndrome to chromosome 2q31. *Am J Hum Genet* 1999;65:1639–1646.

Calabrese G, Telvi L, Capodiferro F, et al. Narrowing the Duane syndrome critical region at chromosome 8q13 down to 40kb. *Eur J Hum Genet* 2000;8:319–324.

Evans JC, Frayling TM, Ellard S, Gutowski NJ. Confirmation of linkage of Duane's syndrome and refinement of the disease locus to an 8.8cM interval on chromosome 2q31. *Hum Genet* 2000;106:636–638.

Gutowski N. Duane's syndrome. *Eur J Neurol* 2000;7:145–149.

Marshman WE, Schalit G, Jones RB, Lee JP, Matthews TD, McCabe S. Congenital anomalies in patients with Duane retraction syndrome and their relatives. *J AAPOS.* 2000;4:106–109.

RESOURCES

355, 427

7   Eales Disease

*Sara Greenhill, MD,
and Andrew W. Eller, MD*

DEFINITION: Eales disease is an idiopathic periphlebitis/vasculitis of the peripheral retina associated with nonperfusion of the affected capillary beds. This results in retinal neovascularization that leads to vitreous hemorrhage.

SYNONYM: Periphlebitis retinae.

DIFFERENTIAL DIAGNOSIS: Syphilis; Cytomegalovirus retinitis; Lyme borreliosis; Tuberculosis; Behçet disease; Connective tissue disorders (such as systemic lupus erythematosis); Inflammatory bowel disease; Pars planitis or intermediate uveitis; Sarcoidosis; Retinal vasculitis; Systemic and ocular lymphoma; Retinal telangiectasia; Sickle cell anemia; Central and branch retinal vein occlusion; Diabetes mellitus; Radiation retinopathy; Multiple sclerosis.

SYMPTOMS AND SIGNS: The most common presenting symptom is vitreous blood manifesting as "floaters" with blurred or decreased vision. It is believed to begin with a retinal occlusive vasculopathy that may be a result of an inflammatory process or a hypersensitivity reaction. Changes may begin unilaterally, but the disease usually progresses to both eyes. The vasculitis leads to retinal capillary obliteration in the affected areas. Vascular sheathing (not inflammatory cuffing) is noted as the vasoobliterative process advances. Other clinical features include microaneurysms, dot-and-blot hemorrhages, cotton-wool spots, hard exudates, dilated capillaries (intraretinal microvascular abnormalities), and tortuous vessels, usually on the venous side. These latter signs occur in other proliferative retinopathies.

ETIOLOGY/EPIDEMIOLOGY: Although the cause is unknown, hypersensitivity is believed to play a role in the pathogenesis of the disease. Some believe tuberculin protein is the inciting agent, but this is unproven. Eales disease is exceedingly rare in Western countries; however, it is common in southern Asia. It usually begins in the second or third decade of life, although women may have a slightly later onset, and it is more common in men.

DIAGNOSIS: Clinical anamnesis involves a thorough eye examination, slit-lamp biomicroscopy, indirect ophthalmoscopy, and fluorescein angiography. Additional laboratory tests should be directed toward other causes for the vasculitis. Testing may include rapid plasma reagin, CD4 count, Lyme titers, tuberculin skin test, erythrocyte sedimentation rate, chest radiography, and blood sugar or glycosylated hemoglobin.

TREATMENT
Standard Therapies: The treatment of Eales disease is directed at its two different components: medical treatment of the underlying inflammatory process and laser and/or surgical treatment for the retinal neovascularization. Medical treatment includes high-dose steroids for a period of up to 3 months and antituberculin medications for those patients who test positive or are in areas endemic to the disease. These treatments are not universally effective. Standard ophthalmic treatment of retinal neovascularization is focal, sector, or circumferential ablation of the peripheral ischemic retina. If visualization of the retina is adequate, classic scatter laser photocoagulation of the nonperfused retina is preferred. If the retina is obscured by vitreous hemorrhage, transconjunctival cryotherapy may be applied. If a vitreous hemorrhage has not cleared spontaneously after several months, pars plana vitrectomy with endolaser photocoagulation may be beneficial.

REFERENCES

Eller AW, Bontempo FA, Faruki H, et al. Peripheral retinal neovascularization (Eales disease) associated with the factor V Leiden mutation. *Am J Ophthalmol* 1998;126:146–149.

Elliot AJ, Harris GS. The present status of the diagnosis and treatment of periphlebitis retinae (Eales' disease). *Can J Ophthalmol* 1969;4:117–122.

Gieser SC, Murphy RP. Eales disease. In: Schachat AP, Murphy RB, eds. *Retina*. St. Louis: CV Mosby, 1994:1503–1507.

Patnaik B, Nagpal PN, Namperumalsamy P, Kalsi R. Eales disease: clinical features, pathophysiology, etiopathogenesis. *Ophthalmol Clin North Am* 1998;11:601–617.

Renie WA, Murphy RP, Anderson KC, et al. The evaluation of patients with Eales' disease. *Retina* 1983;3:243–248.

RESOURCES

355, 427

8   Acute Posterior Multifocal Placoid Pigment Epitheliopathy

Stephen C. Kaufman, MD, PhD

DEFINITION: Acute posterior multifocal placoid pigment epitheliopathy (APMPPE) is a retinal disorder of unknown etiology characterized by bilateral, acute central vision loss associated with yellow-white lesions at the level of the deep retina or retinal pigment epithelium. Spontaneous visual recovery occurs in most cases.

DIFFERENTIAL DIAGNOSIS: Acute retinal epitheliitis; Birdshot retinochoroidopathy; Multiple evanescent white dot syndrome; Recurrent multifocal choroiditis; DUSN; Ocular histoplasmosis; Reticulum cell sarcoma (large cell lymphoma); Sarcoid; Serpiginous choroiditis.

SYMPTOMS AND SIGNS: The patient may experience a viral prodrome that is followed by acute vision loss. The initial dramatic decrease in visual acuity is often bilateral. Visual acuity may range from 20/20 to hand motion depending on the location of the creamy lesions near or under the fovea. Color vision may also be impaired. Shortly after onset, white-yellow lesions, ranging from one-fifth to one disc diameter in size, can be seen in the posterior pole deep in the retina or the retinal pigmented epithelium (RPE) and may spread toward the equator. Vitreitis or anterior uveitis is rare, as are macular edema, retinal hemorrhages, vasculitis, and papillitis. The electrooculogram may be reduced. After 2–5 weeks, the deep retinal lesions resolve, leaving a mottled RPE appearance. Ninety percent of patients recover 20/30 vision or better; however, final visual recovery may not occur for weeks to months after the disappearance of the white-yellow RPE lesions. Two thirds of patients have residual visual deficits. Rarely, subretinal neovascularization occurs. A significant cerebellar vasculitis may rarely be associated with APMPPE.

ETIOLOGY/EPIDEMIOLOGY: Typically occurring in the third decade of life, the condition has been reported in

individuals from 8 to 57 years of age. Males are affected as commonly as females and there is no predilection for race.

DIAGNOSIS: The diagnosis should be suspected from the symptoms and the clinical finding of cream-colored deep retinal plaques. These multiple, white-yellow placoid lesions exhibit a characteristic appearance during fluorescein angiography. Initial hypofluorescence may be associated with the poor filling of the choriocapillaris. Late hyperfluorescence may be related to leakage from the damaged blood-retinal barrier. A positive tuberculin skin test result has been reported in some patients; however, there are no specific laboratory tests for APMPPE.

TREATMENT
Standard Therapies: No active beneficial treatment exists for APMPPE. Although corticosteroids have been used to treat other "white dot syndromes," they have not been beneficial in APMPPE. Because inflammation (e.g., anterior uveitis) may play a role in the pathogenesis of the disorder, other immunomodulatory drugs may be useful.

REFERENCES
Annesley WH, Tomer TL, Shields JA. Multifocal placoid pigment epitheliopathy. *Am J Ophthalmol* 1973;76:511.
Deutman AF, Oosterhuis JA, Boen-Tan TN, et al. Acute posterior multifocal placoid pigment epitheliopathy: pigment epitheliopathy or choriocapillaritis? *Br J Ophthalmol* 1972;56:863.
Fitzpatrick PJ, Robertson DM. Acute posterior multifocal placoid pigment epitheliopathy. *Arch Ophthalmol* 1973;89:373.
Gass JDM. Acute posterior multifocal placoid pigment epitheliopathy: a long-term follow-up. In: Fine SL, Owens SL, eds. *Management of retinal vascular and macular disorders.* Baltimore: Williams & Wilkins, 1983:176–181.
Holt WS, Regan CD, Trempe C. Acute posterior multifocal placoid pigment epitheliopathy. *Am J Ophthalmol* 1976;81:403.
Savino PJ, Weinberg RJ, Yassin JG, et al. Diverse manifestations of acute posterior multifocal placoid pigment epitheliopathy. *Am J Ophthalmol* 1974;77:659.

RESOURCES
288, 355

9   Horner Syndrome

Rolf Salvesen, MD, PhD

DEFINITION: Horner syndrome consists of the clinical triad miosis, ptosis, and hemifacial anhidrosis. It is caused by a dysfunction of the "oculosympathetic pathway" running from the hypothalamus to the eye and face.

SYNONYM: Claude Bernard-Horner syndrome.

DIFFERENTIAL DIAGNOSIS: Raeder syndrome; Carotid artery aneurysm and dissection.

SYMPTOMS AND SIGNS: With miosis, the difference of pupil diameters exceeds 2 mm and is clearly more conspicuous in darkness. After a light stimulus has constricted the pupils, the Horner pupil demonstrates delayed dilatation. The "psychosensory reflex," i.e., mydriasis to sudden noise or pain, is impaired. With ptosis, a characteristic feature is an "upside-down ptosis" with slight elevation of the lower eyelid due to a dysfunction of smooth muscles within it. This may be more easily demonstrated when the patient looks upward. When the lower part of the cornea of the Horner side touches the lower eyelid, a small part of the white sclera intervenes between the cornea and the lower eyelid on the healthy side. Quantitative evaporimetric studies (measurements of sweat evaporation) demonstrate that hypohidrosis is present, often when not recognized clinically. Anhidrosis is not present in dysfunction of the postganglionary sympathetic neurons. The impression of enophthalmos is due to the ptosis, especially of the lower eyelid. Heterochromia iridum, i.e., a relative deficiency of pigment in the iris of the Horner side, is usually present when the syndrome is congenital or caused by a lesion that has occurred before the age of 1–2 years.

ETIOLOGY/EPIDEMIOLOGY: The syndrome is caused by a lesion or dysfunction of the sympathetic pathway to the eye and adjacent face and orbit. Dysfunction of the central sympathetic neuron may be caused by an infarction in the brainstem (typically a Wallenberg syndrome) or the hypothalamus, a tumor within these regions, a multiple sclerosis plaque, or, rarely, a syringomyelia. The preganglionary neuron may be damaged by a C8 or T1 nerve radiculopathy due to a bulging disc, by a lung cancer infiltrating the paravertebral sympathetic chain, or by lymphomas and other expanding lesions in the mediastinum or lower part of the neck. Perhaps most frequently, an internal carotid artery dissection disturbs the integrity and function of the postganglionic sympathetic neuron located in the adventitia of the vessel. The neuron also may be damaged during infection of the middle ear, by a parasellar tumor located in the middle cranial fossa, or by a process in the orbit. Cluster headache is associated with intermittent Horner syndrome during the attacks of pain. The prevalence of the syndrome relates to the prevalence of the various underlying conditions.

DIAGNOSIS: The diagnosis is suspected when a small pupil, a drooping eyelid, or both are observed. If the patient recognizes asymmetric sweating of the face during stress or exercise, the suspicion is reinforced. Application of cocaine 4% eye drops may establish the diagnosis beyond doubt; the normal pupil will dilate markedly, whereas the Horner pupil will not. Hydroxyamphetamine 1% eye drops will distinguish lesions of the postganglionic neuron; the Horner pupil will dilate when the dysfunction is localized to the central or preganglionic neuron but not in postganglionary neuron dysfunction. Phenylephrine eye drops will bring about dilatation in central and postganglionary neuron dysfunction but not in preganglionary neuron lesions. Measurements of evaporation will disclose reduced sweating in central and preganglionary dysfunction but not in a postganglionary lesion, as far as the lateral supraorbital location is concerned. After the dysfunction has been localized, imaging techniques must be applied to establish the exact anatomic cause of the syndrome.

TREATMENT
Standard Therapies: The underlying condition should be treated as appropriate.

REFERENCES
Cremer SA, Thompson HS, Digre KB, et al. Hydroxyamphetamine mydriais in Horner's syndrome. *Am J Ophthalmol* 1990; 110:71–76.
Salvesen R. Innervation of sweat glands in the forehead. A study in patients with Horner's syndrome. *J Neurol Sci* 2001;183: 39–42.
Salvesen R, Fredriksen T, Bogucki A, et al. Sweat gland and pupillary responsiveness in Horner's syndrome. *Cephalalgia* 1987; 7:135–146.
Thompson HS, Mensher JH. Adrenergic mydriasis in Horner's syndrome. *Am J Ophthalmol* 1971;72:472–480.
Van der Wiel HL, van Gijn J. The diagnosis of Horner's syndrome. Use and limitations of the cocaine test. *J Neurol Sci* 1986; 73:311–316.

RESOURCES
288, 355, 427

10   Iridocorneal Endothelial Syndromes

M. Bruce Shields, MD

DEFINITION: The iridocorneal endothelial (ICE) syndrome is an acquired primary abnormality of the corneal endothelium variably associated with corneal edema, anterior chamber angle changes, alterations in the iris, and glaucoma.

SYNONYMS: Progressive iris atrophy (previously called essential iris atrophy); Chandler syndrome; Cogan-Reese syndrome.

DIFFERENTIAL DIAGNOSIS: Corneal endothelial disorders (posterior polymorphous dystrophy, Fuchs endothelial dystrophy); Distortion of the iris (Axenfeld-Rieger syndrome, aniridia, iridoschisis); Nodular lesions of the iris (melanomas, iris melanosis, nodular inflammatory disorders).

SYMPTOMS AND SIGNS: All clinical variations of the ICE syndrome typically have their onset in early to middle adulthood. Familial cases are rare, and there is no consistent association with systemic diseases. Nearly all cases are clinically unilateral. Clinical findings include a characteristic fine hammered-silver appearance of the posterior cornea, frequent corneal edema, peripheral anterior synechiae of the anterior chamber angle, associated glaucoma in approximately 50% of cases, and variable changes in the iris, ranging from minimal corectopia and atrophy (Chandler syndrome) through extensive iris atrophy with hole formation (progressive iris atrophy) and dark, apparently proliferating, nodules on the iris in association with any degree of atrophy (Cogan-Reese syndrome). The most common presenting manifestations are abnormalities of the iris, reduced visual acuity, and pain.

ETIOLOGY/EPIDEMIOLOGY: The ICE syndromes are believed to be an acquired disorder, possibly of viral etiology. Herpes simplex virus may cause the initial abnormality of the corneal endothelium. The abnormal endothelium is known to be responsible for the corneal edema and also to proliferate as a membrane across the anterior chamber angle and onto the iris, with subsequent contraction that causes the changes in the latter two structures.

The syndromes are a disorder complex of uncertain prevalence, with a predilection for women.

DIAGNOSIS: The clinical workup should include careful biomicroscopic (slit-lamp) evaluation of the posterior cornea, which shows the fine hammered-silver appearance; gonioscopy, which shows the peripheral anterior synechiae; and evaluation of the iris, which shows the spectrum of changes. Confirmation of the diagnosis is best achieved with specular microscopy, which shows pleomorphisms in size and shape of the corneal endothelial cells with virtually pathognomic dark areas within the cells.

TREATMENT
Standard Therapies: Management involves treatment of the corneal edema, the associated glaucoma, or both. Corneal edema may be controlled by lowering the intraocular pressure, instilling hypertonic saline solutions, wearing soft contact lenses, or undergoing corneal transplantation in severe cases. The glaucoma may be controlled with standard medical therapy, although glaucoma filtering surgery is eventually necessary in more than half of cases.

Investigational Therapies: Antiviral agents have been used. Another approach may be to prevent the growth of the endothelial membrane, and an immunotoxin that inhibits the proliferation of human corneal endothelium in tissue culture has been described.

REFERENCES
Alvarado JA, Underwood JL, Green WR, et al. Detection of herpes simplex viral DNA in the iridocorneal endothelial syndrome. *Arch Ophthalmol* 1994;112:1601–1609.

Chandler PA. Atrophy of the stroma of the iris. Endothelial dystrophy, corneal edema and glaucoma. *Am J Ophthalmol* 1956; 41:607–615.

Cogan DG, Reese AB. A syndrome of iris nodules, ectopic Descemet's membrane and unilateral glaucoma. *Doc Ophthalmol* 1969;26:424–433.

Shields MB, Campbell DG, Simmons RJ. The essential iris atrophies. *Am J Ophthalmol* 1978;85:749–759.

Wilson MC, Shields MB. A comparison of the clinical variations of the iridocorneal endothelial syndrome. *Arch Ophthalmol* 1989;107:1465–1468.

RESOURCES
288, 355, 427

11 Essential Iris Atrophy

Stephen C. Kaufman, MD, PhD

DEFINITION: Essential (progressive) iris atrophy is one of three variants of iridocorneal endothelial (ICE) syndrome. ICE syndrome, in each of its forms, is believed to result from an abnormality of the corneal endothelium, which affects the cornea, iris, and anterior chamber angle. Essential iris atrophy is characterized by corectopia, iris thinning, and iris holes.

SYNONYM: Progressive iris atrophy.

DIFFERENTIAL DIAGNOSIS: Chandler syndrome; Iris-nevus syndrome of Cogan-Reese; Trauma; Iris ischemia; Some congenital iris dysplasia.

SYMPTOMS AND SIGNS: Signs appear typically in only one eye, beginning between the third to fifth decades of life. Iris thinning is seen first. As the iris stroma thins in areas, the weakened iris stretches, and the location of the pupil changes (corectopia). The thinned iris stroma progresses to frank hole formation. Peripheral anterior synechiae (PAS) may develop and can gradually zipper closed the anterior chamber angle, producing glaucoma. The corneal endothelium may have a beaten-metal appearance.

ETIOLOGY/EPIDEMIOLOGY: This monocular disorder is more common in females. The iris atrophy may be caused by iris ischemia produced by the PAS; but it is more generally accepted that the neural crest–derived corneal endothelium is abnormal. As the disorder progresses, the corneal endothelium replicates and covers the anterior chamber angle and iris. Over time, the abnormal sheet of endothelium and its newly deposited Descemet membrane contract, which subsequently thins or shreds the iris. Glaucoma can occur as the endothelial cells cover the trabecular meshwork.

DIAGNOSIS: Clinical features suggest the diagnosis. A large, low-energy argon laser burn to the iris is sometimes used. If corneal endothelium covers the iris, the treated area turns white; if not, a dark spot or no color change occurs.

TREATMENT

Standard Therapies: Because essential iris atrophy is the most benign form of ICE syndrome, treatment may not be necessary. Glaucoma can be a complex complication to control, but drugs that decrease aqueous production are more effective than miotics. Ultimately, filtering surgery may be necessary.

REFERENCES

Bourne WM. Partial corneal involvement in the iridocorneal endothelial syndrome. *Am J Ophthalmol* 1982;94:774.

Campbell DG, Shields MB, Smith TR. The corneal endothelium and the spectrum of essential iris atrophy. *Am J Ophthalmol* 1978;86:317.

Eagle RC Jr, Font RL, Yanoff M, et al. The iris naevus (Cogan-Reese) syndrome: light and electron microscopic observations. *Br J Ophthalmol* 1980;64:446.

Hirst LW, Quigley HA, Stark WJ, et al. Specular microscopy of iridocorneal endothelial syndrome. *Am J Ophthalmol* 1980; 89:11.

Rodrigues MM, Streeten BW, Spaeth GL. Chandler's syndrome as a variant of essential iris atrophy: a clinicopathologic study. *Arch Ophthalmol* 1978;96:643.

Shields MB. Progressive essential iris atrophy, Chandler's syndrome, and the iris nevus (Cogan-Reese) syndrome: a spectrum of disease. *Surv Ophthalmol* 1979;24:3.

Shields MB, Campbell DG, Simmons RJ. The essential iris atrophies. *Am J Ophthalmol* 1978;85:749.

Shields MB, Campbell DG, Simmons RJ, et al. Iris nodules in essential iris atrophy. *Arch Ophthalmol* 1976;94:406.

RESOURCES
168, 286, 288, 355

12 Keratoconus

Donna Wicker, OD, Ayad A. Farjo, MD, Bradley Taylor, OD, MPH, and Susan Gromacki, OD, MS

DEFINITION: Keratoconus is characterized by a progressive thinning and distortion of the central and paracentral cornea that is typically bilateral but often asymmetric. Dis-ease severity ranges from mild to dramatic with distorted or blurred vision generally beginning in the second or third decade of life.

SYNONYMS: KC; Conical cornea.

DIFFERENTIAL DIAGNOSIS: Corneal ectasias (keratoglobus, pellucid marginal corneal degeneration); Corneal dystrophies (epithelial basement membrane dystrophy and stromal dystrophies such as granular, lattice, or macular dystrophy); Corneal warpage secondary to rigid contact lens wear or irregular astigmatism.

SYMPTOMS AND SIGNS: Early symptoms in the late teen years include blurred or distorted vision at both distance and near. Frequent changes in glasses or contact lenses may be needed. Monocular diplopia, ghost images, and multiple images may persist despite changes in lens prescription. Photodysphoria and glare sensitivity may accompany the distorted vision. With retinoscopy, a scissoring reflex is commonly observed; keratometry shows distorted and irregular mires. Corneal topographic mapping demonstrates an irregular steepening of the cornea slightly below center. Several slit-lamp biomicroscopic signs may occur. A Fleischer ring is a brownish ring of iron deposits either completely or partially encircling the base of the cone. Vogt striae are vertical stretch marks within the cone apex, which appear as fine white lines in the stroma. Corneal scarring in the stroma near the apex of the cone may occur as the disease progresses. Thinning of the central cornea may be visually evident as well. Late signs of keratoconus may be visible even without the aid of slit-lamp biomicroscopy. Viewing the cornea with an ophthalmoscope may show the outline of the cone as a honey or oil droplet against the background red reflex of the fundus (Charleaux sign). Temporal illumination of the cornea can demonstrate a nasal arrowhead (Rizutti sign). Lastly, the cornea can distend the lower lid in downgaze, demonstrating its conical shape (Munson sign).

ETIOLOGY/EPIDEMIOLOGY: Prevalence estimates vary, and are probably about 55 per 100,000 population. This value likely underestimates the true prevalence because many patients have mild disease and are asymptomatic. There may be a slight female preponderance. Keratoconus is believed to have an autosomal-dominant inheritance pattern. The precise mechanism by which the disease progresses remains unclear—increased activity of proteolytic enzymes, collagen disorders, eye rubbing, and contact lens wear have all been suggested to play a role.

DIAGNOSIS: Diagnosis is based on distorted keratometry mires, characteristic corneal topography showing irregular steepening of the inferonasal cornea, stromal thinning, and/or characteristic biomicroscopic findings.

TREATMENT

Standard Therapies: Corneal curvature changes result in myopia and astigmatism, and glasses correction may be sufficient in the early stages. When this is inadequate, contact lenses are recommended. Although soft contact lenses may be used in mild keratoconus, generally rigid gas-permeable lenses are prescribed. The area between the irregular corneal surface and the back of the contact lens fills with tears and the main refractive surface becomes the front surface of the hard contact lens, resulting in a clearer image. Specialty contact lenses have been developed, but the inferonasal location of the cone's apex complicates a well-centered lens fit. If contact lens correction cannot provide adequate visual acuity or if the lenses become too uncomfortable to tolerate, surgery may be performed. Overall, 10%–20% of these patients will require penetrating keratoplasty (corneal transplantation). The success rate is generally excellent. Keratorefractive procedures that achieve effect through ablation of the central cornea (photorefractive keratectomy, PRK, and laser-assisted *in situ* keratomileusis, LASIK) are contraindicated in these patients because the corneal thinning and steepening may worsen, hastening the need for corneal transplantation.

Investigational Therapies: Procedures that spare the central cornea, such as intracorneal ring segments, are being investigated actively.

REFERENCES

Mandell RB. Keratoconus. In: Mandell, RB, ed. *Contact lens practice.* Springfield, IL: Charles C. Thomas, 1988:732–751.

Zadnik K, Barr JT. Diagnosis, contact lens prescribing and care of the keratoconus patient. In: *Clinical practice in contact lenses.* Boston: Butterworth-Heineman, 1999.

RESOURCES

288, 307, 355

13   Leber Congenital Amaurosis

Richard A. Lewis, MD, MS

DEFINITION: Leber congenital amaurosis (LCA) is a single eponym for a broad group of hereditary ocular disorders characterized by moderate to severe visual impairment identifiable at birth or within the first 3 months of life, infantile nystagmus, a variety of retinal changes, and minimal to absent responses on a standard electroretinogram.

SYNONYMS: Amaurosis congenita of Leber; Congenital amaurosis of retinal origin; Congenital tapetoretinal dysplasia; Dysgenesis neuroepithelialis retinae; Hereditary retinal aplasia; Retinal blindness, congenital.

DIFFERENTIAL DIAGNOSIS: Achromatopsia; Blue cone monochromacy; Complete congenital color blindness; Congenital stationary night blindness; Jeune syndrome; Joubert syndrome; Renal-retinal dysplasia (Senior-Loken syndrome); Rod monochromacy (complete congenital achromatopsia).

SYMPTOMS AND SIGNS: Leber congenital amaurosis is characterized by moderate to severe visual impairment identified at or within a few months of birth, infantile nystagmus, sluggish pupillary responses (and occasionally a paradoxical pupil response), and absent or poorly recordable electroretinographic responses early in life. Additional features include symmetric midfacial hypoplasia with enophthalmos and hypermetropic refractive errors. Although the fundus may be normal initially, irregular retinal pigmentation, attenuated retinal vessels, and pale optic nerves frequently evolve later. Some forms of LCA have been reported in association with systemic conditions including structural abnormalities of the central nervous system (cerebellar hypoplasia), neurologic disorders, developmental and mental retardation, hearing impairment, short stature and other skeletal anomalies, and kidney disease. Considerable intrafamilial similarity occurs in the retinal features, but numerous variations in retinal pathology have been defined, including normal or near normal fundus, "salt and pepper" fundus, pigmentary retinopathy similar to "retinitis pigmentosa," "leopard spots" (round, large pigment clumps throughout the retina, coarser in the periphery), "marbleized" fundus, macular "colobomas," and diffuse optic atrophy. Some children develop cataracts in the latter half of the first decade of life, and rare individuals develop keratoconus.

ETIOLOGY/EPIDEMIOLOGY: Leber congenital amaurosis is the most common hereditary cause of visual impairment in infants and children. No substantive epidemiologic studies report a valid prevalence, but estimates are near 1 in 15,000 in the general population. Rare families with a similar phenotype and dominant pattern of inheritance have been reported, but it is not clear that these represent the same genetic entities.

DIAGNOSIS: The diagnosis is made from the early-onset diminished responsiveness, moving eye movements evolving to infantile nystagmus, poorly reactive pupils, and abnormal electroretinographic responses.

TREATMENT

Standard Therapies: No medical or surgical intervention has been shown to alter the natural course of LCA, nor has any pharmacologic therapy shown any effect on modulating or moderating its progression. Conventional spectacles may benefit some individuals with substantive refractive errors and retainable acuity. However, low vision aids, magnifiers, and closed-circuit television systems are often inappropriate for children who have light perception-only or hand movement-only vision, and alternative training for mobility is necessary. Recent gene therapy experiments in a dog model of Leber amaurosis have shown incomplete correction of the deficit.

REFERENCES
Acland GM, Aguirre GD, Ray J, et al. Gene therapy restores vision in a canine model of childhood blindness. *Nat Genet* 2001;28:92–95.

Heher KL, Traboulsi EI, Maumenee IH. The natural history of Leber's congenital amaurosis. Age-related findings in 35 patients. *Ophthalmology* 1992;99:241–245.

Lotery AJ, Namperumalsamy P, Jacobson SG, et al. Mutation analysis of 3 genes in patients with Leber congenital amaurosis. *Arch Ophthalmol* 2000;118:538–543.

McKusick VA, ed. Online Mendelian Inheritance in Man (OMIM). Baltimore, MD. The Johns Hopkins University. Entry nos. 180069, 204000, 204100, 600179, 602225, 604232, 604392, 604393, and 604537.

Nickel B, Hoyt CS. Leber's congenital amaurosis. Is mental retardation a frequent associated defect? *Arch Ophthalmol* 1982; 100:1089–1092.

Smith D, Oestreicher J, Musarella MA. Clinical spectrum of Leber's congenital amaurosis in the second to fourth decades of life. *Ophthalmology* 1990;97:1156–1161.

RESOURCES
77, 234, 355

14   Leber Hereditary Optic Neuropathy

Valérie Biousse, MD,
and Nancy J. Newman, MD

DEFINITION: Leber hereditary optic neuropathy (LHON) is a mitochondrial disease manifested typically by rapid onset and poor recovery of sequential optic neuropathy, usually in young men.

SYNONYMS: Leber optic neuropathy; Leber optic atrophy.

DIFFERENTIAL DIAGNOSIS: Other hereditary optic neuropathies (autosomal dominant and recessive); Toxic and nutritional optic neuropathies; Compressive optic neuropathy; Optic neuritis; Ischemic optic neuropathy.

SIGNS AND SYMPTOMS: Visual loss is painless, central, and occurs in one eye weeks to months before the second eye. Vision deteriorates to visual acuity of 20/200 or worse. Color vision is affected early and severely, and visual fields typically show central or cecocentral defects. Rarely, patients may experience spontaneous improvement in the vision of one or both eyes even years after initial visual loss. Ophthalmoscopic abnormalities in patients with LHON include hyperemia of the optic nerve head, dilatation and tortuosity of vessels, hemorrhages, or circumpapillary telangiectatic microangiopathy during the acute phase of visual loss. Eventually, the only fundus finding will be optic atrophy. In most patients with LHON, visual loss is the only manifestation of the disease. Some patients have family members with associated cardiac conduction abnormalities, especially preexcitation syndromes. Minor neurologic and skeletal abnormalities have been reported in a few patients, as has disease clinically indistinguishable from multiple sclerosis.

ETIOLOGY/EPIDEMIOLOGY: The disease has been linked to point mutations in the mtDNA and follows a maternal inheritance pattern. Men become symptomatic more frequently than women, evinced by a male predominance of 85%–95%. The onset of visual loss classically occurs between the ages of 15 and 35, but LHON has been noted in patients ranging in age from 1 to 80. Three individual mutations in the mtDNA account for approximately 85%–90% of LHON cases worldwide (11778, 3460, and 14484 mtDNA mutations). They are designated "primary mutations" in that each alone has been associated with LHON and is not found in controls. Thus, they have a primary pathogenic role in LHON.

DIAGNOSIS: The diagnosis of LHON should be considered in any case of unexplained bilateral optic neuropathy, regardless of age of onset, gender, family history, or ophthalmoscopic appearance. Ancillary tests in LHON have limited clinical value. Electrocardiography may show cardiac conduction abnormalities. Formal color vision testing may show defects prior to acuity loss, but these findings are not predictive of who will suffer visual loss. Visual-evoked responses are predictably abnormal after visual loss. Standard flash electroretinograms are typically normal. Electroencephalograms, cerebrospinal fluid, and brain CT and MRI are generally unremarkable. The diagnosis of LHON is confirmed by the detection of one of the three primary point mutations in the mtDNA on whole blood samples or any tissue that contains mitochondria.

TREATMENT

Standard Therapies: Irreversible damage makes optic atrophy difficult to treat; however, patients should probably avoid agents that might stress mitochondrial energy production such as tobacco, cyanide-containing products, excessive alcohol, and environmental toxins. Symptomatic therapies include pacemakers in patients with heart block or serious cardiac conduction defects or arrhythmias, and low vision aids for patients with visual loss from optic atrophy.

Investigational Therapies: As the specific genetic and biochemical abnormalities are better defined, more directed therapies may replace or bypass the genetic or metabolic deficiencies in patients with the disease and in their relatives at risk.

REFERENCES

Biousse V, Newman NJ. Neuro-ophthalmology of mitochondrial diseases. *Semin Neurol* 2001;21:275–291.

Kerrison JB, Newman NJ. Clinical spectrum of Leber's hereditary optic neuropathy. *Clin Neurosci* 1997;4:295–301.

Newman NJ. Leber's hereditary optic neuropathy: new genetic considerations. *Arch Neurol* 1993;50:540–548.

Newman NJ. Hereditary optic neuropathies. In: Miller NR, Newman NJ, eds. *Walsh & Hoyt clinical neuro-ophthalmology*, 5th ed. Vol. 1. Baltimore: Williams & Wilkins, 1999:741–773.

Nikoskelainen EK, Huoponen K, Juvonen V, et al. Ophthalmologic findings in Leber hereditary optic neuropathy with special reference to mtDNA mutations. *Ophthalmology* 1996; 103:504–514.

RESOURCES

204, 288, 355, 478

15   Lenz Microphthalmia Syndrome

John M. Opitz, MD

DEFINITION: Lenz microphthalmia is an X-linked syndrome of multiple congenital anomalies including underdevelopment or lack of development of the eyes and blindness or (severe) visual impairment, developmental delay in most cases, and shortness of stature.

SYNONYMS: Microphthalmia (small eye) or anophthalmos (no eye), with associated anomalies; MMA; Lenz "dysplasia."

DIFFERENTIAL DIAGNOSIS: Any one of a large number of known microphthalmia/anophthalmia syndromes.

SYMPTOMS AND SIGNS: Signs of Lenz microphthalmia include the following: microphthalmia (with microcornea) or anophthalmia, at times with coloboma (cleft) of optic disc, choroid, ciliary body, and iris; head size small/normal or microcephalic; mental retardation in most affected boys; dysgenesis of corpus callosum and dilation of lateral ventricles; hypospadias and cryptorchidism in males, at times associated with renal dysgenesis and hydroureter; unusual body habitus with long cylindrical thorax/trunk, narrow, sloping shoulders, and underdeveloped clavicles; and lumbar hyperlordosis and occasional kyphoscoliosis. Dental abnormalities include the absence of upper lateral incisors, irregular lower incisors, and other defects of size, position, number, and eruption. Carrier mothers may be somewhat short and have a small head and "crooked" fifth fingers.

ETIOLOGY/EPIDEMIOLOGY: All pedigrees to date are compatible with (rare) mutation and/or deletion of an X-linked gene, with occasional mild manifestations in carrier women. Few cases have been reported, and the population prevalence is unknown. The condition may be heterogeneous and complex; severe cases may be deletions (i.e., a contiguous gene syndrome). In one family studied, the condition appears to be linked to a locus in region Xq27-q28.1.

DIAGNOSIS: Diagnosis is made by clinical examination, MRI of the eyes and brain, ultrasonography of the kidneys, and echocardiography of the heart. High-resolution chromosome examination with special emphasis on X markers and fluorescent *in situ* hybridization is also recommended.

TREATMENT
Standard Therapies: Ophthalmologic therapies are used, including eye prosthesis (if indicated). Urologic repair is performed for hypospadias and/or renal involvement. Other treatment includes cardiac support for heart involvement and special pedagogic support for blindness and developmental delay.

REFERENCES

Forrester S, Kovach M, Reynolds N, et al. Manifestations in four males with and an obligate carrier of the Lenz microphthalmia syndrome. *Am J Med Genet* 2001;98:92–100.

Graham CA, Redmond RM, Nevin NC. X-linked clinical anophthalmos: localization of the gene to Xq27-Xq28. *Ophthal Paediatr Genet* 1991;12:43–48.

Herrmann J, Opitz JM. The Lenz microphthalmia syndrome. *Birth Defects Org Art Ser* 1969;5:138–141.

Hoefnagel D, Keenan ME, Allen FH. Heredofamilial bilateral anophthalmia. *Arch Ophthal* 1963;69:760–764.

Lenz W. Recessiv-geschlechtsgebundene Mikrophthalmie mit multiplen Missbildungen. *Z Kinderheilk* 1955;77:384–390.

RESOURCES
199, 295, 355

16   Nance-Horan Syndrome

Annick Toutain, MD

DEFINITION: Nance-Horan syndrome (NHS) is characterized by the association in males of dense congenital cataract with microcornea and distinctive facial and dental anomalies.

SYNONYMS: Cataract-dental syndrome; X-linked cataract with Hutchinsonian teeth; Mesiodens-cataract syndrome.

DIFFERENTIAL DIAGNOSIS: Isolated cataracts; X-linked microphthalmia; Lenz microphthalmia; Oculo-cerebro-renal syndrome of Lowe.

SYMPTOMS AND SIGNS: The congenital cataracts are bilateral, severe, dense, and, most often, total. They are associated with microcornea or even microphthalmia, early-onset nystagmus, and, often, secondary strabismus. Visual impairment is substantial. Distinctive dental abnormalities of both the deciduous and the permanent teeth include diastema and crown-shaped and barrel-shaped anomalies (screwdriver-shaped incisors in which the incisal edge and the gingival edge are distinctly smaller than the body of the tooth; hutchinsonian teeth; globular, mulberry-shaped, bud-shaped, barrel-shaped canines, premolars, and molars; and extra cusps. Both missing teeth and supernumerary and impacted teeth are frequent. A characteristic but not universal finding is mesiodens. Facial dysmorphism, including a long face, a marked and broad chin with prognathism, a distinctive nose with a high ponticulus, a narrow glabella, and a bulbous tip, and prominent and anteverted ears, is sometimes subtle and limited to a suggestive facial gestalt. Approximately 30% of patients have intellectual impairment. It is usually mild or moderate, but profound retardation has occurred. In heterozygous females, structural manifestations are similar to affected males but less severe. Ocular signs present in more than 90% of carriers include bilateral, predominantly posterior, most often Y-sutural opacities, often asymmetric in the lens. Corneal diameters are nearly always less than normal. Cataract surgery for carriers is required infrequently, and visual function is generally good. Dental anomalies are always present, including barrel-shaped incisors, crowded and overlapping teeth, and soft enamel. Facial appearance resembles that of affected males, but is milder.

ETIOLOGY/EPIDEMIOLOGY: Nance-Horan syndrome is an X-linked genetic condition of unknown pathogenesis. The gene has been mapped to the X chromosome at Xp22.13. Fewer than 50 families have been reported but the disorder is probably underdiagnosed.

DIAGNOSIS: The diagnosis should be suspected in any male with congenital cataract, especially with a suggestive family history or with dental disease. Dental anomalies and suggestive facial features should be sought on physical examination and on dental (Panorex) radiographs. Ocular examination of at-risk females in the family is helpful and usually shows posterior sutural lens opacities and mild microcornea.

TREATMENT

Standard Therapies: Treatment is palliative. Cataracts usually require surgery for extraction, although the results may be poor and glaucoma occurs in approximately half of operated eyes. Complications can be treated medically or surgically. Education appropriate for the degree of visual or intellectual handicap or in a special school for the visually impaired may be required. Dental anomalies need orthodontic treatment.

REFERENCES
Lewis RA. Mapping the gene for X-linked cataracts and microcornea with facial, dental, and skeletal features to Xp22; an appraisal of the Nance-Horan syndrome. *Trans Am Ophthalmol Soc* 1989;87:658–728.

Nance WE, Warburg M, Bixler D, et al. Congenital X-linked cataract, dental anomalies and brachymetacarpalia. *Birth Defects Orig Art Ser* 1974;4:285–291.

Toutain A, Ayrault A-D, Moraine CL. Mental retardation in Nance-Horan syndrome: clinical and neuropsychological assessment in four families. *Am J Med Genet* 1997;71:305–314.

Toutain A, Ronce N, Dessay B, et al. Nance-Horan syndrome: linkage analysis in 4 families refines localization in Xp22.31-p22.13 region. *Hum Genet* 1997;99:256–261.

Walpole SM, Ronce N, Grayson C, et al. Exclusion of RAI2 as the causative gene for Nance-Horan syndrome. *Hum Genet* 1999;104:410–411.

RESOURCES
355, 363, 373

---

17   Norrie Disease

Richard A. Lewis, MD

DEFINITION: Norrie disease is a severe X-linked form of congenital or perinatal blindness in males characterized by vascular degenerative and proliferative changes in the neural retina and vitreous, resulting in fibroproliferative tractional retinal disorganization and sequential and progressive atrophy of both eyes.

SYNONYMS: Atrophia bulborum hereditaria; Episkopi (Cyprus) blindness; Microcephaly-vitreoretinal dysplasia; X-linked pseudoglioma.

DIFFERENTIAL DIAGNOSIS: Coats disease; COFS syndrome; Familial exudative vitreoretinopathy; Goltz-Gorlin syndrome; Lenz microphthalmia syndrome; Microphthalmia-microcephaly syndrome; Oculo-dento-digital syndrome; Persistent hyperplastic primary vitreous; (Bilateral) retinoblastoma; Retinopathy of prematurity; Waardenburg anophthalmia.

SYMPTOMS AND SIGNS: The earliest feature is often bilateral and symmetric leukocoria caused by total retinal detachment and secondary retrolental membranes. Over time, the globes shrink (phthisis bulbi or atrophia bulborum). Associated features include cataract, shallowed anterior chamber, vitreoretinal hemorrhages, retinal folds, and tractional retinal detachment. Some individuals have persistent remnants of hyaloid vessels in the vitreous. At least one third of individuals are developmentally delayed disproportionately to their visual handicap; many develop progressive neurosensory hearing loss even to total deafness, but considerable intrafamilial variability occurs. More than half of patients are neither deaf nor retarded. In some families, a microdeletion syndrome incorporating the Norrie gene has associated microcephaly, generalized hypotonia, growth retardation, and gonadal hypoplasia. Rare female carriers may show peripheral retinal vascular anomalies reminiscent of spontaneously involuted retinopathy of prematurity, and a Coats-like picture has been documented.

ETIOLOGY/EPIDEMIOLOGY: Norrie disease is inherited as an X-linked trait. Male-to-male transmission has never been documented, and obligate female carriers are usually healthy. No incidence or prevalence figures are available, although the disorder has been reported from European, African, Asian, and Hispanic lineages. Classic linkage, translocation, and deletion mapping have assigned the *ND* gene to Xp11.3-p11.4. The three exon gene codes for a polypeptide "Norrin" of 133 amino acids whose function is not yet entirely understood, although predicted tertiary structure is similar to transforming growth factor beta.

DIAGNOSIS: In the familial clinical situation, the uncomplicated diagnosis is based on characteristic retinal changes. In an isolated situation of a normal birth weight male presenting with rapidly progressive hemorrhagic retinal degeneration and fibroproliferative tractional retinal detachment, differential confusion with retinopathy of prematurity or exudative vitreoretinopathy may occur. Direct mutational analysis of the Norrie gene (*NDP*) will secure the diagnosis in more than 95% of patients.

TREATMENT
Standard Therapies: Early vitreoretinal surgical intervention may moderate the tractional retinal detachment and the risk of both secondary glaucoma and secondary phthisis, but does not improve central visual prognosis. Cataract surgery may improve appearance of the dense white pupil but seldom improves function. Appropriate monitoring for hearing deficits and intervention with electromechanical amplification and even cochlear implants should be considered for those with progressive hearing impairment. Behavioral modification may be a lifelong challenge even when cognitive impairment is not present.

REFERENCES
Berger W, Meindl A, van de Pol TJR, et al. Isolation of a candidate gene for Norrie disease by positional cloning. *Nat Genet* 1992; 1:199–203.
Berger W, Ropers H-H. Norrie disease. In: Scriver CR, Beaudet AL, Sly WS, et al., eds. *The metabolic and molecular bases of inherited disease,* 8th ed. New York: McGraw-Hill, 2001:5977–5985.
Chen Z-Y, Battellini EM, Fielder A, et al. A mutation in the Norrie disease gene (NDP) associated with X-linked familial vitreoretinopathy. *Nat Genet* 1993;5:180–183.
Meindl A, Lorenz B, Achatz H, et al. Missense mutations in the *NDP* gene in patients with a less severe course of Norrie disease. *Hum Mol Genet* 1995;4:489–490.

RESOURCES
288, 355, 375, 462

---

18   Pars Planitis

Stephen Guest, MD

DEFINITION: Pars planitis is an idiopathic disease of the eye(s) characterized by intraocular inflammation centered about the pars plana and peripheral retina.

SYNONYMS: Intermediate uveitis; Peripheral uveitis; Chronic cyclitis.

DIFFERENTIAL DIAGNOSIS: Sarcoid uveitis; Toxocariasis; Lyme disease; Ocular tuberculosis; Ocular syphilis.

SYMPTOMS AND SIGNS: Pars planitis is classically a condition limited to the eye(s). Symptoms may include floaters and blurred vision; rarely, pain, photophobia, and redness may occur. Often, mild anterior uveitis may manifest as cells and flare in the anterior chamber. The main focus of the inflammation is in the vitreous base overlying the pars plana and peripheral retina. The *sine qua non* of the disease is the presence of an inflammatory white band over the pars plana. This may be in the form of a confluent white "snowbank" or as more patchy condensations often called "snowballs." The anterior vitreous behind the lens usually has a cellular infiltrate, and condensations or clumps in the midvitreous cavity may give rise to the subjective floaters. The retinal vasculature is commonly affected with focal areas of peripheral retinal periphlebitis and sometimes with fronds of new vessels extending into the vitreous. These new vessels can occasionally bleed, causing vitreous hemorrhage. The most common cause of reduced vision is swelling of the central macula caused by leakage of fine macular capillary blood vessels and called cystoid macular edema (CME). This can often be confirmed by fluorescein angiography if not visible clinically. Optic disc edema is usually associated with CME. Retinal detachment may occur in up to 5% of eyes. Other signs related to chronic inflammation may be present, such as cataract, epiretinal membranes, glaucoma, band keratopathy of the cornea, and lens/iris adhesions resulting in a misshapen pupil. The clinical course of the disease is varied, with 10% of patients having a benign self-limiting course, 59% a prolonged smoldering course, and 31% a course characterized by multiple exacerbations.

ETIOLOGY/EPIDEMIOLOGY: The etiology is unknown, but it is widely believed to be a T cell–mediated disorder. Pars planitis is associated with multiple sclerosis approximately 15% of the time. This condition usually affects children or young adults. The diagnosis should be questioned if onset is after age 40. There is no definite gender predilection. Pars planitis accounts for 2.4%–15.4% of uveitis cases. Bilateral disease is present in most cases.

DIAGNOSIS: The diagnosis is made based on the clinical findings, but other possible causes must be ruled out in selected instances. Tests for sarcoidosis, syphilis, and tuberculosis should be performed and, if appropriate, Lyme and *Toxocara* antibodies.

TREATMENT

Standard Therapies: Treatment is multifaceted and can be divided into medical and surgical modalities. Many patients have mild symptoms and require no treatment. Medical treatment is focused on immunosuppression. Topical steroids are the mainstay of treatment for inflammation in the anterior chamber. For clinically significant vitreous inflammation or cystoid macular edema (typically vision less than 20/40 equivalent), periocular steroid injections or systemic steroids are usually the first line of therapy. Typically, periocular injections are reserved for disease that is primarily uniocular. Patients unresponsive to or intolerant of steroids may require other immunosuppressants, including chemotherapy and immunomodulators such as cyclosporine or methotrexate. Surgical treatment includes cryotherapy. Cryotherapy to areas of peripheral exudate associated with retinal new vessels has shown regression of these abnormal blood vessels and also has limited the amount of inflammatory activity in some patients. Retinal laser photocoagulation may perform the same function, but often can be difficult to apply in an eye with an opaque vitreous. Vitrectomy removes visually significant vitreous opacities and is believed to have a long-term beneficial effect on the level of inflammation and the severity of any CME. Cataract surgery may be necessary in severe or long-standing cases.

REFERENCES

Saperstein DA, Capone A Jr, Aaberg TM. Intermediate uveitis (pars planitis). In: Guyer DR, Yannuzzi LA, Chang S, et al., eds. *Retina-vitreous-macula,* 1st ed. Philadelphia: WB Saunders, 1999:599–613.

Malinowski SM, Folk JC, Pulido JS. Pars planitis. *Curr Opin Ophthalmol* 1994;5:72–82.

Nussenblatt RB, Whitcup SM, Palestine AG. Intermediate uveitis. In: *Uveitis: fundamentals and clinical practice,* 2nd ed. St. Louis: CV Mosby, 1996:279–288.

RESOURCES
27, 57, 355, 482

19   Retinal Arterial Occlusion in Young Patients

Neelakshi Bhagat, MD,
and Marco A. Zarbin, MD, PhD

DEFINITION: Central retinal artery occlusion (CRAO) occurs at the level of lamina cribrosa in the optic nerve and leads to widespread (ischemic) infarction of the retina.

Branch retinal artery occlusion (BRAO) results in occlusion of a tributary of the central retinal artery.

DIFFERENTIAL DIAGNOSIS: Ophthalmic artery occlusion; Carotid artery occlusion; Retinal inflammation (e.g., viral retinitis); Neoplastic retinal infiltration (e.g., large cell lymphoma).

SYMPTOMS AND SIGNS: Retinal artery occlusion leads to infarction of the retina in the distribution of the vessel involved. Patients with CRAO present with unilateral acute severe painless visual loss. Two thirds of patients have visual acuity worse than 20/400. If a small arteriole in the macula is occluded (BRAO), the most common presenting symptom is an acute onset of scotoma. Visual acuity ranges from 20/20 to 20/400 depending on the location of the retina served by the involved arteriole. An obstructed arteriole in the peripheral retina may have no symptoms.

ETIOLOGY/EPIDEMIOLOGY: Obstruction of arterial flow occurs primarily through one or a combination of emboli, thrombosis, or arterial spasm. Fewer than 10% of arterial occlusions occur in people younger than 30 years. Hypercoagulable states or embolic conditions are identified in up to 91% of young patients with retinal artery occlusions. Embolic sources can be endogenous or exogenous. In young patients, emboli arise from diseased heart valves from rheumatic fever, congenital valvular dysfunction, patent foramen ovale, mitral valve prolapse, atrial myxoma, and aortic valve papillary fibroelastoma. Long-bone fractures or injury to fatty tissue can give rise to fat emboli. Leukoembolization can occur in disseminated intravascular coagulopathy, acute pancreatitis, collagen-vascular diseases, thrombotic thrombocytopenic purpura, or hemolytic-uremic syndrome. Exogenous emboli include talc, fragments of artificial heart valves, arterial implants, and particles from injection of methylprednisolone acetate into nasal mucosa, face, orbits, and periocular lesions. Retinal arteriolar thrombosis has been reported to occur in association with protein C deficiency, protein S deficiency, antithrombin III deficiency, homocystinuria, hyperhomocystinemia, antiphospholipid antibody syndrome, activated protein C resistance, factor V Leiden deficiency, essential thrombocytopenia, dysproteinemias, polycythemia, pregnancy, and malignancy. Associated inflammatory conditions include aortic arch syndrome (Takayasu disease), Moyamoya disease, Ménière disease, Kawasaki disease, Churg-Strauss syndrome, multiple sclerosis, Crohn disease, sickle cell disease, and Susac syndrome. Associated infectious conditions include cat scratch disease, HIV, herpes zoster, herpes simplex, mucormycosis, syphilis, toxoplasmosis, and Lyme disease. Reflex spasm can lead to retinal artery obstruction in younger patients with history of migraines, inhalation of cocaine, use of amphetamines and other adrenergic agents, excessive use of oxymethazolone hydrochloride (Afrin) nasal spray, and with use of propranolol. Optic disc pathology as drusen, physically small sclerochoroidal rims, or disc edema, may also predispose to CRAO.

DIAGNOSIS: Acutely, results of the retinal examination may appear normal. Retinal edema develops within hours to days. Even at early stages before retinal ischemic retinal whitening has developed, slow flow of blood may lead to ophthalmoscopically visible sludging of blood in retinal vessels, termed box-carring. In BRAO, a focal area of inner retinal whitening is noted with attenuation of the involved arteriole. An embolus may be visible at the site of exit of the central retinal artery from the optic nerve head or at a branch point of the involved artery. Cholesterol emboli appear refractile and appear to be larger than the caliber of the occluded vessel. Platelet-fibrin emboli appear grayish white and tend to have a linear configuration conforming to the shape of the occluded vessel. Calcific emboli can appear chalk white. In CRAO, all the arterioles are attenuated, and the retina appears pale and edematous. The normal foveal reflex appears as the "cherry red spot" in the center of the surrounding pale macular retina, due to perfusion of the subfoveal choroidal vessels visible through the thin foveal retina.

TREATMENT

Standard Therapies: Irreversible damage to neurosensory retina occurs within 90 minutes of total CRAO. Some patients present with partial occlusion, however, and so can demonstrate visual improvement after 24 hours of ischemia. There is no proven therapy for this retinal arterial occlusion. If the patient presents within 24 hours of the occlusion, intervention is directed at increasing perfusion pressure in the central retinal artery and includes ocular massage, anterior chamber paracentesis, and use of oral acetazolamide and aspirin. Some institutions offer radiographically directed intraarterial administration of tissue plasminogen activator to lyse clots in the ophthalmic or central retinal artery. If multiple arterial occlusions occur, one may consider either daily aspirin or anticoagulation with subcutaneous low molecular weight heparin or oral warfarin.

REFERENCES

Ciulla TA, Volpe NA. Retinal arterial occlusion in young patients. *Am J Ophthalmol* 1996;122:134–136.

Cruysberg JR, Deutman AF. Retinal arterial occlusions in young patients. *Am J Ophthalmol* 1996;122:134.

Greven CM. Retinal arterial occlusions in the young. *Curr Opin Ophthalmol* 1997;8:3–7.

Sanborn GE. Retinal artery obstruction in young patients. *Ophthalmology* 1997;115:942.

RESOURCE

355

20 Retinal Vein Occlusion in Young Patients

Marco A. Zarbin, MD, PhD, and Neelakshi Bhagat, MD

DEFINITION: Central retinal vein occlusion (CRVO) occurs with formation of thrombus at the level of lamina cribrosa in the optic nerve. If the thrombosis occurs in a small branch of the central retinal vein, branch retinal vein occlusion (BRVO) results.

DIFFERENTIAL DIAGNOSIS: Carotid artery insufficiency.

SYMPTOMS AND SIGNS: The hallmark of retinal vein occlusion is retinal hemorrhage. Obstruction of a retinal vein causes elevation of venous and capillary pressure, which leads to extravasation of erythrocytes and serous exudation into the retina. In CRVO, dilatation and tortuosity of all the branches of the central retinal vein occur with flame-shaped intraretinal hemorrhages throughout the retina. In BRVO, these signs are noted only in the involved sector. Acute loss of vision occurs due to macular hemorrhage, edema, or parafoveal capillary occlusion. Subsequent capillary endothelial damage leads to retinal ischemia, including macular nonperfusion. The intraretinal hemorrhages and edema usually resolve gradually.

ETIOLOGY/EPIDEMIOLOGY: Only 7.5%–20% of CRVOs occur in patients younger than 50 years. Systemic atherosclerotic and atherogenic diseases, hypertension, and diabetes are the most common contributing factors in the elderly. The artery and vein are bound in a common adventitial sheath. Thickening of the arterial wall compresses the vein, causing distortion of the vein lumen, leading to turbulent blood flow and predisposition to thrombosis. Genetic defects that predispose to retinal venous thrombosis in patients younger than 50 years include activated protein C resistance, protein C or S deficiency, antithrombin III deficiency, prothrombin gene mutations, factor V (e.g., Leiden) mutations, homocystinuria, hyperhomocystinemia, factor XII deficiency, familial hyperlipidemia, plasminogen deficiency, dysplasminogenemia, lipoproteinemia, and plasminogen activator inhibitor. In addition, cardiopulmonary bypass during heart-lung transplantation is associated with disturbances in hemostasis and alterations in platelet function and has been associated with vein occlusions in young patients. Infectious diseases associated with vein occlusions include syphilis, tuberculosis, and AIDS. Associated inflammatory conditions include Behçet disease, Reye syndrome, Crohn disease, Fabry disease psuedotumor cerebri, myasthenia gravis, Sturge-Weber, acute multifocal placoid pigment epitheliopathy, sarcoidosis, serpiginous choroidopathy, Moyamoya disease, cavernous sinus thrombosis, and polycystic ovarian syndrome. Drugs such as oral contraceptives, antiandrogenics, diuretics, and bromocriptine also have been implicated in young patients with CRVO. Other associated conditions include glaucoma, ocular hypertension, retinal vasculitis, retinal arteriovenous communication, optic nerve drusen, and trauma, and systemic disorders including diabetes mellitus, end-stage renal disease, hypercholesterolemia, beta-thalassemia, and hypertension. Bilateral BRVO in young patients has occurred in association with essential hypertension.

TREATMENT
Standard Therapies: In patients younger than 45 years, excluding conditions that predispose to hypercoagulability is important. The patient should undergo a general medical evaluation for associated conditions. If multiple retinal vein occlusions or bilateral vein occlusions are noted, the patient is comanaged with a medical physician to evaluate for a possible treatable underlying cause. One should consider aspirin or anticoagulation with low-molecular-weight heparin or warfarin if a clotting diathesis is identified. No clinically proven treatment exists for retinal vein occlusions.

Investigational Therapies: Experimental surgical treatments include use of tissue-plasminogen activator through retinal vein cannulation for CRVO, and sheathotomy in BRVO.

REFERENCES
Abul el-Asar Am, al-Momen AK, al-Amro S, et al. Hypercoagulable states associated with retinal venous occlusion in young adults. *Int Ophthalmol* 1996–1997;20:197–204.

Bhagat N, Goldberg MF, Gascon P, et al. Central retinal vein occlusion: review of management. *Eur J Ophthalmol* 1999;9:165–180.

Fong ACO, Schatz H. Central retinal vein occlusion in young adults. *Surv Ophthalmol* 1993;37:393–417.

Vine AK, Samama MM. The role of abnormalities in the anticoagulant and fibrinolytic systems in retinal vascular occlusions. *Surv Ophthalmol* 1993.

RESOURCE
355

21 Retinitis Pigmentosa

Richard A. Lewis, MD, MS

DEFINITION: Retinitis pigmentosa (RP) is a descriptive term for a set of hereditary progressive disorders that diffusely and primarily affect photoreceptor and retinal pigment epithelial function, often with a family history of similar disorder, associated with distinctive retinal changes.

SYNONYMS: Retinal heredodegeneration; Photoreceptor dystrophy; Rod-cone dystrophy; Cone or cone-rod dystrophy.

DIFFERENTIAL DIAGNOSIS: Abetalipoproteinemia; Alstrom syndrome; Bardet-Biedl syndrome; Cockayne syndrome; Hyperornithinemia-gyrate atrophy; Infantile Refsum syndrome; Mitochondrial cytopathies; Laurence-Moon syndrome; Loken-Senior syndrome; Pallidal degeneration; Refsum syndrome (phytanic acid storage disorder); Usher syndromes.

SYMPTOMS AND SIGNS: The characteristic initial symptom is loss of dim light (and night) perception, followed by an awareness of loss of peripheral vision. Even with severe restriction of field, central visual acuity may remain good even with advanced disease. The initial ophthalmoscopic changes are seen in the postequatorial retina, where depigmentation of the pigment epithelium precedes migration of pigment-containing macrophages into the retina along small and larger retinal vessels leading to a disseminated bone-spicule distribution. Eventually, the retinal vessels narrow, the inner retina atrophies, and the optic discs become pale. More subtle changes include myopic refractive errors, usually with oblique astigmatism, characteristic posterior cortical and precapsular opacities of the lens, premature syneresis, and liquefaction of the vitreous gel with pigment particles and perhaps other cells.

ETIOLOGY/EPIDEMIOLOGY: RPs unassociated with abnormalities are inherited as autosomal-recessive, autosomal-dominant, and X-linked traits, and rare mitochondrial variants occur. The overall frequency is estimated at approximately 1 in 3,700. At least 29 unique disorders have been assigned specific chromosomal loci, of which only 15 genes have been isolated and cloned. These appear to explain less than half of all RPs, suggesting that many more causative genes remain to be mapped and cloned.

DIAGNOSIS: In the usual situation of a retinal disorder without systemic or constitutional features, ophthalmologic examination will establish the diagnosis from the visual field, biomicroscopic, and ophthalmoscopic examinations. Additional findings in the retina may include macular epiretinal membranes, cystoid macular edema, and macular atrophy. Electroretinography may be useful in problematic situations (e.g., infants or children), but is nonpredictive and the results do not correlate to genetic type.

TREATMENT
Standard Therapies: No medical treatment exists, but several supportive interventions are appropriate for patients with RP. Chronic cystoid macular edema may respond to oral acetazolamide or other carbonic anhydrase inhibitors in some patients. Guidance should be offered for optical aids, field expanders, and sunglasses.

Investigational Therapies: A prospective randomized trial of four regimens of combined supplemental vitamin A and vitamin E among ~600 patients older than 18 years and younger than 49 years with either RP or Usher syndrome type II monitored over ~5 years showed no differences in the rate of decline of visual acuity or the rate of decline in peripheral visual field. An apparently small benefit in slowing the rate of decline of ERG B-wave voltages was interpreted from a subset of data in the groups receiving 15,000 IU of vitamin A palmitate and 50 IU vitamin E, but the interpretation of the data is controversial.

REFERENCES

Berson EL, Rosner B, Sandberg MA, et al. A randomized trial of vitamin A and vitamin E supplementation for retinitis pigmentosa. *Arch Ophthalmol* 1993;111:761–772.

Bromley WC, Hayes RP, Roderick TH. Prevalence of retinitis pigmentosa in Maine. *Am J Ophthalmol* 1984;97:357–365.

Heckenlively JR, Yoser SL, Friedman LH, et al. Clinical findings and common symptoms in retinitis pigmentosa. *Am J Ophthalmol* 1988;105:504–511.

Marmor MF, Aguirre G, Arden G, et al. Retinitis pigmentosa: a symposium on terminology and methods of examination. *Ophthalmology* 1983;90:126–131.

Massof RW, Finkelstein D. Supplemental vitamin A retards loss of ERG amplitude in retinitis pigmentosa (Editorial). *Arch Ophthalmol* 1993;111:751–754.

RESOURCES
161, 288, 355, 419

22   Retinoblastoma

Christopher J. Schwimer, DO,
and Richard A. Prayson, MD

DEFINITION: Retinoblastoma (Rb), although rare, is the most common malignant intraocular neoplasm of the nucleated retinal layers in infants, children, and, rarely, adults. The tumor is of neuroectodermal cell lineage, and a predisposition to form this neoplasm may be inherited.

SYNONYMS: Glioma of the retina; Neuroepithelioma of the retina.

DIFFERENTIAL DIAGNOSIS: Coats disease; Lymphoma; Retinocytoma; Uveitis; Retinal detachment; *Toxocara* endophthalmitis; Persistent hyperplastic primary vitreous; Medulloepithelioma.

SYMPTOMS AND SIGNS: Patients, usually younger than 3 years, with Rb may present with leukocoria, strabismus, decrease in visual acuity, proptosis, and/or metastatic disease. A common parental complaint is that of the so-called "cat's eye" reflex in a flash photograph. Tumor bilaterality is encountered in some patients with the familial form of disease. In this setting, patients are at risk for the development of a variety of nonocular cancers, including, but not limited to, melanoma, osteosarcoma, soft tissue sarcomas, and malignant neoplasms of the central nervous system. The simultaneous occurrence of a pineal or parasellar neoplasm in a patient with bilateral Rbs has been termed trilateral Rb.

ETIOLOGY/EPIDEMIOLOGY: Mutation in the *RB1* gene, located on chromosome 13 (13q14), is known to be involved in the etiology. Heritable disease is clinically transmitted in an autosomal-dominant fashion. The incidence is approximately 1 in 15,000 live births with approximately 23% of patients having bilateral tumors.

DIAGNOSIS: The clinical diagnosis is presumptive, and treatment usually begins with no pathologic diagnosis, although fine-needle aspiration cytology may be useful in making a pretreatment diagnosis. Slit-lamp and fundus examinations with adjunct ultrasonography and radiographic survey (CT and/or MRI) are the mainstay of disease assessment. Histopathology of enucleated tumors shows small blue cells in sheets or forming distinctive structures known as Flexner Wintersteiner rosettes and fleurettes.

TREATMENT

Standard Therapies: Retinoblastoma is treated with sight-sparing modalities when possible; however, enucleation may be necessary. Radiation therapy can be a useful approach, but is avoided when possible, due to the increased risk of the development of secondary nonocular tumors in the prior field of irradiation. In patients with tumors of limited size and extent of spread, ophthalmic plaque brachytherapy, cryotherapy, and transpupillary (laser) thermotherapy, possibly with prior debulking chemoreduction therapy, may provide effective control of Rb. Patients at increased risk for or with metastasis require chemotherapy (commonly cyclosporine), which may be also administered intrathecally. Hematopoetic stem cell rescue is an effective adjunct therapy in patients with distant metastasis. The current cure rate approaches 95% in developed countries.

REFERENCES

Finger PT, Czechonska G, Demirci H, et al. Chemotherapy for retinoblastoma: a current topic. *Drugs* 1999;58:983–996.

McLean IW, Burnier MN, Zimmerman LE, et al. Tumors of the retina. In: Rosal J, Sobin LH, eds. *Atlas of tumor pathology, tumors of the eye and ocular adnexa.* Third Series, Fascicle 12. Washington, DC: Armed Forces Institute of Pathology, 1994: 100–135.

Schwimer CJ, Prayson RA. Clinicopathologic study of retinoblastoma including MIB-1, p53, and CD99 immunohistochemistry. *Ann Diagn Pathol* 2001;5:148–154.

RESOURCES

30, 355

23   X-Linked Juvenile Retinoschisis

*Darin H. Haivala, MD,
and Sumit K. Nanda, MD*

DEFINITION: Juvenile X-linked retinoschisis is an inherited bilateral retinal disease characterized by splitting within the nerve fiber layer of the retina.

SYNONYMS: Congenital hereditary retinoschisis; Congenital vitreous veils; Cystic disease of the retina in children; Sex-linked juvenile retinoschisis.

DIFFERENTIAL DIAGNOSIS: Cystoid macular edema of any cause; Epiretinal macular membrane (macular pucker); Niacin maculopathy; Familial foveal retinoschisis; Retinal detachment; Acquired (senile) retinoschisis; Goldmann-Favre vitreotapetoretinal degeneration; Other retinal dystrophies, including X-linked retinitis pigmentosa and Stargardt disease.

SIGNS AND SYMPTOMS: Young males with juvenile X-linked retinoschisis typically present during the early school years with reading difficulties. Less commonly, a child may present with strabismus, nystagmus, or vitreous hemorrhage or retinal detachment. Progressive visual loss is characteristically rapid during the first decade of life, with stabilization occurring during the second decade at about the 20/50 to 20/100 level. The central visual loss is always associated with foveal schisis, which occurs in 100% of males with the disorder. A peripheral schisis cavity, usually located in the inferotemporal quadrant, occurs in approximately half of patients. A peripheral visual field defect corresponds to the area of schisis. Acute dramatic loss of vision may occur with associated retinal detachment or vitreous hemorrhage. Biomicroscopically, foveal schisis appears as small intraretinal cysts in a coarse stellate or radial pattern centered in the fovea. Peripheral schisis cavities appear as smooth, domelike elevations of the retina. Multiple holes are present in the thin inner layer of the retinoschisis cavity in most patients.

ETIOLOGY/EPIDEMIOLOGY: The X-linked juvenile retinoschisis gene (*XLRS1*) has been mapped to the distal short arm of chromosome X (Xp22.2-22.1). The protein retinoschisin appears to be released by photoreceptors and is found within inner retinal layers. It seems to have a function in cell-to-cell adhesion and in phospolipid binding. The exact pathogenesis of the disease is unknown, but histopathologic and electrophysiologic studies suggest a defect in the Müller cells of the retina.

DIAGNOSIS: The findings of fundus examination are characteristic for the disorder, especially in a younger affected male. Electroretinography may aid in the diagnosis with a near normal a-wave and a selective loss of the b-wave, which reflects the schisis between the inner and outer retina.

TREATMENT
Standard Therapies: No specific treatment exists for X-linked retinoschisis. Scleral buckling and vitrectomy may treat complications such as retinal detachment and vitreous hemorrhage. Prophylactic treatment of the schisis cavity is associated with significant complications and is not recommended.

REFERENCES
Condon GP, Brownstein S, Wang NS, et al. Congenital hereditary (juvenile X-linked) retinoschisis. Histopathologic and ultrastructural findings in three eyes. *Arch Ophthalmol* 1986;104: 576–583.

Eksandh LC, Ponjavic V, Ayyagari R, et al. Phenotypic expression of juvenile X-linked retinoschisis in Swedish families with different mutations in the *XLRS1* gene. *Arch Ophthalmol* 2000; 118:1098–1104.

Grayson C, Reid SNM, Ellis JA. Retinoschisin, the X-linked retinoschisis protein, is a secreted photoreceptor protein, and is expressed and released by Weri-Rb1 cells. *Hum Mol Genet* 2000;9:1873–1879.

Retinoschisis Consortium. Functional implications of the spectrum of mutations found in 234 cases with X-linked juvenile retinoschisis (XLRS). *Hum Mol Genet* 1998;7:1185–1192.

RESOURCES
57, 288, 355

24　Stargardt Disease

Richard A. Lewis MD, MS

DEFINITION: Stargardt disease is a bilateral progressive autosomal-recessive disorder of the retina with characteristic foveal atrophy in the shape of a bull's eye and surrounding deep retinal flecks.

SYNONYM: Fundus flavimaculatus.

DIFFERENTIAL DIAGNOSIS: Central areolar choroidal degeneration; Juvenile macular degeneration; Fundus albipunctatus; Flecked retina of Kandori; Mallattia Leventinese/dominant drusen; Cone dystrophy; Combined rod and cone dystrophy; Central areolar choroidal sclerosis; Retinitis pigmentosa inversa; Kjellin syndrome; Chloroquine or hydroxychloroquine maculopathy; Crystalline maculopathies; Vitamin A deficiency; Neuronal ceroid lipofuscinosis (some forms).

SYMPTOMS AND SIGNS: Beginning with subtle and progressive decreased central acuity, affected patients have few complaints of night blindness, color vision deficiency, or photophobia. Characteristic onset occurs from ages 6 to 15 years, but it is seen as late as the seventh decade of life.

ETIOLOGY/EPIDEMIOLOGY: Stargardt disease is arguably the most common hereditary autosomal-recessive macular disorder and has been reported worldwide; no substantive epidemiologic studies report a valid prevalence, but estimates range near 1 in 15,000 in the general population. Rare families with a similar phenotype and a dominant pattern of inheritance have been reported, but these do not link to markers on chromosome 1p. No evidence suggests a second locus for classic recessive Stargardt disease.

DIAGNOSIS: Beginning as early as age 5 years and peaking in the midteens, affected individuals have evanescent to rapid impairment of central vision, progressive bilateral atrophy of the foveal retinal pigment epithelium and neuroepithelium, and the frequent appearance of yellow-orange flecks distributed around the macula and/or in the midretinal periphery. Typically the flecks do not extend closer than about one-third the disc diameter from the border of the sclerochoroidal rim. The beaten-metal elliptical foveal lesions evolve into geographic atrophy, and the temporal sector of the optic nerve becomes pale, suggesting inner retinal atrophy. Eventually, the flecks atrophy, leaving a faint footprint of thinned RPE and slight powdery granularity of pigment. Approximately 20% of patients develop visual disabilities after age 20. Characteristically, a fluorescein angiogram shows a silent- or dark-choroid sign, in which fluorescence from the deep circulation cannot be visualized where the RPE is intact, and the atrophic fovea appears as a bull's eye transmission defect, as do the flecks as they atrophy. Color vision deteriorates with acuity and is nonspecific. Visual fields and electrophysiologic responses may be abnormal but are nonspecific and generally unnecessary.

TREATMENT

Standard Therapies: No pharmacologic therapy has shown any effect. Conventional spectacles may benefit substantive refractive errors. Low vision aids, magnifiers, and closed circuit television are helpful for both distance and near visual function.

REFERENCES

Allikmets R. Simple and complex: genetic predisposition to retinal disease. *Am J Hum Genet* 2000;67:793–799.

Blacharski PA. Fundus flavimaculatus. In: Newsome DA, ed. *Retinal dystrophies and degenerations.* New York: Raven, 1988: 135–159.

Lewis RA, Lupski JR. Macular degeneration: the emerging genetics. *Hosp Pract* 2000;35:41–58.

Lewis RA, Lupski JR. Inherited macular dystrophies and susceptibility to degeneration. In: Scriver CR, Beaudet AL, Sly WS, et al., eds. *The metabolic and molecular bases of inherited disease,* 8th ed. Columbus, OH: McGraw-Hill, 2001.

Lewis RA, Shroyer NF, Singh N, et al. Genotype/phenotype analysis of a photoreceptor-specific ATP-binding cassette transporter gene, *ABCR,* in Stargardt disease. *Am J Hum Genet* 1999;64:422–434.

Rivera A, White K, Stohr H, et al. A comprehensive survey of sequence variation in the *ABCA4* (*ABCR*) gene in Stargardt disease and age-related macular degeneration. *Am J Hum Genetics* 2000;67:800–813.

RESOURCES

57, 252, 293, 355

25   Tolosa-Hunt Syndrome

Aresu Naderi, MD,
M. Amir Ahmadi, MD,
and Bita Esmaeli, MD

DEFINITION: Tolosa-Hunt syndrome is characterized by painful ophthalmoplegia associated with an idiopathic granulomatous inflammatory process in the cavernous sinus.

SYNONYM: Painful ophthalmoplegia.

DIFFERENTIAL DIAGNOSIS: Vascular and traumatic lesions; Neoplasms; Infectious or specific inflammatory processes involving the anterior portion of the cavernous sinus, orbital apex, or the superior orbital fissure; Ophthalmoplegic migraine and cluster headaches.

SYMPTOMS AND SIGNS: Patients with Tolosa-Hunt syndrome often present with pain in and about the eye (ophthalmic division of the trigeminal nerve). Unilateral ocular motor nerve palsies with ipsilateral periorbital or hemicranial pain, pupillomotor dysfunction, and sensory loss along the distribution of the first and second branches of the trigeminal nerve are hallmarks of this syndrome. The clinical course is characterized by spontaneous remissions and recurrences with prompt response to systemic steroid therapy.

ETIOLOGY/EPIDEMIOLOGY: The etiology of Tolosa-Hunt syndrome remains unknown. This syndrome is a form of idiopathic orbital inflammation with reported age of onset from 3 to 75 years, although most commonly it occurs in middle to late adulthood. There is no sex predilection.

DIAGNOSIS: The diagnosis is made by cerebral MRI with gadolinium enhancement or by CT. Tolosa-Hunt syndrome is a diagnosis of exclusion, and other causes of painful ophthalmoplegia such as neoplasm, infection, or aneurysm must be ruled out.

TREATMENT
Standard Therapies: Treatment of Tolosa-Hunt syndrome consists of systemic corticosteroid therapy for a period of weeks or longer and pain management with analgesics.

Investigational Therapies: Some investigators have advocated acupuncture as an additional method to reduce intractable pain in Tolosa-Hunt syndrome.

REFERENCES
Adams RD, Victor M, Ropper AH. *Principles of neurology,* 6th ed. New York: McGraw-Hill, 1997:181, 271, 1093.

Attout H, Rahmeh F, Ziegler F. Cavernous sinus lymphoma mimicking Tolosa-Hunt syndrome. *Rev Med Intern* 2000;21:795–798.

Glaser JS. *Neuro-ophthalmology,* 3rd ed. Philadelphia: Lippincott Williams & Wilkins, 1999:429–430.

Kline LB. The Tolosa-Hunt syndrome. *Surv Ophthalmol* 1982;27:79–95.

Kline LB. The Tolosa Hunt syndrome. *J Neurol Neurosurg Psychiatry* 2001;71:577–582.

Leigh RJ, Zee DS. *The neurology of eye movements,* 3rd ed. New York: Oxford University Press, 1999:370–371.

Nepp J, Grdser S, Flarrer S, et al. Tolosa-Hunt syndrome—intractable pain treatment with acupuncture? *Acupunct Electrother Res* 2000;25:155–163.

Tessitore E, Tessitore A. Tolosa-Hunt syndrome preceded by facial palsy. *Headache* 2000;40:393–396.

Victor M, Ropper AH. *Adams and victor's principles of neurology,* 7th ed. New York: McGraw-Hill, 2001:288.

RESOURCES
27, 301, 368

26   Usher Syndrome

Richard A. Lewis, MD, MS

DEFINITION: The Usher syndromes are a set of autosomal-recessive clinically and genetically heterogeneous disorders whose cardinal feature is the coinheritance of neurosensory hearing impairment and progressive pigmentary retinopathy similar to retinitis pigmentosa.

SYNONYMS: Hallgren syndrome; Deafness-retinitis pigmentosa; Retinitis pigmentosa-sensorineural deafness.

DIFFERENTIAL DIAGNOSIS: Alstrom syndrome; Cockayne syndrome; Fetal rubella syndrome; Infantile phytanic acid storage disease; Refsum syndrome.

SYMPTOMS AND SIGNS: Three clinical types of Usher syndrome are recognized. Usher syndrome type I is most severe, characterized by profound congenital deafness (classically associated with absence of speech development), early-onset pigmentary retinopathy usually diagnosed in the mid–first decade of life, and absent or severely diminished vestibulocerebellar responses. Usher syndrome type II is characterized by a congenital but moderate to severe hearing impairment characterized by a down-sloping audiogram (of more marked losses in higher frequencies, thus permitting some speech development with electromechanical amplification), and a later onset/discovery of pigmentary retinopathy (usually in the second decade of life), and normal vestibular reflexes. Usher syndrome type III is typified by a progressive hearing loss with variable severity of pigmentary retinopathy and progressive vestibular dysfunction. Types I and II are the most common.

ETIOLOGY/EPIDEMIOLOGY: The frequency of the Usher syndromes depends on the population: in Scandinavia it is approximately 3.5 in 100,000 and in the United States approximately 4.4 in 100,000. The Usher syndromes appear to account for approximately 50% of all individuals who are both hearing impaired and blind, and about 3%–6% of all hearing-impaired children. At least 10 genetic loci for Usher syndromes have been identified: 6 for Usher type I (*USH1A-USH1F*); 3 for Usher type II (*USH2A-USH2C*); and 1 for Usher type III (*USH3A*). The most common form of Usher syndrome type I, Ib, is localized to chromosome 11q13.5. Usher type 2A, the most common of the milder forms, maps to chromosome 1q41.

DIAGNOSIS: Clinical diagnosis requires the coordination of the ophthalmologist, the otolaryngologist, the audiologist, and the geneticist. Recognition of hearing impairment may be delayed until speech is profoundly delayed. Brain-stem auditory evoked responses and interactive audiometry may assist the diagnosis or the documentation of the loss. Pigmentary retinopathy may be subtle, and electroretinography at age 2 or 3 years may be needed to confirm the suspicion. When retinal abnormalities are visible, electrophysiology will be predictably abnormal; the degree of the abnormality is noncategorizing. Vestibular dysfunction in adults with Usher type I is obvious in the swinging and swaying gait (of peripheral origin). Type I patients are also predictably delayed in sitting and walking (usually after age 18 months).

TREATMENT

Standard Therapies: Selective education is needed for the combined sensory losses. Early intervention for auditory stimulation and speech therapy is essential. For patients with type I, cochlear implants may be helpful. Central vision is involved. Conventional ophthalmologic intervention for refractive errors and for low vision aids and magnifiers is age-dependent. Cataract surgery may be necessary in the third and fourth decades.

REFERENCES

Astuto LM, Weston MD, Carney CA, et al. Genetic heterogeneity in Usher syndrome: analysis of 151 families with Usher type I. *Am J Hum Genet* 2000;67:1569–1574.

Boughman JA, Vernon M, Shaver KA. Usher syndrome: definition and estimate of prevalence from two high risk populations. *J Chronic Dis* 1993:36:595–603.

Fishman GA, Kumar A, Joseph ME, et al. Usher's syndrome: ophthalmic and neuro-otologic findings suggesting genetic heterogeneity. *Arch Ophthalmol* 1983;110:1367–1374.

Smith RJ, Berlin CI, Hejtmancik JF, et al. Clinical diagnosis of the Usher syndromes: Usher syndrome consortium. *Am J Med Genet* 1994;50:32–38.

Weston MD, Kelley PM, Overbeck LD, et al. Myosin VIIa screening in 189 Usher syndrome type I patients. *Am J Hum Genet* 1996;59:1074–1083.

RESOURCES

355, 370, 481

27   Posterior Uveitis

N. Kevin Wade, MD,
and Raymond J. Seto, MD

DEFINITION: Posterior uveitis is not a single disorder but a complex of features that involve inflammation of the choroid. Posterior uveitis may be either a primary process or a feature of a systemic disease.

DIFFERENTIAL DIAGNOSIS: Large cell lymphoma; Malignant melanoma; Rhegmatogenous retinal detachment; Retained intraocular foreign body; Retinoblastoma; Leukemia; Various retinal dystrophies such as retinitis pigmentosa.

SYMPTOMS AND SIGNS: Onset of ocular problems is gradual; most complaints include blurred vision, floaters, and scotomata. Occasionally, an acute manifestation occurs with redness, pain, and photophobia. Clinical signs include white blood cells and clumped inflammatory debris in the vitreous, retinal or choroidal infiltrates, retinal or choroidal edema, and cuffing of the retinal blood vessels (either arterioles or venules or both) with inflammatory cells. Other features include optic nerve swelling, retinal hemorrhages or exudates, or anterior segment inflammation with aqueous cells and flare. Conditions such as glaucoma, cataract, choroidal neovascularization, retinal detachment, hypotony, or phthisis bulbi may develop.

ETIOLOGY/EPIDEMIOLOGY: Causes of posterior uveitis include both infectious and noninfectious conditions. Among the former are bacterial, fungal, parasitic, and viral infections. Noninfectious problems include conditions of possible immunologic or allergic origin, those of unknown etiology, and malignancies masquerading as ocular inflammation. Common causes include toxoplasmosis, sarcoidosis, syphilis, ocular histoplasmosis, and idiopathic multifocal choroiditis and panuveitis.

DIAGNOSIS: Posterior uveitis requires an accurate and thorough medical history. Patients with posterior uveitis benefit from examination and investigation by an ophthalmologist because of the high likelihood of detectable associated systemic disease. Exclusion of syphilis, tuberculosis, and sarcoidosis is important. Serologic titers for infectious agents including herpes viruses, toxoplasmosis, toxocariasis, and antibody testing for spirochetal infections are useful. Cultures of blood or intravenous sites may be useful if infectious causes are suspected; chest radiography may be helpful for the detection of sarcoidosis or tuberculosis. Neuroimaging and lumbar puncture are warranted when large cell lymphoma is suspected and when HIV-associated opportunistic infections indicate systemic or central nervous system involvement.

TREATMENT

Standard Therapies: Exclusion or treatment of an infectious or neoplastic cause is imperative before initiating therapy. Corticosteroids are considered the first-line drug of choice when posterior uveitis does not respond to topical steroids but requires either injected or systemic steroid therapy. Immunosuppressive drugs such as cyclosporine, methotrexate, azathioprine, tacrolimus, mycophenolate mofetil, cyclophosphamide, and chlorambucil are adjunctive therapies or corticosteroid-sparing agents for patients whose inflammation may not respond to steroid therapy alone or if side effects (e.g., glaucoma) pose a concern.

Investigational Therapies: Ocular implants, slow-release intravitreous medications, monoclonal antibodies against interleukins, specific antiparasitic and antiviral agents, and oral tolerance therapies are all being explored.

REFERENCES

Pepose JS, Holland GN, Wilhelmus KR. *Ocular infection and immunity.* St. Louis: CV Mosby, 1996.

Rahi AH, Tabbara KF. Laboratory investigations in posterior uveitis. *Int Ophthalmol Clin* 1995;35:59–74.

Sabrosa NA, Pavesio C. Treatment strategies in patients with posterior uveitis. *Int Ophthalmol Clin* 2000;40:153–161.

Wade NK. Diagnostic testing in patients with ocular inflammation. *Int Ophthalmol Clin* 2000;40:37–54.

Whitcup SM, Nussenblatt RB. Immunologic mechanisms of uveitis. New targets for immunomodulation. *Arch Ophthalmol* 1997;115:520–525.

RESOURCES

27, 355, 359, 482

28   Wyburn-Mason Syndrome

Jerry A. Shields, MD

DEFINITION: Wyburn-Mason syndrome is a sporadic, congenital, nonhereditary condition characterized by arteriovenous communications mainly in the retina and the midbrain. It is generally classified as one of the neurooculocutaneous syndromes, or phakomatoses.

SYNONYM: Bonnet-Dechaumme-Blanc syndrome.

DIFFERENTIAL DIAGNOSIS: von Hippel-Lindau syndrome; Sturge-Weber syndrome; Retina and brain cavernous hemangiomatosis; Other conditions associated with retinal and brain vascular malformations.

SYMPTOMS AND SIGNS: Wyburn-Mason syndrome manifests with skin, eye, central nervous system (CNS), and visceral abnormalities. Unlike most other phakomatoses, no major cutaneous changes are associated with Wyburn-Mason syndrome, except for the rare occurrence of small facial angiomas. The classic ocular finding is the arteriovenous communication of the retina called racemose hemangioma. It can be complex and extend into the orbit, mandible, maxilla, pterygoid fossa, and brain. It can also affect the orbit and midbrain without retinal involvement. Patients with retinal involvement are often asymptomatic; those with more extensive lesions can experience severe visual loss. Patients with orbital involvement can present with proptosis, blepharoptosis, displacement of the globe, and oculomotor palsies. CNS lesions also can be asymptomatic or can induce severe symptoms. Although the lesions are congenital, they may not produce symptoms until the second or third decade of life. Spontaneous cerebral or subarachnoid hemorrhages can lead to a variety of neurologic symptoms, including severe headaches, vomiting, and nuchal rigidity. Severe intracranial hemorrhages can cause hemiparesis, hemiplegia, and even death. The bones of the skull frequently can be involved with the vascular malformation. When the mandible or maxilla is affected, excessive bleeding can follow dental work. In rare instances, vascular abnormalities have occurred in other bones, muscle, and kidney.

ETIOLOGY/EPIDEMIOLOGY: The etiology is unknown. It is a developmental abnormality that is characterized by arteriovenous communications. It does not appear to have a hereditary tendency and specific genetic abnormalities are yet to be identified. Estimation of frequency of brain lesions in patients with retinal abnormalities has ranged from 20% to 80%. Estimation of frequency of retinal abnormalities in patients with brain lesions has ranged from 10% to 70%.

DIAGNOSIS: The diagnosis should be suspected in a patient with the aforementioned symptoms and signs. The ocular features should suggest the diagnosis. Imaging studies should be performed (CT or MRI of the skull and the brain to detect potentially dangerous CNS lesions).

TREATMENT

Standard Therapies: In general, no dermatologic or ophthalmic treatment is necessary in patients with racemose hemangiomatosis. The retinal lesions generally require no treatment, but if they produce retinal or vitreal hemorrhage, laser treatment or cryotherapy can be attempted to control the bleeding, and persistent blood in the vitreous can be removed by vitrectomy. The intracranial arteriovenous communications are not usually amenable to surgical resection because of their locations. These patients should be referred to neurosurgeons or radiation oncologists for consideration for embolization techniques or radiotherapy with charged particles, stereotactic radiation, or other methods.

REFERENCES

Archer DM, Deutman A, Ernest JT, et al. Arteriovenous communications of the retina. *Am J Ophthalmol* 1975;75:224–241.

Ebert EM, Boger WP III, Albert DM. Wyburn Mason's syndrome (arteriovenous communication between the retina and midbrain). In: Albert DM, Jakobiec FA, eds. *Principles and practice of ophthalmology.* Philadelphia: WB Saunders, 1994:3317–3320.

Shields JA, Shields CL. Systemic hamartomatoses ("phakomatoses"). In: Shields JA, Shields CL, eds. *Intraocular tumors: a text and atlas.* Philadelphia: WB Saunders, 1992:513–539.

Willinsky RA, Lasjaunais P, Terbrugge K, et al. Multiple cerebral arteriovenous malformations (AVMs). Review of our experience from 203 patients with cerebral vascular lesions. *Neuroradiology* 1990;32:207–210.

Wyburn-Mason R. Arteriovenous aneurysm of midbrain and retina, facial naevi and mental changes. *Brain* 1943;66:163–203.

RESOURCES

284, 355, 368

Pulmonary Disorders

1   Acute Respiratory Distress Syndrome

*Sami I. Said, MD,
and J. Georges Youssef, MD*

DEFINITION: Acute respiratory distress syndrome (ARDS) is a severe injury to most or all of both lungs. The injury results from inflammation, which often starts in one lung, but eventually affects both, involving mainly the pulmonary alveoli and surrounding capillaries. Damaged alveoli collapse or fill up with fluid (lung edema), thus losing their ability to oxygenate the blood and eliminate carbon dioxide.

SYNONYMS: Adult respiratory distress syndrome; Acute lung injury.

DIFFERENTIAL DIAGNOSIS: Cardiogenic (or hydrostatic) pulmonary edema; Extensive, bilateral pneumonia.

SYMPTOMS AND SIGNS: Patients have increasingly severe respiratory distress, associated with decreasing oxygen levels in arterial blood and tissues, stiff lungs, and diffuse densities on chest radiography. Most patients require mechanical ventilation because of respiratory failure. The disorder may also be accompanied or followed by impairment of other vital functions: cardiovascular, renal, hepatic, hematologic, and neurologic, forming the multiorgan dysfunction syndrome, a frequent cause of death. The mortality rate is approximately 40%–50%.

ETIOLOGY/EPIDEMIOLOGY: Risk factors for developing acute respiratory distress syndrome include systemic bacterial infection (sepsis), extensive trauma, severe burns, aspiration of gastric contents, acute pancreatitis, and multiple emergency blood transfusions. The disorder may also follow the inhalation of toxic fumes, or gases such as chlorine, phosgene, and nitrogen dioxide. The incidence of acute respiratory distress syndrome may be as low as 1.5 but is no higher than 4.8 per 100,000 population. Men and women appear to be equally affected.

DIAGNOSIS: The diagnosis is based on the presence of respiratory distress in the setting of sepsis, trauma, or other predisposing conditions, and in the absence of left ventricular failure or other causes of increased pulmonary microvascular pressure. The latter is best ascertained by direct measurement of pulmonary artery wedge pressure during right heart catheterization.

TREATMENT
Standard Therapies: Standard therapy consists of mechanical ventilatory support, supplemental oxygen, and the use of positive end-expiratory pressure to promote alveolar patency and help reduce inspired oxygen concentrations. Ventilation at large tidal volumes can accentuate lung injury; therefore, tidal volumes below those traditionally employed are recommended. Failure of other organ systems calls for measures directed to support those organs.

Investigational Therapies: Recombinant human activated protein C (Xigris) is being investigated, as is the neuropeptide vasoactive intestinal peptide.

REFERENCES
Beal AL, Cerra FB. Multiple organ failure syndrome in the 1990s: systemic inflammatory response and organ dysfunction. *JAMA* 1994;271:226–233.
Bernard GR. Efficacy and safety of recombinant human activated protein C for severe sepsis. *N Engl J Med* 2000;344:699–709.
Said SI, Dickman KG. Pathways of inflammation and cell death in the lung: modulation by vasoactive intestinal peptide. *Reg Pept* 2000;93:21–29.
Tobin MJ. Culmination of an era in research on the acute respiratory distress syndrome. *N Engl J Med* 2000;342:1360–1361.
Villar J, Slutsky AS. The incidence of the adult respiratory distress syndrome. *Am Rev Respir Dis* 1989;140:814–816.
Ware LB, Marthay MA. The acute respiratory distress syndrome. *N Engl J Med* 2000;342:1334–1349.

RESOURCES
40, 51, 52

2   Alpha 1-Antitrypsin Deficiency

James K. Stoller, MD

DEFINITION: Alpha 1-antitrypsin (A1AT) deficiency is characterized by low levels of A1AT in the blood, which confers risk for developing early-onset emphysema and/or bronchiectasis and also may be associated with chronic liver disease, panniculitis, and vasculitis.

SYNONYMS: Alpha 1-antiprotease deficiency; Genetic emphysema; Alpha one.

DIFFERENTIAL DIAGNOSIS: Centriacinar (smoking-related) emphysema; Marfan syndrome; Hypocomplementemic urticarial vasculitis, Ehlers-Danlos syndrome; Intravenous ritalin abuse; Alpha 1-antichymotrypsin deficiency; Salla disease; Asthma; Chronic bronchitis; Cystic fibrosis; Common variable hypogammaglobulinemia; Ciliary dysmotility disorders; Wilson disease; Chronic viral hepatitis; Hemochromatosis; Chronic alcohol use; All causes of prolonged neonatal hepatitis; All causes of lobular panniculitis.

SYMPTOMS AND SIGNS: The most frequent clinical consequence is emphysema, classically of a panacinar type. Affected individuals most frequently present with dyspnea. They commonly have wheezing, phlegm production, and cough. Features that should arouse clinical suspicion include emphysema in a never or minimal smoker, emphysema with predominant hyperlucency at the lung bases on the chest radiograph, bronchiectasis, the co-occurrence in an individual or family of unexplained chronic liver and lung disease, or painful skin nodules suggesting panniculitis. Associated liver disease is less common, and may manifest as childhood hepatitis or adult-onset cirrhosis. Some individuals with severely decreased levels of A1AT do not develop clinical manifestations.

ETIOLOGY/EPIDEMIOLOGY: A1AT deficiency is an autosomal-codominant disease with approximately 100 abnormal alleles identified. Severe deficiency occurs with approximately equal frequency in men and women, although male sex has been characterized as a risk factor for more severe airflow obstruction and for liver disease. The normal allele is M, and the most common deficient phenotype associated with lung disease is the Z homozygote, PI*ZZ. Population screening studies suggest that the frequency of severe deficient phenotypes is 1 in 1,600 in Sweden and 1 in 3,500 to 1 in 5,000 in North America. The Z allele and severe A1AT deficiency are uncommon in non-caucasian groups, although other less common deficient alleles have been described in Asian populations (M_{Siyama}).

DIAGNOSIS: The diagnosis is based on measurement of a serum level of A1AT and, when confirmatory testing or pedigree analysis is needed, by determination of the phenotype. Testing by nephelometry is commonly used to determine serum levels. Phenotype determination is most commonly accomplished by isoelectric focusing.

TREATMENT

Standard Therapies: For patients with emphysema, therapy consists of standard treatment for chronic obstructive pulmonary disease (bronchodilators, supplemental oxygen if indicated, consideration of inhaled corticosteroids, pulmonary rehabilitation, smoking cessation, and routine vaccinations). Specific therapy for A1AT deficiency–related lung disease is augmentation therapy, which consists of weekly infusion of purified pooled human plasma-derived A1AT. Patients with cirrhosis should receive standard therapy for advanced liver disease. Liver transplantation corrects A1AT deficiency and has been reserved for individuals with end-stage liver disease. Intravenous augmentation therapy appears to be the most effective therapy for panniculitis.

Investigational Therapies: Augmentation therapy with different products and by different routes of administration is being investigated, as is gene therapy. Other approaches are evaluating agents to encourage secretion of the abnormal A1AT protein from the hepatocyte.

REFERENCES

Alpha 1-antitrypsin Deficiency Registry Study Group. Survival and FEV1 decline in individuals with severe deficiency of alpha 1-antitrypsin. *Am J Respir Crit Care Med* 1998;158: 49–59.

Dirksen A, Dijkman JK, Madsen F, et al. A randomized clinical trial of alpha 1-antitrypsin augmentation therapy. *Am J Respir Crit Care Med* 1999;160:1468–1472.

Minai OA, Stoller JK. Therapy for alpha 1-antitrypsin deficiency: pharmacology and clinical recommendations. *Biodrugs* 2000;13:135–147.

Stoller JK. Clinical features and natural history of severe alpha 1-antitrypsin deficiency. *Chest* 1997;111(suppl):123–128.

RESOURCES

16, 17, 18, 40

3   Alveolar Capillary Dysplasia

Robin H. Steinhorn, MD

DEFINITION: Alveolar capillary dysplasia (ACD) is a lethal developmental anomaly of the pulmonary vasculature. It is generally described as the failure of formation of the normal air-blood diffusion barrier in the newborn lung. Alveolar capillary dysplasia is usually associated with "misalignment" of the pulmonary veins.

SYNONYM: Misalignment of pulmonary veins.

DIFFERENTIAL DIAGNOSIS: Idiopathic persistent pulmonary hypertension of the newborn; Surfactant protein B deficiency.

SYMPTOMS AND SIGNS: Alveolar capillary dysplasia is a pulmonary disease that presents in early infancy. Infants generally become critically ill in the first days of life with severe hypoxemia and pulmonary hypertension, although presentation has been reported at age 6 weeks in an infant with a patchy distribution of disease. Most patients have other associated anomalies of the cardiovascular, gastrointestinal, urogenital, or musculoskeletal systems. The initial presentation is identical to severe idiopathic pulmonary hypertension of the newborn; however, infants with ACD do not respond, or respond only transiently, to therapies that are usually effective in reversing this condition.

ETIOLOGY/EPIDEMIOLOGY: Fewer than 50 cases of ACD have been reported. No sex predilection has been identified. Although the cause is unknown, 6 cases have been reported in siblings, indicating that in some cases this may be a familial disorder with autosomal-recessive inheritance.

DIAGNOSIS: The diagnosis should be considered in infants who present with severe hypoxemia and idiopathic pulmonary hypertension and who do not respond as expected after 7–10 days of neonatal intensive care treatment. The initial chest radiograph is usually normal. If a cardiac catheterization is performed, the capillary blush phase may be absent. The diagnosis can only be confirmed by lung biopsy or autopsy. Pathologic features include a paucity of alveolar capillaries, widened alveolar septae, and increased muscularization of pulmonary arterioles. Pulmonary veins in the bronchovascular bundle are usually malpositioned, but this finding is not required for the diagnosis. A focal distribution of disease has been described, so examining multiple lung sections is necessary if ACD is suspected.

TREATMENT

Standard Therapies: Standard therapies include mechanical ventilation, high concentrations of inspired oxygen, inhalational nitric oxide, and extracorporeal membrane oxygenation support. These therapies prolong life by days to weeks, but have not led to long-term survival. The longest reported survival is to age 2 months with the use of extracorporeal membrane support followed by inhaled nitric oxide.

Investigational Therapies: Theoretically, ACD could be treated by lung transplantation. Successful transplantation has not yet occurred, and donor availability limits its use for neonatal diseases.

REFERENCES

Boggs S, Harris MC, Hoffman DJ, et al. Misalignment of pulmonary veins with alveolar capillary dysplasia: affected siblings and variable phenotypic expression. *J Pediatr* 1994;124: 125–128.

Cullinane C, Cox PN, Silver MM. Persistent pulmonary hypertension of the newborn due to alveolar capillary dysplasia. *Pediatr Pathol* 1992;12:499–514.

Garola RE, Thibeault DW. Alveolar capillary dysplasia, with and without misalignment of pulmonary veins: an association of congenital anomalies. *Am J Perinatol* 1998;15:103–107.

Steinhorn RH, Cox PN, Fineman JR, et al. Inhaled nitric oxide enhances oxygenation but not survival in infants with alveolar capillary dysplasia. *J Pediatr* 1997;130:417–422.

RESOURCE

21

4 Idiopathic Congenital Central Hypoventilation Syndrome

Debra E. Weese-Mayer, MD, and Jean M. Silvestri, MD

DEFINITION: Idiopathic congenital central hypoventilation syndrome (CCHS) is characterized by adequate ventilation while awake but alveolar hypoventilation with normal respiratory rates and shallow breathing during sleep. More severely affected children hypoventilate both while awake and while asleep.

DIFFERENTIAL DIAGNOSIS: Congenital myopathy; Myasthenia gravis; Altered airway or intrathoracic anatomy; Diaphragm dysfunction; Congenital cardiac disease; Structural hindbrain or brainstem abnormality; Möbius syndrome; Leigh disease; Pyruvate dehydrogenase deficiency; Discrete carnitine deficiency.

SYMPTOMS AND SIGNS: Patients typically present in the newborn period with duskiness or cyanosis on falling asleep and decreasing arterial blood oxyhemoglobin saturation with increasing carbon dioxide partial pressure, yet no increase in depth or rate of breathing on awakening. Affected children also have absent or negligible ventilatory sensitivity to hypercarbia and hypoxemia during sleep and wakefulness. Associated conditions include Hirschsprung disease, tumors of neural crest origin, lack of heart rate variability with prolonged sinus pauses, constipation, esophageal dysmotility, altered perception of pain, diminished pupillary light response and altered lacrimation, altered perception of anxiety, extreme breath-holding spells, absent perception of dyspnea and asphyxia, altered temperature regulation, and sporadic profuse sweating. During exercise, affected children may be at risk for hypercarbia and hypoxemia.

ETIOLOGY/EPIDEMIOLOGY: Evidence for a genetic basis for CCHS is growing. It is believed that CCHS is the most severe manifestation of a general autonomic nervous system (ANS) dysfunction, with a family pattern consistent with mendelian transmission. A specific candidate genetic loci for CCHS and ANS dysfunction has not yet been identified.

DIAGNOSIS: The initial evaluation should include chest radiography, diaphragm fluoroscopy, bronchoscopy, electrocardiography, Holter recording, echocardiography, MRI of the brain/brainstem, and a detailed neurologic evaluation that may require a muscle biopsy. Serum and urinary carnitine levels should be assessed to rule out an inborn error in fatty acid metabolism. A detailed ophthalmologic evaluation should be performed to assess pupillary reactivity and optic disc anatomy. A rectal biopsy should be considered in the event of abdominal distention and delayed defecation to assess for Hirschsprung disease. Infants should undergo detailed recording in a respiratory physiology laboratory to evaluate spontaneous breathing during sleep and wakefulness.

TREATMENT

Standard Therapies: As soon as the diagnosis is confirmed, a pediatric otolaryngologist should perform a tracheostomy. Arrangement for discharge to home with the primary mechanical ventilator (and back-up ventilator) should be completed, and requests for 24-hour per day care with highly trained registered nurses, a pulse oximeter, and an end-tidal carbon dioxide monitor should be made to optimize management. Typically, the infant who requires ventilatory support 24 hours a day will have a tracheostomy and use a home mechanical ventilator in the pressure-plateau mode. As the infant becomes ambulatory, diaphragm pacing by phrenic nerve stimulation should be considered to allow for increased mobility and improved quality of life. Children who consistently require ventilatory support during sleep only can be considered as candidates for noninvasive ventilation with either bilevel positive airway pressure or a negative pressure ventilator.

REFERENCES

Marazita MM, Maher BS, Cooper ME, et al. Genetic segregation analysis of autonomic nervous system dysfunction in families of probands with congenital central hypoventilation syndrome. *Am J Med Genet* 2001 (in press).

Weese-Mayer DE, Shannon DC, Keens TG, et al. American Thoracic Society statement on the diagnosis and management of idiopathic congenital central hypoventilation syndrome. *Am J Respir Crit Care Med* 1999;160:368–373.

Weese-Mayer DE, Silvestri JM, Huffman AD, et al. Case/control family study of ANS dysfunction in idiopathic congenital central hypoventilation syndrome. *Am J Med Genet* 2001 (in press).

Weese-Mayer DE, Silvestri JM, Kenny AS, et al. Diaphragm pacing with a quadripolar phrenic nerve electrode: an international study. *PACE* 1996;19:1311–1319.

Weese-Mayer DE, Silvestri JM, Menzies LJ, et al. Congenital central hypoventilation syndrome: diagnosis, management, and long-term outcome in thirty-two children. *J Pediatr* 1992; 120:381–387.

RESOURCE

87

5   Churg-Strauss Syndrome

John H. Stone, MD, MPH

DEFINITION: Churg-Strauss syndrome (CSS) is a form of systemic vasculitis associated with atopic phenomena (particularly asthma and rhinitis), peripheral and tissue eosinophilia, extravascular granulomatous inflammation, and necrotizing vasculitis.

SYNONYMS: Allergic angiitis and granulomatosis; Allergic granulomatosis and angiitis; Allergic granulomatosis; Eosinophilic granulomatous vasculitis; Churg-Strauss vasculitis.

DIFFERENTIAL DIAGNOSIS: Hypereosinophil syndrome; Chronic eosinophilic pneumonia; Eosinophilic gastroenteritis; Löffler syndrome; Eosinophilic leukemia; Allergic bronchopulmonary aspergillosis; Polyarteritis nodosa; Microscopic polyangiitis; Wegener granulomatosis; Henoch-Schönlein purpura; Cryoglobulinemic vasculitis.

SYMPTOMS AND SIGNS: Three phases are described: (a) prodromal phase, characterized by the presence of allergic disease (typically asthma or allergic rhinitis), which may last from months to many years; (b) eosinophilia/tissue infiltration phase, in which remarkably high peripheral eosinophilia may occur and tissue infiltration by eosinophils is observed in the lung, gastrointestinal tract, and other tissues; and (c) vasculitic phase, in which systemic vasculitis affects a wide range of organs (Insert Figs. 56 and 57). Symptoms and signs include the following: fatigue, fever, weight loss, allergic rhinitis, nasal polyps, serous otitis media with conductive hearing loss, nonerosive sinusitis, fleeting pulmonary infiltrates, congestive heart failure, glomerulonephritis, mesenteric vasculitis with "intestinal angina" (postprandial abdominal pain) and gastrointestinal hemorrhage, palpable purpura, cutaneous ulcerations, nodules over the elbows that may mimic rheumatoid nodules, migratory inflammatory arthritis, and vasculitic neuropathy of the peripheral nerves, leading classically to mononeuritis multiplex. Peripheral nerve involvement occurs in approximately 75% of patients.

ETIOLOGY/EPIDEMIOLOGY: Etiology is unknown. The condition is hypothesized to result from interactions between a microbial pathogen(s) and an individual with the proper genetic risk factors and (perhaps) other environmental exposures. The gender distribution is approximately equal, with perhaps a slight male predominance. It is most common among middle-aged individuals, but cases are reported in all age groups. The disease may occur in all races, but appears to be more common among caucasians in Western countries.

DIAGNOSIS: Criteria for the classification of CSS include: (a) asthma; (b) eosinophilia; (c) mononeuropathy or polyneuropathy; (d) nonfixed pulmonary infiltrates; (e) abnormality of the paranasal sinuses; and (f) extravascular eosinophils. The presence of four or more of these criteria distinguishes CSS from other forms of vasculitis with a high degree of sensitivity and specificity. In separating the disorder from other eosinophilic conditions, the critical step in diagnosis is the demonstration of vasculitis (often associated with eosinophilic infiltration in the region of inflammation) in an involved organ.

TREATMENT
Standard Therapies: Many patients achieve satisfactory treatment responses with corticosteroids alone; therefore, monotherapy is often a reasonable first approach. However, patients with evidence of rapidly progressive glomerulonephritis, symptoms of mononeuritis multiplex, or other potentially devastating disease complications should be treated promptly with both cyclophosphamide and corticosteroids. The use of interferon-α appears promising, but further studies are required.

REFERENCES
Churg J, Strauss L. Allergic granulomatosis, allergic angiitis, and periarteritis nodosa. *Am J Pathol* 1951;27:277–301.

Guillevin L, Cohen P, Gayraud M, et al. Churg-Strauss syndrome: clinical study and long-term follow-up of 96 patients. *Medicine* 1999;78:26–37.

Lanham J, Elkon K, Pusey C, et al. Systemic vasculitis with asthma and eosinophilia: a clinical approach to the Churg-Strauss syndrome. *Medicine* 1984;63:65–81.

Masi A, Hunder G, Lie J, et al. The American College of Rheumatology 1990 criteria for the classification of Churg-Strauss syndrome (allergic granulomatosis and angiitis). *Arthritis Rheum* 1990;33:1094–1100.

Stirling R, Chung K. Leukotriene antagonists and Churg-Strauss syndrome: the smoking gun? *Thorax* 1999;54:865–866.

RESOURCES
40, 107, 357, 359

6 Primary Ciliary Dyskinesia

Lucia Bartoloni, MD

DEFINITION: Primary ciliary dyskinesia (PCD) is a multisystemic disorder of variable severity caused by dysmotility or complete immotility of cilia and flagella. Lack of proper ciliary and flagellar movement predisposes to recurrent upper respiratory tract infections (leading to bronchiectasis) and male subfertility. Kartagener syndrome is a subgroup of PCD in which patients show anomalies of lateralization ranging from dextrocardia to situs inversus totalis.

SYNONYMS: Immotile cilia syndrome; Kartagener syndrome.

DIFFERENTIAL DIAGNOSIS: Cystic fibrosis; Situs inversus not due to ciliary immotility.

SYMPTOMS AND SIGNS: Symptoms usually begin in the first decade as persistent rhinitis and sinusitis and progress as bronchitis and lung infections that lead to bronchiectasis, irreversible enlargements of bronchi, and severe lung damage. The pace of progression is variable. During infancy, otitis is frequently reported, which may resolve in adult life. Sperm are often immotile, leading to male subfertility. Approximately two thirds of patients experience chronic headaches. In Kartagener syndrome, organ orientation is a random rather than a predetermined event, because monozygotic twins occur with situs inversus in one twin and normal visceral orientation in the other.

ETIOLOGY/EPIDEMIOLOGY: PCD is a genetically heterogeneous disorder usually inherited in an autosomal-recessive manner. A few cases of dominant and X-linked inheritance are described. The incidence is estimated at 1 in 20,000 to 30,000. All ethnic groups are affected. Airway epithelia are covered by numerous short cilia, whereas the spermatozoon has a single long flagellum. The ultrastructure of cilia and flagella is similar. Both have a central circular structure, called an axoneme, which is formed by nine peripheral doublets of microtubules, plus two central microtubules. The doublets are connected to each other and with the central pair by different proteins. The more than 250 different polypeptides forming the axoneme create and coordinate the beating of cilia and flagella. A defect in any one of these proteins may alter the proper movement of the cilium. A different gene encodes for each of these proteins, which underlies the high genetic heterogeneity of PCD. Several axonemal proteins have been described.

DIAGNOSIS: The diagnosis should be suspected based on the presence of recurrent rhinitis, sinusitis, or bronchitis. The presence of situs inversus, seen by radiography, and the immotility of sperm may support the diagnosis of PCD/Kartagener syndrome. Immotility of the respiratory cilia makes the diagnosis. Ciliary motility is determined by (a) saccharine test, (b) nasal brush, and (c) bronchial epithelium biopsy.

TREATMENT

Standard Therapies: Treatment is generally palliative. For control of respiratory tract infections, antibiotics are tailored to individual patients. Tubes are often inserted in children's ears to diminish the frequency of otitis. Physiotherapy and/or exercise are good prophylaxis because they help to clear the bronchi of mucus, thereby reducing the occurrence of infections. If the lungs are severely damaged, surgical removal of one or more lobes might be needed. Lung transplantation may become necessary.

REFERENCES

Afzelius BA, Mossberg B. Immotile-cilia syndrome (primary ciliary dyskinesia), including Kartagener syndrome. In: Scriver CR, Beaudet AL, Sly WS, et al., eds. *The metabolic and molecular bases of inherited disease,* 7th ed. New York: McGraw-Hill, 1995:3943–3954.

Blouin J-L, Meeks M, Radhakrishna U, et al. Primary ciliary dyskinesia: a genome-wide linkage analysis reveals extensive locus heterogeneity. *Eur J Hum Genet* 2000;8:109–118.

Narayan D, Krishnan SN, Upender M, et al. Unusual inheritance of primary ciliary dyskinesia (Kartagener's syndrome). *J Med Genet* 1994;31:493–496.

Noone PG, Bali D, Carson JL, et al. Discordant organ laterality in monozygotic twins with primary ciliary dyskinesia. *Am J Med Genet* 1999;82:155–160.

Olbrich H, Haffner K, Kispert A, et al. Mutations in *DNAH5* cause primary ciliary dyskinesia and randomization of left-right asymmetry. *Nat Genet* 2002;30:143–144.

Pennarun G, Escudier E, Chapelin C, et al. Loss-of-function mutations in a human gene related to *Chlamydomonas reinhardtii* dynein IC78 result in primary ciliary dyskinesia. *Am J Hum Genet* 1999;65:1508–1519.

RESOURCES

40, 106

7   Recurrent Respiratory Papillomatosis

*Craig S. Derkay, MD,
and Ryan P. Hester, MD*

DEFINITION: Recurrent respiratory papillomatosis (RRP) is the most common benign neoplasm of the larynx in children. It is most often associated with exophytic lesions of the larynx, but has the tendency to spread and recur throughout the respiratory tract.

SYNONYMS: Laryngeal papilloma; Juvenile-onset respiratory papilloma.

DIFFERENTIAL DIAGNOSIS: Squamous cell carcinoma; Vocal nodules and polyps; Asthma; Croup.

SYMPTOMS AND SIGNS: The disorder may occur in either childhood or adulthood with two distinct forms generally recognized: an aggressive juvenile form and a less aggressive adult form. The aggressive form, although more prevalent in children, can also occur in adults. Most symptoms are related to airway obstruction resulting in a clinical triad of progressive hoarseness, stridor, and respiratory distress. Some degree of dysphonia is often the initial symptom, followed by inspiratory stridor, which becomes biphasic with progression of disease. Other possible presenting symptoms include chronic cough, recurrent pneumonia, failure to thrive, dyspnea, dysphagia, and acute life-threatening events. Disease course and severity are highly variable, with some patients experiencing spontaneous remission and others suffering from aggressive papillomatous growth, requiring multiple surgical procedures over many years. The latter group is at risk for extralaryngeal spread and malignant transformation.

ETIOLOGY/EPIDEMIOLOGY: The disorder is of viral etiology, induced by human papillomavirus (HPV) types 6 and 11. These are the same HPV types most commonly identified in genital warts, and there is a clear association between maternal cervical HPV infection and childhood-onset RRP. Transmission is believed to be through direct contact in the birth canal. Neonatal papillomatosis has occurred, suggesting that, in at least some cases, development of disease may occur *in utero*. Circumstantial evidence suggests that adult-onset disease is the result of oral-genital contact, although it is also possible that it reflects activation of virus present since birth. The disorder may affect people of any age, although onset does appear to be bimodal in distribution. Childhood-onset RRP is most often diagnosed between 2 and 4 years of age and the adult-onset variety peaks between the ages of 20 and 40 years. Except for a slight male predilection in adult-onset RRP, gender distribution is comparable. The incidence rate is estimated at 4.3 per 100,000 children and 1.8 per 100,000 adults in the United States.

DIAGNOSIS: The preoperative diagnosis of RRP is best made with a flexible fiberoptic nasopharyngoscope facilitating a thorough examination of the aerodigestive tract and biopsy of any indeterminate lesions. Recurrence of these lesions resulting in stridor and a voice change heralds the need for additional surgical management.

TREATMENT

Standard Therapies: No single modality has proven consistently effective in eradication of RRP. The current standard of care is surgical therapy with the goal of complete removal of papillomas and preservation of normal structures. This is often not possible, and thus the goal may be subtotal removal with the clearing of the airway. As many as 10% of patients ultimately require some form of adjuvant therapy. The most commonly recommended is systemic interferon-α. Other adjuvants in use include methotrexate, ribavarin, acyclovir, isotretinoin, indole-3-carbinol, and intralesional injections of cidofovir. Optimal management of gastroesophageal reflux disease and avoidance of tracheostomy unless absolutely necessary may contribute to decreased clinical severity as well as decreased incidence of distal tracheal spread.

REFERENCES

Armstrong LR, Derkay CS, Reeves WC. Initial results from the National Registry for Juvenile-Onset Recurrent Respiratory Papillomatosis. *Arch Otolaryngol Head Neck Surg* 1995;121: 1386–1391.

Derkay CS. Task force on recurrent respiratory papillomas. *Arch Otolaryngol Head Neck Surg* 1999;125:743–748.

Shah K, Kashima H, Polk BF, et al. Rarity of caesarean delivery in cases of juvenile-onset respiratory papillomatosis. *Obstet Gynecol* 1986;68:795–799.

Silver RD, et al. Diagnosis and management of pulmonary metastasis from recurrent respiratory papillomatosis. *Arch Otolaryngol Head Neck Surg* (in press).

RESOURCES

38, 40, 413

8 Pulmonary Alveolar Proteinosis

Josh W. McDonald, MD

DEFINITION: Pulmonary alveolar proteinosis (PAP) is an uncommon lung injury pattern characterized by dyspnea, radiographic infiltrates, and the biopsy finding of a granular precipitate within alveolar spaces.

SYNONYMS: Alveolar lipoproteinosis; Phospholipoproteinosis.

DIFFERENTIAL DIAGNOSIS: Infectious pneumonia; Pulmonary edema; Chronic interstitial lung disease; Pneumoconioses.

SYMPTOMS AND SIGNS: Patients typically present with slowly progressive dyspnea, accompanied by cough, weight loss, and sometimes fever. Fatigue and chest pain may also occur. A few patients are asymptomatic. The cough is usually dry but may produce fragments of gelatinous sputum. Because the symptoms mimic those of infectious pneumonia, patients with PAP are often placed on antibiotics early in their clinical course. Radiographically, bilateral diffuse airspace opacities are seen, characterized by fine nodular infiltrates most prominent in the hilar regions. This appearance typically resembles pulmonary edema. Pulmonary function tests show moderate to marked hypoxemia and mild restrictive changes.

ETIOLOGY/EPIDEMIOLOGY: The disorder occurs more often in males (male:female ratio is approximately 2:1 to 4:1), and at widely varying ages, ranging from newborns to the elderly, but most commonly in individuals aged 20–50 years. Familial occurrence is rare. PAP is a nonspecific injury pattern, and has been reported in a variety of clinical settings and industrial exposures, including toxic gas inhalation, aluminum, silica, and other dust exposures, gastroesophageal reflux, underlying malignancy (especially leukemia or lymphoma), and opportunistic infection. In many patients, the pattern also occurs as an isolated finding, without an associated exposure or clinical condition. PAP may originate from a defect in surfactant generation or metabolism, or a defect in alveolar macrophage function, leading to accumulation and impaired clearance of intraalveolar metabolic products such as surfactant. Altered immunity may play a role in the disorder.

DIAGNOSIS: The diagnosis may be suggested by the clinical and radiographic picture, and by a cloudy appearance in cytologic preparations such as bronchoalveolar lavage, but lung biopsy is required for an unequivocal diagnosis. Microscopically, the biopsy findings differ from infectious pneumonia in that the intraalveolar precipitate is granular and relatively acellular, rather than predominantly neutrophilic as in many bacterial infections. Typically, the interstitial tissues (alveolar septa) are unremarkable or show only mild inflammation and thickening. The intraalveolar precipitate may be associated with scattered cholesterol clefts, foamy macrophages, and reactive alveolar pneumonocytes.

TREATMENT

Standard Therapies: The treatment of choice is pulmonary lavage. This may need to be repeated due to disease recurrence. Steroid therapy is not significantly helpful and may actually predispose to infections. Modification of occupational exposures is advisable where a causal relationship to a toxic exposure is documented. If infection (bacterial, viral, or fungal) complicates the disorder, appropriate cultures, special stains, and/or treatment should be instituted.

Investigational Therapies: Granulocyte-macrophage colony-stimulating factor is being investigated as a potential treatment.

REFERENCES

Blanc PD, Golden JA. Unusual occupationally related disorders of the lung: case reports and a literature review. *Occup Med State Art Rev* 1992;7:413–415.

Dail DH. Metabolic and other disorders. In: Dail DH, Hammar SP, eds. *Pulmonary pathology,* 2nd ed. New York: Springer-Verlag, 1994:745–751.

Katzenstein AA. *Katzenstein and Askin's surgical pathology of nonneoplastic lung disease,* 3rd ed. Philadelphia: WB Saunders, 1997:393–395.

RESOURCES

40, 357

9   Primary Pulmonary Hypertension

Michael D. McGoon, MD

DEFINITION: Pulmonary hypertension (PH) refers to any condition in which systolic pulmonary artery (PA) pressure exceeds 35 mm Hg or mean PA pressure exceeds 25 mm Hg. The disorder can cause symptoms of dyspnea, angina, syncope, and right ventricular failure. Patients with primary pulmonary hypertension (PPH) do not have a specific identifiable cause for the hemodynamic abnormality.

SYNONYMS: Idiopathic PH; PH of unknown etiology; Idiopathic pulmonary vascular disease.

DIFFERENTIAL DIAGNOSIS: Secondary pulmonary hypertension (SPH).

SYMPTOMS AND SIGNS: Nearly 100% of adult patients present with dyspnea, and one third have symptoms of angina or syncope. Syncope tends to be more common in children. Chronic PH leads to right ventricular (RV) failure, with symptoms of leg edema, anorexia due to gut edema, abdominal pain, and distention due to hepatic congestion and ascites. PH can be suspected on physical examination by a loud (i.e., audible at the apex) pulmonic closure component of the second heart sound, an RV (left parasternal) lift, a holosystolic murmur that increases in intensity during inspiration, an RV S4 gallop, and a diastolic murmur of pulmonary regurgitation. When RV failure develops, findings include jugular venous distention, an RV S3 gallop, leg edema, pulsatile hepatomegaly, and ascites.

ETIOLOGY/EPIDEMIOLOGY: PPH has an incidence of approximately 2 per million population, resulting in 500–800 new cases in the United States annually. Women outnumber men by approximately 2:1; mean age is 35–40 years. Most cases appear to be random. Approximately 6% of cases occur in families and have an autosomal-dominant pattern of inheritance; a PPH gene has been identified.

DIAGNOSIS: First, the presence of PH needs to be confirmed and then the diagnoses of SPH must be excluded. After history and physical examination, assessment leading to a diagnosis of PPH includes chest radiography showing RV enlargement, large central pulmonary arteries, and clear peripheral lung fields; electrocardiogram consistent with RV hypertrophy and right atrial enlargement; Doppler echocardiogram showing an elevated RV systolic pressure, RV enlargement and hypocontractility, tricuspid regurgitation, and a flattened interventricular septum producing a compressed D-shaped left ventricle; ventilation/perfusion lung scintigraphy and/or spiral or electron beam CT indicating low probability of chronic pulmonary embolism; complete spirometry excluding obstructive or restrictive pulmonary disease; antinuclear antibody and HIV serology to assess possible associated disease; and right heart hemodynamic catheterization to confirm and quantify pulmonary pressure and assess response to vasodilators.

TREATMENT

Standard Therapies: For patients who exhibit a substantial reduction (i.e., >10 mm Hg) of mean PA pressure in response to an acute vasodilator study with intravenous epoprostenol (prostacyclin) or inhaled nitric oxide, a trial of treatment with nifedipine, amlodipine, or diltiazem is warranted. Otherwise, standard therapy is oral bosentan or continuous infusion of epoprostenol using an indwelling central catheter and portable infusion pump. Either treatment is best initiated and followed at specialized referral centers. Adjunctive therapy includes anticoagulation with warfarin, diuresis, digoxin, and oxygen supplementation. Appropriately selected patients may be candidates for lung or heart-lung transplantation.

Investigational Therapies: Recent investigational treatment includes open-label subcutaneous continuous infusion of Uniprost, an epoprostenol analogue that is under review by the FDA. Investigations of selective endothelin-A receptor blockers are in the initial stages.

REFERENCES
Barst R J, Rubin LJ, et al. A comparison of continuous intravenous epoprostenol (prostacyclin) with conventional therapy for primary pulmonary hypertension. *N Engl J Med* 1996;334: 296–301.

Lilienfeld DE, Rubin LJ. Mortality from primary pulmonary hypertension in the United States, 1979–1996. *Chest* 2000;117: 796–800.

McGoon MD. Pulmonary hypertension. In: Murphy JG, ed. *Mayo Clinic cardiology review*. Philadelphia: Lippincott Williams & Wilkins, 2000.

Rich S, Rubin LJ, et al. Anorexigens and pulmonary hypertension in the United States: results from the Surveillance of North American Pulmonary Hypertension. *Chest* 2000;117:870–874.

Rubin LJ. Primary pulmonary hypertension. *N Engl J Med* 1997; 336:111–117.

RESOURCES
35, 40, 357, 409

Renal Disorders

1 | Alport Syndrome

*Vimal Chadha, MD,
and Bradley A. Warady, MD*

DEFINITION: Alport syndrome is an inherited renal disorder characterized by progressive hematuric nephritis.

SYNONYMS: Hereditary nephritis; Nephritis and nerve deafness.

DIFFERENTIAL DIAGNOSIS: IgA nephropathy; Benign familial hematuria.

SYMPTOMS AND SIGNS: Male patients usually have severe renal disease and females are either asymptomatic carriers or develop mild disease consistent with an X-linked inheritance pattern that characterizes the majority of patients. The cardinal clinical feature is hematuria, which is persistent and occurs early in life in affected males, but may be intermittent and occur late in affected females. Progressive proteinuria typically develops and can lead to nephrotic syndrome in approximately 40% of cases. End-stage renal disease (ESRD) develops in virtually all affected males. Patients with autosomal-dominant inheritance appear to exhibit a slower rate of progression to ESRD than most patients with X-linked Alport syndrome. Approximately 50% of patients have progressive, bilateral, high-frequency sensorineural hearing loss. The progression of hearing loss roughly parallels that of renal impairment. In some families, hematuric nephritis progresses to ESRD without hearing loss. The most common ocular lesion is the pigmentary alteration of the retina, characterized by perimacular yellowish flecks. Anterior lenticonus, leiomyomatosis, and platelet abnormalities may also occur.

ETIOLOGY/EPIDEMIOLOGY: Alport syndrome results from mutations of type IV collagen, which is the major collagenous constituent of basement membranes. The exact pathophysiology and factors responsible for progressive renal disease are unclear. Inheritance is mostly X-linked (85%); a small minority of patients exhibit an autosomal-dominant pattern and the rest are autosomal recessive. Alport syndrome is the cause of approximately 0.6%–2.3% of cases of ESRD. There is no geographic clustering, and all ethnic groups are affected. The gene frequency is estimated to be 1 per 5,000 to 1 per 10,000 population.

DIAGNOSIS: Alport syndrome should be suspected in all patients with glomerular hematuria and normal complement levels. The most rapid method of confirming the diagnosis is by performing a renal biopsy. Diffuse thickening and lamellation of the glomerular basement membrane is the pathognomonic ultrastructural finding. Immunohistochemistry may be useful in confirming the diagnosis in equivocal renal biopsies. Immunohistochemistry of a skin biopsy can also confirm the diagnosis in males with X-linked inheritance. Presymptomatic and prenatal diagnosis is possible by linkage analysis or by direct gene studies in previously tested families.

TREATMENT

Standard Therapies: Hearing aids are required for deafness and corrective surgery for visual problems. Genetic counseling is indicated for patients and their families. No treatment prevents the progression of renal failure. Dialysis and/or transplantation may be initiated when ESRD develops. Selection of a living related donor for transplantation should be made carefully, because some female carriers remain asymptomatic.

Investigational Therapies: Gene therapy is promising. Cyclosporine therapy or angiotensin-converting enzyme inhibition may slow the rate of progression of renal failure.

REFERENCES

Callis L, Vila A, Carrera M, et al. Long-term effects of cyclosporin A in Alport's syndrome. *Kidney Int* 1999;55:1051–1056.

Kashtan CE. Alport's syndromes: phenotypic heterogeneity of progressive hereditary nephritis. *Pediatr Nephrol* 2000;14: 502–512.

Proesmans W, Knockaert H, Trouet D. Enalapril in pediatric patients with Alport's syndrome: 2 years' experience. *Eur J Pediatr* 2000;159:430–433.

Tryggvason K, Martin P. In: Scriver CR, Beaudet AL, Sly WS, et al., eds. *The metabolic and molecular bases of inherited diseases,* 8th ed. New York: McGraw-Hill, 2001:5453–5464.

RESOURCES

19, 179, 372

2   Blue Diaper Syndrome

Uri S. Alon, MD

DEFINITION: Blue diaper syndrome is a rare metabolic disorder caused by the breakdown of unabsorbed tryptophan by intestinal bacteria. It is characterized by irritability, intestinal disturbances, failure to thrive, visual abnormalities, hypercalciuria, nephrocalcinosis, and kidney damage.

SYNONYMS: Drummond syndrome; Hypercalcemia with nephrocalcinosis; Indicanuria.

DIFFERENTIAL DIAGNOSIS: Intestinal infection with *Pseudomonas aeruginosa*.

SYMPTOMS AND SIGNS: The syndrome is suspected in infants when blue urine stains their diaper. Symptoms include irritability, failure to thrive, poor appetite, vomiting, and constipation. Infections and fever are frequently present. Children often have poor vision resulting from ophthalmic abnormalities. Some children develop hypercalcemia, which can result in the development of hypercalciuria, nephrocalcinosis, and, occasionally, impaired kidney function and renal failure.

ETIOLOGY/EPIDEMIOLOGY: Blue diaper syndrome is an autosomal-recessive disorder. Males and females are equally affected. The biochemical nature of the disease is thought to be related to a defect in the intestinal absorption of tryptophan. The excessive trytophan is converted by intestinal bacteria to indole. Indole is absorbed and metabolized to indican, which is excreted in the urine. When exposed to air, indican is hydrolyzed and oxidized to indigo blue, which colors the urine blue.

DIAGNOSIS: The diagnosis is based on the finding of indicanuria in a fresh urine specimen. Intestinal disorders associated with poor absorption of tryptophan such as constipation, blind loop syndrome, biliary obstruction, and malabsorption, as well as metabolic disorders such as Hartnup disorder and phenylketonuria, need to be ruled out. Blue diaper syndrome is not accompanied by aminoaciduria.

TREATMENT
Standard Therapies: Standard treatment is the restriction of foods high in tryptophan. Supplemental nicotinic acid can help to control intestinal infections. Dietary calcium and vitamin D intake may need to be restricted.

REFERENCES
Blue diaper syndrome. New Fairfield, CT: National Organization of Rare Disorders, 1999.
Hwang ST, Shulman RJ. Enzymes and transport defects. In: McMillan JA, DeAngelis CD, Feigin RD, et al., eds. *Oski's pediatrics,* 3rd ed. Philadelphia: Lippincott Williams & Wilkins, 1999:1698–1702.
Levi HL. Hartnup disorder. In: Scriver CR, Beaudet AL, Sly WS, et al., eds. *The metabolic and molecular bases of inherited diseases,* 8th ed. New York: McGraw-Hill, 2001:4957–4969.
Rezvani I. Tryptophan. In: Behrman RE, Kliegman RM, Jenson HB, eds. *Nelson textbook of pediatrics,* 16th ed. Philadelphia: WB Saunders, 2000:353–354.

RESOURCES
108, 196, 308

3   Branchio-Oto-Renal Syndrome

Tarak Srivastava, MD, and Bradley A. Warady, MD

DEFINITION: Branchio-oto-renal (BOR) syndrome is characterized by the presence of a branchial sinus, fistula, or cysts, auricular malformations, preauricular pits, deafness, and renal anomalies.

SYNONYMS: Ear pits–deafness syndrome; Branchio-oto-renal dysplasia; Branchio-oto-ureteral syndrome; Melnick-Fraser syndrome; Preauricular pit–cervical fistula–hearing loss syndrome.

DIFFERENTIAL DIAGNOSIS: Goldenhar syndrome; Treacher-Collins syndrome; Otomandibular dysostosis; Towns-Brocks syndrome; Dysmorphic pinna–hypospadias–renal dysplasia; Dysmorphic pinna–polycystic kidney syndrome; Oto-renal-genital syndrome; Branchio-oculo-facial syndrome; Branchial arch syndrome. The combination of renal failure and deafness is commonly mistaken for Alport syndrome.

SYMPTOMS AND SIGNS: Branchial defects, hearing loss, preauricular pits, pinna anomalies, and renal malformations are characteristic of BOR syndrome. Branchial defects consist of a branchial cleft, cyst, sinus, or fistula that occurs in the middle to lower third of the neck. Otologic manifestations include hearing loss (conductive, sensorineural, or mixed) that ranges from mild to profound and can differ between the two ears. The deafness can be stable or progressive. The external pinna can be malformed, malpositioned, or small. The preauricular pit, tag, or sinus is present near the superior attachment of the helix of the ear. The external auditory canal may be atretic or stenosed. The ossicles of the middle ear are absent, hypoplastic, displaced, or fused, and the cochlea can be absent or underdeveloped. The vestibular apparatus can be absent or have hypoplastic semicircular canals. The renal anomalies seen in BOR syndrome range from severe malformations such as renal agenesis, renal hypoplasia or dysplasia, crossed renal ectopia, and polycystic kidneys to mild defects such as blunting of calyces, calyceal diverticulae, extrarenal or bifid pelvis, megaureter, uretero-pelvic junction obstruction, duplication of the ureter and collecting system, fetal lobulation, and vesico-ureteric reflux.

ETIOLOGY/EPIDEMIOLOGY: The BOR syndrome is an autosomal-dominant disorder. It occurs in 1 in 40,000 live births and is found in 2%–3% of children with profound deafness.

DIAGNOSIS: The diagnosis is made when at least two of five features (branchial defects, hearing loss, preauricular pits, pinna anomalies, and renal malformations) are present in a patient with two or more affected family members, or three features are present in a patient with no affected family members. An audiologic assessment with pure tone audiometry, tympanometry, and threshold auditory brainstem–evoked responses and a CT of the temporal bone to delineate the middle and inner ear defects should be performed. Renal anomaly is investigated by urinalysis, renal function tests, and imaging studies such as renal ultrasonography and CT.

TREATMENT
Standard Therapies: The child with hearing impairment should undergo appropriate aural rehabilitation with annual audiometry. An episode of otitis media should be aggressively managed with consideration for subsequent antibiotic prophylaxis. A middle ear effusion present for more than 3 months should be treated with tube placement for drainage. Surgical exploration of the middle ear should be considered when hearing loss is confined to the lateral ossicular chain, because creation of a neo-oval window may be beneficial. Because branchial cleft deformities have the potential to become easily infected, surgical excision should be performed at the earliest opportunity. A nephrologist should closely monitor the renal impairment, and surgical repair should be undertaken for correctable defects, such as uretero-pelvic junction obstruction. Dialysis and renal transplantation are indicated following the development of end-stage renal failure. Genetic counseling should be offered to the family.

REFERENCES
Chen A, Francis M, Ni L, et al. Phenotypic manifestations of branchio-oto-renal syndrome. *Am J Med Genet* 1995;58: 365–370.
Kumar S, Deffenbacher K, Cremers CWRJ, et al. Branchio-oto-renal syndrome: identification of novel mutations, molecular characterization, mutation distribution, and prospect for genetic testing. *Genet Test* 1997–1998;1:243–251.
Kumar S, Deffenbacher K, Marres HAM, et al. Genomewide search and genetic localization of a second gene associated with autosomal dominant branchio-oto-renal syndrome: clinical and genetic implications. *Am J Hum Genet* 2000;66: 1715–1720.
Melnick M, Bixler D, Nance WE, et al. Familial branchio-oto-renal dysplasia: a new addition to the branchial arch syndromes. *Clin Genet* 1976;9:25–34.
Smith RJH, Schwartz C. Branchio-oto-renal syndrome. *J Commun Disord* 1998;31:411–421.

RESOURCES
37, 308, 365

4 Cystinosis

Vimal Chadha, MD,
and Bradley A. Warady, MD

DEFINITION: Cystinosis is an inherited lysosomal storage disorder in which there is excessive intralysosomal storage of the amino acid cystine in virtually all body cells. Characteristic clinical manifestations include Fanconi syndrome, renal failure, severe growth retardation, hypothyroidism, and photophobia.

SYNONYM: Cystine storage disease.

DIFFERENTIAL DIAGNOSIS: Other causes of Fanconi syndrome (e.g., inherited idiopathic, inborn errors of metabolism such as Wilson disease, tyrosinemia, galactosemia, etc.); Acquired causes such as certain medications (e.g., cidofovir, gentamicin, and azathioprine) and heavy metal poisonings.

SYMPTOMS AND SIGNS: Three different forms of cystinosis can be distinguished; infantile or nephropathic cystinosis is the most common and most severe. The usual presentation begins at 8–12 months, with symptoms related to impaired renal tubular reabsorption of water, phosphate, sodium, potassium, bicarbonate, glucose, and amino acids. Polyuria, polydipsia, hypophosphatemic rickets, acidosis, and hypokalemia result. Severe growth retardation and renal failure develop within the first decade of life. Photophobia generally appears between age 3 and 6 years and is progressive. Hypothyroidism is often present, and hepatosplenomegaly is a common physical finding. After renal transplantation, patients continue to accumulate cystine in the rest of their organs and can develop retinal blindness, corneal erosions, diabetes mellitus, pancreatic insufficiency, distal myopathy, swallowing difficulties, primary hypogonadism in males, and neurologic deterioration. The benign or adult form is associated with cystine crystals in the cornea and bone marrow, but no renal failure. The adolescent form has intermediate symptoms, and renal involvement occurs late and progresses slowly.

ETIOLOGY/EPIDEMIOLOGY: Cystinosis is transmitted as an autosomal-recessive trait. The biochemical defect involves the lysosomal cystine carrier, resulting in the failure of egress of cystine from within lysosomes. The excessive accumulation of cystine results in cellular damage, although the exact mechanism remains unclear. The esti-

mated incidence is 1 in 200,000 live births, with a carrier frequency of 1 in 200 in the general population.

DIAGNOSIS: Diagnosis is made by showing an elevated cystine content in polymorphonuclear leukocytes or by slit-lamp examination showing corneal crystals, which are generally present in patients older than 1 year. In affected families, the diagnosis can be made prenatally by measuring the cystine content of amniotic cells or the cystine content of the placenta at birth.

TREATMENT
Standard Therapies: The supportive management of patients presenting with Fanconi syndrome includes adequate replacement of fluid and electrolytes. Phosphate supplements and vitamin D are required to treat or prevent rickets. Oral L-carnitine replacement is required to correct its deficiency. Levothyroxine and insulin are required for the management of hypothyroidism and diabetes mellitus, respectively. Recombinant human growth hormone has been used to treat growth retardation. Indomethacin usage has been associated with decreased urinary losses of electrolytes and phosphorus. Once end-stage renal disease is reached, dialysis and renal transplantation are required. The specific treatment of cystinosis is aimed at depleting the affected cells of cystine. Cysteamine has been effective accomplishing this. If started early (<2 years age) and given regularly, it slows the progression of renal failure and improves linear growth. However, it does not prevent the accumulation of corneal crystals and the development of Fanconi syndrome. The most common problems associated with cysteamine therapy are nausea, vomiting, and a foul odor and taste. Cysteamine bitartrate (Cystagon), which has significantly fewer side effects, may also be used. Leukocyte cystine levels should be checked every 3–4 months, with the goal of achieving and maintaining a cystine level of below 1 nmol of half cystine/mg protein.

Investigational Therapies: Researchers are exploring the efficacy of cysteamine eye drops.

REFERENCES
Gahl WA. Nephropathic cystinosis. *Pediatr Rev* 1997;18:302–304.
Gahl WA, Thoene JG, Schneider JA. In: Scriver CR, Beaudet AL, Sly WS, et al., eds. *The metabolic and molecular bases of inherited diseases,* 8th ed. New York: McGraw-Hill, 2001:5085–5101.
Markello TC, Bernardini IM, Gahl WA. Improved renal function in children with cystinosis treated with cysteamine. *N Engl J Med* 1993;328:1157–1162.

Schneider JA, Clark KF, Greene AA, et al. Recent advances in the treatment of cystinosis. *J Inherit Metab Disord* 1995;18:387–397.

RESOURCES

34, 109, 129

5   Cystinuria

Uri S. Alon, MD

DEFINITION: Cystinuria is a metabolic disorder characterized by the abnormal transport of cystine and the dibasic amino acids lysine, ornithine, and arginine in the intestine and kidney.

DIFFERENTIAL DIAGNOSIS: Hyperoxaluria.

SYMPTOMS AND SIGNS: The clinical manifestations are those associated with urolithiasis, including renal colic, hematuria, infection, and obstruction of the urinary tract. Frequent recurrence of urolithiasis can result in damage to the kidneys. Patients may pass "gravel" or stones that are usually small with a jagged crystalline surface.

ETIOLOGY/EPIDEMIOLOGY: Cystinuria is inherited in an autosomal-recessive manner. The disorder results from defects in the renal tubular reabsorption transport systems for cystine and the dibasic amino acids. Supersaturation of cystine in the urine, especially when acidic, results in stone formation. Cystinuria occurs in approximately 1 in 7,000 to 1 in 15,000 persons, but may be more prevalent in specific ethnic groups. The disease typically presents between ages 10 and 30, but can start earlier. Both sexes are affected.

DIAGNOSIS: All children with kidney stones should be studied for cystinuria, as should adults with recurrent stones. Cystine stones are faintly radioopaque and can be detected by ultrasonography. The diagnosis can be made by examination of a freshly voided first morning urine specimen for the typical hexagonal crystals. At times, it is necessary to acidify the urine to precipitate the crystals. The diagnosis should also be suspected in a patient with a positive nitroprusside test result in which the urine turns purple-red. The diagnosis is confirmed by quantitative measurement of cystine by amino acid chromatography or other methods; patients usually excrete more than 300 mg cystine/L (1,200 μM). Chemical analysis of a kidney stone can also be used for diagnosis.

TREATMENT
Standard Therapies: Patients with cystinuria should be monitored frequently with renal ultrasonography. A high fluid intake is essential for the prevention of new cystine stone formation. Alkalinization of the urine with bicarbonate or citrate is also recommended, with a target pH of 7.5. A higher urine pH can result in the formation of calcium phosphate salts. The use of a citrate salt may be helpful by chelating urinary calcium, whereas a low-sodium diet may decrease cystine excretion. Although restricting methionine in the diet can decrease cystine production, a severe restriction should be avoided in a growing child. Pharmacologic therapy includes D-penicillamine. The medicine is effective, but can be associated with side effects in up to 67% of patients. The orphan drug α-mercaptopropionylglycine, also known as tiopronin (Thiola, Mission Pharmaceutical, San Antonio, Texas), is also effective, but serious side effects are seen in 33% of patients. Treatment with captopril is controversial and has been reported to be less effective in children than in adults. Treatment of patients with symptoms related to cystine stone formation is similar to that of patients with other urinary tract stones. When end-stage renal disease develops due to cystinuria, renal transplantation is an effective form of therapy, because cystinuria has not been reported to recur in the transplanted kidney.

Investigational Therapies: Meso-2–3-dimercaptosuccinic acid (Succimer) is being studied for its ability to prevent the formation of cystine stones, and tromethamine-E and acetylcysteine-bicarbonate are being studied for their ability to dissolve stones. The drug 2,3-dimercaptosuccinic acid (CHEMET, McNeil, Ft. Washington, PA) is also being tested. Gene therapy is being studied as well.

REFERENCES

Cystinuria. New Fairfield, CT: National Organization of Rare Disorders; 1999.

Gregory MJ, Schwartz GJ. Diagnosis and treatment of renal tubular disorders. *Semin Nephrol* 1998;18:317–329.

Joly D, Rieu P, Mejean A, et al. Treatment of cystinuria. *Pediatr Nephrol* 1999:13:945–950.

Palacin M, Goodyear P, Nunes V, et al. Cystinuria. In: Scriver CR, Beaudet AL, Sly W, et al., eds. *The metabolic and molecular bases of inherited disease,* 8th ed. New York: McGraw-Hill, 2001:4909–4932.

Thoene JG. *Physician's guide to rare diseases,* 2nd ed. Montvale, NJ: Dowden, 1995:189–190.

RESOURCES

37, 130, 308

6 Interstitial Cystitis

Ursula Wesselmann, MD

DEFINITION: Interstitial cystitis (IC) is a chronic inflammatory condition of the bladder wall characterized by pressure and pain above the pubic area, as well as urinary urgency and frequency (up to 50 micturitions/day) and nocturia.

SYNONYM: Hypersensitive bladder disorders.

DIFFERENTIAL DIAGNOSIS: Cystitis; Bladder cancer; Endometriosis; Pelvic inflammatory disease; Chronic prostatitis; Prostatodynia; Reiter syndrome.

SYMPTOMS AND SIGNS: Key symptoms include suprapubic pain/pressure, urinary frequency and urgency, and nocturia. These symptoms are similar to those caused by bladder infection, but in patients with IC a bladder infection cannot be documented and the symptoms do not respond to antibiotic treatment. Patients with IC may also experience perineal pain involving the urethra, vagina, and rectum; pelvic/abdominal pain; and low back pain. Dyspareunia can be so severe that many women abstain from sexual activity. The disease may be associated with other chronic conditions such as fibromyalgia, vulvodynia, migraines, allergic reactions, and gastrointestinal problems.

ETIOLOGY/EPIDEMIOLOGY: The exact cause of IC is unknown. There are an estimated 700,000 cases of IC in the United States, but the disease is underdiagnosed, and the true prevalence is difficult to determine. More than 25% of IC patients are younger than 30 years, and the female:male ratio is estimated to be 9:1. Most patients with IC are white.

DIAGNOSIS: The primary clinical diagnosis pertains to the presence of irritative voiding symptoms along with pain symptoms referable to the lower urinary tract. No IC-specific marker exists; the diagnosis is one of exclusion, confirmed by a thorough clinical evaluation and selected tests to exclude other causes that can mimic the symptoms of IC.

TREATMENT
Standard Therapies: Because the etiology of IC remains unclear, it is difficult to direct treatment against the specific cause or causes of IC. No cure has yet been established. Once diagnosed, however, many treatment options are available. No treatments are uniformly effective for all IC patients. The most successful treatment plans are tailored to the needs of the individual IC patient, and include pain management strategies. Patients with mild cases of IC may be helped by change in diet, stress reduction, and behavioral interventions (including the keeping of voiding diaries and pelvic floor muscle training). Acupuncture and a transcutaneous electrical nerve stimulator have been advocated. For more symptomatic patients, oral medications may be added. Pentosan polysulfate sodium was approved specifically for the treatment of IC in the United States. Other medications that may help include those for chronic pain management, such as tricyclic antidepressants, anticonvulsants, membrane-stabilizing agents, nonsteroidal antiinflammatory drugs, muscle relaxants, and opioids. Hydroxyzine and other antihistamines have been recommended. Bladder instillations of dimethyl sulfoxide or other agents (cortisone, silver nitrate, clorpactin, hyaluronic acid) are also common. For patients with severe symptoms, implantable sacral nerve root stimulation devices or long-acting opioids may be useful.

REFERENCES
Curhan GC, Speizer FE, Hunter DJ, et al. Epidemiology of interstitial cystitis: a population based study. *J Urol* 1999;161:549–552.
Gillenwater JY, Wein AJ. Summary of the National Institute of Arthritis, Diabetes, Digestive and Kidney Diseases Workshop on Interstitial Cystitis. National Institutes of Health, Bethesda, Maryland, August 28–29, 1987. *J Urol* 1988;140:203–206.
Hanno PM, Landis RJ, Matthews-Cook Y, et al., for the Interstial Cystitis Database Study Group. The diagnosis of interstitial cystitis revisited: lessons learned from the National Institutes of health interstitial cystitis data base. *J Urol* 1999;161:553–557.
Jones CA, Nyberg LM. Epidemiology of interstitial cystitis. *Urology* 1997;49(suppl 5A):2–9.
Sant GR, ed. *Interstitial cystitis.* Philadelphia: Lippincott-Raven, 1997.
Wesselmann U, Burnett AL. Genitourinary pain. In: Wall PD, Melzack R, eds. *Textbook of pain,* 4th ed. New York: Churchill Livingstone, 1999:689–709.

RESOURCES

34, 214, 372

7   Denys-Drash Syndrome

Douglas Blowey, MD

DEFINITION: Denys-Drash syndrome is characterized by genital abnormalities, Wilms tumor, and progressive kidney disease leading to kidney failure.

SYNONYMS: Drash syndrome; Nephropathy-pseudohermaphroditism-Wilms tumor.

DIFFERENTIAL DIAGNOSIS: WAGR syndrome; Fraiser syndrome.

SYMPTOMS AND SIGNS: Wilms tumor is a cancer of the kidney and may involve one or both kidneys. An enlargement of the abdomen is usually the first symptom; however, abdominal pain, blood in the urine, or nonspecific symptoms such as weight loss, fever, and fatigue may occur. Kidney disease occurs early in life and is a progressive process resulting in kidney failure. Swelling (edema), high blood pressure, and blood and protein in the urine are common signs of kidney disease. Individuals with Denys-Drash syndrome can have the gonads (testes, ovaries) of one sex and the external appearance of the opposite sex (pseudohermaphroditism). Gonadoblastoma is a cancer of the gonadal cells (testes, ovaries) that occurs in some patients.

ETIOLOGY/EPIDEMIOLOGY: Denys-Drash syndrome results from an abnormality of the Wilms tumor 1 (*WT1*) gene located on chromosome 11p13. Most gene abnormalities are new deficiencies (*de novo*), although familial transmission occurs rarely.

DIAGNOSIS: The diagnosis is based on clinical findings and chromosomal studies.

TREATMENT
Standard Therapies: Early detection of Wilms tumor can greatly improve the outcome, and routine abdominal ultrasonography is recommended. Treatment programs combine surgery, radiation therapy, and chemotherapy. Surgical correction may be required for the genitourinary anomalies. Hormone treatment is required for those individuals who have had the gonads removed. Treatment of the kidney disease is supportive, because drug therapy does not change the progressive nature of the disease. Individuals with very poor kidney function may require dialysis and/or renal transplantation.

REFERENCES
Barratt TM, Avner ED, Harmon WE, eds. *Pediatric nephrology,* 4th ed. Philadelphia: Lippincott Williams & Wilkins, 1999.

Breslow NE, Takashima JR, Ritchey ML, et al. Renal failure in Denys-Drash and Wilms' tumor-aniridia syndromes. *Cancer Res* 2000;60:4030–4032.

Koziell A, et al. Frasier and Denys-Drash syndromes: different disorders or a part of a spectrum? *Arch Dis Child* 1999;81:365–369.

Mueller RF. The Denys-Drash syndrome. *J Med Genet* 1994;31:471–477.

Scriver CR, Beaudet AL, Sly WS, et al., eds. *The metabolic and molecular bases of inherited disease,* 8th ed. New York: McGraw-Hill, 2001.

RESOURCES
30, 37, 84, 308

8   The Bladder Exstrophy–Epispadias–Cloacal Exstrophy Complex

John P. Gearhart, MD, FACS, and Yousef E. Tadros, MD

DEFINITION: Exstrophy of the bladder is part of a spectrum of anomalies involving the urinary tract, genital tract, musculoskeletal system, and sometimes the intestinal tract. In classic bladder exstrophy, most anomalies are related to defects of the abdominal wall, bladder, genitalia, pelvic bones, rectum, and anus.

SYNONYM: Ectopia vesicae.

DIFFERENTIAL DIAGNOSIS: Pseudoexstrophy (Marshall and Muecke); Superior vesical fissure; Duplicate exstrophy; Covered exstrophy.

SYMPTOMS AND SIGNS: The variants of the bladder exstrophy–epispadias–cloacal exstrophy complex of genitourinary malformations can be as simple as a mild glandular epispadias, or can encompass an overwhelming multisystem defect such as cloacal exstrophy.

ETIOLOGY/EPIDEMIOLOGY: Bladder exstrophy, cloacal exstrophy, and epispadias are variants of the exstrophy–epispadias complex (Insert Fig. 58). The etiology of this complex has been attributed to the failure of the cloacal membrane to be reinforced by ingrowth of mesoderm (Muecke). The incidence of bladder exstrophy has been estimated to be between 1 in 10,000 and 1 in 50,000 live births. However, data from the International Clearinghouse for Birth Defects monitoring system estimated the incidence to be 3.3 in 100,000 live births. Two series have reported a 5:1 to 6:1 ratio of male to females born with the syndrome.

DIAGNOSIS: In prenatal ultrasonographic examinations of babies who were subsequently born with classic bladder exstrophy, several observations were made: (a) absence of bladder filling; (b) a low-set umbilicus; (c) widening of the pubic ramus; (d) diminutive genitalia; and (e) a lower abdominal mass that increased in size as the pregnancy progressed and as the intraabdominal viscera increased in size.

TREATMENT
Standard Therapies: The primary objectives in modern surgical management of classic bladder exstrophy are a secure abdominal closure; reconstruction of a functional and cosmetically acceptable penis in the male and of external genitalia in the female; and urinary continence with the preservation of renal function and volitional voiding. Currently, these objectives can best be achieved with newborn primary bladder and posterior urethral closure, early epispadias repair, and, finally, bladder neck reconstruction when the bladder reaches an appropriate volume for an outlet procedure (Insert Fig. 59).

Investigational Therapies: The use of three-dimensional CT to evaluate the bony pelvis and pelvic floor anatomy in classic bladder exstrophy is being explored, and it may provide new insight for long-term issues such as urinary and fecal incontinence and pelvic organ prolapse and help in developing better techniques for pelvic osteotomy in these patients.

REFERENCES
Gearhart JP. Bladder and cloacal exstrophy. In: Gonzales ET, Bauer SB, eds. *Pediatric urology practice.* Philadelphia: Lippincott Williams & Wilkins, 1999:339–364.
Gearhart JP, Jeffs RD. Chapter 63. In: Campbell MF, Retik AB. *Campbell's urology,* 7th ed. Vol. 2. Philadelphia: WB Saunders, 1997:1939–1990.

RESOURCES
34, 285, 372, 480

---

9   Galloway-Mowat Syndrome

*Tarak Srivastava, MD,
and Bradley A. Warady, MD*

DEFINITION: Galloway-Mowat syndrome is characterized by the presence of early-onset (<3 years of age), steroid-resistant nephrotic syndrome and central nervous system anomalies, consisting of microcephaly, developmental delay, and abnormal sulci and gyri of the brain.

SYNONYMS: Microcephaly–hiatal hernia–nephrotic syndrome; Nephrosis–neural dysmigration syndrome; Microcephaly–infantile spasms–psychomotor retardation–nephrotic syndrome.

DIFFERENTIAL DIAGNOSIS: Congenital intrauterine infections causing secondary nephrotic syndrome; Microcephaly, nephrotic syndrome, and developmental delay (MNSDD) with or without spondylorhizomelic short stature; Congenital nephrotic syndrome of the Finnish type; Denys-Drash syndrome; Idiopathic congenital nephrotic syndrome associated with nail-patella syndrome, bupthalmos, or urinary tract anomalies.

SYMPTOMS AND SIGNS: Nephrotic syndrome characterized by edema formation secondary to proteinuria and hypoalbuminemia usually presents during infancy. The glomerular findings on kidney biopsy range from normal to mesangial proliferation, focal segmental glomerulosclerosis, or diffuse mesangial sclerosis. The nephrotic syndrome does not to respond to corticosteroid therapy and progresses to renal failure. Central nervous system disorder is characterized by microcephaly at birth. On follow-up, the child exhibits severe developmental delay, muscle tone abnormalities from hypotonia to spasticity, and a seizure disorder. CT or MRI of the brain demonstrates sulcus and gyrus abnormalities (e.g., microgyria, pachygyria, or lissencephaly), diffuse cortical atrophy, or cerebellar hypoplasia/dysgenesis. Hiatal hernia and ophthalmologic abnormalities such as miosis, corneal opacity, cataract, microopthalmos, hypoplastic iris, or optic atrophy may also be seen. There are no diagnostic dysmorphic features, although a sloping forehead, flat occiput, hypertelorism, large, low-set floppy ears, small midface, small pinched nose, high-arched palate, and micrognathia have been described. Additional findings reported include club feet, campylodactyly, flexion contractures of joints, notched ears, hypoplastic nails, eventration of diaphragm, anteposed anus, thyroid dysplasia, adrenal hypoplasia, ovarian agenesis, atrophic thymus, calcification of the intervertebral disc, platybasia, Dandy-Walker malformation, aqueductal stenosis with hydrocephalus, and central canal malformation.

ETIOLOGY/EPIDEMIOLOGY: Galloway-Mowat syndrome is an autosomal-recessive disorder of unknown etiology. Only 27 cases have been reported in children with different ethnic backgrounds and with no gender predilection. No incidence or prevalence data are available.

DIAGNOSIS: The diagnosis is made in the clinical setting of nephrotic syndrome during the first 3 years of life that is corticosteroid resistant, in association with microcephaly and progressive developmental delay. Neuroimaging of the patient demonstrates gyral abnormalities, and congenital intrauterine infection and other recognizable syndromes are absent. The diagnostic evaluation should include a urinalysis for proteinuria; serum measurements for albumin, blood urea nitrogen, and creatinine; CT or MRI of the brain; electroencephalography; and a barium swallow study to investigate for a hiatal hernia.

TREATMENT

Standard Therapies: Treatment is multidisciplinary and supportive. The corticosteroid-resistant nephrotic syndrome is managed with albumin infusions, diuretic therapy, and thyroid, vitamin, and mineral supplementation. Dialysis therapy has been used in a handful of cases with end-stage renal failure. The severe developmental delay requires nutritional support and rehabilitative therapy from physical, occupational, and speech therapists. Seizures may be controlled by anticonvulsant medications. Surgical repair may be needed for hiatal hernia. The family should be counseled regarding future pregnancies, which carry a 25% risk of recurrence for the disorder.

REFERENCES

Cohen AH, Turner MC. Kidney in Galloway-Mowat syndrome: clinical spectrum with description of pathology. *Kidney Int* 1994;45:1407–1415.

Cooperstone BG, Friedman A, Kaplan BS. Galloway-Mowat syndrome of abnormal gyral patterns and glomerulopathy. *Am J Med Genet* 1993;47:250–254.

Galloway WH, Mowat AP. Congenital microcephaly with hiatus hernia and nephrotic syndrome in two sibs. *J Med Genet* 1968;5:319–321.

Kozlowski PB, Sher JH, Nicastri AD, et al. Brain morphology in the Galloway-Mowat syndrome. *Clin Neuropathol* 1989;8:85–91.

Meyers KEC, Kaplan P, Kaplan BS. Nephrotic syndrome, microcephaly, and developmental delay: three separate syndromes. *Am J Med Genet* 1999;82:257–260.

Srivastava T, Whiting JM, Garola RE, et al. Podocyte proteins in Galloway-Mowat syndrome. *Pediatr Nephrol* 2001;16:1022–1029.

RESOURCES

145, 308, 368, 372

---

10   Benign Familial Hematuria

*Anirut Pattaragam, MD,
and Bradley A. Warady, MD*

DEFINITION: Benign familial hematuria (BFH) is defined by the familial occurrence of persistent microscopic hematuria without proteinuria, progression to renal failure, or extrarenal manifestations. Diffuse attenuation of the glomerular basement membrane (thin GBM) on renal biopsy is usually considered the hallmark of the condition.

SYNONYMS: Thin glomerular basement membrane disease; Thin basement membrane disease (TBMD); Thin membrane nephropathy; Familial thin basement membrane nephropathy.

DIFFERENTIAL DIAGNOSIS: Alport syndrome; IgA nephropathy; Sporadic benign hematuria; Hypercalciuria.

SYMPTOMS AND SIGNS: Hematuria, typically isolated, microscopic, and persistent, is often first detected by routine urinalysis in children. In some cases, microhematuria is intermittent and may not be detected until adulthood. Recurrent episodes of gross hematuria, often associated with upper respiratory tract infection, are not unusual. Some patients may show mild proteinuria, although overt proteinuria has rarely been described.

ETIOLOGY/EPIDEMIOLOGY: Benign familial hematuria is usually transmitted as an autosomal-dominant trait. Gender differences in expression of BFH are not apparent. Currently, the incidence of the disorder has not been clearly determined. Although the incidence of TBMD in different series has varied from 0.8% to 11% of patients, these figures include other clinical conditions (e.g., Alport syndrome) associated with the same ultrastructural lesion. The basic biochemical defect has not been characterized, and the antigenicity of the GBM is normal. However, a linkage to locus COL4A3/COL4A4 on chromosome 2 has been detected in some families, indicating that mutations at type IV collagen loci may be responsible for some cases.

DIAGNOSIS: The diagnosis is based on the presence of isolated hematuria, negative symptoms, the absence of progressive renal disease in family members, and, if necessary, the renal biopsy finding of a diffusely thin GBM by electron microscopy with normal antigenicity. The finding of hematuria in family members can further support the diagnosis. The normal GBM thickness is age- and gender-dependent. At birth, the GBM thickness is about 100–150 nm. It reaches approximately 200 nm at 1 year. The discrimination point between normal and low GBM thickness in children is approximately 200–250 nm. Because other glomerular disorders may occur in patients with a thin GBM, the diagnosis has to be reconsidered if any new signs or symptoms are observed during the subsequent follow-up period. Marked variability of the GBM width within a glomerulus should raise suspicion of Alport syndrome. Immunohistologic evaluation of the GBM type IV collagen may be helpful in differentiating BFH from Alport syndrome. Hypercalciuria can be ruled out by the finding of a random urine calcium:creatinine ratio of less than 0.2:1.

TREATMENT

Standard Therapies: In addition to reassurance, follow-up evaluation is the mainstay of therapy. A reasonable follow-up evaluation includes a urinalysis and measurement of blood pressure and renal function every 1–2 years.

REFERENCES

Frasca GM, Onetti-Muda A, Renieri A. Thin glomerular basement membrane disease. *J Nephrol* 2000;13:15–19.

Gubler MC. Disorders of the basement membrane: thin glomerular basement membrane syndrome, nail-patella syndrome, and collagen type III glomerulopathy. In: Morgan SH, Grunfeld J, eds. *Inherited disorders of the kidney,* 1st ed. New York: Oxford University Press, 1998:215–230.

Gubler MC, Knebelmann B, Antignac C. Inherited glomerular disease. In: Barratt TM, Avner ED, Harmon WE, eds. *Pediatric nephrology,* 4th ed. Philadelphia: Lippincott Williams & Wilkins, 1999:475–495.

Kashtan CE. Alport syndrome and thin glomerular basement membrane disease. *J Am Soc Nephrol* 1998;9:1736–1750.

RESOURCES

34, 308, 372

---

11 Hemolytic-Uremic Syndrome

Bernard S. Kaplan, MD, BCh

DEFINITION: Hemolytic-uremic syndrome (HUS) is characterized by acute hemolytic anemia with fragmented erythrocytes, thrombocytopenia, and acute renal injury.

DIFFERENTIAL DIAGNOSIS: Thrombotic thrombocytopenic purpura.

SYMPTOMS AND SIGNS: Shigatoxin-associated HUS (Stx HUS) must be anticipated in any patient with bloody diarrhea, and in any patient with diarrhea whose urine volume does not increase with adequate rehydration, who becomes pale or edematous during or after bloody diarrhea, and who has seizures during or after bloody diarrhea. All patients have anemia and thrombocytopenia. Approximately 50% of patients are anuric, hypertension is common, and other organs, especially the pancreas, may be affected. The acute mortality rate is less than 5% in Stx HUS; complete recovery occurs in 64% of patients, chronic renal insufficiency with hypertension in 4% of patients, late sequelae in 12% of patients, and end-stage renal disease in 9% of patients. Diabetes mellitus and cholelithiasis are additional complications. Recurrent episodes after recovery from Stx HUS or after transplantation are uncommon.

ETIOLOGY/EPIDEMIOLOGY: *E. coli* 0157:H7 is the Stx-producing bacterium that is the cause of HUS in 80%–90% of cases. Five percent to 15% of children with *E. coli* 0157:H7 infection develop HUS. Stx1 and Stx2 are the two shiga-like toxins that injure glomerular endothelial, epithelial, and tubular cells. Stx HUS occurs in all ages but mainly between 6 months and 4 years, with slightly more females affected. It occurs mainly in summer, sporadically, and in epidemics. Stx HUS follows ingestion of contaminated ground meat, fruit, vegetables, water, apple cider, milk-containing products, and many kinds of undercooked and prepared meats.

TREATMENT

Standard Therapies: Antibiotics do not reduce the risk of developing symptomatic *E. coli* 0157:H7 infection, and antimotility agents should not be used. The importance of washing hands, cooking ground meat well, avoiding contamination of food by uncooked meat, and eating only pasteurized dairy products must be emphasized. Electrolytes and fluid balance are managed carefully. Dialysis is started when there are clinical symptoms of uremia or the patient is anuric. Continuous hemodiafiltration is used for patients with a precarious hemodynamic status. Packed red blood cells are transfused slowly when the hemoglobin concentration falls below 6 g/dL. Platelet transfusions are indicated for active bleeding or for surgery. Hypertension is treated by vasodilators and fluid removal. Adequate nutrition is maintained enterally or parenterally.

Investigational Therapies: Synsorb Pk is being investigated as a treatment for HUS.

REFERENCES

Kaplan BS, et al. The pathogenesis and treatment of hemolytic uremic syndrome. *J Am Soc Nephrol* 1998;9:1126–1133.

Meyers KW, et al. Principles of the treatment of Shigatoxin-associated hemolytic uremic syndrome: pay meticulous attention to detail, and do no harm. In: Kaper JB, O'Brien A, eds. Escherichia coli *0157:H7 and Other Shiga-Toxin–Producing* E. coli *Strains.* Washington, DC: American Society of Microbiology Press, 1998:364–373.

RESOURCES

37, 248, 368, 372

---

12 Inherited Hemolytic-Uremic Syndrome

Bernard S. Kaplan, MD, BCh

DEFINITION: Inherited hemolytic uremic syndrome (HUS) is characterized by acute hemolytic anemia with fragmented erythrocytes, thrombocytopenia, and acute renal injury, in the absence of diarrhea.

DIFFERENTIAL DIAGNOSIS: Thrombotic thrombocytopenic purpura; Shiga toxin–associated hemolytic uremic syndrome.

SYMPTOMS AND SIGNS: In the recessive form of inherited HUS, no recognized precipitating events occur. Most affected individuals are infants and children. Some patients have complete resolution; some may have several episodes. HUS may recur before and after renal transplantation. In the dominant form, adults are affected more often, and pregnancy may be a precipitating event. The mortality rate is high, and complete recovery is uncommon. Recurrent episodes may occur before or after transplantation.

ETIOLOGY/EPIDEMIOLOGY: The pathogenesis of the inherited forms of HUS is unknown; but linkage exists to the factor H locus on chromosome 1. Many patients have decreased serum factor H levels. Inheritance can be autosomal recessive or autosomal dominant; no sex or race preferences exist for either form. Inherited HUS accounts for less than 5% of all cases of HUS.

DIAGNOSIS: Diagnostic criteria of inherited HUS are acute hemolytic anemia with fragmented erythrocytes, thrombocytopenia, and acute renal injury, in the absence of diarrhea, in a patient with a family history of HUS. A diagnosis cannot be made in the absence of a family history.

TREATMENT

Standard Therapies: Electrolyte and fluid balance is managed carefully. Dialysis is started when clinical symptoms of uremia occur or the patient is anuric. Continuous hemodiafiltration is used for patients with a precarious hemodynamic status or colonic gangrene. Packed red blood cells are transfused slowly when the hemoglobin concentration falls below 6 g/dL. Platelet transfusions are indicated for active bleeding or for surgery. Hypertension is treated by vasodilators and fluid removal. Adequate nutrition is maintained enterally or parenterally. Fresh frozen plasma infusions and plasmapheresis are indicated. A waiting period of 6–12 months between the occurrence of HUS and a renal transplant is advisable to be sure the patient is free from active disease. Living related donors and the use of cyclosporine A are associated with a higher rate of recurrences after transplantation.

REFERENCES

Ducloux D, et al. Recurrence of hemolytic-uremic syndrome in renal transplant recipients: a meta-analysis. *Transplantation* 1998;65:1405–1407.

Kaplan BS, et al. Renal transplantation in adults with autosomal recessive inheritance of hemolytic uremic syndrome. *Am J Kidney Dis* 1997;30:760–765.

Kaplan BS, et al. Autosomal dominant hemolytic uremic syndrome: variable phenotypes and transplantation. *Pediatr Nephrol* 2000;14:464–468.

Warwicker P, et al. Familial relapsing haemolytic uraemic syndrome and complement factor H deficiency. *Nephrol Dial Transplant* 1999;14:1229–1233.

RESOURCES

37, 248, 368, 372

---

13 Congenital Hepatic Fibrosis

Ari M. Simckes, MD

DEFINITION: Congenital hepatic fibrosis (CHF) is a hereditary disorder characterized by portal hypertension and histopathologic changes in the liver. It may be isolated, but is most often associated with autosomal-recessive polycystic kidney disease (ARPKD).

SYNONYMS: Biliary dysgenesis; Ductal plate malformation.

DIFFERENTIAL DIAGNOSIS: Caroli disease; Banti disease; Polycystic kidney disease; Nephronophthisis-medullary cystic kidney disease; Gaucher disease; Helminthiasis of the bile ducts; Tumors of the extrahepatic bile ducts.

SYMPTOMS AND SIGNS: Clinical manifestations may be divided into four forms: portal hypertensive, cholangitic, mixed, and latent. The portal hypertensive form often presents with gastrointestinal (GI) bleeding, and the cholangitic form with cholestasis and recurrent cholangitis. The latent form may be detected incidentally later in life. The disease often presents during the first decade of life with hepatomegaly and findings secondary to portal hypertension. Bleeding from the GI tract is a frequent presenting sign. Splenomegaly often occurs along with thrombocytopenia from hypersplenism. Splenorenal and gastrorenal shunts may be detected, and the risk of portal vein thrombosis is increased. Dilatation of the intrahepatic duct is commonly observed. Cholangiocarcinoma and hepatocellular carcinoma are rare yet significant complications of CHF. For patients with both CHF and ARPKD, presentation often occurs in the neonate or young child with palpable nephromegaly, progressive renal dysfunction, and hypertension. Newborns may have compromised respiratory function from pulmonary hypoplasia and fluid retention.

ETIOLOGY/EPIDEMIOLOGY: Congenital hepatic fibrosis results from abnormal prenatal differentiation and development of biliary ducts and hepatocytes, resulting in persistence of ductal plates not usually present in postnatal livers and an increase in portal tract fibrous tissue. It usually is inherited as an autosomal-recessive trait and it occurs equally in males and females, but may occur sporadically. The overall incidence of CHF is not known. Around 50% of those with CHF also have renal involvement. CHF is associated with other liver disorders.

DIAGNOSIS: Diagnosis is made based on the aforementioned clinical observations and radiographic studies, and is confirmed by liver biopsy. Blood tests of liver function are usually normal. Renal function and the presence of metabolic acidosis must be assessed. A blood culture should be obtained if cholangitis is suspected, as well as bacterial culture of hepatic tissue if a liver biopsy or aspirate is performed. Imaging should include Doppler ultrasonography of the liver, portal vasculature, kidneys, and spleen. CT, magnetic resonance cholangiography, and nuclear liver and biliary scans are warranted at times. Kidney biopsy may be helpful if the renal diagnosis is unclear. Prenatal ultrasonography may detect enlarged echogenic kidneys in those with ARPKD.

TREATMENT

Standard Therapies: Treatment is symptomatic and supportive. For portal hypertension, there are surgical procedures such as portosystemic shunting and medical therapies. β-blockers may be useful for treatment of portal hypertension. Sclerotherapy, band ligation, and pharmacologic management are treatment options for varices. Cholangitis requires treatment with antibiotics. Liver transplantation, although curative, is reserved for patients with progressive hepatic failure and chronic cholangitis. Renal dysfunction requires correction of fluid and electrolyte imbalances and hypertension management. Renal osteodystrophy is treated with phosphate binders, calcium, a low-phosphate diet, and vitamin D. Appropriate caloric and protein intake are essential. Hormone therapy with growth hormone and erythropoietin may be required. Dialysis is necessary for end-stage kidney disease, and surgical removal of enlarged cystic kidneys is sometimes required to allow for that. Renal transplantation is the ultimate goal for those with renal failure.

Investigational Therapies: The role of ursodeoxycholic acid, a bile acid oral medication used for the dissolution of gallstones, is being investigated as an agent to prevent cholangitis.

REFERENCES

Lipschitz B, Berdon WE, Defelice AR, et al. Association of congenital hepatic fibrosis with autosomal dominant polycystic kidney disease. Report of a family review of literature. *Pediatr Radiol* 1993;23:131–133.

Schiff L, Schiff ER, eds. *Diseases of the liver,* 7th ed. Philadelphia: JB Lippincott, 1993:1204–1206.

Suchy FJ, Sokol RJ, Balistreri WF, eds. *Liver disease in children,* 2nd ed. Philadelphia: Lippincott Williams & Wilkins, 2001:50–51, 901–902.

Walker A, ed. *Pediatric gastrointestinal disease,* 3rd ed. Hamilton, ON: Decker. 2000:895–900.

Zakim D, Boyer TD, eds. *Hepatology: a textbook of liver disease,* 3rd ed. Philadelphia: WB Saunders, 1996:1640–1643.

RESOURCES

37, 39, 308, 372

14   Loken-Senior Syndrome

Richard A. Lewis, MD, MS

DEFINITION: Loken-Senior syndrome (LSS) is an autosomal-recessive syndrome of nephronophthisis (with or without medullary cystic renal disease) and a progressive pigmentary dystrophy, with onset typically in the first year of life.

SYNONYMS: Juvenile nephronophthisis with Leber amaurosis; Renal dysplasia and retinal aplasia; Renal dysplasia-blindness; Renal-retinal dysplasia; Retinal-renal syndrome; Senior-Loken syndrome.

DIFFERENTIAL DIAGNOSIS: Amaurosis congenital of Leber; Brachymorphism-onychodysplasia-dysphalangism syndrome; Juvenile nephronophthisis–medullary cystic disease; Nephronophthisis 1; Rhyns syndrome; Saldino-Mainzer syndrome.

SYMPTOMS AND SIGNS: Infants with LSS are born with severe visual impairment and develop nystagmus in the first 2 months of life. Electrophysiology demonstrates a poorly recordable or nonrecordable electroretinogram. Progressive pigmentary retinopathy becomes apparent in the first year of life, which is often confused with Leber congenital amaurosis. In LSS, however, an insidious nephronophthisis with or without medullary cystic renal disease also appears in the first year of life. Other features may occur in individual families, suggesting that this clinical phenotype may be genetically heterogeneous, including vasopressin-resistant diabetes insipidus, neurosensory hearing impairment, cerebellar ataxia, and hepatic fibrosis.

ETIOLOGY/EPIDEMIOLOGY: LSS has considerable variability between families, perhaps reflective of genetic heterogeneity. A late-onset form of retinitis pigmentosa occurs in a small fraction of patients with nephronophthisis type 1 mutations without an apparent genotype/phenotype correlation. Another locus for early-onset LSS colocalizes to the nephronophthisis type 3 locus (*NPHP3*) and a fourth form occurs on chromosome 1p36 (*SLSN4*).

DIAGNOSIS: Electrophysiology demonstrates profound dysfunction of the retinal photoreceptors with a nonrecordable or poorly recordable response from both rods and cones. Imaging studies and conventional biochemical assays demonstrate deterioration in renal function with progressive azotemia. Occasionally, onset of renal disease occurs in the latter part of the first decade of life.

TREATMENT

Standard Therapies: Treatment should include supportive care for renal failure. Rarely, renal transplantation has been performed in some patients. Conventional management for the severe visual impairment includes low vision assessment and formal training.

REFERENCES

Loken AC, Hanssen O, Halvorsen S, et al. Hereditary renal dysplasia and blindness. *Acta Paediatr* 1961;50:177–184.

McKusick VA, ed. Online Mendelian Inheritance in Man (OMIM). Baltimore: The Johns Hopkins University. Entry no. 266900; last update March 5, 2001.

Omran H, Sasmaz G, Haffner K, et al. Identification of a gene locus for Senior-Loken syndrome in the region of the nephronophthisis type 3 gene. *J Am Soc Nephrol* 2002;13:75–79.

Scheuermann MJ, Otto E, Becker A, et al. Mapping of gene loci for nephronophthisis type 4 and Senior-Loken syndrome, to chromosome 1p36. *Am J Hum Genet* 2002;70:1240–1246.

Senior B, Friedman AI, Braudo JL. Juvenile familial nephropathy with tapetoretinal degeneration: a new oculorenal dystrophy. *Am J Ophthalmol* 1961;52:625–633.

Warady BA, Cibis G, Alon U, et al. Senior-Loken syndrome: revisited. *Pediatrics* 1994;94:111–112.

RESOURCES

37, 161, 355, 372

---

15 Medullary Cystic Kidney Disease

Ari M. Simckes, MD

DEFINITION: Medullary cystic kidney disease (MCKD) is a complex of inherited kidney disorders that share clinical symptoms and anatomic findings. The two categories of MCKD include nephronophthisis (NPH) and MCKD. Nephronophthisis-MCDK results in progressive loss of kidney function as a result of alterations in the structure of the renal tubules and interstitium, causing dilatation, inflammation, and fibrosis. There are three variants of NPH and two variants of MCKD.

SYNONYMS: Medullary cystic disease (MCD); Familial juvenile nephronophthisis.

DIFFERENTIAL DIAGNOSIS: Renal-retinal dysplasia (syndrome); Renal dysplasia–retinal aplasia; Loken-Senior syndrome; Leber congenital amaurosis; Polycystic kidney disease; Medullary sponge kidney.

SYMPTOMS AND SIGNS: The age of onset varies depending on the variant of the NPH-MCKD complex, yet the symptoms are similar. NPH usually presents during the first or second decade of life. The most common initial feature of NPH is impairment of the ability to concentrate urine. Features in children with NPH include polyuria, polydipsia, secondary enuresis, nocturia, lethargy, pallor, anemia, pruritis, failure to thrive, and growth retardation. Progressive kidney failure often occurs during the second decade. Other manifestations may include ocular, neurologic, and hepatic abnormalities. MCKD presents during adulthood. Hyponatremia secondary to urinary sodium wasting and anemia are often the initial features. Renal failure develops eventually. Extrarenal manifestations include hyperuricemia and gout.

ETIOLOGY/EPIDEMIOLOGY: The three variants of NPH are inherited in an autosomal-recessive pattern, whereas the two variants of MCKD are inherited in an autosomal-dominant pattern. Genes suspected to be responsible for each of the variants have been localized. The incidence of NPH-MCKD varies with geography, and it is more common in Europe than in the United States, where it is 9 patients per 8.3 million population. NPH causes ~1% of pediatric end-stage kidney disease in the United States.

DIAGNOSIS: The diagnosis is based on the characteristic signs and symptoms and on sonography and renal histology. An inability to concentrate urine on a first morning specimen and secondary enuresis are suggestive. Laboratory studies must be performed to assess for anemia, renal function, electrolyte abnormalities, metabolic acidosis, and renal osteodystrophy. Specific tests should include urinalysis, serum urea nitrogen, creatinine, electrolytes, calcium, phosphorous, parathyroid hormone, and complete blood count. Renal sonography usually shows normal or small kidneys with increased echogenicity and decreased corticomedullary differentiation. Kidney biopsy findings are similar in all variants of NPH-MCKD and include cysts, patchy tubular and interstitial fibrosis, atrophy, and inflammation. Assessments for associated abnormalities must be performed, including hepatic function tests, liver sonography, ophthalmologic evaluations, and neurologic assessment. Genetic testing is available for variants of NPH-MCKD.

TREATMENT

Standard Therapies: Therapy for NPH-MCKD is supportive and directed toward the correction of electrolyte, fluid, and acid/base disturbances. Adequate fluid and sodium supplementation is required. Severe polyuria may require nasogastric or gastrostomy tube placement for hydration and supplementary nutrition. As renal function decreases, metabolic acidosis must be corrected. Secondary hyperparathyroidism is treated with calcium supplementation, dietary phosphorous restriction, binders, and vitamin D therapy. Anemia may be treated with iron, folate, and erythopoietin. Short stature is treated with adequate caloric intake and growth hormone. Renal replacement therapy will ultimately be required, with the goal of kidney transplantation. In addition to referral to a nephrologist and assessment by a dietician, psychosocial and genetic counseling is advised. Periodic assessment of asymptomatic siblings of patients with NPH to monitor renal function, urine concentrating ability, and growth is advised.

REFERENCES

Barratt TM, Avner ED, Harmon WE. *Pediatric nephrology*, 4th ed. Philadelphia: Lippincott Williams & Wilkins, 1999:453–458.

Brenner BM, ed. *The kidney*, 5th ed. Philadelphia: WB Saunders, 1996:1845–1847.

Hildebrandt F, Otto E. Molecular genetics of nephronophthisis and medullary cystic kidney disease. *J Am Soc Kidney Dis* 2000;11:1753–1761.

RESOURCES

37, 54, 308, 372

16   Medullary Sponge Kidney

Robert D. Lewis, MD,
and Bradley A. Warady, MD

DEFINITION: Medullary sponge kidney (MSK) refers to a specific structural abnormality of the renal collecting ducts. The characteristic lesion is cystic malformations of the collecting ducts and tubules of one or more renal papillae. The disorder may involve one or both kidneys.

SYNONYMS: Precalyceal canalicular ectasia; Cystic dilatation of renal collecting tubules.

DIFFERENTIAL DIAGNOSIS: Hyperparathyroidism; Tuberculosis; Idiopathic hypercalciuria; Hypervitaminosis D; Milk alkali syndrome; Chronic metabolic acidosis; Sarcoidosis; Metastatic malignancy; Renal papillary necrosis; Polycystic kidney disease.

SYMPTOMS AND SIGNS: In the absence of complications, patients with MSK are asymptomatic. The common presenting complaints when complications develop are bleeding, infection, and stone formation. Acute renal colic and excretion of small stones occur in approximately half of patients with MSK. Hypercalciuria is also common. Infection of the urinary tract is the presenting complaint in some individuals. Frank hematuria occurs less frequently. The most commonly recognized renal functional abnormalities include a decreased ability to concentrate and acidify urine, an elevated fractional excretion of sodium, and systemic acidosis secondary to renal bicarbonate loss; none of these is present in all patients. MSK is associated with several developmental and hereditary disorders, including congenital hypertrophy, Beckwith-Wiedemann syndrome, congenital pyloric stenosis, Caroli syndrome, Ehlers-Danlos syndrome, and Marfan syndrome.

ETIOLOGY/EPIDEMIOLOGY: The etiology of MSK is unknown. Its association with congenital abnormalities, the occasional finding of familial patterns, and the unchanging nature of the cystic lesions over time suggest a developmental cause. The prevalence is difficult to ascertain, because MSK is a benign condition. Estimates of its incidence in the general population range from 1 in 1,000 to 1 in 5,000 persons. Age of detection is usually between the third and fifth decades of life. Among adults, MSK has been found to occur more frequently in women.

DIAGNOSIS: Definitive diagnosis is made by intravenous urography that demonstrates papillary ductal dilatation. Ectatic tubules are imaged as striations radiating from the calyces. The radiographic pattern is referred to as a "brush" pattern. Medullary cyst formations are imaged as round opacifications in the papillae referred to as "bouquets of flowers" or "bunches of grapes." Evidence of nephrocalcinosis may also be found.

TREATMENT

Standard Therapies: The emphasis is on the prevention of complications. Urinary tract infections should be treated as indicated in the absence of MSK. Thiazide diuretics benefit those patients who develop calcium stones by decreasing the quantity of calcium excretion and the risk of intrarenal calcifications. Alkali therapy is not warranted for impaired urinary acidification, unless systemic acidemia exists. In patients with partial renal tubular acidosis, raising the urine pH may promote intraductal precipitation of calcium appetite. In contrast, alkali therapy is recommended in the setting of complete tubular acidosis because it can also help decrease urinary calcium excretion and the frequency of stone passage. Stones within the collecting system may be treated with extracorporeal shock-wave lithotripsy (ESWL). The role of ESWL in treating parenchymal stones has not been determined.

REFERENCES

Alvarado L, Walling AD. Medullary sponge kidney. *Kansas Med* 1996;97:30–32.

Grantham JJ, Nair V, Winklhofer F. Cystic diseases of the kidney. In: Brenner BM, ed. *Brenner & Rector's the kidney*, 6th ed. Philadelphia: WB Saunders, 2000:1717–1719.

Indridason, et al. Medullary sponge kidney and congenital hemi-hypertrophy. *J Am Soc Nephrol* 1996;8:1124–1130.

Nakada SY, Erturk E, Monaghan J, et al. Role of extracorporeal shock-wave lithotripsy in treatment of urolithiasis in patients with medullary sponge kidney. *Urology* 1993;41:331–333.

RESOURCES

34, 37, 308, 372

---

17   MURCS Association

Shama Shakir, MD,
and Bradley A. Warady, MD

DEFINITION: MURCS association is a sometimes lethal condition with an unusual constellation of nonrandom findings that include müllerian duct aplasia, renal aplasia, and cervical-thoracic somite dysplasia.

SYNONYMS: Klippel-Feil malformation sequence; Müllerian duct aplasia, renal aplasia, and cervical-thoracic somite malformation.

DIFFERENTIAL DIAGNOSIS: VACTERL syndrome.

SYMPTOMS AND SIGNS: Characteristically, only female infants are affected. They are born with anomalies such as hypoplasia of the craniofacial bones, rib and limb defects, anal atresia, cleft palate, micrognathia, encephalocele, or hydrocephalus. Renal anomalies such as unilateral renal agenesis, renal dysplasia, and ectopic kidney are less frequently present. Primary amenorrhea may be associated with uterine hypoplasia/aplasia, double-blind vagina, bicornuate uterus, or absence of the proximal two thirds of the vagina. Older patients may present with dyspareunia or sterility. Cervical-thoracic anomalies include hypoplasia of vertebrae, hemivertebrae, butterfly vertebrae, and other anomalies in the C5–T1 region. Rarely, bilateral corneal anesthesia and reduced sensation in the ophthalmic division of the fifth cranial nerve occurs.

ETIOLOGY/EPIDEMOLOGY: Frequency is 1 in 50,000 in females; 3 cases in males have been reported. The phenotype is greatly variable, and the etiopathologic mechanism is unknown.

DIAGNOSIS: Antenatal sonography demonstrates a massive umbilical cord related to the patent urachus, enlarged bladder, single small kidney, or suspicious urethral obstruction in a female. Prenatal MRI by ultrafast single-shot fast-spin echo sequence can show the vertebral defects. Primary amenorrhea leads to a detailed endocrine evaluation with basal and dynamic testing of the pituitary reserve. The persistence of a progesterone value within the follicular phase is diagnostic of chronic anovulation.

TREATMENT

Standard Therapies: Treatment consists of surgical correction for the various anomalies and hormonal treatment, as indicated.

REFERENCES

Kubik-Huch RA, Wisser J, Stallmach T, et al. Prenatal diagnosis of fetal malformations by ultrafast magnetic resonance imaging. *Prenat Diagn* 1998;18:1205–1208.

Lin HJ, Cornford ME, Hu B, et al. Occipital encephalocele and MURCS association. *Am J Med Genet* 1996;61:59–62.

Mahajan P, Kher A, Khungar A, et al. MURCS association: a review of 7 cases. *J Postgrad Med* 1992;38:109–111.

Mendez JP, Ulloa-Aguirre A, Sanchez FJ, et al. Endocrine evaluation in a patient with MURCS association and ovarian agenesis. *Eur J Obstet Gynecol Reprod Biol* 1986;22:161–169.

Pablo Mendez J, Orozco M, Ivan RA, et al. MURCS association and hypothalamic anovulation. *Rev Invest Clin* 1992;44:115–121.

RESOURCES

308, 372

18   Familial Juvenile Hyperuricemic Nephropathy

Anthony J. Bleyer, MD, MS

DEFINITION: Familial juvenile hyperuricemic nephropathy (FJHN) is a condition characterized by a renal tubular defect in the excretion of uric acid. Patients develop hyperuricemia and, frequently, precocious gout. Renal failure also develops over time.

SYNONYMS: Nephropathy, familial, with gout; Familial gouty nephropathy; Juvenile gouty nephropathy.

DIFFERENTIAL DIAGNOSIS: Familial focal and segmental glomerulosclerosis; Alport syndrome; Renal failure; Lesch-Nyhan syndrome; Lead intoxication; Familial intoxication with lead; Autosomal-dominant medullary cystic kidney disease type 2.

SYMPTOMS AND SIGNS: Patients develop hyperuricemia in childhood. Gout or kidney disease is variable within families and between different affected families. Gout frequently develops in the teenage years or early adulthood in both men and women. Severe tophaceous gout involving numerous joints is not uncommon in untreated individuals. Hypertension is commonly present. Laboratory studies show renal insufficiency with a slow, progressive rise in the serum creatinine level. The urinary sediment is bland, suggesting tubulointerstitial disease. The onset of renal failure is variable, with end-stage renal disease beginning sometime between the midtwenties and midsixties, depending on the kindred.

ETIOLOGY/EPIDEMIOLOGY: The predominant abnormality in this condition is a tubular defect in the ability to excrete uric acid in the urine. The cause is unclear. Because the condition is inherited in an autosomal-dominant fashion, a parent and relatives are frequently also affected with gout. The gene for FJHN has been linked to chromosome 16.

DIAGNOSIS: Patients more often present with gout. They may also present with unexplained renal failure. In both types of presentation, a strong, positive family history is frequently present. Laboratory studies are required for correct diagnosis. Patients have a serum uric acid level that is elevated compared with age- and sex-adjusted norms. The serum creatinine is also elevated, unless early in the course of the disease. A 24-hour urine collection should be performed to assess kidney function and uric acid excretion. Recent genetic and clinical evidence suggests that familial juvenile hyperuricemic nephropathy and autosomal-dominant medullary cystic kidney disease type 2 may in fact be the same disease. In medullary cystic kidney disease type 2, medullary cysts are frequently not present, and hyperuricemia is frequently seen. In some family members with familial juvenile hyperuricemic nephropathy, hyperuricemia may not be present. The gene or genes responsible for these two conditions have not been identified but are linked extremely closely on chromosome 16.

TREATMENT
Standard Therapies: Allopurinol, if started early enough, will prevent patients from developing gout. It may also prevent or delay the worsening of renal failure. Probenecid may also be useful.

Investigational Therapies: Allopurinol analogues and other therapeutic agents that metabolize uric acid are being developed.

REFERENCES
Dahan K, Fuchshuber A, Adamis S, et al. Familial juvenile hyperuricemic nephropathy and autosomal dominant medullary cystic kidney disease type 2: two facets of the same disease? *J Am Soc Nephrol* 2001;12:2348–2357.

Kamatani N, Moritani M, Yamanaka H, et al. Localization of a gene for familial juvenile hyperuricemic nephropathy to 16p12 by genome wide linkage analysis of a large family. *Arthritis Rheum* 2000;43:925–929.

McBride MB, Rigden S, Haycock GB, et al. Presymptomatic detection of juvenile hyperuricaemic nephropathy in children. *Pediatr Nephrol* 1998;12:357–364.

McBride MB, Simmonds HA, Ogg CS, et al. Efficacy of allopurinol in ameliorating the progressive renal disease in familial juvenile hyperuricaemic nephropathy (FJHN): a six year update. In: Griesmacher, et al, eds. *Purine and pyrimidine metabolism in man IX*. New York: Plenum, 1998:7–11.

McKusick VA. *Mendelian Inheritance in Man: catalogs of autosomal dominant, autosomal recessive, and x-linked phenotypes*, 12th ed. Baltimore: Johns Hopkins University Press, 1998: 1242–1243.

Puig JG, Miranda ME, Mateos FA, et al. Hereditary nephropathy associated with hyperuricemia and gout. *Arch Intern Med* 1993;153:357–365.

RESOURCES
34, 372

19   Autosomal-Recessive Polycystic Kidney Disease

Kevin E. C. Meyers, MD

DEFINITION: Autosomal-recessive polycystic kidney disease (ARPKD) is a genetic disorder associated with cystic dilatation of the collecting tubules of the kidneys, with bile duct dilatation and fibrosis or scarring of the liver's portal tracts.

DIFFERENTIAL DIAGNOSIS: Autosomal-dominant polycystic kidney disease; Multicystic dysplasia; Glomerulocystic kidney disease; Juvenile nephronophthisis; Meckel-Gruber syndrome; Jeune syndrome; Zellweger syndrome; Ivemark syndrome; Bardet-Biedel syndrome.

SYMPTOMS AND SIGNS: Most children with ARPKD present prenatally or as infants. Features at delivery may include reduced quantity of amniotic fluid or large flank masses that complicate delivery, cause respiratory distress, or lead to feeding difficulties. In severely affected infants, the lungs may be underdeveloped, the eyes deep set, the nose beaked, the jaw small, and the ears low set secondary to oligohydramnios. Children who survive beyond the first year of life do not usually develop renal insufficiency until late childhood or adolescence. Older children with ARPKD may present with abdominal enlargement secondary to increased kidney size or hepatosplenomegaly. Increased drinking and urination are commonly observed, and some children have low-serum sodium concentration. The findings of chronic renal failure (anemia, growth failure, renal osteodystrophy) appear as the child develops chronic renal insufficiency. Hypertension is commonly seen. Urinalysis may show white blood cells in the absence of infection. Older children and adolescents may have problems associated with hepatic fibrosis and splenomegaly. If symptoms become severe, liver transplantation may be needed.

ETIOLOGY/EPIDEMIOLOGY: The disease is inherited in an autosomal-recessive fashion. The gene has been localized to the long arm of chromosome 6. In the general population, ARPKD has an incidence of 1 in 6,000 to 1 in 40,000. Both sexes are affected.

DIAGNOSIS: The diagnosis is suspected on the basis of the clinical findings. Antenatal ultrasonographic diagnosis can be made by the presence of oligohydramnios, a poorly filled urinary bladder, and bilateral renal enlargement as measured by the kidney circumference:abdominal circumference ratio, and the typical hyperechogenic appearance of the kidneys in the disease. The most important indication for DNA testing is prenatal diagnosis in families with at least one affected child. Ultrasonography, endoscopic retrograde cholangiopancreatography, and magnetic resonance cholangiography can be used to diagnose nonobstructive dilatation of the intrahepatic bile ducts.

TREATMENT

Standard Therapies: Treatment is supportive and aimed at preserving renal function. This includes artificial ventilation and neonatal intensive care; sodium bicarbonate for metabolic acidosis; adequate fluid and salt supplementation; appropriate management of systemic and portal hypertension; antibiotic therapy of biliary or urinary infections; and later, treatment for chronic renal insufficiency including dialysis and renal transplantation. Things to avoid include caffeine-containing products because they enlarge the renal cysts; all nonsteroidal antiinflammatory agents because they may precipitate acute kidney failure; and contact sports to prevent damage or rupture of enlarged intraabdominal organs.

Investigational Therapy: Surgical management with removal of one or both kidneys in severely affected neonates with pulmonary hypoplasia or severe feeding difficulties is being explored, as are targeted gene therapy, gene complementation, and specific immunologic or pharmacologic interruption of growth factor pathways.

REFERENCES

Avner ED, Woychik RP, Dell KM, et al. Cellular pathophysiology of cystic kidney disease: insight into future therapies. *Int J Dev Biol* 1999;43:457–461

Hallermann C, Mucher G, Kohlschmidt N, et al. Syndrome of autosomal recessive polycystic kidneys with skeletal and facial anomalies is not linked to the ARPKD gene locus on chromosome 6p. *Am J Med Genet* 2000;90:115–119.

Nakanishi K, Sweeney WE Jr, Zerres K, et al. Proximal tubular cysts in fetal human autosomal recessive polycystic kidney disease. *J Am Soc Nephrol* 2000;11:760–763.

Zerres K, Mucher G, Becker J, et al. Prenatal diagnosis of autosomal recessive polycystic kidney disease (ARPKD): molecular genetics, clinical experience, and fetal morphology. *Am J Med Genet* 1998;76:137–144.

RESOURCES

304, 308, 372, 395

20   Bilateral Renal Agenesis

Anirut Pattaragam, MD,
and Bradley A. Warady, MD

DEFINITION: Bilateral renal agenesis refers to the complete absence of both kidneys without identifiable rudimentary tissue.

DIFFERENTIAL DIAGNOSIS: Bilateral renal hypoplasia; Bilateral renal aplasia; Ectopic kidney.

SYMPTOMS AND SIGNS: Bilateral renal agenesis is a lethal anomaly that results in either fetal loss or perinatal death. In the neonatal period, infants usually die within hours of birth as a result of pulmonary hypoplasia, probably caused by severe oligohydramnios and uterine compression. The pregnancy is always complicated by oligohydramnios in the second trimester (approximately 16 weeks of gestation), when the amniotic fluid volume is more dependent on fetal kidney function. The severe oligohydramnios leads to a restricted amniotic space, causing skeletal deformities and the Potter sequence, the latter characterized by pulmonary hypoplasia and a characteristic facial appearance with flattening of the profile and the nose, low-set ears, underdeveloped chin, and a prominent skin fold. These infants may also have associated nonurinary tract malformations of the eye, ear, and extremities.

ETIOLOGY/EPIDEMIOLOGY: Bilateral renal agenesis has an estimated incidence of 0.1–0.3 in 1,000 births. The pathogenesis is a failure of the formation of the metanephros during a very early stage of development, generally prior to the 5th week of gestation. Observations in both animal and human studies have suggested that the possible mechanism may be a failure of ureteric bud formation, failure of the bud to reach the metanephric blastema, or failure of the bud and the metanephric blastema to mutually influence one another. The condition occurs with a male:female ratio of 2.5:1. Approximately 15%–20% of patients with bilateral renal agenesis and/or dysplasia represent a familial occurrence, which leads researchers to believe this is an autosomal-dominant disorder with incomplete (50%–90%) penetrance and variable expression. The recurrence risk can be determined if the inheritance pattern and/or the recognizable syndrome are known.

DIAGNOSIS: The diagnosis is made by prenatal ultrasonography, demonstrating absence of both kidneys. Identification of the anomaly with transabdominal ultrasonography is difficult before 18 weeks of gestation. High-frequency transvaginal sonography can demonstrate the fetal urinary tract as early as 12–13 weeks of gestation, facilitating earlier diagnosis. Color Doppler ultrasonography can be an adjunct to the diagnostic evaluation.

TREATMENT
Standard Therapies: Early diagnosis and family counseling are the mainstays of management. In all new cases of bilateral renal agenesis, the parents of the affected child should undergo renal ultrasonography. If the parents show no abnormalities, each of their subsequent children has a 3.5% risk of having the disorder; if either parent shows any signs of a renal anomaly, particularly unilateral renal agenesis, the risk may be as high as 15%–20% for each subsequent birth.

REFERENCES
Cramford MA. Chromosomal and development anomalies. In: Morgan SH, Grunfeld J, eds. *Inherited disorders of the kidney,* 1st ed. New York: Oxford University Press, 1998:110–131.
Limwonase C, Clarren SK, Cassidy SB. Syndromes and malformations of the urinary tract. In: Barratt TM, Avner ED, Harmon WE, eds. *Pediatric nephrology,* 4th ed. Philadelphia: Lippincott Williams & Wilkins, 1999:427–452.
Mackenzie FM, Kingston GO, Oppenheimer L. The early prenatal diagnosis of bilateral renal agenesis using transvaginal sonography and color Doppler ultrasonography. *J Ultrasound Med* 1994;13:49–51.
Rascher W, Meyer-Schwickerath M, Olbing H. Congenital anomalies of the urinary tract. In: Davision AM, Cameron JS, Grunfeld JP, et al., eds. *Oxford textbook of clinical nephrology,* 2nd ed. New York: Oxford University Press, 1998:2543–2563.

RESOURCES
26, 34, 308, 365

21 WAGR Syndrome

Douglas Blowey, MD

DEFINITION: WAGR syndrome is a genetic syndrome in which there is a predilection to Wilms tumor, aniridia, gonadoblastoma and genitourinary abnormalities, and mental retardation. A combination of two or more of the conditions must be present for an individual to be diagnosed with WAGR syndrome.

SYNONYMS: WAGR complex; Wilms tumor–aniridia–genitourinary anomalies–mental retardation syndrome; Wilms tumor–aniridia–gonadoblastoma–mental retardation syndrome.

DIFFERENTIAL DIAGNOSIS: Denys-Drash syndrome; Frasier syndrome.

SYMPTOMS AND SIGNS: Wilms tumor is a cancer of the kidney that may involve one or both organs. An enlargement of the abdomen is usually the first symptom; abdominal pain, blood in the urine, or nonspecific symptoms such as weight loss, fever, and fatigue may also occur. Aniridia is characterized by partial or complete absence of the iris. Other disorders of the eye include cataract, nystagmus, and glaucoma. Vision is variably affected. Gonadoblastoma is a cancer of the testes or ovaries. In males, common genitourinary abnormalities include cryptorchidism and hypospadias. Some individuals with WAGR syndrome have the gonads of one sex and the external appearance of the opposite sex (pseudohermaphroditism). Mental retardation is common; however, the severity ranges from near normal intelligence to severe mental retardation. Individuals with WAGR syndrome have an increased risk for progressive kidney disease that may result in renal failure and the need for dialysis.

ETIOLOGY/EPIDEMIOLOGY: WAGR syndrome is caused by defects in the short arm of chromosome 11 at band p13. The defects occur for unknown reasons early in development. In 10% of cases, one of the patient's parents is found to have a balanced translocation.

DIAGNOSIS: The diagnosis of WAGR syndrome is based on clinical findings and chromosomal studies.

TREATMENT

Standard Therapies: Early detection of Wilms tumor can greatly improve outcome, and routine abdominal ultrasonography is recommended. Treatment programs combine surgery, radiation therapy, and chemotherapy. Treatment of the visual problems is aimed at improving vision and facilitating any unique educational needs. Medical and surgical intervention may be needed for the treatment of glaucoma and/or cataracts. Surgical correction may also be required for the genitourinary anomalies. Hormone treatment is required for those individuals who have had the gonads removed. Early and repeated developmental evaluations can identify difficulties in learning, communication, and social skills.

REFERENCES
Breslow NE, Takashima JR, Ritchey ML, et al. Renal failure in Denys-Drash and Wilms' tumor-aniridia syndromes. *Cancer Res* 2000;60:4030–4032.

Hirose M. The role of Wilms' tumor genes. *J Med Invest* 1999;46: 130–140.

Scriver CR, Beaudet AL, Sly WS, et al., eds. *The metabolic and molecular bases of inherited disease.* New York: McGraw-Hill, 2001.

RESOURCES
24, 308, 355, 412

Skeletal Disorders

1 Acheiropodia

Donald Basel, MB, BCh, and Petros Tsipouras, MD

DEFINITION: Acheiropodia is a genetic disorder that results in congenital truncation of the limbs. It is primarily found in individuals of Brazilian descent; only two siblings have been reported outside of Brazil.

SYNONYMS: Acheiropody; Handless and footless families of Brazil.

DIFFERENTIAL DIAGNOSIS: Constricting bands, congenital; Symmetric absent hands and feet.

SYMPTOMS AND SIGNS: The disorder is characterized by congenital absence of the limb components distal to humeral and tibial diaphyses, i.e., bilateral, symmetric truncation defects of the lower arm and shin. The clinical expression shows little variability among affected individuals. Occasionally, finger-like appendages may be noted on the truncated limbs. No systemic manifestations are associated with this disorder, and biochemical investigations should be normal. Intelligence and life expectancy are normal.

ETIOLOGY/EPIDEMIOLOGY: Acheiropodia is caused by a mutation in the gene *C7orf2*, which is located at 7q36 (the murine orthologue is known as Lmbr1). It is believed that the mutation arose from a single carrier and that the incidence in Brazil is approximately 1 in 250,000 births. Both sexes are affected equally.

DIAGNOSIS: The diagnosis is made in the presence of symmetric, congenital truncation defects of the limbs and in the absence of any systemic manifestations. Radiographs show complete absence of the distal epiphyses of the humeri and the components distal to the tibial diaphyses. Aplasia of the radii, ulnae, fibulae, and bony elements of both hands and feet are noted. Occasionally, there may be some rudimentary remnants of the forelimb, and an ectopic bone, the Bohomoletz bone, has been described at the distal end of the humerus.

TREATMENT

Standard Therapies: No specific therapy exists. Antenatal diagnosis may be offered to at-risk carriers where the laboratory facilities are available to identify the genetic defect.

REFERENCES
Escamilla MA, DeMille MC, Benavides E, et al. A minimalist approach to gene mapping: locating the gene for acheiropodia, by homozygosity analysis. *Am J Hum Genet* 2000; 66: 1995–2000.

Freire-Maia A. The extraordinary handless and footless families of Brazil—50 years of acheiropodia. *Am J Med Genet* 1981; 9:31–41.

Horn D, Kolb GP. Two isolated cases with symmetrically absent hands and feet. *Clin Dysmorphol* 1994;3:228–233.

Ianakiev P, van Baren MJ, Daly MJ, et al. Acheiropodia is caused by a genomic deletion in C7orf2, the human orthologue of the *Lmbr1* gene. *Am J Hum Genet* 2001;68:38–45.

Toledo SPA, Saldanha PH. A radiological and genetic investigation of acheiropody in a kindred including six cases. *J Hum Genet* 1969;17:81–94.

RESOURCES
188, 351

2 Acromesomelic Dysplasias Due to Mutations of the *CDMP-1* Gene: Grebe Syndrome and Hunter-Thompson Acromesomelic Dysplasia

Donald Basel, MB, BCh, and Petros Tsipouras, MD

DEFINITION: The acromesomelic dysplasias—Grebe syndrome (AMDG) and Hunter-Thompson acromesomelic dysplasia (AMDH)—are characterized by short-limbed dwarfism. The distal elements of the limbs are shorter than their proximal counterparts, and the hands show variable degrees of shortening.

SYNONYMS: Acromesomelic dysplasia; Acromesomelic dysplasia, Hunter-Thompson type; Acromesomelic dysplasia, Grebe type; Achondrogenesis, Brazilian; Grebe chondrodysplasia; Grebe dysplasia.

DIFFERENTIAL DIAGNOSIS: Acromesomelic dysplasia, Maroteaux type; Pseudoachondroplasia; Acrodysostosis.

SYMPTOMS AND SIGNS: Both AMDH and AMDG cause congenital dwarfism with a proximal-distal gradient of severity. Grebe syndrome tends to be more severe, whereas AMDH shows variable severity and some overlap with AMDG. In both disorders, the humeri and femora are relatively normal. In AMDG, the radii/ulnae and tibiae/fibulae are significantly shortened and deformed, whereas the carpal and tarsal bones are fused. In AMDH, the radii/ulnae and tibiae/fibulae are of variable length, and dislocations of the hips, knees, ankles, and elbows are common. The hands/feet in AMDH show significant shortening of the metacarpals/metatarsals and the phalanges appear almost square. In AMDG, several metacarpal and metatarsal bones are absent, as are the proximal and middle phalanges of the fingers and toes.

ETIOLOGY/EPIDEMIOLOGY: Both AMDG and AMDH are caused by mutations in the *CPMP-1* gene, located on chromosome 20q11.2. Male and female offspring of gene carriers are equally at risk.

DIAGNOSIS: Diagnosis is made based on clinical and radiologic evaluation of the patient. It can be confirmed by the presence of a mutation in the *CDMP-1* gene. Radiographs of the skull and vertebral column are normal, whereas the appendicular skeleton may show many abnormalities. In AMDG, the humerus shows a shallow trochlear depth and a severely malformed middle segment. Hypoplasia of the ulna and angulation of the radius in the middle and at the neck are common, whereas the distal radius is variably formed. The femora may show a decrease in the length of the diaphysis and asymmetry of the femoral condyles. The articular components of the tibia are severely deformed, and both tibial and fibular diaphyses are absent. The lateral malleolus is also absent in most affected individuals, whereas the patellae tend to be hypoplastic. The carpal and tarsal bones are fused, as are the metacarpal and metatarsal bones, which may also be absent. The proximal and middle phalangeal bones are absent in most cases, whereas the distal phalanx is mostly present. In AMDH, the primary differences appear to be quantitative, with AMDG showing a more significant shortening of the bones. Polydactyly is not associated with AMDH, and the carpal/tarsal bones are not all fused, although there may be one fusion. The digits generally have two or three phalanges. The hips show hypoplastic acetabulae and a tendency toward precocious osteoarthritis, often in association with dislocations.

TREATMENT

Standard Therapies: No specific treatment is available. Each patient should be evaluated individually for any potential management. Antenatal diagnosis may be offered to at-risk carriers, either through molecular studies or high-resolution ultrasonography scanning in the second trimester.

REFERENCES

Costa T, Ramsby G, Cassia F, et al. Grebe syndrome: clinical and radiographic findings in affected individuals and heterozygous carriers. *Am J Med Genet* 1998;75:523–529.

Hunter AGW, Thompson MW. Acromesomelic dwarfism: description of a patient and comparison with previously reported cases. *Hum Genet* 1976;34:107–113.

Langer LO, Cervenka J, Camargo M. A severe autosomal recessive acromesomelic dysplasia, the Hunter-Thompson type, and comparison with the Grebe type. *Hum Genet* 1989;81:323–328.

Romeo G, Zonana J, Rimoin DL, et al. Heterogeneity of nonlethal severe short-limbed dwarfism. *J Pediatr* 1977;91:918–923.

Thomas JT, Kilpatrick M, Lin K, et al. Disruption of human limb morphogenesis by a dominant negative mutation in cartilage-derived morphogenetic protein-1. *Nat Genet* 1997;17:58–64.

RESOURCES

246, 253, 351

---

3 Acromesomelic Dysplasia, Maroteaux Type

Donald Basel, MB, BCh,
and Petros Tsipouras, MD

DEFINITION: Acromesomelic dysplasia, Maroteaux type, is a disorder that belongs to a heterogeneous group of skeletal dysplasias that cause disproportionate shortening of the forelimbs and digits.

SYNONYMS: Acromesomelic dwarfism; St. Helena dysplasia.

DIFFERENTIAL DIAGNOSIS: Hunter-Thompson acromesomelic dysplasia; Grebe syndrome; Pseudoachondroplasia; Psuedohypoparathyroidism; Acrodysostosis.

SYMPTOMS AND SIGNS: The primary feature is congenital dwarfism with shortening of the middle and distal segments of the appendicular skeleton. The forearms and shins are primarily shortened, whereas the arm, thigh, and trunk are of normal proportion. Both hands and feet show brachydactyly. Extension of the arm at the elbow may be limited by the bony deformities. The syndrome is associated with dysmorphic features that include frontal bossing, midfacial hypoplasia, and a small nose. The overall head size is usually normal, as is intelligence. Lumbar spinal stenosis has been reported; therefore, an enlarged head circumference should alert the clinician to the possible presence of hydrocephalus. In infancy, the vertebral bodies may be oval shaped; this later evolves into posterior wedging of the vertebral bodies, which has been described in association with kyphosis. The remaining systems are unaffected. Early slowing of growth velocity results in an average adult height of approximately 115 cm. The severity of the disorder may vary among affected individuals.

ETIOLOGY/EPIDEMIOLOGY: Acromesomelic dysplasia, Maroteaux type, is inherited as an autosomal-recessive disorder in which heterozygous carriers are unaffected. The gene responsible for this malformation has been localized to the pericentromeric region of chromosome 9. Both sexes are equally affected.

DIAGNOSIS: The diagnosis is extremely difficult to make in infancy, but should be considered in any infant or individual with mesomelic shortening of the limbs in association with brachydactyly. The radiologic findings include bowed radii and a shortened radius and ulna, often in conjunction with dislocation of the radial head. Hypoplasia of the proximal radius and distal ulna has been reported, whereas the tibia and fibula, although short, are otherwise normal. The tubular bones of the digits become progressively shorter in the first year of life and show characteristic cone-shaped epiphyses. The linear growth of the bones is abnormal. The spine may show wedging with a shortened dorsal margin. The clavicles curve superiorly and appear high in relation to the thorax. In childhood, the pelvis shows hypoplasia of the basilar portion of the ilia and irregular ossification of the superior acetabula. The rest of the skeletal survey is normal. The metabolic screen is normal, as are growth hormone studies.

TREATMENT
Standard Therapies: No specific treatment is available for this skeletal abnormality. Each patient should be appraised individually for management of symptoms.

REFERENCES
Haliloglu M, Ozen H, Unsal M. Acromesomelic dysplasia associated with mild lumbar spine stenosis. *Eur Radiol* 1999;9:103–104.

Ianakiev P, Kilpatrick MW, Daly MJ, et al. Localization of acromesomelic dysplasia on chromosome 9 by homozygosity mapping. *Clin Genet* 2000;57:278–283.

Kant SG, Polinkovsky A, Mundlos S, et al. Acromesomelic dysplasia Maroteaux type maps to human chromosome 9. *Am J Hum Genet* 1998;63:155–162.

Langer LO, Garrett RT. Acromesomelic dysplasia. *Radiology* 1980;137:349–355.

Maroteaux P, Martinelli B, Campailla E. Le nanisme acromesomelique. *Presse Med* 1971;79:1839–1842.

RESOURCES
246, 253, 351

---

4   Antley-Bixler Syndrome

Khalid Khoshhal, MD,
and Mervyn Letts, MD, FRCS(C)

DEFINITION: Antley-Bixler syndrome (ABS) is a disorder of bone and cartilage characterized by craniosynostosis, frontal bossing, depressed nasal bridge, joint contractures, and multiple skeletal fusions.

SYNONYMS: Craniosynostosis; Choanal atresia; Radial humeral synostosis; Multisynostotic osteodysgenesis; Trapezoidcephaly–multiple synostosis.

DIFFERENTIAL DIAGNOSIS: Primary craniosynostosis; Camptomelic dysplasia; Acrocephalosyndactyly syndromes (Apert syndrome, Crouzon disease, Saethre-Chotzen syndrome, Pfeiffer syndrome, Carpenter syndrome, Sakati syndrome, Goodman syndrome, Summitt syndrome); Osteogenesis imperfecta.

SYMPTOMS AND SIGNS: Antley-Bixler syndrome is characterized by craniofacial and skeletal abnormalities. Craniofacial abnormalities include craniosynostosis, frontal bossing, midface hypoplasia, depressed nasal bridge, proptosis, and dysplastic ears (Insert Fig. 60).

Skeletal abnormalities include joint contractures (most commonly elbow contracture due to radiohumeral synostosis, or less commonly due to radioulnar synostosis), arachnodactyly, camptodactylyl and long bone (most commonly the femur then the ulna) bowing, and perinatal fractures. Rocker-bottom feet, clubfeet, synostosis of carpal and tarsal bones, and vertebral body anomalies are less common skeletal abnormalities (Insert Fig. 61). Choanal stenosis or atresia is common and might lead to life-threatening complications. Other common defects are urogenital anomalies. Less commonly seen are cardiac defects, partial cutaneous syndactyly, and narrow chest and pelvis. Mental retardation is not a constant finding (some patients have normal intelligence, and it is likely that brain development is normal if craniectomy is performed to treat sutural synostosis and if secondary factors, such as apnea, are avoided).

ETIOLOGY/EPIDEMIOLOGY: The cause of ABS is unknown, but its occurrence in two pairs of siblings suggests that it is inherited as an autosomal-recessive trait. It also may result from spontaneous (sporadic) mutations (*FGFR2* gene mutations). A phenocopy of the ABS can occur in the offspring of mothers taking the antifungal agent fluconazole during early pregnancy. Males and females are both affected, with a ratio of females:males of 7:1.

DIAGNOSIS: The diagnosis can be made prenatally with utrasonographic examination by observing specific skull and skeletal anomalies. After birth, this diagnosis is usually made based on characteristic clinical findings.

TREATMENT
Standard Therapies: Treatment is symptomatic and supportive. Early deaths are usually caused by upper airway obstruction, which may require tracheostomy. Surgical treatment of choanal atresia or stenosis may be lifesaving. Surgery may also correct certain craniofacial, skeletal, cardiac, urogenital, or other potentially associated abnormalities. Physical therapy is recommended to improve range of movement at certain joints. Genetic counseling is important.

REFERENCES
Antley RM, Bixler D. Trapezoidcephaly, midface hypoplasia, and cartilage abnormalities with multiple synostosis and skeletal fractures. *Birth Defects* 1975;11:397.
Crisponi G, Porcu C, Piu ME. Antley-Bixler syndrome: case report and review of the literature. *Clin Dysmorph* 1997;6:61–68.
DeLozier CD, Antley RM, Williams R, et al. The syndrome of multisynostotic osteodysgenesis with long-bone fractures. *Am J Med Genet* 1980;7:391–403.
Escobar LF, Bixler D, Sadove M, et al. Antley-Bixler syndrome from a prognostic perspective: report of a case and review of the literature. *Am J Med Genet* 1988;29:829–836.
Rumball KM, Pang E, Letts RM. Musculoskeletal manifestations of the Antley-Bixler syndrome. *J Pediatr Orthop* 1999;8:139–143.

RESOURCES
96, 149, 361

5   Borjeson-Forssman-Lehmann Syndrome

Meral Gunay-Aygun, MD, PhD

DEFINITION: Borjeson-Forssman-Lehmann syndrome (BFLS) is characterized by mental retardation, short stature, obesity, hypogonadism, epilepsy, and typical craniofacial features.

SYNONYM: Borjeson syndrome.

DIFFERENTIAL DIAGNOSIS: Prader-Willi syndrome; Coffin-Lowry syndrome; Bardet-Biedl syndrome.

SYMPTOMS AND SIGNS: Typical craniofacial features include large and thick (but normally formed) ears and "grotesque" facial features with prominent supraorbital ridges, deep-set eyes, ptosis, and narrow palpebral fissures. At birth, the ears are large in the long axis, particularly involving the ear lobe. Mental retardation of variable severity is a constant feature of males with BFLS. Microcephaly is common, and electroencephalography results are markedly abnormal with poor alpha rhythms. Seizures may be present. Eye involvement including optic nerve and retinal abnormalities, ptosis, and nystagmus are common. All males have genital hypoplasia and poorly developed secondary sexual characteristics. Both hypothalamic and gonadal abnormalities are shown to contribute to hypogonadism. Other endocrine abnormalities include adult-onset diabetes mellitus and short stature. Size at birth is normal. Deceleration of growth begins at 8–10 years of age, and final adult height ranges from 140 to 150 cm in men and from 125 to 155 cm in women. Truncal obesity starting late in infancy or early in childhood is another common feature. Skeletal radiographic abnormalities in affected males include a steep radiocarpal angle, delayed bone age, vertebral abnormalities, small femoral and/or humeral heads, narrow cervical spinal canal, and hypoplasia of distal phalanges. Carrier females have milder and more variable findings such as mental functions ranging from normal to severely retarded, relatively large ears, obesity, coarse facial appearance, delayed secondary sexual characteristics, and variable radiographic abnormalities.

ETIOLOGY/EPIDEMIOLOGY: Only 5–10 affected families have been reported. The inheritance pattern is X-linked recessive. Males are severely affected. Females can also be severely affected depending on the ratio of the cells with the abnormal X chromosome as the active X chromosome. The syndrome is mapped to Xq26-q27. Candidate genes include *FGF2* (fibroblast growth factor homologous factor 2) and *SOX3* genes.

DIAGNOSIS: The diagnosis is based on clinical findings. Skeletal radiography findings such as feet changes including short toes may be supportive, especially for diagnosing carrier females.

TREATMENT
Standard Therapies: Treatment is symptomatic.

REFERENCES
Ardinger HH, Hanson JW, Zellweger HU. Borjeson-Forssman-Lehmann syndrome: further delineation in five cases. *Am J Med Genet* 1984;19:653–664.
Borjeson M, Forssman H, Lehmann O. An X-linked, recessively inherited syndrome characterized by grave mental deficiency, epilepsy, and endocrine disorder. *Acta Med Scand* 1962; 171:13–21.
Gecz J, Baker E, Donnelly A, et al. Fibroblast growth factor homologous factor 2 (FHF2): gene structure, expression and mapping to the Borjeson-Forssman-Lehmann syndrome region in Xq26 delineated by a duplication breakpoint in a BFLS-like patient. *Hum Genet* 1999;104:56–63.
Gedeon AK, Kozman HM, Robinson H, et al. Refinement of the background genetic map of Xq26-q27 and gene locatisation for Borjeson-Forssman-Lehmann syndrome. *Am J Med Genet* 1996;64:63–68.
Kubota T, Oga S, Ohashi H, et al. Borjeson-Forssman-Lehmann syndrome in a woman with skewed X-chromosome inactivation. *Am J Med Genet* 1999;87:258–261.

RESOURCES
96, 361, 368, 462

---

6   Campomelic Syndrome

John M. Opitz, MD

DEFINITION: The campomelic syndrome is a genetic multiple congenital anomalies syndrome characterized by shortness of stature; congenital bowing of long bones, especially of tibiae, but sometimes also of femurs and/or upper limbs; a characteristic facial appearance of multiple minor anomalies; cleft palate; multiple other skeletal anomalies; developmental delay (not in all patients); tracheobronchial hypoplasia; and incomplete development of external (and at times internal) genitalia in genetic males, making some of them appear like infant girls.

SYNONYMS: Camptomelic syndrome; *SRY-Box 9, SOX9,* mutations syndrome; Autosomal sex reversal (SRA1) syndrome 1; Acampomelic campomelic "dysplasia."

DIFFERENTIAL DIAGNOSIS: Osteogenesis imperfecta; Hypophosphatasia; Nonsyndromal congenital bowing of the legs.

SYMPTOMS AND SIGNS: Intrauterine growth is usually not retarded, but prenatal shortness occurs. Signs of the

disorder include a skull that is relatively large, long, and narrow with high forehead and flat facial profile; anteversion of nostrils and micrognathia; cleft of palate (or of uvula), or submucous cleft with velopharyngeal incompetence; regurgitation of formula through the nose; and predisposition to frequent middle ear infections. Frequent respiratory distress may occur. The tracheobronchial tree may be unstable and/or underdeveloped with a reduced number of incompletely formed, soft cartilage rings associated with more or less severe stridor, impairment of oxygenation, and risk of right heart failure. The cervical and thoracic vertebrae may have absence of ossification or lack of pedicles. Defects of the lower limbs may include dislocated hips and the Middleton triad of anterior bowing of the tibiae, and dimple over the apex of the bowing and clubfoot deformity. Small scapulae are of diagnostic value. Genetic (46,XY) males may have "intersex" or female genitalia. Absence of olfactory lobes and occasional heart and renal malformations may occur.

ETIOLOGY/EPIDEMIOLOGY: The disorder is caused by either mutations in the *SOX9* gene or disturbance (at times through chromosome rearrangements) of regulatory elements of the gene located over a large region upstream (or 5') of *SOX9*. Prevalence of the disorder is unknown.

DIAGNOSIS: Diagnosis is made based on clinical appearance as well as radiographic studies of vertebrae, hips, chest, legs, and feet. Ultrasonography of kidneys and echocardiography of the heart should be performed. Molecular studies may confirm presence of a *SOX9* mutation.

TREATMENT

Standard Therapies: The respiratory system should be supported and stabilized (supplementary oxygen, possibly tracheostomy). With deficiency of cervical vertebral pedicles, early referral to neurosurgery is indicated to consider the need for a collar and/or fusion of neck vertebrae. Other therapies include scoliosis surveillance, closure of cleft palate, and vigorous treatment of middle ear infections to prevent hearing loss. Gastrostomy (G-button) feedings may be helpful. Reassignment of sex should be considered in cases of intersex or female genitalia in a genetic male. Orthopedic treatment for hip dislocation (Pavlick harness) and clubfeet (casts or surgery) is indicated. The bowed tibiae usually straighten spontaneously.

REFERENCES

Foster JW, Dominguez-Steglich MA, Guioli S, et al. Campomelic dysplasia and autosomal sex reversal caused by mutations in an SRY-related gene. *Nature* 1994;37:525–530.

Houston CS, Opitz JM, Spranger JW, et al. The campomelic syndrome: review, report of 17 cases, and follow-up on the currently 17-year-old boy first reported by Maroteaux et al in 1971. *Am J Med Genet* 1983;15:3–28.

Mansour S, Hall CM, Pembrey ME, et al. A clinical and genetic study of campomelic dysplasia. *J Med Genet* 1995;32:415–420.

Marouteaux P, Spranger JW, Opitz JM et al. Le syndrome campomélique. *Presse Med* 1971;22:1157–1162.

Neri G, Opitz JM. Syndromal (and nonsyndromal) forms of male pseudoehrmaphroditism. *Am J Med Genet* 1999;89:201–209.

Olney PN, Kean LS, Graham D, et al. Campomelic syndrome and deletion of *SOX9*. *Am J Med Genet* 1999;84:20–24.

Wunderle VM, Critcher R, Hastie N, et al. Deletion of long-range regulatory elements upstream of *SOX9* causes campomelic dysplasia. *Proc Natl Acad Sci USA* 1998;95:10649–10654.

RESOURCES

188, 246, 351

---

7   Camurati-Engelmann Disease

Katrien Janssens, Wendy Ballemans, and Wim Van Hul, PhD

DEFINITION: Camurati-Engelmann disease (CED) is a bone dysplasia caused by mutations in *TGFB1*. Patients show an increased bone density in the long bones and at the skull base and mainly suffer from pain, claudication, general weakness, and fatigue.

SYNONYMS: Progressive diaphyseal dysplasia; Diaphyseal dysplasia Camurati-Engelmann.

DIFFERENTIAL DIAGNOSIS: Van Buchem disease; Ribbing disease; Craniodiaphyseal dysplasia; Paget disease.

SYMPTOMS AND SIGNS: Patients have pain in the lower and upper limbs, easy fatigability, and muscle weakness. A common symptom is a typical waddling gait, which can be seen as early as when the child starts to walk. Encroachment of nerves in the skull and bony overgrowth in the internal auditory canal can cause facial paralysis, hearing difficulties, imbalance, vertigo, and tinnitus. Similarly, encroachment of sclerotic bone on the orbit or optic nerves can lead to exophthalmos and loss of vision. Occasionally, other symptoms such as reduced subcutaneous fat, poor appetite, headache, and delayed puberty have been described. Systemic manifestations include mild anemia, leukopenia, and hepatosplenomegaly. Radiologically, sclerosis of the cortex of the diaphyses of the long bones is evident. The bones are affected in a fixed order: tibia, femur, fibula, humerus, ulna, radius. Sclerosis can expand to the metaphyses, but the epiphyses are typically spared. Accretion of new bone at the periosteal side causes the diaphyses to become thicker than the epiphyses. At the endosteal side, a narrowing or even complete obliteration of the medullary canal occurs. In the most severe cases, the mandibula, vertebrae, thoracic cage, shoulder girdle, and carpal and tarsal bones are involved. Scintigraphically, accumulation of ^{99m}Tc methylene diphosphonate can be seen at sites of active remodeling.

ETIOLOGY/EPIDEMIOLOGY: The disorder is inherited in an autosomal-dominant mode. Five missense mutations and one small, inframe duplication in *TGFB1* have been described, causing CED in 24 families. Genetic heterogeneity cannot be ruled out, however. The prevalence is estimated to be less than 1 in 1 million. Affected families and sporadic patients are found in Asia, America, and Europe.

DIAGNOSIS: Diagnosis can be made based on radiographs. Bilateral affection of the lower and upper limbs is typical, with a marked thickening of the cortex and a narrowed medullary canal. The lining of the long bones is irregular. Clinically, the waddling gait and painful limbs can give an indication of CED; however, large inter- and intrafamilial variability exists, both in clinical and radiologic symptoms. In some patients, abnormal values in bone formation and resorption markers are present, but this is not generalized.

TREATMENT
Standard Therapies: Reaming of the medullary canal has been performed and results in pain relief, but the obliteration recurs. Another option is resection of the cortex, although this diminishes the strength of the bone. By way of craniotomy, the orbital contents and optic nerves can be decompressed. Glucocorticoids such as prednisolone and dexamethasone can alleviate the symptoms of pain, fatigue, muscle weakness, and headache, but do not alter the radiologic symptoms. It is uncertain whether biphosphonates such as pamidronate are helpful; both relief and worsening of pain have been described.

REFERENCES
Janssens K, Gershoni-Baruch R, Guañabens N, et al. Mutations in the gene encoding the latency-associated peptide of TGF-β1 cause Camurati-Engelmann disease. *Nat Genet* 2000; 26:273–275.
Janssens K, Gershoni-Baruch R, Van Hul E, et al. Localisation of the gene causing diaphyseal dysplasia Camurati-Engelmann to chromosome 19q13. *J Med Genet* 2000;37:245–249.
Kinoshita A, Takashi S, Tomita H, et al. Domain-specific mutations in *TGFB1* result in Camurati-Engelmann disease. *Nat Genet* 2000;26:19–20.
Naveh Y, Kaftori JK, Alon U, et al. Progressive diaphyseal dysplasia: genetics and clinical and radiological manifestations. *Pediatrics* 1984;74:399–405.
Sparkes RS, Graham CB. Camurati-Engelmann disease: genetics and clinical manifestations with a review of the literature. *J Med Genet* 1972;9:73–85.

RESOURCES
347, 351, 462

---

8 Coffin-Siris Syndrome

Eva M. McGhee, PhD

DEFINITION: Coffin-Siris syndrome is a genetic condition characterized by intrauterine growth retardation, developmental delay, coarse face, hypoplastic fifth fingers and nails, hirsutism, and initial difficulties with feeding. Additional findings include ptosis, recurrent respiratory problems, structural brain anomalies, and cardiac anomalies.

SYNONYM: Fifth digit syndrome.

DIFFERENTIAL DIAGNOSIS: Dandy-Walker syndrome.

SYMPTOMS AND SIGNS: Coffin-Siris syndrome is characterized by a combination of coarse features, developmental delay, sparse hair, and facial abnormalities (wide nose or mouth, low nasal bridge, and thick lips). Hypoplastic nails, short stature of prenatal onset, hypotonia, sparse scalp hair, deficient terminal phalanges, feeding difficulties, frequent infections, delayed dentition, and heart defects also may be present.

ETIOLOGY/EPIDEMIOLOGY: The cause of Coffin-Siris syndrome is unknown; its occurrence in siblings of unaffected parents indicates the disease may be autosomal recessive. It is seen in both sexes, but more often in females than males (female:male ratio is approximately 4:1).

DIAGNOSIS: No molecular, cellular, biochemical, or cytogenetic test is available to diagnose Coffin-Siris syndrome. The diagnosis is based on clinical findings. Because some patients have shown a karyotype of chromosomal aberrations, chromosome analysis should be performed.

TREATMENT
Standard Therapies: No treatment is currently available. The most common operations reported in patients with Coffin-Siris syndrome include cardiac surgery, gastric placement fundoplication, hernia repair, ear tube place-

ment, and adenoid removal. Tracheostomy, pulmonary artery banding, eye surgery, and tear duct probing have also been performed.

REFERENCES

Coffin GS, Siris E. Mental retardation with absent fifth fingernail and terminal phalanx. *Am J Dis Child* 1970;119:433–439.

Fleck BJ, Pandya A, Vanner L, et al. Coffin Siris syndrome: review and presentation of new cases from a questionnaire study. *Am J Med Genet* 2001;99:1–7.

McGhee EM, Klump CJ, Bitts SM, et al. Candidate region for Coffin-Siris syndrome at 7q32→34. *Am J Med Genet* 2000;93:241–243.

McKusick VA. *Mendelian Inheritance in Man,* 12th ed. Baltimore: Johns Hopkins University Press, 1998:676–677.

McPherson EW, Laneri G, Clemens MM, et al. Apparently balanced t(1;7)(q21.3;q34) in an infant with Coffin-Siris syndrome. *Am J Med Genet* 1997;71:430–433.

RESOURCES

351, 362, 462

9 Cornelia de Lange Syndrome

Antonie D. Kline, MD

DEFINITION: Cornelia de Lange syndrome (CdLS) is a genetic syndrome of proportionate small stature affecting all systems, but primarily the craniofacial, gastrointestinal, musculoskeletal, and neurodevelopmental systems.

SYNONYMS: de Lange syndrome; Brachmann–de Lange syndrome.

DIFFERENTIAL DIAGNOSIS: Rubinstein-Taybi syndrome; Chromosome abnormality (duplication 3q syndrome); Fetal alcohol syndrome; Scott craniodigital syndrome.

SYMPTOMS AND SIGNS: Paramount in CdLS is growth retardation that is of prenatal onset and persists throughout life, along with microcephaly. Most affected patients have a similar facial appearance (Insert Fig. 62). Synophrys is typical, with an arched appearance. Eyelashes are long and curly. Ears may be thick, dysplastic, low-set, or posteriorly rotated. The midface is flattened. The nose is short with anteverted nares. The philtrum tends to be long and tented. The mouth may have downturned corners, a thin upper lip, high palate, micrognathia, and a bluish discoloration circumferentially. Occasionally, cleft palate is present. Feeding problems and gastroesophageal reflux disease (GERD) are common. Patients can present in infancy with congenital diaphragmatic hernia or later with pyloric stenosis. Congenital heart disease occurs in 25% of patients, typically as septal defects. Typical extremity findings include small hands and feet. Malformations of the upper limbs are present in approximately 30% of patients, and may range from transverse terminal deficiencies to absent forearm bones. Other extremity anomalies include brachydactyly, clinodactyly of the fifth fingers, single transverse palmar creases, proximally placed shortened thumbs, dislocated radial head, hip abnormalities, partial syndactyly of toes 2 and 3, and bunions. Genitourinary malformations include renal anomalies, micropenis, hypospadias and/or cryptorchidism in males, and uterine anomalies in females. Other findings are generalized hirsutism and a low posterior hairline, as well as cutis marmarata. Neurologically, there is a tendency toward hypertonicity. Gait is wide based with a slightly stooped position. Seizures occur in 20% of patients. There may be a low-pitched cry in infancy. Deafness may be present, both sensorineural and conductive. Ophthalmologic findings include high myopia, ptosis, nystagmus, nasolacrimal duct malformations, and blepharitis. Developmental abilities range from normal IQ with learning disabilities to profound mental retardation. Behavioral disorders, such as attention deficit disorder with or without hyperactivity, aggression, defiance, self-injury, and perseveration, are common.

ETIOLOGY/EPIDEMIOLOGY: Most cases are sporadic, although familial cases have been reported, both with affected parents and children, and with affected siblings. Recurrence risk has been estimated at 1.5%. No microdeletion or duplication has been found, although there is some clinical overlap with cases involving duplication of the long arm of chromosome 3 (3q25). The prevalence is estimated to be 1 in 10,000. All ethnic groups are affected.

DIAGNOSIS: The diagnosis is made clinically. PAPP-A has been found to be reduced retrospectively on second trimester maternal blood samples.

TREATMENT

Standard Therapies: Treatment is generally preventative. Growth charts for CdLS are available. A workup for GERD is essential initially and for any suspected symptoms. Developmental assessments should be regular, and services initiated and used. Routine audiology, ophthalmology, and pediatric dentistry visits are recommended.

REFERENCES

Ireland M. Cornelia de Lange syndrome. In: Cassidy SB, Allanson JE, eds. *Management of genetic syndromes.* New York: Wiley-Liss, 2001:85–102.

Jackson L, Kline AD, Barr MA, et al. de Lange syndrome: a clinical review of 310 individuals. *Am J Med Genet* 1993;47:940–946.

Kline AD, Barr M, Jackson LG. Growth manifestations in the Brachmann-de Lange syndrome. *Am J Med Genet* 1993;47: 1042–1049.

Opitz JM. Editorial comment: the Brachmann-de Lange syndrome. *Am J Med Genet* 1985;22:89–102.

RESOURCES

96, 113, 114, 119

10   Crouzon Syndrome

Millie D. Long, MD, and Kant Y. K. Lin, MD

DEFINITION: Crouzon syndrome is characterized by craniosynostosis, maxillary hypoplasia, shallow orbits, and bilateral exorbitism.

DIFFERENTIAL DIAGNOSIS: Simple craniosynostosis; Pfeiffer syndrome; Apert syndrome; Jackson-Weiss syndrome; Saethre-Chotzen syndrome.

SYMPTOMS AND SIGNS: Crouzon syndrome typically involves both the cranium and the face, but variability of expression characterizes the syndrome. Various skull shapes have been reported based on the order, rate, and progression of sutural synostosis. Brachycephaly, scaphocephaly, trigonocephaly, and cloverleaf skull have all been observed. Shallow orbits with ocular proptosis are essential diagnostic criteria. Other associated facial features include hypertelorbitism, divergent strabismus, maxillary midface hypoplasia, and a short upper lip. Abnormalities of the central nervous system include progressive hydrocephalus, chronic cerebellar herniation, and jugular foramen stenosis, which occur with significant frequency. Early closure of the sutures, particularly if multiple sutures are involved, can be responsible for intracranial hypertension, leading to frequent headaches, seizures, and mental deficiency if left untreated. Intelligence is generally normal to low-normal. Vision problems can occur as a result of ocular proptosis. Conjunctivitis is frequently observed, and luxation of the globes has occurred in severe cases. Exotropia, poor vision, and optic atrophy occur. Lateral palatal swellings are common, but cleft lip and cleft palate are less so. Due to the midface hypoplasia, dental arch width is reduced and the maxillary arch is shortened.

Crowding of maxillary teeth and crossbite are therefore common. There is a small incidence of cervical spine abnormalities. Conductive hearing deficit can occur due to atresia of the external auditory canals. Calcification of the stylohyoid ligament is also common. Limb abnormalities such as mild defects in the hands, elbow stiffness, and carpal fusions have been associated with Crouzon syndrome, but they are infrequently seen.

ETIOLOGY/EPIDEMIOLOGY: Crouzon syndrome follows an autosomal-dominant pattern of inheritance, but approximately 30% of cases represent a new mutation. The frequency of the syndrome is estimated to be 1 in 25,000 in the general population. Increased paternal age at conception has been a significant factor in contributing to new mutations. The syndrome accounts for 4.5% of all cases of craniosynostosis. More than 30 variations have been identified, perhaps explaining the variability of expressivity. Most are related to amino acid substitutions located on the fibroblast growth factor receptor (*FGFR*) 2 gene on chromosome 10.

DIAGNOSIS: Diagnosis can be made on physical examination, demonstrating the clinical observation of a brachycephalic anterior cranial vault with shallow, hyperteloric orbits and globe proptosis. Genetic analysis can confirm the diagnosis if one of the known mutations is encountered. The skeletal abnormalities can be better defined by quantitative CT scan analysis.

TREATMENT

Standard Therapies: Treatment is determined by the functional problems encountered in the patient, and is often performed in stages throughout the early years of life. Most treatments are surgical, and early referral to a multidisciplinary craniofacial team, with craniofacial plastic surgeons, neurosurgeons, otolaryngologists, ophthalmologists, pediatric critical care specialists, pediatric anesthesiologists, geneticists, neuroradiologists, speech language pathologists, audiologists, and oral surgeons, is critical. Generally, the skull deformities are addressed during infancy, especially if there is evidence or suspicion of intracranial hypertension or hydrocephalus. Orbital and facial deformities are addressed during early childhood and the jaws are corrected during adolescence.

REFERENCES

Cohen MM, Maclean RE, eds. *Craniosynostosis: diagnosis, evaluation and management,* 2nd ed. New York: Oxford University Press, 2000:86–87, 278–282, 361–365.

Gorlin RJ, Cohen MM, Levin LS, eds. *Syndromes of the head and neck,* 3rd ed. New York: Oxford University Press, 1990:524–526.

RESOURCES

121, 124, 149, 462

---

11 Diastrophic Dysplasia

Andrea Superti-Furga, MD

DEFINITION: Diastrophic dysplasia is a genetic disorder affecting the skeleton, joints, and ligaments. Its main features are short stature, clubfeet, and restriction of movements at large and small joints.

SYNONYM: Diastrophic dwarfism (no longer used).

DIFFERENTIAL DIAGNOSIS: Spondyloepiphyseal dysplasia; Spondyloepimetaphyseal dysplasia; Metatropic dysplasia.

SYMPTOMS AND SIGNS: At birth, affected infants have short limbs, clubfeet, radially deviated thumbs ("hitchhiker thumbs"), cleft palate, transient and painful swelling of the ear pinna, and hemangioma on the forehead. In childhood, the disorder is characterized by short stature with progressive scoliosis or kyphoscoliosis, short ribs, contractures of large and small joints, ulnar deviation of the fingers, and clubfoot with poor response to treatment. Hearing and vision are usually not impaired. In adulthood, patients have stature between 100 and 140 cm (classic diastrophic dysplasia), scoliosis or kyphoscoliosis, joint contractures (hip, knee, fingers, and toes), clubfoot (if not corrected), and arthrosis (hips and knees).

ETIOLOGY/EPIDEMIOLOGY: Diastrophic dysplasia is a genetic, autosomal-recessive disorder caused by mutations in the gene coding for a sulfate transporter of the cell membrane, called *DTDST* or *SLC26A2.* Both sexes are affected. This is part of a spectrum of disorders originating from mutations in the *DTDST* gene that includes two lethal conditions, achondrogenesis 1B and atelosteogenesis 2; the severe but usually nonlethal condition diastrophic dysplasia; and a milder condition with normal stature, recessive multiple epiphyseal dysplasia. The precise incidence of each of these disorders is not known, but as a group they may be relatively frequent.

DIAGNOSIS: Diagnostic assessment of a child with suspected skeletal dysplasia includes measurement of standing height, sitting height, and head circumference; clinical examination including neurologic and orthopedic details; and a complete radiographic survey of the skeleton. The combination of short stature, clubfeet, joint contractures, and proximally deviated thumbs is highly suggestive of diastrophic dysplasia, but the diagnosis must be verified by radiography. Final confirmation should be obtained by mutation analysis of the *DTDST* gene.

TREATMENT

Standard Therapies: Therapy is symptomatic and not causal. The strategy consists of looking for complications and trying to prevent their consequences. Management issues include (a) treatment of cleft palate in the infant when present; (b) treatment of clubfoot either by casting or by surgery; (c) orthopedic assessment, physical therapy, and surgery to prevent and/or reduce joint contractures (feet, hips) as well as scoliosis; (d) assessment of neurologic complications, particularly imaging (MRI, CT scans) of the cervical spine, neurophysiologic evaluation, and spinal surgery when indicated; (e) special precaution during anesthesia and surgery to prevent neck hyperextension and spinal chord compression; (f) physical therapy and analgesic medication to reduce arthrosis-associated pain; (g) counseling for professional education and perspectives within the context of physical handicap; (h) monitoring of psychosocial adjustment and timely interventions to support the affected individual and the family; and (i) genetic counseling.

REFERENCES

Horton WA, Rimoin DL, Lachman RS, et al. The phenotypic variability of diastrophic dysplasia. *J Pediatr* 1978;93:609–613.

Lamy M, Maroteaux P. Le nanisme diastrophique. *Presse Med* 1960;68:1976–1983.

Makitie O, Kaitila I. Growth in diastrophic dysplasia. *J Pediatr* 1997;130:641–646.

Rossi A, Superti-Furga A. Mutations in the diastrophic dysplasia sulfate transporter (DTDST) gene (*SLC26A2*): 22 novel muta-tions, mutation review, associated skeletal phenotypes and diagnostic relevance. *Hum Mutat* 2001;17:159–171.

Superti-Furga A. Defects in sulfate metabolism and skeletal dys-plasias. In: Scriver CR, Beaudet AL, Valle D, et al., eds. *The metabolic and molecular bases of inherited disease,* 8th ed. New York: McGraw-Hill, 2001:5189–5201.

RESOURCES

188, 360, 361

12   Femoral Hypoplasia–Unusual Facies Syndrome

Robert M. Campbell, Jr., MD

DEFINITION: Femoral hypoplasia–unusual facies syndrome is a sporadically inherited disorder characterized by shortened or absent bilateral femurs; pelvic abnormalities; dislocation of the hips; bilateral talipes equinovarus; and unusual facial morphology, a high occurrence of cleft palate, and micrognathia.

SYNONYMS: Femoral-facial syndrome; Kyphomelic dysplasia.

DIFFERENTIAL DIAGNOSIS: Caudal regression syn-drome; Robert syndrome; Pierre Robin syndrome; Prox-imal femoral focal deficiency.

SYMPTOMS AND SIGNS: Shortened lower extremities with joint abnormalities and triangular face with distinct abnormalities of the eyes, nose, and mouth are character-istic. Micrognathia with a thin upper lip is present at birth. Cleft palate is common. The shortened nose is character-istic, with a broad tip and hypoplastic alae nasi. The ver-milion border of the upper lip is thin, but with long philtrum. Up-slanting palpebral fissures are seen. The upper extremities show a variable shortening of the humeri with limited range of motion of the elbows due to either fusion of the joint or dislocation of the radial heads. On ra-diography, the acetabulae are often hypoplastic or absent, with vertical ischial axis and large obturator foramen, with dislocation of the hips. Shortening or absence of both femoral shafts are present with lateral bowing, with dim-ples on the soft tissue at the apex of the deformity. Fibulas may be absent. Talipes equinovarus is common. Congenital abnormalities of the vertebra of the spine occur along with scoliosis. Inguinal hernias may also occur. Other abnor-malities include toe polydactyly, genitourinary tract abnor-mality such as cryptorchidism, hypoplastic labia majora, absent or polycystic kidneys, and abnormal genitourinary collecting system. Cardiovascular system abnormalities in-clude ventriculoseptal defect, pulmonary artery stenosis, and truncus arteriosus.

ETIOLOGY/EPIDEMIOLOGY: The prevalence is un-known. Up to 1993, 55 cases had been reported. There is a slight predominance of males over females. The mode of inheritance appears to be sporadic, but an autosomal-dominant form of inheritance is suggested. One third of cases are associated with maternal diabetes.

DIAGNOSIS: Diagnosis usually can be made based on both clinical examination of the face and radiographic evaluation of the lower extremities. Diagnosis also may be possible based on the presence of bilateral significant femoral hypoplasia with two of four facial findings: (a) up-slanting eyes, (b) hypoplastic alae nasi with a broad nasal tip, (c) long philtrum with a thin upper lip, or (d) small mouth mandible. The syndrome is suggested when the ratio of philtrum to nose length is greater than 0.36:1. Pre-natal diagnosis is possible by ultrasonography.

TREATMENT

Standard Therapies: Treatment involves operative proce-dures. The cleft palate is corrected surgically. Hip disloca-tions have been treated with reduction/open procedures with uncertain outcome. Patients have gone on to become ambulatory, even with complete absence of femurs, al-though with severe limb length discrepancy. Amputation of the feet and fitting with prostheses has also been per-formed to address the severe shortening of the lower ex-tremities. Club feet can be corrected surgically, although recurrence is possible. Anesthesiologists should be aware of the upper airway abnormalities in these children when they undergo surgeries. Physical therapy and other services for the physically disabled may be helpful. Genetic counseling is recommended for both patients and their families.

REFERENCES

Burn J, Winter R, Baraitser M, et al. The femoral hypoplasia-unusual facies syndrome. *J Med Genet* 1984;21:331–340.

Johnson J, Carey J, Manford G, et al. Femoral hypoplasia-unusual facies syndrome in infants of diabetic mothers. *J Pediatr* 1983;866–870.

Jones KL. *Smiths recognizable patterns of human malformation*, 4th ed. Philadelphia: WB Saunders, 1988.

Riedel F, Froster-Iskenius U. Caudal dysplasia and femoral hypoplasia—unusual facies syndrome: different manifestations of the same disorder? *Eur J Pediatr* 1985;144:80–82.

Robinow M, Sonek J, Buttino L, et al. Femoral-facial syndrome—prenatal diagnosis–autosomal dominant inheritance. *Am J Med Genet* 1995;57:397–399.

RESOURCES

108, 149, 360

---

13 Fibrodysplasia Ossificans Progressiva

Frederick S. Kaplan, MD, and Eileen M. Shore, PhD

DEFINITION: Fibrodysplasia ossificans progressiva (FOP) is a disorder of connective tissue characterized by congenital malformation of the great toes and recurrent episodes of painful soft tissue swelling that progress to severely disabling heterotopic ossification.

SYNONYM: Myositis ossificans progressiva.

DIFFERENTIAL DIAGNOSIS: Aggressive juvenile fibromatosis; Progressive osseous heteroplasia.

SYMPTOMS AND SIGNS: The characteristic feature is short great toes caused by malformation of the cartilaginous anlage of the first metatarsal and proximal phalanx. Ectopic ossification progresses in regular patterns of involvement (proximal before distal, axial before appendicular, cranial before caudal, and dorsal before ventral). Paraspinal muscles are involved early in life with subsequent spread to the shoulders and hips. The ankles, wrists, and jaw may be affected in late stages. Typically, episodes of soft tissue swelling begin during the first decade. Painful, tender, and rubbery soft tissue lesions (flare-ups) appear spontaneously or may be precipitated by minor trauma. Once ossification develops, it is permanent. Involvement of the muscles of mastication (frequently the outcome of injection of local anesthetic or overstretching of the jaw during dental procedures) can severely limit movement of the mandible. Ankylosis of the spine and rib cage restricts mobility and may imperil cardiopulmonary function. Restrictive chest wall disease with predisposition to pneumonia may follow.

ETIOLOGY/EPIDEMIOLOGY: The disorder has an estimated incidence of 1 per 2 million live births. Both genders and all races are affected. Autosomal-dominant transmission with variable expression is established. Most cases are sporadic. Gonadal mosaicism has been reported. Dysregulation of *BMP4* gene expression has been reported, but mutational screening and linkage analysis suggest that the primary genetic defect in FOP lies not in *BMP4* itself, but in a gene that affects expression of *BMP4*.

DIAGNOSIS: Misdiagnosis is common, but can be avoided simply by examining the patient's toes. Most children undergo unnecessary lesional biopsies, which exacerbate the condition. Routine biochemical studies of mineral metabolism are normal, although serum alkaline phosphatase activity and urinary basic fibroblast growth factor levels may be increased.

TREATMENT

Standard Therapies: There is no established treatment. Limited benefits have been reported using corticosteroids and disodium etidronate together during flare-ups and by using isotretinoin to prevent disease activation. Medical intervention is supportive. Dental therapy should preclude injections of local anesthetics and stretching of the jaw. Dental techniques for focused administration of local anesthetic are available. All intramuscular injections should be avoided. Prevention of falls is crucial. Measures against recurrent pulmonary infections are important.

Investigational Therapies: Investigational therapies include antiangiogenic agents and BMP antagonists. Corticosteroids, cox-2 inhibitors, leukotriene inhibitors, and thalidomide are also being explored.

REFERENCES

Feldman G, Li M, Martin S, et al. Fibrodysplasia ossification progressiva, a heritable disorder of severe heterotopic ossification, maps to human chromosome 4q 27-31. *Am J Hum Genet* 2000;66:128–135.

Gannon FH, Valentine BA, Shore EM, et al. Acute lymphocytic infiltration in an extremely early lesion of fibrodysplasia ossificans progressiva. *Clin Orthop Rel Res* 1998;346:19–25.

Janoff HB, Zasloff MA, Kaplan FS. Submandibular swelling in patients with fibrodysplasia ossificans progressiva. *Otolaryngol Head Neck Surg* 1996;114:599–604.

Nussbaum BL, O'Hara I, Kaplan FS. Fibrodysplasia ossificans progressiva: report of a case with guidelines for pediatric dental and anesthetic management. *J Dent Child* 1996;63:448–450.

Xu M-Q, Feldman G, Le Merrer M, et al. Linkage exclusion and mutational analysis of the noggin gene in patients with fibrodysplasia ossificans progressiva. *Clin Genet* 2000;58: 291–298.

RESOURCES

203, 351

---

14   Freeman-Sheldon Syndrome

Michael Bamshad, MD

DEFINITION: Freeman-Sheldon syndrome is an autosomal-dominant disorder characterized by multiple, nonprogressive congenital contractures (e.g., clubfeet, camptodactyly); unusual facial characteristics consisting of blepharophimosis, prominent nasolabial and philtral folds, H-shaped dimpling of the chin, and severely pursed lips; and scoliosis.

SYNONYMS: Craniocarpotarsal dystrophy; Whistling face syndrome; Whistling face–windmill vane hand syndrome.

DIFFERENTIAL DIAGNOSIS: Distal arthrogryposis type 1; Variant Freeman-Sheldon syndrome; Multiple pterygium syndrome; Schwartz-Jampel syndrome.

SYMPTOMS AND SIGNS: Freeman-Sheldon syndrome is characterized by multiple, nonprogressive congenital contractures, oropharyngeal abnormalities, scoliosis, and a distinctive face. The most salient characteristics of the face include a very small oral opening (often only a few millimeters in diameter at birth), an H-shaped dimpling of the chin, deep nasolabial folds, and blepharophimosis or narrow palpebral fissures. Infants may fail to thrive because of the inability to feed through such a narrow oral opening, dysphagia, and vomiting. The contractures typically include camptodactyly, ulnar deviation of the wrist, and clubfeet. Males may have an inguinal hernia or cryptorchidism. Low birth weight, small stature, or dislocation of the hip may be present in some children. Scoliosis is a common problem in older children and adolescents. Abnormalities of the muscle have been reported in some cases but are not a consistent feature. Most children with this syndrome have normal muscle tone, stretch reflexes, and muscle strength. Skeletal defects and cleft palate are not typically part of the spectrum of findings.

ETIOLOGY/EPIDEMIOLOGY: No accurate prevalence estimates exist, but more than 100 individuals have been reported. The syndrome is inherited as an autosomal-dominant trait, although most cases are sporadic. It has been described in Africans, Asians, and Europeans. Equal numbers of males and females are affected. A variant has been mapped to chromosome 11p15.5. It is unknown whether classic Freeman-Sheldon syndrome maps to the same location.

DIAGNOSIS: The diagnosis is usually based on clinical findings alone. Ancillary studies include radiographs of the skull, vertebral column, hands, feet, and hips. Electromyography may help to differentiate Freeman-Sheldon syndrome from Schwartz-Jampel syndrome.

TREATMENT

Standard Therapies: Treatment usually involves multiple surgical procedures and/or the use of splints or casts to improve the flexibility of joints. Surgical procedures are often used to enlarge the opening of the mouth and to treat the scoliosis. The proper anesthetic management of children with Freeman-Sheldon syndrome is important to consider because of the apparent increased incidence of malignant hyperthermia and the difficulties of establishing an adequate airway. Services that benefit the physically disabled may be helpful to some individuals. Genetic counseling is recommended for patients and their families. Other treatment is symptomatic and supportive.

REFERENCES

Jones KL. *Smith's recognizable patterns of human malformation,* 4th ed. Philadelphia: WB Saunders, 1988.

Krakowiak PA, Bohnsack JF, Carey JC, et al. Clinical analysis of a variant of Freeman-Sheldon syndrome (DA2B). *Am J Med Genet* 1998;76:93–98.

Krakowiak PA, O'Quinn JR, Watkins WS, et al. A variant of Freeman-Sheldon syndrome maps to chromosome 11p15.5-pter. *Am J Hum Genet* 1997;60:426–432.

Munro HM, Butler PJ, Washington EJ. Freeman-Sheldon (whistling face) syndrome. Anaesthetic and airway management. *Paediatr Anaesth* 1997;7:345–348.

RESOURCES

59, 120, 164, 351

15   Fryns Syndrome

Gregory M. Enns, MD, MB, ChB

DEFINITION: Fryns syndrome is an autosomal-recessive condition with characteristic features that include diaphragmatic hernia, unusually coarse face, and distal limb hypoplasia. Most patients are stillborn or die in the early neonatal period.

DIFFERENTIAL DIAGNOSIS: Tetrasomy 12p (Pallister-Killian syndrome); Other chromosome abnormalities (duplication or deletion 1q, deletion 6p, ring 15, trisomy 22); Other conditions with diaphragmatic hernia (Simpson-Golabi-Behmel syndrome, Beckwith-Wiedemann syndrome, de Lange syndrome, pentalogy of Cantrell).

SYMPTOMS AND SIGNS: A history of polyhydramnios developing in the second trimester is present in approximately 60% of cases. Stillbirth or early neonatal death is typical. Birth weight, length, and head circumference are usually normal, although patients occasionally are large for their gestational age. Affected individuals may have a coarse face, distal digital hypoplasia, diaphragmatic defects, urogenital anomalies, cleft lip and/or palate, gastrointestinal tract anomalies, abnormal lung lobation, cardiac defects, and central nervous system malformations. Craniofacial features include cloudy corneas, abnormal ears, large mouth, microretrognathia, and anteverted nares. Common limb anomalies include hypoplastic or absent nails, contractures, broad terminal digits, and distal phalanx hypoplasia. The diaphragmatic defects are often large, and usually unilateral and left-sided. Gastrointestinal abnormalities include intestinal malrotation, omphalocele, duodenal atresia, ectopic pancreas, accessory spleens, Meckel diverticulum, and anorectal anomalies. Aganglionosis of the colon and ureters may be present. A variety of genitourinary abnormalities may also be seen such as cystic kidney dysplasia, renal agenesis, hydronephrosis, ureteral anomalies, cryptorchidism, hypospadias, bicornuate uterus, vaginal hypoplasia, and uterine atresia. Brain findings include cerebellar abnormalities, Dandy-Walker malformation, agenesis of the corpus callosum, arrhinencephaly, hydrocephalus, heterotopias, and optic nerve hypoplasia. Profound mental retardation is present in the small percentage of patients who survive past the neonatal period. Those patients are less likely to have a diaphragmatic defect, severe lung hypoplasia, or a complex heart defect.

ETIOLOGY/EPIDEMIOLOGY: Fryns syndrome is an autosomal-recessive condition with an estimated prevalence of 1 in 14,000 population. Despite reports of multiple chromosome abnormalities, a candidate gene or gene locus has not been identified.

DIAGNOSIS: Fryns syndrome should be considered in any neonate or stillborn fetus with coarse facial features, diaphragmatic hernia, and distal limb hypoplasia. A detailed family history should be taken. Other genetic syndromes or chromosome abnormalities must be excluded. A skin biopsy for chromosome analysis on cultured fibroblasts may be necessary to detect tetrasomy 12p (Pallister-Killian syndrome). Other diagnostic studies (complete skeletal radiographs, echocardiography, abdominal ultrasonography, neuroimaging) are indicated to search for the associated malformations. Three-dimensional ultrasonography has been used in prenatal diagnosis.

TREATMENT
Standard Therapies: Therapy is supportive only. The use of heroic measures to prolong life should be considered carefully, given the extremely poor prognosis of the disease.

Genetic counseling should be offered to the parents for future pregnancies.

REFERENCES

Enns GM, Cox VA, Goldstein RB, et al. Congenital diaphragmatic defects and associated syndromes, malformations, and chromosome anomalies: a retrospective study of 60 patients and literature review. *Am J Med Genet* 1998;79:215–225.

Fryns JP, Van den Berghe H. Corneal clouding, subvalvular aortic stenosis, and midfacial hypoplasia associated with mental deficiency and growth retardation—a new syndrome? *Eur J Pediatr* 1979;131:179–183.

Jones KL. Fryns syndrome. In: *Smith's recognizable patterns of human malformation,* 5th ed. Philadelphia: WB Saunders, 1997:210–211.

Ramsing M, Gillessen-Kaesbach G, Holzgreve W, et al. Variability in the phenotypic expression of Fryns syndrome: a report of two sibships. *Am J Med Genet* 2000;95:415–424.

Van Hove JLK, Spiridigliozzi GA, Heinz R, et al. Fryns syndrome survivors and neurologic outcome. *Am J Med Genet* 1995;59: 334–340.

RESOURCES

96, 361

---

16   Goldenhar Syndrome

Adele Schneider, MD

DEFINITION: Goldenhar syndrome is a malformation complex involving structures derived from the first and second branchial arches, the first pharyngeal pouch, first branchial cleft, and primordial of the temporal bone. It is a heterogeneous condition with variable manifestations. Cardinal features include auricular appendages, microtia, mandibular hypoplasia, vertebral anomalies, and epibulbar dermoids or lipodermoids.

SYNONYMS: Oculo-auriculo-vertebral (OAV) spectrum; Hemifacial microsomia; First and second branchial arch syndrome; Facio-auriculo-vertebral sequence.

DIFFERENTIAL DIAGNOSIS: Townes-Brock syndrome; Treacher-Collins syndrome.

SYMPTOMS AND SIGNS: Patients show variable combinations of findings, which can be unilateral or bilateral. Some degree of facial asymmetry is seen in 65% of patients; when unilateral, it tends to be right sided. Auricular or preauricular appendages and/or pits occur along a line from the tragus to the angle of the mouth. Microtia, anotia, ear anomalies, and atresia/stenosis of external auditory canal with associated conductive hearing loss occur in most patients. Hypoplasia or aplasia of ossicles may occur. Some patients have sensorineural hearing loss. Most frequent ophthalmic findings include epibulbar dermoids and/or subconjunctival lipoma. Microphthalmia/anophthalmia, microcornea, and coloboma of the eyelid may also occur. High-arched palate, macrostomia (unilateral lateral facial cleft), micrognathia, cleft lip/palate, unilateral malar, and maxillary or mandibular hypoplasia have been described. Malfunction of the soft palate may be present. Skeletal findings include vertebral anomalies with hemi-vertebrae (common), as well as spina bifida and rib and limb anomalies. Cardiovascular and renal anomalies may be present. CNS findings are rare, but more common when associated with microphthalmia. Development is usually normal, although about 13% of patients have an IQ below 85.

ETIOLOGY/EPIDEMIOLOGY: The etiology is unknown. Goldenhar syndrome is usually sporadic; patterns of inheritance have been observed as autosomal dominant with variable expression, autosomal recessive, and multifactorial. Several abnormal karyotypes have been noted, including 22q deletion. The estimated recurrence risk is 2%–3%. Hypotheses regarding the cause of this syndrome include a neurocristopathy and developmental field defect. Another theory suggests vascular pathogenesis around blastogenesis, during the first 4 weeks of gestation.

DIAGNOSIS: The diagnosis is based on clinical features. Studies should include vertebral radiography, renal ultrasonography, hearing test, CT of temporal bones, ophthalmologic evaluation, and echocardiography (if a murmur exists). Chromosome study, G-banding, and fluorescence *in situ* hybridization for 22q deletion should be performed. In some cases, prenatal diagnosis by high-resolution ultrasonography is possible.

TREATMENT

Standard Therapies: Hearing loss should be detected and treated as early as possible. Surgery to repair facial clefts should be performed in infancy if possible. Mandibular hypoplasia should be treated to prevent dental malocclusion and the progression of mandibular asymmetry as the face grows. The patient should have appropriate orthodontic and dental care. Necessary surgery to remove epibulbar dermoids and for ear anomalies should be performed. If anophthalmia or microphthalmia is present, the patient should be referred to an ocularist and oculoplastic surgeon for enlargement of orbit. Patients should receive psychosocial support and appropriate referrals for other manifestations of the disease. Early intervention should occur when necessary.

Investigational Therapies: Chest wall/vertebral abnormalities have been treated by the titanium rib project.

REFERENCES

De Catte L, Laubach M, Legein J, et al. Early prenatal diagnosis of oculoauriculo-vertebral dysplasia or the Goldenhar syndrome. *Ultrasound Obstet Gynecol* 1996;8:422–424.

Gibson AJN, Sillence DO, Taylor TKF. Abnormalities of the spine in Goldenhar syndrome. *J Pediatr Orthop* 1996;16:44–49.

Hathout EH, Elmendorf E, Bartley J. Brief clinical report: hemifacial microsomia an abnormal chromosome 22. *Am J Med Genet* 1998;76:71–73.

Jones KL. *Smith's recognizable patterns of human malformation*, 5th ed. Philadelphia: WB Saunders, 1997.

Nakajima H, Goto G, Tanaka N, et al. Goldenhar syndrome associated with various cardiovascular malformations. *Jpn Circ J* 1998;62:617–620.

RESOURCES

143, 170, 199, 462

---

17   Holt-Oram Syndrome

Michael Bamshad, MD

DEFINITION: Holt-Oram syndrome is a genetic disorder consisting primarily of congenital heart disease and upper limb abnormalities (typically defects of the forearm, fingers, and wrist).

SYNONYMS: Atriodigital dysplasia; Heart-hand syndrome; Upper limb–cardiovascular syndrome.

DIFFERENTIAL DIAGNOSIS: Heart-hand syndrome II; Heart-hand syndrome III; Familial atrial septal defect; Okihiro syndrome.

SYMPTOMS AND SIGNS: Most individuals with Holt-Oram syndrome have heart and skeletal defects. The heart defects range from mitral valve prolapse to left-side hypoplasia. The most common are atrial and ventricular septal defects. However, cardiac abnormalities may be limited to conduction defects such as bradycardia, and some individuals have a normal cardiac examination. Limb defects range from hypoplastic carpal bones to duplication of the thumb (digit 1) to mild shortening of digit 1 to absence of the hand, forearm, and marked shortening of the upper arm. The more anterior elements of the limb (e.g., thumb) are usually affected before the more posterior elements of the limb. Upper limb defects are commonly bilateral and asymmetric. Hypoplasia of the musculature of the upper back (manifested as sloping shoulders) and pectoral girdle are common. The heart and limb defects vary widely within and between families.

ETIOLOGY/EPIDEMIOLOGY: The prevalence is approximately 1 in 100,000 population, and it has been described in Africans, Asians, and Europeans. Males and females are affected in equal numbers. The syndrome is caused by mutations in *TBX5*, a T-box gene, located on chromosome 12q24. It is transmitted as an autosomal-dominant trait. Although the broader category of hand-heart syndromes is genetically heterogeneous, Holt-Oram syndrome has not been mapped to any locus other than the region containing *TBX5*.

DIAGNOSIS: Often, the diagnosis can be based on the clinical examination alone. Ancillary studies that may help confirm the diagnosis include electrocardiography, echocardiography, and skeletal radiography.

TREATMENT
Standard Therapies: Treatment is by surgical correction where necessary, both of heart and skeletal defects. Services that benefit the physically disabled may be helpful to some individuals. Genetic counseling is recommended for patients and their families.

REFERENCES

Basson CT, Bachinsky DR, Lin RC, et al. Mutations in human TBX5 [corrected] cause limb and cardiac malformation in Holt-Oram syndrome. *Nat Genet* 1997;15:30–35.

Basson CT, Cowley GS, Solomon SD, et al. The clinical and genetic spectrum of the Holt-Oram syndrome (heart-hand syndrome). *N Engl J Med* 1996;330:885–891.

Li QY, Newbury-Ecob RA, Terrett JA, et al. Holt-Oram syndrome is caused by mutations in TBX5, a member of the Brachyury (T) gene family. *Nat Genet* 1997;15:21–29.

Newbury-Ecob RA, Leanage R, Raeburn JA, et al. Holt-Oram syndrome: a clinical genetic study. *J Med Genet* 1996;33:300–307.

RESOURCES

60, 185, 351, 357

18   Malignant Hyperthermia

*Sheila M. Muldoon, MD,
and Stephen Holman, MD*

DEFINITION: Malignant hyperthermia (MH) is a genetic disorder of skeletal muscle. When MH-susceptible individuals are given potent inhalation agents and/or succinylcholine, they can develop a hypermetabolic state that can rapidly progress to a high temperature, cardiac arrest, and death.

SYNONYM: Hyperpyrexia.

DIFFERENTIAL DIAGNOSIS: Fever of unknown origin.

SYMPTOMS AND SIGNS: Temperature elevation, for which the syndrome is named, is a late sign. Increased metabolism, manifested as elevated end-tidal carbon dioxide, is the earliest and most sensitive sign in anesthetized patients. Manifestations include increased oxygen consumption, decreased mixed venous oxygen, hypoxia, cyanosis, and skin mottling. Respiratory and metabolic acidosis can ensue rapidly. Skeletal muscle rigidity is the most unique sign of MH. Muscle damage is reflected by increases in serum creatine kinase, potassium, calcium, and phosphate. Rhabdomyolysis with myoglobinuria/myoglobinemia often occurs. The time of onset after induction of general anesthesia may vary from minutes to hours and patients may have had previously uneventful exposure to general anesthetics.

ETIOLOGY/EPIDEMIOLOGY: The estimated incidence varies from 1 in 15,000 in children to 1 in 50,000 in adults. Published reports probably underestimate the true incidence because of the difficulty in defining mild MH events. Demographic data on age and sex distribution of patients referred for testing indicates that 68% are males and 32% are females. MH is distributed worldwide and affects all ethnic groups, with a mean age of 21–23 years. Molecular genetic studies in humans and susceptible pigs have estab-lished the ryanodine receptor gene (*RYR1*) on chromosome 19 as the primary locus for MH. Mutations in *RYR1* have been linked in approximately 50% of cases, and more than 20 mutations have been reported in this gene. The genetic cause of the remaining 50% of cases is unknown, although five other loci have been identified by linkage analysis.

DIAGNOSIS: Many individuals with MH are otherwise unaffected. Thus, identifying these individuals before they are given general anesthesia is difficult. Family history of the disorder is important, as is a history of adverse metabolic response to general anesthesia. Definitive diagnosis is made by caffeine/halothane contracture testing on vastus lateralis muscle specimens. The test is invasive, however, and is done only in specialized MH diagnostic centers.

TREATMENT
Standard Therapies: Successful treatment of an MH episode involves the rapid cessation of the anesthetic triggering agent, cooling, and administration of Dantrolene sodium intravenously. Dantrolene inhibits the calcium release channel in skeletal muscle without affecting neuromuscular transmission and is effective for both prophylaxis and treatment of fulminant MH. The recommended initial dose is 2.4 mg/kg intravenously, with further increments as needed for an acute episode. Oral preparation of the drug is not recommended because of variable absorption.

REFERENCES
Jurkat-Rott K, McCarthy T, Lehmann-Horn F. Genetics and pathogenesis of malignant hyperthermia. *Muscle Nerve* 2000; 23:4–17.
Karen SM, Lojeski EW, Muldoon SM. *Malignant hyperthermia.* New York: Churchill-Livingstone, 1998.
Tremper KK, ed. *Atlas of anesthesia.* Vol IV.

RESOURCES
254, 366, 376

19   Jackson-Weiss Syndrome

*Millie D. Long, MD,
and Kant Y. K. Lin, MD*

DEFINITION: Jackson-Weiss syndrome consists of craniosynostosis, midface hypoplasia, and anomalies of the feet consisting of short, broad first metatarsals and abnormally shaped tarsal bones.

SYNONYM: Adelaide-type craniosynostosis.

DIFFERENTIAL DIAGNOSIS: Apert syndrome; Crouzon syndrome; Pfieffer syndrome; Sathre-Chotzen syndrome.

SYMPTOMS AND SIGNS: The most consistent anomaly associated with Jackson-Weiss is an abnormality in the clinical or radiographic appearance of the feet. These anomalies include syndactyly of the second and third toes, broad medially deviated great toes, fusion of the metatarsals, abnormally shaped tarsal bones, and fusion of the first cuneiform and navicular bones. Craniofacial anomalies include ocular hypertelorbitism, proptosis, and midface deficiency resulting from the affected cranial base sutures. Severe acrocephaly can also occur. Problems with speech and language are common because of the conglomerate craniofacial anomalies affecting the nasopharynx. However, some affected individuals show no abnormalities of the face or skull. Intelligence is normal.

ETIOLOGY/EPIDEMIOLOGY: Jackson-Weiss is an autosomal-dominant syndrome with extremely high penetrance and great variability in expression. The gene mutation believed to be responsible was identified at the fibroblast growth factor receptor (*FGFR*) 2 gene on chromosome 10. Genetic testing for this anomaly is not recommended because of the overlap of this mutation with Crouzon syndrome. Jackson-Weiss is also known to have a fibroblast growth factor receptor (FGFR) 3-associated coronal synostosis.

DIAGNOSIS: Diagnosis can be made clinically with the appropriate findings. Other craniosynostosis syndromes must be ruled out. For example, broad thumbs in addition to broad toes would support a diagnosis of Pfieffer syndrome rather than Jackson-Weiss. CT can help to delineate the deformities of the craniofacial skeleton.

TREATMENT
Standard Therapies: The treatment method is determined by the functional disturbances seen in the patient. Most treatment methods require surgery and may involve correction of the craniosynostosis, midface hypoplasia, and orbital and extremity deformities. Because of the variability in presentation and the widespread involvement of multiple organ systems, early referral to a multidisciplinary craniofacial team with craniofacial plastic surgeons, pediatric neurosurgeons, otolaryngologists, oral surgeons, orthodontists, ophthalmologists, pediatric orthopedic surgeons, pediatric critical care specialists, pediatric anesthesiologists, neuroradiologists, and geneticists is essential.

REFERENCES
Cohen MM, Maclean RE. *Craniosynostosis: diagnosis, evaluation and management,* 2nd ed. New York: Oxford University Press, 2000:197–203; 411–412.
Gorlin RJ, Cohen MM, Levin LS, eds. *Syndromes of the head and neck,* 3rd ed. New York: Oxford University Press, 1990:529–531.

RESOURCES
96, 121, 351

20   Klippel-Feil Syndrome

David J. Driscoll, MD
Daniele Rigamonti, MD,
and Philippe Gailloud, MD

DEFINITION: The Klippel-Feil syndrome is defined as congenital fusion of any two of the seven cervical vertebrae.

SYNONYM: Brevicollis syndrome.

DIFFERENTIAL DIAGNOSIS: Acquired spinal fusion (postinfection, spine inflammatory disorders); Wildervanck (or cervico-oculo-acoustic) syndrome; Mayer-Rokitansky-Kåster syndrome.

SYMPTOMS AND SIGNS: The signs classically associated with the Klippel-Feil syndrome include short neck, low posterior hairline, and restricted mobility of the upper spine. Deafness, usually of the sensorineural type, is present in up to 30% of patients. However, the genetic heterogeneity underlying the Klippel-Feil syndrome can result in less typical clinical presentations. Subgroups defined by their mode of inheritance and associated malformations have been defined, some of which are not associated with a short neck despite the presence of cervical fusion. A wide range of systemic anomalies has been associated with Klippel-Feil syndrome, including skeletal anomalies (short stature, atlantoaxial instability, congenital scoliosis, spina bifida, spinal canal stenosis, and rib, limb, and digital malformations), urogenital (absent vagina, renal agenesis, or malrotation), cardiac (situs inversus), pulmonary (lobar agenesis), vascular (low carotid bifurcations), neurologic (Chiari I malformation, syringomyelia, diastematomyelia, sleep-disordered breathing, dermoid cyst in the posterior fossa, and hereditary neuropathies), craniofacial (facial asymmetry, cleft palate, and craniosynostosis), and laryngeal anomalies. Individuals with Klippel-Feil syndrome can suffer serious neurologic injury from apparently minor neck trauma and should be encouraged to avoid risky activities, such as contact sports. These patients may also represent challenging endotracheal intubations.

ETIOLOGY/EPIDEMIOLOGY: The Klippel-Feil syndrome is caused by a failure of segmentation of the cervical vertebrae during the early weeks of fetal development. Although familial occurrences are now recognized, the Klippel-Feil syndrome is predominantly sporadic, with an incidence reaching up to 0.5% of live births.

DIAGNOSIS: The Klippel-Feil anomaly may be incidentally detected in patients undergoing radiologic investigations for unrelated reasons. It can also be initially discovered during imaging studies performed to evaluate conditions associated with the Klippel-Feil anomaly itself. Although spinal fusion can be documented by plain films and CT, only by combined myelography and CT (myelo-CT), or preferably MRI, can one provide a detailed evaluation of the spinal canal and its content.

TREATMENT
Standard Therapies: No specific treatment exists. Symptomatic treatment includes surgery to correct cervical instability and possible spinal cord compression.

REFERENCES
Clarke RA, Catalan G, Diwan AD, et al. Heterogeneity in Klippel-Feil syndrome: a new classification. *Pediatr Radiol* 1998;28: 967–974.
Taybi H. Klippel Feil syndrome. In: Taybi H, Lachman RS, eds. *Radiology of syndromes, metabolic disorders, and skeletal dysplasias*, 4th ed. St. Louis: CV Mosby, 1996:275–276.

RESOURCES
225, 351

21   Marinesco-Sjögren Syndrome

William R . Wilcox, MD, PhD

DEFINITION: Marinesco-Sjögren syndrome is an autosomal-recessive disorder characterized by cataracts, cerebellar ataxia, mental retardation, muscle weakness, short stature, and hypergonadotropic hypogonadism.

SYNONYMS: Marinesco-Garland syndrome; Cataract and cerebellar atrophy; Hereditary oligophrenic cerebellolentiform degeneration.

DIFFERENTIAL DIAGNOSIS: Mucolipidosis IV; Lowe syndrome; Carbohydrate deficient glycoprotein syndrome; Zellweger syndrome.

SYMPTOMS AND SIGNS: Marinesco-Sjögren syndrome is usually evident at birth because of hypotonia. The cataracts are often not present at birth but may appear rapidly during childhood. Motor milestones are significantly delayed, with ataxia becoming noticeable by the time the child can sit. Most affected individuals are eventually able to ambulate with a walker. Linear growth is poor, and pubertal development may not occur because of hypergonadotropic hypogonadism. Mental retardation is generally mild to moderate in severity. Neurologic deterioration is slow to absent, and prolonged survival is possible, but the muscle weakness tends to be progressive. Less commonly reported features include optic atrophy, brachydactyly, and cone epiphyses.

ETIOLOGY/EPIDEMIOLOGY: Marinesco-Sjögren syndrome is inherited as an autosomal-recessive trait with complete penetrance in both sexes. The genetic defect is unknown. More than 100 cases have been reported. It is panethnic, but rare except in genetic isolates in rural areas.

DIAGNOSIS: The diagnosis should be suspected based on the clinical symptoms. An ophthalmologic examination (cataracts) and MRI of the brain (cerebellar atrophy, particularly involving the vermis) can be helpful. Muscle biopsy findings are generally nonspecific, although ragged red fibers and abnormal mitochondria have been reported. Multilamellar inclusions can be present in muscle and conjunctival biopsy samples as well as in cultured fibroblasts. Results of metabolic testing are normal.

TREATMENT

Standard Therapies: Treatment is supportive and based on symptoms. Removal of the cataracts and placement of a lens implant is often required to preserve vision. Physical and occupational therapy and special education are helpful. Hormone replacement therapy is needed if hypogonadism is present.

REFERENCES

Georgy BA, Snow RD, Brogdon BG, et al. Neuroradiologic findings in Marinesco-Sjögren syndrome. *AJNR* 1998;19:281–283.

Superneau DW, Wertelecki W, Zellweger H, et al. Myopathy in Marinesco-Sjögren syndrome. *Eur Neurol* 1987;26:8–16.

Suzuki Y, Murakami N, Goto Y, et al. Apoptotic nuclear degeneration in Marinesco-Sjögren syndrome. *Acta Neuropathol (Berl)* 1997;94:410–415.

Walker PD, Blitzer MG, Shapira E. Marinesco-Sjögren syndrome: evidence for a lysosomal storage disorder. *Neurology* 1985;35:415–419.

Zimmer C, Gosztonyi G, Cervos-Navarro J, et al. Neuropathy with lysosomal changes in Marinesco-Sjögren syndrome: fine structural findings in skeletal muscle and conjunctiva. *Neuropediatrics* 1992;23:329–335.

RESOURCES

258, 351, 368

---

22 Nail-Patella Syndrome

Elizabeth Sweeney, MB, ChB, and Iain McIntosh, PhD

DEFINITION: Nail-patella syndrome (NPS) is a genetic condition affecting the nails, patellae, elbows, and kidneys. There is also a risk of glaucoma. The severity is variable from person to person, even within the same family.

SYNONYMS: Onycho-osteodysplasia; Hereditary osteoonychodysplasia; Fong disease; Turner-Kieser syndrome; Österreicher-Turner syndrome.

DIFFERENTIAL DIAGNOSIS: Small patella syndrome (ischiopatellar dysplasia); Patella aplasia-hypoplasia; Anonychia.

SYMPTOMS AND SIGNS: The fingernails are affected in 98% of patients in a characteristic manner. The thumbnail is the most severely (and may be the only) affected nail, and the severity of nail involvement decreases toward the fifth finger. Nails may be absent, small, thin, ridged, or split. Some nails may have a longitudinal ridge of skin running through the middle. The lunulae of the nails are often triangular. The toenails are involved in half of patients, typically with a small, dystrophic little toenail, but other nails may be thickened or discolored. There is often loss of the skin creases overlying the distal interphalangeal joints of the fingers, and there may be clinodactyly of the fifth finger and hyperextensibility of the finger joints with swan necking. Pes planus is a frequent occurrence, and congenital talipes is common. The Achilles tendons may be short, leading to toe-walking, and tight hamstring tendons may limit knee extension. The patellae are prone to lateral dislocation. Most patients have hypoplastic patellae; some patients have absent patellae. Most patients have some loss of elbow extension, and often limited pronation and supination of the elbows occurs. Some may have elbow pterygia. The shoulders and hips may also be affected. Back pain occurs in half of patients and may be severe. There may be an increased lumbar lordosis and occasionally spondylolisthesis or vertebral defects. Radiographs of the pelvis show iliac horns in 70% of patients. Renal involvement may be clinically detectable in 30% of patients and may manifest at any age. Renal disease may progress to renal failure in a minority of patients. Raised intraocular pressure or glaucoma affects approximately 20% of patients and may develop at a younger age than in the general population. Irritable bowel syndrome and chronic constipation are more common in patients with NPS. The incidence of Raynaud phenomenon, of paraesthesia of the hands and feet, and of weakened teeth is increased.

ETIOLOGY/EPIDEMIOLOGY: The syndrome is caused by mutations in the gene *LMX1B*, which is located on chromosome 9 at 9q34. *LMX1B* is essential for dorsoventral patterning of the developing limb, regulation of collagen expression in the glomerular basement membrane, development of the anterior chamber of the eye, and differentiation of dopaminergic neurons. The incidence is estimated at 1 in 50,000 people, but this may be an underestimate. The syndrome has been reported in all ethnic groups, and is inherited in an autosomal-dominant manner. Approximately 15% of cases may be the result of a new *LMX1B* mutation, with neither parent being affected.

DIAGNOSIS: Diagnosis is made on clinical features, although gene testing may be of help in difficult cases. Prenatal diagnosis may be possible in the first trimester by means of molecular analysis of a chorionic villus sample.

TREATMENT
Standard Therapies: No specific treatment exists, but joints may benefit from individualized physiotherapy or surgery. Because the joint anatomy is abnormal in NPS, MRI scanning is recommended before physiotherapy or surgery. Particular attention should be directed to the muscle attachment points, because there may be wide variation from normal. Glaucoma may be treated in the standard manner, and kidney involvement may require medical treatment or occasionally dialysis or transplantation. Proteinuria may be controlled using angiotensin-converting enzyme inhibitors. Kidney function should be carefully monitored during pregnancy. It is recommended that patients have yearly urinalysis from birth and regular ophthalmologic examinations to diagnose glaucoma as early as possible.

REFERENCES
Beals RK Eckhardt AL. Hereditary onycho-osteodysplasia (nail-patella syndrome). *J Bone Joint Surg [Am]* 1969;51:505–515.
Chen H, Lun Y, Ovchimnikov D, et al. Limb and kidney defects in Lmx1b mice suggest an involvement of LMX1B in human nail-patella syndrome. *Nat Genet* 1998;19:51–55.
Clough MV, Hamlington JD, McIntosh I. Restricted distribution of loss-of-function mutations within the *LMX1B* genes of nail patella syndrome patients. *Hum Mutat* 1999;14:459–465.
Lichter PR, Richards JE, Downs CA, et al. Cosegregation of open-angle glaucoma and the nail-patella syndrome. *Am J Ophthalmol* 1997:124:506–515.

RESOURCES
276, 277, 308, 351

---

23 | Noonan Syndrome

Judith E. Allanson, MB, ChB

DEFINITION: Noonan syndrome is an autosomal-dominant multiple congenital anomaly syndrome. Features are variable and include short stature, congenital heart defect, broad or webbed neck, chest deformity with pectus carinatum above and pectus excavatum below, developmental delay, undescended testicles, and a characteristic facial appearance.

DIFFERENTIAL DIAGNOSIS: Cardiofaciocutaneous syndrome; Costello syndrome; Multiple lentigines (LEOPARD) syndrome; Watson syndrome; Williams syndrome; Aarskog syndrome.

SYMPTOMS AND SIGNS: The facial appearance of Noonan syndrome is most distinctive in newborns and in middle childhood; it is difficult to recognize in adults. In the neonate, features include a tall forehead, wide-spaced and down-slanting eyes, low-set posteriorly rotated ears with a thickened rim, a well-grooved upper lip, and short neck with excess skin. In infancy, eyes are prominent and lids may be droopy or thickened. The nose has a depressed root, with a wide base and bulbous tip. In childhood, there may be apparent lack of expression or droopy, myopathic appearance. By adolescence, features are fine and the face has lengthened, becoming broad at the temples and tapering down to a small, pointed chin. The neck lengthens, creating a broad or webbed shape. The chest shape is unusual; nipples appear low set and widely spaced. A pectus deformity exists, and the shoulders are rounded. Birth weight may be increased by edema, and failure to thrive may follow, exacerbated by poor suck and slow feeding. Mean height is at the lower end of the range in the general population until puberty but with extended growth, so final adult height approaches the lower limits of normal. Early developmental milestones may be delayed. Congenital heart defects are found in 50%–80% of patients, particularly pulmonary valve dysplasia and cardiomyopathy. Mild ocular findings are among the most common features and include astigmatism, refractive errors, amblyopia, and nystagmus. Two thirds of affected persons have excessive bruising and a variety of coagulation defects. Enlargement of liver and spleen is relatively common. Pubertal development may be delayed. Lymphatic problems occur in approximately 20% of patients. Many different skin changes are described, the most common being hyperkeratosis.

ETIOLOGY/EPIDEMIOLOGY: Noonan syndrome is inherited in an autosomal-dominant fashion. It is reported in 1 in 1,000 to 1 in 2,500 newborns. Because the features are frequently mild, it may be underdiagnosed. A causative gene was identified in 2001. This gene, PTPN11, encodes the nonreceptor protein tyrosine phosphatase SHP-2, which seems essential in several intracellular signaling pathways controlling a variety of developmental processes. It also has a role in modulating cell proliferation, differentiation, and migration.

DIAGNOSIS: Diagnosis should be suspected when the cardinal features listed earlier are found. Research laboratory testing of *PTPN11* is available.

TREATMENT
Standard Therapies: At diagnosis, the physician should search for associated medical complications. Echocardiography, electrocardiography, eye and hearing examination, prothrombin time, partial thromboplastin time and bleeding time, and renal ultrasonography are recommended. Growth and development should be closely monitored, with intervention where appropriate. Some growth specialists recommend growth hormone treatment in any child with Noonan syndrome who is small, irrespective of results, beginning at 7 or 8 years. Other specialists would first evaluate spontaneous production of growth hormone. Beta-blockade or calcium channel blockers are most frequently used to treat obstructive cardiomyopathy. Surgical treatment of this and other structural defects follows standard approaches. Prophylaxis to prevent subacute bacterial endocarditis is required for dental work, surgery, and catheterization. Most ocular defects require standard nonsurgical treatment. Coagulation abnormalities, lymphatic anomalies, and dermatologic changes should all be treated with specific and standard therapies. Aspirin and aspirin-containing medications should be avoided.

REFERENCES
Allanson JE. Noonan syndrome. *J Med Genet* 1987;24:9–13.
Allanson JE, Hall JG, Hughes HE, et al. Noonan syndrome: the changing phenotype. *Am J Med Genet* 1985;21:507–514.
Ishizawa A, Oho S-I, Dodo H, et al. Cardiovascular abnormalities in Noonan syndrome: the clinical findings and treatment. *Acta Paediatr Jpn* 1996;38:84–90.
Lee NB, Kelly L, Sharland M. Ocular manifestations of Noonan syndrome. *Eye* 1992;6:328–334.
Romano AA, Blethen SL, Dana K, et al. Growth hormone treatment in Noonan syndrome: the National Cooperative Growth Study experience. *J Pediatr* 1996;128(suppl):18–21.
Tartaglia M, Mehler EL, Goldberg R, et al. Mutations in *PTPN11*, encoding the protein tyrosine phosphatase SHP-2, cause Noonan syndrome. *Nat Genet* 2001;29:465–468.
Witt DR, Keena BA, Hall JG, et al. Growth curves for height in Noonan syndrome. *Clin Genet* 1986;30:150–153.

RESOURCES
188, 357, 374, 462

---

24   Familial Expansile Osteolysis

Mary Beth Dinulos, MD

DEFINITION: Familial expansile osteolysis (FEO) is a skeletal dysplasia characterized by expansile bone lesions, bone pain and deformity, early-onset deafness, and dental abnormalities.

SYNONYMS: McCabe disease; Hereditary expansile polyostotic osteolytic dysplasia.

DIFFERENTIAL DIAGNOSIS: Paget disease of bone; Generalized enchondromatosis; Genochondromatosis; Polyostotic fibrous dysplasia; Osteofibrous dysplasia.

SYMPTOMS AND SIGNS: The initial symptom may be early-onset deafness in the first decade of life. The hearing loss is typically conductive in nature, but may progress to a mixed conductive or sensorineural type. Dental abnormalities are common and may be present by the second decade. External cervical and apical resorption of the teeth may lead to tooth mobility, fracture, and premature loss. The skeletal manifestations may become apparent within the second to third decade. The individual may present with bone pain, deformity, and pathologic fractures. Radiographs may show both general and focal skeletal changes. The focal lesions are most commonly seen in the extremities, especially the tibia, fibula, humerus, and radius. As the disease progresses, new lesions continue to appear and older lesions tend to "expand" within the bone. Severe bone pain and deformity may necessitate amputation. A biopsy of a focal lesion typically shows active remodeling with increased activity of osteoclasts and osteoblasts.

ETIOLOGY/EPIDEMIOLOGY: The disorder is inherited in an autosomal-dominant manner. A gene for FEO has been identified (*TNFRSF11A*), which resides on the long arm of chromosome 18 (18q21). Mutations in *TNFRSF11A* have been found in individuals with FEO, as well as in several patients with Paget disease of bone. Only a few kindreds with FEO have been reported, and include individuals of Northern Irish, German, and American ancestry.

DIAGNOSIS: The earliest symptom may be hearing loss in childhood. Focal skeletal lesions are typically evident by early adulthood and may be accompanied by pain, deformity, and pathologic fractures as the disease progresses. Skeletal radiographs show the characteristic expansile lesions. Biopsy of a focal lesion will typically show active remodeling. Urinary hydroxyproline and serum alkaline phosphatase levels may be elevated. A history of dental abnormalities (external resorption of the teeth) will aid in diagnosis.

TREATMENT
Standard Therapies: There is no effective treatment for FEO.

Investigational Therapies: Dichloro-methylene-diphosphonate is being investigated.

REFERENCES
Crone MD, Wallace RG. The radiologic features of familial expansile osteolysis. *Skel Radiol* 1990;19:245–250.
Hughes AE, Ralston SH, Marken J, et al. Mutations in *TNFRSF11A*, affecting the signal peptide of RANK, cause familial expansile osteolysis. *Nat Genet* 2000;24:45–48.
Mitchell CA, Kennedy JG, Owens PD. Dental histology in familial expansile osteolysis. *J Oral Pathol Med* 1990;19:65–70.
Osterberg PH, Wallace RG, Adams DA, et al. Familial expansile osteolysis. A new dysplasia. *J Bone Joint Surg [Br]* 1988;70:255–260.
Wallace RG, Barr RJ, Osterberg PH, et al. Familial expansile osteolysis. *Clin Orthop Rel Res* 1989;248:265–277.

RESOURCES
347, 360

---

25 Progeria

W. Ted Brown, MD, PhD

DEFINITION: Progeria is a disease of childhood with striking features resembling premature aging.

SYNONYM: Hutchinson-Gilford progeria syndrome (HGPS).

DIFFERENTIAL DIAGNOSIS: Neonatal progeroid syndrome; Acrogeria; Mandibulo-acral dysplasia; Cockayne syndrome; Hallermann-Streif syndrome; Geroderma osteodysplastica; Congenital generalized lipodystrophy; Petty-Laxova-Weidemann progeroid syndrome; Ehlers-Danlos syndrome, progeroid form.

SYMPTOMS AND SIGNS: Children with progeria usually appear normal in early infancy. However, features such as midfacial cyanosis, "sculpted nose," and sclerodema may suggest the existence of the syndrome at birth. Profound growth failure usually occurs during the first year of life. A characteristic facies, alopecia, loss of subcutaneous fat, abnormal posture, stiffness of joints, and bone and skin changes usually become apparent during the second year of life. Motor and mental development are normal. The clinical manifestations almost always include short stature; weight distinctly low for height; diminished subcutaneous fat; head disproportionately large for face; micrognathia; prominent scalp veins; generalized alopecia; prominent eyes; delayed and abnormal dentition; pyriform thorax; short, dystrophic clavicles; "horse-riding" stance; wide-based shuffling gait; coxa valga; thin limbs; prominent, stiff joints; and failure to complete sexual maturation. Features frequently present are skin that is thin, taut, dry, wrinkled, and brown spotted in various areas; sclerodermatous skin over the lower abdomen, proximal thighs, and buttocks; prominent superficial veins; loss of eyebrows and eyelashes; sculpted, beaked nasal tip; faint nasolabial cyanosis; thin lips; protruding ears;

absence of ear lobules; thin, high-pitched voice; dystrophic nails; and progressive radiolucency of the terminal phalanges and distal clavicles (acroosteolysis). Children with progeria usually have severe atherosclerosis, and death occurs as a result of complications of cardiac or cerebral vascular disease generally between 5 and 20 years, with a median life span of approximately 13 years.

ETIOLOGY/EPIDEMIOLOGY: The condition is believed to represent a sporadic dominant mutation of an as yet unidentified gene. Lack of affected siblings, a paternal age effect, lack of consanguinity, and two sets of affected identical twins suggest it is a dominant mutation. The reported incidence is approximately 1 in 8 million births.

DIAGNOSIS: The earliest signs suggestive of a diagnosis include failure to thrive, alopecia, and subcutaneous skin changes suggesting scleroderma. Variable degrees of insulin resistance, occasionally insulin-dependent diabetes mellitus, abnormalities of collagen, increased metabolic rate, and inconsistent abnormalities of serum cholesterol and other lipids are found, but there are no demonstrable abnormalities of thyroid, parathyroid, pituitary, or adrenal function. Twenty-four-hour growth hormone levels are normal, but reduced levels of insulin-like growth factor I have been noted. Variable abnormalities of DNA repair have also been observed. Dramatically increased levels of hyaluronic acid occur in the urine of affected patients.

TREATMENT
Standard Therapies: No specific treatment exists. Growth hormone therapy has produced increased linear growth but with no effect on the progression of atherosclerosis.

REFERENCES
Abdenur JE, Brown WT, Friedman S, et al. Response to nutritional and growth hormone treatment in progeria. *Metab Clin Exp* 1997;46:851.

Brown WT. Progeria: a human-disease model of accelerated aging. *Am J Clin Nutr* 1992;55(suppl):122.

DeBusk FL. The Hutchinson-Gilford progeria syndrome. *J Pediatr* 1972;80:697.

RESOURCES
96, 351, 357, 404

---

26   Robinow Syndrome

Michael A. Patton, MD,
and Ali R. Afzal, MD

DEFINITION: Robinow syndrome is an inherited skeletal dysplasia characterized by mesomelic limb shortening (middle section), hemivertebrae, and genital hypoplasia.

DIFFERENTIAL DIAGNOSIS: Aarskog syndrome; Leri-Weil dysostosis; Jarcho-Levin syndrome.

SYMPTOMS AND SIGNS: The facial features consist of marked hypertelorism with prominent forehead, midfacial hypoplasia, and a short nose. The facial features have been described as resembling "fetal facies." The affected individual may have a tented upper lip and gum hypertrophy. Tongue tie or ankyloglossia is also occasionally present. The limbs show mesomelic shortening (i.e., shortening of radius/ulna and tibia/fibula). There may also be brachydactyly and ectrodactyly. In the spine, hemivertebrae and rib fusion are present, which cause severe kyphoscoliosis. Overall growth is less than 2 SD below the mean. Genital hypoplasia in boys leads to micropenis and normal size testes and in girls to labial hypoplasia. Congenital heart defects are seen in approximately 15% of patients. Intelligence is normal.

ETIOLOGY/EPIDEMIOLOGY: Both autosomal-recessive and autosomal-dominant inheritance occur. Mutations in the *ROR2* gene on chromosome 9q22 have been reported in the autosomal-recessive cases. No mutations have been reported in the autosomal-dominant cases yet. The syndrome is rare, although it has been reported in increased frequency in some consanguineous populations, for example, in Turkey and Oman.

DIAGNOSIS: Robinow syndrome is diagnosed based on the clinical and radiologic features. Gene analysis may become available for diagnosis in the future.

TREATMENT
Standard Therapies: Relatively little treatment is available other than orthopedic correction for the scoliosis. The micropenis may be treated with testosterone. Growth hor-

mone may be used to treat the short stature, but care must be exercised in the presence of scoliosis.

REFERENCES

Afzal AR, Rajab A, Fenske C, et al. Autosomal recessive Robinow syndrome is allelic to dominant brachydactyly type B and caused by loss of function mutations in *ROR2*. *Nat Genet* 2000;25:419–422.

Robinow M, Silverman FN, Smith HD. A newly recognized dwarfing syndrome. *Am J Dis Child* 1969;117:645–651.

Soliman AT, Rajab A, Alsalmi I, et al. Recessive Robinow syndrome: with emphasis on endocrine functions. *Metabolism* 1998;47:1337–1343.

Webber SA, Wargowski DS, Chitayat D, et al. Congenital heart disease and Robinow syndrome: coincidence or an additional component of the syndrome? *Am J Med Genet* 1990;37:519–521.

RESOURCES

96, 188, 420

27   Rubinstein-Taybi Syndrome

Jack H. Rubinstein, MD

DEFINITION: Rubinstein-Taybi syndrome is characterized by mental retardation, broad thumbs and first toes, retarded height and microcrania, dysmorphic facial features, and cryptorchidism.

SYNONYMS: Broad thumb-hallux syndrome; Rubinstein syndrome; Broad thumbs and great toes, characteristic facies, and mental retardation; Michail-Matsoukas-Theodorou-Rubinstein-Taybi syndrome.

DIFFERENTIAL DIAGNOSIS: Saethre-Chotzen syndrome; Cornelia de Lange syndrome.

SYMPTOMS AND SIGNS: Patients often have a history of feeding difficulties, gastroesophageal reflux, constipation, recurrent respiratory infections, sleep apnea, stridor, and occasional problems with anesthesia. Stature and head circumference are below the 50th percentile. Mental retardation may occur. Autistic-like behaviors, electroencephalographic abnormalities, seizures, tethered spinal cord, rare myelomeningocele, hypotonia, lax ligaments, hyperextensible/dislocated joints and stiff awkward gait, Legg-Perthes, tight heel cords, kyphosis, scoliosis, lordosis, and sternal and rib anomalies may occur. Facial features include prominent forehead, beaked or straight nose, broad nasal bridge, nasal septum extending below nasal alae, "grimacing" smile, apparent hypertelorism, laterally downslanting palpebral fissures, heavy and/or highly arched eyebrows, long lashes, and epicanthi. Ophthalmologic findings may include strabismus, refractive error, ptosis, Duane syndrome, nasolacrimal duct obstruction, colobomata, cataracts, corneal scar, and increased cup to disc ratio with or without glaucoma. Abnormalities in rotation, posi-

tion, or shape of ears, recurrent otitis media, and hearing loss have been reported. A thin upper lip, mild retrognathia, highly arched palate with wide alveolar ridges, dental irregularity/crowding, and talon cusps may occur. The thumbs are broad and flat with short distal phalanx and a small hole or distal notch radiographically. Other fingers tend to have broad, short, or tufted terminal phalanges. The hallux may be wide and flat, with the distal phalanx of the entire ray involved. There may be duplication of the proximal or distal phalanx or both. Congenital heart defects or cardiomyopathy may occur. Renal anomalies, urinary tract infections, nephrosis, and calculi have been reported, as well as incomplete or delayed descent of the testes. Cutaneous findings include dermatoglyphic anomalies, simian crease, deep plantar crease between first and second toes, hirsutism, flat capillary hemangiomata on forehead or elsewhere, ingrown nails or paronychiae, prominent fingertip pads, keloids, and supernumerary nipples. Tumors include leukemia, lymphoma, medulloblastoma, meningioma, neuroblastoma, pilomatrixoma, and rhabdomyosarcoma.

ETIOLOGY/EPIDEMIOLOGY: The incidence and prevalence in the general population are unknown. A birth prevalence of 1 in 100,000 to 1 in 125,000 is estimated for the Netherlands. Most individuals have been caucasian, with fewer cases of African and Asian origin. Other than monozygotic twins, affected siblings occurred in only two or three families. Cases with mother and child involved are not well documented. The recurrence risk for offspring of affected individuals might be as high as 50%.

DIAGNOSIS: The syndrome is identified by the characteristic facies, broad thumb and great toes, and mental retardation. Photographic and radiographic studies, echocardiography, abdominal ultrasonography, CT, and MRI help to document involved systems (Insert Figs. 64–65). Cytogenetic and molecular studies of the CREB-binding protein (CBP) gene area on chromosome 16p13.3 can help confirm the diagnosis in 15%–20% of cases.

TREATMENT

Standard Therapies: An interdisciplinary, coordinated, experienced team is required for early intervention; special education; occupational, physical, and speech/language therapies; and appropriate medical, surgical, and dental care, depending on the systems and pathology identified. Counseling, genetic counseling, and support groups can be helpful.

REFERENCES

Michail J, Matsoukas J, Theodorou S. Pouces bot arque' en fort abduction-extension et autres symptomes concomitants. *Rev Chir Orthop* 1957;43:142–146.

Miller RW, Rubinstein JH. Tumors in Rubinstein-Taybi syndrome. *Am J Med Genet* 1995;56:112–115.

Petrij F, Dauwerse HC, Blough RI, et al. Diagnostic analysis of the Rubinstein-Taybi syndrome: five cosmids should be used for microdeletion detection and low number of protein truncating mutations. *J Med Genet* 2000;37:168–176.

Rubinstein JH. Broad thumb-hallux (Rubinstein-Taybi) syndrome 1957–1988. *Am J Med Genet* 1990;6(suppl):3–16.

RESOURCES

113, 360, 423, 424

---

28   Saethre-Chotzen Syndrome

Millie D. Long, MD,
and Kant Y. K. Lin, MD

DEFINITION: Saethre-Chotzen syndrome is characterized by craniosynostosis, a low-set frontal hairline, ptosis of the eyelids, a deviated nasal septum, facial asymmetry, mild midface hypoplasia, brachydactyly, partial syndactyly, and various other skeletal anomalies.

DIFFERENTIAL DIAGNOSIS: Primary craniosynostosis; Pfieffer syndrome; Crouzon syndrome; Apert syndrome, Jackson-Weiss syndrome.

SYMPTOMS AND SIGNS: The presence of craniosynostosis is not required for the diagnosis. When present, the time of onset, the degree of involvement, and the location of the affected suture are quite variable. Thus, patients have presented with a variety of skull shapes, including brachycephaly, acrocephaly, and trigonocephaly. Defining craniofacial features include facial asymmetry, low-set frontal hairline, and eye abnormalities including ptosis, hypertelorism, strabismus, and tear duct stenosis. The ears can be low set and small, often deviated posteriorly, with an associated hearing deficit (Insert Fig. 63). The nose is flattened or beaked, and often has a deviated septum. Oral anomalies include a narrow or arched palate, occasionally cleft palate, malocclusion, and other dental anomalies such as supernumerary teeth and enamel hypoplasia. Associated abnormalities of the extremities include some degree of brachydactyly and partial cutaneous syndactyly between the second and third fingers and toes. Clinodactyly of the fifth finger has also been noted. Some individuals have broad toes. Intelligence is usually normal, although mild to moderate mental retardation does occur. Epilepsy and schizophrenia have also been noted. Other less frequent findings associated with the syndrome include short stature, cryptorchidism, renal anomalies, congenital heart defects, and an imperforate anus.

ETIOLOGY/EPIDEMIOLOGY: Saethre-Chotzen syndrome is an autosomal-dominant disorder with high penetrance and variable expressivity. The gene mutation believed responsible for causing the syndrome has been found in the *TWIST* gene located on chromosome 7. Mutations have also been found on the fibroblast growth factor receptor (*FGFR*) 2 gene on chromosome 10 and the *FGFR 3* genes on chromosome 4.

DIAGNOSIS: Diagnosis is based on clinical features. It can be confirmed by identifying the *TWIST* mutation by DNA analysis. Prenatal diagnosis can be made by chorionic villus sampling or amniocentesis if the mutation has been identified in an affected parent.

TREATMENT

Standard Therapies: The timing and treatment method are determined by the functional disturbances seen in the individual patient. Most treatments require surgery and may involve correction of the craniosynostosis, midface hypoplasia, and nasal, orbital, and extremity deformities. Because of the variability in presentation and the involvement of multiple organ systems, early referral to a multidisciplinary team with craniofacial plastic surgeons, pediatric neurosurgeons, otolaryngologists, oral surgeons, orthodontists, ophthalmologists, pediatric critical care specialists, pediatric anesthesiologists, neuroradiologists, and geneticists is essential.

REFERENCES
Cohen MM, Maclean RE, eds. *Craniosynostosis: diagnosis, evaluation and management,* 2nd ed. New York: Oxford University Press, 2000:374–376.

Gorlin RJ, Cohen MM, Levin LS, eds. *Syndromes of the head and neck,* 3rd ed. New York: Oxford University Press, 1990:527–529.

RESOURCES
96, 360, 462

---

29   Spondyloepiphyseal Dysplasia Congenita

John Hicks, MD, DDS, PhD

DEFINITION: Spondyloepiphyseal dysplasia (SED) congenita is a type II collagenopathy. It is a rare form of osteochondrodysplasia associated with mild to moderate short stature, platyspondyly with cone-shaped flattened vertebrae, and precocious hip degenerative disease.

SYNONYMS: Spondyloepiphyseal dysplasia, congenital type; Spondyloepiphyseal dysplasia, late-onset.

DIFFERENTIAL DIAGNOSIS: SED tarda; Type II collagenopathies; Hypochondrogenesis; Kniest dysplasia; Stickler syndrome; Achondroplasia type II; Multiple epiphyseal dysplasia 2; Mutations in type IX and X collagen; Metaphyseal chondrodysplasia, Schmid type; Morquoi-Brailsford chondroosteodystrophy; Perthes disease; Bilateral congenital hip dislocation; Traumatic synovitis.

SYMPTOMS AND SIGNS: Characteristic findings include short-trunk dwarfism identifiable at birth; normocephalic head; myopia and retinal detachment; cleft palate; flat facies; platyspondyly, short neck, cervical subluxation, odontoid hypoplasia, kyphoscoliosis, and lumbar lordosis; barrel chest and pectus carinatum; cervical myelopathy, childhood hypotonia, and mental retardation; sensorineural hearing loss; hypoplasia of abdominal muscles; abdominal and inguinal hernias; lack of ossification of os pubis and distal femoral and proximal tibial epiphyses, talus, and calcaneous; and flattening of vertebral bodies. In the mildest forms, a height of up to 140 cm may be reached. Some forms of SED congenita may be so mild that premature hip joint degeneration is the only sign. With microscopic examination, chondrocytes composing the cartilage possess fine granular inclusions in the cisterns of the rough endoplasmic reticulum.

ETIOLOGY/EPIDEMIOLOGY: The disorder arises from a type II collagen gene (*COL2A1*, chromosome 12q13.1-13.2) mutation. There are several different type II collagenopathies. Type II collagen is primarily located in cartilaginous tissues, the tectorial membrane of the inner ear, nucleolus pulposus of intervertebral discs, and the vitreous of the eye. Mutations in the *COL2A1* gene result in distortion of the morphology of collagen's triple helix with adverse effects on tissue properties and functions.

DIAGNOSIS: The disorder may be diagnosed at birth due to short-trunk dwarfism. Clinical symptoms and signs and radiologic findings provide additional definitive diagnostic evidence. Suspicion for SED congenita may be raised by a family history of SED in other kindred. Genetic testing may be performed to evaluate for *COL2A1* (12q13.1-13.2) mutations. Prenatal cytogenetic analysis of amniotic fluid and chorionic villus samples may provide diagnostic information for genetic counseling.

TREATMENT
Standard Therapies: Symptomatic treatment is needed, depending on the phenotype of the proband. Corticosteroid therapy may be helpful in modulating sensorineural hearing loss.

REFERENCES
Baitner A, Maurer S, Gruen M, et al. The genetic basis of the osteochondrodysplasias. *J Pediatr Orthop* 2001;20:594–605.
Gedeon AK, Colley A, Jamieson R, et al. Identification of the gene (*SEDL*) causing X-linked spondyloepiphyseal dysplasia tarda. *Nat Genet* 1999;22:400–404.
Gedeon AK, Tiller GE, LeMerrer M, et al. The molecular basis of X-linked spondyloepiphyseal dysplasia tarda (SEDL). *Am J Hum Genet* 2001;68:1386–1397.
Horton W. Advances in the genetics of human chondroplasias. *Pediatr Radiol* 1997;27:419–421.
Tiller GE, Hannig VL, Dozier DP, et al. A recurrent RNA splicing mutation in the *SEDL* gene causes X-linked spondyloepiphyseal dysplasia tarda (SEDL). *Am J Hum Genet* 2001;68:1398–1407.

RESOURCES
188, 247, 253

30   Spondyloepiphyseal Dysplasia Tarda

John Hicks, MD, DDS, PhD

DEFINITION: Spondyloepiphyseal dysplasia (SED) tarda was first described in the mid-1930s and is a form of osteochondrodysplasia associated with short stature of usually a mild to moderate degree, flat vertebrae, and progressive severe hip disease. This condition is termed tarda because the affected children are clinically and radiographically normal at birth and do not display features until >6 years of age. Inheritance pattern varies from autosomal dominant (SED tarda, classic type) to autosomal recessive (SED, Toledo type) to X-linked (SED, X-linked).

SYNONYMS: Spondyloepiphyseal dysplasia, late; SEDT; SED, X-linked.

DIFFERENTIAL DIAGNOSIS: Type II collagenopathies; Kniest dysplasia; SED congenita; Hypochondrogenesis; Stickler syndrome; Achondroplasia type II; Multiple epiphyseal dysplasia 2; Mutations in type IX and X collagen; Metaphyseal chondrodysplasia, Schmid type; Morquoi-Brailsford chondroosteodystrophy; Perthes disease; Bilateral congenital hip dislocation; Traumatic synovitis.

SYMPTOMS AND SIGNS: The characteristic findings in spondyloepiphyseal dysplasia tarda (autosomal-dominant or Toledo autosomal-recessive form) are (a) short stature, usually identifiable in childhood, but possibly not detected until the third or fourth decade of life; (b) normocephalic head; (c) flat facies; (d) spinal deformities (platyspondyly, short neck, cervical subluxation, odontoid hypoplasia, kyphoscoliosis, and lumbar lordosis); (e) thoracic deformities (barrel chest and pectus carinatum); (f) joint deformities (severe osteoarthritis of hips, multiple loose bodies in various joints, flattened metatarsal and metacarpal heads, symmetrical polyarticular osteoarthritis, and platyspondyly); (g) stiff gait that precedes joint degeneration; (h) bilateral pain and stiffness in hips (most severe), back (most severe), knees, shoulders, and elbows; and (i) normal intelligence. Mean height in men is 141–162 cm and in women 138–149 cm. Laboratory results include absence or severe deficiency of beta-2-globulin in typical SED tarda. In autosomal-recessive SED Toledo type, the abnormalities occur in urinary mucopolysaccharide (chondroitin-6-sulfate), low activity of PAPS-chondroitin sulfate sulfotransferase, and chondroitin sulfate synthesis. In addition, the SED Toledo phenotype includes corneal opacities. The X-linked form of SED tarda has an identical phenotype as that described for the autosomal-dominant classic form of SED.

ETIOLOGY/EPIDEMIOLOGY: The prevalence of the various forms of SED is not known with certainty. The prevalence for the X-linked SED type in a Scottish population is 1 in 100,000 population. The autosomal-dominant (classic) and autosomal-recessive (Toledo) forms of SED have been linked by some to type II collagen gene (*COL2A1*, chromosome 12q13.1-13.2) mutations. These mutations vary from a single base pair substitution to an entire exon deletion to duplication of portions of the gene. These mutations result in delayed secretion or overmodification of procollagen, resulting in defective collagen synthesis, aggregation, assembly, and folding. Type II collagen is primarily located in cartilaginous tissues, the tectorial membrane of the inner ear, nucleus pulposus of intervertebral discs, and the vitreous of the eye. Mutations in the *COL2A1* gene results in distortion of collagen's triple helix of collagen with adverse effects on tissue properties and functions. The X-linked form of SED has been mapped to the short arm of the X chromosome (Xp22.2-p22.1), and the associated gene is known as *Sedlin* (*SEDL*, *SEDT*, 170 kb). The *SEDL* gene product is a 140–amino acid protein with a role in protein transport from the endoplasmic reticulum to Golgi body and protein packaging into vesicles. This protein is critical for transport of type II procollagen to the Golgi for modification prior to packaging into vesicles for release from the cell membrane. *SEDL* protein is expressed widely, particularly in fibroblasts, lymphocytes, and fetal cartilage. The *SEDL* protein has homology with TRAPP (transport protein particle) in other species. TRAPP is responsible for the targeting and fusion of the protein acceptor compartment with the endoplasmic reticulum to the Golgi body transport vesicles. It has been noted that less severe missense mutations of *SEDL* may result in different phenotypic expression, with some probands developing precocious osteoarthritis only.

DIAGNOSIS: The earliest diagnostic clues for SED tarda may be a stiff gait with joint pain being most severe in the hips and back (spine). Clinical signs and symptoms and radiologic findings, as previously outlined, provide definitive diagnostic evidence. Suspicion for SED tarda of various types may be triggered by a family history of SED in other kindred. Genetic testing for diagnosis may be performed to evaluate for *COL2A1* (12q13.1-13.2) and *Sedlin* (Xp22.2-p22.1) mutations. Prenatal cytogenetic analysis of amniotic fluid and chorionic villus samples may provide diagnostic information for genetic counseling, and also indicate the need for parental, sibling, and extended family cytogenetic testing. Identification of mutations in the *COL2A1*

(12q13.1-13.2) or *Sedlin* (Xp22.2-p22.1) locus may provide for prenatal and neonatal diagnosis, parental testing in high-risk families, pregnancy planning, appropriate termination of pregnancy, and *in utero* gene therapy in the future.

TREATMENT
Standard Treatment: Symptomatic treatment is needed depending on the phenotype of the proband. There is no known treatment for SED tarda.

REFERENCES
Baitner A, Maurer S, Gruen M, et al. The genetic basis of the osteochondrodysplasias. *J Pediatr Orthop* 2001;20:594–605.

Gecz J, Hillman M, Gedeon A, et al. Gene structure and expression study of the *SEDL* gene for spondyloepiphyseal dysplasia tarda. *Genomics* 2000;69:242–251.
Gedeon A, Colley A, Jamieson R, et al. Identification of the gene (*SEDL*) causing X-linked spondyloepiphyseal dysplasia tarda. *Nat Genet* 1999;22:400–404.
Gedeon A, Tiller G, LeMerrer M, et al. The molecular basis of X-linked spondyloepiphyseal dysplasia tarda. *Am J Hum Genet* 2001;68:1386–1397.
Grunebaum E, Arpaia E, MacKenzie J, et al. A missense mutation in the *SEDL* gene results in delayed onset of X-linked spondyloepiphyseal dysplasia tarda in a large pedigree. *J Med Genet* 2001;38:409–411.

RESOURCES
188, 247, 253

---

31 Trichorhinophalangeal Syndrome Type I

John Hicks, MD, DDS, PhD

DEFINITION: Trichorhinophalangeal syndrome type I (TRPSI) is a malformation syndrome characterized by distinctive craniofacial and skeletal abnormalities.

DIFFERENTIAL DIAGNOSIS: Trichorhinophalangeal syndrome type III; Trichorhinophalangeal syndrome type II; Perthes-like hip malformation.

SYMPTOMS AND SIGNS: The characteristic findings are short stature; sparse, thin, slow-growing scalp hair; prominent pear-shaped nose; long flat philtrum; thin upper vermillion border; protruding prominent ears; normocephalic head; micrognathia; brachydactyly, short metacarpals, short phalanges; cone-shaped epiphyses at the phalanges, and hip malformations on radiographic studies; and normal intelligence.

ETIOLOGY/EPIDEMIOLOGY: The disorder is predominantly inherited in an autosomal-dominant form, although autosomal-recessive (haploinsufficiency) forms occur. The disorder shares a mutated gene on chromosome 8 (8q24.12, *TRPS1*) with trichorhinophalangeal syndrome types II and III.

DIAGNOSIS: Clinical and radiologic findings support the diagnosis. Additionally, molecular genetic testing for nonsense and in-frame splice mutations in the *TRPS1* gene (8q24.12) provides confirmatory evidence for TRPSI. Pre-natal diagnosis in suspected probands may be identified by chorionic villous sampling and amniotic fluid analysis for the mutated *TRPS1* gene. Diagnosis may also be provided with such testing for the neonate and family members where there is a history of TRPSI. The disorder can be differentiated from TRPSII by the lack of exostoses and from TRPSIII by the lack of severely short stature and severely shortened metacarpals. Mutation analysis can also differentiate TRPSI from TRPSII and from TRPSIII.

TREATMENT
Standard Therapies: Symptomatic treatment depends on the phenotype of the affected individual. No therapy is available.

REFERENCES
Giedion A. Burdea M, Fruchter Z, et al. Autosomal dominant transmission of the trichorhinophalangeal syndrome: report of 4 unrelated families, review of 60 cases. *Helv Paediatr Acta* 1973;28:249–259.
Ludecke J, Schaper J, Meinecke P, et al. Genotypic and phenotypic spectrum in trichorhinophalangeal syndrome types I and III. *Am J Hum Genet* 2001;68:81–91.
McCloud D, Solomon L. The trichorhinophalangeal syndrome. *Br J Dermatol* 1977;96:403–407.
Momeni P, Glockner G, Schmidt O, et al. Mutations in a new gene, encoding a zinc-finger protein, cause trichorhinophalangeal syndrome type I. *Nat Genet* 2000;24:71–74.

RESOURCES
188, 230, 246, 360

32 Trichorhinophalangeal Syndrome Type II

John Hicks, MD, DDS, PhD

DEFINITION: Trichorhinophalangeal syndrome type II (TRPSII) is a short stature syndrome characterized by sparse hair, bulbous nose, short phalanges, mental retardation, and multiple exostoses.

SYNONYM: Langer-Giedion syndrome.

DIFFERENTIAL DIAGNOSIS: Trichorhinophalangeal syndrome type I (TRPSI); Trichorhinophalangeal syndrome type III (TRPSIII; Sugio-Kajii syndrome); Multiple exostoses syndrome.

SYMPTOMS AND SIGNS: Characteristic findings include multiple exostoses that occur during the first decade of life; mental retardation; microcephaly; redundant skin; short stature; brachydactyly, short metacarpals, and short phalanges; sparse, thin, slow-growing scalp hair; bulbous tip of nose; cone-shaped epiphyses at the phalanges and hip malformations; and neonatal hypotonia. Less consistent findings include hyperextensible joints; recurrent upper respiratory infections; and delayed speech development. Features that may occur and are not shared with TRPSI and TRPSIII include tented, thick alae; prominent philtrum; bushy eyebrows; hearing loss; ureteral reflux; persistent cloaca; hydrometrocolpos; hematometra; and prune belly sequence.

ETIOLOGY/EPIDEMIOLOGY: The disorder is inherited in an autosomal-dominant pattern. It is caused by a contiguous deletion (chromosome 8q24.11-q24.13) of the TRPS1 and EXT1 genes. There is a male predilection that is not shared by TRPSI and TRPSIII.

DIAGNOSIS: Clinical and radiologic findings provide support for the diagnosis. Genetic testing for contiguous deletion of *TRPS1* and *EXT1* genes (chromosome 8q24.11-q24.13) confirms the diagnosis. Prenatal diagnosis in suspected probands may be identified by chorionic villus sampling and amniotic fluid analysis. Diagnosis may also be provided with such molecular genetic testing for the neonate and family members where there is a history of TRPSII.

TREATMENT
Standard Therapies: No therapy is available. Symptomatic treatment depends on the phenotype.

REFERENCES
Langer L. The thoracic-pelvic-phalangeal dystrophy. *Birth Defects Orig Art Ser* 1969;5:55–64.
Ludecke H-J, Wagner M, Nardmann J, et al. Molecular dissection of a contiguous gene syndrome: localization of the genes involved in the Langer-Giedion syndrome. *Hum Mol Genet* 1995;4:31–36.
McCloud D, Solomon L. The trichorhinophalangeal syndrome. *Br J Dermatol* 1977;96:403–407.
Parrish J, Wagner M, Hecht J, et al. Molecular analysis of overlapping chromosomal deletions in patients with Langer-Giedion syndrome. *Genomics* 1991;11:54–61.
Wuyts W, van Hul W. Molecular basis of multiple exostoses: mutations in the *EXT1* and *EXT2* genes. *Hum Mutat* 2000;15:220–227.

RESOURCES
230, 246, 360, 371

33 Trichorhinophalangeal Syndrome Type III

John Hicks, MD, DDS, PhD

DEFINITION: Trichorhinophalangeal syndrome type III (TRPSIII) is characterized by features similar to those of Ruvulcaba syndrome, including sparse hair, beaked nose, long upper lip, short stature, and severe metacarpophalangeal shortening. Individuals with the syndrome do not have mental retardation and microcephaly.

SYNONYM: Sugio-Kajii syndrome.

DIFFERENTIAL DIAGNOSIS: Trichorhinophalangeal syndrome type I (TRPSI); Ruvalcaba syndrome; Trichorhinophalangeal syndrome type II (TRPSII; Langer-Giedion syndrome); Perthes-like hip malformation.

SYMPTOMS AND SIGNS: The characteristic findings are severe short stature; severe brachydactyly, severely short metacarpals and short phalanges; sparse, thin, slow-growing scalp hair; bulbous tip of nose; long, flat philtrum; thin upper vermillion border; protruding prominent ears; normocephalic head; micrognathia; cone-shaped epiphyses at the phalanges and hip malformations; and normal intelligence.

ETIOLOGY/EPIDEMIOLOGY: The disorder is caused by several different mutations in the zinc finger transcription factor *TRPS1*, which is located on the long arm of chromosome 8 (8q24.12). This gene is located centromeric (proximal) to the gene *EXT1*, which is mutated in multiple exostoses syndrome and TRPSII.

DIAGNOSIS: Clinical and radiologic findings support the diagnosis. Cytogenetic testing for exon 6 mutations in the *TRPS1* gene (8q24.12) provides confirmatory evidence. Prenatal diagnosis in suspected probands may be identified by chorionic villus sampling and amniotic fluid analysis. Diagnosis may also be provided with such testing for the neonate and family members where there is a history of TRPS.

TREATMENT
Standard Therapies: No therapy is available. Symptomatic treatment depends on the phenotype.

REFERENCES
Ludecke J, Schaper J, Meinecke P, et al. Genotypic and phenotypic spectrum in trichorhinophalangeal syndrome types I and III. *Am J Hum Genet* 2001;68:81–91.

McCloud D, Solomon L. The trichorhinophalangeal syndrome. *Br J Dermatol* 1977;96:403–407.

Momeni P, Glockner G, Schmidt O, et al. Mutations in a new gene, encoding a zinc-finger protein, cause trichorhinophalangeal syndrome type I. *Nat Genet* 2000;24:71–74.

Sugio Y, Kajii T. Ruvalcaba syndrome: autosomal dominant inheritance. *Am J Med Genet* 1984;19:741–753.

RESOURCES
188, 230, 246, 360

---

34   Waardenburg Syndromes

Andrew P. Read, PhD

DEFINITION: The Waardenburg syndromes (WS) are a group of inherited conditions characterized by the combination of hearing loss and patchy pigmentary abnormalities.

DIFFERENTIAL DIAGNOSIS: Piebaldism; Nonsyndromic hearing loss.

SYMPTOMS AND SIGNS: The hearing loss is congenital, nonprogressive, and sensorineural; in approximately 50% of patients it is severe or profound. Pigmentary abnormalities may include iris heterochromia, white forelock, early graying, and white skin patches. These features are variable, even within a family. Dystopia canthorum is a crucial discriminant between the two main types of WS, WS1 (with dystopia canthorum), and WS2 (without dystopia). Apart from dystopia, the features of WS1 and WS2 are similar. Rare subtypes include WS3 (Klein-Waardenburg syndrome, WS1 with limb abnormalities) and WS4 (Waardenburg-Shah syndrome, WS2 with Hirschsprung disease).

ETIOLOGY/EPIDEMIOLOGY: WS1 is a true genetic entity, caused by mutations in the *PAX3* gene and inherited in an autosomal-dominant fashion. It is found in both sexes and all racial groups with a frequency of approximately 1 in 40,000. The other forms are heterogeneous. WS2 is also autosomal dominant. Approximately 15% of families have mutations in the *MITF* gene; the rest have unidentified genetic causes. Most patients with "WS3" have just a variant of WS1; a few are homozygous for *PAX3* mutations and are severely affected. WS4 can be caused by homozygosity for mutations in the *EDN3* (endothelin 3) or *EDNRB* (endothelin receptor B) genes, by heterozygosity for mutations in *SOX10*, or by unknown genetic causes.

DIAGNOSIS: Dystopia canthorum is assessed by computing an index, W, from the inner canthal, interpupillary, and outer canthal distances. A W value greater than 1.95 indicates WS1, which may be confirmed by PAX3 mutation testing. Diagnostic genetic tests are not commonly available for the other types.

TREATMENT
Standard Therapies: There is no specific treatment. Hearing loss is treated by standard means, including hearing aids or cochlear implants. Some patients with WS1 request cosmetic surgery for the dystopia. A weak associa-

tion of neural tube defects exists with WS1 (but not WS2), and therefore folate supplementation in early pregnancy may be worth considering if either parent has WS1.

REFERENCES

Gorlin RJ, Toriello HV, Cohen MM. *Hereditary hearing loss and its syndromes.* New York: Oxford University Press, 1995.

Read AP. Waardenburg syndrome. In: Scriver CR, Beaudet AL, Sly WS, et al., eds. *The metabolic and molecular bases of inherited disease,* 8th ed. New York: McGraw-Hill, 2001.

Read AP, Newton VE. Syndrome of the month: Waardenburg syndrome. *J Med Genet* 1997;34:656–665.

RESOURCES

149, 321, 337, 355

Resources

The following organizations provide help to patients and families affected by rare disorders:

NORD Member Organizations

National Members

Alpha 1 Association
Alpha-1 Foundation
American Brain Tumor Association
American Laryngeal Papilloma Foundation
American Porphyria Foundation
American Syringomyelia Alliance Project
Amyotrophic Lateral Sclerosis Association (ALS)
Aplastic Anemia & MDS International Foundation, Inc.
Association for Glycogen Storage Disease
Association of Gastrointestinal Motility Disorders
Batten Disease Support & Research Association
Benign Essential Blepharospasm Research Foundation
Charcot-Marie-Tooth Association
Chromosome 18 Registry Research Society
Cleft Palate Foundation
Cornelia de Lange Syndrome Foundation
Cystinosis Foundation, Inc.
Dysautonomia Foundation, Inc.
Dystonia Medical Research Foundation
Dystrophic Epidermolysis Bullosa Research of America
  (DEBRA)
Ehlers Danlos National Foundation
Epilepsy Foundation of America
Families of Spinal Muscular Atrophy
Foundation Fighting Blindness
Foundation for Ichthyosis and Related Skin Types
Genetic Alliance
Guillain-Barré Syndrome Foundation International
Hemochromatosis Foundation
Hereditary Colon Cancer Association
Hereditary Disease Foundation
HHT Foundation International, Inc.
Histiocytosis Association of America
Huntington's Disease Society of America
Immune Deficiency Foundation
International FOP Association, Inc.
International Joseph Diseases Foundation, Inc.
International Rett Syndrome Association
Interstitial Cystitis Association
Lowe Syndrome Association, Inc.

Mastocytosis Society (TMS)
Mucolipidosis Type IV Foundation (ML4)
Myasthenia Gravis Foundation of America
Myeloproliferative Disease Research Center
Myositis Association of America, Inc.
Narcolepsy Network, Inc.
National Adrenal Disease Foundation
National Alopecia Areata Foundation
National Ataxia Foundation
National Foundation for Ectodermal Dysplasias
National Hemophilia Foundation
National Marfan Foundation
National MPS Society, Inc.
National Multiple Sclerosis Society
National Neurofibromatosis Foundation
National PKU News
National Spasmodic Torticollis Association
National Tay-Sachs & Allied Diseases
National Urea Cycle Disorder Foundation
Neurofibromatosis, Inc.
Osteogenesis Imperfecta Foundation, Inc.
Parkinson's Disease Foundation, Inc.
Prader-Willi Syndrome Association
Pulmonary Hypertension Association
PXE International, Inc.
Reflex Sympathetic Dystrophy Association
Scleroderma Foundation
Sickle Cell Disease Association of America
Stevens-Johnson Syndrome Foundation
Sturge-Weber Foundation
The Paget Foundation
Tourette Syndrome Association
Trigeminal Neuralgia Association
United Leukodystrophy Foundation
United Mitochondrial Disease Foundation
VHL Family Alliance
Wegener's Granulomatosis Association
Williams Syndrome Assocation
Wilson's Disease Association

Associate Members

Acid Maltase Deficiency Association (AMDA)
Alternating Hemiplegia of Childhood Foundation
A-T Children's Project
American Autoimmune Related Disease Association

American Behçet's Disease Association
American Self-Help Group Clearinghouse
Amyotrophic Lateral Sclerosis of Greater Philadelphia Chapter
Canadian Organization for Rare Disorders (CORD)
Children's PKU Network
Chromosome Deletion Outreach Inc.
Chronic Granulomatous Disease Association
CLIMB
Consortium of MS Centers
Contact A Family
Cooley's Anemia Foundation, Inc.
Cushing Support & Research Foundation, Inc.
Family Caregiver Alliance
Family Support Network of North Carolina
Freeman-Sheldon Parent Support Group
Hydrocephalus Association
Incontinentia Pigmenti International Foundation
K-T Support Group
Late Onset Tay-Sachs Foundation
Les Turner ALS Foundation, Ltd.
National Lymphedema Network, Inc.
National Niemann-Pick Disease Foundation
National Patient Travel Helpline
National Spasmodic Dysphonia Association
Osteoporosis and Related Bone Diseases National Resource Center
Organic Acidemia Association
Parent to Parent New Zealand, Inc.
Rare & Expensive Disease Management Program (REM)
Recurrent Respiratory Papillomatosis Foundation
Restless Legs Syndrome Foundation
Sarcoid Networking Association
Shwachman-Diamond Syndrome International
Society for PSP
Sotos Syndrome Support Association
Taiwan Foundation for Rare Disorders
Takayasu's Arteritis Association
The CDG Family Network Foundation

Umbrella Organizations Covering Many Diseases

March of Dimes
1275 Mamaroneck Avenue
White Plains, NY 10605
(888) 663-4637

Genetic Alliance
4301 Connecticut Avenue NW, Suite 404
Washington, DC 20008
(800) 336-4363

For information regarding free or low-cost travel for treatment or to participate in clinical trials:

National Patient Travel Helpline
4620 Haygood Road, Suite 1
Virginia Beach, VA 23455
(800) 296-1217

Other Resources

1. 11Q Research and Resource Group
6123 A Duncan Road
Petersburg, VA 23803
Tel: 804-863-2114
Fax: 804-828-5343
msjohnso@vcu.edu

2. 22q and You Center
The Department of Clinical Genetics
The Children's Hospital of Philadelphia
One Children's Center
34th Street and Civic Center Boulevard
Philadelphia, PA 19104
Tel: 215-590-2920
Fax: 215-590-3298
lunny@email.chop.edu

3. 49XXXXY
10001 NE 74th Street
Vancouver, WA 98662-3801
Tel: 360-892-7547
kimbj@juno.com

4. 4P-Support Group
2585 Taylor
Longview, WA 98632
Tel: 703-497-2807
fourpminus@4p-supportgroup.org

5. 5p- Society
PMB 502
7108 Katella Ave.
Stanton, CA 90680
Tel: 714-901-1544
Fax: 562-920-5240
Toll free: 888-970-0777
fivepminus@aol.com

6. Aarskog Syndrome Parents Support Group
62 Robin Hill Lane
Levittown, PA 19055-1411
Tel: 215-943-7131

7. AboutFace U.S.A.
P.O. Box 969
Batavia, IL 60510
Tel: 312-337-0742
Fax: 815-444-1943
Toll free: 888-486-1209
AboutFace2000@aol.com

8. Acid Maltase Deficiency Association, Inc.
P.O. Box 700248
San Antonio, TX 78270-0248
Tel: 210-494-6144
Fax: 210-490-7161
tianrama@aol.com

9. Adams-Oliver Syndrome Support Group
16 Kirton Close
Radyr Way
Llandaff, Cardiff
South Glamorean, CF5 2NB
Wales, United Kingdom

10. Adenoid Cystic Carcinoma Foundation
P.O. Box 254
Canandaigua, NY 14424
sharon.lane@mail.acor.org

11. Adult Congenital Heart Association, Inc.
273 Perham St.
West Roxbury, MA 02132
Tel: 617-325-1191
info@adultcongenitalheart.org

12. Agenesis of Corpus Callosum (ACC) Network
5749 Merrill Hall
Room 18
University of Maine
Orono, ME 04469-5749
Tel: 207-581-3119
Fax: 207-581-3120
um-acc@maine.maine.edu

13. Aicardi Syndrome Awareness and Support Group
29 Delavan Avenue
Toronto
Ontario, M5P 1T2
Canada
Tel: 416-481-4095

14. Alagille Syndrome Alliance
10630 SW Garden Park Place
Tigard, OR 97223
Tel: 503-639-6217
cchahn@worldnet.att.net

15. Alexander Graham Bell Association for the Deaf, Inc.
3417 Volta Place, NW
Washington, DC 20007-2778
Tel: 202-337-5220
Fax: 202-337-8314
Toll free: 800-432-7543
agbell2@aol.com

16. Alpha 1 Association
8120 Penn Avenue South
Suite 549
Minneapolis, MN 55431-1326
Tel: 952-703-9979
Fax: 952-703-9977
Toll free: 800-521-3025
aina@alpha1.org

17. Alpha One Foundation
2937 SW 27th Ave.
Suite 302
Miami, FL 33133
Tel: 305-567-9888
Fax: 305-567-0563
Toll free: 888-825-7421
info@alphaone.org

18. Alpha-1-Antitrypsin Deficiency Registry
Cleveland Clinic Foundation
Department of Pulmonary Diseases
9500 Euclid Ave.
Cleveland, OH 44195
Tel: 216-444-4576

19. Alport Syndrome—Hereditary Nephritis Study
Alport Study Department of Physiology
#156
410 Chipeta Way
Salt Lake City, UT 84108-1297
Tel: 801-581-5479
Fax: 801-585-3232
david.f.barker@m.cc.utah.edu

20. Alternating Hemiplegia of Childhood Foundation (IFAHC)
239 Nevada Street
Redwood City, CA 94062
Tel: 650-365-5798
Fax: 650-365-5798
laegan6@sbcglobal.net

21. Alveolar Capillary Dysplasia Association (ACD)
28 West 520 Douglas Road
Naperville, IL 60564-9593
acd-association.com

22. Alzheimer's Association
919 North Michigan Avenue
Suite 1000
Chicago, IL 60611-1676
Tel: 312-335-8700
Fax: 312-335-1110
Toll free: 800-272-3900
info@alz.org

23. Alzheimer's Disease Education and Referral Center
P.O. Box 8250
Silver Spring, MD 20907-8250
Tel: 301-495-3311
Fax: 301-495-3334
Toll free: 800-438-4380
adear@alzheimers.org

24. Ambiguous Genitalia Support Network
P.O. Box 313
Clements, CA 95227-0313
Tel: 209-727-0313
Fax: 209-727-0313
agsn@jps.net

25. American Association for Klinefelter Syndrome Information and Support
2945 West Farwell Ave.
Chicago, IL 60645-2925
Tel: 773-761-5298
Fax: 773-761-5298
Toll free: 888-466-5747
aaksis@aol.com

26. American Association of Kidney Patients
100 South Ashley Drive
Suite 280
Tampa, FL 33602
Tel: 813-223-7099
Fax: 813-223-0001
Toll free: 800-749-2257
aakpnat@aol.com

27. American Autoimmune Related Diseases Association, Inc.
22100 Gratiof Ave.
Eastpointe, MI 48021-2227
Tel: 810-776-3900
Fax: 810-776-3903
Toll free: 800-598-4668
aarda@aol.com

28. American Behçet's Disease Association
P.O. Box 15247
Chattanooga, TN 37415-0247
Toll free: 800-723-4238
shrinkrap2@aol.com

29. American Brain Tumor Association
2720 River Road
Suite 146
Des Plaines, IL 60018
Tel: 847-827-9910
Fax: 847-827-9918
Toll free: 800-886-2282
info@abta.org

30. American Cancer Society, Inc.
1599 Clifton Road NE
Atlanta, GA 30329
Tel: 404-320-3333
Toll free: 800-227-2345

31. American Council of the Blind, Inc.
1155 15th Street
Suite 720
Washington, DC 20005
Tel: 202-467-5081
Fax: 202-467-5085
Toll free: 800-424-8666
info@acb.org

32. American Diabetes Association
National Service Center
1660 Duke St.
Alexandria, VA 22314
Tel: 703-549-1500
Fax: 703-549-6995
Toll free: 800-342-2383

33. American Foundation for the Blind
11 Penn Plaza
Suite 300
New York, NY 10001
Tel: 212-502-7600
Fax: 212-502-7777
Toll free: 800-232-5463
afbinfo@afb.org

34. American Foundation for Urologic Disease
1128 North Charles Street
Baltimore, MD 21201
Tel: 410-468-1800
Fax: 410-468-1808
Toll free: 800-242-2383
admin@afud.org

35. American Heart Association
National Center
7272 Greenville Avenue
Dallas, TX 75231-4596
Tel: 214-373-6300
Fax: 214-373-0268
Toll free: 800-242-8721
inquire@heart.org

36. American Hemochromatosis Society (AHS)
777 East Atlantic Ave.
PMB Z-363
Delray Beach, FL 33483-5352
Tel: 561-266-9037
Fax: 561-266-9038
Toll free: 888-655-4766
ahs@emi.net

37. American Kidney Fund, Inc.
6110 Executive Boulevard
Suite 1010
Rockville, MD 20852
Tel: 301-881-3052
Fax: 301-881-0898
Toll free: 800-638-8299
helpline@akfinc.org

38. American Laryngeal Papilloma Foundation
P.O. Box 6108
Spring Hill, FL 34611-6108
Tel: 352-684-7191
carrie@atlantic.net

39. American Liver Foundation
75 Maiden Lane
Suite 603
New York, NY 10038
Tel: 212-668-1000
Fax: 973-25-63214
Toll free: 800-465-4837
webmail@liverfoundation.org

40. American Lung Association
1740 Broadway
New York, NY 10019
Tel: 212-315-8700
Fax: 212-265-5642
Toll free: 800-586-4872
info@lungusa.org

41. American Porphyria Foundation
P.O. Box 22712
Houston, TX 77024
Tel: 713-266-9617
Fax: 713-871-1788
porphyrus@juno.com

42. American Syringomyelia Alliance Project, Inc.
300 Green Street, Suite 206
P.O. Box 1586
Longview, TX 75606-1586
Tel: 903-236-7079
Fax: 903-757-7456
Toll free: 800-272-7282
info@asap4sm.com

43. Amyotrophic Lateral Sclerosis Association
27001 Agoura Road
Suite 150
Calabasas Hills, CA 91301-5104
Tel: 818-880-9007
Fax: 818-880-9006
Toll free: 800-782-4747
mary@alsa-national.org

44. Androgen Insenitivity Support Group
1191 University Blvd.
No. 507
Denver, CO 80206-4613
Tel: 978-455-2012
aisusgroup.aol.com

45. Anencephaly Support Foundation
30827 Sifton
Spring, TX 77386
Tel: 281-364-9222
Toll free: 888-206-7526
asf@asfhelp.com

46. Angelman Syndrome Foundation, Inc.
414 Plaza Drive
Suite 209
Westmont, IL 60559
Tel: 630-734-9267
Fax: 630-655-0391
Toll free: 800-432-6435
asf@adminsys.com

47. Angelman Syndrome Support and Education Research Trust
P.O. Box 505
Sittingbourne
Kent, ME10 1NE
United Kingdom
Tel: 01795 429061
assert@walburns.freeserve.co.uk

48. Apert Support and Information Network
P.O. Box 1184
Fair Oaks, CA 95628
Tel: 916-961-1092
Fax: 916-961-1092
apertnet@ix.netcom.com

49. Apert Syndrome Support Group
8708 Kathy
St. Louis, MO 63126
Tel: 314-965-3356

50. Aplastic Anemia & MDS International Foundation, Inc.
P.O. Box 613
Annapolis, MD 21404-0613
Tel: 410-867-0242
Fax: 410-867-0240
Toll free: 800-747-2820
help@aamds.org

51. ARDS Support Center Inc.
7172 Regional Street
No. 278
Dublin, CA 94568-2324
www.ards.org

52. ARDSNet (ARDS Clinical Network)
www.ardsnet.org

53. Arthritis Foundation
1330 West Peachtree Street
Atlanta, GA 30309
Tel: 404-872-7100
Fax: 404-872-0457
Toll free: 800-283-7800
info@arthritis.org

54. Arthrogryposis Group
1 The Oaks
Gillingham
Dorset, SP8 4SW
United Kingdom
Tel: 01747 8226555
Fax: 01747 822655
taguk@aol.com

55. Ashermans Syndrome Online Community
7 George Drosini St.
Xylotymbou
Larnaca, 7510
Cyprus
Tel: 04-723716
Fax: 04-724150
krypoly@logos.cy.net

56. Association for Glycogen Storage Disease
P.O. Box 896
Durant, IA 52747
Tel: 563-785-6038
Fax: 563-785-6038
maryc@agsdus.org

57. Association for Macular Diseases, Inc.
210 East 64th Street
New York, NY 10021
Tel: 212-605-3719
Fax: 212-605-3795
macula@macula.org

58. Association for Neuro-Metabolic Disorders
5223 Brookfield Lane
Sylvania, OH 43560-1809
Tel: 419-885-1497
volk4olks@aol.com

59. Association for Spina Bifida and Hydrocephalus
ASBAH House
42 Park Road
Peterborough, PE1 2UQ
United Kingdom

60. Association of Children's Prosthetic/Orthotic Clinics
6300 North River Road
Suite 727
Rosemont, IL 60018-4226
Tel: 847-698-1637
Fax: 847-823-0536
king@aaos.org

61. Association of Gastrointestinal Motility Disorders, Inc.
(AGMD)
11 North St.
Lexington, MA 02420
Tel: 781-861-3874
Fax: 781-861-7834
agmdinc@aol.com

62. A-T (Ataxia-Telangiectasia) Project
3002 Enfield Road
Austin, TX 78703
Tel: 512-472-4892
Fax: 512-472-4892
Toll free: 877-873-2828
mhoward@atproject.org

63. Ataxia-Telangiectasia Children's Project
668 South Military Trail
Deerfield Beach, FL 33442
Tel: 954-481-6611
Fax: 954-725-1153
Toll free: 800-543-5728
bradmargus@atcp.org

64. AVENUES—A National Support Group for Arthrogryposis
Multiplex Congenita
P.O. Box 5192
Sonora, CA 95370
Tel: 209-928-3688
avenues@sonnet.com

65. Awakenings (Parkinson's Disease Information and News)
Web Site on the Internet
editor@parkinsonsdisease.com

66. Barth Syndrome Family Support Network
c/o Kennedy-Krieger Institute
Johns Hopkins Univ.
707 N. Broadway
Baltimore, MD 21205

67. Barth Syndrome Foundation
P.O. Box 23173
Lincoln, NE 68542

68. Batten Disease Support and Research Association
120 Humphries Dr.
Suite 2
Reynoldsburg, OH 43068
Tel: 740-927-4298
Fax: 614-445-4191
Toll free: 800-448-4570
bdsra1@bdsra.com

69. Beckwith Wiedemann Support Network
2711 Colony Rd.
Ann Arbor, MI 48104
Tel: 734-973-0263
Fax: 734-973-9721
Toll free: 800-837-2976
a800bwsn@aol.com

70. Bell's Palsy Research Foundation
9121 East Tanque Verde
Suite 105-286
Tucson, AZ 85749
Tel: 520-749-4614
Fax: 954-337-7803
Toll free: 874-125-5335
bellspalsy@aol.com

71. Bell's Palsy Web Site and Online Support Group
c/o Annette Lemke
65 Calle El Avion
Camarillo, CA 93010
seabee86@aol.com

72. Benign Essential Blepharospasm Research Foundation, Inc.
P.O. Box 12468
Beaumont, TX 77726-2468
Tel: 409-832-0788
Fax: 409-832-0890
bebrf@ih2000.net

73. Bernard-Soulier Syndrome Website and Registry
Royal College of Surgeons in Ireland
123 St. Stephen's Green
Dublin 2
Ireland
Tel: 353-1-4022100
bernard-soulier@rcsi.ie

74. Better Hearing Institute
5021-B Backlick Road
Annandale, VA 22003
Tel: 703-642-0580
Fax: 703-750-9302
Toll free: 800-327-9355
mail@betterhearing.org

75. Birth Defect Research for Children, Inc.
930 Woodcock Rd.
Suite 225
Orlando, FL 32803
Tel: 407-895-0802
Fax: 407-895-0824
abcd@birthdefects.org

76. Blepharophimosis, Ptosis, Epicanthus Inversus Family Network
SE 820 Meadow Vale Drive
Pullman, WA 99163
Tel: 509-332-6628
lschauble@wsu.edu

77. Blind Children's Fund
4740 Okemos Road
Okemos, MI 48864-1637
Tel: 517-347-1357
Fax: 517-347-1459
blindchfnd@aol.com

78. Bloom's Syndrome Registry
Department of Pediatrics
Cornell University Medical College
1300 York Ave.
New York, NY 10021
Tel: 212-746-3956

79. Brain and Pituitary Foundation of America
281 East Moody Avenue
Fresno, CA 93720-1524
Tel: 209-434-0610

80. British Coalition of Heritable Disorders of Connective Tissue
Rochester House
5 Aldershot Road
Fleet
Hampshire, GU13 9NG
United Kingdom
Tel: 01252 810472
Fax: 01252 810473

81. Caitlin Raymond International Registry of Bone Marrow Donor Banks
University of Massachusetts Medical Center
65 Lake Avenue North
Worcester, MA 01655
Tel: 508-792-8969
Fax: 508-792-8972
Toll free: 800-726-2824
info@CRIR.org

82. CancerNet—A service of the National Cancer Institute
www.cancer.net

83. CancerOnline
Web Site on the Internet
cancerinfo@stonecottage.com

84. Candlelighters Childhood Cancer Foundation
3910 Warner St.
Kensington, MD 20895
Tel: 301-962-3520
Fax: 301-962-3521
Toll free: 800-366-2223
info@candlelighters.org

85. Carcinoid Cancer Foundation, Inc.
1751 York Avenue
New York, NY 10128
Tel: 212-722-3132
Fax: 212-831-3031
mwarner@carcinoid.org

86. CARES Foundation, Inc. (Congenital Adrenal Hyperplasia, Research, Education and Support)
P.O. Box 264
Short Hills, NJ 07078
Tel: 973-912-3895
Fax: 973-912-3894
Toll free: 866-227-3737
kelly@caresfoundation.org

87. CCHS (Congenital Central Hypoventilation) Support Network
71 Maple Street
Oneonta, NY 13820
Tel: 607-432-8872
vanderlaanm@hartwick.edu

88. CCMS Support Group
63 Stirrup Way
Burlington, NJ 08016
Tel: 609-239-7831
Fax: 609-239-6916
tmontague@home.com

89. Centers for Disease Control and Prevention
1600 Clifton Road NE
Atlanta, GA 30333
Tel: 404-639-3534

90. Charcot-Marie-Tooth Association
2700 Chestnut St.
Chester, PA 19013
Tel: 610-499-7486
Fax: 610-499-7487
Toll free: 800-606-2682
cmtassoc@aol.com

91. CHARGE Syndrome Foundation, Inc.
2004 Parkade
Columbia, MO 65202-3121
Tel: 573-499-4694
Fax: 573-499-4694
Toll free: 800-442-7604
marion@chargesyndrome.org

92. CHERUBS—The Association of Congenital Diaphragmatic Hernia Research, Advocacy and Support
P.O. Box 1150
Creedmore, NC 27522
Tel: 919-693-8158
Fax: 707-924-1114
dawntorrence@cherubs-cdh.org

93. Children Anguished with Lymphatic Malformations
c/o Tina Marie Baalman
11413 Prestige Dr.
Frisco, TX 75034
Tel: 972-377-4326
staycalm@juno.com

94. Children's Brain Diseases Foundation
350 Parnassus Avenue
Suite 900
San Francisco, CA 94117
Tel: 415-566-5402
Fax: 415-863-3452
jr.der6022@aol.com

95. Children's Brittle Bone Foundation
7701 95th St.
Pleasant Prairie, WI 53158
Tel: 847-433-4981
Fax: 262-947-0724
info@cbbf.org

96. Children's Craniofacial Association
P.O. Box 280297
Dallas, TX 75228
Tel: 972-994-9902
Fax: 972-240-7607
Toll free: 800-535-3643
contactcca@ccakids.com

97. Children's Heart Association for Support and Education
c/o The Cardiac Clinic, Division of Cardiology
The Hospital For Sick Children
555 University Avenue
Toronto
Ontario, M5G 1X8
Canada
Tel: 416-410-2427

98. Children's Liver Alliance
3835 Richmond Avenue
Suite 190
Staten Island, NY 10312-3828
Tel: 718-987-6200
Fax: 718-987-6200
livers4kids@earthlink.net

99. Children's Liver Disease Foundation
AXA Equity & Law House
35-37 Great Charles Street Queensway
Birmingham, B3 3JY
United Kingdom
Tel: 0121-212-3839
Fax: 0121-212-4300

100. Children's PKU Network
3970 Via de la Valle
Suite 120 E
Del Mar, CA 92014
Tel: 858-509-0767
Fax: 858-509-0768
pkunetwork@aol.com

101. Chromosome 18 Registry and Research Society
6302 Fox Head
San Antonio, TX 78247
Tel: 210-657-4968
Fax: 210-657-4968
cody@chromosome18.org

102. Chromosome 22 Central
232 Kent Avenue
Timmins
Ontario, P4N 3C3
Canada
Tel: 705-268-3099
Fax: 705-268-3099
mum2_1@hotmail.com

103. Chromosome 9P- Network
c/o Beverly Udell
675 North Round Table Drive
Las Vegas, NV 89110
Tel: 702-453-0788
Fax: 702-459-4711
beverlyudell9p-@msn.com

104. Chromosome Deletion Outreach, Inc.
P.O. Box 724
Boca Raton, FL 33429-0724
Tel: 561-391-5098
Fax: 561-395-4252
Toll free: 888-236-6880
cdo@att.net

105. Chronic Granulomatous Disease Association, Inc.
2616 Monterey Road
San Marino, CA 91108
Tel: 626-441-4118
cgda@socal.rr.com

106. Chronic Lung Disease Forum
Cheshire Medical Center
580-590 Court St.
Keene, NH 3431
Tel: 603-354-5400

107. Churg-Strauss Syndrome International Support Group
2 Saint Andrews Court
St. Augustine, FL 32084
Tel: 904-824-1083
robbins@aug.com

108. Cleft Palate Foundation
104 South Estes Drive
Suite 204
Chapel Hill, NC 27514
Tel: 919-933-9044
Fax: 919-933-9604
Toll free: 800-242-5338
cleftline@aol.com

109. CLIMB (Children Living with Inherited Metabolic Diseases)
The Quadrangle
Crewe Hall
Weston Road
Crewe
Cheshire, CW1 6UR
United Kingdom
Tel: 44 870 7700 325
Fax: 44 870 7700 327
info@climb.org.uk

110. Cobalamin Network
P.O. Box 174
Thetford Center, VT 05075-0174
Tel: 802-785-4029
SueBee18@valley.net

111. Coffin-Lowry Syndrome Foundation
3045 255th Avenue SE
Sammamish, WA 98075
Tel: 425-427-0939
clsfoundation@yahoo.com

112. Cohen Syndrome Support Group
7 Woods Court
Brackley
Northants, NN13 6HP
United Kingdom
Tel: 01280-704515

113. Congenital Heart Anomalies, Support, Education, & Resources
2112 North Wilkins Road
Swanton, OH 43558
Tel: 419-825-5575
Fax: 419-825-2880
myer106w@wonder.em.cdc.gov or chaser@compuserve.com

114. Congenital Heart Disease Resource Page
Web Site on the Internet
sheri.berger@csun.edu

115. Congenital Heart Information Network
1561 Clark Dr.
Yardley, PA 19067
Tel: 215-493-3068
Fax: 215-493-3068
mb@tchin.org

116. Consortium of Muscuar Sclerosis Centers
c/o Gimbel MS Center
718 Teaneck Road
Teaneck, NJ
Tel: 201-837-0727
Fax: 201-837-8504
jhalper@aol.com

117. Contact Group for Trisomy 9p
11 Durgoyne Drive
Beardsden
Glasgow
Scotland, United Kingdom

118. Cooley's Anemia Foundation, Inc.
129-09 26th Avenue
Suite 203
Flushing, NY 11354-1131
Tel: 718-321-2873
Fax: 718-321-3340
Toll free: 800-522-7222
ncaf@aol.com

119. Cornelia de Lange Syndrome Foundation, Inc.
302 West Main Street
Suite 100
Avon, CT 06001
Tel: 860-676-8166
Fax: 860-676-8337
Toll free: 800-753-2357
info@cdlsusa.org

120. Craniofacial Foundation of America
Tennessee Craniofacial Center
975 East Third Street
Chattanooga, TN 37403
Tel: 423-778-9192
Fax: 423-778-8172
Toll free: 800-418-3223
farmertm@erlanger.org

121. Craniofacial Support Group
44 Helmsdale Road
Leamington Spa, CV32 7DW
United Kingdom
Tel: 44 1926 334629
sjmoody@compuserve.com

122. Creutzfeldt-Jakob Disease Foundation, Inc.
P.O. Box 611625
Miami, FL 33261-1625
Fax: 954-436-7591
crjakob@aol.com

123. Crohn's and Colitis Foundation of America
386 Park Avenue South
17th Floor
New York, NY 10016-9804
Tel: 212-685-3440
Fax: 212-779-4098
Toll free: 800-932-2423
mhda37b@prodigy.com

124. Crouzon's/Meniere's Support Network
3757 North Catherine Drive
Prescott Valley, AZ 86314-8320
katy@northlink.com

125. CRY - Cardiac Risk in the Young
Epsom Downs Metro Centre - Unit 7
Waterfield
Tadworth
Surrey, KT20 5LR
United Kingdom
www.cry.dircon.co.uk

126. Cushing Support and Research Foundation, Inc.
65 East India Row
Suite 22-B
Boston, MA 02110
Tel: 617-723-3674
Fax: 617-723-3674
cushinfo@aol.com

127. Cyclic Vomiting Syndrome Association (CVSA)
3585 Cedar Hill Road NW
Canal Winchester, OH 43110
Tel: 614-837-2586
Fax: 614-837-6543
waitesd@cvsaonline.org

128. Cystic Hygroma and Lymphangioma Support Group
Villa Fontane
Church Road
Worth
Crawley
Sussex, RH10 4RT
United Kingdom

129. Cystinosis Foundation, Inc.
604 Vernon St.
Oakland, CA 94610
Fax: 559-222-7997
Toll free: 800-392-8458

130. Cystinuria Support Network
21001 NE 36th Street
Sammamish, WA 98074
Tel: 425-868-2996
Fax: 425-897-0675
cystinuria@aol.com

131. Dercum's Support
P.O. Box 350
Somis, CA 93066
Tel: 805-386-3125
dercumdata@aol.com

132. Diabetes Insipidus Foundation, Inc.
4533 Ridge Drive
Baltimore, MD 21229
Tel: 410-247-3953
diabetesinsipidus@maxinter.net

133. Diamond Blackfan Anemia Registry
Schneider Children's Hospital
Hematology/Oncology/SCT
269-01 76th Ave.
New Hyde Park, NY 11040
avlachos@lij.edu

134. Diamond Blackfan Anemia Support Group
Ted Gordon Smith, MD
11 Hollyfield Avenue
London, N11 3BY
United Kingdom

135. Digestive Disease National Coalition
507 Capitol Court
Suite 200
Washington, DC 20002
Tel: 202-544-7497
Fax: 202-546-7105
ddirks@aol.com

136. Dr. Joseph Gleeson
Division of Pediatric Neurology
Department of Neuroscience
9500 Gilman Dr.
La Jolla, CA 92093
Tel: 858-822-3535
jogleeson@ucsd.edu

137. Dysautonomia Foundation, Inc.
633 Third Avenue
12th Floor
New York, NY 10017-6706
Tel: 212-949-6644
Fax: 212-682-7625
fdinfo@videobureau.com

138. Dysautonomia Foundation, Inc., Toronto Chapter
343 Clark Avenue West
Suite 1103
Thornhill
Ontario, L4J 7K5
Canada
Tel: 905-882-7725
Fax: 905-764-7752

139. Dystonia Medical Research Foundation
1 East Wacker Drive
Suite 2430
Chicago, IL 60601-1905
Tel: 312-755-0198
Fax: 312-803-0138
Toll free: 800-377-3978
dystonia@dystonia-foundation.org

140. Dystonia Society
46–47 Britton Street
London, EC1M 5UI
United Kingdom
Tel: 0 (171) 490-5671
Fax: 0 (171) 490-5672

141. Dystrophic Epidermolysis Bullosa Research Association of America, Inc. (DEBRA)
40 Rector Street
14th Floor
New York, NY 10006
Tel: 212-513-4090
Fax: 212-513-4099
jcampbell21@nyc.rr.com

142. Dystrophic Epidermolysis Bullosa Research Association-United Kingdom
DEBRA House
13 Wellington Business Park
Dukes Ride
Crowthorne
Berkshire, RG45 6LS
United Kingdom
Tel: +44 134477
admin@debra.org.uk

143. EA/TEF Child and Family Support Connection, Inc.
111 West Jackson Boulevard
Suite 1145
Chicago, IL 60604-3502
Tel: 312-987-9085
Fax: 312-987-9086
eatef2@aol.com

144. Ear Anomalies Reconstructed: Atresia/Microtia Support Group
72 Durand Road
Maplewood, NJ 07040
Tel: 973-761-5438
Fax: 973-378-8930
grossinsco@aol.com

145. Epilepsy Foundation
4351 Garden City Drive
Landover, MD 20785
Tel: 301-459-3700
Fax: 301-577-2684
Toll free: 800-332-1000
postmaster@efa.org

146. Erythromelalgia Association
4343 Roosevelt Way, NE
#305
Seattle, WA 98105
Tel: 206-632-0894
Fax: 206-632-1894
jeanmilt@prodigy.net

147. Erythropoietic Protoporphyria Research and Education Fund
Channing Laboratory, Harvard Medical School
Brigham & Women's Hospital
181 Longwood Ave.
Boston, MA 02115-5804
Tel: 617-525-2249
Fax: 617-731-1541
mmmathroth@bics.bwh.harvard.edu

148. Fabry Support & Information Group
108 NE 2nd St.
Suite C
P.O. Box 510
Concordia, MO 64020
Tel: 660-463-1355
Fax: 660-463-1356
jjohnson@cpgnet.com

149. FACES: The National Craniofacial Association
P.O. Box 11082
Chattanooga, TN 37401
Tel: 423-266-1632
Fax: 423-267-3124
Toll free: 800-332-2373
faces@faces-cranio.org

150. Facio-Scapulo-Humeral Society, Inc.
3 Westwood Road
Lexington, MA 02420
Tel: 781-860-0501
Fax: 781-860-0599
carol.perez@fshsociety.org

151. Fahr Disease Registry
Parkinson's Disease and Movement Disorders Clinic
Southern Illinois University School of Medicine
P.O. Box 19230
Springfield, IL 62794-9230

152. Families of Spinal Muscular Atrophy
P.O. Box 196
Libertyville, IL 60048
Tel: 847-367-7620
Fax: 847-367-7623
Toll free: 800-886-1762
sma@interaccess.com

153. Families with Moyamoya Support Network
4900 McGowan Street SE
Cedar Rapids, IA 52403

154. Family Caregiver's Alliance
690 Market Street
Suite 600
San Francisco, CA 94104
Tel: 415-434-3388

155. FG Syndrome Support Group
66 Ford Road
Dagenham
Essex, RM10 9JR
United Kingdom

156. Fighters for Encephaly Defects Support (FEDS)
3032 Brereton Street
Pittsburgh, PA 15219
Tel: 412-261-5363

157. Floating Harbor Syndrome Support Group
160 Guild NE
Grand Rapids, MI 49505
Tel: 616-447-9175
Fax: 616-447-9175
jdswanson@aol.com

158. FOD (Fatty Oxidation Disorders) Family Support Group
805 Montrose Drive
Greensboro, NC 27410
Tel: 336-547-8682
goulddan@aol.com

159. Food and Drug Administration (FDA) Office of Inquiry & Consumer Information
Office of Inquiry and Consumer Information
5600 Fisher Lane
Room 12-A-40
Rockville, MD 20857
Tel: 301-827-4420
Toll free: 888-463-6332

160. Forward Face, Inc.
317 East 34th Street
Room 901
New York, NY 10016
Tel: 212-684-5860
Fax: 212-684-5864
Toll free: 800-393-3223

161. Foundation Fighting Blindness
11435 Cronhill Dr.
Owings Mills, MD 21117-2220
Fax: 410-363-2393
Toll free: 800-683-5555
jchader@blindness.org

162. Foundation for Ichthyosis & Related Skin Types
650 North Cannon Ave.
Suite 17
Lansdale, PA 19446
Tel: 215-631-1411
Toll free: 800-545-3286
info@scalyskin.org

163. Foundation for Nager and Miller Syndromes
1827 Grove Street, #2
Glenview, IL 60025-2913
Tel: 847-7246449
Fax: 847-724-6449
Toll free: 800-507-3667
fnms@interaccess.com

164. Freeman-Sheldon Parent Support Group
509 East Northmont Way
Salt Lake City, UT 84103
Tel: 801-364-7060
Fax: 801-585-7395
fspsg@aol.com

165. Friedreich's Ataxia Research Alliance
2001 Jefferson Davis Hwy.
Suite 209
Arlington, VA 22202
Tel: 703-413-4468
Fax: 703-413-4467
fara@frda.org

166. Galactosaemia Support Group
31 Cotysmore
Sutton Coldfield
West Midlands, B75 6BJ
United Kingdom

167. Genetic Alliance
4301 Connecticut Avenue NW
Suite 404
Washington, DC 20008-2304
Tel: 202-966-5557
Fax: 202-966-8553
Toll free: 800-336-4363
info@geneticalliance.org

168. Glaucoma Research Foundation
200 Pine Street
Suite 200
San Francisco, CA 94104
Tel: 415-986-3162
Fax: 415-986-3763
Toll free: 800-826-6693
info@glaucoma.org

169. Gluten Intolerance Group of North America
15110 Tenth Avenue SW
Suite A
Seattle, WA 98166-1820
Tel: 206-246-6652
Fax: 206-246-6531
gig@accessone.com

170. Goldenhar Syndrome Support Network Society
9325 163 St.
Edmonton
Alberta, T5R 2P4
Canada
Tel: 780-465-9534
support@goldenharsyndrome.org

171. Guillain-Barré Syndrome Foundation International
P.O. Box 262
Wynnewood, PA 19096
Tel: 610-667-0131
Fax: 610-667-7036

172. Hemangioma Support System
c/o Cynthia Schumerth
1215 Monterey Terrace
DePere, WI 54115
Tel: 920-336-9399

173. Hemochromatosis Foundation, Inc.
P.O. Box 8569
Albany, NY 12208-2569
Tel: 518-489-0972
Fax: 518-489-0227

174. Hepatitis Foundation International
30 Sunrise Terrace
Cedar Grove, NJ 07009-1423
Tel: 973-239-1035
Fax: 973-857-5044
Toll free: 800-891-0707
hfi@intac.com

175. Hereditary Angioedema Association, Inc.
c/o Scott McCoy
950 Alexander Spring Rd.
Carlisle, PA 17013
Tel: 717-249-3438
Fax: 904-658-1322
hae@d3mail.com

176. Hereditary Colon Cancer Association (HCCA)
3601 N 4th Ave.
Suite 201
Sioux Falls, SD 57104
Tel: 605-373-2067
Fax: 605-336-6699
Toll free: 800-264-6783
info@hereditarycc.org

177. Hereditary Disease Foundation, Inc.
11400 West Olympic Blvd.
Suite 855
Los Angeles, CA 90064
Tel: 310-575-9656
Fax: 310-575-9156
cures@hdfoundation.org

178. Hereditary Fructose Intolerance Laboratory
Biology Department
Boston University
Cummington St.
Boston, MA 02215
Tel: 617-353-5310
Fax: 617-353-6340
tolan@bio.bu.edu

179. Hereditary Nephritis Foundation
1390 W 6690 S, #202 H
Murray, UT 84123
Tel: 801-262-5901

180. Hermansky-Pudlak Syndrome Network, Inc.
One South Road
Oyster Bay, NY 11771-1905
Tel: 516-922-3440
Fax: 516-922-4022
Toll free: 800-789-9477
appell@worldnet.att.net or *hpsn@juno.com*

181. HHT (Hereditary Hemorrhagic Telangiectasia) Foundation
International, Inc.
P.O. Box 8087
New Haven, CT 06530
Tel: 410-357-9932
Toll free: 800-448-6389
hhtinfo@hht.org

182. Hidradenitis Information Development and Exchange
Web Site on the Internet
hidecan@globalserve.net

183. Histiocytosis Association of America
302 North Broadway
Pitman, NJ 08071
Tel: 856-548-2758
Fax: 856-589-6614
Toll free: 800-548-2758
histiocyte@aol.com

184. HME Contact Group
3 Linn Drive
Netherlee
Glasgow, G44 3PT
Scotland
Tel: 0141 633 2617
hmecontactgroup@tinyworld.co.uk

185. Holt-Oram Syndrome Support Group
21 Forth Road, Rivers Estate
Redcar
Cleveland, TS10 1PN
United Kingdom
Tel: 164-248-5379
106524.33@compuserve.com

186. Home Page of Dr. J.T. Hain
Web Site on the Internet
www.tchain.com

187. HSPinfo.org (Hereditary Spastic Paraplegia/Familial
Spastic Paraparesis)
Web Site on the Internet
info@hspinfo.org

188. Human Growth Foundation
997 Glen Cove Road
Glen Head, NY 11545
Tel: 516-671-4041
Fax: 516-671-4055
Toll free: 800-451-6434
hgf1@hgfound.org

189. Huntington's Disease Society of America
158 West 29th Street
Seventh Floor
New York, NY 10001-5300
Tel: 212-242-1968
Fax: 212-239-3430
Toll free: 800-345-4372
edonohue@hdsa.org

190. Hydrocephalus Association
870 Market Street
Suite 705
San Francisco, CA 94102
Tel: 415-732-7040
Fax: 415-732-7044
hydroassoc@aol.com

191. Hypoparathyroidism Association, Inc.
2835 Salmon Street
Idaho Falls, ID 83406
Tel: 208-524-3857
Fax: 208-524-2619
hpth@hypoparathyroidism.org

192. IFFGD-Pediatric
158 Pleasant Street
North Andover, MA 01845
Tel: 978-685-4477
Toll free: 800-394-2747
aanastas@iffgd.org

193. Immune Deficiency Foundation
40 West Chesapeake Avenue
Suite 308
Towson, MD 21230
Tel: 410-321-6647
Fax: 410-321-9165
Toll free: 800-296-4433
jb@primaryimmune.org

194. Incontinentia Pigmenti International Foundation
30 East 72nd Street, #16
New York, NY 10021
Tel: 212-452-1231
Fax: 212-452-1406
nipf@pipeline.com

195. Independent Holoprosencephaly Support Site
Web Site on the Internet
tim.smith@gashead.demon.co.uk

196. Infantile Hypercalcaemia Foundation
37 Mulberry Green
Old Harlow
Essex, CM17 OEY
United Kingdom

197. International Agnosia Foundation
C/O Volunteers for the Blind, Inc.
P.O. Box 8061
Calabasas, CA 91302-8061
Tel: 818-996-6464
Fax: 818-222-9124

198. International Bundle Branch Block Association
6631 West 83rd Street
Los Angeles, CA 90045-2899
Tel: 310-670-9132

199. International Children's Anophthalmia Network (ICAN)
(ican) C/O Genetics
Albert Einstein Medical Center, Levy 2 West
5501 Old York Road
Philadelphia, PA 19141
Tel: 215-456-8722
Fax: 215-456-2356
Toll free: 800-580-4226
aemcgenetics@icdc.com

200. International Dyslexia Association
Chester Building
Suite 382
8600 LaSalle Road
Baltimore, MD 21286-2044
Tel: 410-296-0232
Fax: 410-321-5069
Toll free: 800-222-3123
info@interdys.org

201. International Fanconi Registry
Rockefeller University
c/o Arleen Auerbach, PhD
1230 York Avenue
New York, NY 10021
Tel: 212-327-7533
Fax: 212-327-8262
Auerbac@rockvax.rockefeller.edu

202. International Foundation for Functional Gastrointestinal
Disorders (IFFGD)
P.O. Box 170864
Milwaukee, WI 53217-8076
Tel: 414-964-1799
Toll free: 888-964-2001
iffgd@iffgd.org

203. International Fibrodysplasia Ossificans Progressiva
Association
P.O. Box 196217
Winter Springs, FL 32719-6217
Tel: 407-365-4194
Fax: 407-365-3213
together@ifopa.org

204. International Foundation for Optic Nerve Disease
(IFOND)
P.O. Box 777
Cornwall, NY 12518
Tel: 845-534-7250
Fax: 845-534-7250
ifond@aol.com

205. International Joseph Diseases Foundation, Inc.
P.O. Box 2550
Livermore, CA 94551-2550
Fax: 925-371-1288
bashor@earthlink.net

206. International Long QT Syndrome Registry
P.O. Box 653
University of Rochester Medical Center
Rochester, NY 14642-8653
Tel: 716-275-5391
Fax: 716-473-2751
heartjlr@heart.rochester.edu

207. International Myeloma Foundation
12650 Riverside Dr.
Suite 206
North Hollywood, CA 91607
Tel: 818-487-7455
Fax: 818-487-7454
Toll free: 800-452-2873
TheIMF@myeloma.org

208. International Peutz-Jeghers Support Group
Center for Medical Genetics
Johns Hopkins Hospital
Blalock 1008
600 North Wolfe Street
Baltimore, MD 21287-4922

209. International Progeria Registry
Department of Human Genetics
Institute for Basic Research
1050 Forest Hill Road
Staten Island, NY 10314
Tel: 718-494-5333
Fax: 718-494-1026
wtbibr@aol.com

210. International Registry of Werner Syndrome
University of Washington
Department of Pathology
P.O. Box 357470
Health Science Building K543
Seattle, WA 98195
Tel: 206-543-5088
Fax: 206-685-8356
gmmartin@u.washington.edu

211. International Rett Syndrome Association
9121 Piscataway Road
Suite 2-B
Clinton, MD 20735
Tel: 301-856-3334
Fax: 301-856-3336
Toll free: 800-818-7388
irsa@rettsyndrome.org

212. International Waldenstrom's Macroglobulinemia
Foundation
2300 Bee Ridge Road
Suite 301
Sarasota, FL 34239-6226
Tel: 941-927-4963
Fax: 941-927-4467
bdr@tminet.com

213. Intersex Society of North America
P.O. Box 301
Petaluma, CA 94953
Tel: 707-283-2170
Fax: 707-283-2171
info@isna.org

214. Interstitial Cystitis Association of America, Inc.
110 North Washington St.
Suite 340
Rockville, MD 20850
Tel: 301-610-5300
Fax: 301-610-5308
Toll free: 800-435-7422
icamail@ichelp.org

215. Intestinal Disease Foundation
1323 Forbes Avenue
Suite 200
Pittsburgh, PA 15219
Tel: 412-261-5888
Fax: 412-471-2722

216. ITP Association
45/8 Avraham Keren Street
Kfar Saba, 44208
Israel
Tel: 972-9-7657950
Fax: 972-9-7410784
aliuneh@tamam.iai.co.il

217. Ivemark Syndrome Association
71 Milton Rd.
Taunton, TA1 2JQ
United Kingdom
Tel: 01823 257430
ingridgladki@aol.com

218. Jeffrey Modell Foundation
43 West 47th Street
5th Floor
New York, NY 10036
Tel: 212-575-1122
Fax: 212-764-4180
Toll free: 800-533-3844
info@jmfworld.com

219. Joubert Syndrome Foundation
6931 South Carlinda Avenue
Columbia, MD 21046
Tel: 410-997-8084
Fax: 410-992-9184
joubert@up.net

220. Juvenile Diabetes Foundation International
120 Wall Street
19th Floor
New York, NY 10005-4001
Tel: 212-785-9500
Fax: 212-785-9595
Toll free: 800-533-2873
info@jdfcure.org

221. Juvenile Scleroderma Network, Inc.
1204 W. 13th St.
San Pedro, CA 90731
Tel: 310-519-9511
Fax: 310-519-9511
Toll free: 800-369-8309
outreachjsdn@aol.com

222. Kabuki Syndrome Network
8060 Struthers Crescent
Regina, Saskatchewan S4Y 1J3
Tel: 306-543-8715

223. Kawasaki Families' Network
46-111 Nahewai Place
Kaneohe, HI 96744
Tel: 808-525-8053
Fax: 808-525-8055
kawasaki@compuserve.com

224. Kennedy Disease (SBMA) Support Group
1804 Quivira Road
Washington, KS 66968
Tel: 785-32-2629
gryphon@grapevine.net

225. KFS (Klippel-Feil Syndrome) Network Online
Web Site on the Internet
g.catalan@student.murdoch.edu.au

226. Klippel-Trenaunay Support Group
5404 Dundee Road
Edina, MN 55436
Tel: 612-925-2596
Fax: 612-925-4708
jvessey@msn.com

227. Kniest Syndrome Group
4956 Queen Avenue South
Minneapolis, MN 55410
Tel: 612-922-6184
Fax: 612-922-8732
sondrols@aol.com

228. Lactic Acidosis Support Trust
1A Whitley Close
Middlewich
Cheshire, CW10 0NQ
United Kingdom
Tel: 0160 6837198
Fax: 016-068-37198

229. LAM Foundation
10105 Beacon Hills Drive
Cincinnati, OH 45241
Tel: 513-777-6889
Fax: 513-777-4109
lamfoundtn@juno.com

230. Langer-Giedion Syndrome Association
89 Ingham Avenue
Toronto
Ontario, M4K 2W8
Canada
Tel: 416-465-3029
Fax: 416-465-4963
kinross@istar.ca

231. Late Onset Tay-Sachs Foundation
1303 Paper Mill Road
Erdenheim, PA 19038
Tel: 215-836-9426
Fax: 215-836-5438
Toll free: 800-672-2022
mpf@bellatlantic.net

232. Laurence-Moon-Bardet-Biedl Syndrome
c/o The Foundation Fighting Blindness
Executive Plaza 1
11350 McCormick Road
Suite 800
Hunt Valley, MD 21031
Tel: 410-785-1414
Fax: 410-771-9470
Toll free: 888-394-3937
randerson@blindness.org

233. Learning Disabilities Association of America
4156 Library Road
Pittsburgh, PA 15234-1349
idanatl@usaor.net

234. Leber's Links: Leber's Congenital Amaurosis, Blindness, and Visual Impairment
Villa D16
District 2
Thu Duc
Ho Chi Minh City, SR
Vietnam
cheryl@hcm.vnn.vn

235. Lennox-Gastaut Syndrome Group
901 Chantilly Rd.
Los Angeles, CA 90077
Tel: 310-440-2948
andydow@aol.com

236. Lennox-Gastaut Syndrome Support Group
wssg@globalnet.co.uk

237. Les Turner Amyotrophic Lateral Sclerosis Foundation, Ltd.
8142 Lawndale Avenue
Skokie, IL 60076
Tel: 847-679-3311
Fax: 847-679-9103
Toll free: 888-257-1107
info@lesturnerals.org

238. Lesch-Nyhan Disease Association
114 Winchester Way
Chamong, NJ 08088-9398
Tel: 215-677-4206

239. Lesch-Nyhan Syndrome Registry
New York University School of Medicine
Department of Psychiatry
550 First Avenue
New York, NY 10012
Tel: 212-263-6458
Fax: 212-629-9523
andersnl@is2.nyu.edu

240. Let's Face It (USA)
P.O. Box 29972
Bellingham, WA 98228-1972
Tel: 360-676-7325
letsfaceit@faceit.org

241. Leukemia & Lymphoma Society
1311 Mamaroneck Ave.
3rd Floor
White Plains, NY 10605
Tel: 914-949-5213
Fax: 914-949-6691
Toll free: 800-955-4572
infocenter@leukemia.org

242. Leukemia Society of America, Inc
600 Third Avenue
4th Floor
New York, NY 10016
Tel: 212-573-8484
Fax: 212-856-9686

243. Lissencephaly Contact Group
39 Barlows Road
Edgbaston
Birmingham, B15 2PN
United Kingdom
Tel: 0121-455-0981

244. Lissencephaly Network, Inc.
10408 Bitterroot Ct.
Fort Wayne, IN 46804
Tel: 219-432-4310
Fax: 219-432-4310
lta1@is2.nyu.edu

245. Little Hearts
1 Springdale Rd.
Cromwell, CT 06416
Tel: 860-635-3222
Fax: 860-635-1631
lh@littlehearts.net

246. Little People of America, Inc.
P.O. Box 745
Lubbock, TX 79408
Tel: 888-572-2001
Fax: 806-797-8830
Toll free: 888-572-2001
lpadatabase@juno.com

247. Little People's Research Fund, Inc.
80 Sister Pierre Drive
Towson, MD 21204-7534
Tel: 410-494-0055
Fax: 410-494-0062
Toll free: 800-232-5773

248. Lois Joy Galler Foundation for Hemolytic Uremic
Syndrome, Inc.
734 Walt Whitman Road
Melville, NY 11747
Tel: 516-673-3017
Fax: 516-673-3025
bob@loisjoygaller.org

249. Lowe Syndrome Association
222 Lincoln Street
West Lafayette, IN 47906
Tel: 765-743-3634
info@lowesyndrome.org

250. Lupus Foundation of America, Inc.
1300 Piccard Drive
Suite 200
Rockville, MD 20850
Tel: 301-670-9292
Fax: 301-670-9486
Toll free: 800-558-0121

251. Lymphoma Research Foundation
8800 Venice Boulevard
Suite 207
Los Angeles, CA 90034
Tel: 310-204-7040
Fax: 310-204-7043
Toll free: 800-500-9976
lrf@lymphoma.org

252. Macular Degeneration International
6700 N. Oracle Rd.
Suite 505
Tucson, AZ 85704
Tel: 520-797-2525
Fax: 520-797-8018
Toll free: 800-393-7634
tperski@aol.com

253. MAGIC Foundation for Children's Growth
1327 North Harlem Avenue
Oak Park, IL 60302
Tel: 708-383-0808
Fax: 708-383-0899
Toll free: 800-362-4423
mary@magicfoundation.org

254. Malignant Hyperthermia Association of the United States
39 East State Street
P.O. Box 1069
Sherburne, NY 13460-1069
Tel: 607-674-7901
Fax: 607-674-7910
mhaus@norwich.net

255. Mannosidosis Web Site
dagm@fagmed.uit.no

256. Maple Syrup Urine Disease Family Support Group
24806 SR 119
Goshen, IN 46526
Tel: 219-862-2992
Fax: 219-862-2012
msud-support@juno.com

257. March of Dimes Birth Defects Foundation
1275 Mamaroneck Avenue
White Plains, NY 10605
Tel: 914-428-7100
Fax: 914-997-4763
Toll free: 888-663-4637
resourcecenter@modimes.org

258. Marinesco-Sjögren Syndrome Support Group
1640 Crystal View Circle
Newbury Park, CA 91320
Tel: 805-499-7410
marinesco-sjogren@pacbell.net

259. Mastocytosis Society, Inc.
433 East 300 South
Spanish Fork, UT 84660
Tel: 801-798-2032
cybermom@sfcn.org

260. Melnick-Needles Syndrome Support Group
4 Kivner Lane
Bexhill-on-Sea
East Sussex, TN40 2ST
United Kingdom
Tel: 014-242-17790
gill@vcarter.freeserve.co.uk

261. Ménière's Network
1817 Patterson Street
Nashville, TN 37203
Tel: 615-329-7807
Fax: 615-329-7935
Toll free: 800-545-4327
ear@earfoundation.org

262. Menkes Syndrome Foundation
1015 Fox Ridge Ct.
Benton, KY 42025
Tel: 270-527-2035
Fax: 270-527-2035
danigordon72@hotmail.com

263. MHE (Multiple Hereditary Exostoses) Family Support
Group
5316 Winter Moss Court
Columbia, MD 21045
Tel: 410-990-5898
hogue@radix.net

264. MHE and Me—A Support Group for Kids with Multiple
Hereditary Exostoses
14 Stony Brook Dr.
Pine Island, NY 10969
Tel: 914-258-6058
mheandme@yahoo.com

265. Mitochondrial Support Group
5022 Michigan Avenue
West Palm Beach, FL 33415
Tel: 407-641-4712

266. ML 4 (Mucolipidosis Type IV Foundation)
719 East 17th Street
Brooklyn, NY 11230
Tel: 718-434-5067
Fax: 718-859-7371
ml4www@aol.com

267. Moebius Syndrome Support Network
38883 Foxholm Drive
Palmdale, CA 93551
Tel: 805-267-2570
lorit@netport.com

268. Moebius Syndrome Support Network (UK)
41 Westley Ave.
Whitley Bay
Tyne and Wear, NE25 8DF
England
Tel: (0191) 253 2090
Fax: (0191) 253 2090

269. Motor Neuron Disease Association
P.O. Box 246
Northampton, NN1 2PR
United Kingdom
Tel: 44 1604 250505
Fax: 44 1604 62476

270. Muscular Dystrophy Association
3300 E. Sunrise Dr.
Tucson, AZ 85718
Tel: 520-529-2000
Fax: 520-529-5300
Toll free: 800-572-1717
mda@mdausa.org

271. Myasthenia Gravis Foundation of America
5841 Cedar Lake Rd.
Suite 204
Minneapolis, MN 55416
Tel: 952-545-9438
Fax: 952-646-2028
Toll free: 800-541-5454
myastheniagravis@msn.com

272. Myasthenia Gravis Links
Web Site on the Internet
stanley.way@prodigy.net

273. Mycosis Fungoides Network
Department of Dermatology
Pavillion A3
UC Medical Center
Cincinnati, OH 45267-0523
Fax: 513-558-3531

274. Myositis Association of America, Inc.
755 Cantrell Avenue
Suite C
Harrisonburg, VA 22801
Tel: 540-433-7686
Fax: 540-432-0206
maa@myositis.org

275. Myotubular Myopathy Resource Group
2602 Quaker Drive
Texas City, TX 77590
Tel: 409-945-8569
Fax: 409-945-2162
gscoggin@aol.com

276. Nail-Patella Syndrome Networking/Support Group
67 Woodlake Dr.
Holland, PA 18966

277. Nail-Patella Syndrome Web Site
Institute of Genetic Medicine
Johns Hopkins University School of Medicine
Baltimore, MD 21287-4922
Tel: 410-955-7948
Fax: 410-614-2522
imcintos@welchlink.welch.jhu.edu

278. Narcolepsy Institute
Montefiore Medical Center
111 East 210th Street
Bronx, NY 10467
Tel: 718-920-6799
Fax: 718-654-9580

279. Narcolepsy Network, Inc.
277 Fairfield Road
Suite 310B
Fairfield, NJ 07004
Tel: 513-891-3522
Fax: 513-891-3836
narnet@aol.com

280. NASPCS—The Charity for Incontinent and Stoma
Children
51 Anderson Dr.
Valley View Park
Darvel
Ayrshire, KA17 0DE
United Kingdom

281. National Adrenal Diseases Foundation
505 Northern Bloulevard
Great Neck, NY 11021
Tel: 516-487-4992
nadfmail@aol.com

282. National Alliance for the Mentally Ill
200 North Glebe Road
Suite 1015
Arlington, VA 22203-3754
Tel: 703-524-7600
Fax: 703-524-9094
Toll free: 800-950-6264
membership@nami.org

283. National Alopecia Areata Foundation
14 Mitchell Blvd.
San Rafael, CA 94903
Tel: 415-456-4644
Fax: 415-456-4274
info@naaf.org

284. National Aphasia Association
156 Fifth Avenue
Suite 707
New York, NY 10010
Fax: 212-989-7777
Toll free: 800-922-4622
naa@aphasia.org

285. National Association for Continence
P.O. Box 8310
Spartanburg, SC 29305
Tel: 864-579-7900
Fax: 864-579-7902
Toll free: 800-252-3337

286. National Association for Parents of the Visually Impaired
P.O. Box 317
Watertown, MA 02472
Tel: 617-972-7441
Fax: 617-972-7444
Toll free: 800-562-6265
napvi@perkins.pvt.k12.ma.us

287. National Association for Pseudoxanthoma Elasticum
(NAPE)
8772 Bridgeport Ave.
St Louis, MO 63144-1808
Tel: 314-963-9153
Fax: 314-977-3587
benham@slu.edu

288. National Association for Visually Handicapped
22 West 21st Street
New York, NY 10010
Tel: 212-889-3141
Fax: 212-727-2931
staff@navh.org

289. National Ataxia Foundation
2600 Fernbrook Lane
Suite 119
Minneapolis, MN 55447
Tel: 763-553-0020
Fax: 763-553-0167
naf@mr.net

290. National Brain Tumor Foundation
414 Thirteenth Street
Suite 700
Oakland, CA 94612
Tel: 510-839-9777
Fax: 510-839-9779
Toll free: 800-934-2873
nbtf@braintumor.org

291. National Carcinoid Support Group, Inc.
P.O. Box 44233
Madison, WI 53744-4233
Tel: 608-271-0487
jean@mick.com

292. National Center of Chromosome Inversions
1029 Johnson Street
Des Moines, IA 50315
Tel: 515-287-6798
Fax: 515-287-6798
ncfci@msn.com

293. National Childhood Cancer Foundation
440 East Huntington Drive
Suite 300
Arcadia, CA 91066-6012
Tel: 626-447-1674
Fax: 626-447-6359
Toll free: 800-458-6223
nccf-info@nccf.org

294. National Dysautonomia Research Foundation
421 W. 4th St.
Suite 9
Red Wing, MN 55066-2555
Tel: 651-267-0525
Fax: 651-267-0524
ndrf@ndrf.org

295. National Federation of the Blind
1800 Johnson Street
Baltimore, MD 21230
Tel: 410-659-9314
Fax: 410-685-5653
nfb@iamdigex.net

296. National Filippi Syndrome Network
125 Homecrest Rd.
Battlecreek, MI 49017
Tel: 616-968-6227

297. National Foundation for Ectodermal Dysplasias
P.O. Box 114
Mascoutah, IL 62258-0114
Tel: 618-566-2020
Fax: 618-566-4718
nfed1@aol.com

298. National Foundation for Facial Reconstruction
317 East 34th St.
#901
New York, NY 10016
Tel: 212-263-6656
Fax: 212-263-7534
Toll free: 800-422-3223
nffr@earthlink.net

299. National Foundation for Jewish Genetic Diseases
250 Park Avenue
Suite 1000
New York, NY 10177
Tel: 212-371-1030
Fax: 212-319-5808

300. National Gaucher Foundation, Inc.
11140 Rockville Pike
Suite 350
Rockville, MD 20852-3106
Tel: 301-816-1515
Fax: 301-816-1516
Toll free: 800-925-8885
ngf@gaucherdisease.org

301. National Headache Foundation
428 West Saint James Place
Second Floor
Chicago, IL 60614-2750
Tel: 773-388-6399
Fax: 773-525-7357
Toll free: 888-643-5552

302. National Hemophilia Foundation
116 West 32nd Street
11th Floor
New York, NY 10001
Tel: 212-328-3700
Fax: 212-328-3799
Toll free: 800-424-2634
info@hemophilia.org

303. National Hydrocephalus Foundation
12413 Centralia
Lakewood, CA 90715-1623
Tel: 562-402-3523
Fax: 562-924-6666
Toll free: 888-857-3434
hydrobrat@earthlink.net

304. National Hypertension Association, Inc.
324 East 30th Street
New York, NY 10016
Tel: 212-889-3557
Fax: 212-447-7032
Toll free: 800-575-9355

305. National Information Center For Children and Youth with Disabilities (NICHCY)
P.O. Box 1492
Washington, DC 20013
Tel: 202-884-8200
Fax: 202-884-8441
Toll free: 800-695-0285
nichcy@aed.org

306. National Institute of Dental & Craniofasc. Research
Rockville Pike
Bethesda, MD 20892-2190
Tel: 301-496-3570

307. National Keratoconus Foundation
Cedars-Sinai Medical Center
8631 West Third Street
Suite 520E
Los Angeles, CA 90048
Tel: 310-855-6455
Fax: 310-360-9712
Toll free: 800-521-2524
nkcf@csmc.edu

308. National Kidney Foundation
30 East 33rd Street
New York, NY 10016
Tel: 212-889-2210
Fax: 212-689-9261
Toll free: 800-622-9010

309. National Lipid Diseases Foundation
1201 Corbin Street
Elizabeth, NJ 07201
Tel: 908-527-8000
Fax: 908-527-8004
Toll free: 800-527-8005

310. National Lymphatic and Venous Diseases Foundation, Inc.
255 Commandants Way
Chelsea, MA 02150
Tel: 617-889-2103
Fax: 617-887-1089
Toll free: 800-301-2103

311. National Lymphedema Network
Latham Square
1611 Telegraph Ave.
Suite 1111
Oakland, CA 94612-2138
Tel: 510-208-3200
Fax: 510-208-3110
Toll free: 800-541-3259
nln@lymphnet.org

312. National Marden Walker Organization
P.O. Box 239
New Haven, KY 40051
Tel: 502-549-3028
Fax: 270-325-3091
stearnsa@bardstown.com

313. National Marfan Foundation
382 Main Street
Port Washington, NY 11050
Tel: 516-883-8712
Fax: 516-883-8040
Toll free: 800-862-7326
staff@marfan.org

314. National MPS (Mucopolysaccharidoses/Mucolipidoses) Society, Inc.
102 Aspen Drive
Downingtown, PA 19335
Tel: 610-942-0100
Fax: 610-942-7188
info@mpssociety.org

315. National Multiple Sclerosis Society
733 Third Avenue
New York, NY 10017
Tel: 212-476-0411
Fax: 212-986-7981
Toll free: 800-344-4867
info@nmss.org

316. National Narcolepsy Registry
729 15th Street NW
4th Floor
Washington, DC 20005
Tel: 202-347-3471
Fax: 202-347-3472
natsleep@erols.com

317. National Neurofibromatosis Foundation, Inc.
95 Pine Street
16th Floor
New York, NY 10005
Tel: 212-344-6633
Fax: 212-747-0004
Toll free: 800-323-7938
nnff@nf.org

318. National Neutropenia Network
P.O. Box 205
6348 North Milwaukee Avenue
Chicago, IL 60646
Toll free: 800-638-8768
Bolyard@u.washington.edu

319. National Niemann-Pick Disease Foundation, Inc.
P.O. Box 49
415 Madison Ave.
Fort Atkinson, WI 53538
Tel: 920-563-0930
Fax: 920-563-0931
Toll free: 877-287-3672
nnpdf@idcnet.com

320. National Oral Health Information Clearinghouse
1 NOHIC Way
Bethesda, MD 20892-3500
Tel: 301-402-7364

321. National Organization for Albinism and
Hypopigmentation
P.O. Box 959
East Hempstead, NH 03826-0959
Tel: 603-887-2310
Fax: 603-887-2310
Toll free: 800-473-2310
noah@albinism.org

322. National Pediatric Myoclonus Center
SIU School of Medicine
Department of Pediatrics
P.O. Box 19658
Springfield, IL 62702-9658
Tel: 217-782-7635
Fax: 217-557-5834
mpranzatelli@siumed.edu

323. National Pemphigus Foundation
P.O. Box 9606
1098 Euclid Avenue
Berkeley, CA 94709-0606
Tel: 510-527-4970
Fax: 510-527-8497
PVnews@aol.com

324. National PKU News
6869 Woodlawn Avenue NE, #116
Seattle, WA 98115-5469
Tel: 206-525-8140
Fax: 206-525-5023
schuett@pkunews.org

325. National Registry for Ichthyosis and Related Disorders
University of Washington
Dermatology Department, Box 356524
1959 N.E. Pacific
Seattle, WA 98195-6524
Tel: 206-616-3179
Fax: 206-616-4302
Toll free: 800-595-1265
fleck@u.washington.edu or geoff@u.washington.edu

326. National Retinoblastoma Parent Group
P.O. Box 317
Watertown, MA 02471
Fax: 617-972-7444
Toll free: 800-562-6265
napvi@perkins.pvt.k12.ma.us

327. National Reye's Syndrome Foundation, Inc.
426 North Lewis Street
P.O. Box 829
Bryan, OH 43506-0829
Tel: 419-636-2679
Fax: 419-636-3366
Toll free: 800-233-7393
reyessyn@mail.bright.net

328. National Sarcoidosis Resource Center
P.O. Box 1593
Piscataway, NJ 08855-1593
Tel: 732-699-0733
Fax: 732-699-0882
nsrc@microfone.net

329. National Sjogren's Syndrome Association
P.O. Box 22066
Beachwood, OH 44122
Tel: 216-292-3866
Fax: 216-292-4955
Toll free: 800-395-6772
nssa@aol.com

330. National Sleep Foundation
1522 K Street
Suite 500
Washington, D.C. 20005
Tel: 202-347-3471
Fax: 202-347-3472
nsf@sleepfoundation.org

331. National Spasmodic Dysphonia Association
One E. Wacker Drive
Suite 2430
Chicago, IL 60601-1905
Tel: 312-755-0198
Fax: 312-803-0138
Toll free: 800-795-6732
nsda@aol.com

332. National Spasmodic Torticollis Association
9920 Talbert Avenue
Suite 233
Fountain Valley, CA 92708
Tel: 714-378-7837
Fax: 714-378-7830
Toll free: 800-487-8385
nstamail@aol.com

333. National Spinal Cord Injury Association
8300 Colesville Road
Suite 551
Silver Spring, MD 20910
Tel: 301-588-6959
Fax: 301-588-9414
Toll free: 800-962-9629
nscia2@aol.com

334. National Subacute Sclerosing Panencephalitis Registry
P.O. Box 70191
283 Wingfield Drive
Mobile, AL 36670-0191
Tel: 334-471-7834
Fax: 334-476-8277
pdyken@aol.com

335. National Tay-Sachs and Allied Diseases Association, Inc.
2001 Beacon Street
Suite 204
Brookline, MA 02135
Tel: 617-277-4463
Fax: 617-277-0134
Toll free: 800-906-8723
ntsad-boston@att.net

336. National Urea Cycle Disorders Foundation
4841 Hill Street
La Canada, CA 91011
Tel: 818-790-2460
Toll free: 800-386-8233
info@nucdf.org

337. National Vitiligo Foundation, Inc.
611 S. Fleishel Ave.
Tyler, TX 75701
Tel: 903-531-0074
Fax: 903-525-1234
vitiligo@trimofran.org

338. National Women's Health Network
514 10th Street NW
Suite 400
Washington, D.C. 20004
Tel: 202-628-7814
Fax: 202-347-1168

339. National Women's Health Resource Center
120 Albany Street
Suite 820
New Brunswick, NJ 08901
Tel: 732-828-8575
Fax: 732-249-4671
Toll free: 877-986-9472
natlwhrc@aol.com

340. Nephrogenic Diabetes Insipidus Network
2 Beechwood Heights
Columbus, GA 31904
Tel: 706-323-7576
Fax: 215-590-3705
mom2awirlwynd@aol.com

341. Neurofibromatosis, Inc.
8855 Annapolis Road
Suite 110
Lanham, MD 20706-2924
Tel: 301-577-8984
Fax: 301-577-0016
Toll free: 800-942-6825
nfinc1@aol.com

342. Neuromuscular Disease Center
Washington University School of Medicine
St. Louis, MO 63110
Tel: 314-362-6981
Fax: 314-362-2826

343. Neutropenia Support Association, Inc.
P.O. Box 243
905 Corydon Avenue
Winnepeg
Manitoba, R3M 3S7
Canada
Tel: 204-489-8454
Toll free: 800-663-8876
stevensl@neutropenia.ca

344. Nevus Network
The Congenital Nevus Support Group
P.O. Box 1981
Woodbridge, VA 22193
Tel: 703-492-0253
nevusnet@bigfoot.com

345. Nevus Outreach, Inc.
1601 Madison Blvd.
Bartlesville, OK 74006
Tel: 918-331-0595
Fax: 918-331-0595
info@nevus.org

346. NF Clinic—MGH
Massachusetts General Hospital
Fruit Street
Boston, MA 02114
Tel: 617-726-5732
Fax: 617-726-5736
maccollin@helix.mgh.harvard.edu

347. NIH Osteoporosis & Related Bone Diseases National Resource Center Website
1232 22nd Street, NW
Washington, DC 20037-1292
Tel: 202-223-0344
Toll free: 800-624-2663
www.osteo.org

348. NIH Osteoporosis and Related Bone Diseases National Resource Center
1232 22nd St. NW
Washington, DC 20037-1292
Tel: 202-223-0344
Fax: 202-293-2356
Toll free: 800-624-2663
orbdnrc@nof.org

349. NIH/Developmental Endocrinology Branch
Building 10, Room 10N262
10 Center Drive
Bethesda, MD 20892
Tel: 301-496-4686
Fax: 301-402-0574

350. NIH/Hematology Branch, National Heart, Lung and Blood Institute (NHLBI)
Tel: 301-402-0764
Fax: 301-402-3088
zamaniw@nhlbi.nih.gov

351. NIH/National Arthritis and Musculoskeletal and Skin Diseases Information Clearinghouse
One AMS Circle
Bethesda, MD 20892-3675
Tel: 301-495-4484
Fax: 301-587-4352

352. NIH/National Cancer Institute
Public Inquiries Office
31 Center Dr., MSC 2580
Building 31, Rm 10A03
Bethesda, MD 20892-2580
Tel: 301-435-3848
Toll free: 800-422-6237

353. NIH/National Diabetes Information Clearinghouse
1 Information Way
Bethesda, MD 20892-3560
Tel: 301-654-3327
Fax: 301-907-8906
Toll free: 800-891-5388
DDIC@info.niddk.nih.gov

354. NIH/National Digestive Diseases Information Clearinghouse
2 Information Way
Bethesda, MD 20892-3570
Tel: 301-654-3810
Fax: 301-907-8906
Toll free: 800-891-5389
nddic@info.niddk.nih.gov

355. NIH/National Eye Institute
Building 31, Room 6A32
31 Center Dr., MSC 2510
Bethesda, MD 20892-2510
Tel: 301-496-5248
Fax: 301-402-1065
2020@nei.nih.gov

356. NIH/National Heart, Lung and Blood Institute
31 Center Drive, MSC 2480
Building 31A, Rm 4A16
Bethesda, MD 20892-2480
Tel: 301-592-8573
Fax: 301-480-4907
nhlbiinfo@rover.nhlbi.nih.gov

357. NIH/National Heart, Lung and Blood Institute Information Center
P.O. Box 30105
Bethesda, MD 20824-0105
Tel: 301-592-8573
Fax: 301-251-1223
nhlbiinfo@rover.nhlbi.nih.gov

358. NIH/National Human Genome Research Institute
31 Center Dr.
Building 31, Rm 4B09
Bethesda, MD 20892
Tel: 301-402-0911

359. NIH/National Institute of Allergy and Infectious Diseases
9000 Rockville Pike
Building 31A
Bethesda, MD 20892
Tel: 301-496-5717
Fax: 301-402-0120

360. NIH/National Institute of Arthritis and Musculoskeletal and Skin Diseases
1 AMS Circle
Bethesda, MD 20892-3675
Tel: 301-496-8188
Fax: 301-718-6366
Toll free: 877-226-4267
NAMSIC@mail.nih.gov

361. NIH/National Institute of Child Health & Human Development
Pregnancy and Perinatology Branch
6100 Executive Blvd., Rm 4B03
Bethesda, MD 20892-7510
Tel: 301-496-5575
bockr@mail.nih.gov

362. NIH/National Institute of Child Health and Human Development
31 Center Dr.
Building 31, Room 2A32
MSC2425
Bethesda, MD 20892
Tel: 301-496-5133
Fax: 301-496-7101

363. NIH/National Institute of Dental and Craniofacial Research
45 Center Dr.
Building 45, Rm 4AS19
Bethesda, MD 20892-6400
Tel: 301-496-4261
Fax: 301-496-9988

364. NIH/National Institute of Diabetes, Digestive & Kidney Diseases
Endocrine Diseases Metabolic Diseases Branch
2 Information Way
Bethesda, MD 20892-3570
Tel: 301-654-3810
Fax: 301-496-7422
nddic@info.niddk.nih.gov

365. NIH/National Institute of Diabetes, Digestive and Kidney Diseases
31 Center Dr.
Building 31, Rm 9A04
Bethesda, MD 20892-2560
Tel: 301-496-3583
Fax: 301-496-7422

366. NIH/National Institute of General Medical Sciences
45 Center Dr., MSC 6200
Bethesda, MD 20892-6200
Tel: 301-496-7301
Fax: 301-402-0224

367. NIH/National Institute of Mental Health
6001 Executive Blvd.
Rm 8184, MSC 9663
Rockville, MD 20892-9663
Tel: 301-443-4513
nimhinfo@nih.gov

368. NIH/National Institute of Neurological Disorders and Stroke
Brain Resources and Information Network (BRAIN)
P.O. Box 5801
Bethesda, MD 20824
Tel: 301-496-5751
Fax: 301-402-2186
Toll free: 800-352-9424

369. NIH/National Institute on Aging
P.O. Box 8057
Gaithersburg, MD 20892-8057
Tel: 301-496-1752
Toll free: 800-222-2225

370. NIH/National Institute on Deafness and Other Communication Disorders (Balance)
National Temporal Bone Hearing
and Balance Pathology Resource Registry
243 Charles Street
Boston, MA 02114-3096
Tel: 617-573-3711
Fax: 617-573-3838
Toll free: 800-822-1327
tbregistry@meei.harvard.edu

371. NIH/National Institute on Deafness and Other Communication Disorders Information Clearinghouse
9000 Rockville Pike
Building 31, Room 3C02
Bethesda, MD 20852
Tel: 301-402-0900
Fax: 301-907-8830
Toll free: 800-241-1044
nidcdinfo@nidcd.nih.gov

372. NIH/National Kidney and Urologic Diseases Information Clearinghouse
9000 Rockville Pike
Building 31, Room 8A52A
Bethesda, MD 20852
Tel: 301-651-4415
Fax: 301-907-8906
Toll free: 800-891-5390

373. NIH/National Oral Health Information Clearinghouse
1 NOHIC Way
Bethesda, MD 20892-3500
Tel: 301-402-7364
Fax: 301-907-8830
nohic@nidcr.nih.gov

374. Noonan Syndrome Support Group, Inc.
P.O. Box 145
Upperco, MD 21155
Tel: 410-374-5245
Toll free: 888-686-2224
wandar@bellatlantic.net

375. Norrie Disease Association
Massachusetts General Hospital
E. #6217
149 13th Street
Charlestown, MA 02129
Tel: 617-726-5718
Fax: 617-724-9620
helix.mgh.harvard.edu

376. North American Malignant Hyperthermia Registry of MHAUS
Children's Hospital of Pittsburgh
Room #7449
3705 Fifth Ave. at DeSoto St.
Pittsburgh, PA 15213-2583
Toll free: 888-274-7899
bwb+@pitt.edu

377. NYS Institute Basic Research in Developmental Disabilities
1050 Forest Hill Road
Staten Island, NY 10314
Tel: 718-494-0600

378. Ollier/Maffucci Self-Help Group
1824 Millwood Road
Sumter, SC 29150
Tel: 803-775-1757
Fax: 803-934-0347
olliers@aol.com

379. OncoLink: The University of Pennsylvania Cancer Center Resource
Web Site on the Internet
editors@oncolink.upenn.edu

380. Opitz G/BBB Family Network, Inc.
P.O. Box 515
Grand Lake, CO 80447
Tel: 970-627-8935
Fax: 970-627-8818
opitznet@mac.com

381. Opsoclonus-Myoclonus Support Network, Inc.
725 North Street
Jim Thorpe, PA 18229
Tel: 570-325-3302
clquinn@ptdprolog.net

382. Organic Acidemia Association
13210 35th Avenue North
Plymouth, MN 55441
Tel: 763-559-1797
Fax: 763-694-0017
oaanews@aol.com

383. Organic Acidemias (UK)
5 Saxon Road
Ashford
Middlesex, TW15 1QL
United Kingdom
Tel: 178-424-5989
dbpriddy@aol.com

384. Osteogenesis Imperfecta Foundation, Inc.
804 West Diamond Avenue
Suite 210
Gaithersburg, MD 20878
Tel: 301-947-0083
Fax: 301-947-0456
Toll free: 800-981-2663
bonelink@oif.org

385. Oxalosis and Hyperoxaluria Foundation
5727 Westcliffe Drive
St. Louis, MO 63129
Tel: 314-846-3645
Fax: 314-846-6779
secy@ohf.org

386. Pallister-Hall Syndrome Family Support Network
125 Knox Rd.
Fairlee, VT 05045
Tel: 802-3333717
messer@sover.net

387. Pallister-Killian Family Support Group
3700 Wyndale Court
Fort Worth, TX 76109
Tel: 817-927-8854
Fax: 817-927-2073

388. Parents of Infants and Children with Kernicterus
517 Brentwood Dr.
Birmingham, AL 35226
Tel: 205-979-2021
Fax: 205-975-7928
ktdixon1@home.com

389. Parkinson's Disease Foundation, Inc.
710 West 168th Street
New York, NY 10032-9982
Tel: 212-923-4700
Fax: 212-923-4778
Toll free: 800-457-6676
relliott@pdf.org

390. Pediatric Cardiomyopathy Registry
Tel: 716-275-2238

391. Phenylalanine Hydroxylase Locus Database (PAHdb)
Home Page
Web Site on the Internet
pahdb@www.debelle.mcgill.ca

392. Pierre Robin Network
P.O. Box 3274
Quincy, IL 62305
prn@pierrerobin.org

393. Pituitary Tumor Network Association
16350 Ventura Boulevard
Suite 231
Encino, CA 91436
Tel: 805-499-2262
Fax: 805-499-1523
ptna@pituitary.com

394. Pityriasis Rubra Pilaris (PRP) Online Support Group
Web Site on the Internet
prp-l@tip.net.au

395. PKR (Polycystic Kidney Research) Foundation
4901 Main St.
Suite 200
Kansas City, MO 64112-2634
Tel: 816-931-2600
Fax: 816-931-8655
Toll free: 800-753-2873
pkdcure@pkrfoundation.org

396. Platelet Disorder Support Association
P.O. Box 61533
Potomac, MD 20859
Tel: 301-294-5967
Fax: 301-294-5967
Toll free: 877-528-3538
pdsa@pdsa.org

397. PMP (Pseudomyxoma Peritonei) Pals
P.O. Box 6484
Salinas, CA 93912
Tel: 831-424-4545
Fax: 831-424-4545
pmppals@yahoo.com

398. Polycystic Ovarian Syndrome Association
P.O. Box 7007
Rosemont, IL 60018-7007
Tel: 630-585-3690
info@pcosupport.org

399. Prader-Willi Syndrome Association, National Headquarters
5700 Midnight Pass Road
Suite 6
Sarasota, FL 34242
Tel: 941-312-0400
Fax: 941-312-0142
Toll free: 800-926-4797
pwsausa@aol.com

400. Premature Ovarian Failure Support Group
P.O. Box 23643
Alexandria, VA 22304
Tel: 703-913-4787
www.pofsupport.org

401. PRISMS (Parents & Researchers Interested in Smith-Magenis Syndrome)
76 S. New Boston Rd.
Francestown, NH 03043-3511
Tel: 603-547-8384
Fax: 603-547-3043
cbessette@monad.net

402. Prof. John A. McGrath, MD
St. John's Institute for Dermatology
The Guy's, King's College
St. Thomas' Hospitals' Med School
London, United Kingdom

403. K. Michael Gibson, PhD
Molecular and Medical Genetics
Oregon Health Science Center
Portland, OR 97201

404. Progeria Research Foundation
P.O. Box 3453
Peabody, MA 01961-3453
Tel: 978-535-2594
Fax: 978-535-5849
progeria@netzero.net

405. Progressive Osseous Heteroplasia Association
33 Stonehearth Square
Indian Head Park, IL 60525
Tel: 708-246-9410

406. Proteus Syndrome Foundation
6235 Whetstone Dr.
Colorado Springs, CO 80918
Tel: 719-264-8445
abscit@aol.com

407. Pseudotumor Cerebri Support Network
4916 St. Andrews Circle
Westerville, OH 43032
Tel: 614-794-0442
Fax: 614-837-5913

408. Pull-thru Network
2312 Savoy St.
Hoover, AL 35226
Tel: 205-978-2930
pullthru@bellsouth.net

409. Pulmonary Hypertension Association
850 Sligo Ave.
Suite 800
Silver Spring, MD 20910
Tel: 301-565-3004
Fax: 301-565-3994
Toll free: 800-748-7274
rino@phassociation.org

410. PXE International, Inc.
23 Mountain Street
Sharon, MA 02067
Fax: 781-784-6672
pxe@pxe.org

411. Ramon Brugada Senior Foundation
www.crtia.be

412. Reaching Out—The WAGR/Aniridia Network
2063 Regina
Lincoln Park, MI 48146
Tel: 313-381-4302
ReachingoutNet@aol.com

413. Recurrent Respiratory Papillomatosis Foundation
P.O. Box 6643
Lawrenceville, NJ 08648-0643
www.rrpf.org

414. Reflex Sympathetic Dystrophy Network
Web Site on the Internet
info@rsdnet.org

415. Reflex Sympathetic Dystrophy Syndrome Association of America
P.O. Box 502
Milford, CT 06460
Tel: 203-877-3790
Fax: 203-882-8362
jwbroatch@aol.com

416. Renewal TMAU (Trimethylaminuria) Support Group
P.O. Box 1606
Grand Central Station
New York, NY 10163
Tel: 212-678-2506
trimeth411@aol.com

417. Restless Legs Syndrome Foundation, Inc.
819 Second St. SW
Rochester, MN 55902
Tel: 507-287-6465
Fax: 507-28-76312
rlsfoundation@rls.org

418. Restricted Growth Association
P.O. Box 4744
Dorchester, DT2 9FA
United Kingdom
Tel: 01308 898445
rga1@talk21.com

419. Retinitis Pigmentosa International
23241 Ventura Boulevard
Suite 117
Woodland Hills, CA 91364
Tel: 818-992-0500
Fax: 818-992-3265
Toll free: 800-344-4877
rpint@pacbell.net

420. Robinow Syndrome Foundation
15955 Uplander Street NW
Andover, MN 55304-2501
Tel: 612-421-4444
Fax: 612-434-3691
kmkruger@uswest.net

421. Rombergs Connection
c/o T. Hildebrand
4106 W. 87th St.
Chicago, IL 60652
rombergs@hotmail.com

422. RSDHope Group
P.O. Box 875
Harrison, ME 04040-0875
Tel: 207-583-4589
roomblue@megalink.net

423. Rubinstein-Taybi Parent Group USA
P.O. Box 146
Smith Center, KS 66967-0146
Tel: 785-697-2984
Fax: 785-697-2985
lbaxter@ruraltel.net

424. Rubinstein-Taybi Support Group
c/o Rosemary Robertson
Appledore Cottage
Knapton
Dilwyn
Herefordshire, HR4 8EU
United Kingdom
Tel: 01568 720350

425. Sarcoid Networking Association
6424 151st Ave. East
Sumner, WA 98390-2601
Tel: 253-891-6886
Fax: 253-891-6886
sarcoidosis_netwrk@prodigy.net

426. Sarcoidosis Network Foundation, Inc.
13337 East South Street
Suite 420
Cerritos, CA 90703
Tel: 714-391-398
Fax: 714-739-1398

427. Schepens Eye Research Institute
20 Staniford Street
Boston, MA 02114-2500
Tel: 617-912-0100
Fax: 617-523-3463
geninfo@vision.eri.harvard.edu

428. Scleroderma Foundation, Inc.
12 Kent Way
Suite 101
Byfield, MA 01922
Tel: 978-463-5843
Fax: 978-463-5809
Toll free: 800-722-4673
erotolo@scleroderma.org

429. Scleroderma Research Foundation
2320 Bath Street
Suite 315
Santa Barbara, CA 93105
Tel: 805-563-9133
Fax: 805-563-2402
Toll free: 800-441-2873
srfcure@srfcure.org

430. Septo-Optic Dysplasia/Optic Nerve Hypoplasia Support Group
228 E. Palomino Ct.
Gilbert, AZ 85296
Tel: 480-926-1627
support@focusfamilies.org

431. Severe Chronic Neutropenia International Registry
Puget Sound Plaza
Suite 620
1325 4th Avenue
Seattle, WA 98101-2509
Tel: 206-543-9749
Fax: 206-543-3668
Toll free: 800-726-4463
registry@u.washington.edu

432. Sexuality Information and Education Council of the U.S.
130 West 42nd Street
Suite 350
New York, NY 10010
Tel: 212-819-9770
Fax: 212-819-9776
siecus@siecus.org

433. Share and Care Cockayne Syndrome Network, Inc.
P.O. Box 570618
Dallas, TX 75357
Tel: 972-613-6273
Fax: 972-613-4590
j93082@aol.com

434. Shwachman-Diamond Syndrome International
5195 Hampstead Village Center Way
PMB #162
New Albany, OH 43054
Fax: 614-934-0752
Toll free: 877-737-4685
4sskids@shwachman-diamond.org

435. Sickle Cell Disease Association of America, Inc.
200 Corporate Pointe
Suite 495
Culver City, CA 90230-8727
Tel: 310-216-6363
Fax: 310-215-3722
Toll free: 800-421-8453

436. Sjögren's Syndrome Foundation, Inc.
333 North Broadway
Jericho, NY 11753
Tel: 516-933-6365
Fax: 516-933-6368
Toll free: 800-475-6473
ssf@idt.net

437. Skin Cancer Foundation
245 Fifth Avenue
Suite 1403
New York, NY 10016
Tel: 212-725-5176
Fax: 212-725-5751
Toll free: 800-754-6490
info@skincancer.org

438. Smith-Lemli-Opitz/RSH Advocacy and Exchange
32 Ivy Lane
Glen Mills, PA 19342
Tel: 610-361-9663
bhook@erols.com

439. Smith-Magenis Syndrome Foundation
81 Cedar Ridge
Dungannon, BT71 6UD
United Kingdom
Tel: 028 8775 0050
gmc@yolger.fsnet.co.uk

440. Society for Mucopolysaccharide (MPS) Diseases
46 Woodside Road
Amersham
Buckinghamshire, HP6 6AJ
United Kingdom
Tel: 149-443-4156
Fax: 149-443-4252
mpsuk@compuserve.com

441. Society for Muscular Dystrophy Information International
P.O. Box 479
Bridgewater
Nova Scotia, B4V 2X6
Canada
Tel: 902-685-3961
Fax: 902-685-3962
smdi@auracom.com

442. Society for Progressive Supranuclear Palsy
Woodholme Medical Building
Suite 515
1838 Greene Tree Road
Baltimore, MD 21208
Tel: 410-486-3330
Fax: 410-486-4283
Toll free: 800-457-4777
spsp@erols.com

443. Sotos Syndrome Support Association
3 Danada Square East
Suite 235
Wheaton, IL 60187-8484
Tel: 630-682-8815
Toll free: 888-246-7772
sssa@well.com

444. Sotos Syndrome Support Group of Great Britain
c/o Child Growth Foundation
4 Mayfield Avenue
London, W4 1PW
United Kingdom

445. Spina Bifida Association of America
4590 MacArthur Boulevard NW
Suite 250
Washington, DC 20007-4226
Tel: 202-944-3285
Fax: 202-944-3295
Toll free: 800-621-3141
sbaa@sbaa.org

446. Spotlight 6
2617 Ted Toad Road
Rising Sun, MD 21911
Tel: 410-658-6264

447. Stevens-Johnson Syndrome Foundation and Support
Group
9285 North Utica Street
Westminster, CO 80030
Tel: 303-430-9559
Fax: 303-487-9359
sjsupport@aol.com

448. Strang-Cornell Hereditary Colon Cancer Program
428 East 72nd Street
New York, NY 10021
Tel: 212-746-5656
Fax: 212-746-8765
mbertag@mail.med.cornell.edu

449. Stratford Orthopedics & Rehabilitation
231 South Gary Avenue
Bloomington, IL 60108
Tel: 630-529-7708

450. Sturge-Weber Foundation
P.O. Box 418
Mt. Freedom, NJ 07970-0418
Tel: 973-895-4445
Fax: 973-895-4846
Toll free: 800-627-5482
swf@sturge-weber.com

451. Sudden Arrhythmia Death Syndromes Foundation
508 E. South Temple, #20
Salt Lake City, UT 84102
Tel: 801-531-0937
Fax: 801-531-0945
Toll free: 800-786-7723
sads@aros.net

452. Superkids, Inc. (newsletter for families and friends of
children with limb differences)
60 Clyde Street
Newton, MA 02460-2250

453. Support Network for Pachygyria, Agyria, Lissencephaly
2410 South 24th Street, #9102
Kansas City, KS 66106
Tel: 913-432-7453

454. Support Organization for Trisomy 13/18 and Related
Disorders, UK
7 Orwell Road
Petersfield
Hampshire, GU31 4LQ
United Kingdom
Tel: 0121-351-3122
enquiries@soft.org.uk

455. Support Organization for Trisomy 18, 13, and Related
Disorders
2982 South Union Street
Rochester, NY 14624-1926
Tel: 716-594-4621
Fax: 716-594-4621
Toll free: 800-716-7638
barbv@trisomy.org

456. Support Report
P.O. Box 506
Somerton, AZ 85360
thesupportreportyahoogroups.com or *skyfireranch@digipax.com*

457. Takayasu's Arteritis Association
16 Rose Lane
Bedford, NH 03110
Tel: 603-641-2774
Fax: 603-641-2774
dpatsos@taa.mv.com

458. Takayasu's Arteritis Foundation, International
P.O. Box 280
1500 Meeting House Rd.
Sea Girt, NJ 08750
Tel: 732-449-0550
Fax: 732-974-6726
pkgrigg@takayasu.org

459. TAR Syndrome Association
212 Sherwood Drive
Linwood, NJ 08234-7658
Tel: 609-927-0418
Fax: 609-653-8639
spp212@aol.com

460. Tardive Dyskinesia/Tardive Dystonia National Association
4424 University Way NE
P.O. Box 45732
Seattle, WA 98145-0732
Tel: 206-522-3166

461. TEF/VATER/VACTRL National Support Network
15301 Grey Fox Road
Upper Marlboro, MD 20772
Tel: 301-952-6837
Fax: 301-952-9152
tefvater@ix.netcom.com

462. The Arc (a national organization on mental retardation)
1010 Wayne Ave.
Suite 650
Silver Spring, MD 20910
Tel: 301-565-3842
Fax: 301-565-3843
Toll free: 800-433-5255
thearc@metronet.com

463. The CDG Family Network Foundation
27047 Spring Valley Rd.
Shannon, IL 61078
Tel: 815-864-2554
springvalliacres@yahoo.com

464. The Paget Foundation
120 Wall Street
Suite 1602
New York, NY 10005
Tel: 212-509-5335
Fax: 212-509-8492
Toll free: 800-237-2438
pagetfdn@aol.com

465. THRESHOLD Newsletter (for uncontrolled seizure disorders)
Family Support Center of New Jersey
2150 Highway 35 North
Suite 207C
Sea Girt, NJ 08750
Tel: 732-9741-144
Fax: 732-974-0940
Toll free: 800-372-6510
fscnj@aol.com

466. Thyroid Foundation of America, Inc.
Ruth Sleeper Hall
RSL 350
40 Parkman Street
Boston, MA 02114-2698
Tel: 617-726-8500
Fax: 617-726-4136
Toll free: 800-832-8321
info@tsh.org

467. Tourette Syndrome Association, Inc.
42-40 Bell Boulevard
Bayside, NY 11361-2861
Tel: 718-224-2999
Fax: 718-279-9596
Toll free: 888-486-8738
ts@tsa-usa.org

468. Treacher-Collins Foundation
P.O. Box 683
Norwich, VT 05055-0683
Tel: 802-649-3050
Toll free: 800-823-2055
tcnet@geocities.com

469. Trigeminal Neuralgia Association
2801 SW Archer Rd.
Suite C
Gainesville, FL 32608
Tel: 352-376-9955
Fax: 352-376-8688
tnanational@tna-support.org

470. Trisomy 9 International Parent Support
Children's Hospital
Div. Gen. & Met.
3901 Beaubien Boulevard
Detroit, MI 48201-2196
Tel: 909-862-4470
atoddna@sprynet.com

471. Tuberous Sclerosis Alliance
801 Roeder Rd., #750
Silver Spring, MD 20910-4487
Tel: 301-459-9888
Fax: 301-459-0394
Toll free: 800-225-6872
ntsa@ntsa.org

472. Turner's Syndrome Society
814 Glencairn Avenue
North York
Ontario, M6B 2A3
Canada
Tel: 416-781-2086
Fax: 416-781-7245
Toll free: 800-465-6744
tssincan@web.net

473. Turner's Syndrome Society of the United States
14450 TC Jester
Suite 260
Houston, TX 77014
Tel: 832-249-9988
Fax: 832-249-9987
Toll free: 800-365-9944
shel@turner-syndrome-us.org

474. Twin Hope (Twin-Twin Transfusion Syndrome)
2592 West 14th Street
Cleveland, OH 44113
Tel: 216-228-8887
twinhope@mail.ohio.net

475. Twin to Twin Transfusion Syndrome Foundation
National Office
411 Longbeach Parkway
Bay Village, OH 44140
Tel: 440-899-8887
Fax: 440-899-1184
info@tttsfoundation.org

476. UNIQUE—Rare Chromosome Disorder Support Group
P.O. Box 2189
Caterham
Surrey, CR3 5GN
United Kingdom
Tel: 4401-883 330766
info@rarechromo.org

477. United Leukodystrophy Foundation
2304 Highland Drive
Sycamore, IL 60178
Tel: 815-895-3211
Fax: 815-895-2432
Toll free: 800-728-5483
ulf@tbcnet.com

478. United Mitochondrial Disease Foundation
8085 Saltsburg Rd.
Suite 201
Pittsburgh, PA 15239
Tel: 412-793-8077
Fax: 412-793-6477
info@umdf.org

479. United Ostomy Association, Inc.
19772 MacArthur Boulevard
Suite 200
Irvine, CA 92612-2405
Tel: 949-660-8624
Fax: 949-660-9262
Toll free: 800-826-0826
uoa@deltanet.com

480. Ureterosigmoidostomy Association
690 Pleasant Hill Rd.
Brunswick, ME 04011
Tel: 207-725-2753
Fax: 320-213-0729
Kascar@yahoo.com

481. Usher Family Support
4918 42nd Avenue South
Minneapolis, MN 55417
Tel: 612-724-6982
kadbmn@aol.com

482. Uveitis/Ocular Inflammatory Disease Support Group
Massachusetts Eye and Ear Infirmary
243 Charles St.
Boston, MA 02114
Tel: 617-573-3968
Fax: 617-573-3181
sfoster@mediaone.net

483. Vascular AnomaliesCenter
Boston Children's Hospital
Longwood Ave.
Boston, MA

484. Vascular Birthmarks Foundation
P.O. Box 106
Latham, NY 12110
Tel: 518-782-9637
linda@birthmark.org

485. Vestibular Disorders Association
P.O. Box 4467
Portland, OR 97208-4467
Tel: 503-2297705
Fax: 503-229-8064
Toll free: 800-837-8428
veda@vestibular.org

486. VHL Family Alliance
171 Clinton Road
Brookline, MA 02445-5815
Tel: 617-232-5946
Fax: 617-734-8233
Toll free: 800-767-4845
info@vhl.org

487. WE MOVE (Worldwide Education and Awareness for Movement Disorders)
Mt. Sinai Medical Center
One Gustave L. Levy Place Box 1052
New York, NY 10029
Tel: 212-241-8567
Fax: 212-987-7363
Toll free: 800-437-6682
wemove@wemove.org

488. Weaver Syndrome Network
4357 153rd Avenue SE
Belluvue, WA 98006
Tel: 425-747-5382
Fax: 425-235-6225

489. Website - Spine University
www.spineuniversity.com

490. Wegener's Granulomatosis Association
P.O. Box 28660
Kansas City, MO 64188-8660
Tel: 816-436-8211
Fax: 816-43-8211
Toll free: 800-277-9474
wgsg@wgsg.org

491. West Syndrome Support Group
wssg@globalnet.co.uk

492. Wide Smiles
P.O. Box 5153
Stockton, CA 95205-0153
Tel: 209-942-2812
Fax: 209-464-1497
webmaster@widesmiles.org

493. Williams Syndrome Association
1316 North Campbell
Suite 16
Royal Oak, MI 48067
Tel: 248-541-3630
Fax: 248-541-3631
Toll free: 800-806-1871
tmonkaba@aol.com or *wsaoffice@aol.com*

494. Wilson's Disease Association
4 Navaho Drive
Brookfield, CT 06804-3124
Tel: 203-775-9666
Toll free: 800-399-0266
hasellner@worldnet.att.net

495. Wolf-Hirschhorn Syndrome Support Group
2B Harvesters Close
Rainham
Gillingham, ME8 8PA
United Kingdom
Tel: 0163 4372218
Fax: 016-343-72218

496. Women's Health, UK
Web Site on the Internet
www.womens-health.co.uk

497. World Health Organization (WHO) Regional Office for the Americas (AMRO)
Pan American Health Organization (PAHO)
525 23rd Street NW
Washington, DC 20037
Tel: 202-974-3000
Fax: 202-974-3663
postmaster@paho.org

498. XLH Network
3517 Mase Lane
Bowie, MD 20715
Tel: 301-262-8850
elaine@xlhnetwork.org

List of Orphan Products Approved for Marketing by the U.S. Food and Drug Administration* Through Friday, April 12, 2002

Total Approvals in 230

Generic Name:	**Albendazole**	Trade Name:	Albenza
Designated Indication:	Treatment of neurocysticercosis due to *Taenia solium* as (a) chemotherapy of parenchymal, subarachnoidal, and racemose (cysts in spinal fluid) neurocysticercosis in symptomatic cases and (b) prophylaxis of epilepsy and other sequelae in asymptomatic neurocysticercosis.		
		Date Designated:	1/18/1996
		Market Approval Date:	6/11/1996

Generic Name:	**Albendazole**	Trade Name:	Albenza
Designated Indication:	Treatment of hydatid disease (cystic echinococcosis due to *Echinococcus granulosus* larvae or alveolar echinococcosis due to *E. multilocularis* larvae).		
		Date Designated:	1/17/1996
		Market Approval Date:	6/11/1996

Generic Name:	**Aldesleukin**	Trade Name:	Proleukin
Designated Indication:	Treatment of metastatic renal cell carcinoma.		
		Date Designated:	9/14/1988
		Market Approval Date:	5/5/1992

---

*Provided by the Office of Orphan Products Development, U.S. Food and Drug Administration.

Generic Name:	**Aldesleukin**	Trade Name:	Proleukin
Designated Indication:	Treatment of metastatic melanoma.		
		Date Designated:	9/10/1996
		Market Approval Date:	1/9/1998

Generic Name:	**Alemtuzumab**	Trade Name:	Campath
Designated Indication:	Treatment of chronic lymphocytic leukemia.		
		Date Designated:	10/20/1997
		Market Approval Date:	5/7/2001

Generic Name:	**Alglucerase injection**	Trade Name:	Ceredase
Designated Indication:	For replacement therapy in patients with Gaucher disease type I.		
		Date Designated:	3/11/1985
		Market Approval Date:	4/5/1991

Generic Name:	**Alitretinoin**	Trade Name:	Panretin
Designated Indication:	Topical treatment of cutaneous lesions in patients with AIDS-related Kaposi sarcoma.		
		Date Designated:	3/24/1998
		Market Approval Date:	2/2/1999

Generic Name:	**Allopurinol sodium**	Trade Name:	Zyloprim for Injection
Designated Indication:	Management of patients with leukemia, lymphoma, and solid tumor malignancies who are receiving cancer therapy, which causes elevations of serum and urinary uric acid levels and who cannot tolerate oral therapy.		
		Date Designated:	10/16/1992
		Market Approval Date:	5/17/1996

Generic Name:	**Alpha1-proteinase inhibitor (human)**	Trade Name:	Prolastin
Designated Indication:	For replacement therapy in the alpha-1-proteinase inhibitor congenital deficiency state.		
		Date Designated:	12/7/1984
		Market Approval Date:	12/2/1987

Generic Name:	**Altretamine**	Trade Name:	Hexalen
Designated Indication:	Treatment of advanced adenocarcinoma of the ovary.		
		Date Designated:	2/9/1984
		Market Approval Date:	12/26/1990

Generic Name:	**Amifostine**	Trade Name:	Ethyol
Designated Indication:	Reduction of the incidence of moderate to severe xerostomia in patients undergoing postoperative radiation treatment for head and neck cancer.		
		Date Designated:	5/12/1998
		Market Approval Date:	6/24/1999

Generic Name:	**Amifostine**	Trade Name:	Ethyol
Designated Indication:	For use as a chemoprotective agent for cisplatin in the treatment of advanced ovarian carcinoma.		
		Date Designated:	5/30/1990
		Market Approval Date:	12/8/1995

Generic Name:	**Aminosalicylic acid**	Trade Name:	Paser Granules
Designated Indication:	Treatment of tuberculosis infections.		
		Date Designated:	2/19/1992
		Market Approval Date:	6/30/1994

Generic Name:	**Amiodarone HCl**	Trade Name:	Cordarone
Designated Indication:	For the acute treatment and prophylaxis of life-threatening ventricular tachycardia or ventricular fibrillation.		
		Date Designated:	3/16/1994
		Market Approval Date:	8/3/1995

Generic Name:	**Amphotericin B lipid complex**	Trade Name:	Abelcet
Designated Indication:	Treatment of invasive fungal infections.		
		Date Designated:	12/3/1996
		Market Approval Date:	10/18/1996

Generic Name:	**Anagrelide**	Trade Name:	Agrylin
Designated Indication:	Treatment of essential thrombocythemia.		
		Date Designated:	1/27/1988
		Market Approval Date:	3/14/1997

Generic Name:	**Antihemophilic factor (recombinant)**	Trade Name:	ReFacto
Designated Indication:	For the control and prevention of hemorrhagic episodes and for surgical prophylaxis in patients with hemophilia A (congenital factor VIII deficiency or classic hemophilia).		
		Date Designated:	2/8/1996
		Market Approval Date:	Not currently approved

Generic Name:	**Antihemophilic factor (recombinant)**	Trade Name:	Kogenate
Designated Indication:	Prophylaxis and treatment of bleeding in individuals with hemophilia A or for prophylaxis when surgery is required in individuals with hemophilia A.		
		Date Designated:	9/25/1989
		Market Approval Date:	2/25/1993

Generic Name:	**Antihemophilic factor/von Willebrand factor complex (human), dried, pasteurized**	Trade Name:	Humate-P
Designated Indication:	Treatment and prevention of bleeding in hemophilia A (classical hemophilia) in adult patients; and treatment of spontaneous and trauma-induced bleeding episodes in severe von Willebrand disease, and in mild and moderate von Willebrand disease where use of desmopressin is known or suspected to be inadequate in adult and pediatric patients.		
		Date Designated:	10/16/1992
		Market Approval Date:	4/1/1999

Generic Name:	**Antithrombin III (human)**	Trade Name:	ATnativ
Designated Indication:	For the treatment of patients with hereditary antithrombin III deficiency in connection with surgical or obstetric procedures or when they suffer from thromboembolism.		
		Date Designated:	2/8/1985
		Market Approval Date:	12/13/1989

Generic Name:	**Antithrombin III (human)**	Trade Name:	Thrombate III
Designated Indication:	For replacement therapy in congenital deficiency of AT-III for prevention and treatment of thrombosis and pulmonary emboli.		
		Date Designated:	11/26/1984
		Market Approval Date:	12/30/1991

Generic Name:	**Antivenin, crotalidae polyvalent immune Fab (ovine)**	Trade Name:	CroFab
Designated Indication:	Treatment of envenomations inflicted by North American crotalid snakes.		
		Date Designated:	1/12/1994
		Market Approval Date:	10/2/2000

Generic Name:	**Aprotinin**	Trade Name:	Trasylol
Designated Indication:	For prophylactic use to reduce perioperative blood loss and the homologous blood transfusion requirement in patients undergoing cardiopulmonary bypass surgery in the course of repeat coronary artery bypass graft surgery, and in selected cases of primary coronary artery bypass graft surgery where the risk of bleeding is especially high (impaired hemostasis) or where transfusion is unavailable or unacceptable.		
		Date Designated:	11/17/1993
		Market Approval Date:	12/29/1993

Generic Name:	**Arsenic trioxide**	Trade Name:	Trisenox
Designated Indication:	Treatment of myelodysplastic syndrome.		
		Date Designated:	7/17/2000
		Market Approval Date:	9/25/2000

Generic Name:	**Arsenic trioxide**	Trade Name:	Trisenox
Designated Indication:	Treatment of acute promyelocytic leukemia.		
		Date Designated:	3/3/1998
		Market Approval Date:	9/25/2000

Generic Name:	**Atovaquone**	Trade Name:	Mepron
Designated Indication:	Treatment of AIDS-associated *Pneumocystis carinii* pneumonia.		
		Date Designated:	9/10/1990
		Market Approval Date:	11/25/1992

Generic Name:	**Atovaquone**	Trade Name:	Mepron
Designated Indication:	Prevention of *Pneumocystis carinii* pneumonia (PCP) in high-risk, HIV-infected patients defined by a history of one or more episodes of PCP and/or a peripheral CD4+ (T4 helper/inducer) lymphocyte count less than or equal to		
		Date Designated:	8/14/1991
		Market Approval Date:	1/5/1999

Generic Name:	**Baclofen**	Trade Name:	Lioresal Intrathecal
Designated Indication:	Treatment of intractable spasticity caused by spinal cord injury, multiple sclerosis, and other spinal diseases (including spinal ischemia, spinal tumor, transverse myelitis, cervical spondylosis, and degenerative myelopathy).		
		Date Designated:	11/10/1987
		Market Approval Date:	6/25/1992

Generic Name:	**Basiliximab**	Trade Name:	Simulect
Designated Indication:	Prophylaxis of solid organ rejection.		
		Date Designated:	12/12/1997
		Market Approval Date:	5/12/1998

Generic Name:	**Benzoate and phenylacetate**	Trade Name:	Ucephan
Designated Indication:	For adjunctive therapy in the prevention and treatment of hyperammonemia in patients with urea cycle enzymopathy due to carbamylphosphate synthetase, ornithine, transcarbamylase, or argininosuccinate synthetase.		
		Date Designated:	1/21/1986
		Market Approval Date:	12/23/1987

Generic Name:	**Beractant**	Trade Name:	Survanta Intratracheal Suspension
Designated Indication:	Treatment of neonatal respiratory distress syndrome.		
		Date Designated:	2/5/1986
		Market Approval Date:	7/1/1991

Generic Name:	**Beractant**	Trade Name:	Survanta Intratracheal Suspension
Designated Indication:	Prevention of neonatal respiratory distress syndrome.		
		Date Designated:	2/5/1986
		Market Approval Date:	7/1/1991

Generic Name:	**Betaine**	Trade Name:	Cystadane
Designated Indication:	Treatment of homocystinuria.		
		Date Designated:	5/16/1994
		Market Approval Date:	10/25/1996

Generic Name:	**Bexarotene**	Trade Name:	Targretin
Designated Indication:	Treatment of cutaneous manifestations of cutaneous T-cell lymphoma in patients who are refractory to at least one prior systemic therapy.		
		Date Designated:	6/18/1999
		Market Approval Date:	12/29/1999

Generic Name:	**Bleomycin sulfate**	Trade Name:	Blenoxane
Designated Indication:	Treatment of malignant pleural effusion.		
		Date Designated:	9/17/1993
		Market Approval Date:	2/20/1996

Generic Name:	**Bosentan**	Trade Name:	Tracleer
Designated Indication:	Treatment of pulmonary arterial hypertension.		
		Date Designated:	10/6/2000
		Market Approval Date:	11/20/2001

Generic Name:	**Botulinum toxin type A**	Trade Name:	Botox
Designated Indication:	Treatment of blepharospasm associated with dystonia in adults (patients 12 years of age and above).		
		Date Designated:	3/22/1984
		Market Approval Date:	12/29/1989

Generic Name:	**Botulinum toxin type A**	Trade Name:	Botox
Designated Indication:	Treatment of cervical dystonia.		
		Date Designated:	8/20/1986
		Market Approval Date:	12/21/2000

Generic Name:	**Botulinum toxin type A**	Trade Name:	Botox
Designated Indication:	Treatment of strabismus associated with dystonia in adults (patients 12 years of age and above).		
		Date Designated:	3/22/1984
		Market Approval Date:	12/29/1989

Generic Name:	**Botulinum toxin type B**	Trade Name:	NeuroBloc
Designated Indication:	Treatment of cervical dystonia.		
		Date Designated:	1/16/1992
		Market Approval Date:	12/8/2000

Generic Name:	**Buffered intrathecal electrolyte/dextrose injection**	Trade Name:	Elliotts B Solution
Designated Indication:	For use as a diluent in the intrathecal administration of methotrexate and cytarabine for the prevention or treatment of meningeal leukemia and lymphocytic lymphoma.		
		Date Designated:	8/24/1994
		Market Approval Date:	9/27/1996

Generic Name:	**Busulfan**	Trade Name:	Busulfex
Designated Indication:	As preparative therapy in the treatment of malignancies with bone marrow transplantation.		
		Date Designated:	7/28/1994
		Market Approval Date:	2/4/1999

Generic Name:	**Caffeine**	Trade Name:	Cafcit
Designated Indication:	Treatment of apnea of prematurity.		
		Date Designated:	9/20/1988
		Market Approval Date:	9/21/1999

Generic Name:	**Calcitonin-human for injection**	Trade Name:	Cibacalcin
Designated Indication:	Treatment of symptomatic Paget disease (osteitis deformans).		
		Date Designated:	1/20/1987
		Market Approval Date:	10/31/1986

Generic Name:	**Calcium acetate**	Trade Name:	Phos-Lo
Designated Indication:	Treatment of hyperphosphatemia in end-stage renal failure.		
		Date Designated:	12/22/1988
		Market Approval Date:	12/10/1990

Generic Name:	**Chenodiol**	Trade Name:	Chenix
Designated Indication:	For patients with radiolucent stones in well-opacifying gallbladders, in whom elective surgery would be undertaken except for the presence of increased surgical risk due to systemic disease or age.		
		Date Designated:	9/21/1984
		Market Approval Date:	7/28/1983

Generic Name:	**Citric acid, glucono-delta-lactone and magnesium carbonate**	Trade Name:	Renacidin Irrigation
Designated Indication:	Treatment of renal and bladder calculi of the apatite or struvite variety.		
		Date Designated:	8/28/1989
		Market Approval Date:	10/2/1990

Generic Name:	**Cladribine**	Trade Name:	Leustatin Injection
Designated Indication:	Treatment of hairy cell leukemia.		
		Date Designated:	11/15/1990
		Market Approval Date:	2/26/1993

Generic Name:	**Clofazimine**	Trade Name:	Lamprene
Designated Indication:	Treatment of lepromatous leprosy, including dapsone-resistant lepromatous leprosy and lepromatous leprosy complicated by erythema nodosum leprosum.		
		Date Designated:	6/11/1984
		Market Approval Date:	12/15/1986

Generic Name:	**Clonidine**	Trade Name:	Duraclon
Designated Indication:	For continous epidural administration as adjunctive therapy with intraspinal opiates for the treatment of pain in cancer patients tolerant to, or unresponsive to, intraspinal opiates.		
		Date Designated:	1/24/1989
		Market Approval Date:	10/2/1996

Generic Name:	**Coagulation factor IX**	Trade Name:	Mononine
Designated Indication:	Replacement treatment and prophylaxis of the hemorrhagic complications of hemophilia B.		
		Date Designated:	6/27/1989
		Market Approval Date:	8/20/1992

Generic Name:	**Coagulation factor IX (human)**	Trade Name:	AlphaNine
Designated Indication:	For use as replacement therapy in patients with hemophilia B for the prevention and control of bleeding episodes, and during surgery to correct defective hemostasis.		
		Date Designated:	7/5/1990
		Market Approval Date:	12/31/1990

Generic Name:	**Coagulation factor IX (recombinant)**	Trade Name:	BeneFix
Designated Indication:	Treatment of hemophilia B.		
		Date Designated:	10/3/1994
		Market Approval Date:	2/11/1997

Generic Name:	**Coagulation factor VIIa (recombinant)**	Trade Name:	NovoSeven
Designated Indication:	Treatment of bleeding episodes in hemophilia A or B patients with inhibitors to factor VIII or factor IX.		
		Date Designated:	6/6/1988
		Market Approval Date:	3/25/1999

Generic Name:	**Colfosceril palmitate, cetyl alcohol, tyloxapol**	Trade Name:	Exosurf Neonatal for Intratracheal Suspension
Designated Indication:	Treatment of established hyaline membrane disease at all gestational ages.		
		Date Designated:	10/20/1989
		Market Approval Date:	8/2/1990

Generic Name:	**Colfosceril palmitate, cetyl alcohol, tyloxapol**	Trade Name:	Exosurf Neonatal for Intratracheal Suspension
Designated Indication:	Prevention of hyaline membrane disease, also known as respiratory distress syndrome, in infants born at 32 weeks' gestation or less.		
		Date Designated:	10/20/1989
		Market Approval Date:	8/2/1990

Generic Name:	**Corticorelin ovine triflutate**	Trade Name:	Acthrel
Designated Indication:	For use in differentiating pituitary and ectopic production of ACTH in patients with ACTH-dependent Cushing syndrome.		
		Date Designated:	11/24/1989
		Market Approval Date:	5/23/1996

Generic Name:	**Cromolyn sodium**	Trade Name:	Gastrocrom
Designated Indication:	Treatment of mastocytosis.		
		Date Designated:	3/8/1984
		Market Approval Date:	12/22/1989

Generic Name:	**Cromolyn sodium 4% ophthalmic solution**	Trade Name:	Opticrom 4% Ophthalmic Solution
Designated Indication:	Treatment of vernal keratoconjunctivitis.		
		Date Designated:	7/24/1985
		Market Approval Date:	10/3/1984

Generic Name:	**Cysteamine**	Trade Name:	Cystagon
Designated Indication:	Treatment of nephropathic cystinosis.		
		Date Designated:	1/25/1991
		Market Approval Date:	8/15/1994

Generic Name:	**Cytarabine liposomal**	Trade Name:	DepoCyt
Designated Indication:	Treatment of neoplastic meningitis.		
		Date Designated:	6/2/1993
		Market Approval Date:	4/1/1999

Generic Name:	**Cytomegalovirus immune globulin (human)**	Trade Name:	CytoGam
Designated Indication:	Prevention or attenuation of primary cytomegalovirus disease in immunosuppressed recipients of organ transplants.		
		Date Designated:	8/3/1987
		Market Approval Date:	12/4/1998

Generic Name:	**Daclizumab**	Trade Name:	Zenapax
Designated Indication:	Prevention of acute renal allograft rejection.		
		Date Designated:	3/5/1993
		Market Approval Date:	12/10/1997

Generic Name:	**Daunorubicin citrate liposome injection**	Trade Name:	DaunoXome
Designated Indication:	Treatment of patients with advanced HIV-associated Kaposi sarcoma.		
		Date Designated:	5/14/1993
		Market Approval Date:	4/8/1996

Generic Name:	**Denileukin diftitox**	Trade Name:	Ontak
Designated Indication:	Treatment of patients with persistent or recurrent cutaneous T-cell lymphoma whose malignant cells express the CD25 component of the IL-2 receptor.		
		Date Designated:	8/21/1996
		Market Approval Date:	2/5/1999

Generic Name:	**Desmopressin acetate**	Trade Name:	NONE ASSIGNED
Designated Indication:	Treatment of mild hemophilia A and von Willebrand disease.		
		Date Designated:	1/22/1991
		Market Approval Date:	3/7/1994

Generic Name:	**Dexrazoxane**	Trade Name:	Zinecard
Designated Indication:	For the prevention of cardiomyopathy associated with doxorubicin administration.		
		Date Designated:	12/17/1991
		Market Approval Date:	5/26/1995

Generic Name:	**Diazepam viscous solution for rectal administration**	Trade Name:	NONE ASSIGNED
Designated Indication:	For the management of selected, refractory patients with epilepsy on stable regimens of antiepileptic drugs (AEDs), who require intermittent use of diazepam to control bouts of increased seizure activity.		
		Date Designated:	2/25/1992
		Market Approval Date:	7/29/1997

Generic Name:	**Diethyldithiocarbamate**	Trade Name:	Imuthiol
Designated Indication:	Treatment of AIDS.		
		Date Designated:	4/3/1986
		Market Approval Date:	Not currently approved

Generic Name:	**Digoxin immune FAB (Ovine)**	Trade Name:	Digibind
Designated Indication:	Treatment of potentially life-threatening digitalis intoxication in patients who are refractory to management by conventional therapy.		
		Date Designated:	11/1/1984
		Market Approval Date:	4/22/1986

Generic Name:	**Dornase-α**	Trade Name:	Pulmozyme
Designated Indication:	To reduce mucous viscosity and enable the clearance of airway secretions in patients with cystic fibrosis.		
		Date Designated:	1/16/1991
		Market Approval Date:	12/30/1993

Generic Name:	**Doxorubicin liposome**	Trade Name:	Doxil
Designated Indication:	Treatment of ovarian cancer.		
		Date Designated:	11/4/1998
		Market Approval Date:	6/28/1999

Generic Name:	**Dronabinol**	Trade Name:	Marinol
Designated Indication:	For the stimulation of appetite and prevention of weight loss in patients with a confirmed diagnosis of AIDS.		
		Date Designated:	1/15/1991
		Market Approval Date:	12/22/1992

Generic Name:	**Eflornithine HCl**	Trade Name:	Ornidyl
Designated Indication:	Treatment of Trypanosoma brucei gambiense infection (sleeping sickness).		
		Date Designated:	4/23/1986
		Market Approval Date:	11/28/1990

Generic Name:	**Epirubicin**	Trade Name:	Ellence
Designated Indication:	Treatment of breast cancer.		
		Date Designated:	9/14/1999
		Market Approval Date:	9/15/1999

Generic Name:	**Epoetin-α**	Trade Name:	Epogen
Designated Indication:	Treatment of anemia associated with end-stage renal disease.		
		Date Designated:	4/10/1986
		Market Approval Date:	6/1/1989

Generic Name:	**Epoetin-α**	Trade Name:	Epogen
Designated Indication:	Treatment of anemia associated with HIV infection or HIV treatment.		
		Date Designated:	7/1/1991
		Market Approval Date:	12/31/1990

Generic Name:	**Epoprostenol**	Trade Name:	Flolan
Designated Indication:	Treatment of primary pulmonary hypertension.		
		Date Designated:	9/25/1985
		Market Approval Date:	9/20/1995

Generic Name:	**Epoprostenol**	Trade Name:	Flolan
Designated Indication:	Treatment of secondary pulmonary hypertension due to intrinsic precapillary pulmonary vascular disease.		
		Date Designated:	3/22/1999
		Market Approval Date:	4/14/2000

Generic Name:	**Etanercept**	Trade Name:	Enbrel
Designated Indication:	Reduction in signs and symptoms of moderately to severely active, polyarticular-course, juvenile rheumatoid arthritis in patients who have had an inadequate response to one or more disease-modifying antirheumatic drugs.		
		Date Designated:	10/27/1998
		Market Approval Date:	5/27/1999

Generic Name:	**Ethanolamine oleate**	Trade Name:	Ethamolin
Designated Indication:	Treatment of patients with esophageal varices that have recently bled to prevent rebleeding.		
		Date Designated:	3/22/1984
		Market Approval Date:	12/22/1988

Generic Name:	**Etidronate disodium**	Trade Name:	Didronel
Designated Indication:	Treatment of hypercalcemia of malignancy inadequately managed by dietary modification and/or oral hydration.		
		Date Designated:	3/21/1986
		Market Approval Date:	4/21/1987

Generic Name:	**Exemestane**	Trade Name:	Aromasin
Designated Indication:	Treatment of advanced breast cancer in postmenopausal women whose disease has progressed following tamoxifen therapy.		
		Date Designated:	9/19/1991
		Market Approval Date:	10/21/1999

Generic Name:	**Felbamate**	Trade Name:	Felbatol
Designated Indication:	Treatment of Lennox-Gastaut syndrome.		
		Date Designated:	1/24/1989
		Market Approval Date:	7/29/1993

Generic Name:	**Filgrastim**	Trade Name:	Neupogen
Designated Indication:	Treatment of patients with severe chronic neutropenia (absolute neutrophil count less than 500/mm^3).		
		Date Designated:	11/7/1990
		Market Approval Date:	12/19/1994

Generic Name:	**Filgrastim**	Trade Name:	Neupogen
Designated Indication:	Treatment of neutropenia associated with bone marrow transplants.		
		Date Designated:	10/1/1990
		Market Approval Date:	6/15/1994

Generic Name:	**Filgrastim**	Trade Name:	Neupogen
Designated Indication:	For use in the mobilization of peripheral blood progenitor cells for collection in patients who will receive myeloablative or myelosuppressive chemotherapy.		
		Date Designated:	7/17/1995
		Market Approval Date:	12/28/1995

Generic Name:	**Filgrastim**	Trade Name:	Neupogen
Designated Indication:	Reduction in the duration of neutropenia, fever, antibiotic use, and hospitalization, following induction and consolidation treatment for acute myeloid leukemia.		
		Date Designated:	11/7/1996
		Market Approval Date:	4/2/1998

Generic Name:	**Fludarabine phosphate**	Trade Name:	Fludara
Designated Indication:	Treatment of chronic lymphocytic leukemia (CLL), including refractory CLL.		
		Date Designated:	4/18/1989
		Market Approval Date:	4/18/1991

Generic Name:	**Follitropin-α, recombinant**	Trade Name:	Gonal-F
Designated Indication:	For the initiation and reinitiation of spermatogenesis in adult males with reproductive failure due to hypothalamic or pituitary dysfunction, or hypogonadotropic hypogonadism. AMENDED indication 6/27/00: for the induction of spermatogenesis in men with primary and secondary hypogonadotropic hypogonadism in whom the cause of infertility is not due to primary testicular failure.		
		Date Designated:	12/21/1998
		Market Approval Date:	5/24/2000

Generic Name:	**Fomepizole**	Trade Name:	Antizole
Designated Indication:	Treatment of methanol or ethylene glycol poisoning.		
		Date Designated:	12/22/1988
		Market Approval Date:	12/8/2000

Generic Name:	**Fomepizole**	Trade Name:	Antizole
Designated Indication:	Treatment of methanol or ethylene glycol poisoning.		
		Date Designated:	12/22/1988
		Market Approval Date:	12/4/1997

Generic Name:	**Fosphenytoin**	Trade Name:	Cerebyx
Designated Indication:	For the acute treatment of patients with status epilepticus of the grand mal type.		
		Date Designated:	6/4/1991
		Market Approval Date:	8/5/1996

Generic Name:	**Gallium nitrate injection**	Trade Name:	Ganite
Designated Indication:	Treatment of hypercalcemia of malignancy.		
		Date Designated:	12/5/1988
		Market Approval Date:	1/17/1991

Generic Name:	**Ganciclovir intravitreal implant**	Trade Name:	Vitrasert Implant
Designated Indication:	Treatment of cytomegalovirus retinitis.		
		Date Designated:	6/7/1995
		Market Approval Date:	3/4/1996

Generic Name:	**Ganciclovir sodium**	Trade Name:	Cytovene
Designated Indication:	Treatment of cytomegalovirus retinitis in immunocompromised patients with AIDS.		
		Date Designated:	10/31/1985
		Market Approval Date:	6/23/1989

Generic Name:	**Gemtuzumab zogamicin**	Trade Name:	Mylotarg
Designated Indication:	Treatment of CD33-positive acute myeloid leukemia.		
		Date Designated:	11/24/1999
		Market Approval Date:	5/17/2000

Generic Name:	**Glatiramer acetate**	Trade Name:	Copaxone
Designated Indication:	Treatment of multiple sclerosis.		
		Date Designated:	11/9/1987
		Market Approval Date:	12/20/1996

Generic Name:	**Gonadorelin acetate**	Trade Name:	Lutrepulse
Designated Indication:	For induction of ovulation in women with hypothalamic amenorrhea due to a deficiency or absence in the quantity or pulse pattern of endogenous GnRH secretion.		
		Date Designated:	4/22/1987
		Market Approval Date:	10/10/1989

Generic Name:	**Halofantrine**	Trade Name:	Halfan
Designated Indication:	Treatment of mild to moderate acute malaria caused by susceptible strains of *Plasmodium falciparum* and *P. vivax*.		
		Date Designated:	11/4/1991
		Market Approval Date:	7/24/1992

Generic Name:	**Hemin**	Trade Name:	Panhematin
Designated Indication:	Amelioration of recurrent attacks of acute intermittent porphyria (AIP) temporarily related to the menstrual cycle in susceptible women and similar symptoms which occur in other patients with AIP, porphyria variegata, and hereditary coproporphyria.		
		Date Designated:	3/16/1984
		Market Approval Date:	7/20/1983

Generic Name:	**Histrelin acetate**	Trade Name:	Supprelin Injection
Designated Indication:	Treatment of central precocious puberty.		
		Date Designated:	8/10/1988
		Market Approval Date:	12/24/1991

Generic Name:	**Hydroxyurea**	Trade Name:	Droxia
Designated Indication:	Treatment of patients with sickle cell anemia as shown by the presence of hemoglobin S.		
		Date Designated:	10/1/1990
		Market Approval Date:	2/25/1998

Generic Name:	**Idarubicin HCl for injection**	Trade Name:	Idamycin
Designated Indication:	Treatment of acute myelogenous leukemia, also referred to as acute nonlymphocytic leukemia.		
		Date Designated:	7/25/1988
		Market Approval Date:	9/27/1990

Generic Name:	**Ifosfamide**	Trade Name:	Ifex
Designated Indication:	Treatment of testicular cancer.		
		Date Designated:	1/20/1987
		Market Approval Date:	12/30/1988

Generic Name:	**Imatinib**	Trade Name:	Gleevec
Designated Indication:	Treatment of chronic myelogenous leukemia.		
		Date Designated:	1/31/2001
		Market Approval Date:	5/10/2001

Generic Name:	**Imatinib mesylate**	Trade Name:	Gleevec
Designated Indication:	Treatment of gastrointestinal stromal tumors.		
		Date Designated:	11/1/2001
		Market Approval Date:	2/1/2002

Generic Name:	**Imiglucerase**	Trade Name:	Cerezyme
Designated Indication:	Replacement therapy in patients with types I, II, and III Gaucher disease.		
		Date Designated:	11/5/1991
		Market Approval Date:	5/23/1994

Generic Name:	**Immune globulin intravenous, human**	Trade Name:	Gamimune N
Designated Indication:	Infection prophylaxis in pediatric patients affected with the human immunodeficiency virus.		
		Date Designated:	2/18/1993
		Market Approval Date:	12/27/1993

Generic Name:	**Infliximab**	Trade Name:	Remicade
Designated Indication:	Treatment of moderately to severely active Crohn disease for the reduction of the signs and symptoms, in patients who have an inadequate response to conventional therapy; and treatment of patients with fistulizing Crohn disease for the reduction in the number of draining enterocutaneous fistula(s).		
		Date Designated:	11/14/1995
		Market Approval Date:	8/24/1998

Generic Name:	**Interferon-α2a**	Trade Name:	Roferon A
Designated Indication:	Treatment of chronic myelogenous leukemia.		
		Date Designated:	6/6/1989
		Market Approval Date:	10/19/1995

Generic Name:	**Interferon-α2a (recombinant)**	Trade Name:	Roferon-A
Designated Indication:	Treatment of AIDS-related Kaposi sarcoma.		
		Date Designated:	12/14/1987
		Market Approval Date:	11/21/1988

Generic Name:	**Interferon-α2b (recombinant)**	Trade Name:	Intron A
Designated Indication:	Treatment of AIDS-related Kaposi sarcoma.		
		Date Designated:	6/24/1987
		Market Approval Date:	11/21/1988

Generic Name:	**Interferon-β1a**	Trade Name:	Avonex
Designated Indication:	Treatment of multiple sclerosis.		
		Date Designated:	12/16/1991
		Market Approval Date:	5/17/1996

Generic Name:	**Interferon-β1b**	Trade Name:	Betaseron
Designated Indication:	Treatment of multiple sclerosis.		
		Date Designated:	11/17/1988
		Market Approval Date:	7/23/1993

Generic Name:	**Interferon-γ1b**	Trade Name:	Actimmune
Designated Indication:	Treatment of chronic granulomatous disease.		
		Date Designated:	9/30/1988
		Market Approval Date:	12/20/1990

Generic Name:	**Interferon-γ1b**	Trade Name:	Actimmune
Designated Indication:	Delaying time to disease progression in patients with severe, malignant osteopetrosis.		
		Date Designated:	9/30/1996
		Market Approval Date:	2/10/2000

Generic Name:	**Iobenguane sulfate I 131**	Trade Name:	NONE ASSIGNED
Designated Indication:	For use as a diagnostic adjunct in patients with pheochromocytoma.		
		Date Designated:	11/14/1984
		Market Approval Date:	3/21/1990

Generic Name:	**Lamotrigine**	Trade Name:	Lamictal
Designated Indication:	Treatment of Lennox-Gastaut syndrome.		
		Date Designated:	8/23/1995
		Market Approval Date:	8/24/1998

Generic Name:	**Lepirudin**	Trade Name:	Refluden
Designated Indication:	Treatment of heparin-associated thrombocytopenia type II.		
		Date Designated:	2/13/1997
		Market Approval Date:	3/6/1998

Generic Name:	**Leucovorin**	Trade Name:	Leucovorin Calcium
Designated Indication:	For use in combination with 5-fluorouracil for the treatment of metastatic colorectal cancer.		
		Date Designated:	12/8/1986
		Market Approval Date:	12/12/1991

Generic Name:	**Leucovorin**	Trade Name:	Leucovorin Calcium
Designated Indication:	For rescue use after high-dose methotrexate therapy in the treatment of osteosarcoma.		
		Date Designated:	8/17/1988
		Market Approval Date:	8/31/1988

Generic Name:	**Leuprolide acetate**	Trade Name:	Lupron Injection
Designated Indication:	Treatment of central precocious puberty.		
		Date Designated:	7/25/1988
		Market Approval Date:	4/16/1993

Generic Name:	**Levocarnitine**	Trade Name:	Carnitor
Designated Indication:	Treatment of genetic carnitine deficiency.		
		Date Designated:	2/28/1984
		Market Approval Date:	4/10/1986

Generic Name:	**Levocarnitine**	Trade Name:	Carnitor
Designated Indication:	Treatment of primary and secondary carnitine deficiency of genetic origin.		
		Date Designated:	7/26/1984
		Market Approval Date:	12/16/1992

Generic Name:	**Levocarnitine**	Trade Name:	Carnitor
Designated Indication:	Treatment of manifestations of carnitine deficiency in patients with end-stage renal disease who require dialysis.		
		Date Designated:	9/6/1988
		Market Approval Date:	12/15/1999

Generic Name:	**Levomethadyl acetate hydrochloride**	Trade Name:	Orlaam
Designated Indication:	Treatment of heroin addicts suitable for maintenance on opiate agonists.		
		Date Designated:	1/24/1985
		Market Approval Date:	7/9/1993

Generic Name:	**Lidocaine patch 5%**	Trade Name:	Lidoderm Patch
Designated Indication:	For relief of allodynia (painful hypersensitivity), and chronic pain in postherpetic neuralgia.		
		Date Designated:	10/24/1995
		Market Approval Date:	3/19/1999

Generic Name:	**Liothyronine sodium injection**	Trade Name:	Triostat
Designated Indication:	Treatment of myxedema coma/precoma.		
		Date Designated:	7/30/1990
		Market Approval Date:	12/31/1991

Generic Name:	**Liposomal amphotericin B**	Trade Name:	AmBisome
Designated Indication:	Treatment of cryptococcal meningitis.		
		Date Designated:	12/10/1996
		Market Approval Date:	8/11/1997

Generic Name:	**Liposomal amphotericin B**	Trade Name:	AmBisome
Designated Indication:	Treatment of visceral leishmaniasis.		
		Date Designated:	12/6/1996
		Market Approval Date:	8/11/1997

Generic Name:	**Lodoxamide tromethamine**	Trade Name:	Alomide Ophthalmic Solution
Designated Indication:	Treatment of vernal keratoconjunctivitis.		
		Date Designated:	10/16/1991
		Market Approval Date:	9/23/1993

Generic Name:	**Mafenide acetate solution**	Trade Name:	Sulfamylon Solution
Designated Indication:	For use as an adjunctive topical antimicrobial agent to control bacterial infection when used under moist dressings over meshed autografts on excised burn wounds.		
		Date Designated:	7/18/1990
		Market Approval Date:	6/5/1998

Generic Name:	**Mefloquine HCl**	Trade Name:	Lariam
Designated Indication:	Treatment of acute malaria due to *Plasmodium falciparum* and *P. vivax*.		
		Date Designated:	4/13/1988
		Market Approval Date:	5/2/1989

Generic Name:	**Mefloquine HCl**	Trade Name:	Lariam
Designated Indication:	Prophylaxis of *Plasmodium falciparum* malaria which is resistant to other available drugs.		
		Date Designated:	4/13/1988
		Market Approval Date:	5/2/1989

Generic Name:	**Megestrol acetate**	Trade Name:	Megace
Designated Indication:	Treatment of patients with anorexia, cachexia, or significant weight loss (≥10% of baseline body weight) and confirmed diagnosis of AIDS.		
		Date Designated:	4/13/1988
		Market Approval Date:	9/10/1993

Generic Name:	**Melphalan**	Trade Name:	Alkeran for Injection
Designated Indication:	Treatment of patients with multiple myeloma for whom oral therapy is inappropriate.		
		Date Designated:	2/24/1992
		Market Approval Date:	11/18/1992

Generic Name:	**Mesna**	Trade Name:	Mesnex
Designated Indication:	For use as a prophylactic agent in reducing the incidence of ifosfamide-induced hemorrhagic cystitis.		
		Date Designated:	11/14/1985
		Market Approval Date:	12/30/1988

Generic Name:	**Methotrexate sodium**	Trade Name:	Methotrexate
Designated Indication:	Treatment of osteogenic sarcoma.		
		Date Designated:	10/21/1985
		Market Approval Date:	4/7/1988

Generic Name:	**Metronidazole (topical)**	Trade Name:	Metrogel
Designated Indication:	Treatment of acne rosacea.		
		Date Designated:	10/22/1987
		Market Approval Date:	11/22/1988

Generic Name:	**Midodrine HCl**	Trade Name:	Amatine
Designated Indication:	Treatment of patients with symptomatic orthostatic hypotension.		
		Date Designated:	12/5/1996
		Market Approval Date:	9/6/1996

Generic Name:	**Mitoxantrone**	Trade Name:	Novantrone
Designated Indication:	Treatment of secondary-progressive multiple sclerosis.		
		Date Designated:	8/13/1999
		Market Approval Date:	10/13/2000

Generic Name:	**Mitoxantrone**	Trade Name:	Novantrone
Designated Indication:	Treatment of hormone refractory prostate cancer.		
		Date Designated:	8/21/1996
		Market Approval Date:	11/13/1996

Generic Name:	**Mitoxantrone**	Trade Name:	Novantrone
Designated Indication:	Treatment of progressive-relapsing multiple sclerosis.		
		Date Designated:	8/13/1999
		Market Approval Date:	10/13/2000

Generic Name:	**Mitoxantrone HCl**	Trade Name:	Novantrone
Designated Indication:	Treatment of acute myelogenous leukemia, also referred to as acute nonlymphocytic leukemia.		
		Date Designated:	7/13/1987
		Market Approval Date:	12/23/1987

Generic Name:	**Modafinil**	Trade Name:	Provigil
Designated Indication:	Treatment of excessive daytime sleepiness in narcolepsy.		
		Date Designated:	3/15/1993
		Market Approval Date:	12/24/1998

Generic Name:	**Monooctanoin**	Trade Name:	Moctanin
Designated Indication:	For dissolution of cholesterol gallstones retained in the common bile duct.		
		Date Designated:	5/30/1984
		Market Approval Date:	10/31/1985

Generic Name:	**Morphine sulfate concentrate (preservative free)**	Trade Name:	Infumorph
Designated Indication:	For use in microinfusion devices for intraspinal administration in the treatment of intractable chronic pain.		
		Date Designated:	7/12/1990
		Market Approval Date:	7/19/1991

Generic Name:	**Nafarelin acetate**	Trade Name:	Synarel Nasal Solution
Designated Indication:	Treatment of central precocious puberty.		
		Date Designated:	7/20/1988
		Market Approval Date:	Not currently approved

Generic Name:	**Naltrexone HCl**	Trade Name:	Trexan
Designated Indication:	For blockade of the pharmacological effects of exogenously administered opioids as an adjunct to the maintenance of the opioid-free state in detoxified, formerly opioid-dependent individuals.		
		Date Designated:	3/11/1985
		Market Approval Date:	11/30/1984

Generic Name:	**Nitisinone**	Trade Name:	Orfadin
Designated Indication:	Treatment of tyrosinemia type 1.		
		Date Designated:	5/16/1995
		Market Approval Date:	1/18/2002

Generic Name:	**Nitric oxide**	Trade Name:	INOmax
Designated Indication:	Treatment of persistent pulmonary hypertension in the newborn.		
		Date Designated:	6/22/1993
		Market Approval Date:	12/23/1999

Generic Name:	**Octreotide**	Trade Name:	Sandostatin LAR
Designated Indication:	Treatment of acromegaly.		
		Date Designated:	8/24/1998
		Market Approval Date:	11/25/1998

Generic Name:	**Octreotide**	Trade Name:	Sandostatin LAR
Designated Indication:	Treatment of diarrhea associated with vasoactive intestinal peptide tumors (VIPoma).		
		Date Designated:	8/24/1998
		Market Approval Date:	11/25/1998

Generic Name:	**Octreotide**	Trade Name:	Sandostatin LAR
Designated Indication:	Treatment of severe diarrhea and flushing associated with malignant carcinoid tumors.		
		Date Designated:	8/24/1998
		Market Approval Date:	11/25/1998

Generic Name:	**Ofloxacin**	Trade Name:	Ocuflox Ophthalmic Solution
Designated Indication:	Treatment of bacterial corneal ulcers.		
		Date Designated:	4/18/1991
		Market Approval Date:	5/22/1996

Generic Name:	**Oprelvekin**	Trade Name:	Neumega
Designated Indication:	Prevention of severe chemotherapy-induced thrombocytopenia.		
		Date Designated:	12/17/1996
		Market Approval Date:	11/25/1997

Generic Name:	**Paclitaxel**	Trade Name:	Taxol
Designated Indication:	Treatment of AIDS-related Kaposi sarcoma.		
		Date Designated:	3/25/1997
		Market Approval Date:	8/4/1997

Generic Name:	**Pegademase bovine**	Trade Name:	Adagen
Designated Indication:	For enzyme replacement therapy for ADA deficiency in patients with severe combined immunodeficiency.		
		Date Designated:	5/29/1984
		Market Approval Date:	3/21/1990

Generic Name:	**Pegaspargase**	Trade Name:	Oncaspar
Designated Indication:	Treatment of acute lymphocytic leukemia.		
		Date Designated:	10/20/1989
		Market Approval Date:	2/1/1994

Generic Name:	**Pentamidine isethionate**	Trade Name:	Pentam 300
Designated Indication:	Treatment of *Pneumocystis carinii* pneumonia.		
		Date Designated:	2/28/1984
		Market Approval Date:	10/16/1984

Generic Name:	**Pentamidine isethionate**	Trade Name:	Nebupent
Designated Indication:	Prevention of *Pneumocystis carinii* pneumonia in patients at high risk for developing this disease.		
		Date Designated:	1/12/1988
		Market Approval Date:	6/15/1989

Generic Name:	**Pentastarch**	Trade Name:	Pentaspan
Designated Indication:	As an adjunct in leukapheresis to improve the harvesting and increase the yield of leukocytes by centrifugal means.		
		Date Designated:	8/28/1985
		Market Approval Date:	5/19/1987

Generic Name:	**Pentosan polysulfate sodium**	Trade Name:	Elmiron
Designated Indication:	Treatment of interstitial cystitis.		
		Date Designated:	8/7/1985
		Market Approval Date:	9/26/1996

Generic Name:	**Pentostatin for injection**	Trade Name:	Nipent
Designated Indication:	Treatment of hairy cell leukemia.		
		Date Designated:	9/10/1987
		Market Approval Date:	10/11/1991

Generic Name:	**Pilocarpine**	Trade Name:	Salagen
Designated Indication:	Treatment of xerostomia induced by radiation therapy for head and neck cancer.		
		Date Designated:	9/24/1990
		Market Approval Date:	3/22/1994

Generic Name:	**Pilocarpine HCl**	Trade Name:	Salagen
Designated Indication:	Treatment of xerostomia and keratoconjunctivitis sicca in Sjögren syndrome patients.		
		Date Designated:	2/28/1992
		Market Approval Date:	2/11/1998

Generic Name:	**Polifeprosan 20 with carmustine**	Trade Name:	Gliadel
Designated Indication:	Treatment of malignant glioma.		
		Date Designated:	12/13/1989
		Market Approval Date:	9/23/1996

Generic Name:	**Porfimer sodium**	Trade Name:	Photofrin
Designated Indication:	For the photodynamic therapy of patients with primary or recurrent obstructing (either partially or completely) esophageal carcinoma.		
		Date Designated:	6/6/1989
		Market Approval Date:	12/27/1995

Generic Name:	**Potassium citrate**	Trade Name:	Urocit-K
Designated Indication:	Prevention of uric acid nephrolithiasis.		
		Date Designated:	11/1/1984
		Market Approval Date:	8/30/1985

Generic Name:	**Potassium citrate**	Trade Name:	Urocit-K
Designated Indication:	For avoidance of the complication of calcium stone formation in patients with uric lithiasis.		
		Date Designated:	9/12/1985
		Market Approval Date:	8/30/1985

Generic Name:	**Potassium citrate**	Trade Name:	Urocit-K
Designated Indication:	Prevention of calcium renal stones in patients with hypocitraturia.		
		Date Designated:	9/16/1985
		Market Approval Date:	8/30/1985

Generic Name:	**Pulmonary surfactant replacement, porcine**	Trade Name:	Curosurf
Designated Indication:	For the treatment and prevention of respiratory distress syndrome in premature infants.		
		Date Designated:	8/2/1993
		Market Approval Date:	Not currently approved

Generic Name:	**Respiratory syncytial virus immune globulin (human)**	Trade Name:	Respigam
Designated Indication:	Prophylaxis of respiratory syncytial virus lowers respiratory tract infections in infants and young children at high risk of RSV disease.		
		Date Designated:	9/27/1990
		Market Approval Date:	1/18/1996

Generic Name:	**Rho (D) immune globulin intravenous (human)**	Trade Name:	WinRho SD
Designated Indication:	Treatment of immune thrombocytopenic purpura.		
		Date Designated:	11/9/1993
		Market Approval Date:	3/24/1995

Generic Name:	**Rifabutin**	Trade Name:	Mycobutin
Designated Indication:	Prevention of disseminated *Mycobacterium avium* complex disease in patients with advanced HIV infection.		
		Date Designated:	12/18/1989
		Market Approval Date:	12/23/1992

Generic Name:	**Rifampin**	Trade Name:	Rifadin I.V.
Designated Indication:	For antituberculosis treatment where use of the oral form of the drug is not feasible.		
		Date Designated:	12/9/1985
		Market Approval Date:	5/25/1989

Generic Name:	**Rifampin, isoniazid, pyrazinamide**	Trade Name:	Rifater
Designated Indication:	For the short-course treatment of tuberculosis.		
		Date Designated:	9/12/1985
		Market Approval Date:	5/31/1994

Generic Name:	**Rifapentine**	Trade Name:	Priftin
Designated Indication:	Treatment of pulmonary tuberculosis.		
		Date Designated:	6/9/1995
		Market Approval Date:	6/22/1998

Generic Name:	**Riluzole**	Trade Name:	Rilutek
Designated Indication:	Treatment of amyotrophic lateral sclerosis.		
		Date Designated:	3/16/1993
		Market Approval Date:	12/12/1995

Generic Name:	**Rituximab**	Trade Name:	Rituxan
Designated Indication:	Treatment of non-Hodgkin B-cell lymphoma.		
		Date Designated:	6/13/1994
		Market Approval Date:	11/26/1997

Generic Name:	**Sacrosidase**	Trade Name:	Sucraid
Designated Indication:	Treatment of congenital sucrase-isomaltase deficiency.		
		Date Designated:	12/10/1993
		Market Approval Date:	4/9/1998

Generic Name:	**Sargramostim**	Trade Name:	Leukine
Designated Indication:	To reduce neutropenia and leukopenia and decrease the incidence of death due to infection in patients with acute myelogenous leukemia.		
		Date Designated:	3/6/1995
		Market Approval Date:	9/15/1995

Generic Name:	**Sargramostim**	Trade Name:	Leukine
Designated Indication:	Treatment of neutropenia associated with bone marrow transplant, for the treatment of graft failure and delay of engraftment, and for the promotion of early engraftment.		
		Date Designated:	5/3/1990
		Market Approval Date:	3/5/1991

Generic Name:	**Satumomab pendetide**	Trade Name:	Oncoscint CR/OV
Designated Indication:	Detection of ovarian carcinoma.		
		Date Designated:	9/25/1989
		Market Approval Date:	12/29/1992

Generic Name:	**Selegiline HCl**	Trade Name:	Eldepryl
Designated Indication:	As an adjuvant to levodopa and carbidopa treatment of idiopathic Parkinson disease (paralysis agitans), postencephalitic parkinsonism, and symptomatic parkinsonism.		
		Date Designated:	11/7/1984
		Market Approval Date:	6/5/1989

Generic Name:	**Sermorelin acetate**	Trade Name:	Geref
Designated Indication:	Treatment of idiopathic or organic growth hormone deficiency in children with growth failure.		
		Date Designated:	9/14/1988
		Market Approval Date:	9/26/1997

Generic Name:	**Sodium phenylbutyrate**	Trade Name:	Buphenyl
Designated Indication:	Treatment of urea cycle disorders: carbamylphosphate synthetase deficiency, ornithine transcarbamylase deficiency, and arginiosuccinic acid synthetase deficiency.		
		Date Designated:	11/22/1993
		Market Approval Date:	4/30/1996

Generic Name:	**Somatrem for injection**	Trade Name:	Protropin
Designated Indication:	For long-term treatment of children who have growth failure due to a lack of adequate endogenous growth hormone secretion.		
		Date Designated:	12/9/1985
		Market Approval Date:	10/17/1985

Generic Name:	**Somatropin**	Trade Name:	Humatrope
Designated Indication:	Treatment of short stature associated with Turner syndrome.		
		Date Designated:	5/8/1990
		Market Approval Date:	12/30/1996

Generic Name:	**Somatropin**	Trade Name:	Genotropin
Designated Indication:	Treatment of adults with growth hormone deficiency.		
		Date Designated:	9/6/1994
		Market Approval Date:	10/31/1997

Generic Name:	**Somatropin**	Trade Name:	Nutropin
Designated Indication:	For use in the long-term treatment of children who have growth failure due to a lack of adequate endogenous growth hormone secretion.		
		Date Designated:	3/6/1987
		Market Approval Date:	10/17/1985

Generic Name:	**Somatropin (rDNA origin)**	Trade Name:	Saizen
Designated Indication:	Treatment of idiopathic or organic growth hormone deficiency in children with growth failure.		
		Date Designated:	3/6/1987
		Market Approval Date:	Not currently approved

Generic Name:	**Somatropin (rDNA origin)**	Trade Name:	Nutropin Depot
Designated Indication:	Long-term treatment of children who have growth failure due to a lack of adequate endogenous growth hormone secretion.		
		Date Designated:	10/28/1999
		Market Approval Date:	Not currently approved

Generic Name:	**Somatropin (rDNA origin) injection**	Trade Name:	Norditropin
Designated Indication:	Treatment of growth failure in children due to inadequate growth hormone secretion.		
		Date Designated:	7/10/1987
		Market Approval Date:	Not currently approved

Generic Name:	**Somatropin (rDNA)**	Trade Name:	Genotropin
Designated Indication:	Treatment of short stature in patients with Prader-Willi syndrome.		
		Date Designated:	7/6/1999
		Market Approval Date:	6/20/2000

Generic Name:	**Somatropin (rDNA)**	Trade Name:	Genotropin
Designated Indication:	Treatment of growth failure in children who were born small for gestational age.		
		Date Designated:	12/27/2000
		Market Approval Date:	7/25/2001

Generic Name:	**Somatropin for injection**	Trade Name:	Serostim
Designated Indication:	Treatment of AIDS-associated catabolism/weight loss.		
		Date Designated:	11/15/1991
		Market Approval Date:	8/23/1996

Generic Name:	**Somatropin for injection**	Trade Name:	Nutropin
Designated Indication:	Treatment of growth retardation associated with chronic renal failure.		
		Date Designated:	8/4/1989
		Market Approval Date:	11/17/1993

Generic Name:	**Somatropin for injection**	Trade Name:	Nutropin
Designated Indication:	As replacement therapy for growth hormone deficiency in adults after epiphyseal closure.		
		Date Designated:	11/18/1996
		Market Approval Date:	12/15/1997

Generic Name:	**Somatropin for injection**	Trade Name:	Humatrope
Designated Indication:	For the long-term treatment of children who have growth failure due to inadequate secretion of normal endogenous growth hormone.		
		Date Designated:	6/12/1986
		Market Approval Date:	3/8/1987

Generic Name:	**Somatropin for injection**	Trade Name:	Nutropin
Designated Indication:	Treatment of short stature associated with Turner syndrome.		
		Date Designated:	3/23/1989
		Market Approval Date:	12/30/1996

Generic Name:	**Sotalol HCl**	Trade Name:	Betapace
Designated Indication:	Treatment of life-threatening ventricular tachyarrhythmias.		
		Date Designated:	9/23/1988
		Market Approval Date:	10/30/1992

Generic Name:	**Sterile talc powder**	Trade Name:	Sclerosol Intrapleural Aerosol
Designated Indication:	Treatment of malignant pleural effusion.		
		Date Designated:	9/18/1995
		Market Approval Date:	12/24/1997

Generic Name:	**Succimer**	Trade Name:	Chemet Capsules
Designated Indication:	Treatment of lead poisoning in children.		
		Date Designated:	5/9/1984
		Market Approval Date:	12/22/1988

Generic Name:	**Sulfadiazine**	Trade Name:	NONE ASSIGNED
Designated Indication:	For use in combination with pyrimethamine for the treatment of *Toxoplasma gondii* encephalitis in patients with and without AIDS.		
		Date Designated:	3/14/1994
		Market Approval Date:	7/29/1994

Generic Name:	**Surface active extract of saline lavage of bovine lungs**	Trade Name:	Infasurf
Designated Indication:	Treatment and prevention of respiratory failure due to pulmonary surfactant deficiency in preterm infants.		
		Date Designated:	6/7/1985
		Market Approval Date:	Not currently approved

Generic Name:	**Synthetic porcine secretin**	Trade Name:	NONE ASSIGNED
Designated Indication:	For use in the diagnosis of gastrinoma associated with Zollinger-Ellison syndrome.		
		Date Designated:	6/18/1999
		Market Approval Date:	4/4/2002

Generic Name:	**Synthetic porcine secretin**	Trade Name:	NONE ASSIGNED
Designated Indication:	For use in conjunction with diagnostic procedures for pancreatic disorders to increase pancreatic fluid secretion.		
		Date Designated:	3/7/2000
		Market Approval Date:	4/4/2002

Generic Name:	**Temozolomide**	Trade Name:	Temodar
Designated Indication:	Treatment of recurrent malignant glioma.		
		Date Designated:	10/5/1998
		Market Approval Date:	8/11/1999

Generic Name:	**Teniposide**	Trade Name:	Vumon for Injection
Designated Indication:	Treatment of refractory childhood acute lymphocytic leukemia.		
		Date Designated:	11/1/1984
		Market Approval Date:	7/14/1992

Generic Name:	**Teriparatide**	Trade Name:	Parathar
Designated Indication:	Diagnostic agent to assist in establishing the diagnosis in patients presenting with clinical and laboratory evidence of hypocalcemia due to either hypoparathyroidism or pseudohypoparathyroidism.		
		Date Designated:	1/9/1987
		Market Approval Date:	12/23/1987

Generic Name:	**Thalidomide**	Trade Name:	Thalomid
Designated Indication:	Treatment of erythema nodosum leprosum.		
		Date Designated:	7/26/1995
		Market Approval Date:	7/16/1998

Generic Name:	**Thyrotropin alpha**	Trade Name:	Thyrogen
Designated Indication:	As an adjunct in the diagnosis of thyroid cancer.		
		Date Designated:	2/24/1992
		Market Approval Date:	11/30/1998

Generic Name:	**Tiopronin**	Trade Name:	Thiola
Designated Indication:	Prevention of cystine nephrolithiasis in patients with homozygous cystinuria.		
		Date Designated:	1/17/1986
		Market Approval Date:	8/11/1988

Generic Name:	**Tobramycin for inhalation**	Trade Name:	TOBI
Designated Indication:	Treatment of bronchopulmonary infections of *Pseudomonas aeruginosa* in cystic fibrosis patients.		
		Date Designated:	10/13/1994
		Market Approval Date:	12/22/1997

Generic Name:	**Topiramate**	Trade Name:	Topamax
Designated Indication:	Treatment of Lennox-Gastaut syndrome.		
		Date Designated:	11/25/1992
		Market Approval Date:	8/28/2001

Generic Name:	**Toremifene**	Trade Name:	Fareston
Designated Indication:	Hormonal therapy of metastatic carcinoma of the breast.		
		Date Designated:	9/19/1991
		Market Approval Date:	5/29/1997

Generic Name:	**Tranexamic acid**	Trade Name:	Cyklokapron
Designated Indication:	Treatment of patients with congenital coagulopathies who are undergoing surgical procedures (e.g., dental extractions).		
		Date Designated:	10/29/1985
		Market Approval Date:	12/30/1986

Generic Name:	**Tretinoin**	Trade Name:	Vesanoid
Designated Indication:	Treatment of acute promyelocytic leukemia.		
		Date Designated:	10/24/1990
		Market Approval Date:	11/22/1995

Generic Name:	**Trientine HCl**	Trade Name:	Syprine
Designated Indication:	Treatment of patients with Wilson disease who are intolerant, or inadequately responsive to penicillamine.		
		Date Designated:	12/24/1984
		Market Approval Date:	11/8/1985

Generic Name:	**Trimetrexate glucuronate**	Trade Name:	Neutrexin
Designated Indication:	Treatment of *Pneumocystis carinii* pneumonia in AIDS patients.		
		Date Designated:	5/15/1986
		Market Approval Date:	12/17/1993

Generic Name:	**Urofollitropin**	Trade Name:	Metrodin
Designated Indication:	For induction of ovulation in patients with polycystic ovarian disease who have an elevated LH:FSH ratio and who have failed to respond to adequate clomiphene citrate therapy.		
		Date Designated:	11/25/1987
		Market Approval Date:	9/18/1986

Generic Name:	**Ursodiol**	Trade Name:	URSO
Designated Indication:	Treatment of patients with primary biliary cirrhosis.		
		Date Designated:	6/20/1991
		Market Approval Date:	12/10/1997

Generic Name:	**Valrubicin**	Trade Name:	Valstar
Designated Indication:	Treatment of carcinoma *in situ* of the urinary bladder.		
		Date Designated:	5/23/1994
		Market Approval Date:	9/25/1998

Generic Name:	**Zalcitabine**	Trade Name:	Hivid
Designated Indication:	Treatment of AIDS.		
		Date Designated:	6/28/1988
		Market Approval Date:	6/19/1992

Generic Name:	**Zidovudine**	Trade Name:	Retrovir
Designated Indication:	Treatment of AIDS.		
		Date Designated:	7/17/1985
		Market Approval Date:	3/19/1987

Generic Name:	**Zidovudine**	Trade Name:	Retrovir
Designated Indication:	Treatment of AIDS-related complex.		
		Date Designated:	5/12/1987
		Market Approval Date:	3/19/1987

Generic Name:	**Zinc acetate**	Trade Name:	Galzin
Designated Indication:	Treatment of Wilson disease.		
		Date Designated:	11/6/1985
		Market Approval Date:	1/28/1997

Generic Name:	**Zoledronate**	Trade Name:	Zometa, Zabel
Designated Indication:	Treatment of tumor-induced hypercalcemia.		
		Date Designated:	8/18/2000
		Market Approval Date:	8/20/2001

Index

A

Aarskog-Scott syndrome, 142
Aarskog syndrome, 142
    and KBG syndrome, 210
    and Noonan syndrome, 722
    and Rieger syndrome, 243–244
    and Robinow syndrome, 725–726
Aase-Smith syndrome, and Gordon
        syndrome, 199
Aase-Smith syndrome II, 143
Aase syndrome, 143, 365
    and thrombocytopenia and absent
        radius syndrome, 260
Abdominal angiomyolipomas, and
        lymphangioleiomyomatosis, 395
Abdominal enlargement, and Denys-
        Drash syndrome, 686
    and WAGR syndrome, 699
Abdominal hernia, and gastroschisis, 197
Abdominal migraine, 525–526
Abdominal pain, and acute intermittent
        porphyria, 490–491
    and ALA-dehydratase–deficient
        porphyria, 492
    and Churg-Strauss syndrome, 674
    and cyclic vomiting syndrome, 525
    and familial lipoprotein lipase
        deficiency, 465–466
    and Henoch-Schönlein purpura,
        414–415
    and sickle cell anemia, 372–373
    and small bowel diverticulosis, 339
    and WAGR syndrome, 699
    and Zollinger-Ellison syndrome, 330
Abdominal swelling, and
        abetalipoproteinemia, 358
Abdominal tumors, and
        pheochromocytoma, 409–410
Abetalipoproteinemia, 358
    and ataxia with vitamin E deficiency,
        606
    and chylomicron retention disease, 380

and congenital disorders of
        glycosylation, 457
    and Friedreich ataxia, 602
    and retinitis pigmentosa, 660
ABO incompatibility, and hereditary
        spherocytosis, 370–371
Abortion, and Asherman syndrome,
        308–309
Abscess formation, and erysipelas, 285
Acalculia, and Gerstmann syndrome, 534
Acalvaria, and anencephaly, 151–152
Acanthosis nigricans, and HAIR-AN
        syndrome, 315–316
Acetazolamide, and myotonia congenita,
        633
    and progressive myoclonus epilepsy,
        531–532
    and pseudotumor cerebri, 582
    and retinal arterial occlusion, 658
    and retinitis pigmentosa, 660
Achard-Thiers syndrome, 300
Acheiropodia, 702
    and Hanhart syndrome, 203
Achilles tendon contractures, and Emery-
        Dreifuss muscular dystrophy, 624
Achondrogenesis, 703
    and achondroplasia, 144
Achondrogenesis type II, and Kniest
        dysplasia, 213
Achondroplasia, 144
    and Kniest dysplasia, 213
    and metatropic dysplasia, 20
    and multiple epiphyseal dysplasia,
        187
    and 3-M syndrome, 259
Achromatopsia, and Leber congenital
        amaurosis, 652
Acid ceramidase deficiency, 443
Acid-maltase deficiency, 452
Acidemia, glutaric type I, 426
    glutaric type II, 426–427
    isovaleric, 427–428

methylmalonic, 429
    propionic, 428
Acidosis, and multiple carboxylase
        deficiency, 483
Acitretin, and Darier disease, 101
    and erythrokeratodermia variabilis,
        112
    and lichen planus, 125
Acne, and HAIR-AN syndrome, 315–316
    and precocious puberty, 325
    and transient acantholytic dermatosis,
        104
    and tuberous sclerosis, 596
Acne inversa, 118–119
Acoustic neuroma, and Ménière disease,
        558
    and neurofibromatosis type 2, 565
Acquired adrenogenital syndrome, and
        Achard-Thiers syndrome, 300
Acquired agranulocytosis, 361–362
Acquired aplastic anemia, 364
    and Fanconi anemia, 366
Acquired dietary deficiency of zinc, and
        acrodermatitis enteropathica, 94
Acquired epileptiform aplasia, 547
Acquired generalized lipodystrophy,
        320–321
Acquired hemolytic anemia, and
        congenital nonspherocytic
        hemolytic anemia, 369
Acquired hypothalamic insufficiency, and
        Prader-Willi syndrome, 237–238
Acquired immunodeficiency syndrome,
        and ACTH deficiency, 302
    and common variable
        immunodeficiency, 13
    and hyper-IgM syndrome, 393
    and Korsakoff syndrome, 546
    and Nezelof syndrome, 408
    and X-linked agammaglobulinemia,
        360
Acquired partial lipodystrophy, 321

Acquired pure red cell aplasia, 413–414
and Diamond-Blackfan anemia, 365
Acquired QT prolongation, and Romano-
Ward long QT syndrome, 54
Acrania, and anencephaly, 151–152
Acrocallosal syndrome, and Greig
cephalopolysyndactyly syndrome,
201
Schinzel type, 145
Acrocephalopolysyndactylia, and Bardet-
Biedl syndrome, 158
and Laurence-Moon syndrome, 215
Acrocephalosyndactyly, 154–155
Acrocephalosyndactyly syndromes, and
Antley-Bixler syndrome, 704–705
Acrodermatitis enteropathica, *fig. 6*, 94
Acro-dermato-ungual-lachrymal-tooth
syndrome, and split hand/split
foot malformation, 256
Acrodynia, and pheochromocytoma,
409
Acrodysostosis, 146
and acrosomelic dysplasia, 702–703
and dyschondrosteosis, 181
Acrofacial dysostosis, and Miller
syndrome, 222–223
and Nager syndrome, 226
and Treacher-Collins syndrome, 263
Acrogeria, and progeria, 724
Gottron type, *figs. 23–24*, 147
Acrokeratosis verruciformis of Hopf, and
Darier disease, 101
Acromegaloidism, and acromegaly, 301
Acromegaly, 301
and HAIR-AN syndrome, 315–316
and pachydermoperiostosis, 129
and Weaver syndrome, 266–267
Acromesomelic dysplasia, Maroteaux
type, 703–704
Acromicric dysplasia, and Leri
pleonosteosis, 217
Acroosteolysis, and Hajdu-Cheney
syndrome, 11
and hereditary sensory neuropathy,
570–571
Acrosomelic dysplasia, 702–704
ACTH, and infantile spasms, 541
and opsoclonus-myoclonus syndrome,
573
ACTH deficiency, 302
Active collagen vascular disease, and
idiopathic thrombocytosis, 421
Acupuncture, and interstitial cystitis,
685
and Tolosa-Hunt syndrome, 664
Acute chorea, 522

Acute disseminated encephalomyelitis,
and encephalitides, 284
Acute febrile neutrophilic dermatosis,
138–139
Acute guttale parapsoriasis, 128–129
Acute intermittent porphyria, 490–491
and ALA-dehydratase–deficient
porphyria, 492
Acute necrotizing encephalitis, 284–285
Acute posterior multifocal placoid
pigment epitheliopathy, 642
Acute respiratory distress syndrome, 670
Acyclovir, and encephalitides, 284
and recurrent respiratory
papillomatosis, 676
and TORCH syndrome, 295
Adamantiades-Behçet syndrome, 4
Adams-Oliver syndrome, 148
and amniotic bands, 150
and aplasia cutis congenita, 96
and cutis marmorata telangiectatica
congenita, 100
Adapalene, and Darier disease, 101
Addison disease, and congenital adrenal
hyperplasia, 304
and methylmalonic acidemias, 429
Addison-Schilder disease, 430
Adducted thumbs, and MASA syndrome,
220
Adducted thumbs syndrome, 220
Adelaide-type craniosynostosis, 719
Adenoid cystic carcinoma, 359
Adenoma-associated virilism, and
Achard-Thiers syndrome, 300
Adenomatous polyposis coli, 352–353
Adenosine deaminase excess, and
congenital nonspherocytic
hemolytic anemia, 369
Adenosylcobalamin deficiency, 429
Adhesive capsulitis, and Parsonage-
Turner syndrome, 577
Adiposis dolorosa, 303
Adrenal hyperplasia,congenital, 304
and HAIR-AN syndrome, 315–316
and primary aldosteronism, 305
and true hermaphroditism, 316–317
Adrenal hypoplasia, and Kallmann
syndrome, 318
Adrenal insufficiency, 302
Adrenalectomy, and primary
aldosteronism, 305
Adrenergic agonists, and congenital
complete heart block, 50
Adrenocorticotropic hormone, and
ACTH deficiency, 302
Adrenogenital syndrome, 304

Adrenoleukodystrophy, and Alexander
disease, 510
and Allan-Herndon-Dudley syndrome,
149
and ataxia-telangiectasia, 605–606
and metachromatic leukodystrophy,
552
and multiple sclerosis, 560
and Pelizaeus-Merzbacher disease, 578
and spinal muscular atrophy, 637
X-linked, 430
Adrenomyeloneuropathy, and adult
polyglucosan body disease, 580
and hereditary spastic paraplegia, 575
Adult polyglucosan body disease,
580–581
Adult respiratory distress syndrome, 670
Advanced bone age, and congenital
generalized lipodystrophy, 322
and Marshall-Smith syndrome, 219
and Sotos syndrome, 255
and Weaver syndrome, 266–267
Aedes aegypti mosquito, and dengue
fever, 281
Aerophagia, and intestinal
pseudoobstruction, 348
Affective disorders, and Kluver-Bucy
syndrome, 545
Afibrinogenemia, congenital, 359–360
and Glanzmann thrombasthenia, 383
Afterload reducers, and Barth syndrome,
44
Aganglionosis, and Hirschsprung disease,
345
Agelman syndrome, and Rett syndrome,
584
Agenesis of corpus callosum, 508
Aglossia adactylia, 203
Agnosia, primary visual, 508–509
Agraphia, and Gerstmann syndrome, 534
Ague, 291
Agyria, and classic lissencephaly, 553–554
Aicardi syndrome, *fig. 50*, 509–510
and acrocallosal syndrome (Schinzel
type), 145
Aicardi-Goutières syndrome, and
Pelizaeus-Merzbacher disease,
578
Airway disease, and situs inversus, 55
Airway obstruction, and recurrent
respiratory papillomatosis, 676
Akinetic mutism, and locked-in
syndrome, 554
Akinetic seizures, and narcolepsy, 562
Al Khumrah hemorrhagic fever, and Rift
Valley fever, 294

ALA-dehydratase–deficient porphyria, 491–492

Alagille syndrome, 332–333
and deletion of the short arm of chromosome 1, 58
and idiopathic neonatal hepatitis, 288

Albinism, and Chédiak-Higashi syndrome, 379
and Hermansky-Pudlak syndrome, 391–392

Albright hereditary osteodystrophy, and acrodysostosis, 146
and Kenny-Caffey syndrome, 211
and Prader-Willi syndrome, 237–238
and progressive osseous heteroplasia, 203

Albuterol, and facioscapulohumeral muscular dystrophy, 625

Alcohol abuse, and alpha 1-antitrypsin deficiency, 671

Alcoholic dementia, and Korsakoff syndrome, 546

Alcoholic pellagra encephalopathy, and Korsakoff syndrome, 546

Alcoholic psychosis, and Korsakoff syndrome, 546

Alcoholism, and Cushing syndrome, 312–313
and Korsakoff syndrome, 546

Aldolase deficiency, and congenital nonspherocytic hemolytic anemia, 369

Aldosteronism, primary, 305

Alexander disease, 510–511
and leukodystrophy, 550–552
and metachromatic leukodystrophy, 552
and Pelizaeus-Merzbacher disease, 578

Alkaptonuria, 431

Alkylating agents, and Waldenström macroglobulinemia, 38

Allan-Herndon-Dudley syndrome, 149
and Wieacker-Wolff syndrome, 638

Allan-Herndon syndrome, 149

Allergic angiitis, and Churg-Strauss syndrome, 674

Allergic angioedema, and hereditary angioedema, 375

Allergic disorders, and eosinophilic gastroenteritis, 342

Allergic enteropathy, 342

Allergic eosinophilic gastroenteropathy, 342

Allodynia, and thalamic pain syndrome, 593

Allopurinol, and familial juvenile hyperuricemic nephropathy, 696
and Lesch-Nyhan syndrome, 465

Alopecia, and Cronkhite-Canada syndrome, 338
and multiple carboxylase deficiency, 482–483
and progeria, 724

Alopecia areata, *fig. 7*, 95

Alopecia neoplastica, and alopecia areata, 95

Alopecia-poliosis-uveitis-vitiligo-deafness-cutaneous-uveo-oto syndrome, 36–37

Alpers disease, and congenital lactic acidosis, 462–464
and Tay-Sachs disease, 501

Alpers-Huttenlocher syndrome, 511–512

Alpers syndrome, 511–512

Alpha 1-antitrypsin deficiency, 671
and biliary atresia, 334
and congenital disorders of glycosylation, 457
and idiopathic neonatal hepatitis, 288
and Niemann-Pick disease, 485

Alpha-fucosidosis, and sialidosis, 498

Alpha-mannosidosis, 467–468

Alpha-mercaptopropionylglycine, and cystinuria, 684

Alpha-thalassemia mental retardation, 274
and Coffin-Lowry syndrome, 171–172

Alpha-thalassemia syndrome, and Fountain syndrome, 196

Alpha-tocopherol, and ataxia with vitamin E deficiency, 607

Alport syndrome, 680
and benign familial hematuria, 688
and brachio-oto-renal syndrome, 682
and familial juvenile hyperuricemic nephropathy, 696
and megalocornea, 556

Alström-Halgren syndrome, 305–306

Alström syndrome, 305–306
and Bardet-Biedl syndrome, 158
and Laurence-Moon syndrome, 215
and retinitis pigmentosa, 660
and Usher syndrome, 665

Alternating hemiplegia of childhood, 512–513

Alveolar capillary dysplasia, 672

Alveolar lipoproteinosis, 677

Alzheimer disease, and Binswanger disease, 519
and corticobasal degeneration, 524–525

and Creutzfeldt-Jakob disease, 608
and frontotemporal dementia, 534
and Gerstmann syndrome, 534
and Korsakoff syndrome, 546
and methylmalonic acidemias, 429
and Whipple disease, 297

Amantadine, and Kleine-Levin syndrome, 544
and multiple system atrophy, 561

Amaurosis congenita of Leber, 651–652

Amegakaryocytic thrombocytopenia, and Fanconi anemia, 366

Amelanotic melanoma, and Bowen disease, 97

Ameloblastoma, 363–364

Ameloblastomic fibromas, and ameloblastoma, 363

Amelogenesis imperfecta, 149–150

Amenorrhea, and autoimmune premature ovarian failure, 30–31
and Sheehan syndrome, 328

Amenorrhea traumatica-atretica, 308–309

Amiloride, and Bartter syndrome, 310–311

Aminoacidopathies, and Cockayne syndrome, 170–171

Amitriptyline, and cyclic vomiting syndrome, 526
and hereditary sensory neuropathy, 570

Amlodipine, and primary pulmonary hypertension, 678

Amnesia, and Korsakoff syndrome, 546

Amniocentesis, and twin-twin transfusion syndrome, 422

Amnion band/rupture sequence, 150–151

Amniotic adhesion malformation syndrome, 150–151

Amniotic band disruption complex, 150–151

Amniotic band disruption sequence, and anencephaly, 151–152

Amniotic band sequence, and Adams-Oliver syndrome, 148

Amniotic band syndrome, 150–151

Amniotic bands, *fig. 25*, 150–151

Amniotic constriction bands, 150–151

Amniotic deformity-adhesion-mutilation syndrome, 150–151

Amphetamines, and narcolepsy, 562

Ampicillin, and listeriosis, 290

Amputation, and thromboangiitis obliterans, 36

Amyloidosis, and benign
    lymphoepithelial lesion, 17
    and familial Mediterranean fever, 19
    and scleromyxedema, 136
    and Sjögren syndrome, 34
Amylopectinosis, 454
Amyoplasia, and arthrogryposis
    multiplex congenita, 155
Amyotrophic lateral sclerosis, 513–514
    and Creutzfeldt-Jakob disease, 608
    and limb girdle muscular dystrophy,
        625
    and myasthenia gravis, 626–627
    and Parsonage-Turner syndrome, 577
    and primary lateral sclerosis, 548–549
    and spinal bulbar muscular atrophy,
        636
Amyotrophy, and neuroacanthocytosis,
    633–634
Anagen effluvium, and alopecia areata, 95
Anal atresia, 153
Anal defects, and cat eye syndrome,
    164–165
Anaphylactoid purpura, 414–415
Anasarca, and congenital complete heart
    block, 49
Anderson disease, 380, 454
Anderson-Fabry disease, 442
Androgen deficiency, and autoimmune
    premature ovarian failure, 30–31
Androgen excess, and Achard-Thiers
    syndrome, 300
Androgen insensitivity, and spinal bulbar
    muscular atrophy, 636
Androgen insensitivity syndrome,
    306–307
Androgens, and dyskeratosis congenita,
    105
Anemia, and Aase syndrome, 143
    acquired aplastic, 364
    and acquired pure red cell aplasia,
        413–414
    autoimmune hemolytic, 367
    and autosomal-recessive osteopetrosis,
        228–229
    congenital nonspherocytic hemolytic,
        369
    Diamond-Blackfan, 365
    and Ewing sarcoma of bone, 381
    Fanconi, 366
    and Gaucher disease, 447
    hereditary spherocytic hemolytic,
        370–371
    and medullary cystic kidney disease,
        693
    and Ménière disease, 558
    and multiple myeloma, 407

and pyruvate kinase deficiency, 496
sickle cell, 372–373
and thalassemia major, 419
and thalassemia minor, 420
and triphalangeal thumb, 143
warm antibody hemolytic, 371–372
X-linked sideroblastic, 373–375
Anencephaly, 151–152
Anesthesia, and Eisenmenger syndrome,
    47
Anetoderma, and Degos disease, 102
Aneurysm, and Korsakoff syndrome, 546
Aneurysmal bone cysts, and
    ameloblastoma, 363
Angelmann syndrome, 152–153
    and deletion of the short arm of
        chromosome 1, 58
Angiocentric immunoproliferative lesion,
    48–49
Angioedema, and erysipelas, 285
    and familial eosinophilic cellulitis, 99
Angioedema, hereditary, 375–376
Angioimmunoblastic lymphadenopathy-
    type T-cell lymphoma, 398–399
Angiokeratoma corporis diffusum
    universale, 442
Angiomatosis retinae, 265–266
Angioneurotic edema, and Melkersson-
    Rosenthal syndrome, 557
Angiotensin-converting enzyme
    inhibitors, and Bartter syndrome,
        311
    and endomyocardial fibrosis, 48
Anhidrosis, and hereditary sensory
    neuropathy
Anhydramnios, and twin-twin
    transfusion syndrome, 421–422
Aniridia, 640
    and WAGR syndrome, 699
Anisometropic amblyopia, and Duane
    syndrome, 645
Ankyloblepharon, and popliteal
    pterygium syndrome, 242
Ankyloblepharon-ectodermal dysplasia-
    facial clefting syndrome, 116–117
Ankylosing spondylitis, and alkaptonuria,
    431
    and diffuse idiopathic skeletal
        hyperostosis, 10
Annular elastolytic giant cell granuloma,
    and granuloma annulare, 116
Annular lichen planus, and granuloma
    annulare, 116
Anodontia, 261
Anomalous pulmonary venous
    connection, and atrial septal
    defects, 43

Anomalous pulmonary venous return,
    and cor triatriatum, 46
Anonychia, and nail-patella syndrome,
    721–722
Anophthalmos, 654
Anorectal malformations, 153–154
Anorexia nervosa, and ACTH deficiency,
    302
    and Cushing syndrome, 312–313
Anosmia, and Kallmann syndrome,
    318–319
Anovulation, and Asherman syndrome,
    308–309
    and polycystic ovary syndrome,
        323–324
Anterior chamber angle changes, and
    iridocorneal endothelial
    syndromes, 649
Anterior cord syndrome, and Brown-
    Séquard syndrome, 520
Anteverted nares, and Marshall-Smith
    syndrome, 219
Anthrax, 278
Antibiotics, and hyper-IgE syndrome, 12
    and Leiner disease, 123
    and mesenteric panniculitis, 350
    and severe chronic neutropenia, 23
Anticardiolipin antibodies, and
    antiphospholipid syndrome, 2
Anticardiolipin syndrome, and idiopathic
    thrombocytopenic purpura, 415
Anticholinergic syndromes, and
    neuroleptic malignant syndrome,
        566
Anticoagulation agents, and
    antiphospholipid syndrome, 2
Anticonvulsant drugs, and chromosome
    14 ring, 64
Anti-copper therapy, and Wilson disease,
    506
Anticytokine therapy, and Langerhans
    cell histiocytosis, 393
Antifungal agents, and Meleda disease,
    128
Antihistamines, and Gianotti-Crosti
    syndrome, 115
    and transient acantholytic dermatosis,
        104
Antimalarial agents, and Sjögren
    syndrome, 34
Antioxidants, and ataxia-telangiectasia,
    605–606
Antiphospholipid antibodies, 2
Antiphospholipid antibody syndrome, 2
    and Asherman syndrome, 308–309
    and thromboangiitis obliterans, 36
Antiphospholipid syndrome, 2

Antiplatelet agents, and antiphospholipid syndrome, 2
Antipsychotic drugs, and tardive dyskinesia, 591
Antipyretics, and neuroleptic malignant syndrome, 566
Antithrombin III deficiency, congenital, 376–377
Anti–tumor necrosis factor, and Behçet disease, 4
  and Takayasu arteritis, 35
Antley-Bixler syndrome, 704–705
Anus, hand, and ear syndrome, 262
Anxiety, and pheochromocytoma, 409
Aortic atresia, 50–51
Aortic calcification, and Singleton-Merten syndrome, 252
Aortopulmonary septal defect, and persistent truncus arteriosus, 56
Apak ataxia–spastic diplegia, and Wieacker-Wolff syndrome, 638
Apartylglucosaminuria, and sialidosis, 498
Apert syndrome, 154–155
  and chromosome 6, partial trisomy 6q, 79
  and Crouzon syndrome, 710
  and Jackson-Weiss syndrome, 719
  and Pfeiffer syndrome type I, 234
  and primary craniosynostosis, 174
  and Saethre-Chotzen syndrome, 727–728
Aphasia, and frontotemporal dementia, 533–534
  and MASA syndrome, 220
Aphonia, and locked-in syndrome, 554
Aphthous stomatitis, major recurrent, 138
Aphthous ulcers, major, 138
  minor, and Sutton disease, 138
Aplasia, and bilateral renal agenesis, 698
Aplasia cutis congenita, 96
  and Adams-Oliver syndrome, 148
Aplastic anemia
  acquired, and dyskeratosis congenita, 104–105
  and acquired agranulocytosis, 361
  and autoimmune hemolytic anemia, 367
  and Diamond-Blackfan anemia, 365
  and paroxysmal nocturnal hemoglobinuria, 389–390
  and sickle cell anemia, 372–373
  and X-linked lymphoproliferative syndrome, 400
Apnea, and Glut-1 deficiency syndrome, 448
  and PEPCK deficiency, 486

Apocrine glands, and Fox-Fordyce disease, 114
  and hidradenitis suppurativa, 118–119
  and Schinzel syndrome, 246–247
Apocrine miliaria, 114
Appendiceal cancer, 412–413
Appetite, strong, and congenital generalized lipodystrophy, 322
Apple-peel syndrome, 349
Apraxia, 515
  and Gerstmann syndrome, 534
Aqueductal stenosis, and Allan-Herndon-Dudley syndrome, 149
  and hydrocephalus, 539
Arachnodactyly, congenital contractual, 3
Arachnoid villi seeding, and hydrocephalus, 539
Areflexia, and congenital hypomyelination neuropathy, 568
  and Dejerine-Sottas syndrome, 527–528
  and Friedreich ataxia, 602–603
  and Lowe syndrome, 466–467
Arena syndrome, and Wieacker-Wolff syndrome, 638
Arenaviridae infection, 282
Areolar choroidal degeneration, and Stargardt disease, 663
Argentine hemorrhagic fever, 282
Arginase deficiency, 506–506
Argininosuccinic aciduria, and Björnstad syndrome, 97
  and Menkes disease, 470
Arima syndrome, and Joubert syndrome, 542
Arm deformities, and Holt-Oram syndrome, 717
Arm weakness, and chronic inflammatory demyelinating polyradiculoneuropathy, 581–582
  and Parsonage-Turner syndrome, 577–578
Armadillo syndrome, 635
Arnold-Chiari syndrome, 515–516
Aromatase deficiency, and congenital adrenal hyperplasia, 304
Aromatase inhibitors, and precocious puberty, 325
Arrhythmias, and X-linked sideroblastic anemia, 373
Arrhythmogenic right ventricular dysplasia, and Brugada syndrome, 45
Arsenic, and Banti syndrome, 377
Artemisinin, and malaria, 291
Arterial disease, and MELAS, 469

Arterial thromboses, and antiphospholipid syndrome, 2
Arteriohepatic dysplasia, 332
Arteriovenous fistulae, and Parkes-Weber syndrome, 232
Arteriovenous malformations, and hereditary hemorrhagic telangiectasia, 418
Arteritis, young female, 35
Arthritis, and alkaptonuria, 431
  and cervical dystonia, 611
  and Cushing syndrome, 312–313
  and eosinophilic fasciitis, 8
  and Henoch-Schönlein purpura, 414–415
  and hereditary hemochromatosis, 387–388
  juvenile rheumatoid, and Kawasaki disease, 15
  and Legg-Calve-Perthes disease, 16
  and microscopic polyangiitis, 27
  and multiple epiphyseal dysplasia, 188
  and restless legs syndrome, 583
  rheumatoid, and Felty syndrome, 8–9
Arthrogryposis, distal, and congenital contractual arachnodactyly, 3
  and Marden-Walker syndrome, 18
  and obstetric brachial plexus palsy, 571
Arthrogryposis multiplex congenita, 155, 199
Arthropod bites, and familial eosinophilic cellulitis, 99
  and Mucha-Habermann disease, 129
Artificial tears, and mucolipidosis, 473–474
Arylsulfatase A deficiency, 552–553
Ascites, and endomyocardial fibrosis, 48
  and hepatorenal syndrome, 344
  and Niemann-Pick disease, 485
  and pseudomyxoma peritonei, 412
Ascorbic acid, and Chédiak-Higashi syndrome, 379
Asherman syndrome, 308–309
Ashkenazi Jews, and familial dysautonomia, 529–530
Aspartoacylase deficiency, 550–551
Aspartylglucosaminuria, 432
  and Fabry disease, 442
  and fucosidosis, 445
Asperger syndrome, and methylmalonic acidemias, 429
Asphyxiating thoracic dysplasia, 155–156
Asphyxiating thoracic dystrophy, 155–156
Aspirin, and antiphospholipid syndrome, 2
  and erythromelalgia, 113
  and retinal arterial occlusion, 658

Aspirin, *(continued)*
  and Sturge-Weber syndrome, 258
Asplenia with cardiovascular anomalies,
    and situs inversus, 55
Asthma, and alpha 1-antitrypsin
      deficiency, 671
  and Churg-Strauss syndrome, 674
  and Cushing syndrome, 312–313
  and lymphangioleiomyomatosis, 395
  and recurrent respiratory
      papillomatosis, 676
Astigmatism, and keratoconus, 651
  and retinitis pigmentosa, 660
Astrocytoma, and glioblastoma
      multiforme, 384–385
  and medulloblastoma, 404–405
Ataxia, 600–607
  and Arnold-Chiari syndrome, 516
  and Baltic/Mediterranean/Unverrich-
      Lundborg myoclonic epilepsy,
      600
  and Creutzfeldt-Jakob disease, 608
  episodic type I, 600–601
  episodic type II, 601–602
  and Joubert syndrome, 542
  and megalocornea, 556
  and metachromatic leukodystrophy,
      552–553
  and myoclonus, 628
  and opsoclonus-myoclonus syndrome,
      572–573
  and Pelizaeus-Merzbacher disease, 578
  and progressive myoclonus epilepsy,
      531–532
  and progressive symmetric
      erythrokeratodermia, 111–112
  and Rett syndrome, 584
  and succinic semialdehyde
      dehydrogenase deficiency, 499
  with vitamin E deficiency, 606–607
Ataxia-telangiectasia, 605–606
  and congenital disorders of
      glycosylation, 457
  and hereditary hemorrhagic
      telangiectasia, 418
  and severe combined
      immunodeficiency, 14
Ataxic gait, and hydrocephalus, 539
Atelosteogenesis type III, 156–157
  and oto-palato-digital syndrome, 229
Atenolol, and Jervell and Lange-Nielsen
      syndrome, 52
  and Romano-Ward long QT
      syndrome, 54
Atherosclerosis, and erythromelalgia, 113
  and thromboangiitis obliterans, 36

Atherosclerotic aortic disease, and
      Singleton-Merten syndrome, 252
Athetoid movements, and oculocerebral
      syndrome, 226–227
Athetosis, and glutaric acidemia type I,
      426
  and tardive dyskinesia, 591
Athetotic cerebral palsy, and Tourette
      syndrome, 594
Atopic dermatitis, and ichthyosis, 120
  and Leiner disease, 123
Atovaquone, and malaria, 291
Atrial septal defects, 42–43
Atriodigital dysplasia, 717
Atrioventricular canal defects, 43–44
Atrioventricular septal defects, 43–44
Atrophia bulborum hereditaria, 655–
      656
Atropine, and congenital complete heart
      block, 50
Attention deficit disorder, and
      carnosinemia, 435
  and methylmalonic acidemias, 429
  and Smith-Magenis syndrome, 254
Attenuated familial adenomatous
      polyposis, 352–353
Atypical Peters anomaly, and
      chromosome 5, trisomy 5p, 78
Auricular appendages, and Goldenhar
      syndrome, 716
Auricular malformations, and brachio-
      oto-renal syndrome, 681–682
Auriculotemporal syndrome, 533
Autism, and fetal valproate syndrome,
      192–193
  and Landau-Kleffner syndrome, 547
  and methylmalonic acidemias, 429
  and phenylketonuria, 488
  and Rett syndrome, 584
  and tuberous sclerosis, 596
Autofluorescing lipidosis, 517
Autoimmune and connective tissue
      disorders, 2–39
Autoimmune hemolytic anemia, 367
  and Diamond-Blackfan anemia, 365
  and hereditary spherocytosis, 370–371
Autoimmune inner ear disease, and
      Ménière disease, 558
Autoimmune oophoritis, 30–31
Autoimmune premature ovarian failure,
      30–31
Autoimmune thrombocytopenia, and
      Bernard-Soulier syndrome, 378
Autoimmune thyroiditis, 329
Autonomic dysfunction, and familial
      dysautonomia, 529–530

  and Lambert-Eaton myasthenic
      syndrome, 621
Autonomic failure, and multiple system
      atrophy, 561
Autosomal-dominant long QT
      syndrome, 54
Autosomal-dominant macrocephaly, and
      Sotos syndrome, 255
Autosomal-dominant "Opitz" GBBB
      syndrome, and chromosome
      22q11 deletion spectrum, 70
Autosomal-dominant trigonocephaly,
      and C syndrome, 162
Autosomal-recessive long QT syndrome,
      51–52
Autosomal-recessive osteopetrosis,
      228–229
Autosomal-recessive polycystic kidney
      disease, 697
Autosomal-recessive pseudoprogeria, and
      Hallermann-Streiff syndrome, 202
Autumnal fever, 289
Axenfelt-Rieger anomaly, and Rieger
      syndrome, 243–244
Axenfelt-Rieger syndrome, 243–244
Axial dystonia, and progressive
      supranuclear palsy, 573–574
Azathioprine, and autoimmune
      hemolytic anemia, 367
  and Banti syndrome, 377
  and Behçet disease, 4
  and chronic inflammatory
      demyelinating
      polyradiculoneuropathy, 582
  and cicatricial pemphigoid, 131
  and Erdheim-Chester disease, 441
  and Henoch-Schönlein purpura, 415
  and idiopathic thrombocytopenic
      purpura, 415–416
  and mesenteric panniculitis, 350
  and microscopic polyangiitis, 28
  and neuromyelitis optica, 567
  and neuromyotonia, 635
  and polyarteritis nodosa, 29
  and posterior uveitis, 666
  and relapsing polychondritis, 30
  and sarcoidosis, 32
  and Takayasu arteritis, 35
Azoospermia, and partial androgen
      insensitivity syndrome, 307–308
Azorean neurologic disease, 555

B

Baar-Gabriel syndrome, and Wieacker-
      Wolff syndrome, 638
Babesiosis, and ehrlichiosis, 283

Bacillary dysentery, and viral hemorrhagic fevers, 282

Bacillus anthracis infection, 278

Back pain, and spondyloepiphyseal dysplasia tarda, 729–730

and twin-twin transfusion syndrome, 421–422

Baclofen, and embouchure dystonia, 613

and Hallervorden-Spatz syndrome, 620

and hereditary spastic paraplegia, 576

and mucolipidosis, 473–474

and oromandibular dystonia, 615

and primary lateral sclerosis, 549

and stiff person syndrome, 589

and Tourette syndrome, 594

Bacterial endocarditis, and Eisenmenger syndrome, 47

Bacterial infections, and anthrax, 278

and botulism, 279

and brucellosis, 280

and chronic granulomatous disease, 386–387

and ehrlichiosis, 283

and erysipelas, 285

and Felty syndrome, 8–9

and giant hypertrophic gastritis, 341

and hyper-IgM syndrome, 393–394

and listeriosis, 290

and severe chronic neutropenia, 22–23

and severe combined immunodeficiency, 14

and Wegener granulomatosis, 422

and Whipple disease, 297–298

Bacterial meningitis, and encephalitides, 284

Bacterial overgrowth, and small bowel diverticulosis, 339

Bacterial sepsis, and dengue fever, 281

and hantavirus pulmonary syndrome, 287

and viral hemorrhagic fevers, 282

Bacterial vesicular infections, and incontinentia pigmenti, 121

Balance problems, and neurofibromatosis type 2, 564–565

Balanitis xerotica obliterans, 126

Baller-Gerold syndrome, 157–158

and Roberts pseudothalidomide syndrome, 244–245

and Townes-Brocks syndrome, 262

Balo concentric sclerosis, 560

Baltic/Mediterranean/Unverrich-Lundborg myoclonic epilepsy, 600

Bang disease, 280

Bannanyan-Zonana syndrome, and PTEN hamartoma tumor syndrome, 240

Bannayan-Riley-Ruvalcaba syndrome, 354

and PTEN hamartoma tumor syndrome, 240

and Sotos syndrome, 255

Banti disease, and congenital hepatic fibrosis, 691

Banti syndrome, 377

Baraitser-Reardon syndrome, and TORCH syndrome, 295

Bardet-Biedl syndrome, 158–159

and Alström syndrome, 306

and autosomal-recessive polycystic kidney disease, 697

and Borjeson-Forssman-Lehmann syndrome, 705

and Cohen syndrome, 172

and Laurence-Moon syndrome, 215

and Pallister-Hall syndrome, 230

and Prader-Willi syndrome, 237–238

and retinitis pigmentosa, 660

Baroreflex failure, and pheochromocytoma, 410

Barraquer-Simons syndrome, 321

Barrett esophagus, 333

Barth syndrome, 44–45

and congenital lactic acidosis, 462–464

Bartsocas-Papas syndrome, and popliteal pterygium syndrome, 242

Bartter syndrome, 309–311

Basal cell carcinoma, and Bowen disease, 97

and melanoma, 405

Basal ganglia calcification, and Fahr disease, 532

Basaloid squamous carcinoma, and adenoid cystic carcinoma, 359

Basilar impression, and Arnold-Chiari syndrome, 516

Bassen-Kornzweig disease, and neuroacanthocytosis, 633

Bassen-Kornzweig syndrome, 358

Batten disease, 516–517

and Kuf disease, 547

Battered child syndrome, and Menkes disease, 470

BBB syndrome, 198–199

Beals syndrome, 3

Bean syndrome, 160

Becker disease, 632–633

Becker muscular dystrophy, 622

Beckwith-Wiedemann syndrome, 518

and Fryns syndrome, 715

and medullary sponge kidney, 694

and Simpson dysmorphia syndrome, 251

and Sotos syndrome, 255

Beemer-Langer syndrome, and Pallister-Hall syndrome, 230

Béguez-César disease, 379

Behavioral disturbances, and Kleine-Levin syndrome, 544

and Landau-Kleffner syndrome, 547

and metachromatic leukodystrophy, 552–553

and methylmalonic acidemias, 429

and phenylketonuria, 488

and Prader-Willi syndrome, 237–238

and Sanfilippo disease, 479

and subacute sclerosing panencephalitis, 574–575

Behçet disease, 4

and Eales disease, 646

and Sutton disease, 138

and Sweet syndrome, 139

and Takayasu arteritis, 35

Benign cystic teratoma, and cystic hygroma, 175

Benign familial hematuria, 688–689

Benign lymphoepithelial lesion, 17

Benign mixed tumor, and adenoid cystic carcinoma, 359

Benign nevus, and melanoma, 405

Benign recurrent intrahepatic cholestasis, and Dubin-Johnson syndrome, 340

Benign symmetric lipomatosis, and adiposis dolorosa, 303

Bent fingers, and chromosome 4 ring, 76

Benzodiazepines, and Huntington disease, 538

and Landau-Kleffner syndrome, 548

and Lennox-Gastaut syndrome, 550

and neuroleptic malignant syndrome, 566

and stiff person syndrome, 588

and Sydenham chorea, 522

and X-linked dystonia-parkinsonism, 619

Benztropine, and myoclonic dystonia, 615

and writer's cramp, 618

Berardinelli lipodystrophy syndrome, and leprechaunism, 216

Berardinelli-Seip syndrome, and neonatal progeroid syndrome, 238

Bernard-Soulier syndrome, 378

and Glanzmann thrombasthenia, 383

and May-Hegglin anomaly, 403

Beta-adrenergic blocking agents, and
  Jervell and Lange-Nielsen
  syndrome, 52
  and Romano-Ward long QT
  syndrome, 54
Beta-blockers, and congenital hepatic
  fibrosis, 692
  and LEOPARD syndrome, 124
  and Marfan syndrome, 219
  and Noonan syndrome, 722
Beta carotene, and congenital
  erythropoietic porphyria, 492–493
  and erythropoietic protoporphyria,
  496
Beta-mannosidosis, and alpha-
  mannosidosis, 467–468
Bexarotene, and mycosis fungoides, 406
Bickers-Adams syndrome, and MASA
  syndrome, 220
Biemond syndrome type II, and Bardet-
  Biedl syndrome, 158
Bifid epiglottis, and Pallister-Hall
  syndrome, 230
Bilateral renal agenesis, 698
Bilateral striopallidodentate calcinosis,
  532
Bile acid synthesis, and idiopathic
  neonatal hepatitis, 288
Bile duct dilatation, and autosomal-
  recessive polycystic kidney disease,
  697
Bile stagnation, and Caroli disease, 336
Bile stones, and Caroli disease, 336
Bilharzia, and liver fluke disease, 286
Biliary atresia, 334
  and Alagille syndrome, 332
  and Byler disease, 335
  and idiopathic neonatal hepatitis, 288
  and Niemann-Pick disease, 485
Biliary dilatation, and Caroli syndrome,
  336
Biliary dysgenesis, 691–692
Biliary tract obstruction, and Dubin-
  Johnson syndrome, 340
Bilious vomiting, and jejunal atresia, 349
Bilirubin encephalopathy, 543
Bilirubin toxicity, and kernicterus, 543
Binder type syndrome, 186–187
Binswanger disease, 519
  and hydrocephalus, 539
Biotin, and multiple carboxylase
  deficiency, 482–483
Biotin deficiency, and Menkes disease, 470
Biotinidase deficiency, 482
  and multiple carboxylase deficiency,
  483
  and propionic acidemia, 428

Birdshot retinochoroidopathy, and acute
  posterior multifocal placoid
  pigment epitheliopathy, 642
Bisphosphonates, and Camurati-
  Engelmann disease, 708
  and Jansen metaphyseal
  chondrodysplasia, 207
  and osteogenesis imperfecta, 227
  and Paget disease, 25
Björnstad syndrome, 97
Black baine, 278
Black death, 292
Blackfan-Diamond anemia, 365
Bladder cancer, and interstitial cystitis, 685
Bladder disturbance, and multiple system
  atrophy, 561
Bladder exstrophy–epispadias–cloacal
  exstrophy complex, *figs. 58–59*,
  686–687
Blake pouch, and Dandy-Walker
  syndrome, 526
Blalock-Taussig shunt, and Ivemark
  syndrome, 205
  and pentalogy of Cantrell, 233–234
Bleeding, and antiphospholipid
  syndrome, 2
  and thrombocytopenia and absent
  radius syndrome, 260
Bleeding diathesis, and Chédiak-Higashi
  syndrome, 379
  and Glanzmann thrombasthenia,
  383–384
Bleeding disorders, and factor IX
  deficiency, 381–382
  and hemophilia, 390–391
  and Hermansky-Pudlak syndrome,
  391–392
Bleomycin, and cystic hygroma, 175
Blepharitis, and blepharospasm, 610
Blepharophimosis, and Marden-Walker
  syndrome, 18
Blepharophimosis-ptosis-epicanthus
  inversus syndrome, 641
Blepharospasm, 610
  and oromandibular dystonia, 615–616
Blindness, and Alström syndrome,
  305–306
  and leukodystrophy, 551–552
  and methylmalonic acidemias, 429
  and neuromyelitis optica, 567
Blinking, and blepharospasm, 610
Blisters, and porphyria cutanea tarda,
  493–494
  and variegate porphyria, 494–495
Bloch-Siemens incontinentia pigmenti
  melanoblastosis cutis linearis,
  121–122

Bloch-Siemens-Sulzberger syndrome,
  121–122
Bloch-Sulzberger syndrome, 121–122
Blood coagulation, and congenital
  antithrombin III deficiency,
  376–377
Blood transfusion, and thalassemia
  major, 419
Bloom syndrome, 159–160
  and Fanconi anemia, 366
  and Rothmund-Thomson syndrome,
  135
  and 3-M syndrome, 259
Blue cone monochromacy, and Leber
  congenital amaurosis, 652
Blue diaper syndrome, 681
Blue rubber bleb nevus syndrome, 160
  and Maffucci syndrome, 217
Blue sclera, and osteogenesis imperfecta,
  227
Body asymmetry, and chromosome 22,
  trisomy mosaic, 72
Body odor, and isovaleric acidemia, 427
Body stalk anomaly syndrome, and
  pentalogy of Cantrell, 233–234
Boeck sarcoid, 32–33
Boehme disease, and Kuf disease, 547
Bohring-Opitz syndrome, and C
  syndrome, 162
Bolivian hemorrhagic fever, 282
Bone cyst, and Langerhans cell
  histiocytosis, 392
Bone disease, and multiple myeloma, 407
  and Q fever, 293
Bone dysplasia, and Dyggve-Melchior-
  Clausen syndrome, 180–181
  and Yunis-Varaaon syndrome, 275
Bone dystrophy, 204–205
Bone hypertrophy, and Klippel-
  Trenaunay syndrome, 212
Bone marrow dysfunction, and
  paroxysmal nocturnal
  hemoglobinuria, 389–390
  and Shwachman-Diamond syndrome,
  417
Bone marrow failure, and acquired
  aplastic anemia, 364
  and dyskeratosis congenita, 104–105
  and Fanconi anemia, 366
Bone marrow infiltration, and large
  granular lymphocyte leukemia,
  394
Bone marrow obliteration, and
  autosomal-recessive osteopetrosis,
  228–229
Bone marrow transplantation, 432
  and Aase syndrome, 143

allogeneic, and Wiskott-Aldrich syndrome, 39
and alpha-mannosidosis, 467–468
and autosomal-recessive osteopetrosis, 229
and chronic granulomatous disease, 387
and Farber disease, 443
and Gaucher disease, 447
and graft-versus-host disease, 10–11
and hemophagocytic lymphohistiocytosis, 397
and Hurler disease, 477
and metachromatic leukodystrophy, 553
and Nezelof syndrome, 408
and polycythemia vera, 411–412
and Sandhoff disease, 497
and Santavuori disease, 585–586
and severe combined immunodeficiency, 14
and Shwachman-Diamond syndrome, 417
and X-linked lymphoproliferative syndrome, 400
Bone modeling abnormalities, and Melnick-Needles syndrome, 221–222
Bone overgrowth, and Proteus syndrome, 239
Bone pain, and familial expansile osteolysis, 723–724
and multiple myeloma, 407
and Paget disease, 24–25
and sickle cell anemia, 372–373
and X-linked hypophosphatemic rickets, 326–327
Bone remodeling, and Paget disease, 24–25
Bonnet-Dechaumme-Blanc syndrome, 667
Bony deformities, and Schwartz-Jampel syndrome, 586–587
Bony encroachment of the nerves, and autosomal-recessive osteopetrosis, 228–229
Bony lesions, and neurofibromatosis type I, 563–564
Borjeson-Forssman-Lehmann syndrome, 705–706
and Prader-Willi syndrome, 237–238
Borjeson syndrome, 705
Borreliosis, and viral hemorrhagic fevers, 282
Bosentan, and primary pulmonary hypertension, 678
Botox, and corticobasal degeneration, 524–525

Botulinum toxin, and blepharospasm, 610
and cervical dystonia, 611
and dystonia, 609
and embouchure dystonia, 613
and Frey syndrome, 533
and laryngeal dystonia, 613–614
and oromandibular dystonia, 615
and paroxysmal dystonia, 617
and tardive dyskinesia, 591
and writer's cramp, 618
Botulism, 279
and Lambert-Eaton myasthenic syndrome, 621
Bowel bypass syndrome, and Sweet syndrome, 139
Bowel obstruction, and jejunal atresia, 349
Bowen-Conradi-Hutterite syndrome, 161
Bowen-Conradi syndrome, 161
Bowen disease, 97–98
Bowen-Hutterite syndrome, 161
Bowenoid papulosis, 98–99
Brachial neuritis, and Parsonage-Turner syndrome, 577–578
Brachial plexitis, and Parsonage-Turner syndrome, 577–578
Brachial radiculitis, and Parsonage-Turner syndrome, 577–578
Brachio-oto-renal syndrome, 681–682
Brachmann-de Lange syndrome, 709
Brachycephaly, and Gorlin-Chaudhry-Moss syndrome, 200
and Weill-Marchesani syndrome, 267–268
Brachyclinodactyly, and Russel-Silver syndrome, 245–246
Brachydactyly, and acrodysostosis, 146
and Saethre-Chotzen syndrome, 727–728
and trichorhinophalangeal syndrome, 732
Brachytherapy, and retinoblastoma, 661
Bradycardia, and Jervell and Lange-Nielsen syndrome, 51–52
and Romano-Ward long QT syndrome, 54
Bradykinesia, and Parkinson disease, 576–577
Brain abnormalities, and chromosome 9, trisomy mosaic, 85–86
and septooptic dysplasia, 188–189
Brain abscess, and encephalitides, 284
and glioblastoma multiforme, 384
Brain aneurysm, and brain arteriovenous malformations, 596
Brain arteriovenous malformations, 596

Brain damage, and galactosemia, 446
Brain destruction, and hydranencephaly, 538
Brain development, and GBBB syndrome, 198–199
Brain dysfunction, and Gerstmann syndrome, 534
Brain growth failure, and Cockayne syndrome, 170–171
Brain hamartomas, and tuberous sclerosis, 595–596
Brain hemorrhagic stroke, and brain arteriovenous malformations, 596
Brain heterotopias, and aplasia cutis congenita, 96
Brain inflammation, and encephalitides, 284–285
Brain injury, and Kluver-Bucy syndrome, 545
Brain tumor, and ataxia-telangiectasia, 605–606
and brain arteriovenous malformations, 596
and Ménière disease, 558
and methylmalonic acidemias, 429
and Von Hippel-Lindau disease, 265–266
Brainstem lesions, and episodic ataxia, 600–601
Brainstem neoplasms, and cyclic vomiting syndrome, 525
Brainstem syrinx, 589–590
Brainstem tumors, and locked-in syndrome, 554
and myasthenia gravis, 626–627
Branched chain amino acid catabolism, and maple syrup urine disease, 468–469
Branched chain ketoacidemia, 468–469
Branchial arch syndrome, and brachio-oto-renal syndrome, 682
Branchial defects, and brachio-oto-renal syndrome, 682
Branchio-oculo-facial syndrome, 161–162
Branchio-oto-renal syndrome, and branchio-oculo-facial syndrome, 161–162
Brandywine type dentinogenesis imperfecta, 177–178
Brazil, and acheiropodia, 702
Breakbone fever, 281
Breast development retardation, and Poland syndrome, 236–237
Breast-feeding, and acrodermatitis enteropathica, 94
and glucose-galactose malabsorption, 343

Breast milk jaundice, and kernicterus, 543

Breast tumors, and PTEN hamartoma tumor syndrome, 240

Breath-holding, and idiopathic congenital central hypoventilation syndrome, 673

Breathing difficulties, and chromosome 4, trisomy 4p, 77–78

Breech birth, and central core disease, 607–608

Brevicollis syndrome, 720

Brittle bone disease, 227–229

Brittle bones, and autosomal-recessive osteopetrosis, 228–229

Broad thumb-hallux syndrome, 726–727

Bromocriptine, and Hallervorden-Spatz syndrome, 620

Bronchiectasis, and alpha 1-antitrypsin deficiency, 671

and primary ciliary dyskinesia, 675

Bronchitis, and alpha 1-antitrypsin deficiency, 671

Bronchodilators, and situs inversus, 55

Bronchopulmonary aspergillosis, and Churg-Strauss syndrome, 674

Bronze diabetes, 387–388

Brown-Séquard syndrome, 520

Brucella melitensis infection, and brucellosis, 280

Brucellosis, 280

and Q fever, 293

Brugada syndrome, 45

Bruising, and Fanconi anemia, 366

Bruton agammaglobulinemia, 360–361

Bubonic plague, 292

Buerger disease, 36

and Takayasu arteritis, 35

Bullous congenital ichthyosiform erythroderma, 109–110

and acrodermatitis enteropathica, 94

and Hay-Wells syndrome, 117

and McGrath syndrome, 127

Bullous impetigo, and pemphigus foliaceus, 132

and pemphigus vulgaris, 132

Bullous lupus erythematosus, and cicatricial pemphigoid, 131

Bullous pemphigoid, 130–131

and alopecia areata, 95

and cicatricial pemphigoid, 131

and dermatitis herpetiformis, 103

and pemphigus foliaceus, 132

and pemphigus vulgaris, 132

Bunyaviridae infection, 282

Burning feet, and hereditary sensory neuropathy, 570

Burns, and epidermolytic epidermolysis bullosa, 108

Byler disease, 335

and hereditary fructose intolerance, 444

C

C syndrome, 162–163

and chromosome 11, partial monosomy 11q, 60

and chromosome 13, partial monosomy 13q, 62

C trigonocephaly syndrome, 162–163

Cachexia, and Cockayne syndrome, 170–171

Café-au-lait spots, and neurofibromatosis type I, 563–564

Caffey disease, and cherubism, 168

CAHMR syndrome, and Cockayne syndrome, 170–171

Calcific aortic stenosis, and Singleton-Merten syndrome, 252

Calcific tendonitis, and Parsonage-Turner syndrome, 577

Calcitonin, and Paget disease, 25

Calcium channel blockers, and LEOPARD syndrome, 124

and Noonan syndrome, 722

and scleroderma, 33

Calcium pyrophosphate dihydrate deposition disease, 169–170

Callosal agenesis, 508

CAMFAK syndrome, and Cockayne syndrome, 170–171

Camp[t]omelic dwarfism, and achondroplasia, 144

and Kniest dysplasia, 213

Camp[t]omelic syndrome, 706–707

Camptodactyly, and Freeman-Sheldon syndrome, 714

and Gordon syndrome, 199

and Weaver syndrome, 266–267

Camptomelic dysplasia, and Antley-Bixler syndrome, 704–705

Campylobacter jejuni infection, and Guillain-Barré syndrome, 535

Camurati-Engelmann disease, 707–708

Canada-Cronkhite syndrome, 338

Canavan disease, 550–551

and Alexander disease, 510

and metachromatic leukodystrophy, 552

and Pelizaeus-Merzbacher disease, 578

Canavan-Van Bogaert-Bertrand disease, 550–551

Cancer, and ACTH deficiency, 302

and ataxia-telangiectasia, 605–606

and common variable immunodeficiency, 13

and dyskeratosis congenita, 104–105

and Lambert-Eaton myasthenic syndrome, 621

and MELAS, 469

and PTEN hamartoma tumor syndrome, 240

Candida albicans diaper dermatitis, and acrodermatitis enteropathica, 94

Candida infection, and Langerhans cell histiocytosis, 392

Candidiasis, mucocutaneous, and severe combined immunodeficiency, 14

Cane fever, 289

Canthoplasty, and blepharophimosis-ptosis-epicanthus inversus syndrome, 641

Cantrell deformity, 233–234

Cantrell pentalogy, 233–234

Cantrell syndrome, 233–234

Captopril, and cystinuria, 684

Carbamazepine, and diabetes insipidus, 314

and episodic ataxia, 600–601

and Fabry disease, 442

and Hallervorden-Spatz syndrome, 620

and hereditary sensory neuropathy, 570

and Kleine-Levin syndrome, 544

and Kluver-Bucy syndrome, 545

and neuromyotonia, 635

and Schwartz-Jampel syndrome, 586

and subacute sclerosing panencephalitis, 574–575

Carbamazepene embryopathy, and fetal hydantoin syndrome, 192

Carbamyl phosphate synthetase I deficiency, 506–506

Carbohydrate-deficient glycoprotein deficiency type III, and hypomelanosis of Ito, 119

Carbohydrate-deficient glycoprotein syndrome, and neonatal progeroid syndrome, 238

Carbohydrate metabolism, and hereditary fructose intolerance, 444

Carbonic anhydrase II deficiency syndrome, and autosomal-recessive osteopetrosis, 228–229

Carbonic anhydrase inhibitors, and episodic ataxia, 600–601

and episodic ataxia type II, 602

Carcinoid, and giant hypertrophic gastritis, 341

Carcinoid apudoma, 311–312

Carcinoid cancer, 311–312

Carcinoid disease, 311–312

Carcinoid syndrome, 311–312
  chronic, and eosinophilic fasciitis, 8
  and mastocytosis, 402

Carcinoma, and giant hypertrophic gastritis, 341

Cardiac defects, and Rieger syndrome, 243–244

Cardiac glycosides, and Barth syndrome, 44

Cardiac output, and hypoplastic left heart syndrome, 50

Cardiac sarcoidosis, 52

Cardiac shunt, unrepaired, and Eisenmenger syndrome, 46–47

Cardioauditory syndrome, 51–52

Cardiocutaneous lentiginosis syndrome, 124–125

Cardiofaciocutaneous syndrome, 163–164
  and Noonan syndrome, 722

Cardiomyopathic lentiginosis, 124–125

Cardiomyopathy, and ataxia with vitamin E deficiency, 606–607
  and Barth syndrome, 44
  and Becker muscular dystrophy, 622
  and carnitine deficiency syndromes, 432
  and Emery-Dreifuss muscular dystrophy, 624
  and hypoplastic left heart syndrome, 50
  and type IV glycogen storage disease, 454

Cardiovascular disorders, 41–56

Cardioverter defibrillator implantation, and Brugada syndrome, 45
  and Romano-Ward long QT syndrome, 54

Carmustine, and mycosis fungoides, 406

Carney complex, and acromegaly, 301
  and LEOPARD syndrome, 124

Carnitine, and facioscapulohumeral muscular dystrophy, 625
  and glutaric acidemia type I, 426
  and glutaric acidemia type II, 426–427

Carnitine acylcarnitine translocase, and medium-chain acyl-CoA dehydrogenase deficiency, 437

Carnitine deficiency, and idiopathic congenital central hypoventilation syndrome, 673

Carnitine deficiency syndromes, 432–433

Carnitine insufficiency, 432–433

Carnitine palmitoyl transferase I deficiency, 433–434

Carnitine palmitoyl transferase II deficiency, 434

Carnitine transporter deficiency, 432–433

Carnosinase deficiency, and carnosinemia, 435

Carnosinemia, 435

Carnosinuria, 435

Caroli disease, 336
  and congenital hepatic fibrosis, 691

Caroli syndrome, 336
  and medullary sponge kidney, 694

Carotid artery insufficiency, 659

Carotid artery occlusion, and retinal arterial occlusion, 657

Carpal tunnel syndrome, and eosinophilic fasciitis, 8
  and writer's cramp, 618

Carpenter syndrome, and Apert syndrome, 154
  and Bardet-Biedl syndrome, 158
  and Laurence-Moon syndrome, 215

Cartilage inflammation, and relapsing polychondritis, 29–30

Castleman disease, and POEMS syndrome, 26

Castration, and androgen insensitivity syndrome, 306

Cat cry syndrome, 175

Cat eye syndrome, 164–165

Cat scratch disease, and bubonic plague, 292

Cataplexy, and narcolepsy, 561–562

Cataract-dental syndrome, 654–655
  and Rieger syndrome, 243–244

Cataracts, and aniridia, 640
  and Conradi-Hünermann syndrome, 173
  and Cronkhite-Canada syndrome, 338
  and De Barsy syndrome, 6
  and hereditary spastic paraplegia, 575–576
  and Lowe syndrome, 466–467
  and Marinesco-Sjögren syndrome, 720–721
  and megalocornea, 556
  and Nance-Horan syndrome, 654–655
  and Norrie disease, 656
  and Rothmund-Thomson syndrome, 135–136
  and Usher syndrome, 665

Catatonia, and locked-in syndrome, 554

CATCH22, 70–71

Catel-Manzke syndrome, 165

Catlike cry, and cri-du-chat syndrome, 175

Caudal dysgenesis, 166

Caudal dysplasia, 166

Caudal regression syndrome, 166
  and femoral hypoplasia–unusual facies syndrome, 712

Cauliflower ears, and relapsing polychondritis, 29

Causalgia, 523

CAVE complex, 230

Cavernous angioma, 117–118

Cavernous hemangioma, 117–118

Cayler cardiofacial syndrome, and chromosome 22q11 deletion spectrum, 70

Cayler syndrome, 178–179

Ceftriaxone, and Whipple disease, 297

Celecoxib, and Lynch syndromes, 401

Celiac disease, and abetalipoproteinemia, 358
  and Cronkhite-Canada syndrome, 338
  and giant hypertrophic gastritis, 341
  and sucrase-isomaltase deficiency, 354

Cellulitis, and erysipelas, 285

Cellulitis phlegmon, 285

Central cord syndrome, and Brown-Séquard syndrome, 520

Central core disease, 607–608
  and limb girdle muscular dystrophy, 625
  and spinal muscular atrophy, 637

Central hypoventilation syndrome, idiopathic congenital, 673

Central nervous system abnormalities, and Wyburn-Mason syndrome, 667

Central nervous system damage, and glutathione synthetase deficiency, 449

Central nervous system demyelination, and Pelizaeus-Merzbacher disease, 578–579

Central nervous system tumors, and Von Hippel-Lindau disease, 265–266

Centrofacial lentiginosis, 124–125

Centronuclear myopathy, 628–629

Cephalic neural tube closure, and anencephaly, 151–152

Cephalosporin, and Whipple disease, 297

Ceramide accumulation, and Farber disease, 443

Ceramide trihexosidase deficiency, 442

Cerebellar ataxia, and congenital disorders of glycosylation, 457–458
  and Hartnup disease, 458
  and Loken-Senior syndrome, 692
  and Machado-Joseph disease, 555
  and Marinesco-Sjögren syndrome, 720–721

Cerebellar ataxia, *(continued)*
  and X-linked sideroblastic anemia, 374–375
Cerebellar dysfunction, and neurofibromatosis type 2, 564–565
Cerebellar hypoplasia, 515–516
  and Dandy-Walker syndrome, 526–527
Cerebellar infarcts, and hydrocephalus, 539
Cerebellar vermian hypoplasia, and Joubert syndrome, 542
Cerebellar vermis agenesis, 542
Cerebral anastomosis, and moyamoya syndrome, 559
Cerebral arteritis, and moyamoya syndrome, 559
Cerebral artery dissection, and moyamoya syndrome, 559
Cerebral calcification, and Fahr disease, 532
Cerebral defects, and oculocerebral syndrome, 226–227
Cerebral dysgenesis, 508
Cerebral gigantism, 255
Cerebral palsy, and Alexander disease, 510
  and congenital disorders of glycosylation, 457
  and dopa-responsive dystonia, 612
  and dystonia, 609
  and hyperekplexia, 540
Cerebral venous thrombosis, and pseudotumor cerebri, 582
Cerebrocostomandibular syndrome, 166–167
Cerebrofaciogenital syndrome, 274
Cerebrohepatorenal syndrome, 487
Cerebromacular degeneration, 501
Cerebromedullospinal disconnection, 554
Cerebro-oculo-facial syndrome, and Neu-Laxova syndrome, 562
Cerebro-oculo-facial-skeletal syndrome, 520–521
  and acrocallosal syndrome (Schinzel type), 145
  and Bowen-Conradi syndrome, 161
Cerebrooculomuscular syndrome, 597–598
Cerebroside sulfate accumulation, and metachromatic leukodystrophy, 552–553
Cerebrospinal fluid, and hydranencephaly, 538
  and hydrocephalus, 539
Cerebrospinal fluid rhinorrhea, 530

Cerebrovascular accident, and botulism, 279
Cerebrovascular ferrocalcinosis, and Fahr disease, 532
Ceroid-lipofuscin accumulation, and Kuf disease, 547
Cervical disk disease, and Parsonage-Turner syndrome, 577
Cervical dystonia, 611
Cervical incompetence, and Asherman syndrome, 308–309
Cervical lymphocele, 175–176
Cervical meningocele, and cystic hygroma, 175
Cervical rhizotomy, and cervical dystonia, 611
Cervical spondylotic myeloradiculopathy, and amyotrophic lateral sclerosis, 513
Cervical-thoracic somite dysplasia, and MURCS association, 695
Cetirizine, and familial eosinophilic cellulitis, 99
  and transient acantholytic dermatosis, 104
Chanarin-Dorfman syndrome, and progressive symmetric erythrokeratodermia, 111
Chandler syndrome, 649–650
  and Cogan-Reese syndrome, 644
Charcot disease, 513–514
Charcot-Marie-Tooth disease, and chronic inflammatory demyelinating polyradiculoneuropathy, 581
  and Dejerine-Sottas syndrome, 527
  and Friedreich ataxia, 602
  and Refsum disease, 604–605
Charcot-Marie-Tooth polyneuropathy syndrome, *fig. 51,* 521–522
Charcot-Marie-Tooth syndrome, and hereditary sensory neuropathy, 570–571
  and Rosenbert-Chutorian syndrome, 585
CHARGE association, 167
  and DiGeorge syndrome, 178
  and Joubert syndrome, 542
CHARGE syndrome, 167–168
  and trisomy 18 syndrome, 88
Charleaux sign, and keratoconus, 651
Charlie M. syndrome, and Möbius syndrome, 223–224
Chédiak-Higashi anomaly, 379
Chédiak-Higashi disease, and Hermansky-Pudlak syndrome, 391

Chédiak-Higashi syndrome, 379
  and acquired agranulocytosis, 361
  and Glanzmann thrombasthenia, 383
Chédiak-Steinbrinck-Higashi syndrome, 379
Cheiloplasty, and Melkersson-Rosenthal syndrome, 557
Chemically induced alopecia, and alopecia areata, 95
Chemotherapy, and angioimmunoblastic lymphadenopathy-type T-cell lymphoma, 398
  and Denys-Drash syndrome, 686
  and Erdheim-Chester disease, 441
  and Ewing sarcoma of bone, 381
  and glioblastoma multiforme, 385
  and lymphomatoid granulomatosis, 49
  and multiple myeloma, 407
  and pars planitis, 657
  and WAGR syndrome, 699
Cherry red spot, and Sandhoff disease, 497
  and sialidosis, 498
  and Tay-Sachs disease, 501
Cherubism, 168–169
Chest pain, and lymphomatoid granulomatosis, 48
Cheyne-Stokes breathing, and leukodystrophy, 550
Chiari malformations, 515–516
  and corpus callosum absence, 508
  and cyclic vomiting syndrome, 525
  and primary lateral sclerosis, 548
Child abuse, and osteogenesis imperfecta, 227
CHILD syndrome, and Conradi-Hünermann syndrome, 173
Childbirth, and Sheehan syndrome, 328
Childhood disintegrative disorder, and Landau-Kleffner syndrome, 547
Chitayat syndrome, and Filippi syndrome, 194–195
  and Scott craniodigital syndrome, 249–250
Chlorambucil, and Behçet disease, 4
  and posterior uveitis, 666
Chloramphenicol, and plague, 292
Chloroquine, and malaria, 291
  and porphyria cutanea tarda, 493–494
  and Q fever, 293
  and variegate porphyria, 494–495
Chlorproguanil, and malaria, 291
Chlorpropamide, and diabetes insipidus, 314
Choanal atresia, 704–705
  and CHARGE syndrome, 167–168
  and Marshall-Smith syndrome, 219

Choanal atresia multiple anomalies syndrome, 167
Cholangitis, and Caroli disease, 336
and liver fluke disease, 286
Cholecystitis, and liver fluke disease, 286
Choledochal cyst, and biliary atresia, 334
and Caroli disease, 336
and idiopathic neonatal hepatitis, 288
Cholestasis, and Alagille syndrome, 332
and idiopathic neonatal hepatitis, 288
Cholestasis of pregnancy, and Dubin-Johnson syndrome, 340
Cholesterol synthesis, and Smith-Lemli-Opitz syndrome, 253
Cholestyramine, and Byler disease, 335
and idiopathic neonatal hepatitis, 288
Cholinesterase inhibitors, and Binswanger disease, 519
and progressive supranuclear palsy, 574
Chondritis, rheumatic, 29–30
Chondroblastoma, and dysplasia epiphysealis hemimelica, 186
Chondrocalcinosis articularis, 169–170
Chondrodysplasia, and Kniest dysplasia, 213
metaphyseal, and Ollier disease, 23–24
Chondrodysplasia punctata, and Conradi-Hünermann syndrome, 173
and maxillonasal dysplasia, 186–187
Chondrodystrophic myotonia, 586–587
Chondroectodermal dysplasia, and asphyxiating thoracic dystrophy, 155
Chondromalacia, systemic, 29–30
Chondrosarcoma, and Ewing sarcoma of bone, 380–381
Chordee, without hypospadias, and Peyronie disease, 25
Chorea, and myoclonus, 628
and neuroacanthocytosis, 633–634
and tardive dyskinesia, 591
Chorea-acanthocytosis, and Huntington disease, 537
Chorea minor, 522
Choreoacanthocytosis, 633–634
Choreoathetosis, and Hallervorden-Spatz syndrome, 620
and Lesch-Nyhan syndrome, 464–465
and Pelizaeus-Merzbacher disease, 578
Chorioangiopagus twins, 421–422
Chorioretinal degeneration, and Cohen syndrome, 172
Chorioretinal lacunae, and Aicardi syndrome, 509–510

Choroid inflammation, and posterior uveitis, 666
Choroid plexus carcinoma, and medulloblastoma, 404–405
Choroid plexus papilloma, and hydrocephalus, 539
and medulloblastoma, 404–405
Choroidal sclerosis, 642
Choroideremia, 642
Choroidoretinal degeneration, 642
Christ-Siemens-Touraine syndrome, 185
Christmas disease, 381–382
Christmas tree syndrome, 349
Chromosomal abnormalities, and holoprosencephaly, 536
Chromosomal anomalies, and leprechaunism, 216
Chromosomal disorders, 57–91
Chromosome 1, deletion of the short arm of, 58
Chromosome 1p36 deletion syndrome, 58
Chromosome 3, distal 3p monosomy, 73
Chromosome 3, distal 3q2 duplication, 73–74
Chromosome 3, distal 3q2 trisomy, 73–74
Chromosome 3, monosomy 3p2, 73
Chromosome 3, trisomy 3q2, 73–74
Chromosome 3 deletion of distal 3p, 73
Chromosome 4, deletion 4q31-qter syndrome, 75
Chromosome 4, deletion 4q32-qter syndrome, 75
Chromosome 4, deletion 4q33-qter syndrome, 75
Chromosome 4, monosomy distal 4q, 75
Chromosome 4, monosomy 4q, 74–75
Chromosome 4, partial monosomy of distal 4q, 75
Chromosome 4, partial trisomies 4q2 and 4q3, 76
Chromosome 4, partial trisomy 4 (q26 or q27-qter), 76
Chromosome 4, partial trisomy 4 (q31 or q32-qter), 76
Chromosome 4, partial trisomy 4 (q25-qter), 76
Chromosome 4, partial trisomy distal 4q, 76
and chromosome 15, distal trisomy 15q, 65
Chromosome 4, partial trisomy 4p, 77–78
Chromosome 4, 4q terminal deletion syndrome, 75
Chromosome 4, trisomy 4p, 77–78
Chromosome 4 long arm deletion, 74–75
Chromosome 4 ring, 76–77
Chromosome 4p-, 272

Chromosome 4q- syndrome, 74–75
Chromosome 5, trisomy 5p, 78
Chromosome 6, partial trisomy 6q, 79
Chromosome 6, partial trisomy 6q2, 79
Chromosome 6 ring, 80
Chromosome 7, monosomy 7p2, 80–81
Chromosome 7, partial deletion of short arm (7p2-), 80–81
Chromosome 7, terminal 7p deletion, 80–81
Chromosome 8, monosomy 8p2, 81–82
Chromosome 8, monosomy 8p21-pter, 81–82
Chromosome 8, partial deletion (short arm), 81–82
Chromosome 8, partial monosomy 8p2, 81–82
Chromosome 9, complete trisomy 9p, 84
Chromosome 9, partial monosomy 9p, 82–83
Chromosome 9, partial monosomy 9p22, 82–83
Chromosome 9, partial monosomy 9p22-pter, 82–83
Chromosome 9, partial trisomy 9p, 84
Chromosome 9, tetrasomy 9p, 83–84
Chromosome 9, tetrasomy 9p mosaicism, 83–84
Chromosome 9, trisomy 9p, and chromosome 9, tetrasomy 9p, 83
Chromosome 9, trisomy 9p (multiple variants), 84–85
Chromosome 9, trisomy mosaic, 85–86
Chromosome 9 ring, 83
and chromosome 9, partial monosomy 9p, 82
Chromosome 10, distal trisomy 10q, 59
Chromosome 10, monosomy 10p, 60
Chromosome 10, 10p- partial, 60
Chromosome 10, partial deletion, 60
Chromosome 10, partial trisomy 10q24-qtr, 59
Chromosome 10, trisomy 10q2, 59
Chromosome 11, monosomy 11q, and chromosome 4, monosomy 4q, 74
Chromosome 11, partial monosomy 11q, 60–61
Chromosome 11, partial trisomy 11q, 61–62
Chromosome 11, partial trisomy 11q13-qtr, 61–62
Chromosome 11 partial trisomy 11q21-qtr, 61–62
Chromosome 11 partial trisomy 11q23-qter, 61–62
Chromosome 11 ring, and chromosome 11, partial monosomy 11q, 60

Chromosome 13, partial monosomy 13q, 62–63

Chromosome 13 ring, and chromosome 13, partial monosomy 13q, 62

Chromosome 14, trisomy mosaic, 64–65

Chromosome 14 ring, 63–64

Chromosome 15, distal trisomy 15q, 65–66

Chromosome 15, trisomy 15q2, 65–66

Chromosome 15 ring, 66
and Russel-Silver syndrome, 245–246

Chromosome 15q deletion, and chromosome 15 ring, 66

Chromosome 18, monosomy 18p, 67

Chromosome 18, monosomy 18q, 67–68
and chromosome 18, monosomy 18p, 67

Chromosome 18, tetrasomy 18p, 69

Chromosome 18 long arm deletion syndrome, 67–68

Chromosome 18 ring, 68–69

Chromosome 18q- syndrome, 67–68

Chromosome 21 monosomy, and chromosome 21 ring, 70

Chromosome 21 ring, 70

Chromosome 22, inverted duplication, 164–165

Chromosome 22, monosomy 22q, and chromosome 10, monosomy 10p, 60

Chromosome 22, partial tetrasomy, 164–165

Chromosome 22, partial trisomy, 164–165

Chromosome 22, trisomy mosaic, and chromosome 22 ring, 72

Chromosome 22 ring, 71–72

Chromosome 22q deletion, and chromosome 22 ring, 71

Chromosome 22q11 deletion spectrum, 70–71

Chromosome 22q11 deletion syndrome, 178–179

Chromosome X pentasomy, 86–87

Chromosome XXXXX syndrome, 86–87

Chronic atrophic polychondritis, 29–30

Chronic dysphagocytosis, 386

Chronic granulomatous disease, 386–387

Chronic inflammatory demyelinating polyradiculoneuropathy, 581–582

Chronic lymphocytic thyroiditis, 329

Chronic mucocutaneous candidiasis, and acrodermatitis enteropathica, 94

Chronic progressive external ophthalmoplegia, 603–604

Chronic sinusitis, and cyclic vomiting syndrome, 525

Churg-Strauss syndrome, *figs. 56–57*, 674
and eosinophilic gastroenteritis, 342
and hypersensitivity myocarditis, 53
and lymphomatoid granulomatosis, 48
and microscopic polyangiitis, 27
and polyarteritis nodosa, 28
and Wegener granulomatosis, 422

Chylomicron retention disease, 380
and abetalipoproteinemia, 358

Cicatricial pemphigoid, 131–132
and bullous pemphigoid, 130–131

Cidofovir, and recurrent respiratory papillomatosis, 676

Ciliary dyskinesia, primary, 675

Ciprofloxacin, and anthrax, 278
and plague, 292
and small bowel diverticulosis, 339

Cirrhosis, and Banti syndrome, 377
and hereditary hemochromatosis, 387–388
and type IV glycogen storage disease, 454
and Wilson disease, 506

Classic lissencephaly, 553–554

Claude Bernard-Horner syndrome, 648

Claudicatio intermittens, and lumbar spinal stenosis, 587

Claudication, and restless legs syndrome, 583

Clavicular abnormalities, and cleidocranial dysplasia, 182
and hyperostosis corticalis generalisata, 204–205

Cleft lip, and popliteal pterygium syndrome, 242

Cleft palate, and camp[t]omelic syndrome, 706–707
and cerebrocostomandibular syndrome, 166–167
and chromosome 4, monosomy distal 4q, 75
and chromosome 4, monosomy 4q, 74
and chromosome 9, trisomy 9p, 84
and chromosome 9 ring, 83
and chromosome 22q11 deletion spectrum, 70–71
and deletion of the short arm of chromosome 1, 58
and diastrophic dysplasia, 711
and Duane syndrome, 645
and femoral hypoplasia–unusual facies syndrome, 712–713
and Fraser syndrome, 196–197
and Gordon syndrome, 199
and Hajdu-Cheney syndrome, 11–12
and holoprosencephaly, 536–537
and Marden-Walker syndrome, 18

and oto-palato-digital syndrome, 229
and Pierre Robin sequence, 235–236
and popliteal pterygium syndrome, 242
and spondyloepiphyseal dysplasia congenita, 728

Cleidocranial dysostosis, 182
and pyknodysostosis, 242

Cleidocranial dysplasia, 182–183
and Melnick-Needles syndrome, 222
and Yunis-Varaaon syndrome, 275

Clindamycin, and hidradenitis suppurativa, 119

Clinodactyly, and Filippi syndrome, 194–195

Clitoral enlargement, and partial androgen insensitivity syndrome, 307–308

Clobazam, and hyperekplexia, 540

Clobetasol, and lichen sclerosis, 126

Clofazimine, and Melkersson-Rosenthal syndrome, 557

Clofibrate, and diabetes insipidus, 314

Clomiphene citrate, and polycystic ovary syndrome, 324

Clonazepam, and Baltic/Mediterranean/Unverrich-Lundborg myoclonic epilepsy, 600
and embouchure dystonia, 613
and hyperekplexia, 540
and myoclonic dystonia, 615
and myoclonus, 628
and oromandibular dystonia, 615
and progressive myoclonus epilepsy, 531–532
and stiff person syndrome, 588

Clonidine, and Tourette syndrome, 594

Clonidine withdrawal, and pheochromocytoma, 410

Clostridial sepsis, and warm antibody hemolytic anemia, 371–372

Clostridium botulinum infection, and botulism, 279

Clotting factor deficiency, and hemophilia, 390–391

Clubfeet, and caudal regression syndrome, 166
and chromosome 5, trisomy 5p, 78
and diastrophic dysplasia, 711
and dystonia, 609
and Freeman-Sheldon syndrome, 714
and Hajdu-Cheney syndrome, 11–12

COACH syndrome, and Joubert syndrome, 542

Coagulopathy, and hemophagocytic lymphohistiocytosis, 397–398
and MELAS, 469

Coats disease, 643
  and Norrie disease, 655
  and retinoblastoma, 661
Coats syndrome, and
    facioscapulohumeral muscular
    dystrophy, 625
Cobalamin, and methylmalonic
    acidemias, 429
Cobblestone lissencephaly, and classic
    lissencephaly, 553
Cochicine, and Behçet disease, 4
  and pachydermoperiostosis, 129
Cochlear implantation, and Norrie
    disease, 656
  and Rosenbert-Chutorian syndrome,
    585
  and Usher syndrome, 665
Cockayne syndrome, 170–171
  and cerebro-oculo-facio-skeletal
    syndrome, 520–521
  and De Barsy syndrome, 6
  and neonatal progeroid syndrome, 238
  and Pelizaeus-Merzbacher disease, 578
  and progeria, 724
  and retinitis pigmentosa, 660
  and Usher syndrome, 665
Coenzyme Q10, and chronic progressive
    external ophthalmoplegia, 604
  and Friedreich ataxia, 602
  and Kearns-Sayre syndrome, 604
Coffin-Lowry syndrome, 171–172
  and Borjeson-Forssman-Lehmann
    syndrome, 705
  and Fountain syndrome, 196
  and Williams syndrome, 270
  and XLMR-hypotonic facies
    syndrome, 274
Coffin-Siris syndrome, 708–709
COFS syndrome, and Cockayne
    syndrome, 170–171
  and Norrie disease, 655
  and trisomy 18 syndrome, 88
Cogan-Reese syndrome, *figs. 54–55*, 644,
    649
Cogan syndrome, and Takayasu arteritis,
    35
Cognitive decline, and Huntington
    disease, 537–538
  and metachromatic leukodystrophy,
    552–553
Cognitive impairment, and
    Baltic/Mediterranean/Unverrich-
    Lundborg myoclonic epilepsy, 600
Cohen syndrome, 172–173
  and Bardet-Biedl syndrome, 158
  and Laurence-Moon syndrome, 215
  and Prader-Willi syndrome, 237–238

Colchicine, and familial eosinophilic
    cellulitis, 99
  and familial Mediterranean fever, 19
  and idiopathic thrombocytopenic
    purpura, 416
  and mesenteric panniculitis, 350
  and Peyronie disease, 26
Cold agglutinin disease, 368
  and warm antibody hemolytic anemia,
    371–372
Cold hemolytic anemia syndromes, 368
Cold intolerance, and chronic
    lymphocytic thyroiditis, 329
  and Sheehan syndrome, 328
Cole-Carpenter syndrome, and
    osteogenesis imperfecta, 227
Colectomy, and familial adenomatous
    polyposis, 352–353
  and Lynch syndromes, 401
Collagenopathy, type II, 213
  and achondroplasia, 144
Colloid degeneration, and
    scleromyxedema, 136
Colloid goiter, and chronic lymphocytic
    thyroiditis, 329
Coloboma, and CHARGE syndrome,
    167–168
  and Joubert syndrome, 542
  and Lenz microphthalmia syndrome,
    654
Colon cancer, and pseudomyxoma
    peritonei, 412
Colonic atresia, and Hirschsprung
    disease, 345
Color blindness, and Leber congenital
    amaurosis, 652
  and Leber hereditary optic neuropathy,
    653
Colorado tick fever, and ehrlichiosis,
    283
Colorectal cancer, and familial
    adenomatous polyposis, 352–353
  and Lynch syndromes, 401
Colostomy, and anorectal malformations,
    153–154
  and Hirschsprung disease, 345
Coma, and carnitine palmitoyl
    transferase I deficiency, 433
  and carnitine palmitoyl transferase II
    deficiency, 434
  and isovaleric acidemia, 427
  and malaria, 291
  and maple syrup urine disease, 468
  and methylmalonic acidemias, 429
  and multiple carboxylase deficiency,
    483
  and PEPCK deficiency, 486

  and propionic acidemia, 428
  and short-chain acyl-CoA
    dehydrogenase deficiency, 438–439
  and West Nile fever, 296
Combined hyperlipidemia, and familial
    dysbetalipoproteinemia, 440
Combined variable immunodeficiency,
    and hyper-IgM syndrome, 393
Common arterial trunk, 55–56
Common atrioventricular orifice, 43
Common variable immunodeficiency,
    13–14
Complete androgen insensitivity
    syndrome, 307
Complex aphthosis, and Behçet disease, 4
Complex IV deficiency, 436
Complex regional pain syndrome,
    523–524
Condyloma accuminata, and bowenoid
    papulosis, 98
Cone dystrophy, and Stargardt disease,
    663
Congenital adrenal hyperplasia, 304
  and Weaver syndrome, 266–267
Congenital adrenal insufficiency, and
    Beckwith-Wiedemann syndrome,
    518
Congenital afibrogenemia, 359–360
Congenital alopecia, and alopecia areata,
    95
Congenital amputation, 150–151
Congenital antithrombin III deficiency,
    376–377
Congenital bilateral perisylvian
    syndrome, 579–580
Congenital chloride diarrhea, and
    microvillus inclusion disease, 351
Congenital clasped thumbs, 220
Congenital complete atrioventricular
    block, 49–50
Congenital complete heart block, 49–50
Congenital constricting bands, 150–151
Congenital contractual arachnodactyly, 3
Congenital defect of the scalp, 96
Congenital disorders of glycosylation,
    457–458
Congenital dysphagocytosis, 386
Congenital erythropoietic porphyria,
    492–493
Congenital esophageal obstruction, 190
Congenital facial diplegia syndrome,
    223–224
Congenital facial paralysis, 223–224
Congenital generalized lipodystrophy,
    322
Congenital heart anomalies, and cor
    triatriatum, 45–46

Congenital heart disease, and chromosome 22q11 deletion spectrum, 70
and Eisenmenger syndrome, 47
and maternal phenylketonuria, 489
Congenital hemidysplasia, and Conradi-Hünermann syndrome, 173
Congenital hepatic fibrosis, 691–692
Congenital high scapula, 257
Congenital hypomyelination neuropathy, 568
Congenital hypothalamic hamartoblastoma syndrome, 230
Congenital infections, and Cockayne syndrome, 170–171
Congenital lactic acidosis, 462–464
Congenital mesodermal dystrophy, 267–268
Congenital microvillus atrophy, 351
Congenital myopathy with fiber-type disproportion, 629–630
Congenital nonspherocytic hemolytic anemia, 369
Congenital oculofacial paralysis, 223–224
Congenital reticulohistiocytosis, and incontinentia pigmenti, 121
Congenital retinal telangiectasias, 643
Congenital scalp defect, 96
Congenital sodium diarrhea, and microvillus inclusion disease, 351
Congenital third-degree atrioventricular block, 49–50
Congenital thrombocytopenia, and Bernard-Soulier syndrome, 378
Congenital tonsillar ectopia, 515–516
Congenital undescended scapula, 257
Congenital varicella, and incontinentia pigmenti, 121
Congestive heart failure, and atrial septal defects, 42
and Churg-Strauss syndrome, 674
and Diamond-Blackfan anemia, 365
and giant cell myocarditis, 52
and MULIBREY nanism, 224–225
and Singleton-Merten syndrome, 252
and very-long-chain acyl-CoA dehydrogenase deficiency, 439–440
and X-linked sideroblastic anemia, 373
Conical cornea, 650–651
Conjunctivitis, and Wegener granulomatosis, 422
Conn syndrome, 305
Conotruncal anomaly face syndrome, 70–71, 178–179
Conradi-Hünermann syndrome, 173–174

Constipation, and FG syndrome, 193–194
and idiopathic congenital central hypoventilation syndrome, 673
Constricting bands, and acheiropodia, 702
Contact dermatitis, and epidermolytic epidermolysis bullosa, 108
and erysipelas, 285
and mycosis fungoides, 406
Contractures, and Wieacker-Wolff syndrome, 638
Convulsions, and multiple carboxylase deficiency, 482
and PEPCK deficiency, 486
Cooley anemia, 419
Copper deficiency, and X-linked sideroblastic anemia, 373
Copper histidine, and Menkes disease, 470
Coproporphyria, hereditary, 494–495
Cor triatriatum, 45–46
Corectopia, and Cogan-Reese syndrome, 644
and essential iris atrophy, 650
Cori disease, 453
Corneal clouding, and Hurler disease, 477
and Maroteaux-Lamy disease, 481
and Morquio disease, 480
and mucolipidosis, 473–474
and Scheie disease, 478
Corneal dystrophies, and keratoconus, 651
Corneal ectasias, and keratoconus, 650
Corneal edema, and Cogan-Reese syndrome, 644
and iridocorneal endothelial syndromes, 649
Corneal opacification, and aniridia, 640
congenital, and De Barsy syndrome, 6
Corneal transplantation, and Cogan-Reese syndrome, 644
and iridocorneal endothelial syndromes, 649
and keratoconus, 651
and Scheie disease, 478
Corneal warpage, and keratoconus, 651
Cornelia de Lange syndrome, *fig. 62,* 709–710
and chromosome 3, trisomy 3q2, 73
and Fryns syndrome, 715
and Gorlin-Chaudhry-Moss syndrome, 200
and Rubinstein-Taybi syndrome, 726–727

Coronal synostosis, and craniofrontonasal syndrome, 183
Coronary insufficiency syndrome, and pheochromocytoma, 409
Corpus callosum absence, 508
and acrocallosal syndrome (Schinzel type), 145
Corpus callosum agenesis, and Aicardi syndrome, 509–510
and cerebro-oculo-facio-skeletal syndrome, 520
and Dubowitz syndrome, 179–180
and FG syndrome, 193–194
Corpus callosum dysgenesis, and Lenz microphthalmia syndrome, 654
Corticobasal degeneration, 524–525
and multiple system atrophy, 561
and progressive supranuclear palsy, 573
Corticobasilar degeneration, and Parkinson disease, 576
Corticosteroids, and alopecia areata, 95
and alpha 1-antitrypsin deficiency, 671
and angioimmunoblastic lymphadenopathy-type T-cell lymphoma, 398
and autoimmune hemolytic anemia, 367
and autosomal-recessive osteopetrosis, 229
and Becker muscular dystrophy, 622
and Behçet disease, 4
and cicatricial pemphigoid, 131
and congenital adrenal hyperplasia, 304
and Cronkhite-Canada syndrome, 338
and Duchenne muscular dystrophy, 623
and endomyocardial fibrosis, 48
and eosinophilia-myalgia syndrome, 7
and eosinophilic gastroenteritis, 342
and Erdheim-Chester disease, 441
and fibrodysplasia ossificans progressiva, 713
and Gianotti-Crosti syndrome, 115
and Henoch-Schönlein purpura, 415
and hypersensitivity myocarditis, 53
and large granular lymphocyte leukemia, 395
and Leiner disease, 123
and lichen planus, 125
and lymphomatoid granulomatosis, 49
and mastocytosis, 402
and Melkersson-Rosenthal syndrome, 557
and microscopic polyangiitis, 28

and Mucha-Habermann disease, 129
and multiple sclerosis, 560
and myasthenia gravis, 627
and POEMS syndrome, 27
and polyarteritis nodosa, 29
and posterior uveitis, 666
and pyoderma gangrenosum, 135
and scleromyxedema, 137
and Sjögren syndrome, 34
and spondyloepiphyseal dysplasia
    congenita, 728
and Sweet syndrome, 139
and tarsal tunnel syndrome, 592
and Tolosa-Hunt syndrome, 664
and viral hemorrhagic fevers, 282
and Vogt-Koyanagi-Harada syndrome,
    37
and warm antibody hemolytic anemia,
    371–372
and Wegener granulomatosis, 423
Corticosterone methyloxidase deficiency,
    and congenital adrenal
    hyperplasia, 304
Cortisol excess, and Cushing syndrome,
    312–313
Costello syndrome, and
    aspartylglucosaminuria, 432
and cardiofaciocutaneous syndrome,
    163–164
and leprechaunism, 216
and Noonan syndrome, 722
Cotrimexasole, and Q fever, 293
Cotton-wool spots, and Eales disease,
    646
Cough, and alpha 1-antitrypsin
    deficiency, 671
and lymphangioleiomyomatosis, 395
and pulmonary alveolar proteinosis,
    677
Coumadin, and congenital antithrombin
    III deficiency, 376–377
and paroxysmal nocturnal
    hemoglobinuria, 389–390
Cowden disease, and adiposis dolorosa,
    303
Cowden syndrome, and Laband
    syndrome, 214
and PTEN hamartoma tumor
    syndrome, 240
and Ruvalcaba-Myhre-Smith
    syndrome, 354
Coxiellosis, and Q fever, 293
Coxoauricular syndrome, and
    ear–patella–short stature
    syndrome, 189
Cranial-cervical dystonia, 615

Cranial malformations, and Greig
    cephalopolysyndactyly syndrome,
    201
Cranial nerve, and CHARGE syndrome,
    167–168
Cranial nerve entrapment, and
    sclerosteosis, 248–249
Cranial nerve palsy, and
    neurofibromatosis type 2, 564–565
Craniectomy, and sclerosteosis, 249
Craniocarpotarsal dystrophy, 714
Craniodiaphyseal dysplasia, and
    Camurati-Engelmann disease,
    707–708
and hyperostosis corticalis
    generalisata, 204–205
Craniodigital syndrome of Scott, 249–250
Craniofacial malformations, and Antley-
    Bixler syndrome, 704–705
and Apert syndrome, 154–155
and Borjeson-Forssman-Lehmann
    syndrome, 705
and branchio-oculo-facial syndrome,
    161–162
and C syndrome, 162–163
and cardiofaciocutaneous syndrome,
    163–164
and cerebro-oculo-facio-skeletal
    syndrome, 520
and chromosome 3, trisomy 3q2,
    73–74
and chromosome 4, monosomy distal
    4q, 75
and chromosome 4, monosomy 4q, 74
and chromosome 4, partial trisomy
    distal 4q, 76
and chromosome 4, trisomy 4p, 77–78
and chromosome 5, trisomy 5p, 78
and chromosome 6, partial trisomy 6q,
    79
and chromosome 6 ring, 80
and chromosome 7, monosomy 7p2,
    80–81
and chromosome 8, monosomy 8p2,
    81–82
and chromosome 9, partial monosomy
    9p, 82
and chromosome 9, tetrasomy 9p, 84
and chromosome 9, trisomy 9p, 84
and chromosome 9, trisomy mosaic,
    85–86
and chromosome 9 ring, 83
and chromosome 10, monosomy 10p,
    60
and chromosome 11, partial
    monosomy 11q, 60–61

and chromosome 11, partial trisomy
    11q, 61–62
and chromosome 14 ring, 63–64
and chromosome 15, distal trisomy
    15q, 65–66
and chromosome 15 ring, 66
and chromosome 18, monosomy 18p,
    67
and chromosome 18, tetrasomy 18p,
    69
and chromosome 18 ring, 68–69
and chromosome 18q- syndrome,
    67–68
and chromosome 21 ring, 70
and congenital lactic acidosis, 462–464
and Cornelia de Lange syndrome, 709
and Crouzon syndrome, 710
and De Barsy syndrome, 6
and epidermal nevus syndrome, 105
and Goldenhar syndrome, 716
and Hajdu-Cheney syndrome, 11
and Hallermann-Streiff syndrome, 202
and holoprosencephaly, 536
and Hunter disease, 478–479
and hyperostosis corticalis
    generalisata, 204–205
and Jackson-Weiss syndrome, 719
and Jarcho-Levin syndrome, 207–208
and Joubert syndrome, 542
and Kabuki make-up syndrome,
    209–210
and KBG syndrome, 210
and Klippel-Feil syndrome, 720
and megalocornea, 556
and pentasomy X, 86–87
and primary craniosynostosis, 174
and pyknodysostosis, 242
and Roberts pseudothalidomide
    syndrome, 244–245
and Rubinstein-Taybi syndrome,
    726–727
and Saethre-Chotzen syndrome,
    727–728
and Scott craniodigital syndrome,
    249–250
and Smith-Magenis syndrome, 254
and Sotos syndrome, 255
and spondyloepiphyseal dysplasia
    tarda, 729–730
and Townes-Brocks syndrome, 262
and Treacher-Collins syndrome,
    262–263
and trichorhinophalangeal syndrome,
    730
and trisomy 18 syndrome, 88
and Wolf-Hirschhorn syndrome, 272

Craniofacial malformations, *(continued)*
    and XLMR-hypotonic facies
        syndrome, 274
Craniofrontonasal dysostosis, 183
Craniofrontonasal dysplasia, 183
    and chromosome 4, partial trisomy
        distal 4q, 76
Craniofrontonasal syndrome, 183
Craniometaphyseal dysplasia, 184
Craniorachischisis, and anencephaly,
    151–152
Craniosynostosis, and achondroplasia,
    144
    and Antley-Bixler syndrome, 704–705
    and Apert syndrome, 154–155
    and Baller-Gerold syndrome, 157–158
    and Crouzon syndrome, 710
    and Jackson-Weiss syndrome, 719
    and Pfeiffer syndrome type I, 234–
        235
    primary, 174
        and chromosome 7, monosomy 7p2,
            80
        and Saethre-Chotzen syndrome,
            727–728
Craniovertebral decompression, and
    syringobulbia, 589
    and syringomyelia, 591
CRASH syndrome, 220
Creatine kinase elevation, and Duchenne
    muscular dystrophy, 623
Creatine phosphokinase elevation, and
    neuroleptic malignant syndrome,
    566
CREST syndrome, and hereditary
    hemorrhagic telangiectasia, 418
Creutzfeldt-Jakob disease, 608
    and progressive supranuclear palsy,
        573
Cri-du-chat syndrome, 175
Crigler-Najjar syndrome, 337
    and kernicterus, 543
Crimean-Congo fever, 282
    and Rift Valley fever, 294
Critical aortic stenosis and coarctation of
        the aorta, and hypoplastic left
        heart syndrome, 50
Crohn disease, and Behçet disease, 4
Cronkhite-Canada syndrome, 338
Cross syndrome, 226–227
    and Laband syndrome, 214
Croup, and recurrent respiratory
    papillomatosis, 676
Crouzon syndrome, 710–711
    and Apert syndrome, 154

    and Gorlin-Chaudhry-Moss
        syndrome, 200
    and Jackson-Weiss syndrome, 719
    and Pfeiffer syndrome type I, 234
    and primary craniosynostosis, 174
    and Saethre-Chotzen syndrome,
        727–728
Cryoglobins, and mixed
    cryoglobulinemia, *fig. 2*, 5
Cryoglobulinemia, essential mixed, 5
Cryoglobulinemic vasculitis, and Churg-
    Strauss syndrome, 674
Cryopathic hemolytic syndromes, 368
Cryosurgery, and bowenoid papulosis, 98
    and granuloma annulare, 116
    and pars planitis, 657
    and retinoblastoma, 661
    and Von Hippel-Lindau disease, 266
Cryptophthalmos, and Fraser syndrome,
    196–197
Cryptophthalmos-syndactyly syndrome,
    196–197
Cryptophthalmos syndrome, 196–197
Cryptorchidism, and chromosome 3,
        trisomy 3q2, 73–74
    and Lenz microphthalmia syndrome,
        654
    and Rubinstein-Taybi syndrome,
        726–727
Crystalline maculopathies, and Stargardt
    disease, 663
Cumulative trauma disorder, and
        complex regional pain syndrome,
        523
Curly hair-ankyloblepharon-nail
        dysplasia syndrome, and Hay-
        Wells syndrome, 117
Cushing syndrome, 312–313
    and familial partial lipodystrophy,
        323
    and HAIR-AN syndrome, 315–316
Cutaneous capillary vascular
        malformations, and Klippel-
        Trenaunay syndrome, 212
Cutaneous focal mucinosis, and
        scleromyxedema, 136
Cutaneous Hodgkin disease, and
        bowenoid papulosis, 98
Cutaneous lipoatrophy, and congenital
        disorders of glycosylation,
        457–458
Cutaneous lipohypertrophy, and
        congenital disorders of
        glycosylation, 457–458

Cutaneous vasculitis, and Sjögren
        syndrome, 34
Cutaneous venous-like anomalies, and
        Maffucci syndrome, 217–218
Cutis laxa, and De Barsy syndrome, 6
    and pseudoxanthoma elasticum,
        133–134
Cutis marmorata telangiectatica
        congenita, *fig. 8*, 100
Cyanosis, and Eisenmenger syndrome, 47
    and Glut-1 deficiency syndrome, 448
    and idiopathic congenital central
        hypoventilation syndrome, 673
    and Ivemark syndrome, 205
    and malignant hyperthermia, 718
    and persistent truncus arteriosus, 56
Cyclic hematopoiesis, 21–22
Cyclic neutropenia, 21–22
Cyclic vomiting syndrome, 525–526
    and intestinal pseudoobstruction, 347
Cyclitis, and pars planitis, 656–657
Cyclooxygenase inhibitors, and Bartter
        syndrome, 311
Cyclophosphamide, and
        antiphospholipid syndrome, 2
    and autoimmune hemolytic anemia,
        367
    and Behçet disease, 4
    and chronic inflammatory
        demyelinating
        polyradiculoneuropathy, 582
    and Henoch-Schönlein purpura, 415
    and idiopathic thrombocytopenic
        purpura, 415–416
    and large granular lymphocyte
        leukemia, 395
    and mantle cell lymphoma, 399
    and mesenteric panniculitis, 350
    and microscopic polyangiitis, 28
    and mixed cryoglobulinemia
        syndrome, 5
    and opsoclonus-myoclonus syndrome,
        573
    and polyarteritis nodosa, 29
    and posterior uveitis, 666
    and relapsing polychondritis, 30
    and scleroderma, 33
    and Takayasu arteritis, 35
    and Wegener granulomatosis, 423
Cyclosporine, and angioimmunoblastic
        lymphadenopathy-type T-cell
        lymphoma, 398
    and autoimmune hemolytic anemia,
        367
    and Behçet disease, 4

and chronic inflammatory demyelinating polyradiculoneuropathy, 582
and dermatitis herpetiformis, 103
and Erdheim-Chester disease, 441
and hemophagocytic lymphohistiocytosis, 397
and hidradenitis suppurativa, 119
and idiopathic thrombocytopenic purpura, 416
and lichen planus, 125
and microscopic polyangiitis, 28
and pars planitis, 657
and posterior uveitis, 666
and retinoblastoma, 661
and Takayasu arteritis, 35
and Vogt-Koyanagi-Harada syndrome, 37
and warm antibody hemolytic anemia, 371–372
Cyproheptadine, and cyclic vomiting syndrome, 526
Cysteamine, and cystinosis, 683
Cystic dysplasia of the kidneys, and Meckel syndrome, 221
Cystic fibrosis, and alpha 1-antitrypsin deficiency, 671
and biliary atresia, 334
and jejunal atresia, 349
and Johanson-Blizzard syndrome, 208
and lymphangioleiomyomatosis, 395
and primary ciliary dyskinesia, 675
and Shwachman-Diamond syndrome, 417
and sucrase-isomaltase deficiency, 354
Cystic hygroma, 175–176
Cystinosis, 683–684
and oculocerebral syndrome, 226–227
Cystinuria, 684–685
Cystitis, interstitial, 685
Cystoid macular edema, and X-linked juvenile retinoschisis, 662
Cystoperitoneal shunt, and Dandy-Walker syndrome, 526
Cytochrome oxidase deficiency, and congenital lactic acidosis, 462–464
Cytochrome oxidase deficiency, human, 436
Cytomegalovirus, and Guillain-Barré syndrome, 535
and TORCH syndrome, 295
Cytomegalovirus retinitis, and Eales disease, 646
Cytopenia, and large granular lymphocyte leukemia, 394

and Shwachman-Diamond syndrome, 417
Cytoskeletal protein abnormalities, and giant axonal neuropathy, 569
Cytotoxic agents, and antiphospholipid syndrome, 2
and microscopic polyangiitis, 28
Cytoxan, and cicatricial pemphigoid, 131
and warm antibody hemolytic anemia, 371–372

D
D-penicillamine, and cystinuria, 684
Da Silva syndrome, and acrocallosal syndrome (Schinzel type), 145
Dacrocystitis, and Wegener granulomatosis, 422
Dacryosialoadenopathy, 17
Danazol, and autoimmune hemolytic anemia, 367
and idiopathic thrombocytopenic purpura, 416
Danbolt-Closs syndrome, 94
Dancing eyes–dancing feet, 572–573
Dandy-Walker cysts, and corpus callosum absence, 508
Dandy-Walker malformation, and hydrocephalus, 539
and Joubert syndrome, 542
Dandy-Walker syndrome, 526–527
and Arnold-Chiari syndrome, 516
Dantrolene, and malignant hyperthermia, 718
and neuroleptic malignant syndrome, 566
Dapsone, and Behçet disease, 4
and cicatricial pemphigoid, 131
and dermatitis herpetiformis, 103
and Henoch-Schönlein purpura, 415
and malaria, 291
and Melkersson-Rosenthal syndrome, 557
and Mucha-Habermann disease, 129
and pyoderma gangrenosum, 135
and transient acantholytic dermatosis, 104
Darier disease, *fig. 9*, 101
and transient acantholytic dermatosis, 104
Darier-White disease, 101
and PTEN hamartoma tumor syndrome, 240
Davies disease, 47–48
Dawson disease, 574–575
De Barsy-Moens-Dierckx syndrome, 6

De Barsy syndrome, 6
and neonatal progeroid syndrome, 238
de Lange syndrome, 709
De Morsier syndrome, 188–189
De Vivo disease, 448
Deafness, and familial expansile osteolysis, 723–724
and Fountain syndrome, 196
and Jervell and Lange-Nielsen syndrome, 51–52
and Johanson-Blizzard syndrome, 208
and Landau-Kleffner syndrome, 547
and Leber congenital amaurosis, 652
and LEOPARD syndrome, 124–125
and methylmalonic acidemias, 429
and mucolipidosis, 472
and Townes-Brocks syndrome, 262
and Treacher-Collins syndrome, 262–263
and Usher syndrome, 664–665
and Wolfram syndrome, 273
Deafness-retinitis pigmentosa, 664–665
Debrancher enzyme deficiency, and type III glycogen storage disease, 453
Decongestive therapy, and hereditary lymphedema, 396
Deefferented state, 554
Deep hemangioma, and cavernous hemangioma, 117
Deep vein thrombosis, and idiopathic thrombocytosis, 421
Deflazacort, and Duchenne muscular dystrophy, 623
Degos disease, 102
Degos syndrome, 102
Dehydration, and ACTH deficiency, 302
and cyclic vomiting syndrome, 525
and glucose-galactose malabsorption, 343
and multiple carboxylase deficiency, 483
and urea cycle disorders, 506–506
Dehydrogenase deficiency, long-chain acyl-CoA, 437
medium-chain acyl-CoA, 437–438
short-chain acyl-CoA, 438–439
very-long-chain acyl-CoA, 439–440
Dejerine-Roussy syndrome, 593
Dejerine-Sottas disease, and infantile neuroaxonal dystrophy, 634
Dejerine-Sottas syndrome, 521–522, 527–528
and congenital hypomyelination neuropathy, 568
and hereditary sensory neuropathy, 570–571

Delayed bone age, and Laron dwarfism, 319–320

Deletion of chromosome 10p, and DiGeorge syndrome, 178

Deletion of the short arm of chromosome 1, 58

Deletion 5p syndrome, 175

Deletion 9p syndrome, partial, 82–83

Deletion 11q syndrome, 60–61

Deletion 13q syndrome, partial, 62–63

Delirium tremens, and Korsakoff syndrome, 546

Dementia, and adult polyglucosan body disease, 580–581

 and Batten disease, 517

 and Binswanger disease, 519

 and carnosinemia, 435

 and corticobasal degeneration, 524–525

 and Creutzfeldt-Jakob disease, 608

 and Hallervorden-Spatz syndrome, 620

 and Kuf disease, 547

 and MELAS, 469

 and myoclonus, 628

 and progressive supranuclear palsy, 573–574

Demyelinating peripheral neuropathy, and congenital disorders of glycosylation, 457–458

Demyelination, segmental, and POEMS syndrome, 26

Dengue fever, 281

 and leptospirosis, 289

 and Q fever, 293

 and Rift Valley fever, 294

Dengue hemorrhagic fever, 281–282

Dengue shock syndrome, 281

Dental abscesses, and X-linked hypophasphatemic rickets, 326–327

Dental anomalies, and dentin dysplasia, 176–177

 and dentinogenesis imperfecta type III, 177–178

 and familial expansile osteolysis, 723–724

 and Gorlin-Chaudhry-Moss syndrome, 200

 and hypomelanosis of Ito, 119–120

 and Johanson-Blizzard syndrome, 208

 and KBG syndrome, 210

 and Lenz microphthalmia syndrome, 654

 and Nance-Horan syndrome, 654–655

 and neonatal progeroid syndrome, 238

 and Rieger syndrome, 243–244

 and Schinzel syndrome, 246–247

 and tooth agenesis, 261

 and Williams syndrome, 270

Dental caries, and trigeminal neuralgia, 595

Dental discoloration, and congenital erythropoietic porphyria, 492–493

Dental dysplasia, and Singleton-Merten syndrome, 252

Dental enamel, and amelogenesis imperfecta, 149–150

Dental fluorosis, and amelogenesis imperfecta, 149

Dentatorubropallidoluysian atrophy, and Baltic/Mediterranean/Unverrich-Lundborg myoclonic epilepsy, 600

 and Huntington disease, 537

 and MERRF, 469

Dentin dysplasia, 176–177

 and dentinogenesis imperfecta type III, 177

Dentinogenesis imperfecta type III, 177–178

Denys-Drash syndrome, 686

 and Galloway-Mowat syndrome, 687

 and WAGR syndrome, 699

Deoxyspergualin, and polyarteritis nodosa, 29

Depression, and ACTH deficiency, 302

 and Cushing syndrome, 312–313

 and Kleine-Levin syndrome, 544

 and narcolepsy, 562

 and progressive myoclonus epilepsy, 531–532

 and Wilson disease, 506

Dercum disease, 303

Dermal ossification, and progressive osseous heteroplasia, 203–204

Dermatitis, and acrodermatitis enteropathica, 94

 and familial eosinophilic cellulitis, 99

 and Hartnup disease, 458

 and Leiner disease, 123–124

 nonspecific, and Bowen disease, 97

Dermatitis herpetiformis, 103

 and transient acantholytic dermatosis, 104

Dermatoglyphic abnormalities, and Kabuki make-up syndrome, 209–210

Dermatologic abnormalities, and De Barsy syndrome, 6

Dermatologic disorders, 93–140

Dermatomyositis, and limb girdle muscular dystrophy, 625

Dermatosis, and multiple carboxylase deficiency, 483

Dermolytic epidermolysis bullosa, 106–107

DeSactis-Cacchione syndrome, and Cockayne syndrome, 170–171

Desbuquois skeletal dysplasia syndrome, and Catel-Manzke syndrome, 165

Desferrioxamine, and Friedreich ataxia, 602

Desmin myopathy, and limb girdle muscular dystrophy, 625

Desmin-related myopathy, 630–631

Desmopressin, and Bernard-Soulier syndrome, 378

Developmental deficits, and infantile neuroaxonal dystrophy, 634

Developmental delays, and Angelman syndrome, 152–153

 and C syndrome, 162–163

 and and camp[t]omelic syndrome, 706–707

 central core disease, 607–608

 and chromosome 3, trisomy 3q2, 73–74

 and chromosome 4, monosomy distal 4q, 75

 and chromosome 4, monosomy 4q, 74

 and chromosome 4, partial trisomy distal 4q, 76

 and chromosome 4 ring, 76

 and chromosome 9, tetrasomy 9p, 84

 and chromosome 10, monosomy 10p, 60

 and classic lissencephaly, 553–554

 and congenital disorders of glycosylation, 457–458

 and Coffin-Siris syndrome, 708–709

 and cri-du-chat syndrome, 175

 and DiGeorge syndrome, 178–179

 and Dubowitz syndrome, 179–180

 and Duchenne muscular dystrophy, 623

 and familial dysautonomia, 529–530

 and Galloway-Mowat syndrome, 687–688

 and Hartnup disease, 458

 and holoprosencephaly, 536–537

 and homocystinuria, 459

 and isovaleric acidemia, 427

 and Joubert syndrome, 542

 and KBG syndrome, 210

 and Laurence-Moon syndrome, 215

 and Marinesco-Sjögren syndrome, 720–721

 and Menkes disease, 470

and methylmalonic acidemias, 429

and mucolipidosis, 472

and Noonan syndrome, 722–723

and Norrie disease, 656

and oculocerebral syndrome, 226–227

and Pelizaeus-Merzbacher disease, 578

and propionic acidemia, 428

and Ruvalcaba-Myhre-Smith
syndrome, 354

and Sandhoff disease, 497

and Sanfilippo disease, 479

and Schinzel Giedion syndrome, 247

and Scott craniodigital syndrome,
249–250

and Smith-Magenis syndrome, 254

and tuberous sclerosis, 596

and Weaver syndrome, 266–267

Developmental disabilities, and Prader-
Willi syndrome, 237–238

Deviant behavior, and Creutzfeldt-Jakob
disease, 608

Devic disease, 567

Devic syndrome, 560

Dexamethasone, and Camurati-
Engelmann disease, 708

and congenital adrenal hyperplasia,
304

and congenital complete heart block,
50

and hemophagocytic
lymphohistiocytosis, 397

and polycystic ovary syndrome, 324

Dextroamphetamine, and narcolepsy, 562

Dextrocardia, and Poland syndrome,
236–237

and primary ciliary dyskinesia, 675

and situs inversus, 55

DHCR7 gene abnormality, 253

Diabetes, and familial partial
lipodystrophy, 323

and HAIR-AN syndrome, 315–316

and hereditary hemochromatosis,
387–388

Diabetes insipidus, 313–314

and holoprosencephaly, 536

and Loken-Senior syndrome, 692

Diabetes mellitus, and Achard-Thiers
syndrome, 300

and acquired generalized
lipodystrophy, 320–321

and Alström syndrome, 305–306

childhood-onset, and Wolfram
syndrome, 273

and chronic inflammatory
demyelinating
polyradiculoneuropathy, 581

and Eales disease, 646

and Johanson-Blizzard syndrome, 208

and Ménière disease, 558

Diabetes of bearded women, 300

Diabetic neuropathy, and tarsal tunnel
syndrome, 592

Dialysis, and Alport syndrome, 680

and autosomal-recessive polycystic
kidney disease, 697

and congenital hepatic fibrosis, 692

and cystinosis, 683

and Denys-Drash syndrome, 686

and hemolytic-uremic syndrome, 690

and inherited hemolytic-uremic
syndrome, 690–691

and Korsakoff syndrome, 546

and maple syrup urine disease, 468

peritoneal, and Reye syndrome, 31

Diaminodiphenylsulfone, and relapsing
polychondritis, 30

and Sjögren syndrome, 34

Diamond-Blackfan anemia, 365

and Aase syndrome, 143

and acquired pure red cell aplasia, 413

Diaphragm dysfunction, and idiopathic
congenital central hypoventilation
syndrome, 673

Diaphragmatic hernia, and Fryns
syndrome, 715

Diaphragmatic pericardium, and
pentalogy of Cantrell, 233–234

Diaphyseal aclasia, 191

Diaphyseal dysplasia, and Camurati-
Engelmann disease, 707–708

Diarrhea, and abetalipoproteinemia,
358

and aspartylglucosaminuria, 432

bloody, and Wiskott-Aldrich
syndrome, 39

and Chronkhite-Canada syndrome,
338

and eosinophilic gastroenteritis, 342

and giant hypertrophic gastritis, 341

and glucose-galactose malabsorption,
343

and graft-versus-host disease, 11

and hemolytic-uremic syndrome,
689–690

in infancy, and Leiner disease, 123–124

and intestinal lymphangiectasia, 346

and microvillus inclusion disease, 351

and sucrase-isomaltase deficiency, 354

Diastrophic dysplasia, 711–712

Diazepam, and oromandibular dystonia,
615

and stiff person syndrome, 588

Dichloro-methylene-diphosphonate, and
familial expansile osteolysis, 723

Dichloroacetate, and congenital lactic
acidosis, 462

and MELAS, 470

Diencephalic seizure, and
pheochromocytoma, 409

Diencephalic syndrome, 528–529

Difficulty breathing, and cor triatriatum,
46

Diffuse fasciitis, with eosinophilia, and
scleroderma, 33

Diffuse idiopathic skeletal hyperostosis,
9–10

Diffuse Lewy body disease, and
progressive supranuclear palsy, 573

Diffuse osteoporosis, and multiple
myeloma, 407

Diffuse perichondritis, 29–30

Diffuse pulmonary lymphangiomatosis,
and lymphangioleiomyomatosis,
395

DiGeorge sequence, and CHARGE
syndrome, 167

DiGeorge syndrome, 70–71, 178–179

and chromosome 10, monosomy 10p,
60

and chromosome 22 ring, 71

and severe combined
immunodeficiency, 14

Digoxin, and endomyocardial fibrosis, 48

and persistent truncus arteriosus, 56

and primary pulmonary hypertension,
678

Dilantin, and fetal hydantoin syndrome,
192

Dilantin embryopathy, 192

Dilated cardiomyopathy, and Alström
syndrome, 305–306

Dilation and curettage, and triploidy
syndrome, 263–264

Diltiazem, and primary pulmonary
hypertension, 678

Diphenylcyclopropenone, and alopecia
areata, 95

Diphenylhydantoin, and Fabry disease, 442

Diploid-triploid mixoploidy, and Russel-
Silver syndrome, 245–246

Diplopia, and hydrocephalus, 539

and keratoconus, 651

and syringobulbia, 589

Dipyridamole, and Degos disease, 102

Dishface, 186–187

Disodium etidronate, and Fahr disease, 532

and fibrodysplasia ossificans
progressiva, 713

Disseminated epidermal necrosis, and toxic epidermal necrolysis, 139

Distal amyotrophy, and hereditary spastic paraplegia, 575–576

Distal aphalangia, and Yunis-Varaaon syndrome, 275

Distal arthrogryposis, and Freeman-Sheldon syndrome, 714

and Gordon syndrome, 199

Distal duplication 6q, 79

Distal duplication 10q, 59

Distal duplication 15q, 65–66

Distal monosomy 9p, 82–83

Distal trisomy 10q, 59

Distal trisomy 10q syndrome, 59

Distal trisomy 11q, 61–62

Distal trisomy 6q, 79

Diuresis, and primary pulmonary hypertension, 678

Diuretics, and Barth syndrome, 44

and Bartter syndrome, 310–311

and congenital complete heart block, 50

and endomyocardial fibrosis, 48

and intestinal lymphangiectasia, 346

and Ménière disease, 558

and persistent truncus arteriosus, 56

and primary aldosteronism, 305

and pseudotumor cerebri, 582

Divalproex, and Landau-Kleffner syndrome, 548

and progressive myoclonus epilepsy, 531–532

Donath-Landsteiner hemolytic anemia, 388–389

Donohue syndrome, 215–216

Dopa-responsive dystonia, 612

and hereditary spastic paraplegia, 576

and Niemann-Pick disease, 485

Dopamine, and Tourette syndrome, 594

Dopamine agonists, and multiple system atrophy, 561

and myoclonic dystonia, 615

and rapid-onset dystonia-parkinsonism, 618

and X-linked dystonia-parkinsonism, 619

Dopaminergic agents, and restless legs syndrome, 583

Doss porphyria, 491–492

Double-outlet right ventricle, and persistent truncus arteriosus, 56

Double vision, and myasthenia gravis, 626–627

Down syndrome, and chromosome 4, monosomy 4q, 74

and chromosome 9, partial monosomy 9p, 82

and chromosome 18, monosomy 18p, 67

and chromosome 21 ring, 70

and chronic lymphocytic thyroiditis, 329

and Johanson-Blizzard syndrome, 208

and megalocornea, 556

and pentasomy X, 86

and Smith-Magenis syndrome, 254

Doxycycline, and anthrax, 278

and brucellosis, 280

and ehrlichiosis, 283

and leptospirosis, 289

and malaria, 291

and Q fever, 293

Drash syndrome, 686

Drug eruption, and Gianotti-Crosti syndrome, 115

and Mucha-Habermann disease, 129

and transient acantholytic dermatosis, 104

Drug exposure, and Guillain-Barré syndrome, 535

Drug-induced cholestasis, and Dubin-Johnson syndrome, 340

Drug reaction, and familial eosinophilic cellulitis, 99

and Kawasaki disease, 15

and neuroleptic malignant syndrome, 566

Drug toxicity, and encephalitides, 284

and intestinal pseudoobstruction, 348

Drug withdrawal, and narcolepsy, 562

Drummond syndrome, 681

Duane retraction syndrome, 645

Duane syndrome, 645

Dubin-Johnson syndrome, 340

and Crigler-Najjar syndrome, 337

Dubowitz syndrome, 179–180

and blepharophimosis-ptosis-epicanthus inversus syndrome, 641

and Fanconi anemia, 366

and 3-M syndrome, 259

Duchenne muscular dystrophy, 623

and Becker muscular dystrophy, 622

Ductal plate malformation, 691–692

Duhring disease, 103

Duncan disease, 400

Dup (10q) syndrome, 59

Duplication 4p syndrome, 77–78

Duplication 6q, partial, 79

Duroplasty, and syringobulbia, 589

and syringomyelia, 591

Dwarfism, 144, 319–320

and acromesomelic dysplasia, 703–704

and acrosomelic dysplasia, 702–703

and Bloom syndrome, 159–160

and Byler disease, 335

and diastrophic dysplasia, 711

and Dyggve-Melchior-Clausen syndrome, 180–181

and Jansen metaphyseal chondrodysplasia, 206–207

and Kniest dysplasia, 213

and Leri pleonosteosis, 216–217

and megalocornea, 556

and MULIBREY nanism, 224–225

and pyknodysostosis, 242

and spondyloepiphyseal dysplasia congenita, 728

and 3-M syndrome, 259

Dwyer osteotomy, and Singleton-Merten syndrome, 252

Dyggve-Melchior-Clausen syndrome, 180–181

Dysarthria, and Friedreich ataxia, 602–603

and myasthenia gravis, 627

and Pelizaeus-Merzbacher disease, 578

and primary lateral sclerosis, 548

Dysautonomia, familial, 529–530

and hereditary sensory neuropathy, 570

Dysbetalipoproteinemia, familial, 440

Dyscephaly, and Hallermann-Streiff syndrome, 202

Dyschondrosteosis, 181–182

Dysencephalia splanchnocystica, 221

Dysentery, and anthrax, 278

Dysfibrinogenemia, and congenital afibrogenemia, 359–360

and Glanzmann thrombasthenia, 383

Dysgenetic male pseudohermaphroditism, and partial androgen insensitivity syndrome, 307–308

Dyshydrotic eczema, and epidermolytic epidermolysis bullosa, 108

Dyskeratosis congenita, 104–105

and acquired agranulocytosis, 361

and Fanconi anemia, 366

Dyskeratosis follicularis, 101

Dyskinesia, and myoclonus, 628

paroxysmal, 616–617

Dyslipidemia, and familial partial lipodystrophy, 323

Dysmorphic disorders, 141–275

Dysmorphic facial features, and chromosome 5, trisomy 5p, 78

Dysmorphic features, and peroxisomal biogenesis disorders, 487

Dysmorphic pinna–hypospadias–renal dysplasia, and brachio-oto-renal syndrome, 681–682

Dysmorphism, and Neu-Laxova syndrome, 563

Dysmyelinogenic leukodystrophy, 510–511

Dyspepsia, and eosinophilic gastroenteritis, 342

Dysphagia, and Barrett esophagus, 333
    and diffuse idiopathic skeletal hyperostosis, 10
    and inclusion body myositis, 631
    and leukodystrophy, 550
    and myasthenia gravis, 627
    and primary lateral sclerosis, 548
    and syringobulbia, 589

Dysphonia, and recurrent respiratory papillomatosis, 676
    and syringobulbia, 589

Dysplasia, cleidocranial, 182
    craniofrontonasal, 183
    craniometaphyseal, 184
    ectodermal, 185
    fibrous, and Ollier disease, 23–24
    maxillonasal, 186–187
    metatropic, 20
    multiple epiphyseal, 187–188
    septooptic, 188–189

Dysplasia epiphysealis hemimelica, 186

Dysplastic mole, and melanoma, 405

Dyspnea, and alpha 1-antitrypsin deficiency, 671
    and atrial septal defects, 43
    and lymphangioleiomyomatosis, 395
    and lymphomatoid granulomatosis, 48
    and primary pulmonary hypertension, 678
    and pulmonary alveolar proteinosis, 677

Dystonia, 609–619
    cervical, 611
    dopa-responsive, 612
    embouchure, 613
    and episodic ataxia, 600–601
    and glutaric acidemia type I, 426
    laryngeal, 613–614
    and Lesch-Nyhan syndrome, 464–465
    laryngeal, 613–614
    and neuroacanthocytosis, 633–634
    oromandibular, 615–616
    paroxysmal, 616–617
    and stiff person syndrome, 588
    and tardive dyskinesia, 591

and Tourette syndrome, 594

Dystonia-parkinsonism, rapid-onset, 617–618
    X-linked, 619

Dystonic gait, and dopa-responsive dystonia, 612

Dystonic posturing, and Hallervorden-Spatz syndrome, 620

Dystosis multiplex, and sialidosis, 498

Dystrophic epidermolysis bullosa, 106–107

Dystrophic epidermolysis bullosa, recessive, *fig. 10*, 106–107

Dystrophinopathy, 622–623

E

Eales disease, 646

Ear, nose, and throat disorders, and DiGeorge syndrome, 178–179

Ear abnormalities, and CHARGE syndrome, 167–168
    and Laband syndrome, 214
    and Miller syndrome, 222–223
    and Nager syndrome, 226
    and Townes-Brocks syndrome, 262
    and Treacher-Collins syndrome, 262–263

Ear cartilage, and relapsing polychondritis, 29

Ear infections, and Hunter disease, 478–479
    and Hurler disease, 477
    and Wiskott-Aldrich syndrome, 39

Ear–patella–short stature syndrome, 189

Ear pinna swelling, and diastrophic dysplasia, 711

Ear pits-deafness syndrome, 681–682

Early amnion rupture sequence, 150–151

Early amnion rupture spectrum, 150–151

Early repolarization syndrome, and Brugada syndrome, 45

Eaton-Lambert syndrome, 621

Ebola, 282
    and Rift Valley fever, 294

Ectodermal abnormalities, and cardiofaciocutaneous syndrome, 163–164
    and Yunis-Varaaon syndrome, 275

Ectodermal dysplasia, 185
    and dyskeratosis congenita, 104–105
    and tooth agenesis, 261

Ectopia cordis, and pentalogy of Cantrell, 233–234

Ectopia vesicae, 686–687

Ectopic kidney, and bilateral renal agenesis, 698

Ectrodactyly, 256

Ectrodactyly-ectodermal dysplasia-clefting, 185

Ectropion uveae, and Cogan-Reese syndrome, 644

Eczema, and Dubowitz syndrome, 179–180
    and hyper-IgE syndrome, 12–13
    and phenylketonuria, 488
    severe atopic, and Wiskott-Aldrich syndrome, 38–39

Eczematous dermatitis, and mycosis fungoides, 406

Edema, and endomyocardial fibrosis, 48
    and hepatorenal syndrome, 344
    and intestinal lymphangiectasia, 346
    and Neu-Laxova syndrome, 562–563

Edward syndrome, and chromosome 18, monosomy 18p, 67

Edwards syndrome, 88

Ehlers-Danlos syndrome, and acrogeria (Gottron type), 147
    and alpha 1-antitrypsin deficiency, 671
    and medullary sponge kidney, 694
    and progeria, 724
    and Takayasu arteritis, 35
    and Weill-Marchesani syndrome, 267–268

Ehrlichia infection, 283

Ehrlichiosis, 283

8p deletion syndrome (partial), 81–82

8p- syndrome (partial), 81–82

18q- syndrome, 67–68

Eisenmenger reaction or complex, 46–47

Eisenmenger syndrome, 46–47

Ekborn syndrome, 583

Ekman-Lobstein disease, 227–228

Elastosis perforans serpiginosa, and granuloma annulare, 116

Elbow contractures, and Emery-Dreifuss muscular dystrophy, 624

Electrocardiograph conduction abnormalities, and LEOPARD syndrome, 124–125

Electroconvulsive therapy, and neuroleptic malignant syndrome, 566

Electrodessication, and bowenoid papulosis, 98

Elejalde syndrome, and Marshall-Smith syndrome, 219

11-β hydroxylase deficiency, and congenital adrenal hyperplasia, 304

11p deletions, and Russel-Silver syndrome, 245–246

11q partial trisomy, 61–62

11q syndrome, partial, 60–61

Ellis-van Creveld syndrome, and Meckel syndrome, 221

Emaciation, and diencephalic syndrome, 528–529

Embolism, and congenital antithrombin III deficiency, 376–377

Embolization, and brain arteriovenous malformations, 596

and Parkes-Weber syndrome, 232

and Wyburn-Mason syndrome, 667

Embouchure dystonia, 613

Embryonal tumors, and Simpson dysmorphia syndrome, 251

Emerging/infectious diseases, 277–298

Emery-Dreifuss muscular dystrophy, 624

Emotional lability, and Sydenham chorea, 522

Emphysema, and alpha 1-antitrypsin deficiency, 671

and lymphangioleiomyomatosis, 395

Empty sella syndrome, and Achard-Thiers syndrome, 300

and MULIBREY nanism, 224–225

primary, 530

Enamel hypoplasia, and amelogenesis imperfecta, 149

Encephalitides, 284–285

and galactosemia, 446

and West Nile fever, 296

Encephaloceles, and corpus callosum absence, 508

Encephalocraniocutaneous lipomatosis, 239

Encephalomyelitis, and stiff person syndrome, 588

Encephalopathy, and carnitine deficiency syndromes, 432

and opsoclonus-myoclonus syndrome, 572–573

and Reye syndrome, 31

and urea cycle disorders, 506–506

Enchondromas, and Maffucci syndrome, 217–218

Enchondromatosis, 23–24, 217–218

and familial expansile osteolysis, 723

and Proteus syndrome, 239

End-stage renal disease, and Alport syndrome, 680

and cystinosis, 683

and cystinuria, 684

Endocardial cushion defects, 43

Endocardial fibroelastosis, 44

Endocrine disorders, 299–330

Endocrinopathy, and POEMS syndrome, 26–27

Endogenous hypertriglyceridemia, 460

Endolymphatic hydrops, 558

Endometrial cancer, and Lynch syndromes, 401

Endometrial polyps, and Asherman syndrome, 308–309

Endometrial tumors, and PTEN hamartoma tumor syndrome, 240

Endometriosis, and interstitial cystitis, 685

Endomyocardial fibrosis, 47–48

Endosteal hyperostosis, 204–205, 248–249

Enteroviral diseases, and ehrlichiosis, 283

Enteroviruses, and West Nile fever, 296

Enthesopathy, and X-linked hypophasphatemic rickets, 326–327

Entrapment neuropathy, and tarsal tunnel syndrome, 592

Enucleation, and retinoblastoma, 661

Enuresis, and diabetes insipidus, 313–314

and medullary cystic kidney disease, 693

Enzyme deficiency, and autoimmune hemolytic anemia, 367

and congenital nonspherocytic hemolytic anemia, 369

Enzyme replacement therapy, and Gaucher disease, 447

Eosinophilia, and Churg-Strauss syndrome, 674

and hypersensitivity myocarditis, 53

Eosinophilia-myalgia syndrome, 7

and eosinophilic fasciitis, 8

and scleroderma, 33

Eosinophilic fasciitis, 8

and eosinophilia-myalgia syndrome, 7

Eosinophilic gastroenteritis, 342

and Churg-Strauss syndrome, 674

Eosinophilic granuloma, 392–393

and eosinophilic gastroenteritis, 342

and lymphangioleiomyomatosis, 395

Epibulbar dermoids, and Duane syndrome, 645

and Goldenhar syndrome, 716

Epidermal nevus, and Darier disease, 101

Epidermal nevus syndrome, 105–106

Epidermodysplasia verruciformis, and Darier disease, 101

Epidermolysis bullosa, and acrodermatitis enteropathica, 94

acquisita, and bullous pemphigoid, 130–131

and cicatricial pemphigoid, 131

and aplasia cutis congenita, 96

atrophicans, 107–108

dystrophic, 106–107

and epidermolytic hyperkeratosis, 109

and Hay-Wells syndrome, 116

and incontinentia pigmenti, 121

junctional, 107–108

letalis, 107–108

and McGrath syndrome, 127

simplex, 108–109

Weber-Cockayne variant, *fig. 12*, 108–109

Epidermolytic epidermolysis bullosa, 108–109

Epidermolytic hyperkeratosis, 109–110

Epididymal lesions, and Von Hippel-Lindau disease, 266

Epidural infection, and syringomyelia, 590

Epigastric distention, and jejunal atresia, 349

Epigastric pain, and giant hypertrophic gastritis, 341

Epilepsy, and Alpers syndrome, 512

Baltic/Mediterranean/Unverrich-Lundborg myoclonic, 600

and Borjeson-Forssman-Lehmann syndrome, 705–706

and corpus callosum absence, 508

and epidermal nevus syndrome, 106

and Glut-1 deficiency syndrome, 448

and hyperekplexia, 540

and Korsakoff syndrome, 546

and Laband syndrome, 214

and Landau-Kleffner syndrome, 547

and Lennox-Gastaut syndrome, 549–550

and narcolepsy, 562

progressive myoclonus, 531–532

and Romano-Ward long QT syndrome, 54

and Sturge-Weber syndrome, 258

Epileptic encephalopathy, and succinic semialdehyde dehydrogenase deficiency, 499

Epinephrine, and mastocytosis, 402

Epiphyseal arrest, and Parkes-Weber syndrome, 232

Episkopi blindness, 655–656

Episodic ataxia type I, 600–601

Episodic ataxia type II, 601–602

Epistaxis, and Bernard-Soulier syndrome, 378

and congenital afibrogenemia, 359–360

and Glanzmann thrombasthenia, 383

and hereditary hemorrhagic telangiectasia, 418

Epithelial odontogenic tumors, and ameloblastoma, 363

Epitheliopathy, acute posterior multifocal placoid pigment, 642

Epoendyoma, and medulloblastoma, 404–405

Epoprostenol, and primary pulmonary hypertension, 678

Epstein anomaly, and chromosome 11, partial trisomy 11q, 61

Epstein-Barr virus, and Guillain-Barré syndrome, 535

and lymphomatoid granulomatosis, 48–49

and X-linked lymphoproliferative syndrome, 400

Epstein syndrome, and May-Hegglin anomaly, 403

Equine antitoxin, and botulism, 279

Erb-Duchenne paralysis, and obstetric brachial plexus palsy, 571

Erdheim-Chester disease, 441

Erectile dysfunction, and multiple system atrophy, 561

Ergotism, and Takayasu arteritis, 35

Eruptive xanthomas, and pseudoxanthoma elasticum, 133–134

Erysipelas, 285

Erysipeloid, and erysipelas, 285

Erythema, and epidermolytic hyperkeratosis, 109–110

and pityriasis rubra pilaris, 133

Erythema annulare centrifugum, and granuloma annulare, 116

Erythema elevatum et diutinum, and Sweet syndrome, 138

Erythema multiforme, *figs. 13–16*, 110–111

and bullous pemphigoid, 130–131

and Mucha-Habermann disease, 129

and Sweet syndrome, 138

Erythema multiforme major, and toxic epidermal necrolysis, 139

Erythema nodosum, and Sweet syndrome, 138

Erythermalgia, 113–114

Erythralgia, 113–114

Erythrocytosis, and polycythemia vera, 411–412

Erythrocytospheresis, and warm antibody hemolytic anemia, 371–372

Erythroderma, and Leiner disease, 123–124

Erythrodermic psoriasis, and ichthyosis, 120

Erythrogenesis imperfecta, 365

Erythroid hypoplasia, 365

Erythroid-specific 5-aminolevulinate synthase deficiency, and X-linked sideroblastic anemia, 373

Erythrokeratodermia, progressive symmetric, 111–112

Erythrokeratodermia figurata variabilis mendes de costa, 112–113

Erythrokeratodermia progressiva symmetrica, 111–112

Erythrokeratodermia variabilis, *fig. 17*, 112–113

and progressive symmetric erythrokeratodermia, 111

Erythrokeratolysis hiemalis, and erythrokeratodermia variabilis, 112

Erythromelalgia, 113–114

and Fabry disease, 442

Erythromycin, and leptospirosis, 289

and Q fever, 293

Erythropoietic protoporphyria, 495–496

Escobar syndrome, 241

and popliteal pterygium syndrome, 242

Esophageal adenocarcinoma, and Barrett esophagus, 333

Esophageal atresia, 190

Esophageal dysmotility, and idiopathic congenital central hypoventilation syndrome, 673

Esophagitis, and Zollinger-Ellison syndrome, 330

Essential iris atrophy, 650

Essential thrombocythemia, 420–421

Essential thrombocytosis, 420–421

Essential tremor, and laryngeal dystonia, 613–614

and Parkinson disease, 576

and Wilson disease, 506

Estradiol, and septooptic dysplasia, 188–189

Estren-Dameshek anemia, 366

Estrogen, and true hermaphroditism, 316–317

Estrogen deficiency, and autoimmune premature ovarian failure, 30–31

Estrogen hormones, and Fox-Fordyce disease, 114

Estrogen therapy, and lichen sclerosis, 126

and Turner syndrome, 264

Ethosuximide, and Landau-Kleffner syndrome, 548

Ethylmalonic aciduria, and short-chain acyl-CoA dehydrogenase deficiency, 438–439

Etoposide, and hemophagocytic lymphohistiocytosis, 397

Etretinate, and bowenoid papulosis, 98

and pityriasis rubra pilaris, 133

Ewing sarcoma, and Langerhans cell histiocytosis, 392

of bone, 380–381

Ewing tumor, 380–381

Exanthema, nonspecific, and Kawasaki disease, 15

Exanthematous disease, and Q fever, 293

Exchange transfusion, and kernicterus, 543

and Reye syndrome, 31

Exercise intolerance, and type V glycogen storage disease, 454–455

and type VII glycogen storage disease, 456–457

Exfoliative dermatitis, and pityriasis rubra pilaris, 133

Exogenous gonadotropin, and polycystic ovary syndrome, 324

Exogenous sex steroid exposure, and precocious puberty, 324

Exomphalos-macroglossia-gigantism syndrome, 518

Exophthalmos, and Camurati-Engelmann disease, 707–708

Exostoses, multiple hereditary, 191

Exstrophy, 686–687

Extra digits, and Pallister-Hall syndrome, 230

Extracorporeal membrane oxygenation, and hantavirus pulmonary syndrome, 287

Extramedullary hematopoiesis, and polycythemia vera, 411–412

Extranodal NK/T-cell lymphoma, and lymphomatoid granulomatosis, 48

Extrapyramidal dysfunction, and Hallervorden-Spatz syndrome, 620

Extrapyramidal movement disorder, and glutaric acidemia type I, 426

Exudative retinopathy, 643

Exudativum, and toxic epidermal necrolysis, 139

Eye movement disorders, and locked-in syndrome, 554

F

Fabry disease, 442

and fucosidosis, 445

Facial abnormalities, and Aarskog
        syndrome, 142
    and acrodysostosis, 146
    and Alagille syndrome, 332
    and Allan-Herndon-Dudley syndrome,
        149
    and camp[t]omelic syndrome,
        706–707
    and cat eye syndrome, 164–165
    and Coffin-Lowry syndrome, 171–172
    and Coffin-Siris syndrome, 708–709
    and cri-du-chat syndrome, 175
    and DiGeorge syndrome, 178–179
    and femoral hypoplasia–unusual facies
        syndrome, 712–713
    and fetal valproate syndrome, 192–193
    and FG syndrome, 193–194
    and Filippi syndrome, 194–195
    and floating harbor syndrome, 195
    and Fountain syndrome, 196
    and Fraser syndrome, 196–197
    and Freeman-Sheldon syndrome, 714
    and GBBB syndrome, 198–199
    and Marshall-Smith syndrome, 219
    and maxillonasal dysplasia, 186–187
    and Melnick-Needles syndrome,
        221–222
    and multiple pterygium syndrome, 241
    and Myhre syndrome, 225
    and Nance-Horan syndrome, 654–655
    and neonatal progeroid syndrome, 238
    and Noonan syndrome, 722–723
    and oto-palato-digital syndrome, 229
    and Pallister-Killian syndrome, 231
    and Pfeiffer syndrome type I, 234–235
    and Prader-Willi syndrome, 237–238
    and progeria, 724
    and Rieger syndrome, 243–244
    and Robinow syndrome, 725–726
    and Schinzel Giedion syndrome, 247
    and Schwartz-Jampel syndrome,
        586–587
    and sclerosteosis, 248–249
    and Setleis syndrome, 137
    and SHORT syndrome, 250
    and Simpson dysmorphia syndrome,
        251
    and 3-M syndrome, 259
    and Williams syndrome, 270
Facial coarsening, and Fryns syndrome,
        715
    and fucosidosis, 445
    and mucolipidosis, 472
    and multiple sulfatase deficiency, 484
Facial dysmorphism, and maternal
        phenylketonuria, 489

Facial ectodermal dysplasia, and aplasia
        cutis congenita, 96
Facial edema, and hereditary
        angioedema, 375
Facial erythema, and Bloom syndrome,
        159–160
Facial-genito-popliteal syndrome, 242
Facial gestalt, and Russel-Silver
        syndrome, 245–246
Facial grimacing, and tardive dyskinesia,
        591
Facial pain, and trigeminal neuralgia, 595
Facial palsy, and aplasia cutis congenita,
        96
    and syringobulbia, 589
Facial paralysis, and Camurati-
        Engelmann disease, 707–708
    and Melkersson-Rosenthal syndrome,
        557
Facies, immobile, and Marden-Walker
        syndrome, 18
Faciodigitogenital syndrome, 142
Faciogenital dysplasia, 142
Faciolabial edema, and Melkersson-
        Rosenthal syndrome, 557
Facioscapulohumeral muscular
        dystrophy, 624–625
Factitious hypoglycemia, and pancreatic
        islet cell tumors, 408–409
Factor IX deficiency, 381–382
    and Glanzmann thrombasthenia, 383
Factor XII deficiency, 382–383
Fahr disease, *fig. 52*, 532
Failure to thrive, and acrodermatitis
        enteropathica, 94
    and blue diaper syndrome, 681
    and Bowen-Conradi syndrome, 161
    and Byler disease, 335
    and cardiofaciocutaneous syndrome,
        163–164
    and carnitine deficiency syndromes,
        432
    and cor triatriatum, 46
    and corpus callosum absence, 508
    and cri-du-chat syndrome, 175
    and diencephalic syndrome, 528–529
    and familial dysautonomia, 529–530
    and FG syndrome, 193–194
    and hydrocephalus, 539
    and idiopathic neonatal hepatitis, 288
    and isovaleric acidemia, 427
    and Leiner disease, 123–124
    and maple syrup urine disease, 468
    and Marshall-Smith syndrome, 219
    and medullary cystic kidney disease,
        693

    and methylmalonic acidemias, 429
    and Niemann-Pick disease, 485
    and propionic acidemia, 428
    and short-chain acyl-CoA
        dehydrogenase deficiency, 438–439
    and thalassemia major, 419
Faintness on standing, and multiple
        system atrophy, 561
Fairbank syndrome, 187–188
Falling episodes, and Duchenne muscular
        dystrophy, 623
    and hyperekplexia, 540
    and inclusion body myositis, 631
Familial adenomatous polyposis,
        352–353
Familial articular chondrocalcinosis,
        169–170
Familial cutaneous-mucosal venous
        malformation, and Maffucci
        syndrome, 217
Familial dysautonomia, 529–530
    and pheochromocytoma, 409
Familial dysbetalipoproteinemia, 440
Familial ectopia lentis, and Marfan
        syndrome, 218
Familial eosinophilic cellulitis, 99
Familial erythrophagocytic
        lymphohistiocytosis, 397–398
Familial expansile osteolysis, 723–724
Familial glomuvenous malformations,
        and Maffucci syndrome, 217
Familial hamartomatous polyposis,
        351–352
Familial hemophagocytic
        lymphohistiocytosis, 397–398
Familial high-density lipoprotein
        deficiency, 500
Familial holoprosencephaly, and Pallister-
        Hall syndrome, 230
Familial hypophosphatemia, and
        hypophosphatasia, 317–318
Familial jaundice, 337
Familial juvenile hyperuricemic
        nephropathy, 696
Familial lipomatosis syndrome, and
        adiposis dolorosa, 303
Familial lipoprotein lipase deficiency,
        465–466
Familial Mediterranean fever, 19
Familial partial lipodystrophy, 323
Familial thoracic aortic aneurysm, and
        Marfan syndrome, 218
Familial visceral myopathy, and small
        bowel diverticulosis, 339
Familial visceral neuropathy, and small
        bowel diverticulosis, 339

Familial Wells syndrome, 99

Fanconi anemia, 366
  and Aase syndrome, 143
  and acquired agranulocytosis, 361
  and acquired aplastic anemia, 364
  and Diamond-Blackfan anemia, 365
  and dyskeratosis congenita, 104–105
  and Rothmund-Thomson syndrome, 135

Fanconi pancytopenia, 366
  and Baller-Gerold syndrome, 157

Fanconi syndrome, and cystinosis, 683
  and Dubowitz syndrome, 179–180
  and thrombocytopenia and absent radius syndrome, 260
  and X-linked hypophasphatemic rickets, 326–327

Farber disease, 443
  and Winchester syndrome, 271

Farber lipogranulomatosis, 443

Faschiola infection, and liver fluke disease, 286

Faschioliasis, 286

Fasciculations, and adult polyglucosan body disease, 580
  and spinal bulbar muscular atrophy, 636

Fasciitis, diffuse, with eosinophilia, 8
  eosinophilic, 8
  and erysipelas, 285

Fasciolosis, 286

Fat loss, and acquired partial lipodystrophy, 321
  and congenital generalized lipodystrophy, 322
  and familial partial lipodystrophy, 323

Fat malabsorption, and abetalipoproteinemia, 358
  and chylomicron retention disease, 380

Fat-soluble vitamins, and abetalipoproteinemia, 358
  and Alagille syndrome, 332
  and biliary atresia, 334
  and Byler disease, 335
  and idiopathic neonatal hepatitis, 288
  and Shwachman-Diamond syndrome, 417

Fatty acid oxidation defects, and carnitine deficiency syndromes, 432
  and urea cycle disorders, 506–506

Fatty acid oxidation disorders, and cyclic vomiting syndrome, 525

Fatty degeneration, and mesenteric panniculitis, 350
  and Reye syndrome, 31

Fatty liver, and congenital generalized lipodystrophy, 322

Fatty tissue overgrowth, and Proteus syndrome, 239

FBN2 gene, and congenital contractual arachnodactyly, 3

Fechtner syndrome, and May-Hegglin anomaly, 403

Feeding difficulties, and chromosome 4, trisomy 4p, 77–78
  and chromosome 22q11 deletion spectrum, 70

Feet, absence of, and acheiropodia, 702

Felbamate, and Landau-Kleffner syndrome, 548
  and Lennox-Gastaut syndrome, 550

Felty syndrome, 8–9

Feminization, and androgen insensitivity syndrome, 306–307

Feminization syndromes, and androgen insensitivity syndrome, 306

Femoral-facial syndrome, 712–713

Femoral hypoplasia–unusual facies syndrome, 712–713
  and multiple pterygium syndrome, 241

Fetal akinesia sequence, and multiple pterygium syndrome, 241
  and trisomy 18 syndrome, 88

Fetal akinesia syndrome, and Neu-Laxova syndrome, 562

Fetal alcohol syndrome, and Cornelia de Lange syndrome, 709
  and fetal hydantoin syndrome, 192
  and maternal phenylketonuria, 489
  and Pierre Robin sequence, 235–236
  and 3-M syndrome, 259
  and Williams syndrome, 270

Fetal hydantoin syndrome, 192

Fetal loss, and antiphospholipid syndrome, 2
  and bilateral renal agenesis, 698

Fetal membrane rupture, and amniotic bands, 150–151

Fetal rubella syndrome, and Usher syndrome, 665

Fetal valproate syndrome, 192–193

Fetal warfarin syndrome, and maxillonasal dysplasia, 186–187

Fetofetal transfusion, 421–422

Fever of unknown origin, and ectodermal dysplasia, 185
  and hemophagocytic lymphohistiocytosis, 397
  and malignant hyperthermia, 718

Fevers, 277–298
  and Churg-Strauss syndrome, 674

and hemophagocytic lymphohistiocytosis, 397
  and neuroleptic malignant syndrome, 566
  and pulmonary alveolar proteinosis, 677

Fexofenadine, and transient acantholytic dermatosis, 104

FG syndrome, 193–194

Fiber-type atrophy, 629–630

Fibrinogen deficiency, and congenital afibrogenemia, 359–360

Fibrinoid leukodystrophy, 510–511

Fibrodysplasia ossificans progressiva, 713–714
  and progressive osseous heteroplasia, 203

Fibroids, and Asherman syndrome, 308–309

Fibromuscular dysplasia, and moyamoya syndrome, 559
  and Takayasu arteritis, 35

Fibromyalgia, and complex regional pain syndrome, 523
  and eosinophilia-myalgia syndrome, 7

Fibrosis, and Erdheim-Chester disease, 441
  and scleroderma, 33–34

Filippi syndrome, 194–195
  and Scott craniodigital syndrome, 249–250

Filoviridae infection, 282

Finger clubbing, and pachydermoperiostosis, 129–130

Finger contractures, and central core disease, 607–608

Finger deformities, and chromosome 15, distal trisomy 15q, 65–66
  and Miller syndrome, 222–223
  and oto-palato-digital syndrome, 229
  and popliteal pterygium syndrome, 242

Finger webbing, and Scott craniodigital syndrome, 249–250

Fish eye disease, and Tangier disease, 500

Fish-odor syndrome, 503

5 fluorouracil, and bowenoid papulosis, 98

5-oxoprolinuria, and glutathione synthetase deficiency, 449

5α-reductase 2 deficiency, and partial androgen insensitivity, 307

5α-reductase deficiency, and true hermaphroditism, 316–317

5p minus syndrome, 175

Flat facial hemangiomata, 258

Flaviviridae infection, 282

Flecainide, and Romano-Ward long QT syndrome, 54

Flecked retina of Kandori, and Stargardt disease, 663

Fleischer ring, and keratoconus, 651

Flexion contractures, and arthrogryposis multiplex congenita, 155

Flexion deformities, and Neu-Laxova syndrome, 562–563

Floaters, and Eales disease, 646
  and pars planitis, 656–657
  and posterior uveitis, 666

Floating harbor syndrome, 195
  and 3-M syndrome, 259

Fludrocortisone, and congenital adrenal hyperplasia, 304
  and multiple system atrophy, 561

Flunarizine, and alternating hemiplegia of childhood, 513

Fluoxetine, and Kluver-Bucy syndrome, 545
  and narcolepsy, 562

Flurandrenolone, and lichen planus, 125

Focal dermal hypoplasia, and incontinentia pigmenti, 121

Focal facial dermal dysplasia, and aplasia cutis congenita, 96

Focal facial dermal dysplasia syndrome, and Setleis syndrome, 137

Folic acid, and sickle cell anemia, 372–373

Folic acid replacement, and congenital nonspherocytic hemolytic anemia, 369
  and hereditary spherocytosis, 370–371

Follicular indolent lymphoma, and mantle cell lymphoma, 399

Follicular mucinosis, and alopecia areata, 95
  and scleromyxedema, 136

Folliculitis, and alopecia areata, 95
  and transient acantholytic dermatosis, 104

Fong disease, 721–722

Food-borne bacteria, and listeriosis, 290

Foot deformities, and Apert syndrome, 154–155
  and Bowen-Conradi syndrome, 161
  and Charcot-Marie-Tooth Polyneuropathy syndrome, 521–522
  and chromosome 4, trisomy 4p, 77–78
  and chromosome 7, monosomy 7p2, 80–81

and chromosome 9, partial monosomy 9p, 82

and chromosome 9, trisomy 9p, 85

and chromosome 10, distal trisomy 10q, 59

and Jackson-Weiss syndrome, 719

and Laband syndrome, 214

and split hand/split foot malformation, 256

and Townes-Brocks syndrome, 262

and trisomy 18 syndrome, 88

and Weill-Marchesani syndrome, 267–268

Foot pain, and erythromelalgia, 113
  and hereditary sensory neuropathy, 570
  and navicular osteochondritis, 21
  and tarsal tunnel syndrome, 592
  and thromboangiitis obliterans, 36

Forbes disease, 453

Forceps marks syndrome, 137

Forebrain underdevelopment, and septooptic dysplasia, 188–189

Forehead hemangioma, and diastrophic dysplasia, 711

Forestier disease, 9–10

Fort Bragg fever, 289

49,XXXXX syndrome, 86–87
  and pentasomy X, 86

Foscarnet, and encephalitides, 284

Fountain syndrome, 196

4-Hydroxybuturic aciduria, 499

Foveal atrophy, and Stargardt disease, 663

Foveal schisis, and X-linked juvenile retinoschisis, 662

Foveolar hyperplasia, and giant hypertrophic gastritis, 341

Fox-Fordyce disease, 114

Fragile X chromosome, and Sotos syndrome, 255

Fragile X syndrome, and Angelman syndrome, 152–153
  and FG syndrome, 193–194
  and Prader-Willi syndrome, 237–238
  and Smith-Magenis syndrome, 254
  and triple X syndrome, 89
  and XYY syndrome, 90

Fraiser syndrome, and Denys-Drash syndrome, 686

Franceschetti-Jadassohn syndrome, 121

Franceschetti-Klein syndrome, 262–263

François syndrome, 202

Fraser cryptophthalmos syndrome, 196–197

Fraser syndrome, 196–197

Freckling, and neurofibromatosis type I, 563–564

Fredrickson type IV hyperlipidemia, 460

Freeman-Sheldon syndrome, 714–715
  and Gordon syndrome, 199
  and Marden-Walker syndrome, 18

Frey-Baillarger syndrome, 533

Frey syndrome, 533

Friedreich ataxia, 602–603
  and ataxia-telangiectasia, 605–606
  and ataxia with vitamin E deficiency, 606–607
  and giant axonal neuropathy, 569
  and Huntington disease, 537
  and Machado-Joseph disease, 555
  and Refsum disease, 604–605

Froehlich syndrome, and Prader-Willi syndrome, 237–238

Frontofacionasal dysostosis, and craniofrontonasal syndrome, 183

Frontometaphyseal dysplasia, and craniometaphyseal dysplasia, 184

Frontonasal dysplasia, and craniofrontonasal syndrome, 183

Frontotemporal dementia, 533–534
  and Binswanger disease, 519
  and progressive supranuclear palsy, 573

Fructose-1,6-diphosphatase deficiency, and PEPCK deficiency, 486

Fructose intolerance, hereditary, 444
  and idiopathic neonatal hepatitis, 288

Fructosemia, 444

Fructosuria, 444–445

Fryns syndrome, 715–716
  and Pallister-Killian syndrome, 231

Fucosidosis, 445–446
  and Fabry disease, 442

Fugue states, and narcolepsy, 562

Fukuyama muscular dystrophy, and Walker-Warburg syndrome, 597

Fumarylacetoacetase deficiency, 504

Functional GnRH deficiency, and Kallmann syndrome, 318

Functionally univentricular anomalies, and persistent truncus arteriosus, 56

Functioning argentaffinoma, 311–312

Functioning carcinoid, 311–312

Fundus albipunctatus, and Stargardt disease, 663

Fundus flavimaculatus, 663

Fungal infections, and chronic granulomatous disease, 386–387
  and encephalitides, 284
  and Felty syndrome, 8–9

and giant hypertrophic gastritis, 341
and sarcoidosis, 32
and Wegener granulomatosis, 422

G

G syndrome, 198–199
GABA agonists, and hyperekplexia, 540
and Santavuori disease, 585–586
Gabapentin, and hereditary sensory
neuropathy, 570
and spinal muscular atrophy, 637
and thalamic pain syndrome, 593
Gait abnormalities, and stiff person
syndrome, 588–589
Gait apraxia, and Rett syndrome, 584
Gait ataxia, and Friedreich ataxia,
602–603
Gait disturbances, and Binswanger
disease, 519
and Charcot-Marie-Tooth
Polyneuropathy syndrome,
521–522
and Dandy-Walker syndrome, 526
and giant axonal neuropathy, 569
and hereditary spastic paraplegia, 576
and sialidosis, 498
Galactocerebrosidase deficiency, and
leukodystrophy, 551–552
Galactose-1 phosphate accumulation,
and galactosemia, 446
Galactosemia, 446
and biliary atresia, 334
and congenital disorders of
glycosylation, 457
and hereditary fructose intolerance, 444
and idiopathic neonatal hepatitis, 288
and phenylketonuria, 488
Galactosialidosis, and sialidosis, 498
Galactosylceramide lipidosis, 551–552
Galloway-Mowat syndrome, 687–688
Gallstones, and hereditary spherocytosis,
370–371
Gamma-hydroxybuterate, and
narcolepsy, 562
Gamma-hydroxybuturic aciduria, 499
Gammaglobulin, and antiphospholipid
syndrome, 2
Ganciclovir, and TORCH syndrome, 295
Gangrene, and erysipelas, 285
Gardner syndrome, and adiposis
dolorosa, 303
Garner syndrome, 352–353
Gastric acid hypersecretion, and
Zollinger-Ellison syndrome, 330
Gastric carcinoma, and Korsakoff
syndrome, 546

Gastric hyposecretory states, and
Zollinger-Ellison syndrome, 330
Gastric outlet obstruction, and Zollinger-
Ellison syndrome, 330
Gastric placement fundoplication, and
Coffin-Siris syndrome, 708–709
Gastrinoma, 330
and pancreatic islet cell tumors, 408–409
Gastritis, giant hypertrophic, 341
Gastroenteritis, and Reye syndrome, 31
Gastroenteritis, eosinophilic, 342
Gastroenterologic disorders, 331–355
Gastroesophageal reflux, and Barrett
esophagus, 333
and hereditary spastic paraplegia,
575–576
Gastroesophageal reflux disease, and
Barrett esophagus, 333
Gastrointestinal bleeding, and Henoch-
Schönlein purpura, 414–415
Gastrointestinal disease, and diencephalic
syndrome, 528–529
Gastrointestinal disorders, and Cornelia
de Lange syndrome, 709
Gastrointestinal polyposis syndrome, and
Cronkhite-Canada syndrome, 338
Gastroplasty, and Korsakoff syndrome,
546
Gastroschisis, 197–198
Gastrostomy tube placement, and
deletion of the short arm of
chromosome 1, 58
Gaucher disease, *fig. 47*, 447
and congenital hepatic fibrosis, 691
and Erdheim-Chester disease, 441
and ichthyosis, 120
and Kuf disease, 547
and Singleton-Merten syndrome, 252
and Tangier disease, 500
Gaze palsy, and chronic progressive
external ophthalmoplegia,
603–604
GBBB syndrome, 198–199
Gelineau syndrome, 561–562
Gelophysic dysplasia, and Leri
pleonosteosis, 217
Gemcitabine, and adenoid cystic
carcinoma, 359
and Ewing sarcoma of bone, 381
GEMSS syndrome, 267–268
and Leri pleonosteosis, 217
Gene therapy, and Alport syndrome, 680
and autosomal-recessive polycystic
kidney disease, 697
and congenital erythropoietic
porphyria, 492–493

and Crigler-Najjar syndrome, 337
and cystinuria, 684
and Duchenne muscular dystrophy,
623
and dystrophic epidermolysis bullosa,
107
and epidermolytic epidermolysis
bullosa, 109
and glioblastoma multiforme, 385
and graft-versus-host disease, 11
and hemophilia, 390–391
and hereditary spherocytosis, 370–371
and hyper-IgM syndrome, 394
and junctional epidermolysis bullosa,
108
and Leber congenital amaurosis, 652
and Leber hereditary optic neuropathy,
653
and maple syrup urine disease, 469
and metachromatic leukodystrophy,
553
and multiple hereditary exostoses, 191
and phenylketonuria, 488
and severe combined
immunodeficiency, 14
and Sjögren syndrome, 34
and type II glycogen storage disease,
452
Genee-Weidemann syndrome, 222–223
Generalized atrophic benign
epidermolyis bullosa, 107–108
Generalized lichen myxedematosus,
136–137
Genital abnormalities, and Aarskog
syndrome, 142
and androgen insensitivity syndrome,
306–307
and camp[t]omelic syndrome,
706–707
and caudal regression syndrome, 166
and chromosome 9, partial monosomy
9p, 82
and chromosome 9, trisomy mosaic,
85–86
and chromosome 15, distal trisomy
15q, 65–66
and Denys-Drash syndrome, 686
and Fraser syndrome, 196–197
and GBBB syndrome, 198–199
and LEOPARD syndrome, 124–125
and popliteal pterygium syndrome,
242
and Schinzel Giedion syndrome, 247
and Townes-Brocks syndrome, 262
and trisomy 18 syndrome, 88
and true hermaphroditism, 316–317

Genital abnormalities, *(continued)*
  and XLMR-hypotonic facies
    syndrome, 274
Genital hypoplasia, and Gorlin-
    Chaudhry-Moss syndrome, 200
  and Robinow syndrome, 725–726
Genital keratinocytic dysplasia, 98–99
Genital lesions, and lichen sclerosis, 126
Genital papules, and bowenoid papulosis,
    98–99
Genitourinary abnormalities, and cat eye
    syndrome, 164–165
  and Denys-Drash syndrome, 686
  and DiGeorge syndrome, 178–179
  and Ewing sarcoma of bone, 381
  and Schinzel syndrome, 246–247
  and WAGR syndrome, 699
Genochondromatosis, and familial
    expansile osteolysis, 723
Gentamicin, and brucellosis, 280
  and listeriosis, 290
  and plague, 292
Geroderma osteodysplastica, and De
    Barsy syndrome, 6
  and progeria, 724
Gerstmann syndrome, 534–535
Gianotti-Crosti syndrome, 115
  and Mucha-Habermann disease,
    129
Giant axonal disease, 569
Giant axonal neuropathy, 569
  and congenital hypomyelination
    neuropathy, 568
Giant cell arteritis, and Takayasu arteritis,
    35
Giant cell granuloma, and cherubism,
    168
Giant cell hepatitis, 288
Giant cell lesions, and ameloblastoma,
    363
Giant cell myocarditis, *fig. 5,* 52–53
  and hypersensitivity myocarditis, 53
Giant cell tumor, and cherubism, 168
Giant hypertrophic gastritis, 341
Giant limb of Robertson, 232
Giant platelets, and Bernard-Soulier
    syndrome, 378
  and May-Hegglin anomaly, 403
Giardia lamblia infection, and common
    variable immunodeficiency, 13
Giardiasis, and Whipple disease, 297
Gigantism, and acromegaly, 301
  and sclerosteosis, 248–249
  and Sotos syndrome, 255
Gilbert syndrome, and Crigler-Najjar
    syndrome, 337
  and kernicterus, 543

Gingival bleeding, and Bernard-Soulier
    syndrome, 378
  and congenital afibrogenemia,
    359–360
  and Glanzmann thrombasthenia, 383
Gingival fibromatosis, and cherubism,
    168
  and Laband syndrome, 214
  and oculocerebral syndrome, 226–227
Gingival hyperplasia, and mucolipidosis,
    472
Gingivitis, and cyclic neutropenia, 21–22
  and severe chronic neutropenia, 22
Giroux-Barbeau syndrome, 111–112
  and erythrokeratodermia variabilis,
    112
GLA deficiency, 442
Glanzmann thrombasthenia, 383–384
Glaucoma, and aniridia, 640
  and Cogan-Reese syndrome, 644
  and essential iris atrophy, 650
  and iridocorneal endothelial
    syndromes, 649
  and megalocornea, 556
  and nail-patella syndrome, 721–722
  and Rieger syndrome, 243–244
  and Scheie disease, 478
  and Sturge-Weber syndrome, 258
  and Weill-Marchesani syndrome,
    267–268
Glioblastoma multiforme, 384–385
Glioma, and neuromyelitis optica, 567
Globoid cell leukodystrophy, 551–552
Glomerular basement membrane, thin,
    and benign familial hematuria,
    688–689
Glomerulocystic kidney disease, and
    autosomal-recessive polycystic
    kidney disease, 697
Glomus tumors, and Bowen disease, 97
Gloomy face syndrome, and
    ear–patella–short stature
    syndrome, 189
Glossitis, and Cronkhite-Canada
    syndrome, 338
Glossopalatine ankylosis syndrome, and
    Möbius syndrome, 223–224
Glossoptosis, and
    cerebrocostomandibular
    syndrome, 166–167
  and Pierre Robin sequence, 235–236
Glucagonoma, and pancreatic islet cell
    tumors, 408–409
Glucocerebrosidase deficiency, and
    Gaucher disease, 447
Glucocorticoid replacement, and ACTH
    deficiency, 302

Glucocorticoids, and antiphospholipid
    syndrome, 2
  and familial eosinophilic cellulitis, 99
  and mixed cryoglobulinemia
    syndrome, 5
  and Takayasu arteritis, 35
Glucose-6-phosphatase deficiency, and
    PEPCK deficiency, 486
Glucose-6-phosphate deficiency, and
    congenital nonspherocytic
    hemolytic anemia, 369
Glucose-6-phosphate dehydrogenase
    deficiency, 385–386
  and pyruvate kinase deficiency, 496
Glucose delivery, and type I glycogen
    storage disease, 450–451
  and type III glycogen storage disease,
    453
Glucose-galactose malabsorption, 343
Glucose intolerance, and familial
    dysbetalipoproteinemia, 440
  and SHORT syndrome, 250
  and type III glycogen storage disease,
    453
  and X-linked sideroblastic anemia, 373
Glucose phosphate isomerase deficiency,
    and congenital nonspherocytic
    hemolytic anemia, 369
Glucose transporter defect, 448
Glut-1 deficiency syndrome, 448
Glutaric acidemia type I, 426
Glutaric acidemia type II, 426–427
Glutaric aciduria, 426
Glutaric aciduria type II, and medium-
    chain acyl-CoA dehydrogenase
    deficiency, 437
Glutathione reductase deficiency, and
    congenital nonspherocytic
    hemolytic anemia, 369
Glutathione synthetase deficiency, 449
  and congenital nonspherocytic
    hemolytic anemia, 369
Gluten-sensitive sprue, and Whipple
    disease, 297
Glycine encephalopathy, and Niemann-
    Pick disease, 485
Glycogen storage disease, and congenital
    lactic acidosis, 462
  and severe chronic neutropenia, 22
Glycogen storage disease type 0, 450
Glycogen storage disease type I, 450–451
Glycogen storage disease type II, 452
Glycogen storage disease type III, 453
Glycogen storage disease type IV, 454
Glycogen storage disease type V, 454–455
Glycogen storage disease type VII,
    456–457

Glycogen storage disease types VI and IX, 455–456

Glycogeneses, and limb girdle muscular dystrophy, 625

Glycogenosis type X, 489–490

Glycoprotein neuraminidase deficiency, 498

Glycosphingolipid catabolism, and Fabry disease, 442

Glycosylation, congenital disorders of, 457–458

Golabi-Rosen syndrome, 251

Goldblatt spastic paraplegia, and Wieacker-Wolff syndrome, 638

Goldblatt syndrome, and Kniest dysplasia, 213

Goldenhar syndrome, 716–717
  and brachio-oto-renal syndrome, 681
  and chromosome 9, trisomy mosaic, 85
  and Parry-Romberg syndrome, 232–233

Goltz-Gorlin syndrome, and Norrie disease, 655

Goltz syndrome, and Aicardi syndrome, 509

GOMBO syndrome, and Myhre syndrome, 225

Gonadal dysgenesis, and androgen insensitivity syndrome, 306

Gonadectomy, and partial androgen insensitivity, 307

Gonadoblastoma, and WAGR syndrome, 699

Gonadotropin-releasing hormone, and precocious puberty, 325

Gonadotropin-releasing hormone deficiency, and Kallmann syndrome, 318–319

Goniotomy, and Sturge-Weber syndrome, 258

Goodpasture syndrome, and Wegener granulomatosis, 422

Gordon syndrome, 199–200

Gorlin-Chaudhry-Moss syndrome, 200

Gottron syndrome, 111–112, 147

Gout, and familial articular chondrocalcinosis, 169–170

Graft-versus-host disease, 10–11
  chronic, and scleroderma, 33
    and severe combined immunodeficiency, 14

Granisetron, and cyclic vomiting syndrome, 526

Granulocyte colony-stimulating factor, and Barth syndrome, 44
  and cyclic neutropenia, 21–22

and Felty syndrome, 9
and severe chronic neutropenia, 23

Granulocyte-macrophage colony-stimulating factor, and pulmonary alveolar proteinosis, 677

Granulocytopenia, and Cohen syndrome, 172

Granuloma annulare, 115–116

Granulomatosis, 386
  and Churg-Strauss syndrome, 674
  lymphomatoid, 48–49

Granulomatous colitis, and Hermansky-Pudlak syndrome, 391–392

Granulomatous disease, chronic, 386–387

Granulomatous disorders, and alopecia areata, 95
  and giant hypertrophic gastritis, 341

Granulomatous infection, and mesenteric panniculitis, 350

Granulomatous lesions of unknown significance, and sarcoidosis, 32

Graves disease, and chronic lymphocytic thyroiditis, 329

Gray platelet syndrome, and Bernard-Soulier syndrome, 378
  and Glanzmann thrombasthenia, 383
  and May-Hegglin anomaly, 403

Grebe syndrome, 702–703
  and acromesomelic dysplasia, 703–704

Greig cephalopolysyndactyly syndrome, 201
  and acrocallosal syndrome (Schinzel type), 145
  and chromosome 4, monosomy 4q, 74
  and craniofrontonasal syndrome, 183
  and Pallister-Hall syndrome, 230

Greither disease, and erythrokeratodermia variabilis, 112
  and progressive symmetric erythrokeratodermia, 111

Groin pain, and Legg-Calve-Perthes disease, 16

Grönblad-Strandberg syndrome, 133–134

Grover disease, 104

Growth acceleration, and congenital generalized lipodystrophy, 322
  and precocious puberty, 325

Growth deficits, and acrocallosal syndrome (Schinzel type), 145
  and acrodysostosis, 146
  and Bowen-Conradi syndrome, 161
  and chromosome 3, monosomy 3p2, 73
  and chromosome 4, monosomy 4q, 74
  and chromosome 4 ring, 76

and chromosome 5, trisomy 5p, 78
and chromosome 6 ring, 80
and chromosome 9, trisomy 9p, 84
and chromosome 9, trisomy mosaic, 85–86
and chromosome 11, partial monosomy 11q, 60–61
and chromosome 13, partial monosomy 13q, 62–63
and chromosome 14 ring, 63–64
and chromosome 15, distal trisomy 15q, 65–66
and chromosome 15 ring, 66
and chromosome 22, trisomy mosaic, 72
and chylomicron retention disease, 380
and Coffin-Siris syndrome, 708–709
and congenital erythropoietic porphyria, 492–493
and Cornelia de Lange syndrome, 709
and cystinosis, 683
and deletion of the short arm of chromosome 1, 58
and distal trisomy 10q, 59
and Filippi syndrome, 194–195
and fucosidosis, 445
and Hartnup disease, 458
and Johanson-Blizzard syndrome, 208
and LEOPARD syndrome, 124–125
and medullary cystic kidney disease, 693
and mucolipidosis, 472
and progeria, 724
and Roberts pseudothalidomide syndrome, 244–245
and Rubinstein-Taybi syndrome, 726–727
and Russel-Silver syndrome, 245–246
and Scott craniodigital syndrome, 249–250
and SHORT syndrome, 250
and Sly disease, 481
and 3-M syndrome, 259
and trisomy 18 syndrome, 88
and Wolf-Hirschhorn syndrome, 272
and X-linked hypophasphatemic rickets, 326–327
and X-linked sideroblastic anemia, 373

Growth hormone deficiency, 314–315
  and Russel-Silver syndrome, 245–246

Growth hormone excess, and acromegaly, 301

Growth hormone receptor dysfunction, and Laron dwarfism, 319–320

Growth hormone therapy, and achondroplasia, 144
  and carnosinemia, 435

Growth hormone therapy, *(continued)*
  and Prader-Willi syndrome, 237–238
  and Russel-Silver syndrome, 245–246
  and Turner syndrome, 264
Guillain-Barré syndrome, 535–536
  and acute intermittent porphyria, 490
  and botulism, 279
  and locked-in syndrome, 554
  and neuromyotonia, 635
  and spinal muscular atrophy, 637
Gum disease, and trigeminal neuralgia, 595
Günther disease, 492–493
Gustatory sweating, 533
Gynecomastia, and spinal bulbar muscular atrophy, 636

H
Habermann disease, 128–129
Hageman trait, 382–383
Hagemoser syndrome, and Rosenbert-Chutorian syndrome, 585
Hailey-Hailey disease, and acrodermatitis enteropathica, 94
  and Darier disease, 101
Hair, kinky, and giant axonal neuropathy, 569
HAIR-AN syndrome, 315–316
Hair hypopigmentation, and oculocerebral syndrome, 226–227
Hair loss, and alopecia areata, 95
Hair sparseness, and cardiofaciocutaneous syndrome, 163–164
  and trichorhinophalangeal syndrome, 730–732
Hajdu-Cheney syndrome, 11–12
  and cleidocranial dysplasia, 182
Hall-Hittner syndrome, 167
Hall-Pallister syndrome, 230
Hallermann-Streiff syndrome, 202
  and neonatal progeroid syndrome, 238
  and progeria, 724
Hallervorden-Spatz disease, and Machado-Joseph disease, 555
Hallervorden-Spatz syndrome, 620
Hallgren syndrome, 664–665
Hallux duplication syndrome, 145
Halofantrine, and malaria, 291
Haloperidol, and neuroacanthocytosis, 633
  and Sydenham chorea, 522
  and Tourette syndrome, 594
Hamartoma, and Peutz-Jeghers syndrome, 351–352

and PTEN hamartoma tumor syndrome, 240
Hand deformities, and Aase syndrome, 143
  and acrodysostosis, 146
  and Apert syndrome, 154–155
  and chromosome 4, trisomy 4p, 77–78
  and chromosome 7, monosomy 7p2, 80–81
  and chromosome 9, partial monosomy 9p, 82
  and chromosome 9, tetrasomy 9p, 84
  and chromosome 9, trisomy 9p, 85
  and chromosome 10, distal trisomy 10q, 59
  and Coffin-Lowry syndrome, 171–172
  and FG syndrome, 193–194
  and Holt-Oram syndrome, 717
  and Laband syndrome, 214
  and Pfeiffer syndrome type I, 234–235
  and Poland syndrome, 236–237
  and Singleton-Merten syndrome, 252
  and split hand/split foot malformation, 256
  and thrombocytopenia and absent radius syndrome, 260
  and Townes-Brocks syndrome, 262
  and Weill-Marchesani syndrome, 267–268
Hand dystonia, and writer's cramp, 618
Hand movement disorders, and Rett syndrome, 584
Hand pain, and erythromelalgia, 113
  and thromboangiitis obliterans, 36
Hand posturing, and trisomy 18 syndrome, 88
Hand-Schuller-Christian syndrome, 392–393
Handless and footless families of Brazil, 702
Hands, absence of, and acheiropodia, 702
Hanhart syndrome, 203
  and Möbius syndrome, 223–224
Hantavirus infection, and anthrax, 278
Hantavirus pulmonary syndrome, 282, 287
Harada syndrome, 36–37
Harding disease, and neuromyelitis optica, 567
HARP syndrome, and neuroacanthocytosis, 633
Hartnup disease, 458
  and ataxia-telangiectasia, 605–606
Hashimoto thyroiditis, 329
Hawkensinosis, and tyrosinemia, 504
Hay-Wells syndrome, 116–117

and popliteal pterygium syndrome, 242
Head enlargement, and Hurler disease, 477
  and hydranencephaly, 538
Head thrusts, and Glut-1 deficiency syndrome, 448
Head trauma, and Korsakoff syndrome, 546
Headache, and brain arteriovenous malformations, 596
  and glioblastoma multiforme, 384–385
  and pseudotumor cerebri, 582
Hearing deficits, and deletion of the short arm of chromosome 1, 58
Hearing loss, and acrodysostosis, 146
  and alpha-mannosidosis, 467–468
  and Alport syndrome, 680
  and Alström syndrome, 305–306
  and Arnold-Chiari syndrome, 516
  and Björnstad syndrome, 97
  and brachio-oto-renal syndrome, 682
  and Camurati-Engelmann disease, 707–708
  and carnosinemia, 435
  and Churg-Strauss syndrome, 674
  and Cockayne syndrome, 170–171
  and Goldenhar syndrome, 716
  and Ménière disease, 558
  and neurofibromatosis type 2, 564–565
  and Norrie disease, 656
  and Refsum disease, 604–605
  and Rosenbert-Chutorian syndrome, 585
  and SHORT syndrome, 250
  and spondyloepiphyseal dysplasia congenita, 728
  and syringobulbia, 589
  and Townes-Brocks syndrome, 262
  and Waardenburg syndromes, 732–733
Heart block, congenital complete, 49–50
Heart defects, and cardiofaciocutaneous syndrome, 163–164
  and cat eye syndrome, 164–165
  and CHARGE syndrome, 167
  and chromosome 3, trisomy 3q2, 73–74
  and chromosome 4, monosomy distal 4q, 75
  and chromosome 4, monosomy 4q, 74
  and chromosome 5, trisomy 5p, 78
  and chromosome 7, monosomy 7p2, 80–81
  and chromosome 9, trisomy mosaic, 85–86
  and chromosome 9 ring, 83

and chromosome 10, monosomy 10p, 60

and chromosome 11, partial monosomy 11q, 60–61

and chromosome 15, distal trisomy 15q, 65–66

and chromosome 22q11 deletion spectrum, 70–71

and Coffin-Siris syndrome, 708–709

and DiGeorge syndrome, 178–179

and GBBB syndrome, 198–199

and Holt-Oram syndrome, 717

and Klippel-Feil syndrome, 720

and Noonan syndrome, 722–723

and pentalogy of Cantrell, 233–234

and pentasomy X, 86–87

and trisomy 18 syndrome, 88

Heart defibrillator implantation, and giant cell myocarditis, 52

Heart disease, childhood, and Kawasaki disease, 15

and Glanzmann thrombasthenia, 383

and Holt-Oram syndrome, 717

and idiopathic congenital central hypoventilation syndrome, 673

and pentalogy of Cantrell, 233–234

and Tangier disease, 500

Heart failure, and Barth syndrome, 44

and hereditary hemochromatosis, 387–388

Heart hamartomas, and tuberous sclerosis, 595–596

Heart-hand syndrome, 717

Heart-lung transplantation, and primary pulmonary hypertension, 678

Heart murmur, and Eisenmenger syndrome, 47

and persistent truncus arteriosus, 56

Heart muscle cell death, and giant cell myocarditis, 52

Heart transplantation, and giant cell myocarditis, 52

and hypoplastic left heart syndrome, 51

Heat stroke, and neuroleptic malignant syndrome, 566

Helicobacter pylori infection, and giant hypertrophic gastritis, 341

and Zollinger-Ellison syndrome, 330

Helminthiasis, and congenital hepatic fibrosis, 691

Hemangioblastomas, and Von Hippel-Lindau disease, 265–266

Hemangiomas, and ameloblastoma, 363

Hemangiomatosis, and Wyburn-Mason syndrome, 667

Hemangiomatosis osteolytica, 217–218

Hematologic malignancy, and Banti syndrome, 377

Hematologic/oncologic disorders, 357–423

Hematopoiesis, cyclic, 21–22

Hematuria, and Alport syndrome, 680

benign familial, 688–689

and cystinuria, 684

Hematuric nephritis, and Alport syndrome, 680

Hemiatrophy, and Parry-Romberg syndrome, 232–233

Hemichoreoathetosis, and thalamic pain syndrome, 593

Hemifacial anhidrosis, and Horner syndrome, 648

Hemifacial atrophy, and Parry-Romberg syndrome, 232–233

Hemifacial microsomia, 716

and Möbius syndrome, 223–224

and Parry-Romberg syndrome, 232–233

Hemifacial spasm, and blepharospasm, 610

Hemihyperplasia, and Proteus syndrome, 239

Hemihypertrophy, and Beckwith-Wiedemann syndrome, 518

and Russel-Silver syndrome, 245–246

Hemihypesthesia, and thalamic pain syndrome, 593

Hemimegalencephaly, and epidermal nevus syndrome, 106

Hemiparesis, and epidermal nevus syndrome, 106

and thalamic pain syndrome, 593

Hemiplegia, and moyamoya syndrome, 559

Hemiplegic migraine, and alternating hemiplegia of childhood, 512

and moyamoya syndrome, 559

Hemispherectomy, and epidermal nevus syndrome, 106

and Sturge-Weber syndrome, 258

Hemivertebrae, and Robinow syndrome, 725–726

Hemochromatosis, and alpha 1-antitrypsin deficiency, 671

and benign lymphoepithelial lesion, 17

hereditary, 387–388

and idiopathic neonatal hepatitis, 288

and type IV glycogen storage disease, 454

and X-linked sideroblastic anemia, 373

Hemodialysis, and hepatorenal syndrome, 344

Hemoglobin H inclusions, and XLMR-hypotonic facies syndrome, 274

Hemoglobinopathies, and autoimmune hemolytic anemia, 367

Hemoglobinopathy-associated hemolytic anemias, and cold hemolytic anemia syndromes, 368

Hemoglobinuria, paroxysmal cold, 388–389

paroxysmal nocturnal, 389–390

Hemolysis, and Crigler-Najjar syndrome, 337

Hemolytic anemia, and Banti syndrome, 377

and congenital erythropoietic porphyria, 492–493

and glutathione synthetase deficiency, 449

and hemolytic-uremic syndrome, 689–690

and inherited hemolytic-uremic syndrome, 690–691

and phosphoglycerate kinase deficiency, 489–490

and type VII glycogen storage disease, 456–457

Hemolytic-uremic syndrome, 689–691

inherited, 690–691

and thrombotic thrombocytopenic purpura, 416

Hemophagocytic lymphohistiocytosis, 397–398

Hemophagocytic syndrome, and X-linked lymphoproliferative syndrome, 400

Hemophilia, 390–391

Hemophilia B, 381–382

Hemoptysis, and lymphangioleiomyomatosis, 395

Hemorrhage, and brain arteriovenous malformations, 596

and moyamoya syndrome, 559

Henoch-Schönlein purpura, 414–415

and Churg-Strauss syndrome, 674

and idiopathic thrombocytopenic purpura, 415

and microscopic polyangiitis, 27

and Wegener granulomatosis, 422

Heparin, and antiphospholipid syndrome, 2

and carotid artery insufficiency, 659

and congenital antithrombin III deficiency, 376–377

Hepatic carcinoma, and type III glycogen storage disease, 453

Hepatic cysts, and type III glycogen storage disease, 453

Hepatic dysfunction, and Beckwith-Wiedemann syndrome, 518
and carnitine deficiency syndromes, 432

Hepatic failure, and type III glycogen storage disease, 453

Hepatic fibrosis, congenital, 691–692
and Loken-Senior syndrome, 692

Hepatic fibrosis syndrome, and Joubert syndrome, 542

Hepatic fructokinase, and fructosuria, 444–445

Hepatic fructokinase deficiency, 444–445

Hepatic glycogen phosphorylase deficiency, 455–456

Hepatic glycogen synthase deficiency, and type 0 glycogen storage disease, 450

Hepatic sarcoidosis, and Banti syndrome, 377

Hepatitis, and alpha 1-antitrypsin deficiency, 671
and Byler disease, 335
and chronic inflammatory demyelinating polyradiculoneuropathy, 581
and hereditary fructose intolerance, 444
idiopathic neonatal, 288
and leptospirosis, 289
and Q fever, 293
and Rift Valley fever, 294
and TORCH syndrome, 295
and Wilson disease, 506

Hepatitis C virus infection, 5
and mixed cryoglobulin syndrome, 5

Hepatoblastoma, and trisomy 18 syndrome, 88

Hepatocyte transplantation, and Crigler-Najjar syndrome, 337

Hepatoerythropoietic porphyria, and congenital erythropoietic porphyria, 492–493

Hepatojejunostomy, and Caroli disease, 336

Hepatolenticular degeneration, 506

Hepatomegaly, and carnitine palmitoyl transferase I deficiency, 433
and carnitine palmitoyl transferase II deficiency, 434
and congenital complete heart block, 49

and congenital hepatic fibrosis, 691
and idiopathic neonatal hepatitis, 288
and Morquio disease, 480
and mucolipidosis, 472
and PEPCK deficiency, 486
and peroxisomal biogenesis disorders, 487
and POEMS syndrome, 26
and type II glycogen storage disease, 452
and types VI and IX glycogen storage disease, 455–456

Hepatorenal syndrome, 344

Hepatosplenomegaly, and autosomal-recessive polycystic kidney disease, 697
and Laband syndrome, 214
and large granular lymphocyte leukemia, 394
and Niemann-Pick disease, 485

Heredipathia atactica polyneuritiformis, 604–605

Hereditary angioedema, 375–376

Hereditary coproporphyria, 494–495

Hereditary dystrophic lipidosis, 442

Hereditary fructose intolerance, 444
and congenital disorders of glycosylation, 457

Hereditary hemochromatosis, 387–388

Hereditary hemorrhagic telangiectasia, 418

Hereditary hypohydrotic ectodermal dysplasia, and keratitis-ichthyosis-deafness syndrome, 122

Hereditary lymphedema, 396–397

Hereditary multiple exostoses, 191

Hereditary myotonias, and neuromyotonia, 635

Hereditary nonpolyposis colorectal cancer, 401

Hereditary nonspherocytic hemolytic anemia, and glucose-6-phosphate dehydrogenase deficiency, 385

Hereditary pyropoikilocytosis, and thalassemia major, 419

Hereditary sensory neuropathy type I, 570

Hereditary sensory neuropathy type II, 571

Hereditary spastic paraparesis, and amyotrophic lateral sclerosis, 513
and primary lateral sclerosis, 548

Hereditary spastic paraplegia, 575–576
and adult polyglucosan body disease, 580

Hereditary spherocytic hemolytic anemia, 370–371

Hereditary spherocytosis, 370–371
and thalassemia major, 419
and warm antibody hemolytic anemia, 371–372

Hereditary stomatocytosis, and hereditary spherocytosis, 370–371

Hereditary tyrosinemia, and ALA-dehydratase–deficient porphyria, 492

Hermansky-Pudlak syndrome, 391–392
and Glanzmann thrombasthenia, 383

Hermaphroditism, and congenital adrenal hyperplasia, 304
true, 316–317

Hernias, and aspartylglucosaminuria, 432
and Hunter disease, 478–479
and Hurler disease, 477
and mucolipidosis, 472
and pseudomyxoma peritonei, 412
and Williams syndrome, 270

Herpes, and anthrax, 278

Herpes encephalitis, and Korsakoff syndrome, 546

Herpes gestationes, and bullous pemphigoid, 130–131

Herpes simplex infection, and dystrophic epidermolysis bullosa, 106
and epidermolytic epidermolysis bullosa, 108
and junctional epidermolysis bullosa, 108

Herpes simplex virus, and TORCH syndrome, 295

Herpes simplex virus type 1, and encephalitides, 284–285

Herpes viruses, and West Nile fever, 296

Herpes zoster, and erysipelas, 285
and Parsonage-Turner syndrome, 577

Herpesvirus infection, and Behçet disease, 4

Herpetic stomatitis, primary, and Sutton disease, 138

Hers disease, 455–456

Heteroplasia, progressive osseous, 203–204

Heterotopic ossification, and fibrodysplasia ossificans progressiva, 713
and progressive osseous heteroplasia, 203–204

Hexokinase deficiency, and congenital nonspherocytic hemolytic anemia, 369

and glucose-6-phosphate
dehydrogenase deficiency, 385
Hexosaminidase A deficiency, 501
HHHO syndrome, 237–238
Hidradenitis suppurativa, 118–119
Hip degeneration, and Laron dwarfism,
319–320
Hip degenerative disease, and
spondyloepiphyseal dysplasia
congenita, 728
Hip disease, and spondyloepiphyseal
dysplasia tarda, 729–730
Hip dislocation, and femoral
hypoplasia–unusual facies
syndrome, 712–713
and spondyloepiphyseal dysplasia
tarda, 729–730
Hip fracture, and Legg-Calve-Perthes
disease, 16
Hip joint, septic, and Legg-Calve-Perthes
disease, 16
Hip pain, and Legg-Calve-Perthes
disease, 16
and spondyloepiphyseal dysplasia
tarda, 729–730
Hippel-Lindau syndrome, 265–266
Hippotherapy, and Rett syndrome, 584
Hirschsprung disease, 345
and idiopathic congenital central
hypoventilation syndrome, 673
Hirsutism, and HAIR-AN syndrome,
315–316
and Laband syndrome, 214
Histamine-induced angioedema, and
hereditary angioedema, 375
Histamine receptor blockers, and
mastocytosis, 402
Histidase deficiency, 459
Histidinemia, 459
Histiocytosis, Langerhans cell, 392–
393
and Niemann-Pick disease, 485
Histiocytosis-X, 392–393
HIV encephalopathy, and frontotemporal
dementia, 534
Holoanencephaly, 151–152
Holocarboxylase synthetase deficiency,
483
and multiple carboxylase deficiency,
482
Holoprosencephaly, 536–537
and hydranencephaly, 538
and septooptic dysplasia, 188–189
Holotelencephaly, 536–537
Holt-Oram syndrome, 717
and Aase syndrome, 143

and thrombocytopenia and absent
radius syndrome, 260
Homocarnosinemia, 435
Homocystinemia, 459–460
Homocystinuria, 459–460
and congenital contractual
arachnodactyly, 3
and congenital disorders of
glycosylation, 457
and Marfan syndrome, 218
and MELAS, 469
and Weill-Marchesani syndrome,
267–268
Hormone replacement therapy, and
Achard-Thiers syndrome, 300
and septooptic dysplasia, 188–189
Horner syndrome, 648
and syringobulbia, 589
HPS, and Hermansky-Pudlak syndrome,
391–392
Hughes syndrome, 2
Human cytochrome oxidase deficiency,
436
Human ehrlichiosis, 283
Human immunodeficiency virus,
neonatal infection, and severe
combined immunodeficiency, 14
Human immunodeficiency virus
infection, and Behçet disease, 4
and chronic inflammatory
demyelinating
polyradiculoneuropathy, 581
and primary lateral sclerosis, 548
and Sutton disease, 138
and TORCH syndrome, 295
Hunter disease, 478–479
and multiple sulfatase deficiency, 484
Hunter syndrome, and mucolipidosis,
472
Hunter-Thompson acromelic dysplasia,
702–703
Huntington chorea, 537–538
Huntington disease, 537–538
and Creutzfeldt-Jakob disease, 608
and frontotemporal dementia, 534
and Hallervorden-Spatz syndrome,
620
and neuroacanthocytosis, 633
and tardive dyskinesia, 591
Hurler disease, 477
and Gaucher disease, 447
Hurler syndrome, and Dyggve-Melchior-
Clausen syndrome, 180
and mucolipidosis, 472
Hutchinson-Gilford progeria syndrome,
724–725

Hutchinson-Gilford syndrome, and
acrogeria (Gottron type), 147
and De Barsy syndrome, 6
and neonatal progeroid syndrome, 238
Hydantoin embryopathy, and Aarskog
syndrome, 142
Hydatid cyst, and Caroli disease, 336
Hydranencephaly, 538
and hydrocephalus, 539
Hydration, and neuroleptic malignant
syndrome, 566
Hydrocephalus, 539
and Arnold-Chiari syndrome, 516
and classic lissencephaly, 553
and Crouzon syndrome, 710
and Dandy-Walker syndrome, 526
and holoprosencephaly, 536
and hydranencephaly, 538
and leukodystrophy, 550
and MASA syndrome, 220
and medulloblastoma, 404–405
and Walker-Warburg syndrome,
597–598
Hydrocortisone, and congenital adrenal
hyperplasia, 304
and septooptic dysplasia, 188–189
and Sheehan syndrome, 328
Hydrolethalus syndrome, and trisomy 13
syndrome, 87
Hydronephrosis, and cyclic vomiting
syndrome, 525
Hydropic changes of placenta, and
triploidy syndrome, 263–264
Hydrops fetalis, and type IV glycogen
storage disease, 454
Hydrops labyrinthi, 558
Hydrotherapy, and Rett syndrome, 584
Hydroxyurea, and congenital
erythropoietic porphyria, 492–493
and idiopathic thrombocytosis, 421
and thalassemia major, 419
Hydroxyzine, and interstitial cystitis, 685
and transient acantholytic dermatosis,
104
Hyper-beta carnosinemia, 435
Hyper-IgE syndrome, 12–13
Hyper-IgM syndrome, 393–394
and common variable
immunodeficiency, 13
and severe combined
immunodeficiency, 14
and X-linked agammaglobulinemia,
360
Hyper-reninism, and Bartter syndrome,
309–311
Hyperactivity, and megalocornea, 556

Hyperacusis, and Tay-Sachs disease, 501

Hyperaldosteronism, and Bartter syndrome, 309–311

Hyperammonemia, and carnitine deficiency syndromes, 432
and urea cycle disorders, 506–506

Hyperandrogenic chronic anovulation, 323–324

Hyperandrogenism, and HAIR-AN syndrome, 315–316
and polycystic ovary syndrome, 323–324

Hyperbilirubinemia, and Crigler-Najjar syndrome, 337
and Dubin-Johnson syndrome, 340
and idiopathic neonatal hepatitis, 288

Hypercalcemia, and blue diaper syndrome, 681
and Jansen metaphyseal chondrodysplasia, 206–207
and Williams syndrome, 270

Hypercalciuria, and benign familial hematuria, 688
and blue diaper syndrome, 681
and medullary sponge kidney, 694

Hyperchloremia, and glucose-galactose malabsorption, 343

Hyperekplexia, 540

Hyperemesis gravidarum, and Korsakoff syndrome, 546

Hypereosinophil syndrome, and Churg-Strauss syndrome, 674

Hypereosinophilic syndrome, and eosinophilic gastroenteritis, 342

Hypergonadotropic hypogonadism, and Marinesco-Sjögren syndrome, 720–721

Hyperhidrosis, and Frey syndrome, 533
and Meleda disease, 128

Hyperhistidinemia, 459

Hyperimmunoglobulin M syndrome, and severe chronic neutropenia, 22

Hyperinsulinemia, and acquired generalized lipodystrophy, 320–321

Hyperinsulinemic hypoglycemia, and congenital disorders of glycosylation, 457

Hyperkeratosis, and Darier disease, 101
and Rothmund-Thomson syndrome, 135–136

Hyperkeratosis palmoplantaris striata-pili torti-hypodontia-sensorineural hearing loss syndrome, and Björnstad syndrome, 97

Hyperlacticacidemia, and type 0 glycogen storage disease, 450
and type I glycogen storage disease, 450–451

Hyperleucine, and maple syrup urine disease, 468

Hyperlipidemia type IV, 460

Hyperlipoproteinemia, type III, 440

Hyperlipoproteinemic liver disease, and warm antibody hemolytic anemia, 371–372

Hypermetamorphosis, and Kluver-Bucy syndrome, 545

Hypermethioninemia, 471–472

Hypermetropia, and Kenny-Caffey syndrome, 211

Hypernatremia, and glucose-galactose malabsorption, 343
and holoprosencephaly, 536

Hyperorality, and Kluver-Bucy syndrome, 545

Hyperornithinemia-gyrate atrophy, and retinitis pigmentosa, 660

Hyperostosis, diffuse idiopathic skeletal, 9–10

Hyperostosis corticalis generalista, and hyperostosis corticalis generalisata, 204–205

Hyperostosis cranialis interna, and hyperostosis corticalis generalisata, 204–205

Hyperostosis interna, and hyperostosis corticalis generalisata, 204–205

Hyperoxaluria, and cystinuria, 684
primary, 461–462

Hyperparathyroidism, and hypophosphatasia, 317–318
and Kenny-Caffey syndrome, 211
and medullary sponge kidney, 694

Hyperpathia, and thalamic pain syndrome, 593

Hyperphagia, and Kleine-Levin syndrome, 544

Hyperphalangism of the index finger, and Catel-Manzke syndrome, 165

Hyperphenylalaninemia, 488

Hyperphosphatemia tarda, 204–205

Hyperpigmentation, and porphyria cutanea tarda, 493–494

Hyperplasia, nodular lymphoid, and common variable immunodeficiency, 13

Hyperplastic gastropathy, and giant hypertrophic gastritis, 341

Hyperplastic polyps, and Cronkhite-Canada syndrome, 338

Hyperpnea, and multiple carboxylase deficiency, 483

Hyperprostaglandin E2 syndrome, 309–311

Hyperpyrexia, 718

Hyperreflexia, and Batten disease, 517
and hyperekplexia, 540
and pheochromocytoma, 409
and primary lateral sclerosis, 548
and short-chain acyl-CoA dehydrogenase deficiency, 438–439

Hypersalivation, and tetrahydrobiopterin deficiency, 502

Hypersensitive bladder disorders, 685

Hypersensitivity myocarditis, 52–53

Hypersomnia, and Kleine-Levin syndrome, 544

Hypersplenism, and Glanzmann thrombasthenia, 383

Hyperstosis corticalis generalisata, 204–205

Hypertelorism, 198–199
and acrocallosal syndrome (Schinzel type), 145
and craniofrontonasal syndrome, 183
and Greig cephalopolysyndactyly syndrome, 201
and Pfeiffer syndrome type I, 234–235
and XLMR-hypotonic facies syndrome, 274

Hypertension, and acute intermittent porphyria, 490
and alveolar capillary dysplasia, 672
and autosomal-recessive polycystic kidney disease, 697
and Caroli syndrome, 336
and familial juvenile hyperuricemic nephropathy, 696
and hemolytic-uremic syndrome, 689–690
and inherited hemolytic-uremic syndrome, 690
and pheochromocytoma, 409
and primary aldosteronism, 305
and primary empty sella syndrome, 530
and primary pulmonary hypertension, 678

Hyperthyroidism, and Johanson-Blizzard syndrome, 208
and pheochromocytoma, 409

Hypertonia, and kernicterus, 543

Hypertrichosis, and chromosome 3, monosomy 3p2, 73
and Gorlin-Chaudhry-Moss syndrome, 200

and Marshall-Smith syndrome, 219
and porphyria cutanea tarda, 493–494
and precocious puberty, 324
Hypertriglyceridemia, and acquired generalized lipodystrophy, 320–321
and congenital generalized lipodystrophy, 322
Hypertrophic lymphocytic gastritis, 341
Hypertrophic neuropathy, 521–522
and Dejerine-Sottas syndrome, 527
Hypertrophic osteoarthropathy, secondary, and pachydermoperiostosis, 129
Hypertrophy, and medullary sponge kidney, 694
Hyperuricemia, and familial juvenile hyperuricemic nephropathy, 696
and Lesch-Nyhan syndrome, 464–465
and type I glycogen storage disease, 450–451
Hypervalinemia, and maple syrup urine disease, 468
Hyperviscosity, and polycythemia vera, 411–412
Hypervitaminosis D, and medullary sponge kidney, 694
Hypnagogic hallucinations, and narcolepsy, 561–562
Hypoalbuminemia, and intestinal lymphangiectasia, 346
Hypobetalipoproteinemia, and abetalipoproteinemia, 358
and chylomicron retention disease, 380
Hypocalcemia, and DiGeorge syndrome, 178
and Kenny-Caffey syndrome, 211
Hypochondrogenesis, and Kniest dysplasia, 213
and spondyloepiphyseal dysplasia congenita, 728
Hypochondroplasia, 144
and dyschondrosteosis, 181
and Kniest dysplasia, 213
Hypocomplementemic urticarial vasculitis, and alpha 1-antitrypsin deficiency, 671
Hypocortisolism, 302
Hypodontia, 261
Hypodysfibrinogenemia, and congenital afibrogenemia, 359–360
Hypofibrinogenemia, and congenital afibrogenemia, 359–360
Hypogammaglobulinemia, and alpha 1-antitrypsin deficiency, 671

common variable, and common variable immunodeficiency, 13–14
and intestinal lymphangiectasia, 346
and X-linked lymphoproliferative syndrome, 400
Hypogenitalism, and Bardet-Biedl syndrome, 158–159
Hypoglossia-hypodactylia syndrome, and Möbius syndrome, 223–224
Hypoglycemia, and Beckwith-Wiedemann syndrome, 518
and carnitine palmitoyl transferase I deficiency, 433
and carnitine palmitoyl transferase II deficiency, 434
and glutaric acidemia type II, 426–427
and narcolepsy, 562
and pancreatic islet cell tumors, 408–409
and pheochromocytoma, 410
and type 0 glycogen storage disease, 450
and type I glycogen storage disease, 450–451
and type III glycogen storage disease, 453
and type IV glycogen storage disease, 454
and types VI and IX glycogen storage disease, 455–456
Hypoglycemic encephalopathy, and Glut-1 deficiency syndrome, 448
Hypogonadism, and autoimmune premature ovarian failure, 30–31
and Borjeson-Forssman-Lehmann syndrome, 705–706
and Prader-Willi syndrome, 237–238
and XXY syndrome, 89–90
Hypokalemia, and intestinal pseudoobstruction, 348
and primary aldosteronism, 305
Hypokalemic metabolic alkalosis, and Bartter syndrome, 309–311
Hypoketotic hypoglycemia, and carnitine deficiency syndromes, 432
and glutaric acidemia type II, 426–427
Hypomegakaryocytic thrombocytopenia, and thrombocytopenia and absent radius syndrome, 260
Hypomelanosis of Ito, 119–120
and chromosome 14, trisomy mosaic, 64
and incontinentia pigmenti, 121
Hypoparathyroidism, and Fahr disease, 532
and pseudohypoparathyroidism, 325–326

and Singleton-Merten syndrome, 252
Hypophosphatasia, 317–318
and camp[t]omelic syndrome, 706–707
Hypophosphatemia, and X-linked hypophasphatemic rickets, 326–327
Hypopituitarism, and idiopathic neonatal hepatitis, 288
and Russel-Silver syndrome, 245–246
and septooptic dysplasia, 188–189
and Sheehan syndrome, 328
Hypoplasia, and bilateral renal agenesis, 698
and Leber congenital amaurosis, 652
muscular, and congenital contractual arachnodactyly, 3
Hypoplastic anemia, 365
Hypoplastic left heart syndrome, 50–51
and chromosome 7, monosomy 7p2, 80
Hypoplastic left ventricle syndrome, 50–51
Hypoplastic nails, and Coffin-Siris syndrome, 708–709
Hyposmia, and Kallmann syndrome, 318–319
Hypospadias, and Lenz microphthalmia syndrome, 654
and true hermaphroditism, 316–317
Hypospadias dysphagia syndrome, 198–199
Hypothalamic hamartoma, and Pallister-Hall syndrome, 230
Hypothalamic-pituitary dysfunction, and Asherman syndrome, 308–309
Hypothalamic-pituitary mass lesions, and Kallmann syndrome, 318
Hypothyroidism, and chronic lymphocytic thyroiditis, 329
and cystinosis, 683
and deletion of the short arm of chromosome 1, 58
and kernicterus, 543
and narcolepsy, 562
Hypotonia, and carnitine deficiency syndromes, 432
and carnosinemia, 435
and central core disease, 607–608
and cerebro-oculo-facio-skeletal syndrome, 520
and chromosome 3, trisomy 3q2, 73–74
and chromosome 4, monosomy distal 4q, 75
and Coffin-Siris syndrome, 708–709

Hypotonia, *(continued)*
and congenital hypomyelination neuropathy, 568
and Dejerine-Sottas syndrome, 527–528
and FG syndrome, 193–194
and giant axonal neuropathy, 569
and glutaric acidemia type I, 426
and hydranencephaly, 538
and isovaleric acidemia, 427
and Joubert syndrome, 542
and kernicterus, 543
and leukodystrophy, 550
and Marinesco-Sjögren syndrome, 720–721
and methylmalonic acidemias, 429
muscular, and Marden-Walker syndrome, 18
and propionic acidemia, 428
and Santavuori disease, 585–586
and short-chain acyl-CoA dehydrogenase deficiency, 438–439
and type II glycogen storage disease, 452
and very-long-chain acyl-CoA dehydrogenase deficiency, 439–440
Hypotonic facies, and XLMR-hypotonic facies syndrome, 274
Hypotony, and megalocornea, 556
Hypotrichosis, and neonatal progeroid syndrome, 238
Hypoxanthine-guanine phosphoribosyl transferase deficiency, and Lesch-Nyhan syndrome, 464–465
Hypoxemia, and alveolar capillary dysplasia, 672
and pulmonary alveolar proteinosis, 677
Hypoxia, and malignant hyperthermia, 718
Hysteria, and narcolepsy, 562

I
Iatrogenic hypothyroidism, and chronic lymphocytic thyroiditis, 329
Ibandronate, and Paget disease, 25
Ichthyosis, 120–121
and Neu-Laxova syndrome, 562–563
Ichthyosis, X-linked, *fig. 18*, 120
Ichthyosis linearis circumflexa, and erythrokeratodermia variabilis, 112
Icteric sclerae, and hereditary spherocytosis, 370–371
Icterus, and Crigler-Najjar syndrome, 337

Icterus neonatorum, and kernicterus, 543
Idebenone, and Friedreich ataxia, 602
Idiopathic ambiguous genitalia, and true hermaphroditism, 316–317
Idiopathic angioedema, and hereditary angioedema, 375
Idiopathic congenital central hypoventilation syndrome, 673
Idiopathic epilepsy, and tuberous sclerosis, 596
Idiopathic granulomatous myocarditis, 52
Idiopathic hemochromatosis, and X-linked sideroblastic anemia, 373
Idiopathic hypercalciuria, and medullary sponge kidney, 694
Idiopathic hypermethioninemia, and methylmalonate semialdehyde dehydrogenase deficiency, 471
Idiopathic hypersomnolence, and narcolepsy, 562
Idiopathic hypogonadotropic hypogonadism, and Kallmann syndrome, 318–319
Idiopathic multicentric osteolysis, and Winchester syndrome, 271
Idiopathic neonatal hepatitis, 288
Idiopathic peptic ulcer disease, and Zollinger-Ellison syndrome, 330
Idiopathic polyneuritis, 535–536
Idiopathic portal hypertension, 377
Idiopathic primary hypertrophic osteoarthropathy, 129–130
Idiopathic thrombocytopenia, and May-Hegglin anomaly, 403
Idiopathic thrombocytopenic purpura, 415–416
Idiopathic thrombocytosis, 420–421
Idiopathic torsion dystonia, and Niemann-Pick disease, 485
Idiopathic vasculitis, and Sjögren syndrome, 34
Idiopathic ventricular fibrillation, 45
and Brugada syndrome, 45
and Romano-Ward long QT syndrome, 54
IgA nephropathy, and benign familial hematuria, 688
and Henoch-Schönlein purpura, 414
Ileal atresia, and Hirschsprung disease, 345
Ileorectal anastomosis, and familial adenomatous polyposis, 352–353
Iloprost, and scleroderma, 33
Imbalance, and Camurati-Engelmann disease, 707–708

Immotile cilia syndrome, 675
ImmTher, and Ewing sarcoma of bone, 381
Immune thrombocytopenia, and Glanzmann thrombasthenia, 383
Immune thrombocytopenic purpura, and Wiskott-Aldrich syndrome, 38
Immunobullous disease, and familial eosinophilic cellulitis, 99
Immunodeficiency, and Bloom syndrome, 159–160
common variable, 13–14
and hyper-IgE syndrome, 12–13
and hyper-IgM syndrome, 393
and ichthyosis, 120
and intestinal lymphangiectasia, 346
and Leiner disease, 123–124
and Nezelof syndrome, 408
severe combined, 14–15
Immunoglobulin, and acquired pure red cell aplasia, 414
Immunosuppression, and acquired aplastic anemia, 364
and graft-versus-host disease, 11
and pars planitis, 657
Immunosuppressive drugs, and antiphospholipid syndrome, 2
Imperforate anus, 153
and Pallister-Hall syndrome, 230
and Townes-Brocks syndrome, 262
Imuran, and Lambert-Eaton myasthenic syndrome, 621
Inborn errors of metabolism, 425–506
and Beckwith-Wiedemann syndrome, 518
Inclusion body myositis, 631–632
and amyotrophic lateral sclerosis, 513
Incontinence, and Binswanger disease, 519
and neuromyelitis optica, 567
Incontinentia pigmenti, *fig. 19*, 121–122
and chromosome 14, trisomy mosaic, 64
and hypomelanosis of Ito, 119
Incontinentia pigmenti achromians, 119–120
and incontinentia pigmenti, 121
Incoordination, and chromosome 22 ring, 71–72
and methylmalonic acidemias, 429
and tetrahydrobiopterin deficiency, 502
and X-linked sideroblastic anemia, 374–375
Increased height, and triple X syndrome, 89
and XXY syndrome, 89–90
and XYY syndrome, 90–91

Indicanuria, and blue diaper syndrome, 681

Indole-3-carbinol, and recurrent respiratory papillomatosis, 676

Infant death, and trisomy 13 syndrome, 87

and trisomy 18 syndrome, 88

Infant of diabetic mother, and Beckwith-Wiedemann syndrome, 518

Infant septicemia, and hypoplastic left heart syndrome, 50

Infantile anorexia, and diencephalic syndrome, 528–529

Infantile esotropia, and Duane syndrome, 645

Infantile facioscapulohumoral dystrophy, and centronuclear myopathy, 629

and myotubular myopathy, 628–629

Infantile hypotonia, and Prader-Willi syndrome, 237–238

Infantile malignant osteopetrosis, 228–229

Infantile neuroaxonal dystrophy, 634

and congenital hypomyelination neuropathy, 568

and Dejerine-Sottas syndrome, 527–528

and giant axonal neuropathy, 569

Infantile neuronal ceroid lipofuscinosis, and infantile neuroaxonal dystrophy, 634

Infantile nystagmus, and Leber congenital amaurosis, 651–652

Infantile polycystic kidneys, and Meckel syndrome, 221

Infantile Refsum disease, and peroxisomal biogenesis disorders, 486

Infantile spasms, 541

and Aicardi syndrome, 509–510

Infectious perichondritis, and relapsing polychondritis, 29

Infertility, and androgen insensitivity syndrome, 306–307

and Asherman syndrome, 308–309

and autoimmune premature ovarian failure, 30–31

and Bloom syndrome, 159–160

and primary ciliary dyskinesia, 675

and pseudomyxoma peritonei, 412

and spinal bulbar muscular atrophy, 636

Inflammatory bowel disease, and common variable immunodeficiency, 13

and Eales disease, 646

and eosinophilic gastroenteritis, 342

and intestinal pseudoobstruction, 347

and mesenteric panniculitis, 350

and small bowel diverticulosis, 339

Inflammatory pseudotumor, and mesenteric panniculitis, 350

Influenza, and anthrax, 278

and dengue fever, 281

and leptospirosis, 289

and Q fever, 293

Inguinal hernia, and SHORT syndrome, 250

Inherited hemolytic-uremic syndrome, 690–691

Inner ear infection, and ataxia-telangiectasia, 605–606

Inosiplex, and subacute sclerosing panencephalitis, 575

Inotropic agents, and congenital complete heart block, 50

Inpingement syndromes, and Parsonage-Turner syndrome, 577

Insect bites, and dermatitis herpetiformis, 103

and transient acantholytic dermatosis, 104

Insomnia, and Creutzfeldt-Jakob disease, 608

Inspiratory stridor, and recurrent respiratory papillomatosis, 676

Insulin, and Achard-Thiers syndrome, 300

and leprechaunism, 216

Insulin-like growth factor, and Laron dwarfism, 319–320

Insulin receptor, and leprechaunism, 215

Insulin replacement, and Wolfram syndrome, 273

Insulin resistance, and acquired generalized lipodystrophy, 320–321

and congenital generalized lipodystrophy, 322

and familial partial lipodystrophy, 323

and growth hormone deficiency, 314–315

and HAIR-AN syndrome, 315–316

Insulinoma, and pancreatic islet cell tumors, 408–409

Insulinopenic diabetes, and SHORT syndrome, 250

Interferon, and angioimmunoblastic lymphadenopathy-type T-cell lymphoma, 398

and idiopathic thrombocytopenic purpura, 416

and mycosis fungoides, 406

and polycythemia vera, 411–412

Interferon-α, and Behçet disease, 4

and bowenoid papulosis, 98

and Churg-Strauss syndrome, 674

and encephalitides, 284

and familial Mediterranean fever, 19

and lymphomatoid granulomatosis, 49

and recurrent respiratory papillomatosis, 676

and Sjögren syndrome, 34

and subacute sclerosing panencephalitis, 575

Interferon-α2a, and Bowen disease, 98

and Erdheim-Chester disease, 441

Interferon-α2b, and adiposis dolorosa, 303

Interferon-γ, and autosomal-recessive osteopetrosis, 229

and chronic granulomatous disease, 387

and hyper-IgE syndrome, 13

and Whipple disease, 297

Intermittent porphyria, and cyclic vomiting syndrome, 525

Interruption of the aortic arch, and hypoplastic left heart syndrome, 50

Interstitial cystitis, 685

Interstitial deletion 17p11.2, 254

Intestinal disturbances, and blue diaper syndrome, 681

Intestinal ganlioneuromatosis, and Ruvalcaba-Myhre-Smith syndrome, 354

Intestinal lymphangiectasia, 346

Intestinal metaplasia of the esophagus, 333

Intestinal polyposis, and PTEN hamartoma tumor syndrome, 240

Intestinal polyps, and Ruvalcaba-Myhre-Smith syndrome, 354

Intestinal pseudoobstruction, 347–349

Intestinal transplantation, and microvillus inclusion disease, 351

Intraabdominal embryonal tumors, and Beckwith-Wiedemann syndrome, 518

Intracranial lesions, and pheochromocytoma, 409

Intracranial pressure elevation, and Arnold-Chiari syndrome, 516

and medulloblastoma, 404–405

and pseudotumor cerebri, 582–583

and sclerosteosis, 248–249

Intraepidermal epithelioma, and Bowen disease, 97

Intraepithelial squamous cell carcinoma, and bowenoid papulosis, 98–99

Intrahepatic cholestasis, 288

Intraocular foreign body, and posterior uveitis, 666

Intraocular inflammation, and pars planitis, 656–657

Intraocular neoplasms, and retinoblastoma, 661

Intrauterine adhesions, and Asherman syndrome, 308–309

Intrauterine growth retardation, and Neu-Laxova syndrome, 562–563

Intrauterine infections, and Galloway-Mowat syndrome, 687

and hydrocephalus, 539

and kernicterus, 543

Intrauterine supraventricular tachycardia, and hypoplastic left heart syndrome, 50

Intravenous gammaglobulin, and Lambert-Eaton myasthenic syndrome, 621

and pemphigus foliaceus, 132

and pemphigus vulgaris, 132

Intravenous immunoglobulin, and autoimmune hemolytic anemia, 367

and bullous pemphigoid, 131

and chronic inflammatory demyelinating polyradiculoneuropathy, 582

and common variable immunodeficiency, 13

and encephalitides, 284

and erythema multiforme, 110

and Guillain-Barré syndrome, 535

and hyper-IgM syndrome, 393–394

and hypersensivity myocarditis, 53

and Kawasaki disease, 15

and multiple sclerosis, 560

and severe combined immunodeficiency, 14

and X-linked agammaglobulinemia, 360–361

and X-linked lymphoproliferative syndrome, 400

Intravenous immunoglobulins, and opsoclonus-myoclonus syndrome, 573

Intraventricular hemorrhage, and hydrocephalus, 539

Irideremia, 640

Iridocorneal dysgenesis, and megalocornea, 556

Iridocorneal-endothelial syndrome, 644, 649–650

Iridogoniodysgenesis, and aniridia, 640

Iridogoniodysgenesis syndrome, 243–244

Iris abnormalities, and iridocorneal endothelial syndromes, 649

Iris agenesis, and aniridia, 640

Iris alterations, and iridocorneal endothelial syndromes, 649

Iris atrophy, essential, 650

Iris hypoplasia, and megalocornea, 556

and Rieger syndrome, 243–244

Iris ischemia, 650

Iris nevus syndrome, 644

Iron deficiency anemia, and autoimmune hemolytic anemia, 367

and thalassemia minor, 420

and X-linked sideroblastic anemia, 374–375

Iron deposition, and Hallervorden-Spatz syndrome, 620

Iron overload, 387–388

Irradiation, and POEMS syndrome, 27

Irritable bowel syndrome, and intestinal pseudoobstruction, 347–348

Isaacs syndrome, 635

Ischemia, and Takayasu arteritis, 35

Islet cell tumors of the pancreas, 408–409

Isochromosome 12p mosaicism, 231

Isolated cryptophthalmos, and Fraser syndrome, 196–197

Isolated supravalaortic stenosis, and Williams syndrome, 270

Isolated thoracic cardiac ectopy, and pentalogy of Cantrell, 233–234

Isoleucinemia, and maple syrup urine disease, 468

Isotretinoin, and Bowen disease, 98

and Darier disease, 101

and erythrokeratodermia variabilis, 112

and fibrodysplasia ossificans progressiva, 713

and hidradenitis suppurativa, 119

and pityriasis rubra pilaris, 133

and recurrent respiratory papillomatosis, 676

and transient acantholytic dermatosis, 104

Isovaleric acidemia, 427–428

Isovaleric acidosis, and ataxia-telangiectasia, 605–606

Isovaleric aciduria, 427

Isovaleryl CoA dehydrogenase deficiency, 427

Ito syndrome, 119–120

Ittrium 90, and carcinoid syndrome, 311–312

Ivemark syndrome, 205–206

and autosomal-recessive polycystic kidney disease, 697

and situs inversus, 55

Iwashita syndrome, and Rosenbert-Chutorian syndrome, 585

J

Jackson-Weiss syndrome, 719

and Apert syndrome, 154

and Crouzon syndrome, 710

and Pfeiffer syndrome type I, 234

and primary craniosynostosis, 174

and Saethre-Chotzen syndrome, 727–728

Jacobi stomatitis neurotica chronica, 138

Jacobsen syndrome, 60–61

Jaeken disease, 457–458

Jansen disease, 206–207

Jansen dysostosis, 206–207

Jansen metaphyseal chondrodysplasia, 206–207

Jansky-Bielschowsky disease, and Kuf disease, 547

Japanese encephalitis virus, 284–285

Japanese type spondylo-metaphyseal dysplasia, 248

Jarcho-Levin syndrome, 207–208

and Robinow syndrome, 725–726

Jaundice, and autoimmune hemolytic anemia, 367

and biliary atresia, 334

and Byler disease, 335

and cold hemolytic anemia syndromes, 368

and congenital nonspherocytic hemolytic anemia, 369

and Dubin-Johnson syndrome, 340

and galactosemia, 446

and graft-versus-host disease, 11

and hepatorenal syndrome, 344

and hereditary spherocytosis, 370–371

and idiopathic neonatal hepatitis, 288

and Niemann-Pick disease, 485

and paroxysmal cold hemoglobinuria, 388–389

and phosphoglycerate kinase deficiency, 489–490

and thalassemia major, 419

and tyrosinemia, 504

Jaw contractions, and oromandibular dystonia, 615–616

Jaw dystonia, 615–616

Jaw tumors, and ameloblastoma, 363–364

Jejunal atresia, 349

Jelly belly, 412–413

Jervell and Lange-Nielsen syndrome, 51–52

Jeune syndrome, 155–156
  and autosomal-recessive polycystic kidney disease, 697
  and Leber congenital amaurosis, 652

Johanson-Blizzard syndrome, 208–209
  and Shwachman-Diamond syndrome, 417

Joint contractures, and Antley-Bixler syndrome, 704–705
  and caudal regression syndrome, 166
  and congenital contractual arachnodactyly, 3
  and Marden-Walker syndrome, 18
  and metatropic dysplasia, 20
  and multiple pterygium syndrome, 241
  and Schwartz-Jampel syndrome, 586–587
  and Weaver syndrome, 266–267
  and Williams syndrome, 270

Joint deformities, and Bowen-Conradi syndrome, 161
  and familial articular chondrocalcinosis, 169–170
  and nail-patella syndrome, 721–722
  and spondyloepiphyseal dysplasia tarda, 729–730

Joint destruction, and alkaptonuria, 431

Joint hyperextensibility, and Laband syndrome, 214
  and SHORT syndrome, 250

Joint laxity, and chromosome 10, distal trisomy 10q, 59
  and Morquio disease, 480

Joint masses, and multiple hereditary exostoses, 191

Joint mobility deficits, and diastrophic dysplasia, 711
  and Leri pleonosteosis, 216–217
  and mucolipidosis, 472
  and Weill-Marchesani syndrome, 267–268

Joint pain, and Farber disease, 443
  and Maroteaux-Lamy disease, 481
  and multiple epiphyseal dysplasia, 187–188
  and Scheie disease, 478

Joint stiffness, and progeria, 724

Joseph disease, 555

Joubert-Boltshauser syndrome, 542

Joubert syndrome, 542
  and Leber congenital amaurosis, 652
  and Meckel syndrome, 221

Jugular lymphatic obstruction, 175–176

Jumping Frenchmen of Maine, and hyperekplexia, 540

Junctional epidermolysis bullosa, 107–108

Junctional epidermolysis bullosa, Herlitz, fig. 11, 107–108

Juvenile amaurotic familial idiocy, 516–517

Juvenile amaurotic idiocy, and carnosinemia, 435

Juvenile chorea, 522

Juvenile dystonic lipidosis, 485

Juvenile hyaline fibromatosis, and Winchester syndrome, 271

Juvenile idiopathic osteoporosis, and osteogenesis imperfecta, 227

Juvenile periodontitis, and hypophosphatasia, 317–318

Juvenile polyposis, and PTEN hamartoma tumor syndrome, 240
  and Ruvalcaba-Myhre-Smith syndrome, 354

Juvenile polyps, and Cronkhite-Canada syndrome, 338

Juvenile rheumatoid arthritis, and Farber disease, 443
  and Winchester syndrome, 271

K

Kabuki make-up syndrome, 209–210
  and C syndrome, 162

Kabuki syndrome, 209–210

Kallmann syndrome, 318–319

Karatoconjunctivitis sicca, 34

Kartagener syndrome, and Ivemark syndrome, 205
  and primary ciliary dyskinesia, 675
  and situs inversus, 55

Kasai portoenterostomy, and biliary atresia, 334

Kawasaki disease, 15–16
  and polyarteritis nodosa, 28
  and Takayasu arteritis, 35

KBG syndrome, 210

Kearns-Sayre syndrome, 462, 603–604

Keller syndrome, 193–194

Kelly syndrome, and Filippi syndrome, 194–195
  and Scott craniodigital syndrome, 249–250

Kenalog, and lichen planus, 125

Kennedy disease, and amyotrophic lateral sclerosis, 513

Kennedy syndrome, 636

Kenny-Caffey syndrome, 211

Kenny syndrome, 211

Keratinization, and pityriasis rubra pilaris, 133

Keratitis-ichthyosis-deafness syndrome, fig. 20, 122–123
  and Baller-Gerold syndrome, 157

Keratoconus, 650–651

Keratocysts, and ameloblastoma, 363

Keratoderma, and Meleda disease, 128

Keratosis follicularis, 101
  and transient acantholytic dermatosis, 104

Keratosis follicularis spinulosa decalvans, and keratitis-ichthyosis-deafness syndrome, 122

Keratosis palmoplantaris, 128

Keratosis palmoplantaris transgrediens, and erythrokeratodermia variabilis, 112
  and progressive symmetric erythrokeratodermia, 111

Keratosis rubra figurate, 112–113

Kernicterus, 543

Ketoacidosis, and multiple carboxylase deficiency, 482–483

Ketotifen, and eosinophilic gastroenteritis, 342

Kidney agenesis, and Fraser syndrome, 196–197
  and Kallmann syndrome, 318–319

Kidney damage, and galactosemia, 446

Kidney disease, and Glanzmann thrombasthenia, 383
  and porphyria cutanea tarda, 493–494
  and thrombotic thrombocytopenic purpura, 416

Kidney failure, and Alström syndrome, 305–306
  and cystinosis, 683
  and Denys-Drash syndrome, 686
  and familial juvenile hyperuricemic nephropathy, 696
  and Galloway-Mowat syndrome, 687
  and malaria, 291
  and pancreatic islet cell tumors, 408–409
  and pseudohypoparathyroidism, 325–326
  and type V glycogen storage disease, 455
  and X-linked sideroblastic anemia, 373

Kidney hamartomas, and tuberous sclerosis, 595–596
Kidney malformations, and Bardet-Biedl syndrome, 158–159
   and brachio-oto-renal syndrome, 681–682
   and branchio-oculo-facial syndrome, 161–162
   and cat eye syndrome, 164–165
   and caudal regression syndrome, 166
   and chromosome 9, trisomy mosaic, 85–86
   and Pallister-Hall syndrome, 230
   and Schinzel Giedion syndrome, 247
   and Townes-Brocks syndrome, 262
Kidney stones, and Lesch-Nyhan syndrome, 465
   and medullary sponge kidney, 695
Kidney transplantation, and Alport syndrome, 680
   and autosomal-recessive polycystic kidney disease, 697
   and cystinosis, 683
   and cystinuria, 684
   and Denys-Drash syndrome, 686
   and inherited hemolytic-uremic syndrome, 690–691
   and Loken-Senior syndrome, 692
   and medullary cystic kidney disease, 694
Kindler syndrome, and Rothmund-Thomson syndrome, 135
Kinesigenic paroxysmal ataxia, 600–601
Kinky hair disease, 470
Kinsbourne syndrome, 572–573
Kjellin syndrome, and Stargardt disease, 663
Kleine-Levin syndrome, 544
Klinefelter syndrome, 89–90
   and Johanson-Blizzard syndrome, 208
   and XYY syndrome, 90
Klippel-Feil anomaly, and Poland syndrome, 236–237
Klippel-Feil syndrome, 720
   and Sprengel deformity, 257
Klippel-Trenaunay syndrome, 212
   and amniotic bands, 150
   and Parkes-Weber syndrome, 232
   and Proteus syndrome, 239
Klippel-Trenaunay-Weber syndrome, 212
   and Sturge-Weber syndrome, 258
Klumpke paralysis, and obstetric brachial plexus palsy, 571
Kluver-Bucy syndrome, 545
Kniest dysplasia, 213
   and metatropic dysplasia, 20

and spondyloepiphyseal dysplasia congenita, 728
Kobberling-Dunnigan syndrome, 323
Kohler disease, 21
Korsakoff syndrome, 546
Kostmann syndrome, and acquired agranulocytosis, 361
   and Barth syndrome, 44
   and severe chronic neutropenia, 22–23
   and Shwachman-Diamond syndrome, 417
Krabbe disease, 551–552
   and metachromatic leukodystrophy, 552
   and Pelizaeus-Merzbacher disease, 578
Krabbe leukodystrophy, 551
Kramer syndrome, 226–227
Kraurosis vulvae, 126
Kuf disease, 547
   and Tay-Sachs disease, 501
Kugelberg-Welander disease, 637
Külmeier-Degos disease, 102
Kunjin fever, 296
Kyphoketosis, and carnitine palmitoyl transferase I deficiency, 433
Kyphomelic dysplasia, 712–713
Kyphoscoliosis, and metatropic dysplasia, 20
   and multiple pterygium syndrome, 241
   and spondyloepiphyseal dysplasia congenita, 728
Kyrle disease, and Darier disease, 101

L
L-carnitine, and medium-chain acyl-CoA dehydrogenase deficiency, 437
L-cysteine, and erythropoietic protoporphyria, 496
L-tryptophan syndrome, 7
La Peste, 292
Laband syndrome, 214
Labial fusion, and partial androgen insensitivity syndrome, 307–308
Labyrinthectomy, and Ménière disease, 558
Labyrinthitis, and Ménière disease, 558
Lacrimal glands, enlargement of, *fig. 3*, 17
Lactase deficiency, and sucrase-isomaltase deficiency, 354
Lactate accumulation, and congenital lactic acidosis, 462–464
Lactate dehydrogenase deficiency, and type V glycogen storage disease, 455
Lactic acidosis, and congenital complete heart block, 49
   and MELAS, 469

Lactic acidosis, congenital, 462–464
Lactosylceramidosis, 485
Lacunar infarcts, and locked-in syndrome, 554
Lafora body disease, and Baltic/Mediterranean/Unverrich-Lundborg myoclonic epilepsy, 600
   and MERRF, 469
Lambert-Eaton myasthenic syndrome, 621
Lamellar ichthyosis, and epidermolytic hyperkeratosis, 109
   and Hay-Wells syndrome, 117
Laminectomy, and diffuse idiopathic skeletal hyperostosis, 10
   and syringobulbia, 589
   and syringomyelia, 591
Lamotrigine, and Landau-Kleffner syndrome, 548
   and Lennox-Gastaut syndrome, 550
Landau-Kleffner syndrome, 547–548
Landouzy-Dejerine muscular dystrophy, 625
Landry-Guillain-Barré-Strohl syndrome, 535–536
Landry-Guillain-Barré syndrome, 535–536
Langer-Giedion syndrome, and trichorhinophalangeal syndrome, 731
Langer mesomelic dysplasia syndrome, and dyschondrosteosis, 181
Langerhans cell histiocytosis, 392–393
   and Erdheim-Chester disease, 441
Language dysfunction, and frontotemporal dementia, 533–534
Large arteriovenous fistulae, and hypoplastic left heart syndrome, 50
Large cell lymphoma, and posterior uveitis, 666
Large granular lymphocyte leukemia, 394–395
Large plaque parapsoriasis, and mycosis fungoides, 406
Laron dwarfism, 319–320
Laron syndrome, 319–320
Larsen syndrome, and atelosteogenesis type III, 156
Laryngeal abnormalities, and Fraser syndrome, 196–197
Laryngeal cartilage, and relapsing polychondritis, 29
Laryngeal dystonia, 613–614
Laryngeal edema, and hereditary angioedema, 375

Laryngeal papilloma, and recurrent respiratory papillomatosis, 676

Laryngeal stenosis, and Leri pleonosteosis, 216–217

Laryngotracheal stenosis, and Leri pleonosteosis, 217

Laser therapy, and Barrett esophagus, 333
  and Bowen disease, 98
  and bowenoid papulosis, 98
  and Coats disease, 643
  and Darier disease, 101
  and Eales disease, 646
  and hidradenitis suppurativa, 119
  and keratoconus, 651
  and pars planitis, 657
  and retinoblastoma, 661
  and Rothmund-Thomson syndrome, 136
  and Sturge-Weber syndrome, 258
  and Von Hippel-Lindau disease, 266
  and Weill-Marchesani syndrome, 267–268

Lassa fever, 282
  and Rift Valley fever, 294

Latah, and hyperekplexia, 540

Lateral sclerosis, primary, 548–549

Lathyrism, and primary lateral sclerosis, 548

Laurence-Moon-Bardet-Biedl syndrome, 158–159, 215

Laurence-Moon-Biedl syndrome, 158–159

Laurence-Moon syndrome, 215
  and Alström syndrome, 306
  and retinitis pigmentosa, 660

Lawrence syndrome, 320–321

Lead intoxication, and familial juvenile hyperuricemic nephropathy, 696

Learning disabilities, and neurofibromatosis type I, 563–564
  and triple X syndrome, 89
  and XXY syndrome, 89–90

Leber amaurosis, and Loken-Senior syndrome, 692–693

Leber congenital amaurosis, 651–652
  and Alström syndrome, 306
  and medullary cystic kidney disease, 693

Leber hereditary optic neuropathy, 653

Leber miliary aneurysms, 643

Left atrial membrane, 45–46

Left sympathectomy, and Jervell and Lange-Nielsen syndrome, 52
  and Romano-Ward long QT syndrome, 54

Leg discomfort, and restless legs syndrome, 583

Leg pain, and lumbar spinal stenosis, 587–588

Leg weakness, and chronic inflammatory demyelinating polyradiculoneuropathy, 581–582

Legg-Calve-Perthes disease, 16

Leigh disease, and idiopathic congenital central hypoventilation syndrome, 673
  and infantile neuroaxonal dystrophy, 634
  and leukodystrophy, 551–552
  and Pelizaeus-Merzbacher disease, 578
  and Tay-Sachs disease, 501

Leigh encephalopathy, and Alexander disease, 510

Leigh syndrome, and human cytochrome oxidase deficiency, 436

Leiner disease, 123–124

Leishmaniasis, and anthrax, 278

Lennox-Gastaut syndrome, 549–550

Lentigines, and LEOPARD syndrome, 124–125

Lentiginosis profusa syndrome, 124–125

Lenz dysplasia, 654

Lenz microphthalmia, and Nance-Horan syndrome, 654

Lenz microphthalmia syndrome, 654

Lenz syndrome, and oculocerebral syndrome, 226–227

Leonhard syndrome, and Gerstmann syndrome, 534

Leontiasis ossea, 204–205

LEOPARD syndrome, 124–125
  and Aarskog syndrome, 142
  and multiple pterygium syndrome, 241
  and Noonan syndrome, 722

Leprechaunism, 215–216
  and neonatal progeroid syndrome, 238
  and SHORT syndrome, 250

Leprosy, and relapsing polychondritis, 29

Leptomeningeal angioma, and Sturge-Weber syndrome, 258

Leptomeningeal carcinomatosis, and pseudotumor cerebri, 582

Leptospira infection, 289

Leptospirosis, 289
  and dengue fever, 281
  and ehrlichiosis, 283
  and hantavirus pulmonary syndrome, 287
  and Kawasaki disease, 15
  and Q fever, 293
  and Rift Valley fever, 294
  and viral hemorrhagic fevers, 282

Leri pleonosteosis, 216–217

Leri-Weill dyschondrosteosis, 181
  and Turner syndrome, 264

Leri-Weill dysostosis, and Robinow syndrome, 725–726

Lesch-Nyhan syndrome, 464–465
  and Allan-Herndon-Dudley syndrome, 149
  and familial juvenile hyperuricemic nephropathy, 696

Letterer-Siwe disease, 392–393
  and incontinentia pigmenti, 121

Leucine catabolism, and isovaleric acidemia, 427

Leukemia, and acquired agranulocytosis, 361
  and acquired aplastic anemia, 364
  chronic lymphatic, and Waldenström macroglobulinemia, 38
  and Churg-Strauss syndrome, 674
  and Erdheim-Chester disease, 441
  and hemophagocytic lymphohistiocytosis, 397
  and idiopathic thrombocytosis, 420–421
  and Langerhans cell histiocytosis, 392
  large granular lymphocyte, 394–395
  and mastocytosis, 402
  and Niemann-Pick disease, 485
  and posterior uveitis, 666
  and Sjögren syndrome, 34
  and TORCH syndrome, 295

Leukemia cutis, and Sweet syndrome, 139

Leukocoria, and Coats disease, 643
  and Norrie disease, 656
  and retinoblastoma, 661

Leukocyte adhesion deficiency, and chronic granulomatous disease, 386

Leukocyte inclusions, and May-Hegglin anomaly, 403

Leukocytoclastic vasculitis, and Mucha-Habermann disease, 129

Leukocytosis, and Ewing sarcoma of bone, 381

Leukodystrophy, 550–552
  metachromatic, 552
  and primary lateral sclerosis, 548

Leukoencephalopathy, 552–553

Leukomelanoderma, and hypomelanosis of Ito, 119

Leukopenia, and Gaucher disease, 447

Leuprolide, and Kluver-Bucy syndrome, 545

Levetiracetam, and progressive myoclonus epilepsy, 531–532

Levodopa, and dopa-responsive dystonia, 612

Levodopa, *(continued)*
    and Hallervorden-Spatz syndrome,
        620
    and multiple system atrophy, 561
    and Parkinson disease, 576
Levodopa/carbidopa, and rapid-onset
    dystonia-parkinsonism, 618
Levothyroxine, and chronic lymphocytic
    thyroiditis, 329
Levulosuria, 444–445
Lewis-Sumner syndrome, and chronic
        inflammatory demyelinating
        polyradiculoneuropathy, 581–582
Lewy body disease, and frontotemporal
        dementia, 534
Lichen amyloidosis, and lichen planus,
        125
Lichen nitidus, 125–126
Lichen planopilaris, 125–126
    and alopecia areata, 95
Lichen planus, *fig. 21*, 125–126
    and Behçet disease, 4
    and Bowen disease, 97
    and bowenoid papulosis, 98
    and lichen sclerosis, 126
    and Mucha-Habermann disease, 129
Lichen sclerosis, 126
Lichen simplex chronicus, and bowenoid
        papulosis, 98
    and lichen sclerosis, 126
Liddle syndrome, and primary
        aldosteronism, 305
Lidocaine, and adiposis dolorosa, 303
    and Romano-Ward long QT
        syndrome, 54
Ligaments, ossification of, and diffuse
        idiopathic skeletal hyperostosis,
        9–10
Limb ataxia, and Friedreich ataxia,
        602–603
Limb-body wall defect, and amniotic
        bands, 150
Limb deficiency, and Adams-Oliver
        syndrome, 148
    and Conradi-Hünermann syndrome,
        173
    and diastrophic dysplasia, 711
    and dyschondrosteosis, 181
    and femoral hypoplasia–unusual facies
        syndrome, 712–713
    and multiple epiphyseal dysplasia,
        187–188
    and Robinow syndrome, 725–726
    and Schmid metaphyseal
        chondrodysplasia, 248

Limb deficiency-splenogonadal fusion
        syndrome, and Möbius syndrome,
        223–224
Limb deformities, and acromesomelic
        dysplasia, 704
    and acrosomelic dysplasia, 702–703
    and chromosome 4, monosomy distal
        4q, 75
    and chromosome 4, partial trisomy
        distal 4q, 76
    and craniofrontonasal syndrome, 183
    and Hanhart syndrome, 203
    and Leri pleonosteosis, 216–217
    and Möbius syndrome, 223–224
    and oto-palato-digital syndrome, 229
    and Parkes-Weber syndrome, 232
    and Roberts pseudothalidomide
        syndrome, 244–245
    and Weismann-Netter-Stuhl
        syndrome, 268
Limb dysfunction, and corticobasal
        degeneration, 524–525
Limb edema, and hereditary angioedema,
        375
    and hereditary lymphedema, 396
Limb girdle muscular dystrophy, 625–626
Limb hypoplasia, and Fryns syndrome,
        715
Limb-mammary syndrome, and Schinzel
        syndrome, 246
    and split hand/split foot
        malformation, 256
Limb movement disorder, and Kleine-
        Levin syndrome, 544
Limb pain, and Camurati-Engelmann
        disease, 707–708
Limb spasms, and rapid-onset dystonia-
        parkinsonism, 617
Limb weakness, and Charcot-Marie-
        Tooth Polyneuropathy syndrome,
        521–522
    and Guillain-Barré syndrome, 535
Lindau disease, 265–266
Linear epidermal nevus syndrome,
        105–106
Linear IgA dermatosis, and cicatricial
        pemphigoid, 131
    and dermatitis herpetiformis, 103
Linear scleroderma, and Parry-Romberg
        syndrome, 232–233
Lipedema, and hereditary lymphedema,
        396
Lipemia retinalis, and familial lipoprotein
        lipase deficiency, 465–466
Lipid exudation, and Coats disease, 643

Lipoatrophy, and neonatal progeroid
        syndrome, 238
Lipodermoids, and Goldenhar syndrome,
        716
Lipodystrophy, acquired generalized,
        320–321
    acquired partial, 321
    congenital generalized, 322
    familial partial, 323
    and progeria, 724
    and SHORT syndrome, 250
Lipogranulomatosis, 441
Lipoid adrenal hyperplasia, and
        congenital adrenal hyperplasia,
        304
Lipoid granulomatosis, 441
Lipoid proteinosis, and Winchester
        syndrome, 271
Lipomas, painful, and adiposis dolorosa,
        303
    and PTEN hamartoma tumor
        syndrome, 240
Lipomatosis of pancreas, 417
Lipoprotein disorders, and MELAS, 469
Lipoprotein lipase deficiency, familial,
        465–466
Liposclerotic mesenteritis, 350
Liposuction, and adiposis dolorosa, 303
Lisch nodules, and Cogan-Reese
        syndrome, 644
Lissencephaly, classic, 553–554
    and Walker-Warburg syndrome,
        597–598
Listeria monocytogenes infection, 290
Listerial infection, and TORCH
        syndrome, 295
Listeriosis, 290
Livedo reticularis, congenital, 100
Liver cirrhosis, and alpha 1-antitrypsin
        deficiency, 671
    and biliary atresia, 334
    and X-linked sideroblastic anemia, 373
Liver disease, and alpha 1-antitrypsin
        deficiency, 671
    and biliary atresia, 334
    and Byler disease, 335
    and carnitine palmitoyl transferase I
        deficiency, 433
    and Caroli disease, 336
    and Crigler-Najjar syndrome, 337
    and galactosemia, 446
    and Glanzmann thrombasthenia, 383
    and hepatorenal syndrome, 344
    and hereditary hemorrhagic
        telangiectasia, 418

and liver fluke disease, 286
and Tangier disease, 500
and tyrosinemia, 504
Liver diseases, and Dubin-Johnson
    syndrome, 340
Liver dysfunction, and porphyria cutanea
    tarda, 493–494
and Shwachman-Diamond syndrome,
    417
and very-long-chain acyl-CoA
    dehydrogenase deficiency, 439–440
Liver failure, and Caroli syndrome, 336
and hemophagocytic
    lymphohistiocytosis, 397–398
and hepatorenal syndrome, 344
and Wilson disease, 506
Liver fluke disease, 286
Liver lobectomy, and Caroli disease, 336
Liver transplantation, and alpha 1-
    antitrypsin deficiency, 671
and biliary atresia, 334
and carnitine palmitoyl transferase I
    deficiency, 433
and carnitine palmitoyl transferase II
    deficiency, 434
and Caroli disease, 336C
and Crigler-Najjar syndrome, 337
and hepatorenal syndrome, 344
and propionic acidemia, 428
Lobar atrophy, and frontotemporal
    dementia, 533–534
Loblowitz ulcus neuroticum ori, 138
Lobster claw anomaly, 256
Locked-in syndrome, 554
Löffler endomyocarditis, 47–48
Löffler myocarditis, and hypersensitivity
    myocarditis, 53
Löffler syndrome, and Churg-Strauss
    syndrome, 674
Löfgren syndrome, 32–33
Loken-Senior syndrome, 692–693
and medullary cystic kidney disease,
    693
and retinitis pigmentosa, 660
Long bone cortical thickening, and
    Kenny-Caffey syndrome, 211
Long bone diaphysis, and hyperostosis
    corticalis generalisata, 204–205
Long bone metaphyseal widening, and
    craniometaphyseal dysplasia, 184
Long-chain acyl-CoA dehydrogenase
    deficiency, 437
Long QT syndrome, autosomal-recessive,
    51–52
and Brugada syndrome, 45

Loose body, and dysplasia epiphysealis
    hemimelica, 186
Lopez Hernandez syndrome, and Gorlin-
    Chaudhry-Moss syndrome, 200
Loratidine, and transient acantholytic
    dermatosis, 104
Lorazepam, and cyclic vomiting
    syndrome, 526
Lou Gehrig disease, 513–514
Louis-Bar syndrome, 605–606
Low birth weight, and chromosome 4
    ring, 76
and chromosome 14 ring, 63–64
and floating harbor syndrome, 195
and maternal phenylketonuria, 489
and X-linked sideroblastic anemia,
    374–375
Low-density gb-lipoprotein deficiency,
    358
Low hairline, and Gorlin-Chaudhry-
    Moss syndrome, 200
and Klippel-Feil syndrome, 720
and Saethre-Chotzen syndrome,
    727–728
Low intracranial pressure, and Arnold-
    Chiari syndrome, 516
Lowe syndrome, 466–467
and Marinesco-Sjögren syndrome,
    720–721
and oculocerebral syndrome, 226–
    227
Lower extremity weakness, and
    hereditary spastic paraplegia,
    575–576
Lubag, 619
Lubs syndrome, 307–308
Lumbar lordosis, and spondyloepiphyseal
    dysplasia congenita, 728
Lumbar pain, and lumbar spinal stenosis,
    587–588
Lumbar spinal stenosis, 587–588
Lung disease, and sarcoidosis, 32–33
Lung edema, and acute respiratory
    distress syndrome, 670
Lung hamartomas, and tuberous
    sclerosis, 595–596
Lung transplantation, and alveolar
    capillary dysplasia, 672
and primary ciliary dyskinesia, 675
and primary pulmonary hypertension,
    678
Lupus, 522
Lupus anticoagulant, and
    antiphospholipid syndrome, 2
Lupus anticoagulant syndrome, 2

Lupus erythematosus, and alopecia
    areata, 95
and Degos disease, 102
and erythema multiforme, 110
and lichen planus, 125
Lutembacher syndrome, and atrial septal
    defects, 42
Lyell syndrome, 139–140
Lyme borreliosis, and Eales disease, 646
Lyme disease, and ehrlichiosis, 283
and granuloma annulare, 116
and pars planitis, 656–657
and primary lateral sclerosis, 548
Lymphadenitis, and bubonic plague, 292
Lymphadenopathy, and
    angioimmunoblastic
    lymphadenopathy-type T-cell
    lymphoma, 398–399
Lymphangioleiomyomatosis, 395–396
Lymphangioma, 175–176
Lymphatic disease, and sarcoidosis, 32–33
Lymphatic filariasis, and bubonic plague,
    292
Lymphatic malformation, and cavernous
    hemangioma, 117
Lymphedema, hereditary, 396–397
and Klippel-Trenaunay syndrome, 212
Lymphocutaneous syndrome, and
    Kawasaki disease, 15
Lymphocytic gastritis, 341
Lymphocytic infiltration, and
    autoimmune premature ovarian
    failure, 30–31
Lymphocytic myocarditis, 52
Lymphoepithelial cysts, benign, and
    benign lymphoepithelial lesion, 17
Lymphoepithelial lesion, benign, 17
Lymphogranulomatosis X, 398–399
Lymphohistiocytosis, hemophagocytic,
    397–398
Lymphoid hyperplasia, and hyper-IgM
    syndrome, 393
Lymphoid infiltration, and Waldenström
    macroglobulinemia, 37–38
Lymphoma, angioimmunoblastic
    lymphadenopathy-type T-cell,
    398–399
and Cushing syndrome, 312–313
and Eales disease, 646
and Erdheim-Chester disease, 441
and Ewing sarcoma of bone, 380–381
and giant hypertrophic gastritis, 341
and Langerhans cell histiocytosis, 392
and mastocytosis, 402
and Niemann-Pick disease, 485

Lymphoma, *(continued)*
  and retinoblastoma, 661
  and sarcoidosis, 32
  and Wegener granulomatosis, 422
Lymphoma-like syndrome, and Chédiak-Higashi syndrome, 379
Lymphomatoid granulomatosis, 48–49
  and Wegener granulomatosis, 422
Lymphomatoid papulosis, and Mucha-Habermann disease, 129
Lymphomatous infiltration, and Guillain-Barré syndrome, 535
Lymphoproliferative syndrome, X-linked, 400
Lynch syndromes, 401
Lysinuric protein intolerance, and urea cycle disorders, 506–506
Lysosomal storage disease(s), and aspartylglucosaminuria, 432
  and Hajdu-Cheney syndrome, 11
Lytic destruction, and multiple myeloma, 407

M
Machado-Joseph disease, 555
Macrocephaly, and acrocallosal syndrome (Schinzel type), 145
  and FG syndrome, 193–194
  and Greig cephalopolysyndactyly syndrome, 201
  and neonatal progeroid syndrome, 238
  and PTEN hamartoma tumor syndrome, 240
  and Russel-Silver syndrome, 245–246
  and Ruvalcaba-Myhre-Smith syndrome, 354
Macrocrania, and Dandy-Walker syndrome, 526
Macrodactyly, and amniotic bands, 150
Macroglobulinemia, 37–38
Macroglossia, and Beckwith-Wiedemann syndrome, 518
  and type II glycogen storage disease, 452
Macrosomia, and Beckwith-Wiedemann syndrome, 518
Macular degeneration, and Stargardt disease, 663
Macular hypoplasia, and aniridia, 640
Madelung deformity, and dyschondrosteosis, 181
Madelung disease, and adiposis dolorosa, 303
Maffucci syndrome, 217–218
  and Proteus syndrome, 239

Magnesium deficiency, and pseudohypoparathyroidism, 325–326
Malabsorption, and intestinal lymphangiectasia, 346
  and mastocytosis, 402
  and Shwachman-Diamond syndrome, 417
  and small bowel diverticulosis, 339
Malabsorption syndrome, and common variable immunodeficiency, 13
Malar hypoplasia, and Miller syndrome, 222–223
  and Nager syndrome, 226
  and Treacher-Collins syndrome, 262–263
Malaria, 291
  and dengue fever, 281
  and leptospirosis, 289
  and Niemann-Pick disease, 485
  and Q fever, 293
  and Rift Valley fever, 294
  and viral hemorrhagic fevers, 282
Male factor infertility, and Asherman syndrome, 308–309
Malignancy, and HAIR-AN syndrome, 315–316
Malignant atrophic papulosis, 102
Malignant catatonia, 566
Malignant edema, 278
Malignant histiocytosis, and Erdheim-Chester disease, 441
Malignant hyperphenylalaninemia, 502
Malignant hyperthermia, 718
  and neuroleptic malignant syndrome, 566
Malignant hypothermia, and central core disease, 607–608
Malignant lymphoma, and Whipple disease, 297
  and X-linked lymphoproliferative syndrome, 400
Malignant melanoma, and Cogan-Reese syndrome, 644
  and posterior uveitis, 666
Malignant pustule, 278
Mallattia Leventinese/dominant drusen, and Stargardt disease, 663
Malnourishment, and Korsakoff syndrome, 546
Malocclusion, and Williams syndrome, 270
Malrotation, and cyclic vomiting syndrome, 525
Malta fever, 280
Mandibular dysostosis, 262–263

Mandibular hypoplasia, and Goldenhar syndrome, 716
  and Hanhart syndrome, 203
  and pyknodysostosis, 242
  and Treacher-Collins syndrome, 262–263
Mandibular malformations, and cherubism, 168–169
Mandibuloacral dysplasia, and acrogeria (Gottron type), 147
  and cleidocranial dysplasia, 182
  and progeria, 724
Mandibulofacial dysostosis, and Hallermann-Streiff syndrome, 202
Mannose, and congenital disorders of glycosylation, 458
Mantle cell lymphoma, 399
Maple syrup urine disease, 468–469
  and Niemann-Pick disease, 485
Marburg disease, and Rift Valley fever, 294
Marburg hemorrhagic fever, 282
Marden-Walker syndrome, 18
  and blepharophimosis-ptosis-epicanthus inversus syndrome, 641
  and Schwartz-Jampel syndrome, 586
Marfan-like appearance, and congenital contractual arachnodactyly, 3
Marfan syndrome, 218–219
  and alpha 1-antitrypsin deficiency, 671
  and congenital contractual arachnodactyly, 3
  and homocystinuria, 459
  and medullary sponge kidney, 694
  and megalocornea, 556
  and Sotos syndrome, 255
  and Takayasu arteritis, 35
  and triple X syndrome, 89
  and Weill-Marchesani syndrome, 267–268
  and XYY syndrome, 90
Marie ataxia, and Machado-Joseph disease, 555
Marie disease, 301
Marinesco-Garland syndrome, 720–721
Marinesco-Sjögren syndrome, 720–721
Marked edema, and Cronkhite-Canada syndrome, 338
Maroteaux-Lamy disease, 480–481
Maroteaux-Lamy syndrome, and mucolipidosis, 472
Marshall-Smith syndrome, *figs. 31–32,* 219–220
Marshall syndrome, and Weaver syndrome, 266–267
Martorell syndrome, 35

MASA syndrome, 220

Masculinization, and androgen insensitivity syndrome, 306–307

MASS phenotype, and Marfan syndrome, 218

Mast cell excess, and mastocytosis, 402

Mastocytosis, 402–403

Maternal isoimmune disease, and Beckwith-Wiedemann syndrome, 518

Maternal lupus, and Conradi-Hünermann syndrome, 173

Maternal phenylketonuria, *fig. 48*, 489
and fetal hydantoin syndrome, 192

Maternal valproic acid, and fetal valproate syndrome, 192–193

Maternal vitamin K deficiency, and Conradi-Hünermann syndrome, 173

Maxillary hypoplasia, and Crouzon syndrome, 710

Maxillary retrusion/mandibular protrusion, and maxillonasal dysplasia, 186–187

Maxillonasal dysplasia, 186–187

May-Hegglin anomaly, 403–404
and Bernard-Soulier syndrome, 378

Mayer-Rokitansky-Karaster syndrome, and Klippel-Feil syndrome, 720

Mayer-Rokitansky-Küster-Hauser syndrome, and caudal regression syndrome, 166

Maypole syndrome, 349

McArdle disease, and phosphoglycerate kinase deficiency, 489

McArdle syndrome, and carnitine palmitoyl transferase II deficiency, 434

McCabe disease, 723–724

McCardle disease, 454–455

McCune-Albright syndrome, and acromegaly, 301
and cherubism, 168
and neurofibromatosis type I, 564

McGrath syndrome, 127

McKusick-Kaufman syndrome, and Bardet-Biedl syndrome, 158
and Laurence-Moon syndrome, 215
and Pallister-Hall syndrome, 230

Measles, and dengue fever, 281
and Kawasaki disease, 15
and subacute sclerosing panencephalitis, 574–575

Mechanical intestinal obstruction, and intestinal pseudoobstruction, 348

Mechanically induced alopecia, and alopecia areata, 95

Meckel-Gruber syndrome, 221
and autosomal-recessive polycystic kidney disease, 697
and Bardet-Biedl syndrome, 158
and trisomy 13 syndrome, 87

Meckel syndrome, 221

Meconium ileus, and Hirschsprung disease, 345

Meconium plug syndrome, and Hirschsprung disease, 345

Mediterranean fever, 280
familial, 19

Medium-chain acyl-CoA dehydrogenase deficiency, 437–438

Medullary cystic kidney disease, 693–694

Medullary sponge kidney, 694
and medullary cystic kidney disease, 693

Medulloblastoma, 404–405
and Ewing sarcoma of bone, 380–381

Medulloepithelioma, and retinoblastoma, 661

Mefloquine, and malaria, 291

Mega cisterna magna, and Dandy-Walker syndrome, 526

Megacolon, and Hirschsprung disease, 345

Megaloblastic anemia, and autoimmune hemolytic anemia, 367

Megalocornea, 556

Meier-Gorlin syndrome, 189

Meige disease, 396–397

Meige syndrome, 615–616
and tardive dyskinesia, 591

Melanocytic nevi, and bowenoid papulosis, 98

Melanoma, 405
and bowenoid papulosis, 98
superficial spreading, and Bowen disease, 97

MELAS, 469–470
and Pelizaeus-Merzbacher disease, 578

Melatonin, and Kleine-Levin syndrome, 544

Meleda disease, 128

Melkersson-Rosenthal syndrome, 557
and Fountain syndrome, 196

Melnick-Fraser syndrome, 681–682

Melnick-Needles osteodysplasty, 221–222

Melnick-Needles syndrome, *figs. 33–34*, 221–222

Melphalan, and scleromyxedema, 137

Meltzer triad, and mixed cryoglobulin syndrome, 5

Memory impairment, and Korsakoff syndrome, 546

Menaline myopathy, and spinal muscular atrophy, 637

Ménétrier disease, and giant hypertrophic gastritis, 341

Ménière disease, 558

Meningeal hemangiomata, 258

Meningitis, and hydrocephalus, 539
and listeriosis, 290
and pseudotumor cerebri, 582
and Q fever, 293
and syringomyelia, 590

Meningocele, and aplasia cutis congenita, 96

Meningococcemia, and dengue fever, 281

Meningomyelocele, and cystic hygroma, 175

Menkes disease, 470–471

Menkes kinky hair syndrome, and Björnstad syndrome, 97

Menopause, and Achard-Thiers syndrome, 300
and pheochromocytoma, 409

Menorrhagia, and Bernard-Soulier syndrome, 378
and congenital afibrogenemia, 359–360

Menstrual irregularities, and Asherman syndrome, 308–309
and chronic lymphocytic thyroiditis, 329
and polycystic ovary syndrome, 323–324

Mental retardation, and acrocallosal syndrome (Schinzel type), 145
and acrodysostosis, 146
and Aicardi syndrome, 509–510
and Allan-Herndon-Dudley syndrome, 149
and alpha-mannosidosis, 467–468
and Borjeson-Forssman-Lehmann syndrome, 705–706
and cardiofaciocutaneous syndrome, 163–164
and carnosinemia, 435
and cat eye syndrome, 164–165
and cerebro-oculo-facio-skeletal syndrome, 520
and chromosome 3, monosomy 3p2, 73
and chromosome 3, trisomy 3q2, 73–74
and chromosome 4, monosomy distal 4q, 75
and chromosome 4, trisomy 4p, 77–78

Mental retardation, *(continued)*
  and chromosome 4 ring, 76
  and chromosome 5, trisomy 5p, 78
  and chromosome 6, partial trisomy 6q, 79
  and chromosome 6 ring, 80
  and chromosome 9, partial monosomy 9p, 82
  and chromosome 9, tetrasomy 9p, 84
  and chromosome 9, trisomy 9p, 84
  and chromosome 9 ring, 83
  and chromosome 10, distal trisomy 10q, 59
  and chromosome 10, monosomy 10p, 60
  and chromosome 11, partial monosomy 11q, 60–61
  and chromosome 11, partial trisomy 11q, 61
  and chromosome 13, partial monosomy 13q, 62–63
  and chromosome 14 ring, 63–64
  and chromosome 15, distal trisomy 15q, 65–66
  and chromosome 15 ring, 66
  and chromosome 18, monosomy 18p, 67
  and chromosome 18 ring, 68–69
  and chromosome 18q- syndrome, 67–68
  and chromosome 21 ring, 70
  and chromosome 22, trisomy mosaic, 72
  and chromosome 22 ring, 71–72
  and chylomicron retention disease, 380
  and classic lissencephaly, 553–554
  and Coffin-Lowry syndrome, 171–172
  and Cohen syndrome, 172
  and congenital bilateral perisylvian syndrome, 579–580
  and corpus callosum absence, 508
  and De Barsy syndrome, 6
  and deletion of the short arm of chromosome 1, 58
  and Dyggve-Melchior-Clausen syndrome, 180–181
  and FG syndrome, 193–194
  and Filippi syndrome, 194–195
  and Fountain syndrome, 196
  and fucosidosis, 445
  and giant axonal neuropathy, 569
  and hereditary spastic paraplegia, 575–576
  and histidinemia, 459

  and homocystinuria, 459
  and Joubert syndrome, 542
  and Kabuki make-up syndrome, 209–210
  and Kenny-Caffey syndrome, 211
  and Laband syndrome, 214
  and Leber congenital amaurosis, 652
  and Lennox-Gastaut syndrome, 549–550
  and Lenz microphthalmia syndrome, 654
  and Marinesco-Sjögren syndrome, 720–721
  and MASA syndrome, 220
  and maternal phenylketonuria, 489
  and megalocornea, 556
  and Myhre syndrome, 225
  and Pallister-Killian syndrome, 231
  and pentasomy X, 86–87
  and phenylketonuria, 488
  and phosphoglycerate kinase deficiency, 489–490
  and Roberts pseudothalidomide syndrome, 244–245
  and Rubinstein-Taybi syndrome, 726–727
  and sialidosis, 498
  and Sly disease, 481
  and Smith-Lemli-Opitz syndrome, 253
  and Smith-Magenis syndrome, 254
  and Sotos syndrome, 255
  and spondyloepiphyseal dysplasia congenita, 728
  and succinic semialdehyde dehydrogenase deficiency, 499
  and Townes-Brocks syndrome, 262
  and trichorhinophalangeal syndrome, 731
  and tuberous sclerosis, 596
  and WAGR syndrome, 699
  and Wieacker-Wolff syndrome, 638
  and Williams syndrome, 270
  and Wolf-Hirschhorn syndrome, 272
  and XLMR-hypotonic facies syndrome, 274
6-Mercaptopurine, and idiopathic thrombocytopenic purpura, 415–416
  and Langerhans cell histiocytosis, 393
Meroanencephaly, 151–152
Meropenem, and Whipple disease, 297
MERRF, 469–470
Merten syndrome, 635
Mesenteric fibromatosis, 350
Mesenteric lipodystrophy, 350
Mesenteric lipogranuloma, 350

Mesenteric panniculitis, 350
Mesiodens-cataract syndrome, 654–655
Mesodermal tissue growth failure, and MULIBREY nanism, 224–225
Mesomelic dwarfism, 181
Metabolic acidosis, and glucose-galactose malabsorption, 343
  and glutaric acidemia type II, 426–427
  and glutathione synthetase deficiency, 449
  and medullary sponge kidney, 694
  and propionic acidemia, 428
  and short-chain acyl-CoA dehydrogenase deficiency, 438–439
Metabolic disturbances, and encephalitides, 284
Metabolic myopathy, and Becker muscular dystrophy, 622
Metabolic rate, increased, and congenital generalized lipodystrophy, 322
Metabolism disorders, 425–506
Metabolism increase, and malignant hyperthermia, 718
Metacarpophalangeal shortening, and trichorhinophalangeal syndrome, 732
Metachromatic leukodystrophy, 552
  and adult polyglucosan body disease, 580
  and infantile neuroaxonal dystrophy, 634
  and multiple sulfatase deficiency, 484
Metachromic leukodystrophy, and Alexander disease, 510
Metaphyseal anadysplasias, and Schmid metaphyseal chondrodysplasia, 248
Metaphyseal chondrodysplasia, and multiple epiphyseal dysplasia, 187
Metaphyseal chondroplasia, and Shwachman-Diamond syndrome, 417
Metastatic carcinoma, and Bowen disease, 97
Metatropic dwarfism, and asphyxiating thoracic dystrophy, 155
Metatropic dwarfism type II, 213
Metatropic dysplasia, 20
Metatropic dysplasia type II, 213
Metformin, and HAIR-AN syndrome, 315–316
  and polycystic ovary syndrome, 324
Methamphetamines, and narcolepsy, 562
Methotrexate, and Behçet disease, 4
  and eosinophilia-myalgia syndrome, 7
  and Felty syndrome, 9

and Langerhans cell histiocytosis, 393

and large granular lymphocyte leukemia, 395

and Mucha-Habermann disease, 129

and mycosis fungoides, 406

and opsoclonus-myoclonus syndrome, 573

and pars planitis, 657

and pityriasis rubra pilaris, 133

and posterior uveitis, 666

and recurrent respiratory papillomatosis, 676

and sarcoidosis, 32

and Takayasu arteritis, 35

and Wegener granulomatosis, 423

Methylmalonate semialdehyde dehydrogenase deficiency, 471–472

Methylmalonic acidemias, 429

Methylmalonic aciduria, 429

Methylphenidate, and narcolepsy, 562

Methylprednisolone, and Henoch-Schönlein purpura, 415

and microscopic polyangiitis, 28

Methylprednisone, and graft-versus-host disease, 11

Metoclopramide, and small bowel diverticulosis, 339

Metronidazole, and botulism, 279

Mexilitine, and myotonia congenita, 633

and Romano-Ward long QT syndrome, 54

Michail-Matsoukas-Theodorou-Rubinstein-Taybi syndrome, 726–727

Michels syndrome, and blepharophimosis-ptosis-epicanthus inversus syndrome, 641

Microangiopathic hemolytic anemia, and autoimmune hemolytic anemia, 367

Microcephaly, and Bowen-Conradi syndrome, 161

and chromosome 3, monosomy 3p2, 73

and chromosome 6, partial trisomy 6q, 79

and Cornelia de Lange syndrome, 709

and Dyggve-Melchior-Clausen syndrome, 180–181

and Filippi syndrome, 194–195

and Galloway-Mowat syndrome, 687–688

and leukodystrophy, 550

and maternal phenylketonuria, 489

and Neu-Laxova syndrome, 562–563

and phenylketonuria, 488

and tetrahydrobiopterin deficiency, 502

and XLMR-hypotonic facies syndrome, 274

Microcephaly–hiatal hernia–nephrotic syndrome, 687–688

Microcephaly–infantile spasms–psychomotor retardation–nephrotic syndrome, 687–688

Microcephaly-vitreoretinal dysplasia, 655–656

Micrognathia, and cerebrocostomandibular syndrome, 166–167

and femoral hypoplasia–unusual facies syndrome, 712–713

and Marshall-Smith syndrome, 219

and neonatal progeroid syndrome, 238

and Pierre Robin sequence, 235–236

and SHORT syndrome, 250

Microhematuria, and benign familial hematuria, 689

Microorchidism, and Kenny-Caffey syndrome, 211

Microphthalmia, 654

Microphthalmia/anophthalmia, and trisomy 13 syndrome, 87

Microphthalmia-linear skin defects syndrome, and Aicardi syndrome, 509

Microphthalmia-microcephaly syndrome, and Norrie disease, 655

Microscopic polyangiitis, 27–27

and polyarteritis nodosa, 28

and Wegener granulomatosis, 422

Microscopic polyarteritis, 27–27

Microtia, and ear–patella–short stature syndrome, 189

and Goldenhar syndrome, 716

Microvillus inclusion disease, 351

Middle aortic syndrome, 35

Middle interhemispheric fusion, 536–537

Midface hypoplasia, and Gorlin-Chaudhry-Moss syndrome, 200

and Jackson-Weiss syndrome, 719

Midodrine, and multiple system atrophy, 561

Migraine, and cyclic vomiting syndrome, 526

and episodic ataxia type II, 601–602

and Sturge-Weber syndrome, 258

and Tolosa-Hunt syndrome, 664

Mikulicz aphthae, 138

Mikulicz syndrome, 17

Mild androgen insensitivity syndrome, 307

Miliaria rubra, and transient acantholytic dermatosis, 104

Milk alkali syndrome, and medullary sponge kidney, 694

Milk allergy, and sucrase-isomaltase deficiency, 354

Milky plasma, and familial lipoprotein lipase deficiency, 465–466

Miller-Fisher syndrome, and Guillain-Barré syndrome, 535–536

Miller syndrome, 222–223

and Nager syndrome, 226

and Treacher-Collins syndrome, 263

Minocycline ingestion, and alkaptonuria, 431

Miosis, and Horner syndrome, 648

Miscarriage, and twin-twin transfusion syndrome, 421–422

Mitochondrial cytopathies, and Niemann-Pick disease, 485

Mitochondrial disease, and Cockayne syndrome, 170–171

Mitochondrial encephalopathies, 469–470

and cyclic vomiting syndrome, 525

Mitochondrial myopathies, and deletion of the short arm of chromosome 1, 58

Mitochondrial myopathy, 462

and Barth syndrome, 44

and type V glycogen storage disease, 454

Mitomycin C, and pseudomyxoma peritonei, 413

Mitral atresia, 50–51

Mitral stenosis, and cor triatriatum, 46

Mitral valve prolapse syndrome, and Marfan syndrome, 218

Mixed connective tissue disease, and scleroderma, 33

Mixed cryoglobulin syndrome, 5

Mixed gonadal dysgenesis, 316–317

Miyoshi distal myopathy, and myofibrillar myopathy, 630

Möbius syndrome, 223–224

and Duane syndrome, 645

and facioscapulohumeral muscular dystrophy, 625

and idiopathic congenital central hypoventilation syndrome, 673

Modafinil, and narcolepsy, 562

Moersch-Woltman syndrome, 588–589

Mofetil, and myasthenia gravis, 627

Mohr syndrome, and Joubert syndrome, 542

Molar pregnancy, and triploidy syndrome, 263–264

Molluscum contagiosum, and granuloma
annulare, 116
Monilethrix, and Björnstad syndrome, 97
Monoclonal protein, and
scleromyxedema, 136–137
Monoclonal protein band, and POEMS
syndrome, 26–27
Mononucleosis, infectious, and Kawasaki
disease, 15
and X-linked lymphoproliferative
syndrome, 400
Monosomy 1p36, 58
Monosomy 3p2, 73
Monosomy 9p, partial, 82–83
Monosomy 10p, and chromosome 10,
distal trisomy 10q, 59
Monosomy 18q syndrome, 67–68
Monozygotic twinning, and GBBB
syndrome, 198–199
Mood disorder, and Wilson disease, 506
Moore-Federman syndrome, and Leri
pleonosteosis, 217
Morbus Behçet, 4
Morphea, and familial eosinophilic
cellulitis, 99
and lichen sclerosis, 126
Morquio disease, 480
and Schwartz-Jampel syndrome, 586
Morquio syndrome, and Dyggve-
Melchior-Clausen syndrome, 180
Morquio-type mucopolysaccharidosis,
and metatropic dysplasia, 20
Morvan disease, and hereditary sensory
neuropathy, 570
Mosaic corneal dystrophy, and
megalocornea, 556
Mosaic tetrasomy 9p, 83–84
Moschcowitz disease, 416
Mosquito-borne diseases, and dengue
fever, 281
and encephalitides, 284
and Rift Valley fever, 294
and West Nile fever, 296
Motor delays, and Dejerine-Sottas
syndrome, 527–528
Motor disturbances, and Kuf disease, 547
Motor neuron disease, 513–514
Motor neuron dysfunction, and adult
polyglucosan body disease,
580–581
and amyotrophic lateral sclerosis, 513
Motor tics, and blepharospasm, 610
and Tourette syndrome, 594
Motor weakness, and hydranencephaly,
538

and Marinesco-Sjögren syndrome,
720–721
and neuromyelitis optica, 567
and Sandhoff disease, 497
Movement, slowness of, and rapid-onset
dystonia-parkinsonism, 617
Movement disorders, and Fahr disease,
532
and Huntington disease, 537–538
and tardive dyskinesia, 591
Movement disturbances, and Sydenham
chorea, 522
Moyamoya disease, and alternating
hemiplegia of childhood, 512
and MELAS, 469
Moyamoya syndrome, 559
Moynahan syndrome, 124–125
Mucha-Habermann disease, 128–129
Mucinous peritoneal carcinomatosis,
412–413
Mucocutaneous bleeding, and Bernard-
Soulier syndrome, 378
Mucocutaneous lymph node syndrome,
and Kawasaki disease, 15
Mucoepidermoid carcinoma, and
adenoid cystic carcinoma, 359
Mucoid fluid, and pseudomyxoma
peritonei, 412
Mucolipidosis, 472–474
and Marinesco-Sjögren syndrome,
720–721
and megalocornea, 556
Mucopolysaccharide storage diseases,
474–481
Mucopolysaccharidosis, and
aspartylglucosaminuria, 432
and Coffin-Lowry syndrome, 171–172
and hydrocephalus, 539
and mucolipidosis, 473
and sialidosis, 498
and Winchester syndrome, 271
Mucosal bleeding, and Wiskott-Aldrich
syndrome, 39
Mucosal leukoplakia, and dyskeratosis
congenita, 105
Mucosal pemphigoid, benign, 131–132
Mucosulfatidosis, 484
Mucous cysts, and popliteal pterygium
syndrome, 242
Mucous membrane bleeding, and
idiopathic thrombocytopenic
purpura, 415
Mucous membrane pemphigoid, and
Behçet disease, 4
Mud fever, 289

Muir-Torre syndrome, and Lynch
syndromes, 401
MULIBREY nanism, 224–225
and Russel-Silver syndrome, 245–246
and 3-M syndrome, 259
Müllerian anomalies, and Asherman
syndrome, 308–309
Müllerian duct aplasia, and MURCS
association, 695
Multicore disease, and limb girdle
muscular dystrophy, 625
Multicore myopathy, and short-chain
acyl-CoA dehydrogenase
deficiency, 438–439
Multicystic dysplasia, and autosomal-
recessive polycystic kidney disease,
697
Multifocal motor neuropathy, and
Charcot-Marie-Tooth
polyneuropathy syndrome, 521–522
and chronic inflammatory
demyelinating
polyradiculoneuropathy, 581–582
Multiple carboxylase deficiency, 482–483
and Leiner disease, 123
Multiple exostoses, cartilaginous, 191
hereditary, figs. 26–30, 191
and trichorhinophalangeal syndrome,
731
Multiple congenital anomaly syndromes,
and Hajdu-Cheney syndrome, 11
Multiple endocrine neoplasia, and
acromegaly, 301
Multiple epiphyseal dysplasia, and
Melnick-Needles syndrome, 222
Multiple epiphyseal dysplasia type I,
187–188
Multiple hamartoma syndrome, and
Cowden syndrome, 240
Multiple hereditary
osteochondromatosis, 191
Multiple lentigines syndrome, 124–125
Multiple myeloma, 407
and POEMS syndrome, 26
and Waldenström macroglobulinemia,
38
Multiple pterygium syndrome, 241
and chromosome 6, partial trisomy 6q,
79
and Freeman-Sheldon syndrome, 714
and Neu-Laxova syndrome, 562
Multiple schwannomatosis, and
neurofibromatosis type 2, 565
Multiple sclerosis, and Alexander disease,
510

and Arnold-Chiari syndrome, 516
and Binswanger disease, 519
and chronic inflammatory
    demyelinating
    polyradiculoneuropathy, 581
and Eales disease, 646
and hereditary spastic paraplegia, 575
and Korsakoff syndrome, 546
Marburg variant, 560
and Ménière disease, 558
and methylmalonic acidemias, 429
and neuromyelitis optica, 567
and Pelizaeus-Merzbacher disease, 578
and primary lateral sclerosis, 548
rare variants of, 560
and Whipple disease, 297
Multiple sulfatase deficiency, 484
Multiple system atrophy, 561
    and Parkinson disease, 576
    and progressive supranuclear palsy,
        573
Multisynostotic osteodysgenesis, 704
Multisystem atrophy, and amyotrophic
    lateral sclerosis, 513
Mumps, and benign lymphoepithelial
    lesion, 17
Munson sign, and keratoconus, 651
MURCS association, 695
Murray-Puretic-Drescher syndrome, and
    Laband syndrome, 214
Muscle atrophy, and spinal bulbar
    muscular atrophy, 636
    and Wieacker-Wolff syndrome, 638
Muscle cramps, and Becker muscular
    dystrophy, 622
    and myotonia congenita, 632
    and neuromyotonia, 635
    and type VII glycogen storage disease,
        456–457
Muscle-eye-brain disease, and Walker-
    Warburg syndrome, 597
Muscle hyperactivity, and
    neuromyotonia, 635
Muscle hypertrophy, and Duchenne
    muscular dystrophy, 623
    and Myhre syndrome, 225
Muscle hypoplasia, and Allan-Herndon-
    Dudley syndrome, 149
Muscle pain, and Becker muscular
    dystrophy, 622
    and sickle cell anemia, 372–373
Muscle phosphofructokinase deficiency,
    456–457
    and phosphoglycerate kinase
        deficiency, 489

Muscle phosphorylase deficiency, and
    type V glycogen storage disease,
    454–455
Muscle rigidity, and neuroleptic
    malignant syndrome, 566
Muscle stiffness, and myotonia congenita,
    632
Muscle tone deficits, and chromosome
    10, distal trisomy 10q, 59
    and chromosome 14 ring, 63–64
    and chromosome 15 ring, 66
    and chromosome 18 ring, 68–69
    and chromosome 18q- syndrome,
        67–68
    and chromosome 22 ring, 71–72
    and tetrahydrobiopterin deficiency,
        502
Muscle tone loss, and infantile
    neuroaxonal dystrophy, 634
Muscle weakness, and acute intermittent
    porphyria, 490–491
    and Camurati-Engelmann disease,
        707–708
    and carnitine deficiency syndromes,
        432
    and congenital hypomyelination
        neuropathy, 568
    and Duchenne muscular dystrophy,
        623
    and facioscapulohumeral muscular
        dystrophy, 624–625
    and Lambert-Eaton myasthenic
        syndrome, 621
    and Marinesco-Sjögren syndrome,
        720–721
    and myasthenia gravis, 626–627
    and myofibrillar myopathy, 630
    and Rosenbert-Chutorian syndrome,
        585
    and spinal bulbar muscular atrophy,
        636
    and Sydenham chorea, 522
Muscular appearance, and congenital
    generalized lipodystrophy, 322
Muscular dystrophy, 622–626
    Becker, 622
    Duchenne, 623
    Emery-Dreifuss, 623
    facioscapulohumeral, 624–625
    and Lambert-Eaton myasthenic
        syndrome, 621
    limb girdle, 625–626
    and spinal muscular atrophy, 637
    and Walker-Warburg syndrome,
        597–598

Muscular hypotonia, and Lowe
    syndrome, 466–467
Musculoskeletal abnormalities, and
    Cornelia de Lange syndrome, 709
Music therapy, and Rett syndrome, 584
Musicians, and embouchure dystonia,
    613
Mutilating acropathy, and hereditary
    sensory neuropathy
Myalgia, 7
Myasthenia gravis, 626–627
    and botulism, 279
    and idiopathic congenital central
        hypoventilation syndrome, 673
    and Lambert-Eaton myasthenic
        syndrome, 621
    and locked-in syndrome, 554
    and neuromyotonia, 635
    and spinal muscular atrophy, 637
Myasthenic syndrome, 621
Mycobacterial disease, and anthrax, 278
Mycophenolate, and cicatricial
    pemphigoid, 131
    and posterior uveitis, 666
    and warm antibody hemolytic anemia,
        371–372
Mycophenolate mofetil, and microscopic
    polyangiitis, 28
    and polyarteritis nodosa, 29
    and Takayasu arteritis, 35
Mycoplasma infection, and
    encephalitides, 284
Mycoplasma pneumoniae infection, and
    Guillain-Barré syndrome, 535
Mycosis fungoides, 406
Myelinoclastic diffuse sclerosis, 560
Myelodysplasia, and acquired aplastic
    anemia, 364
    and acquired pure red cell aplasia, 413
Myelodysplastic syndrome, and acquired
    agranulocytosis, 361
Myelofibrosis, and acquired aplastic
    anemia, 364
Myelogenous leukemia, and Chédiak-
    Higashi syndrome, 379
Myelokathexis, and acquired
    agranulocytosis, 361
Myeloma, multiple, 407
Myelopathy, and primary lateral sclerosis,
    548
    and stiff person syndrome, 588
Myelotomy, and Arnold-Chiari
    syndrome, 516
    and syringobulbia, 589
    and syringomyelia, 590

Myhre syndrome, 225
Myocardial infarction, and factor XII
	deficiency, 382
Myocarditis, acute necrotizing
	eosinophilic, 53
	and Barth syndrome, 44
	giant cell, 52–53
	hypersensitivity, 53
Myoclonic astatic epilepsy, and Lennox-
	Gastaut syndrome, 549
Myoclonic dystonia, 614–615
Myoclonic epilepsy, and progressive
	myoclonus epilepsy, 531–532
Myoclonic jerk, 627–628
Myoclonus, 627–628
	and Tourette syndrome, 594
Myoclonus epilepsy, and MERRF, 469
Myoclonus syndrome, 498
Myofibrillar myopathy, desmin and
	desmin-related, 630–631
Myoglobinuria, and paroxysmal cold
	hemoglobinuria, 388–389
	and type VII glycogen storage disease,
	456–457
Myokymia, and episodic ataxia, 600–
	601
	and neuromyotonia, 635
Myopathies, and Lambert-Eaton
	myasthenic syndrome, 621
	and Prader-Willi syndrome, 237–238
Myopathy, centronuclear, 628–629
	congenital, 629–630
	and idiopathic congenital central
	hypoventilation syndrome, 673
	and inclusion body myositis, 631
	and limb girdle muscular dystrophy,
	625
	and myasthenia gravis, 626–627
	myofibrillar, 630–631
	myotubular, 628–629
	and Schwartz-Jampel syndrome,
	586–587
	and type II glycogen storage disease,
	452
Myophosphorylase deficiency, and
	phosphoglycerate kinase
	deficiency, 489
Myopia, and homocystinuria, 459
	and spondyloepiphyseal dysplasia
	congenita, 728
Myositis, and eosinophilia-myalgia
	syndrome, 7
	inclusion body, 631–632
Myotonia, and Schwartz-Jampel
	syndrome, 586–587
Myotonia congenita, 632–633

Myotonic dystrophy, and Marden-Walker
	syndrome, 18
	and Prader-Willi syndrome, 237–238
Myotubular myopathy, 628–629
Myriachit, and hyperekplexia, 540
Myxedema, and hereditary lymphedema,
	396
	and pachydermoperiostosis, 129
Myxomas, and ameloblastoma, 363

N
Nadolol, and Jervell and Lange-Nielsen
	syndrome, 52
	and Romano-Ward long QT
	syndrome, 54
Naegeli type ectodermal dysplasia
	syndrome, and hypomelanosis of
	Ito, 119
Nager acrofacial dysostosis, 226
Nager syndrome, 226
	and Miller syndrome, 222–223
	and Treacher-Collins syndrome, 263
Nail dystrophy, and dyskeratosis
	congenita, 105
Nail hypoplasia, and Laband syndrome,
	214
Nail-patella syndrome, *fig. 63*, 721–722
Nance-Horan syndrome, 654–655
Nanukayami, 289
Narcolepsy, 561–562
	and Kleine-Levin syndrome, 544
Nasal abnormalities, and Laband
	syndrome, 214
Nasal cartilage, and relapsing
	polychondritis, 29
Nasal congestion, and Hunter disease,
	478–479
	and Hurler disease, 477
Nasal hypoplasia, and acrodysostosis,
	146
Nasal polyps, and Churg-Strauss
	syndrome, 674
Nasal septum deviation, and Saethre-
	Chotzen syndrome, 727–728
Nasal tip bifidity, and craniofrontonasal
	syndrome, 183
Nasomaxillary hypoplasia, 186–187
Navicular osteochondritis, 21
Neck edema, and cystic hygroma, 175
Neck lesions, and cystic hygroma,
	175–176
Necrobiotic granuloma, 115–116
Necrotizing enterocolitis, and
	Hirschsprung disease, 345
Necrotizing vasculitis, and Henoch-
	Schönlein purpura, 414

Nemaline rod myopathy, and limb girdle
	muscular dystrophy, 625
Neonatal adrenoleukodystrophy, and
	peroxisomal biogenesis disorders,
	486–487
Neonatal bacterial sepsis, and TORCH
	syndrome, 295
Neonatal convulsions, and Glut-1
	deficiency syndrome, 448
Neonatal hepatitis, and biliary atresia,
	334
	and galactosemia, 446
Neonatal hepatitis syndrome, 288
Neonatal hyperbilirubinemia, 543
Neonatal progeroid syndrome, 238–239
	and acquired generalized
	lipodystrophy, 320–321
	and congenital generalized
	lipodystrophy, 322
Neonatal sleep myoclonus, 541
Neoplasms, and Bloom syndrome,
	159–160
	and mesenteric panniculitis, 350
	and Tolosa-Hunt syndrome, 664
Neoplastic diseases, and eosinophilic
	gastroenteritis, 342
Neoplastic retinal infiltration, and retinal
	arterial occlusion, 657
Nephritis, and Henoch-Schönlein
	purpura, 414–415
Nephrocalcinosis, and blue diaper
	syndrome, 681
Nephronophthisis, and Loken-Senior
	syndrome, 692–693
	and medullary cystic kidney disease,
	693–694
Nephropathy, familial juvenile
	hyperuricemic, 696
Nephrosis–neural dysmigration
	syndrome, 687–688
Nephrotic syndrome, and chronic
	lymphocytic thyroiditis, 329
	and Galloway-Mowat syndrome, 687
Neridronate, and Paget disease, 25
Nerve conduction velocity decline, and
	congenital hypomyelination
	neuropathy, 568
	and Dejerine-Sottas syndrome,
	527–528
Nerve deafness, and Björnstad syndrome,
	97
Neu-Laxova syndrome, 562–563
	and acrocallosal syndrome (Schinzel
	type), 145
	and cerebro-oculo-facio-skeletal
	syndrome, 520

Neuhauser syndrome, 556

Neural entrapment, and diffuse idiopathic skeletal hyperostosis, 10

Neuraminidase deficiency, 498

Neuritis leprosy, and hereditary sensory neuropathy, 570

Neuroacanthocytosis, 633–634

Neuroblastoma, and Ewing sarcoma of bone, 381
    and Langerhans cell histiocytosis, 392
    and pheochromocytoma, 409

Neurodegeneration, and Niemann-Pick disease, 485

Neurodevelopmental deficits, and Cornelia de Lange syndrome, 709

Neuroendocrine tumors, 408–411
    and carcinoid syndrome, 311–312
    and Zollinger-Ellison syndrome, 330

Neurofibromatosis, and Takayasu arteritis, 35

Neurofibromatosis type 1, 563–564
    and epidermal nevus syndrome, 105

Neurofibromatosis type 2, 564–565

Neurogenic arthrogryposis, 520–521

Neuroleptic malignant syndrome, 566

Neuroleptics, and Huntington disease, 538
    and myoclonic dystonia, 615

Neurologic degeneration, and Cockayne syndrome, 170–171

Neurologic disease, and Q fever, 293

Neurologic disorders, 507–598

Neurologic disturbances, and Binswanger disease, 519
    and De Barsy syndrome, 6
    and tetrahydrobiopterin deficiency, 502

Neuromuscular disorders, 599–638

Neuromyelitis optica, 560, 567

Neuromyotonia, 635
    and stiff person syndrome, 588

Neuronal ceroid lipofuscinosis, 516–517, 547, 584–586
    and Baltic/Mediterranean/Unverrich-Lundborg myoclonic epilepsy, 600
    and Hallervorden-Spatz syndrome, 620
    and MERRF, 469
    and Niemann-Pick disease, 485
    and Stargardt disease, 663

Neuronal storage diseases, and Farber disease, 443

Neuropathy, acute motor and sensory axonal, 535–536
    acute motor axonal, 535–536
    congenital hypomyelination, 568

and Dejerine-Sottas syndrome, 527–528
    and Guillain-Barré syndrome, 535–536
    hereditary sensory type I, 570
    hereditary sensory type II, 571
    and Parsonage-Turner syndrome, 577–578
    and Prader-Willi syndrome, 237–238
    and Rosenbert-Chutorian syndrome, 585

Neurosyphilis, and encephalitides, 284
    and primary lateral sclerosis, 548

Neurotic excoriations, and dermatitis herpetiformis, 103

Neurotoxicity, and giant axonal neuropathy, 569

Neurotropic viruses, and West Nile fever, 296

Neuroxonal dystrophy, infantile, 634

Neutropenia, and acquired agranulocytosis, 361–362
    and Barth syndrome, 44
    cyclic, 21–22
    and Felty syndrome, 8–9
    and large granular lymphocyte leukemia, 394
    periodic, 21–22
    severe chronic, 22–23

Neutrophil degranulation, and Chédiak-Higashi syndrome, 379

Neville-Lake disease, 485

Nevus comedonicus syndrome, 105–106

Nevus vascularis reticularis, 100

Nezelof syndrome, 408

Niacin maculopathy, and X-linked juvenile retinoschisis, 662

Nicotine, and Tourette syndrome, 594

Nicotinic acid, and blue diaper syndrome, 681

Niemann-Pick disease, 485
    and Erdheim-Chester disease, 441
    and Gaucher disease, 447
    and Kuf disease, 547

Niemann-Pick syndrome, and ataxia-telangiectasia, 605–606

Nievergelt syndrome, and dyschondrosteosis, 181

Nifedipine, and primary pulmonary hypertension, 678
    and scleroderma, 33

Night blindness, and choroideremia, 642
    and Leber congenital amaurosis, 652
    and Refsum disease, 604–605

Night sweats, and angioimmunoblastic lymphadenopathy-type T-cell lymphoma, 398

Nigmegen breakage syndrome, and Dubowitz syndrome, 179–180

Nigrospinodentatal degeneration, 555

Niikawa-Kuroki syndrome, 209–210

9p partial monosomy, 82–83

9p syndrome, partial, 82–83

Nitrates, and scleroderma, 33

Nitric oxide, and alveolar capillary dysplasia, 672

Nitrogen mustard, and mycosis fungoides, 406

Nocturia, and diabetes insipidus, 313–314
    and interstitial cystitis, 685
    and medullary cystic kidney disease, 693

Node enlargement, and mantle cell lymphoma, 399

Nodular regenerative hyperplasia, and Banti syndrome, 377

Non-Hodgkin lymphoma, and angioimmunoblastic lymphadenopathy-type T-cell lymphoma, 398–399
    and Waldenström macroglobulinemia, 38

Nonaka distal myopathy, and myofibrillar myopathy, 630

Nonbullous ichthyosiform erythroderma, and epidermolytic hyperkeratosis, 109

Noncirrhotic portal fibrosis, 377

Nonhemolytic unconjugated hyperbilirubinemia, 337

Noninfectious hematologic syndromes, and ehrlichiosis, 283

Nonketotic hyperglycinemia, and hydrocephalus, 539

Nonne-Milroy disease, 396–397

Nonspecific aorto-arteritis, 35

Nonspecific thoracic outlet syndrome, and complex regional pain syndrome, 523

Nonsteroidal antiinflammatory drugs, and erythromelalgia, 113
    and Legg-Calve-Perthes disease, 16
    and lumbar spinal stenosis, 587–588
    and relapsing polychondritis, 30
    and tarsal tunnel syndrome, 592

Noonan-like multiple giant cell lesion syndrome, and cherubism, 168

Noonan syndrome, 722–723
    and Aarskog syndrome, 142
    and blepharophimosis-ptosis-epicanthus inversus syndrome, 641

Noonan syndrome, *(continued)*
    and cardiofaciocutaneous syndrome,
        163–164
    and chromosome 22, trisomy mosaic,
        72
    and KBG syndrome, 210
    and LEOPARD syndrome, 124
    and multiple pterygium syndrome, 241
    and Turner syndrome, 264
    and type II glycogen storage disease,
        452
    and Williams syndrome, 270
Normochromic normocytic anemia, and
    multiple myeloma, 407
Norrie disease, 655–656
Nystagmus, and Duane syndrome, 645
    and Loken-Senior syndrome, 692
    and Pelizaeus-Merzbacher disease, 578
    and syringobulbia, 589
    and X-linked juvenile retinoschisis, 662

O

Obesity, and adiposis dolorosa, 303
    and Alström syndrome, 305–306
    and Borjeson-Forssman-Lehmann
        syndrome, 705–706
    and Cohen syndrome, 172
    and Cushing syndrome, 312–313
    and familial dysbetalipoproteinemia,
        440
    and HAIR-AN syndrome, 315–316
    and Laurence-Moon syndrome, 215
    and polycystic ovary syndrome,
        323–324
    postnatal, and Bardet-Biedl syndrome,
        158–159
    and Prader-Willi syndrome, 237–238
    and progressive myoclonus epilepsy,
        531–532
    and pseudotumor cerebri, 582
Obsessive compulsive disorder, and
    Smith-Magenis syndrome, 254
Obstetric brachial plexus palsy, 571–572
Obstructive cardiac neoplasms, and
    hypoplastic left heart syndrome,
    50
Occipital encephalocele, and Joubert
    syndrome, 542
    and Meckel syndrome, 221
Occipital-facial-cervical-thoracic-
    abdominal-digital dysplasia,
    207–208
Occlusive thrombo-aortopathy, 35
Ochronosis, 431
Octreotide, and intestinal
    lymphangiectasia, 346

Ocular abnormalities, and Alagille
    syndrome, 332
    and cat eye syndrome, 164–165
    and chromosome 3, trisomy 3q2,
        73–74
    and chromosome 21 ring, 70
    and De Barsy syndrome, 6
    and homocystinuria, 459
    and oculocerebral syndrome, 226–
        227
    and Rieger syndrome, 243–244
    and Schwartz-Jampel syndrome,
        586–587
    and Sturge-Weber syndrome, 258
    and Walker-Warburg syndrome,
        597–598
    and Weill-Marchesani syndrome,
        267–268
    and Wyburn-Mason syndrome, 667
Ocular depression, and SHORT
    syndrome, 250
Ocular hypertelorism, and LEOPARD
    syndrome, 124–125
Ocular implantation, and posterior
    uveitis, 666
Ocular pain, 649
    and Tolosa-Hunt syndrome, 664
Ocular palsy, and Tolosa-Hunt syndrome,
    664
Ocular pemphigoid, 131–132
Oculo-auriculo-vertebral spectrum, 716
Oculo-cerebro-cutaneous syndrome, and
    branchio-oculo-facial syndrome,
    161–162
Oculo-cerebro-renal syndrome of Lowe,
    466–467
Oculocerebrorenal syndrome, and
    megalocornea, 556
Oculo-dento-digital syndrome, and
    Norrie disease, 655–656
Oculoauriculovertebral spectrum, and
    Townes-Brocks syndrome, 262
Oculocerebral syndrome with
    hypopigmentation, 226–227
Oculocutaneous albinism, and Chédiak-
    Higashi syndrome, 379
    and Hermansky-Pudlak syndrome,
        391–392
    and oculocerebral syndrome, 226–227
Oculomandibulodyscephaly, 202
Oculomotor abnormalities, and Joubert
    syndrome, 542
Oculomotor apraxia, and Wieacker-Wolff
    syndrome, 638
Odor, fishlike, and trimethylaminuria,
    503

Odor of maple syrup, and maple syrup
    urine disease, 468
OEIS complex, and caudal regression
    syndrome, 166
Oflaxacin, and Q fever, 293
Ohdo blepharophimosis syndrome, and
    blepharophimosis-ptosis-
    epicanthus inversus syndrome, 641
OK-432, and cystic hygroma, 175
Okihiro syndrome, and Holt-Oram
    syndrome, 717
Olfactogenital syndrome, 318–319
Olfactory deficits, and Refsum disease,
    604–605
Oligodontia, 261
Oligohydramnios, and autosomal-
    recessive polycystic kidney disease,
    697
    and bilateral renal agenesis, 698
Oligohydramnios deformation sequence,
    and amniotic bands, 150
Oligoovulation, and Asherman
    syndrome, 308–309
Oligophrenia, and Joubert syndrome, 542
Oligosaccharidosis, and
    aspartylglucosaminuria, 432
Oligospermia, and partial androgen
    insensitivity syndrome, 307–308
Olivopontocerebellar atrophy, and
    Machado-Joseph disease, 555
Olivopontocerebellar hypoplasia, and
    congenital disorders of
    glycosylation, 457–458
Ollier disease, 23–24
    and Maffucci syndrome, 217
Olpadronate, and Paget disease, 25
Omenn syndrome, and severe combined
    immunodeficiency, 14
Omental torsion, and mesenteric
    panniculitis, 350
Omphalocele, and Beckwith-Wiedemann
    syndrome, 518
    and gastroschisis, 197
Ondansetron, and cyclic vomiting
    syndrome, 526
1p36 deletion, and Prader-Willi
    syndrome, 237–238
Onycho-osteodysplasia, 721–722
Onychodystrophy, and Cronkhite-
    Canada syndrome, 338
Oophoritis, autoimmune, 30–31
Opalescent dentin, 176–177
Ophthalmia, sympathetic, and Vogt-
    Koyanagi-Harada syndrome, 37
Ophthalmic artery occlusion, and retinal
    arterial occlusion, 657

Ophthalmologic abnormalities, and mucolipidosis, 473–474
Ophthalmologic disorders, 639–667
Ophthalmoplegia, chronic progressive external, 603–604
  and Kearns-Sayre syndrome, 603–604
  and Machado-Joseph disease, 555
  and Tolosa-Hunt syndrome, 664
Opisthotonous, and leukodystrophy, 551–552
Opitz (BBBG) syndrome, and chromosome 22 ring, 71
Opitz-Fraaias syndrome, 198–199
Opitz-G syndrome, 198–199
Opitz GBBB syndrome, 178–179
Opitz-Kaveggia syndrome, 193–194
Opitz syndrome, 198–199
Opitz trigonocephaly syndrome, 162–163
Opsoclonus-myoclonus, and Glut-1 deficiency syndrome, 448
Opsoclonus-myoclonus syndrome, 572
Optic aphasia, 508–509
Optic atrophy, and hereditary spastic paraplegia, 575–576
  and Leber hereditary optic neuropathy, 653
  and metachromatic leukodystrophy, 552–553
  and Pelizaeus-Merzbacher disease, 578
  and Wolfram syndrome, 273
Optic glioma, and neurofibromatosis type I, 563–564
Optic nerve atrophy, and Rosenbert-Chutorian syndrome, 585
Optic nerve compression, and pseudotumor cerebri, 583
Optic nerve hypoplasia, and septooptic dysplasia, 188–189
Optic neuritis, and Leber hereditary optic neuropathy, 653
Oral contraceptives, and Achard-Thiers syndrome, 300
  and congenital antithrombin III deficiency, 376–377
  and HAIR-AN syndrome, 315–316
  and progressive myoclonus epilepsy, 531–532
Oral-facial-digital syndrome(s), and Gordon syndrome, 199
  and Greig cephalopolysyndactyly syndrome, 201
  and Pallister-Hall syndrome, 230
Oral ulcerations, and Sutton disease, 138
Organ structural abnormalities, and fetal valproate syndrome, 192–193
  and Wolf-Hirschhorn syndrome, 272

Organic acidemias, and urea cycle disorders, 506–506
Organic aciduria, and carnitine deficiency syndromes, 432
  and maple syrup urine disease, 468
Organomegaly, and Beckwith-Wiedemann syndrome, 518
  and hemophagocytic lymphohistiocytosis, 397–398
  and POEMS syndrome, 26–27
  and sialidosis, 498
Ornipressin, and hepatorenal syndrome, 344
Ornithine transcarbamylase deficiency, 506–506
  and Allan-Herndon-Dudley syndrome, 149
Orofacial clefts, and trisomy 13 syndrome, 87
Orofacial digital syndrome II, and acrocallosal syndrome (Schinzel type), 145
Orofacial dyskinesia(s), and neuroacanthocytosis, 633–634
  and tardive dyskinesia, 591
Orofacial malformations, and Johanson-Blizzard syndrome, 208
Oromandibular dystonia, 615–616
Oromandibular-limb hypoplasia complex, 203
Oropharyngeal abnormalities, and Freeman-Sheldon syndrome, 714
Osler-Weber-Rendu disease, 418
Osteitis deformans, 24–25
Osteitis fibrosa cystica, and craniometaphyseal dysplasia, 184
Osteoarthritis, and familial articular chondrocalcinosis, 169–170
  and Hunter disease, 478–479
  and Scheie disease, 478
  and Sly disease, 481
Osteochondritis, of the navicular, 21
Osteochondritis dissecans, and dysplasia epiphysealis hemimelica, 186
Osteochondrodysplasia, and spondyloepiphyseal dysplasia congenita, 728
  and spondyloepiphyseal dysplasia tarda, 729–730
  and Yunis-Varaaon syndrome, 275
Osteochondroma, and dysplasia epiphysealis hemimelica, 186
  and Ewing sarcoma of bone, 380–381
Osteochondromatosis, 191
  and Ollier disease, 23–24
Osteodental dysplasia, 182

Osteofibrous dysplasia, and familial expansile osteolysis, 723
Osteogenesis imperfecta, 227–228
  and achondroplasia, 144
  and Antley-Bixler syndrome, 704–705
  and camp[t]omelic syndrome, 706–707
  and cleidocranial dysplasia, 182
  and megalocornea, 556
  and Weill-Marchesani syndrome, 267–268
Osteolysis, familial expansile, 723–724
Osteomalacia, and hypophosphatasia, 317–318
  and Weismann-Netter-Stuhl syndrome, 268
  and X-linked hypophasphatemic rickets, 326–327
Osteonecrosis, idiopathic, 16
Osteopathia striata, and craniometaphyseal dysplasia, 184
Osteopenia, and growth hormone deficiency, 314–315
  and osteogenesis imperfecta, 227–228
Osteopetrosis, autosomal-recessive, 228–229
  and hyperostosis corticalis generalisata, 204–205
  and pyknodysostosis, 242
  and sclerosteosis, 248–249
Osteoporosis, and Hajdu-Cheney syndrome, 11
  and lymphangioleiomyomatosis, 395–396
  and Singleton-Merten syndrome, 252
Osteopsathyrosis, 227–228
Osteosarcoma, and Ewing sarcoma of bone, 380–381
  and Rothmund-Thomson syndrome, 135–136
Osteosclerosis, and hyperostosis corticalis generalisata, 204–205
Osteosclerotic myeloma, 26–27
Osteotomy, and Ollier disease, 23–24
Österreicher-Turner syndrome, 721–722
Ostrich foot, 256
Otitis media, and situs inversus, 55
Otomandibular dysostosis, and brachio-oto-renal syndrome, 681
Otopalatodigital syndrome, 229–230
  and Catel-Manzke syndrome, 165
Otopalatodigital syndrome type II, and acrocallosal syndrome (Schinzel type), 145
  and atelosteogenesis type III, 156

Ovarian cancer, and Lynch syndromes, 401
  and pseudomyxoma peritonei, 412
Ovarian failure, and Asherman
    syndrome, 308–309
  autoimmune premature, 30–31
Ovatestes, 316–317
Overgrowth, and Hunter disease,
    478–479
  and Proteus syndrome, 239
  and Simpson dysmorphia syndrome,
    251
  and Sotos syndrome, 255
  and Weaver syndrome, 266–267
Overuse syndrome, and complex regional
    pain syndrome, 523
Oxandrolone, and Duchenne muscular
    dystrophy, 623
Oxidative phosphorylation defects, and
    short-chain acyl-CoA
    dehydrogenase deficiency, 438–439

P
Pacemaker implantation, and congenital
    complete heart block, 50
  and giant cell myocarditis, 52
Pachydermoperiostosis, 129–130
Pachygyria, and classic lissencephaly,
    553–554
  and Yunis-Varaaon syndrome, 275
Paclitaxel, and adenoid cystic carcinoma,
    359
Paget disease, and Camurati-Engelmann
    disease, 707–708
  and diffuse idiopathic skeletal
    hyperostosis, 10
  and Erdheim-Chester disease, 441
  and familial expansile osteolysis, 723
  and Weismann-Netter-Stuhl
    syndrome, 268
Paget disease of bone, 24–25
Pain dysfunction syndrome, and complex
    regional pain syndrome, 523
Pain insensitivity, and hereditary sensory
    neuropathy
Palatal palsy, and syringobulbia, 589
Pallidal degeneration, and retinitis
    pigmentosa, 660
Pallido-dentate calcifications, and Fahr
    disease, 532
Pallidotomy, and dystonia, 609
  and Parkinson disease, 576
Pallister-Hall syndrome, 230–231
Pallister-Killian syndrome, 231–232
  and Fryns syndrome, 715
  and Simpson dysmorphia syndrome,
    251

Pallister-ulnar-mammary syndrome,
    246–247
Palpebral fissure widening, and Duane
    syndrome, 645
Palsy, progressive supranuclear, 573–574
Panchondritis, 29–30
Pancreas absence, and leprechaunism,
    216
Pancreatectomy, and pancreatic islet cell
    tumors, 409
Pancreatic acinar dysfunction, and
    Shwachman-Diamond syndrome,
    417
Pancreatic agenesis, and Johanson-
    Blizzard syndrome, 208
Pancreatic enzyme replacement, and
    Johanson-Blizzard syndrome, 208
Pancreatic hypoplasia, and Johanson-
    Blizzard syndrome, 208
Pancreatic insufficiency, 417
  and Johanson-Blizzard syndrome, 208
Pancreatic islet cell tumors, 408–409
  and Von Hippel-Lindau disease, 266
Pancreaticoduodenectomy, and
    pancreatic islet cell tumors, 409
Pancreatitis, and familial lipoprotein
    lipase deficiency, 465–466
  and isovaleric acidemia, 427
  and mesenteric panniculitis, 350
  and propionic acidemia, 428
Pancytopenia, and hemophagocytic
    lymphohistiocytosis, 397–398
PANDAS, and Sydenham chorea, 522
Panencephalitis, subacute sclerosing,
    574–575
Panic attacks, and pheochromocytoma,
    409
Panniculitis, and alpha 1-antitrypsin
    deficiency, 671
Papilledema, and pseudotumor cerebri,
    582–583
Papillomatosis, recurrent respiratory, 676
Papillon-Lefevre keratoderma, and
    Meleda disease, 128
Papular acrodermatitis of childhood, 115
Papular articaria, and transient
    acantholytic dermatosis, 104
Papular eruption of axillae, 114
Papular mucinosis, 136–137
  and granuloma annulare, 116
Papulonecrotic tuberculid, and Mucha-
    Habermann disease, 129
Papulovesicular acrolocated syndrome,
    115
Para-aminobenzoic acid, and Peyronie
    disease, 26

Paraganglioma, 409–410
Paralysis, and Batten disease, 517
Paralysis agitans, 576–577
Paralytic ileus, and intestinal
    pseudoobstruction, 348
Paralytic neuritis, and Parsonage-Turner
    syndrome, 577–578
Paramedial pits, and popliteal pterygium
    syndrome, 242
Paraneoplastic pemphigus, and cicatricial
    pemphigoid, 131
Paraplegia, and Creutzfeldt-Jakob disease,
    608
  hereditary spastic, 575–576
Paraproteinemia, and scleroderma, 33
Paraproteinemia-associated
    polyneuropathy syndromes, and
    POEMS syndrome, 26
Parapsoriasis, and Mucha-Habermann
    disease, 128–129
Parapsoriasis lichenoides, 128–129
Parapsoriasis varioliformis acuta,
    128–129
Parasitic diseases, and eosinophilic
    gastroenteritis, 342
  and liver fluke disease, 286
  and malaria, 291
Parathyroid glands, and DiGeorge
    syndrome, 178–179
Paresis, and Batten disease, 517
Paresthesia(s), and Creutzfeldt-Jakob
    disease, 608
  and Guillain-Barré syndrome, 535
Parkes-Weber syndrome, 232
  and Klippel-Trenaunay syndrome,
    212
Parkinson disease, 576–577
  and Binswanger disease, 519
  and corticobasal degeneration,
    524–525
  and frontotemporal dementia, 534
  and Hallervorden-Spatz syndrome, 620
  and hydrocephalus, 539
  and laryngeal dystonia, 613–614
  and multiple system atrophy, 561
  and progressive supranuclear palsy,
    573
  and rapid-onset dystonia-
    parkinsonism, 617
Parkinsonism, and Fahr disease, 532
  and multiple system atrophy, 561
  and myoclonus, 628
  and neuroacanthocytosis, 633–634
  and progressive supranuclear palsy,
    573–574
  and Wilson disease, 506

Parotid glands, and benign lymphoepithelial lesion, 17
Parotidectomy, and Frey syndrome, 533
Paroxysmal cold hemoglobinuria, *figs. 43–44*, 388–389
Paroxysmal dyskinesia, 616–617
Paroxysmal dystonia, 616–617
Paroxysmal hypertension, and pheochromocytoma, 409–410
Paroxysmal nocturnal hemoglobinuria, 389–390
    and acquired agranulocytosis, 361
    and autoimmune hemolytic anemia, 367
    and cold hemolytic anemia syndromes, 368
Paroxysmal tachycardia, and pheochromocytoma, 409
Parry-Romberg syndrome, 232–233
Pars plana vitrectomy, and Eales disease, 646
Pars planitis, 656–657
Parsonage-Turner syndrome, 577–578
Partial 1q duplication, and Russel-Silver syndrome, 245–246
Partial androgen insensitivity, and true hermaphroditism, 316–317
Partial androgen insensitivity syndrome, 307–308
Partial 15q deletion, and Russel-Silver syndrome, 245–246
Partial deletion of the short arm of chromosome 9, 82–83
Partial duplication 3q syndrome, 73–74
Partial duplication 15q syndrome, 65–66
Partial epilepsy, and episodic ataxia, 600–601
Partial hydatiform mole, 263–264
Partial lipodystrophy, and Parry-Romberg syndrome, 232–233
Partial molar pregnancy, 263–264
Partial monosomy of the long arm of chromosome 11, 60–61
Partial monosomy of the long arm of chromosome 13, 62–63
Partial trisomy 3q syndrome, 73–74
Partial trisomy 11q, 61–62
Partial trisomy 14, trisomy 13 syndrome, and chromosome 18, monosomy 18p, 67
Parvoviral infection, and TORCH syndrome, 295
Parvovirus B19 infection, and Diamond-Blackfan anemia, 365

Patau syndrome, 87–88
    and chromosome 18, monosomy 18p, 67
Patella absence, and ear–patella–short stature syndrome, 189
Paternal chromosome 15(q11-q13) deficiency, 237–238
Pathergic granulomatosis, 422–423
Paucity of interlobular bile ducts, 332
Pavlick harness, and camp[t]omelic syndrome, 706–707
PAX2 abnormalities, and CHARGE syndrome, 167
Pearson marrow-pancreas syndrome, and Shwachman-Diamond syndrome, 417
Pearson syndrome, 462
    and chronic progressive external ophthalmoplegia, 603–604
    and X-linked sideroblastic anemia, 373
Peau d'orange, and eosinophilic fasciitis, 8
Pectoral muscle deformity, and Poland syndrome, 236–237
Pegvisomant, and acromegaly, 301
Pelizaeus-Merzbacher disease, 578–579
    and adult polyglucosan body disease, 580
    and Cockayne syndrome, 170–171
    and leukodystrophy, 551–552
    and metachromatic leukodystrophy, 552
Pelizaeus-Merzbacher syndrome, and Allan-Herndon-Dudley syndrome, 149
Pelletier-Leisti syndrome, 195
Pelvic abnormalities, and femoral hypoplasia–unusual facies syndrome, 712–713
Pelvic inflammatory disease, and interstitial cystitis, 685
Pelvic tumors, and Ewing sarcoma of bone, 380–381
    and pheochromocytoma, 409–410
Pemoline, and narcolepsy, 562
Pemphigoid, bullous, 130–131
Pemphigus, and bullous pemphigoid, 130–131
Pemphigus foliaceus, 132
Pemphigus vulgaris, 132
    and cicatricial pemphigoid, 131
    and Sutton disease, 138
Pena-Shokeir II syndrome, 520–521
Pendular nystagmus, and infantile neuroaxonal dystrophy, 634
Penicillamine, and Wilson disease, 506

Penicillin, and erysipelas, 285
    and leptospirosis, 289
    and Sydenham chorea, 522
Penicillin G, and anthrax, 278
    and botulism, 279
Penile carcinoma *in situ*, 98–99
Penile fibromatosis, 25–26
Penile macules, and PTEN hamartoma tumor syndrome, 240
    and Ruvalcaba-Myhre-Smith syndrome, 354
Penile malignancy, and Peyronie disease, 25
Penile pain, and Peyronie disease, 25–26
Penis, acquired curvature of, 25–26
    congenital curvature of, and Peyronie disease, 25
    inflammation of, and Peyronie disease, 25–26
    plastic induration of, 25–26
Penta-X syndrome, 86–87
Pentalogy of Cantrell, 233–234
    and Fryns syndrome, 715
Pentasomy X, 86–87
Pentosan polysulfate sodium, and interstitial cystitis, 685
Pentoxyphylline, and scleroderma, 33
PEP syndrome, 26–27
PEPCK deficiency, 486
Pepper syndrome, 172
Peptic disease, and Zollinger-Ellison syndrome, 330
Peptic disorders, and cyclic vomiting syndrome, 525
Peradenitis mucosa necrotica recurrens, 138
Percutaneous balloon compression, and trigeminal neuralgia, 595
Percutaneous glycerol rhizotomy, and trigeminal neuralgia, 595
Percutaneous radiofrequency rhizotomy, and trigeminal neuralgia, 595
Perforating collagenosis, and granuloma annulare, 116
Perforating sarcoid, and granuloma annulare, 116
Pergolide, and Parkinson disease, 576
Perheentupa syndrome, 224–225
Perianal fistula, and hidradenitis suppurativa, 118
Periarteritis nodosa, 28–29
    infantile, and Kawasaki disease, 15
Pericardiectomy, and MULIBREY nanism, 224–225
Pericarditis, and MULIBREY nanism, 224–225

Perichondritis, diffuse, 29–30
  infectious, and relapsing
    polychondritis, 29
Perineal fistula, 153
Periodic disease, and familial
    Mediterranean fever, 19
Periodic neutropenia, 21–22
Periodic peritonitis, and familial
    Mediterranean fever, 19
Periodic syndrome, 525–526
Perioral erythema, and Meleda disease,
    128
Perioral paresthesias, and syringobulbia,
    589
Peripheral blood eosinophilia, and
    familial eosinophilic cellulitis, 99
Peripheral dysostosis, 146
Peripheral eosinophilia, and eosinophilic
    gastroenteritis, 342
Peripheral nerve tumors, and
    neurofibromatosis type I, 563–
    564
Peripheral neurofibromatosis, 563–564
Peripheral neuropathy, and ALA-
    dehydratase–deficient porphyria,
    492
  and Chédiak-Higashi syndrome, 379
  and erythromelalgia, 113
  and restless legs syndrome, 583
  and Tangier disease, 500
Periphlebitis retinae, 646
Perisylvian polymicrogyria, 579–580
Perisylvian syndrome, congenital
    bilateral, 579–580
Peritoneal mesothelioma, and
    pseudomyxoma peritonei, 412
Peritonitis, benign paroxysmal, and
    familial Mediterranean fever, 19
Perlman nephroblastosis syndrome, and
    Beckwith-Wiedemann syndrome,
    518
Perlman syndrome, and Simpson
    dysmorphia syndrome, 251
Peromelia with micrognathism, 203
Peroneal muscular dystrophy, 521–522
Peroxisomal biogenesis disorders,
    486–487
Peroxisomal disorders, and congenital
    disorders of glycosylation, 457
Persistent truncus arteriosus, 55–56
Personality changes, and frontotemporal
    dementia, 533–534
Perspiration, and ectodermal dysplasia,
    185
Perthes disease, and spondyloepiphyseal
    dysplasia congenita, 728

and spondyloepiphyseal dysplasia
    tarda, 729–730
Pervasive developmental disorder, and
    Smith-Magenis syndrome, 254
Pes cavus, and ataxia with vitamin E
    deficiency, 606–607
  and Friedreich ataxia, 602–603
Pes cavus deformity, and Singleton-
    Merten syndrome, 252
Pestilential fever, 292
Petechia(e), and idiopathic
    thrombocytopenic purpura, 415
  and Wiskott-Aldrich syndrome, 39
Peter anomaly, and aniridia, 640
Peter plus syndrome, and Rieger
    syndrome, 243–244
Pette-Doring panencephalomyelitis,
    574–575
Petty-Laxova-Weidemann progeroid
    syndrome, and progeria, 724
Peutz-Jeghers syndrome, 351–352
  and LEOPARD syndrome, 124
  and PTEN hamartoma tumor
    syndrome, 240
  and Ruvalcaba-Myhre-Smith
    syndrome, 354
Peyronie disease, 25–26
Pfeiffer syndrome, and Apert syndrome,
    154
  and Crouzon syndrome, 710
  and Jackson-Weiss syndrome, 719
  and primary craniosynostosis, 174
  and Saethre-Chotzen syndrome,
    727–728
Pfeiffer syndrome type I, 234–235
Phakomatoses, and Wyburn-Mason
    syndrome, 667
Phalangeal abnormalities, and Filippi
    syndrome, 194–195
Phenobarbital, and Byler disease, 335
  and hyperekplexia, 540
  and idiopathic neonatal hepatitis, 288
  and kernicterus, 543
  and progressive myoclonus epilepsy,
    531–532
Phenylalanine hydroxylase deficiency,
    and phenylketonuria, 488
Phenylephrine eye drops, and Horner
    syndrome, 648
Phenylketonuria, 488
  and carnosinemia, 435
  maternal, 489
  and tetrahydrobiopterin deficiency,
    502
Phenytoin, and episodic ataxia, 600–601
  and Hallervorden-Spatz syndrome, 620

and myotonia congenita, 633
  and neuromyotonia, 635
  and Schwartz-Jampel syndrome, 586
Phenytoin embryopathy, 192
Pheochromocytoma(s), 409–410
  and mastocytosis, 402
  and Von Hippel-Lindau disease, 266
Phillipines, and X-linked dystonia-
    parkinsonism, 619
Phlebectasia, congenital generalized, 100
Phlebothrombosis, and hereditary
    lymphedema, 396
Phlebotomy, and hereditary
    hemochromatosis, 387–388
  and polycythemia vera, 411–412
  and porphyria cutanea tarda, 493–494
  and variegate porphyria, 494–495
  and X-linked sideroblastic anemia, 373
Phosphate, low reabsorption of, and X-
    linked hypophasphatemic rickets,
    326–327
Phosphofructokinase deficiency, and
    congenital nonspherocytic
    hemolytic anemia, 369
  and type V glycogen storage disease,
    455
Phosphoglycerate kinase deficiency,
    489–490
  and type V glycogen storage disease,
    454–455
Phosphoglycerate mutase deficiency, and
    type V glycogen storage disease,
    455
Phospholipoproteinosis, 677
Phosphorylase kinase deficiency, 455–456
Photodynamic therapy, and Barrett
    esophagus, 333
  and Bowen disease, 98
Photodysphoria, and keratoconus, 651
Photopheresis, and mycosis fungoides,
    406
Photophobia, and Chédiak-Higashi
    syndrome, 379
  and cystinosis, 683
  and posterior uveitis, 666
Photoreceptor dystrophy, 660
Photorefractive keratectomy, and
    keratoconus, 651
Photosensitivity, and Cockayne
    syndrome, 170–171
  and Rothmund-Thomson syndrome,
    135–136
Phototherapy, and Crigler-Najjar
    syndrome, 337
  and kernicterus, 543
  and mycosis fungoides, 406

Phthisis bulbi, and Norrie disease, 656

Physical therapy, and congenital contractual arachnodactyly, 3

Phytanic acid accumulation, and Refsum disease, 604–605

Pick disease, 533–534
  and corticobasal degeneration, 524–525
  and Creutzfeldt-Jakob disease, 608

Piebaldism, and Waardenburg syndromes, 732

Pierre Robin sequence, 235–236
  and Catel-Manzke syndrome, 165
  and chromosome 4, monosomy distal 4q, 75

Pierre Robin syndrome, and femoral hypoplasia–unusual facies syndrome, 712

Pigment deposition, and alkaptonuria, 431

Pigmentary abnormalities, and Waardenburg syndromes, 732

Pigmentary dystrophy, and Loken-Senior syndrome, 692–693

Pigmentary retinal dystrophy, and Laurence-Moon syndrome, 215

Pigmentary retinopathy, and Alström syndrome, 305–306
  and Usher syndrome, 664–665

Pigmented dermatosis, 121–122

Pigmented hairy epidermal nevus syndrome, 105–106

Pigmented lesions, and melanoma, 405

Pigmented penile papules, 98–99

Pili torti, and Björnstad syndrome, 97

Pilonidal sinus, and hidradenitis suppurativa, 118

Pimozide, and Sydenham chorea, 522
  and Tourette syndrome, 594

Pinnae, abnormal, and congenital contractual arachnodactyly, 3

Pioglitazone, and HAIR-AN syndrome, 315–316

Piracetam, and Baltic/Mediterranean/Unverrich-Lundborg myoclonic epilepsy, 600
  and myoclonus, 628

Pirfenidone, and Hermansky-Pudlak syndrome, 392

Pitt-Rogers-Danks syndrome, and Wolf-Hirschhorn syndrome, 272

Pituitary dwarfism, 319–320

Pituitary failure, and chronic lymphocytic thyroiditis, 329

Pituitary gigantism, and Sotos syndrome, 255

Pituitary gland tumors, and acromegaly, 301

Pituitary gland underdevelopment, and septooptic dysplasia, 188–189

Pituitary necrosis, and Sheehan syndrome, 328

Pituitary tumor hemorrhage, and primary empty sella syndrome, 530

Pityriasis lichenoides et varioliformis acuta, 128–129
  and granuloma annulare, 116

Pityriasis rosea, and Mucha-Habermann disease, 129

Pityriasis rubra pilaris, *fig. 22*, 133

Placidity, and Kluver-Bucy syndrome, 545

Plague, 292
  and anthrax, 278

Plantar fasciitis, and tarsal tunnel syndrome, 592

Plasma cautery, and Barrett esophagus, 333

Plasma cell dyscrasia, and POEMS syndrome, 26–27

Plasma cell myeloma, 407

Plasma discoloration, and familial dysbetalipoproteinemia, 440

Plasma exchange, and autoimmune hemolytic anemia, 367
  and Guillain-Barré syndrome, 535

Plasma infusion, and thrombotic thrombocytopenic purpura, 416

Plasmapheresis, and bullous pemphigoid, 131
  and chronic inflammatory demyelinating polyradiculoneuropathy, 582
  and congenital complete heart block, 50
  and Crigler-Najjar syndrome, 337
  and erythema multiforme, 110
  and Henoch-Schönlein purpura, 415
  and Kawasaki disease, 15
  and Lambert-Eaton myasthenic syndrome, 621
  and microscopic polyangiitis, 28
  and multiple sclerosis, 560
  and pemphigus foliaceus, 132
  and pemphigus vulgaris, 132
  and polyarteritis nodosa, 29
  and Sjögren syndrome, 34
  and warm antibody hemolytic anemia, 371–372

Plasmodium infection, and malaria, 291

Plastyspondyly, and spondyloepiphyseal dysplasia congenita, 728

Platelet bleeding disorder, and Bernard-Soulier syndrome, 378

Platelet count elevation, and idiopathic thrombocytosis, 420–421

Platelet disorders, and Wiskott-Aldrich syndrome, 38–39

Platelet transfusions, and Bernard-Soulier syndrome, 378
  and Glanzmann thrombasthenia, 383

Pneumoconioses, and pulmonary alveolar proteinosis, 677

Pneumocystis carinii, and severe combined immunodeficiency, 14
  and pulmonary alveolar proteinosis, 677
  and Q fever, 293
  and severe chronic neutropenia, 22

Pneumocystis carinii pneumonia, and hyper-IgM syndrome, 393
  and severe combined immunodeficiency, 14

Pneumonia(s), and acute respiratory distress syndrome, 670
  and anthrax, 278
  and Churg-Strauss syndrome, 674
  and hantavirus pulmonary syndrome, 287
  and hyper-IgE syndrome, 12

POEMS syndrome, 26–27
  and scleroderma, 33

Poikiloderma, and Rothmund-Thomson syndrome, 135–136

Poikiloderma congenitale, 135–136

Pointed fifth finger and nail, and chromosome 4, monosomy 4q, 74

Poland syndrome, 236–237
  and Schinzel syndrome, 246–247

Poliodystrophy, and Alpers syndrome, 511–512

Poliomyelitis, and locked-in syndrome, 554
  and Parsonage-Turner syndrome, 577

Pollicization, and split hand/split foot malformation, 256

Pollitt syndrome, and Menkes disease, 470

Polyangiitis, and Churg-Strauss syndrome, 674
  microscopic, 27–27
  and polyarteritis nodosa, 28

Polyarteritis, microscopic, 27–27

Polyarteritis nodosa, 28–29
  and Churg-Strauss syndrome, 674
  and lymphomatoid granulomatosis, 48
  and microscopic polyangiitis, 27
  and Wegener granulomatosis, 422

Polychondritis, relapsing, 29–30

Polyclonal IgG, and mixed cryoglobulin syndrome, 5

Polycystic kidney disease, autosomal-recessive, 697
  and congenital hepatic fibrosis, 691–692
  and medullary cystic kidney disease, 693
  and medullary sponge kidney, 694

Polycystic kidneys, and Meckel syndrome, 221

Polycystic liver, and Caroli disease, 336

Polycystic ovary syndrome, 323–324
  and Achard-Thiers syndrome, 300
  and Asherman syndrome, 308–309
  and HAIR-AN syndrome, 315–316

Polycythemia vera, 411–412
  and idiopathic thrombocytosis, 421

Polydactyly, and acrocallosal syndrome (Schinzel type), 145
  and Greig cephalopolysyndactyly syndrome, 201
  and Meckel syndrome, 221
  and Pallister-Hall syndrome, 230
  and trisomy 13 syndrome, 87

Polydipsia, and diabetes insipidus, 313–314
  and medullary cystic kidney disease, 693

Polyglucosan body disease, adult, 580–581

Polyglucosan disease, 580–581

Polyhydramnios, and Fryns syndrome, 715
  and twin-twin transfusion syndrome, 421–422

Polymicrogyria, and classic lissencephaly, 553–554

Polymorphous light eruption, and erythropoietic protoporphyria, 495

Polymorphous low-grade adenocarcinoma, and adenoid cystic carcinoma, 359

Polymyositis, and facioscapulohumeral muscular dystrophy, 625
  and inclusion body myositis, 631
  and scleroderma, 33

Polyneuritis, acute febrile, 535–536
  acute infective, 535–536
  and locked-in syndrome, 554

Polyneuropathy(ies), and Lambert-Eaton myasthenic syndrome, 621
  and POEMS syndrome, 26–27

Polyostotic fibrous dysplasia, and familial expansile osteolysis, 723

Polyostotic osteolytic dysplasia, and familial expansile osteolysis, 723–724

Polyposis, familial adenomatous, 352–353

Polyradiculoneuropathy, chronic inflammatory demyelinating, 581–582

Polyradiculopathy, acute inflammatory demyelinating, 535–536

Polyserositis, and familial Mediterranean fever, 19

Polysplenia syndrome, and Ivemark syndrome, 205

Polysyndactyly, 201

Polyuria, and diabetes insipidus, 313–314
  and medullary cystic kidney disease, 693

Pompe disease, 452
  and Gaucher disease, 447
  and spinal muscular atrophy, 637

Popliteal pterygium syndrome, 242
  and Hay-Wells syndrome, 117
  and multiple pterygium syndrome, 241

Porphyria, acute intermittent, 490–491
  ALA-dehydratase–deficient, 491–492
  congenital erythropoietic, 492–493
  and dystrophic epidermolysis bullosa, 106
  and epidermolytic epidermolysis bullosa, 108
  and Guillain-Barré syndrome, 535
  and junctional epidermolysis bullosa, 108
  variegate, 494–495

Porphyria cutanea tarda, *fig. 49*, 493–494

Port-wine stain, and Sturge-Weber syndrome, 258

Portal hypertension, and Banti syndrome, 377
  and congenital hepatic fibrosis, 691–692
  and Langerhans cell histiocytosis, 392

Portal vein thrombosis, and Banti syndrome, 377

Positional skull molding, and primary craniosynostosis, 174

Positive end-expiratory pressure, and acute respiratory distress syndrome, 670

Postaxial acrofacial dysostosis, 222–223

Postaxial polydactyly, and Bardet-Biedl syndrome, 158–159

Posterior encephalocele, and cystic hygroma, 175

Posterior fossa arachnoid cysts, and Dandy-Walker syndrome, 526

Posterior fossa tumors, and Arnold-Chiari syndrome, 516

Posterior uveitis, 666

Postherpetic neuralgia, and complex regional pain syndrome, 523

Postictal paralysis, and alternating hemiplegia of childhood, 512

Postpartum hypopituitarism, 328

Postpartum thyroiditis, and Sheehan syndrome, 328

Posttraumatic atrophy, and Parry-Romberg syndrome, 232–233

Posttraumatic pain syndrome, 523

Postural instability, and Parkinson disease, 576–577
  and progressive supranuclear palsy, 573–574

Potassium supplementation, and Bartter syndrome, 311

Potter sequence, and bilateral renal agenesis, 698
  and caudal regression syndrome, 166

Potter syndrome, and Meckel syndrome, 221

Prader-Willi syndrome, 237–238
  and Bardet-Biedl syndrome, 158
  and Borjeson-Forssman-Lehmann syndrome, 705
  and Cohen syndrome, 172
  and deletion of the short arm of chromosome 1, 58
  and Laurence-Moon syndrome, 215
  and Smith-Magenis syndrome, 254
  and spinal muscular atrophy, 637

Pramipexole, and Parkinson disease, 576

Prazosin, and scleroderma, 33

Preaxial acrofacial dysostosis, 226

Precalyceal canalicular ectasia

Precancerous adenomas, and familial adenomatous polyposis, 352–353

Precocious gout, and familial juvenile hyperuricemic nephropathy, 696

Precocious puberty, 324–325
  and Pallister-Hall syndrome, 230

Prednisolone, and Camurati-Engelmann disease, 708

Prednisone, and Aase syndrome, 143
  and chronic inflammatory demyelinating polyradiculoneuropathy, 582
  and congenital complete heart block, 50

and Diamond-Blackfan anemia, 365
and Duchenne muscular dystrophy, 623
and eosinophilic fasciitis, 8
and eosinophilic gastroenteritis, 342
and idiopathic thrombocytopenic purpura, 415–416
and inclusion body myositis, 631
and Lambert-Eaton myasthenic syndrome, 621
and Langerhans cell histiocytosis, 393
and lichen planus, 125
and myasthenia gravis, 627
and sarcoidosis, 32
and Sheehan syndrome, 328
and Sweet syndrome, 139
and transient acantholytic dermatosis, 104
Pregnancy, and antiphospholipid syndrome, 2
and chronic lymphocytic thyroiditis, 329
and congenital antithrombin III deficiency, 376–377
and congenital complete heart block, 50
and Eisenmenger syndrome, 47
and Fox-Fordyce disease, 114
and listeriosis, 290
and maternal phenylketonuria, 489
Prekallikrein deficiency, and factor XII deficiency, 382
Premature aging, and acrogeria (Gottron type), *fig. 23*, 147
and progeria, 724–725
Premature labor, and twin-twin transfusion syndrome, 421–422
Premature menarche, and precocious puberty, 324
Premature pubarche, and precocious puberty, 324
Premature thelarche, and precocious puberty, 324
Prematurity, and Beckwith-Wiedemann syndrome, 518
Pretibial myxedema, and scleromyxedema, 136
Primaquine, and malaria, 291
Primary aldosteronism, 305
Primary ciliary dyskinesia, 675
and situs inversus, 55
Primary craniosynostosis, 174
Primary empty sella syndrome, 530
Primary hyperoxaluria, 461–462
Primary lateral sclerosis, 548–549

Primary pulmonary hypertension, 678
and Eisenmenger syndrome, 47
Primary visual agnosia, 508–509
Primidone, and progressive myoclonus epilepsy, 531–532
Primitive neuroectodermal tumor, 404–405
Prion disease, 608
Prion protein abnormalities, and Creutzfeldt-Jakob disease, 608
Probenecid, and familial juvenile hyperuricemic nephropathy, 696
Progeria, 724–725
and Hallermann-Streiff syndrome, 202
and Singleton-Merten syndrome, 252
and Werner syndrome, 269
Progeria infantum, and acrogeria (Gottron type), 147
Progeroid syndrome, 269
neonatal, 238–239
Progesterone, and lichen sclerosis, 126
and mesenteric panniculitis, 350
Progressive facial hemiatrophy, 232–233
Progressive familial intrahepatic cholestasis, 335
Progressive hemifacial atrophy, 232–233
Progressive iris atrophy, 649–650
Progressive myoclonus epilepsy, 531–532
Progressive osseous heteroplasia, 203–204
Progressive supranuclear palsy, 573–574
Progressive symmetric erythrokeratodermia, 111–112
and erythrokeratodermia variabilis, 112
Progressive systemic sclerosis, 33–34
Proguanil, and malaria, 291
Propionic acidemia, 428
and multiple carboxylase deficiency, 483
Propionic aciduria, 428
Propranolol, and cyclic vomiting syndrome, 526
and Jervell and Lange-Nielsen syndrome, 52
and Kluver-Bucy syndrome, 545
and Romano-Ward long QT syndrome, 54
Proptosis, and retinoblastoma, 661
Prostacyclin, and Eisenmenger syndrome, 47
and scleroderma, 33
Prostaglandin E_1, and hypoplastic left heart syndrome, 51
Prostaglandins, and scleroderma, 33
Prostatitis, and interstitial cystitis, 685

Prostatodynia, and interstitial cystitis, 685
Proteinuria, and Alport syndrome, 680
Proteus syndrome, 239
and adiposis dolorosa, 303
and Klippel-Trenaunay syndrome, 212
and PTEN hamartoma tumor syndrome, 240
Proton pump inhibitors, and Barrett esophagus, 333
and Zollinger-Ellison syndrome, 330
Protoporphyria, erthropoietic, 495–496
Protriptyline, and narcolepsy, 562
Proximal femoral focal deficiency, and femoral hypoplasia–unusual facies syndrome, 712
Prurigo nodularis, and lichen planus, 125
Pruritis, and angioimmunoblastic lymphadenopathy-type T-cell lymphoma, 398
and Byler disease, 335
and idiopathic neonatal hepatitis, 288
and lichen sclerosis, 126
and medullary cystic kidney disease, 693
Pseudo-Hurler polydystrophy, and mucolipidosis, 473
Pseudobulbar palsy, and primary lateral sclerosis, 548
and progressive supranuclear palsy, 573–574
Pseudobulbar paresis, and congenital bilateral perisylvian syndrome, 579–580
Pseudoclaudication, 587–588
Pseudocoma, 554
Pseudogout, 169–170
Pseudohermaphroditism, and congenital adrenal hyperplasia, 304
Pseudohypertrophic myopathy, 622
Pseudohypoparathyroidism, 325–326
and Aarskog syndrome, 142
and acromesomelic dysplasia, 704
Pseudomyxoma peritonei, 412–413
Pseudoobstruction, and small bowel diverticulosis, 339
Pseudoobstruction syndrome, 348
Pseudopelade, and alopecia areata, 95
Pseudorheumatoid nodule, 115–116
Pseudothalidomide syndrome, 244–245
and thrombocytopenia and absent radius syndrome, 260
Pseudotrisomy 13 syndrome, and acrocallosal syndrome (Schinzel type), 145

Pseudotumor cerebri, 582–583
    and primary empty sella syndrome,
        530
Pseudoxanthoma elasticum, 133–134
Psoralen-UV-A, and granuloma
        annulare, 116
Psoriasis, and Bowen disease, 97
    and bowenoid papulosis, 98
    and erythrokeratodermia variabilis,
        112
    and Leiner disease, 123
    and lichen planus, 125
    and Mucha-Habermann disease, 129
    and mycosis fungoides, 406
Psorospermose folliculaire vegetante, 101
Psychiatric disorders, and DiGeorge
        syndrome, 178–179
Psychomotor deficits, and megalocornea,
        556
Psychomotor delay, and peroxisomal
        biogenesis disorders, 487
Psychomotor deterioration, and
        congenital lactic acidosis, 462–
        464
Psychomotor regression, and Santavuori
        disease, 585–586
Psychomotor retardation, and
        carnosinemia, 435
    and chromosome 6 ring, 80
    and chromosome 9, trisomy 9p, 84
    and chromosome 11, partial
        monosomy 11q, 60–61
    and chromosome 14 ring, 63–64
    and Lowe syndrome, 466–467
    and mucolipidosis, 473–474
    and pentasomy X, 86–87
    and trisomy 13 syndrome, 87
    and trisomy 18 syndrome, 88
Psychosis, and methylmalonic acidemias,
        429
Psychosis polyneurotica, 546
PTEN hamartoma tumor syndrome, *fig.
        35*, 240
Pterygia, and multiple pterygium
        syndrome, 241
Pterygium colli, and Sprengel deformity,
        257
Pterygium syndrome, multiple, 241
Pterygium syndrome, popliteal, 242
Ptosis, and blepharospasm, 610
    and chronic progressive external
        ophthalmoplegia, 603–604
    and Duane syndrome, 645
    and Horner syndrome, 648
    and myasthenia gravis, 627

and Saethre-Chotzen syndrome,
        727–728
    and syringobulbia, 589
Puberty, delayed, and growth hormone
        deficiency, 314–315
    and Kallmann syndrome, 318
    precocious, 324–325
Puerperal curettage, and Asherman
        syndrome, 308–309
Pulmonary alveolar proteinosis, 677
Pulmonary congestion, and
        endomyocardial fibrosis, 48
Pulmonary disease, and Marshall-Smith
        syndrome, 219
Pulmonary disorders, 669–678
Pulmonary edema, and pulmonary
        alveolar proteinosis, 677
Pulmonary emboli, and idiopathic
        thrombocytosis, 421
Pulmonary embolism, and warm
        antibody hemolytic anemia,
        371–372
Pulmonary failure, and malaria, 291
Pulmonary fibrosis, and Hermansky-
        Pudlak syndrome, 391–392
Pulmonary hypertension, primary, 678
Pulmonary lavage, and pulmonary
        alveolar proteinosis, 677
Pulmonary sinus malformation, 45–46
Pulmonary stenosis, and LEOPARD
        syndrome, 124–125
Pulmonary vascular obstructive disease,
        46–47
Pulmonary vein misalignment, 672
Pulpless teeth, 176–177
Pulseless disease, 35
Pupillary inequality, and Duane
        syndrome, 645
Pure red cell aplasia, acquired, 413–414
Purine nucleoside analogues, and
        Waldenström macroglobulinemia,
        38
Purpura, and Bernard-Soulier syndrome,
        378
    and Glanzmann thrombasthenia, 383
    and Henoch-Schönlein purpura,
        414–415
    idiopathic thrombocytopenic, 415–416
    immune thrombocytopenic, and
        Wiskott-Aldrich syndrome, 38
    palpable, and mixed cryoglobulin
        syndrome, *fig. 1*, 5
    and Sjögren syndrome, 34
    thrombotic thrombocytopenic, 416
Purtilo syndrome, 400

Pyknodysostosis, 242–243
    and cleidocranial dysplasia, 182
Pyle disease, and craniometaphyseal
        dysplasia, 184
Pyoderma fistulans, and hidradenitis
        suppurativa, 118
Pyoderma gangrenosum, 134–135
    and Sweet syndrome, 139
Pyridostigmine bromide, and myasthenia
        gravis, 627
Pyridoxine, and homocystinuria, 459
    and primary hyperoxaluria, 462
    and X-linked sideroblastic anemia, 373
Pyrimethamine, and malaria, 291
    and TORCH syndrome, 295
Pyrimidine nucleotidase deficiency, and
        congenital nonspherocytic
        hemolytic anemia, 369
Pyroglutamic aciduria, 449
Pyrroloporphyria, 490
Pyruvate carboxylase deficiency, and
        PEPCK deficiency, 486
Pyruvate dehydrogenase deficiency, and
        idiopathic congenital central
        hypoventilation syndrome, 673
Pyruvate kinase deficiency, 369, 496–
        497
    and thalassemia major, 419

Q

Q fever, 293
QT interval prolongation, and Jervell and
        Lange-Nielsen syndrome, 51–52
    and Romano-Ward long QT
        syndrome, 54
QT prolongation, 54
Quadriplegia, and locked-in syndrome,
        554
Quantal squander, 635
Quartan fever, 291
Quinacrine ingestion, and alkaptonuria,
        431
Quinidine, and Brugada syndrome, 45
    and malaria, 291
Quinine, and malaria, 291
Quinolone, and Q fever, 293
Quintuple-X syndrome, 86–87

R

Rabson-Mendenhall syndrome, and
        leprechaunism, 215
Racemose hemangioma, and Wyburn-
        Mason syndrome, 667
Radial aplasia, and Baller-Gerold
        syndrome, 157–158

Radial club hand, and thrombocytopenia and absent radius syndrome, 260
Radial humeral synostosis, 704
Radiation, and mesenteric panniculitis, 350
Radiation fibrosis, and Takayasu arteritis, 35
Radiation necrosis, and syringobulbia, 589
Radiation retinopathy, and Eales disease, 646
Radiation therapy, and Denys-Drash syndrome, 686
    and Erdheim-Chester disease, 441
    and medulloblastoma, 404–405
    and multiple myeloma, 407
    and WAGR syndrome, 699
    and Wyburn-Mason syndrome, 667
Raeder syndrome, 648
Ragged red fibers, and MERRF, 469
Ragpicker disease, 278
Ramon syndrome, and cherubism, 168
Ramsay-Hunt syndrome, 600
    and MERRF, 469
Rapamycin, and polyarteritis nodosa, 29
Rapid-onset dystonia-parkinsonism, 617–618
Rapp-Hodgkin syndrome, and Hay-Wells syndrome, 116
Rasmussen syndrome, 284–285
Rat-bite fever, and anthrax, 278
Raynaud phenomenon, and scleroderma, 33
Raynaud syndrome, and Fabry disease, 442
Reactive hypoglycemia, and pancreatic islet cell tumors, 408–409
Reactive lymphocytosis, and large granular lymphocyte leukemia, 394
Reactive mast cell hyperplasia, and mastocytosis, 402
Recombinant factor VIIa, and Bernard-Soulier syndrome, 378
    and Glanzmann thrombasthenia, 383
Recombinant human activated protein C, and acute respiratory distress syndrome, 670
Recurrent respiratory papillomatosis, 676
Red blood cell, aberrant shape of, and hereditary spherocytosis, 370–371
    and sickle cell anemia, 372–373
Red blood cell aplasia, and Diamond-Blackfan anemia, 365

Red blood cell transfusion, and warm antibody hemolytic anemia, 371–372
Reflex sympathetic dystrophy, 523
    and erythromelalgia, 113
    and tarsal tunnel syndrome, 592
Refsum disease, 604–605
    and ataxia with vitamin E deficiency, 606
    and congenital disorders of glycosylation, 457
    and Friedreich ataxia, 602
    and progressive symmetric erythrokeratodermia, 111
Refsum syndrome, and retinitis pigmentosa, 660
    and Usher syndrome, 665
Reifenstein syndrome, 307–308
Reinhardt-Pfeiffer syndrome, and dyschondrosteosis, 181
Reiter syndrome, and interstitial cystitis, 685
Relapsing polychondritis, 29–30
Remnant removal disease, 440
Renal agenesis, bilateral, 698
Renal aplasia, and MURCS association, 695
Renal cell carcinomas, and Von Hippel-Lindau disease, 265–266
Renal colic, and cystinuria, 684
Renal cysts, and peroxisomal biogenesis disorders, 487
    and Von Hippel-Lindau disease, 265–266
Renal disorders, 679–699
Renal dysplasia, and Loken-Senior syndrome, 692–693
    and medullary cystic kidney disease, 693–694
Renal-ear-anal-radial syndrome, 262
Renal insufficiency, and homocystinuria, 459
    and multiple myeloma, 407
Renal-retinal dysplasia, and Leber congenital amaurosis, 652
Renal transplantation, and congenital hepatic fibrosis, 692
Renal tubular acidosis, and giant axonal neuropathy, 569
    and Lowe syndrome, 466–467
Repetitive strain injury, and complex regional pain syndrome, 523
Resection, and diffuse idiopathic skeletal hyperostosis, 10
Reserpine, 633, and Huntington disease, 538

and tardive dyskinesia, 591
Respiratory alkalosis, and urea cycle disorders, 506–506
Respiratory chain disorders, and congenital disorders of glycosylation, 457
Respiratory distress, and methylmalonic acidemias, 429
Respiratory distress syndrome, and hypoplastic left heart syndrome, 50
Restless legs syndrome, 583
Restrictive cardiomyopathy, and MULIBREY nanism, 224–225
Rethore syndrome, 84
Reticular dysgenesis, and acquired agranulocytosis, 361
    and severe combined immunodeficiency, 14
Reticulate hyperpigmentation, and dyskeratosis congenita, 104–105
Reticulum cell sarcoma, and acute posterior multifocal placoid pigment epitheliopathy, 642
Retinal angiomas, and Von Hippel-Lindau disease, 265–266
Retinal aplasia, and Loken-Senior syndrome, 692–693
    and medullary cystic kidney disease, 693–694
Retinal arterial occlusion, 657–658
Retinal blindness, 651–652
Retinal degeneration, and Cockayne syndrome, 170–171
Retinal detachment, and Coats disease, 643
    and Norrie disease, 656
    and posterior uveitis, 666
    and spondyloepiphyseal dysplasia congenita, 728
    and Vogt-Koyanagi-Harada syndrome, *fig. 4*
    and X-linked juvenile retinoschisis, 662
Retinal dystrophy, and Bardet-Biedl syndrome, 158–159
    and choroideremia, 642
    and Joubert syndrome, 542
Retinal folds, and Norrie disease, 656
Retinal heredodegeneration, 660
Retinal inflammation, and retinal arterial occlusion, 657
Retinal lesions, and acute posterior multifocal placoid pigment epitheliopathy, 642

Retinal neovascularization, and Eales disease, 646

Retinal telangiectasia, and Eales disease, 646

Retinal vasculitis, and Eales disease, 646

Retinal vein occlusion, 659

Retinitis pigmentosa, 517, 660
  and ataxia with vitamin E deficiency, 606–607
  and carnosinemia, 435
  and choroideremia, 642
  and hereditary spastic paraplegia, 575–576
  and posterior uveitis, 666

Retinitis pigmentosa inversa, and Stargardt disease, 663

Retinoblastoma, 661
  and Coats disease, 643
  and posterior uveitis, 666

Retinocerebellar angiomatosis, 265–266

Retinocytoma, and retinoblastoma, 661

Retinoic acid, and bowenoid papulosis, 98

Retinoic acid embryopathy, and CHARGE syndrome, 167
  and DiGeorge syndrome, 178

Retinoids, and epidermolytic hyperkeratosis, 110
  and erythrokeratodermia variabilis, 112
  and Fox-Fordyce disease, 114
  and ichthyosis, 121
  and keratitis-ichthyosis-deafness syndrome, 123
  and pachydermoperiostosis, 129
  and pityriasis rubra pilaris, 133
  and progressive symmetric erythrokeratodermia, 112
  and transient acantholytic dermatosis, 104

Retinopathy of prematurity, and Norrie disease, 656

Retinoschisis, X-linked juvenile, 662

Retractile mesenteritis, 350

Retroperitoneal fibrosis, and mesenteric panniculitis, 350

Rett syndrome, *fig. 53*, 584
  and chromosome 11, partial trisomy 11q, 61
  and infantile neuroaxonal dystrophy, 634
  and Joubert syndrome, 542

Reversible prerenal azotemia, and hepatorenal syndrome, 344

Reye syndrome, 31–32
  and carnitine deficiency syndromes, 432

and carnitine palmitoyl transferase I deficiency, 433
and carnitine palmitoyl transferase II deficiency, 434
and medium-chain acyl-CoA dehydrogenase deficiency, 437

Rhabdomyolysis, and malignant hyperthermia, 718

Rheumatic carditis, and endomyocardial fibrosis, 48

Rheumatic chondritis, 29–30

Rheumatic chorea, 522

Rheumatoid arthritis, and chronic inflammatory demyelinating polyradiculoneuropathy, 581
  and Fabry disease, 442
  and familial articular chondrocalcinosis, 169–170
  and Felty syndrome, 8–9
  juvenile, and Kawasaki disease, 15
  and Legg-Calve-Perthes disease, 16

Rheumatoid factor, and mixed cryoglobulin syndrome, 5

Rheumatoid nodule, and granuloma annulare, 116

Rheumatoid vasculitis, and thromboangiitis obliterans, 36

Rhinitis, and Churg-Strauss syndrome, 674

Rhizomelic chondrodysplasia punctata, and Conradi-Hünermann syndrome, 173

Rhyns syndrome, and Loken-Senior syndrome, 692

Rib abnormalities, and hyperostosis corticalis generalisata, 204–205
  and Jarcho-Levin syndrome, 207–208
  and Poland syndrome, 236–237
  and 3-M syndrome, 259

Rib cage constriction, and asphyxiating thoracic dystrophy, 155–156

Rib fracture, and multiple myeloma, 407

Rib gap defects, and cerebrocostomandibular syndrome, 166–167

Ribavirin, and hantavirus pulmonary syndrome, 287
  and recurrent respiratory papillomatosis, 676
  and viral hemorrhagic fevers, 282
  and West Nile fever, 296

Ribbing disease, and Camurati-Engelmann disease, 707–708

Riboflavin, and glutaric acidemia type I, 426
  and glutaric acidemia type II, 426–427

and trimethylaminuria, 503

Rickets, 326–327
  and Schmid metaphyseal chondrodysplasia, 248
  and Weismann-Netter-Stuhl syndrome, 268

Rickettsial diseases, and viral hemorrhagic fevers, 282

Rickettsial infections, and dengue fever, 281
  and Q fever, 293

Rickettsioses, and hantavirus pulmonary syndrome, 287

Rieger anomaly, and SHORT syndrome, 250

Rieger syndrome, 243–244
  and aniridia, 640
  and SHORT syndrome, 250

Rifampin, and Alagille syndrome, 332
  and brucellosis, 280
  and Byler disease, 335

Rift Valley fever, 282, 294

Right isomerism sequence

Rigid spine syndrome, and Emery-Dreifuss muscular dystrophy, 624

Rigidity, and Hallervorden-Spatz syndrome, 620
  and Parkinson disease, 576–577

Rigors, and malaria, 291

Riley-Day syndrome, 529–530

Riley-Smith syndrome, and PTEN hamartoma tumor syndrome, 240

Riluzole, and amyotrophic lateral sclerosis, 513
  and spinal muscular atrophy, 637

Ring 4, 76–77

Ring 6, 80

Ring 9, 83

Ring 15, 66

Ring 18, 68–69

Ring 21, 70

Ring 22, 71–72

Ring constriction syndrome, 150–151

Risperidone, and Tourette syndrome, 594

Ritalin abuse, and alpha 1-antitrypsin deficiency, 671

Ritscher-Schinzel syndrome, and Joubert syndrome, 542

Rituxan, and chronic inflammatory demyelinating polyradiculoneuropathy, 581–582

Rituximab, and Waldenström macroglobulinemia, 38

Roberts pseudothalidomide syndrome, *figs. 36–37*, 244–245

Roberts syndrome, 244–245
  and Baller-Gerold syndrome, 157
  and femoral hypoplasia–unusual facies
    syndrome, 712
Robin anomaly, and
    cerebrocostomandibular
    syndrome, 167
Robinow syndrome, 725–726
  and Aarskog syndrome, 142
  and dyschondrosteosis, 181
  and Kabuki make-up syndrome, 209
  and MULIBREY nanism, 224–225
  and Rieger syndrome, 243–244
Rocky Mountain spotted fever, and
    ehrlichiosis, 283
  and Kawasaki disease, 15
Rod-cone dystrophy, 660
Rod monochromacy, and Leber
    congenital amaurosis, 652
Rodent-borne viruses, and hantavirus
    pulmonary syndrome, 287
Romano-Ward long QT syndrome, 54
Romberg syndrome, 232–233
Rootless teeth, 176–177
Ropinerole, and Parkinson disease, 576
Rosenbert-Chutorian syndrome, 585
Rosenfeld-Kloepfer syndrome, 129–
    130
Rosenthal fibers, and Alexander disease,
    510–511
Rosiglitazone, and HAIR-AN syndrome,
    315–316
Rotational osteotomy, and Schmid
    metaphyseal chondrodysplasia,
    248
  and split hand/split foot
    malformation, 256
Rotator cuff tear, and Parsonage-Turner
    syndrome, 577
Rothmund-Thomson syndrome,
    135–136
  and Baller-Gerold syndrome, 157
  and Cockayne syndrome, 170–171
  and megalocornea, 556
Rotor syndrome, and Dubin-Johnson
    syndrome, 340
Rough endoplasmic reticulum, and
    Dyggve-Melchior-Clausen
    syndrome, 180–181
Roussy-Levy syndrome, 521–522
  and hereditary sensory neuropathy,
    570
RSH syndrome, 253
Rubella, and dengue fever, 281
Rubella virus, and TORCH syndrome,
    295

Rubeola virus, and subacute sclerosing
    panencephalitis, 574–575
Rubinstein syndrome, 726–727
Rubinstein-Taybi syndrome, *figs. 64–66*,
    726–727
  and Cornelia de Lange syndrome,
    709
Rudiger syndrome, and Schinzel Giedion
    syndrome, 247
Russell-Silver dwarfism, and Bloom
    syndrome, 159–160
Russell-Silver syndrome, 245–246
  and ear–patella–short stature
    syndrome, 189
  and MULIBREY nanism, 224–225
  and SHORT syndrome, 250
  and 3-M syndrome, 259
Russell syndrome, 528–529
Rutherford syndrome, and Laband
    syndrome, 214
Ruvalcaba-Myhre-Smith syndrome, 354
  and PTEN hamartoma tumor
    syndrome, 240
Ruvulcaba syndrome, and
    trichorhinophalangeal syndrome,
    732

S
Saalam seizures, 541
Sacral tumors, and Ewing sarcoma of
    bone, 380–381
SADDAN dysplasia, 144
  and Kniest dysplasia, 213
Saethre-Chotzen syndrome, 727–728
  and Apert syndrome, 154
  and Baller-Gerold syndrome, 157
  and chromosome 7, monosomy 7p2,
    80
  and Crouzon syndrome, 710
  and Gorlin-Chaudhry-Moss
    syndrome, 200
  and Pfeiffer syndrome type I, 234
  and primary craniosynostosis, 174
Saldino-Mainzer syndrome, and Loken-
    Senior syndrome, 692
Salicylic acid, and Darier disease, 101
Salivary gland neoplasm, and adenoid
    cystic carcinoma, 359
Salivary glands, enlargement of, *fig. 3*, 17
  tumors of, and benign
    lymphoepithelial lesion, 17
Salla disease, and alpha 1-antitrypsin
    deficiency, 671
Sandhoff disease, 497–498
  and Tay-Sachs disease, 501
Sanfilippo disease, 479

Sanjad-Sakati syndrome, 211
Santavuori disease, 585–586
Santavuori-Haltia disease, 585–586
Sarcoglycanopathies, 625
Sarcoid, and acute posterior multifocal
    placoid pigment epitheliopathy,
    642
Sarcoid uveitis, and pars planitis,
    656–657
Sarcoidosis, 32–33
  and chronic granulomatous disease,
    386
  and chronic inflammatory
    demyelinating
    polyradiculoneuropathy, 581
  and Eales disease, 646
  and encephalitides, 284
  and Erdheim-Chester disease, 441
  and Farber disease, 443
  and granuloma annulare, 116
  and lymphangioleiomyomatosis, 395
  and medullary sponge kidney, 694
  and neuromyelitis optica, 567
  and relapsing polychondritis, 29
  and Sjögren syndrome, 34
  and Takayasu arteritis, 35
  and Vogt-Koyanagi-Harada syndrome,
    37
  and Wegener granulomatosis, 422
Sarcosine accumulation, and glutaric
    acidemia type II, 426
Sathre-Chotzen syndrome, and Jackson-
    Weiss syndrome, 719
SC-phocomelia syndrome, 244–245
Scabies, and dermatitis herpetiformis,
    103
  and transient acantholytic dermatosis,
    104
Scalp-ear-nipple syndrome, and aplasia
    cutis congenita, 96
  and Schinzel syndrome, 246
Scalp lesions, and aplasia cutis congenita,
    96
Scaphoid face, 186–187
Scapula elevata, 257
Scapular deformities, and Sprengel
    deformity, 257
Scheie disease, 477–478
Scheie syndrome, and Winchester
    syndrome, 271
Scheuthauer-Marie-Sainton syndrome,
    182
Schilder disease, 430, 560
Schinzel acrocallosal syndrome, 145
Schinzel Giedion syndrome, 247
Schinzel syndrome, 246–247

Schizophrenia, and frontotemporal
  dementia, 534
 and Kluver-Bucy syndrome, 545
Schmid-Fraccaro syndrome, 164–165
Schmid metaphyseal chondrodysplasia,
  248
Schwachman-Diamond-Oski syndrome,
  and acquired agranulocytosis, 361
Schwachman syndrome, and Johanson-
  Blizzard syndrome, 208
Schwartz-Jampel-Aberfeld syndrome,
  586–587
Schwartz-Jampel syndrome, 586–587
 and blepharophimosis-ptosis-
  epicanthus inversus syndrome, 641
 and Freeman-Sheldon syndrome, 714
 and Marden-Walker syndrome, 18
Sciatica, and tarsal tunnel syndrome, 592
Scleral buckling, and X-linked juvenile
  retinoschisis, 662
Scleritis, and Wegener granulomatosis,
  422
Sclerodactyly, and scleroderma, 33
Scleroderma, 33–34
 and alopecia areata, 95
 and eosinophilia-myalgia syndrome, 7
 and eosinophilic fasciitis, 8
 and scleromyxedema, 136
 and small bowel diverticulosis, 339
 and thromboangiitis obliterans, 36
Scleroderma-like skin changes, and
  eosinophilia-myalgia syndrome, 7
Scleroderma-like syndromes, and
  eosinophilic fasciitis, 8
Scleromyxedema, 136–137
 and scleroderma, 33
Sclerosing mesenteritis, 350
Sclerosing osteochondrodysplasia, and
  pyknodysostosis, 242–243
Sclerosing panencephalitis, and multiple
  sclerosis, 560
Sclerosis, progressive systemic, 33–34
Sclerosteosis, 248–249
 and craniometaphyseal dysplasia, 184
 and hyperostosis corticalis
  generalisata, 204–205
Sclerotherapy, and cavernous
  hemangioma, 118
 and congenital hepatic fibrosis, 692
 and Parkes-Weber syndrome, 232
Scoliosis, and ataxia with vitamin E
  deficiency, 606–607
 and chromosome 15, distal trisomy
  15q, 65–66
 and Duchenne muscular dystrophy,
  623

 and dystonia, 609
 and Freeman-Sheldon syndrome, 714
 and Friedreich ataxia, 602–603
Scotomata, and posterior uveitis, 666
 and retinal arterial occlusion, 658
Scott craniodigital syndrome, 249–250
 and Cornelia de Lange syndrome,
  709
 and Filippi syndrome, 194–195
Scrub typus, and leptospirosis, 289
Sea-blue histiocytosis, 485
Seathre-Chotzen syndrome, and
  Rubinstein-Taybi syndrome,
  726–727
Sebaceous nevus of Jadassohn, and
  aplasia cutis congenita, 96
Sebastian syndrome, and May-Hegglin
  anomaly, 403
Seborrheic dermatitis, and Darier disease,
  101
 and Leiner disease, 123
Seborrheic keratoses, and Bowen disease,
  97
 and bowenoid papulosis, 98
 and melanoma, 405
Seckel bird-headed dwarfism, and 3-M
  syndrome, 259
Seckel syndrome, and cerebro-oculo-
  facio-skeletal syndrome, 520
 and chromosome 4 ring, 76
 and Fanconi anemia, 366
 and SHORT syndrome, 250
Secundum/primum atrial septal defect,
  and atrial septal defects, 43
Segawa disease, 612
Segmental vitiligo, and hypomelanosis of
  Ito, 119
Seitelberger disease, 634
Seizure disorders, and
  pseudohypoparathyroidism,
  325–326
Seizures, and acrocallosal syndrome
  (Schinzel type), 145
 and Aicardi syndrome, 510
 and alternating hemiplegia of
  childhood, 512
 and Angelman syndrome, 152–153
 and Baltic/Mediterranean/Unverrich-
  Lundborg myoclonic epilepsy, 600
 and Beckwith-Wiedemann syndrome,
  518
 and brain arteriovenous
  malformations, 596
 and carnosinemia, 435
 and chromosome 14 ring, 63–64
 and classic lissencephaly, 553–554

 and congenital bilateral perisylvian
  syndrome, 579–580
 and congenital disorders of
  glycosylation, 457–458
 and corpus callosum absence, 508
 and encephalitides, 284–285
 and Galloway-Mowat syndrome,
  687–688
 and giant axonal neuropathy, 569
 and glioblastoma multiforme, 384–385
 and holoprosencephaly, 536–537
 and hydrocephalus, 539
 and infantile spasms, 541
 and kernicterus, 543
 and Kleine-Levin syndrome, 544
 and Kuf disease, 547
 and Lennox-Gastaut syndrome,
  549–550
 and leukodystrophy, 550
 and Lowe syndrome, 466–467
 and megalocornea, 556
 and MELAS, 469
 and Menkes disease, 470
 and MERRF, 469
 and moyamoya syndrome, 559
 and Niemann-Pick disease, 485
 and paroxysmal dystonia, 616–617
 and Pelizaeus-Merzbacher disease, 578
 and PEPCK deficiency, 486
 and peroxisomal biogenesis disorders,
  487
 and phenylketonuria, 488
 and progressive myoclonus epilepsy,
  531–532
 and Rett syndrome, 584
 and Sanfilippo disease, 479
 and Santavuori disease, 585–586
 and Schinzel Giedion syndrome, 247
 and Sturge-Weber syndrome, 258
 and succinic semialdehyde
  dehydrogenase deficiency, 499
 and tetrahydrobiopterin deficiency,
  502
 and tuberous sclerosis, 596
Selegiline, and tetrahydrobiopterin
  deficiency, 502
Self-injury, and Smith-Magenis
  syndrome, 254
Self-mutilation, and Lesch-Nyhan
  syndrome, 464–465
Semantic dementia, 508–509
 and frontotemporal dementia,
  533–534
Senior-Loken syndrome, 692–693
 and Joubert syndrome, 542
 and Leber congenital amaurosis, 652

Sensory dysfunction, and familial dysautonomia, 529–530

Sensory impairment, and neuromyelitis optica, 567

Sensory loss, and adult polyglucosan body disease, 580–581

Sepsis, and Caroli disease, 336
and ehrlichiosis, 283
and hemophagocytic lymphohistiocytosis, 397
and idiopathic neonatal hepatitis, 288
and listeriosis, 290
and persistent truncus arteriosus, 56

Septic shock, and erysipelas, 285

Septicemia, and biliary atresia, 334

Septicemic plague, and viral hemorrhagic fevers, 282

Septooptic dysplasia, 188–189
and Kallmann syndrome, 318

Serotonin syndrome, and neuroleptic malignant syndrome, 566

Serpiginous choroiditis, and acute posterior multifocal placoid pigment epitheliopathy, 642

Sertraline, and Kluver-Bucy syndrome, 545

Servelle-Martorell syndrome, and Klippel-Trenaunay syndrome, 212

Setleis syndrome, 137

7p2 monosomy syndrome, 80–81

7p2- syndrome, 80–81

17-α hydroxylase deficiency, and congenital adrenal hyperplasia, 304

17-β hydroxysteroid dehydrogenase deficiency, and congenital adrenal hyperplasia, 304
and partial androgen insensitivity, 307

17,20 lyase deficiency, and partial androgen insensitivity, 307

Seventh nerve palsy, and Möbius syndrome, 223–224

Severe chronic neutropenia, 22–23

Severe combined immunodeficiency, 14–15
and Leiner disease, 123
and Nezelof syndrome, 408

Sex chromosome abnormalities, and Turner syndrome, 264–265

Sexual behavior, increased, and Kluver-Bucy syndrome, 545

Sexual development abnormalities, and androgen insensitivity syndrome, 306–307

Sezary syndrome, and mycosis fungoides, 406

Shaking palsy, 576–577

Sheathotomy, and carotid artery insufficiency, 659

Sheehan syndrome, 328
and primary empty sella syndrome, 530

Shields type III, 177–178

Shiga toxin–associated hemolytic uremic syndrome, 690

Shimmelpinning syndrome, 105–106

Shimpo, Crow-Fukase, and Takatsukis syndrome, 26–27

Shock, and hantavirus pulmonary syndrome, 287
and hypoplastic left heart syndrome, 50

Short arm 18 deletion syndrome, 67

Short-chain acyl-CoA dehydrogenase deficiency, 438–439

Short chest, and Jarcho-Levin syndrome, 207–208

Short neck, and C syndrome, 162–163
and chromosome 3, trisomy 3q2, 73–74
and chromosome 9, tetrasomy 9p, 84
and chromosome 15, distal trisomy 15q, 65–66
and Klippel-Feil syndrome, 720
and Morquio disease, 480
and spondyloepiphyseal dysplasia congenita, 728

Short rib-polydactyly syndrome, and asphyxiating thoracic dystrophy, 155
and Meckel syndrome, 221
and Pallister-Hall syndrome, 230

Short stature, and Aarskog syndrome, 142
and Borjeson-Forssman-Lehmann syndrome, 705–706
and C syndrome, 162–163
and camp[t]omelic syndrome, 706–707
and cardiofaciocutaneous syndrome, 163–164
and chromosome 9, trisomy 9p, 84
and chromosome 13, partial monosomy 13q, 62–63
and chromosome 18q- syndrome, 67–68
and cleidocranial dysplasia, 182
and Coffin-Lowry syndrome, 171–172
and Coffin-Siris syndrome, 708–709
and Conradi-Hünermann syndrome, 173
and diastrophic dysplasia, 711

and Dyggve-Melchior-Clausen syndrome, 180–181
and dyschondrosteosis, 181
and ear–patella–short stature syndrome, 189
and Fanconi anemia, 366
and Gorlin-Chaudhry-Moss syndrome, 200
and growth hormone deficiency, 314–315
and Kabuki make-up syndrome, 209–210
and KBG syndrome, 210
and Kenny-Caffey syndrome, 211
and Laron dwarfism, 319–320
and Leri pleonosteosis, 216–217
and Marinesco-Sjögren syndrome, 720–721
and Maroteaux-Lamy disease, 481
and multiple hereditary exostoses, 191
and multiple pterygium syndrome, 241
and Myhre syndrome, 225
and neurofibromatosis type I, 563–564
and Noonan syndrome, 722–723
and pentasomy X, 86–87
and Prader-Willi syndrome, 237–238
and progeria, 724
and Russel-Silver syndrome, 245–246
and Scheie disease, 478
and Schmid metaphyseal chondrodysplasia, 248
and Schwartz-Jampel syndrome, 586–587
and SHORT syndrome, 250
and Shwachman-Diamond syndrome, 417
and Sly disease, 481
and spondyloepiphyseal dysplasia congenita, 728
and spondyloepiphyseal dysplasia tarda, 729–730
and trichorhinophalangeal syndrome, 730–732
and Turner syndrome, 264–265
and types VI and IX glycogen storage disease, 455–456
and Weill-Marchesani syndrome, 267–268
and X-linked hypophasphatemic rickets, 326–327
and XLMR-hypotonic facies syndrome, 274

Short sternum, and trisomy 18 syndrome, 88

SHORT syndrome, 250
and Rieger syndrome, 243–244

SHORT syndrome, *(continued)*
   and Russel-Silver syndrome, 245–246
Shoulder pain, and Parsonage-Turner
      syndrome, 577–578
Shoulder weakness, and central core
      disease, 607–608
Shprintzen velo-cardio-facial syndrome,
      178–179
Shuffling gait, and MASA syndrome, 220
Shulman syndrome, 8
Shwachman-Bodian syndrome, 417
Shwachman-Diamond-Oski syndrome,
      417
Shwachman-Diamond syndrome, 417
   and Barth syndrome, 44
   and severe chronic neutropenia, 22
Shwachman syndrome, 417
Shy-Drager syndrome, 561
Sialidase deficiency, 498
Sialidosis, 498
   and Baltic/Mediterranean/Unverrich-
      Lundborg myoclonic epilepsy, 600
   and Fabry disease, 442
   and MERRF, 469
   and mucolipidosis, 473
Sialoadenitis, and benign
      lymphoepithelial lesion, 17
Sialogogues, and benign lymphoepithelial
      lesion, 17
Sialolithiasis, and benign
      lymphoepithelial lesion, 17
Siberian plague, 278
Sicca syndrome, 34
Sickle cell anemia, 372–373
   and Eales disease, 646
   and Legg-Calve-Perthes disease, 16
   and MELAS, 469
   and phosphoglycerate kinase
      deficiency, 489
   and thalassemia major, 419
Sildenafil, and multiple system atrophy,
      561
Silver-Russell syndrome, 245–246
Simpson dysmorphia syndrome, 251–252
Simpson-Golabi-Behmel syndrome, 251
   and Beckwith-Wiedemann syndrome,
      518
   and Fryns syndrome, 715
   and Marshall-Smith syndrome, 219
   and Sotos syndrome, 255
Singleton-Merten syndrome, 252
Sinopulmonary infections, and X-linked
      agammaglobulinemia, 360–361
Sinusitis, and situs inversus, 55
Sirenomelia, and caudal regression
      syndrome, 166

Situs inversus, 54–55
Situs inversus totalis, 54–55
   and primary ciliary dyskinesia, 675
Situs inversus viscerum, 54–55
6q deletion, and Prader-Willi syndrome,
      237–238
6q+ syndrome, partial, 79
Sixth nerve palsy, and Duane syndrome,
      645
   and Möbius syndrome, 223–224
Sjögren-Larsson disease, and Pelizaeus-
      Merzbacher disease, 578
Sjögren-Larsson syndrome, and
      progressive symmetric
      erythrokeratodermia, 111
Sjögren syndrome, and chronic
      inflammatory demyelinating
      polyradiculoneuropathy, 581
   and congenital complete heart block,
      50
   and cutaneous vasculitis, 34
Skeletal abnormalities, and Aarskog
      syndrome, 142
   and Alagille syndrome, 332
   and alpha-mannosidosis, 467–468
   and camp[t]omelic syndrome,
      706–707
   and cat eye syndrome, 164–165
   and central core disease, 607–608
   and chromosome 9, trisomy mosaic,
      85–86
   and chromosome 9 ring, 83
   and chromosome 21 ring, 70
   and Coffin-Lowry syndrome, 171–172
   and De Barsy syndrome, 6
   and diastrophic dysplasia, 711
   and Dubowitz syndrome, 179–180
   and Dyggve-Melchior-Clausen
      syndrome, 180–181
   and epidermal nevus syndrome, 106
   and Ewing sarcoma of bone, 381
   and familial expansile osteolysis,
      723–724
   and Fountain syndrome, 196
   and Holt-Oram syndrome, 717
   and homocystinuria, 459
   and Hunter disease, 478–479
   and Kabuki make-up syndrome,
      209–210
   and KBG syndrome, 210
   and Klippel-Feil syndrome, 720
   and Maroteaux-Lamy disease, 481
   and Morquio disease, 480
   and mucolipidosis, 472
   and multiple sulfatase deficiency, 484
   and Ollier disease, 23–24

   and pentasomy X, 86–87
   and Saethre-Chotzen syndrome,
      727–728
   and Scheie disease, 478
   and Schinzel syndrome, 246–247
   and Schmid metaphyseal
      chondrodysplasia, 248
   and Shwachman-Diamond syndrome,
      417
   and Simpson dysmorphia syndrome,
      251
   and Sly disease, 481
   and trichorhinophalangeal syndrome,
      730
   and Weill-Marchesani syndrome,
      267–268
   and Yunis-Varaaon syndrome, 275
Skeletal development delay, and
      ear–patella–short stature
      syndrome, 189
Skeletal disease, and fucosidosis, 445
Skeletal disorders, 701–733
Skeletal dysplasia, 144
   and Cockayne syndrome, 170–171
   and dyschondrosteosis, 181
   and multiple hereditary exostoses, 191
   and Robinow syndrome, 725–726
   and Schinzel Giedion syndrome, 247
Skeletal fusion, and Antley-Bixler
      syndrome, 704–705
Skeletal growth disorders, and metatropic
      dysplasia, 20
Skeletal mineralization, and
      hypophosphatasia, 317–318
Skeletal muscle rigidity, and malignant
      hyperthermia, 718
Skeletal overgrowth, and sclerosteosis,
      248–249
Skin abnormalities, and Wyburn-Mason
      syndrome, 667
Skin cancer, and melanoma, 405
Skin changes, and Conradi-Hünermann
      syndrome, 173
   and POEMS syndrome, 26–27
Skin fragility, and epidermolyis bullosa,
      106–109
   and McGrath syndrome, 127
Skin fragility-ectodermal dysplasia
      syndrome, 127
Skin hamartomas, and tuberous sclerosis,
      595–596
Skin hyperpigmentation, and Cronkhite-
      Canada syndrome, 338
Skin hypopigmentation, and
      oculocerebral syndrome, 226–
      227

Skin mottling, and malignant
hyperthermia, 718

Skin overgrowth, and Proteus syndrome, 239

Skin pain, and erysipelas, 285

Skin rash, and graft-versus-host disease, 11

Skin redness, and erysipelas, 285

Skull abnormalities, and Adams-Oliver syndrome, 148

and cleidocranial dysplasia, 182

Skull deformities, and Hajdu-Cheney syndrome, 11

Skull sclerosis, and craniometaphyseal dysplasia, 184

Sleep, excessive daytime, and narcolepsy, 561–562

Sleep apnea, and diffuse idiopathic skeletal hyperostosis, 10

and Kleine-Levin syndrome, 544

and narcolepsy, 562

Sleep disorders, and Kleine-Levin syndrome, 544

and Smith-Magenis syndrome, 254

Sleep paralysis, and narcolepsy, 561–562

Slender bone nanism, 259

Slow virus diseases, and subacute sclerosing panencephalitis, 574–575

Sly disease, 481

Small bowel cancer, and Lynch syndromes, 401

Small bowel diverticulosis, *fig. 42*, 339

Small brain, and chromosome 11, partial trisomy 11q, 61–62

Small cell carcinoma, and Ewing sarcoma of bone, 380–381

Small head, and chromosome 4, partial trisomy distal 4q, 76

and chromosome 4 ring, 76

and chromosome 6 ring, 80

and chromosome 9, trisomy mosaic, 85–86

and chromosome 9 ring, 83

and chromosome 13, partial monosomy 13q, 62–63

and chromosome 15 ring, 66

and chromosome 18 ring, 68–69

and chromosome 18q- syndrome, 67–68

and classic lissencephaly, 553–554

and Rett syndrome, 584

and Rubinstein-Taybi syndrome, 726–727

Small intestine infection, and Whipple disease, 297–298

Small lymphocytic lymphoma, and mantle cell lymphoma, 399

Small patella syndrome, and nail-patella syndrome, 721–722

Small stature, and Cornelia de Lange syndrome, 709

and Williams syndrome, 270

Smith-Lemli-Opitz syndrome, 253

and blepharophimosis-ptosis-epicanthus inversus syndrome, 641

and holoprosencephaly, 536

and Meckel syndrome, 221

and trisomy 13 syndrome, 87

Smith-Magenis syndrome, 254

and Angelman syndrome, 152–153

Smith-McCort syndrome, 180–181

Snoring, and Hunter disease, 478–479

and Hurler disease, 477

Sodium benzoate, and urea cycle disorders, 506–506

Sodium channel blocking agents, and Romano-Ward long QT syndrome, 54

Sodium cromoglycate, and eosinophilic gastroenteritis, 342

Sodium phenylacetate, and urea cycle disorders, 506–506

Sodium valproate, and hyperekplexia, 540

and Kleine-Levin syndrome, 544

Soft contact lenses, and iridocorneal endothelial syndromes, 649

and keratoconus, 651

Soft tissue hypertrophy, and Klippel-Trenaunay syndrome, 212

Soft tissue swelling, and fibrodysplasia ossificans progressiva, 713

Solar elastosis, and pseudoxanthoma elasticum, 133–134

Solar sensitivity, and Chédiak-Higashi syndrome, 379

Solar urticaria, and erythropoietic protoporphyria, 495

Solitary osteochondromas, and multiple hereditary exostoses, 191

Solumedrol, and bullous pemphigoid, 131

Sotos syndrome, *fig. 38*, 255–256

and Beckwith-Wiedemann syndrome, 518

and PTEN hamartoma tumor syndrome, 240

and Weaver syndrome, 266–267

and XYY syndrome, 90

Spasmodic dysphonia, 613–614

Spasmodic torticollis, 611

Spastic ataxia, and Glut-1 deficiency syndrome, 448

Spastic motor loss, and Brown-Séquard syndrome, 520

Spastic paraparesis, and carnosinemia, 435

and methylmalonic acidemias, 429

and multiple carboxylase deficiency, 482

Spastic paraplegia, and Allan-Herndon-Dudley syndrome, 149

and dopa-responsive dystonia, 612

and Laurence-Moon syndrome, 215

and MASA syndrome, 220

Spastic quadriplegia, and metachromatic leukodystrophy, 552

Spastic spinal paralysis, 548–549

Spasticity, and corpus callosum absence, 508

and giant axonal neuropathy, 569

and hydranencephaly, 538

and hydrocephalus, 539

and metachromatic leukodystrophy, 552–553

and mucolipidosis, 473–474

and oculocerebral syndrome, 226–227

and Pelizaeus-Merzbacher disease, 578

and primary lateral sclerosis, 548

Speech deficits, and Angelman syndrome, 152–153

and chromosome 4 ring, 77

and chromosome 8, monosomy 8p2, 81–82

and chromosome 11, partial monosomy 11q, 60

and chromosome 18, monosomy 18p, 67

and chromosome 22q11 deletion spectrum, 70–71

and deletion of the short arm of chromosome 1, 58

and floating harbor syndrome, 195

and histidinemia, 459

and Jackson-Weiss syndrome, 719

and mucolipidosis, 473–474

and phenylketonuria, 488

and Sanfilippo disease, 479

and SHORT syndrome, 250

and triple X syndrome, 89

and XXY syndrome, 89–90

and XYY syndrome, 90–91

Speilmeyer-Vogt disease, and Refsum disease, 604–605

Spherocytic hemolytic anemia, 370–371

Spherocytosis, 370–371

Spheroid bodies, and Hallervorden-Spatz syndrome, 620

Spherophakia-brachymorphia syndrome, 267–268

Sphingolipidosis, 447
  and congenital disorders of glycosylation, 457

Spinal abnormalities, and Lenz-microphthalmia syndrome, 654

Spinal bulbar muscular atrophy, 636

Spinal cord compression, and diffuse idiopathic skeletal hyperostosis, 10

Spinal cord disorders, and chronic inflammatory demyelinating polyradiculoneuropathy, 581

Spinal cord infarction, and syringobulbia, 589

Spinal cord tumors, and Parsonage-Turner syndrome, 577
  and primary lateral sclerosis, 548
  and Von Hippel-Lindau disease, 265–266

Spinal deformity, and metatropic dysplasia, 20

Spinal hemiplegia, and Brown-Séquard syndrome, 520

Spinal mobility deficits, and Klippel-Feil syndrome, 720

Spinal muscular atrophy, 637
  and amyotrophic lateral sclerosis, 513
  and infantile neuroaxonal dystrophy, 634
  and Prader-Willi syndrome, 237–238

Spinal pain, and multiple myeloma, 407

Spinal stenosis, lumbar, 587–588

Spindle cell hemangioendothelioma, 217–218

Spinobulbar spasticity, and primary lateral sclerosis, 548–549

Spinocerebellar ataxia, 555
  and Huntington disease, 537
  and X-linked sideroblastic anemia, 374–375

Spinocerebellar atrophy, 555

Spinopontine atrophy, 555

Spiramycin, and TORCH syndrome, 295

Spironolactone, and Bartter syndrome, 310–311
  and HAIR-AN syndrome, 315–316
  and primary aldosteronism, 305

Splenectomy, and autoimmune hemolytic anemia, 367
  and congenital nonspherocytic hemolytic anemia, 369
  and Felty syndrome, 9
  and hereditary spherocytosis, 370–371

and Proteus syndrome, 239
  and pyruvate kinase deficiency, 496
  and thalassemia major, 419

Splenic agenesis, primary, and Ivemark syndrome, 205

Splenogonadal fusion complex, and Hanhart syndrome, 203

Splenomegaly, and autoimmune hemolytic anemia, 367
  and Banti syndrome, 377
  and congenital erythropoietic porphyria, 492–493
  and congenital hepatic fibrosis, 691
  and hereditary spherocytosis, 370–371
  and Morquio disease, 480
  and phosphoglycerate kinase deficiency, 489–490
  and polycythemia vera, 411–412
  and pyruvate kinase deficiency, 496
  and Tangier disease, 500
  and thalassemia major, 419

Split hand/split foot malformation, 256

Spondylo-humero-femoral hypoplasia, 156–157

Spondyloarthropathies, with aortitis, and Takayasu arteritis, 35

Spondylocostal dysostosis, 207–208

Spondylocostal dysplasia, 207–208

Spondyloepimetaphyseal dysplasia, and metatropic dysplasia, 20

Spondyloepimetaphyseal dysplasia congenital, and Kniest dysplasia, 213

Spondyloepiphyseal dysplasia, and diastrophic dysplasia, 711
  and Dyggve-Melchior-Clausen syndrome, 180
  and multiple epiphyseal dysplasia, 187

Spondyloepiphyseal dysplasia congenita, 728–729

Spondyloepiphyseal dysplasia tarda, 729–730

Spondylothoracic dysostosis, 207–208

Spondylothoracic dysplasia, 207–208

Sprengel deformity, 257
  and Poland syndrome, 236–237

Squamous cell carcinoma, and Bowen disease, 97–98
  and bowenoid papulosis, 98
  and melanoma, 405
  and recurrent respiratory papillomatosis, 676

Squinting, and infantile neuroaxonal dystrophy, 634

St. Anthony's fire, 285

St. Helena dysplasia, 703–704

St. Vitus dance, 522

Staphylococcal disease, and anthrax, 278

Staphylococcal scalded skin syndrome, and erythema multiforme, 110
  and McGrath syndrome, 127
  and toxic epidermal necrolysis, 139

Staphylococcus aureus infection, and hyper-IgE syndrome, 12–13

Stargardt disease, 663
  and X-linked juvenile retinoschisis, 662

Startle disease, 540

Startle epilepsy, and hyperekplexia, 540

Startle response, and hyperekplexia, 540

Static cerebral palsy, and glutaric acidemia type I, 426

Steatorrhea, and chylomicron retention disease, 380

Steele-Richardson-Olszewski syndrome, 573–574

Stein-Leventhal syndrome, 323–324

Stem cell transplantation, 373
  and acquired aplastic anemia, 364
  and Diamond-Blackfan anemia, 365
  and dyskeratosis congenita, 105
  and Ewing sarcoma of bone, 381
  and Fanconi anemia, 366
  and mantle cell lymphoma, 399
  and multiple myeloma, 407
  and mycosis fungoides, 406
  and pyruvate kinase deficiency, 496
  and severe combined immunodeficiency, 14
  and Shwachman-Diamond syndrome, 417
  and thalassemia major, 419
  and Waldenström macroglobulinemia, 38

Stenosis, of the common pulmonary vein, 45–46
  segmental, and Takayasu arteritis, 35

Stereotactic radiation, and Wyburn-Mason syndrome, 667

Stereotypies, and Smith-Magenis syndrome, 254
  and Tourette syndrome, 594

Sternum defects, and pentalogy of Cantrell, 233–234

Steroid 21-hydroxylase deficiency, and congenital adrenal hyperplasia, 304

Steroid hydroxylase deficiency, 304

Steroids, and adiposis dolorosa, 303
  and bullous pemphigoid, 131
  and Eales disease, 646
  and granuloma annulare, 116

and hantavirus pulmonary syndrome, 287

and idiopathic thrombocytopenic purpura, 415–416

and infantile spasms, 541

and methylmalonic acidemias, 429

and pars planitis, 657

and pemphigus foliaceus, 132

and pemphigus vulgaris, 132

and sarcoidosis, 32

and Sjögren syndrome, 34

and Sutton disease, 138

Stevens-Johnson syndrome, and Behçet disease, 4

and erythema multiforme, 110–111

and Kawasaki disease, 15

Stickler dysplasia, and Kniest dysplasia, 213

Stickler syndrome, and congenital contractual arachnodactyly, 3

and Pierre Robin sequence, 235–236

and spondyloepiphyseal dysplasia congenita, 728

Stiff baby syndrome, 540

Stiff gait, and spondyloepiphyseal dysplasia tarda, 729–730

Stiff man syndrome, 540, 588–589

Stiff neck, and cervical dystonia, 611

Stiff person syndrome, 588–589

and neuromyotonia, 635

Still disease, and Winchester syndrome, 271

Stomach cancer, and Lynch syndromes, 401

Stomatitis necrotica, 138

Stool absence, and jejunal atresia, 349

Storage disease, and Langerhans cell histiocytosis, 392

and Yunis-Varaaon syndrome, 275

Storage disorders, and Schinzel Giedion syndrome, 247

Strabismus, and Coats disease, 643

and Duane syndrome, 645

and retinoblastoma, 661

and Williams syndrome, 270

and X-linked juvenile retinoschisis, 662

Streeter anomaly, 150–151

Streptococcal staphylococcus scarlatiniform eruptions, and Kawasaki disease, 15

Streptomycin, and brucellosis, 280

and plague, 292

Striatonigral degeneration, 561

Stroke, and glioblastoma multiforme, 384

and moyamoya syndrome, 559

Strokelike episodes, and MELAS, 469

Struma lymphomatosa, 329

Strumpell-Lorrain syndrome, 575–576

Sturge-Weber-Krabbe disease, 258

Sturge-Weber syndrome, 258

and Klippel-Trenaunay syndrome, 212

and Wyburn-Mason syndrome, 667

Stuttering, and laryngeal dystonia, 613–614

Stuve-Wiedemann syndrome, and Schwartz-Jampel syndrome, 586

Subacute cutaneous lupus, and granuloma annulare, 116

Subacute cutaneous lupus erythematosus, and Sjögren syndrome, 34

Subacute sclerosing panencephalitis, 574–575

Subarachnoid hemorrhage, and syringomyelia, 590

Subcortical arteriosclerotic encephalopathy, 519

Subcutaneous granuloma, 115–116

Subcutaneous palisading granuloma, 115–116

Subdural effusions, and hydranencephaly, 538

Subdural hematoma, and Binswanger disease, 519

Submucous fibroid, and Asherman syndrome, 308–309

Suboccipital decompression, and Arnold-Chiari syndrome, 516

Substance abuse, and Wilson disease, 506

Succinic semialdehyde dehydrogenase deficiency, 499

Succinylcholine, and malignant hyperthermia, 718

Sucrase-isomaltase deficiency, 354–355

Sudanophilic leukodystrophy, 578–579

Sudation parotidienne, 533

Sudden death, and congenital complete heart block, 49

and Jervell and Lange-Nielsen syndrome, 51–52

and Romano-Ward long QT syndrome, 54

Sudden death during sleep, and Brugada syndrome, 45

Sudeck atrophy, 523

Sugio-Kajii syndrome, 732

Sulfadiazine, and TORCH syndrome, 295

Sulfadoxine, and malaria, 291

Sulfamethoxazole, and chronic granulomatous disease, 387

Sulfasalazine, and Melkersson-Rosenthal syndrome, 557

and pyoderma gangrenosum, 135

Sulfatide lipidosis, 552–553

Sulfatidosis, 552–553

Sulfazopyridine, and Melkersson-Rosenthal syndrome, 557

Sun exposure, and Cockayne syndrome, 171

and Rothmund-Thomson syndrome, 136

and transient acantholytic dermatosis, 104

Sunlight avoidance, and congenital erythropoietic porphyria, 492–493

and erythropoietic protoporphyria, 496

Supernumerary teeth, and cleidocranial dysplasia, 182

Supranuclear palsy, and multiple system atrophy, 561

Suprapubic pain, and interstitial cystitis, 685

Supraumbilical abdominal wall, and pentalogy of Cantrell, 233–234

Supravalvular mitral ring, and cor triatriatum, 46

Surdocardiac syndrome, 51–52

Surfactant protein B deficiency, and alveolar capillary dysplasia, 672

Surgical contracture release, and congenital contractual arachnodactyly, 3

Surgical reconstruction, and atrial septal defects, 43

Sutton disease, 138

Swamp fever, 289

Sweating, and Frey syndrome, 533

and hereditary sensory neuropathy type II, 571

and idiopathic congenital central hypoventilation syndrome, 673

and mantle cell lymphoma, 399

and neuromyotonia, 635

Swedish porphyria, 490

Sweet syndrome, 138–139

and Sjögren syndrome, 34

Swiss-cheese cartilage dysplasia, and metatropic dysplasia, 20

Sydenham chorea, 522

and Huntington disease, 537

and Tourette syndrome, 594

Sydenham disease, 522

Symbrachydactyly, and amniotic bands, 150

and Poland syndrome, 236–237

Sympathetic ophthalmia, and Vogt-Koyanagi-Harada syndrome, 37

Sympatholytic agents, and scleroderma, 33

Syncope, and Brugada syndrome, 45
    and congenital complete heart block, 49
    and Jervell and Lange-Nielsen syndrome, 51
    and primary pulmonary hypertension, 678
    and Romano-Ward long QT syndrome, 54

Syndactyly, and Apert syndrome, 154–155
    and Filippi syndrome, 194–195
    and Fraser syndrome, 196–197
    and Greig cephalopolysyndactyly syndrome, 201
    and Saethre-Chotzen syndrome, 727–728
    and sclerosteosis, 248–249
    and Scott craniodigital syndrome, 249–250
    and split hand/split foot malformation, 256

Syndactyly type I, 194–195

Syndrome of erythroderma, 123–124

Syndrome of ST elevation and right bundle branch block, 45

Syndromic bile duct paucity, 332

Synechiae, and Cogan-Reese syndrome, 644
    and essential iris atrophy, 650

Syngnathia, and popliteal pterygium syndrome, 242

Synkinesia, and Kallmann syndrome, 318–319

Synophyrs, and chromosome 3, monosomy 3p2, 73

Synovial chondromatosis, and dysplasia epiphysealis hemimelica, 186

Synovitis, toxic, and Legg-Calve-Perthes disease, 16

Syphilis, and alopecia areata, 95
    and anthrax, 278
    and Eales disease, 646
    and granuloma annulare, 116
    and idiopathic neonatal hepatitis, 288
    and Ménière disease, 558
    and Mucha-Habermann disease, 129
    and pars planitis, 656–657
    and relapsing polychondritis, 29
    and TORCH syndrome, 295
    and Weismann-Netter-Stuhl syndrome, 268

Syphilitic aortitis, and Singleton-Merten syndrome, 252

Syphilitic chancre, and Sutton disease, 138

Syringobulbia, 589–590

Syringomyelia, 590–591
    and Arnold-Chiari syndrome, 516

Syrinx, 590–591

Systematized nevus depigmentosus, and hypomelanosis of Ito, 119

Systemic carnitine deficiency, and very-long-chain acyl-CoA dehydrogenase deficiency, 439–440

Systemic chondromalacia, 29–30

Systemic lupus erythematosus, and antiphospholipid syndrome, 2
    and chronic inflammatory demyelinating polyradiculoneuropathy, 581
    and congenital complete heart block, 49
    and Eales disease, 646
    and encephalitides, 284
    and scleroderma, 33
    and Wegener granulomatosis, 422

Systemic mastocytosis, and eosinophilic gastroenteritis, 342

Systemic panniculitis, and mesenteric panniculitis, 350

Systemic vasculitis, and Churg-Strauss syndrome, 674

T

T-cell chronic lymphocytic leukemia, 394–395

T-cell immunodeficiency, and Nezelof syndrome, 408

T-cell leukemia, and mycosis fungoides, 406

T-cell lymphomas, and mycosis fungoides, 406

T-lymphocytes, impaired function of, and severe combined immunodeficiency, 14

T-lymphoproliferative disease, 394–395

T-wave abnormalities, and Romano-Ward long QT syndrome, 54

Tachycardia, and acute intermittent porphyria, 490
    and neuroleptic malignant syndrome, 566

Tacrolimus, and posterior uveitis, 666
    and Takayasu arteritis, 35

Tafenoquine, and malaria, 291

Tails, and metatropic dysplasia, 20

Takayasu arteritis, 35

Talipes, and Gordon syndrome, 199

Talipes equinovarus, and femoral hypoplasia–unusual facies syndrome, 712–713

Tamoxifen, and mesenteric panniculitis, 350
    and Peyronie disease, 26
    and precocious puberty, 325

Tangier disease, 500
    and Refsum disease, 604–605

Tapetochoroidal dystrophy, 642

TAR syndrome, 260

Tardive dyskinesia, 591–592

TARK4 syndrome, 260

Tarsal tunnel syndrome, 592

Tarsoepiphyseal aclasia, 186

Tarsomegalie, 186

Tauri disease, 456–457
    and phosphoglycerate kinase deficiency, 489

Tay-Sachs disease, 501
    and Alexander disease, 510
    and Farber disease, 443
    and Refsum disease, 604–605
    and Sandhoff disease, 497

Tazarotene, and Darier disease, 101

Teebi hypertelorism syndrome, and craniofrontonasal syndrome, 183

Telangiectasia(s), hereditary hemorrhagic, 418
    and Rothmund-Thomson syndrome, 135–136

Telecanthus, with associated anomalies, 198–199
    and SHORT syndrome, 250

Telecanthus hypospadias syndrome, 198–199

Telogen effluvium, and alopecia areata, 95

Temporal lobe infarctions, and Korsakoff syndrome, 546

Temporolimbic disorders, and Kluver-Bucy syndrome, 545

Temporomandibular joint disease, and oromandibular dystonia, 615

Tendon reflex deficits, and X-linked sideroblastic anemia, 374–375

Tennis elbow, and complex regional pain syndrome, 523

10q deletion syndrome, and Coffin-Lowry syndrome, 171–172

10p deletion syndrome, partial, 60

Tentorial herniation, and locked-in syndrome, 554

Terbinafine, and Meleda disease, 128

Terrorism, and anthrax, 278
    and botulism, 279

Tertian fever, 291

Testicular atrophy, and spinal bulbar muscular atrophy, 636

Testicular enlargement, and precocious puberty, 324

Testicular feminization, 306–307

Testosterone, and Robinow syndrome, 726

and septooptic dysplasia, 188–189

and true hermaphroditism, 316–317

Testosterone biosynthesis, and androgen insensitivity syndrome, 306

Tetany, and Cronkhite-Canada syndrome, 338

Tetrabenazine, and Huntington disease, 538

and myoclonus, 628

and oromandibular dystonia, 615

and tardive dyskinesia, 591

Tetracycline, and Cronkhite-Canada syndrome, 338

and ehrlichiosis, 283

and malaria, 291

and plague, 292

and Q fever, 293

and small bowel diverticulosis, 339

and Whipple disease, 297

Tetracycline staining, and amelogenesis imperfecta, 149

Tetrahydrobiopterin deficiency, 502

Tetralogy of Fallot, and chromosome 14, trisomy mosaic, 64–65

and chromosome 22q11 deletion spectrum, 70

and Eisenmenger syndrome, 47

and persistent truncus arteriosus, 56

Tetrasomy, short arm of chromosome 9, 83–84

short arm of chromosome 18, 69

Tetrasomy 9p, 83–84

and chromosome 9, trisomy 9p, 84

Tetrasomy 12p, 231

and Fryns syndrome, 715

Tetrathiomolybdate, and Wilson disease, 506

Thalamic pain syndrome, 593

Thalamic stroke, and thalamic pain syndrome, 593

Thalamic tumor, and thalamic pain syndrome, 593

Thalamotomy, and dystonia, 609

and Parkinson disease, 576

Thalassemia, and autoimmune hemolytic anemia, 367

and phosphoglycerate kinase deficiency, 489

Thalassemia major, 419

and sickle cell anemia, 372–373

Thalassemia minor, 420

Thalassemia trait, 420

Thalidomide, and Behçet disease, 4

and carcinoid syndrome, 311–312

and fibrodysplasia ossificans progressiva, 714

and mesenteric panniculitis, 350

Thanatophoric dysplasia, 144

and Jarcho-Levin syndrome, 207–208

Thevenard disease, 570

Thiamine, and Korsakoff syndrome, 546

Thiazide diuretics, and medullary sponge kidney, 694

Thiazolidinediones, and HAIR-AN syndrome, 315–316

and polycystic ovary syndrome, 324

Thirst, and diabetes insipidus, 313–314

13q syndrome, partial, 62–63

Thistle tube teeth, 176–177

Thomsen disease, 632–633

and Schwartz-Jampel syndrome, 586

Thoracic abnormalities, and Lenz microphthalmia syndrome, 654

and spondyloepiphyseal dysplasia tarda, 729–730

Thoracic deformities, and Morquio disease, 480

and Noonan syndrome, 722–723

Thoracic-pelvic-phalangeal dystrophy, 155–156

Thorax deformity, and cerebrocostomandibular syndrome, 166–167

3-β hydroxysteroid dehydrogenase deficiency, and congenital adrenal hyperplasia, 304

and partial androgen insensitivity, 307

3-hydroxyisobutyric aciduria, and methylmalonate semialdehyde dehydrogenase deficiency, 471

3-M slender boned dwarfism, 259

3-M syndrome, 259

and ear–patella–short stature syndrome, 189

and Russel-Silver syndrome, 245–246

3-methylglutaconic aciduria, and Barth syndrome, 44

3,4-diaminopyradine, and Lambert-Eaton myasthenic syndrome, 621

3C syndrome, and Joubert syndrome, 542

Thrombate III, and congenital antithrombin III deficiency, 376–377

Thromboangiitis obliterans, 36

Thrombocytopenia, and Aase syndrome, 143

and absent radius syndrome, 260

and antiphospholipid syndrome, 2

and Bernard-Soulier syndrome, 378

and Gaucher disease, 447

and hemolytic-uremic syndrome, 689–690

and idiopathic thrombocytopenic purpura, 415–416

and inherited hemolytic-uremic syndrome, 690–691

and May-Hegglin anomaly, 403

Thrombocytopenia absent radii, and Fanconi anemia, 366

Thrombocytopenic purpura, and hemolytic-uremic syndrome, 689–690

and inherited hemolytic-uremic syndrome, 690

Thrombocytosis, and polycythemia vera, 411–412

Thrombophilic disorders, and antiphospholipid syndrome, 2

Thrombosis, and antiphospholipid syndrome, 2

and congenital antithrombin III deficiency, 376–377

Thrombotic thrombocytopenic purpura, 416

Thumb abnormalities, and Nager syndrome, 226

Thumb deformities, and Pfeiffer syndrome type I, 234–235

and Rubinstein-Taybi syndrome, 726–727

Thymic dysplasia, and Nezelof syndrome, 408

Thymic tumor, and neuromyotonia, 635

Thymus defects, and DiGeorge syndrome, 178–179

Thyroid-binding globulin, and chronic lymphocytic thyroiditis, 329

Thyroid cancer, and chronic lymphocytic thyroiditis, 329

Thyroid disease, and Ménière disease, 558

Thyroid tumors, and PTEN hamartoma tumor syndrome, 240

Thyroiditis, chronic lymphocytic, 329

Thyroxine, and septooptic dysplasia, 188–189

and Sheehan syndrome, 328

Tibioperoneal toxopachyosteosis, 268

Tic disorder, and myoclonus, 628

Tic doloureux, 595

Tics, and neuroacanthocytosis, 633–634
and tardive dyskinesia, 591
Tigroid leukoencephalopathy, 578–579
Tin mesoporphyrin, and acute
intermittent porphyria, 490
and Crigler-Najjar syndrome, 337
Tinea capitis, and alopecia areata, 95
Tinea corporis, and granuloma annulare,
116
and mycosis fungoides, 406
Tinnitus, and Camurati-Engelmann
disease, 707–708
and Ménière disease, 558
and syringobulbia, 589
Tiopronin, and cystinuria, 684
Tizanidine, and primary lateral sclerosis,
549
Tobacco use, and thromboangiitis
obliterans, 36
Toe deformities, and chromosome 15,
distal trisomy 15q, 65–66
and fibrodysplasia ossificans
progressiva, 713
and Miller syndrome, 222–223
and Pfeiffer syndrome type I, 234–235
and Rubinstein-Taybi syndrome,
726–727
Toe webbing, and Scott craniodigital
syndrome, 249–250
Tolosa-Hunt syndrome, 664
Tongue contractions, and oromandibular
dystonia, 615–616
Tongue fissuring, and Melkersson-
Rosenthal syndrome, 557
Tongue hypoplasia, and Hanhart
syndrome, 203
Tonsillar herniation, and Arnold-Chiari
syndrome, 516
Tonsils, orange-yellow, and Tangier
disease, 500
Tooth agenesis, 261
Tooth eruption delay, and cleidocranial
dysplasia, 182
and SHORT syndrome, 250
Topical 5, and Bowen disease, 98
Topiramate, and Lennox-Gastaut
syndrome, 550
and progressive myoclonus epilepsy,
531–532
TORCH syndrome, 295
Toriello-Carey syndrome, and
acrocallosal syndrome (Schinzel
type), 145
Total body irradiation, and Ewing
sarcoma of bone, 381
and mantle cell lymphoma, 399

Total parenteral nutrition, and intestinal
pseudoobstruction, 347–348
and maple syrup urine disease,
468–469
and microvillus inclusion disease, 351
Totally anomalous pulmonary venous
return, and persistent truncus
arteriosus, 56
Touraine-Solente-Gole syndrome,
129–130
Tourette syndrome, 594
and Sydenham chorea, 522
Townes-Brocks syndrome, 262
and brachio-oto-renal syndrome, 681
and cat eye syndrome, 164–165
and Goldenhar syndrome, 716
Townes syndrome, 262
Toxemia of pregnancy, and
pheochromocytoma, 409
Toxic epidermal necrolysis, 139–140
and erythema multiforme, *fig. 14*,
110–111
Toxic exposures, and West Nile fever, 296
Toxic myocarditis, and hypersensitivity
myocarditis, 53
Toxic oil syndrome, and eosinophilia-
myalgia syndrome, 7
and eosinophilic fasciitis, 8
and scleroderma, 33
Toxic shock syndrome, and Kawasaki
disease, 15
Toxic synovitis, and Legg-Calve-Perthes
disease, 16
Toxin exposure, and Guillain-Barré
syndrome, 535
Toxocariasis, and pars planitis, 656–657
Toxoplasma gondii infection, and TORCH
syndrome, 295
Toxoplasmosis, and Aicardi syndrome,
509
and Coats disease, 643
and glioblastoma multiforme, 384
Trabeculectomy, and Cogan-Reese
syndrome, 644
Trabeculotomy, and Sturge-Weber
syndrome, 258
Tracheal cartilage, and relapsing
polychondritis, 29
Tracheobronchial hypoplasia, and
camp[t]omelic syndrome, 706–707
Tracheoesophageal fistula, and
esophageal atresia, 190
Tracheomalacia, and esophageal atresia,
190
Tracheostomy, and camp[t]omelic
syndrome, 706–707

and chromosome 4, monosomy distal
4q, 75
and Coffin-Siris syndrome, 709
and idiopathic congenital central
hypoventilation syndrome, 673
Traction alopecia, and alopecia areata, 95
Trans-scleral cryotherapy, 643
Trans-sphenoidal adenomectomy, and
acromegaly, 301
and Cushing syndrome, 312–313
Transcutaneous electrical nerve
stimulation, and interstitial
cystitis, 685
Transferase deficiency galactosemia, 446
Transgrediens of Siemens, 128
Transient acantholytic dermatosis, 104
Transient erythroblastopenia of
childhood, and Diamond-Blackfan
anemia, 365
Transient ischemic attacks, and
moyamoya syndrome, 559
Transjugular intrahepatic portosystemic
shunt, and hepatorenal syndrome,
345
Transmissible spongiform
encephalopathy, 608
Transposition of the great arteries, and
persistent truncus arteriosus, 56
Transverse myelitis, and syringobulbia,
589
Traumatic synovitis, and
spondyloepiphyseal dysplasia
congenita, 728
Traumatic ulcers, and Sutton disease, 138
Treacher-Collins syndrome, 262–263
and brachio-oto-renal syndrome, 681
and Goldenhar syndrome, 716
and Miller syndrome, 222–223
and Nager syndrome, 226
Tremor(s), and acute intermittent
porphyria, 490
and carnosinemia, 435
and Hallervorden-Spatz syndrome, 620
and Parkinson disease, 576–577
Tretinoin, and Darier disease, 101
Trevors disease, 186
Triamcinolone, and lichen planus, 125
and transient acantholytic dermatosis,
104
Triamterene, and Bartter syndrome,
310–311
Trichodystrophies, and alopecia areata,
95
Trichopoliodystrophy, 470
Trichorhinophalangeal syndrome type I,
730–731

Trichorhinophalangeal syndrome type II, 731

Trichorhinophalangeal syndrome type III, 732

Trichothiodystrophy, and ichthyosis, 120
and Menkes disease, 470
and progressive symmetric erythrokeratodermia, 111

Trichotillomania, and alopecia areata, 95

Triclabendazole, and liver fluke disease, 286

Trifacial neuralgia, 595

Trifunctional protein, and medium-chain acyl-CoA dehydrogenase deficiency, 437

Trigeminal neuralgia, 595

Trihexyphenidyl, and embouchure dystonia, 613
and Hallervorden-Spatz syndrome, 620
and oromandibular dystonia, 615
and writer's cramp, 618

Trimethoprim, and chronic granulomatous disease, 387

Trimethoprim-sulfamethoxazole, and brucellosis, 280
and listeriosis, 290
and Whipple disease, 297

Trimethylaminuria, 503

Triosephosphate isomerase deficiency, and congenital nonspherocytic hemolytic anemia, 369

Triple X syndrome, 89

Triploidy syndrome, 263–264

Triptans, and cyclic vomiting syndrome, 526

Trisomy 4p, and chromosome 4, partial trisomy distal 4q, 76

Trisomy 6q, partial, 79

Trisomy 6q syndrome, partial, 79

Trisomy 9 mosaic, 85–86
and chromosome 9, trisomy 9p, 84

Trisomy 9p syndrome (partial), 84

Trisomy 11q, partial, 61–62

Trisomy 13, and Meckel syndrome, 221

Trisomy 13 syndrome, 87–88

Trisomy 14 mosaic, 64–65

Trisomy 14 mosaicism syndrome, 64–65

Trisomy 18, and Bowen-Conradi syndrome, 161
and chromosome 18, monosomy 18p, 67
and chromosome 18, tetrasomy 18p, 69

Trisomy 18 syndrome, 88

Trisomy 22, and chromosome 22, trisomy mosaic, 72

Trisomy 22 mosaic, 72

Trisomy 22 mosaicism syndrome, 72

Trisomy D syndrome, 87–88

Trisomy E syndrome, 88

Trisulfapyrimidine, and TORCH syndrome, 295

Tropheryma whippelii infection, and Whipple disease, 297–298

Tropical ulcer, and anthrax, 278

True hermaphroditism, 316–317

Truncal adiposity, and growth hormone deficiency, 314–315

Truncus arteriosus, persistent, 55–56

Truncus arteriosus communis, 55–56

Tryptophan malabsorption, and blue diaper syndrome, 681

Tryptophan syndrome, 7

Tubal pelvic factor infertility, and Asherman syndrome, 308–309

Tuberculoma, and glioblastoma multiforme, 384

Tuberculosis, and ACTH deficiency, 302
and Eales disease, 646
and Langerhans cell histiocytosis, 392
and medullary sponge kidney, 694
and pars planitis, 656–657
and relapsing polychondritis, 29
and sarcoidosis, 32
and Sutton disease, 138
and syringomyelia, 590

Tuberous sclerosis, 595–596
and epidermal nevus syndrome, 105
and hypomelanosis of Ito, 119
and neurofibromatosis type I, 564

Tuberous sclerosis complex, and lymphangioleiomyomatosis, 395

Tularemia, and anthrax, 278
and ehrlichiosis, 283
and plague, 292

Tumor, and Korsakoff syndrome, 546

Tumor-induced osteomalacia, and X-linked hypophosphatemic rickets, 326–327

Tumor obstructing lymph flow, and hereditary lymphedema, 396

Turcot syndrome, 352–353

Turner-Kieser syndrome, 721–722

Turner syndrome, 264–265
and chromosome 22, trisomy mosaic, 72
and cystic hygroma, 175
and dyschondrosteosis, 181
and Kabuki make-up syndrome, 209
and multiple pterygium syndrome, 241

21-hydroxylase deficiency, and congenital adrenal hyperplasia, 304

Twin-twin transfusion syndrome, 421–422

TWIST mutation syndrome, and Baller-Gerold syndrome

Type 0 glycogen storage disease, 450

Type A syndrome, and Achard-Thiers syndrome, 300

Type B syndrome, and Achard-Thiers syndrome, 300

Type I glycogen storage disease, 450–451

Type II glycogen storage disease, 452

Type III glycogen storage disease, 453

Type IV glycogen storage disease, 454

Type IV hyperlipidemia, 460

Type V glycogen storage disease, 454–455

Type VII glycogen storage disease, 456–457

Types VI and IX glycogen storage disease, 455–456

Typhoid fever, and dengue fever, 281
and viral hemorrhagic fevers, 282

Tyrosine kinase inhibitors, and idiopathic thrombocytosis, 421

Tyrosinemia, 504
and hereditary fructose intolerance, 444
and Niemann-Pick disease, 485
and phenylketonuria, 488
and type IV glycogen storage disease, 454

U

Ulcer disease, and mastocytosis, 402

Ulcers, of the mouth, and Barth syndrome, 44
and Behçet disease, 4
and cyclic neutropenia, 21–22
and severe chronic neutropenia, 22
and Zollinger-Ellison syndrome, 330

Ulerythema ophryogenes, and Darier disease, 101

Ullrich-Turner syndrome, 264–265

Ulnar-mammary syndrome, 246–247

Ultraviolet light, and alopecia areata, 95

Umbilical anomalies, and Rieger syndrome, 243–244

Umbilical cord hemorrhage, and congenital afibrogenemia, 359–360

Undescended testicles, and Noonan syndrome, 722–723

Undulant fever, 280

Undulating myokymia, 635

Unstable hemoglobin syndromes, and glucose-6-phosphate dehydrogenase deficiency, 385

Unverrich-Lundborg disease, and MERRF, 469

UPD chromosome 14, and chromosome 14, trisomy mosaic, 64
Upper airway resistance syndrome, and narcolepsy, 562
Upper arm pain, and Parsonage-Turner syndrome, 577–578
Upper motor neuron disease, 548–549
Urea cycle defects, and carnitine deficiency syndromes, 432
  and carnosinemia, 435
  and congenital disorders of glycosylation, 457
  and cyclic vomiting syndrome, 525
  and methylmalonic acidemias, 429
  and propionic acidemia, 428
Urea cycle disorders, 505–506
Urinary blood, and Denys-Drash syndrome, 686
  and WAGR syndrome, 699
Urinary excretion of fructose, and fructosuria, 444–445
Urinary tract obstruction, and cystinuria, 684
Urinary urgency, and Binswanger disease, 519
  and hereditary spastic paraplegia, 575–576
  and interstitial cystitis, 685
Urine, dark, and alkaptonuria, 431
Urogenital abnormalities, and Klippel-Feil syndrome, 720
Urolithiasis, and cystinuria, 684
  and primary hyperoxaluria, 461–462
Ursodeoxycholic acid, and Alagille syndrome, 332
  and Byler disease, 335
  and Caroli disease, 336
  and congenital hepatic fibrosis, 692
Urticaria, and erythema multiforme, 110
Urticaria pigmentosa, and mastocytosis, 402
Urticarial drug reactions, and bullous pemphigoid, 130–131
Urticarial vasculitis, and erythema multiforme, 110
Usher syndrome, 664–665
  and Alström syndrome, 306
Uveitis, and pars planitis, 656–657
  posterior, 666
  and retinoblastoma, 661
Uveomeningitic syndrome, 36–37
Uveomeningoencephalitic syndrome, 36–37
Uveoparotid fever, and benign lymphoepithelial lesion, 17

V
VACTERL, and caudal regression syndrome, 166
  and Townes-Brocks syndrome, 262
VACTERL association, and Baller-Gerold syndrome, 157
VACTERL syndrome, and MURCS association, 695
Vacuolating leukoencephalopathy, and Alexander disease, 510
Vaginal enlargement, and partial androgen insensitivity, 307
Valproate, and Lennox-Gastaut syndrome, 550
Valproic acid, and Alpers syndrome, 512
  and Baltic/Mediterranean/Unverrich-Lundborg myoclonic epilepsy, 600
  and myoclonus, 628
Valproic acid embryopathy, 192–193
Valvular heart disease, and antiphospholipid syndrome, 2
Van Bogaert-Dawson disease, 574–575
van Buchem disease, 204–205
  and Camurati-Engelmann disease, 707–708
  and sclerosteosis, 248–249
van Lohuizen syndrome, 100
Varicella, and Mucha-Habermann disease, 129
  and Reye syndrome, 31
Varicella-zoster, and TORCH syndrome, 295
Variegate porphyria, 494–495
  and erythropoietic protoporphyria, 495
Varioliform gastritis, 341
Vascular disease, and homocystinuria, 459
Vascular embolization, and thromboangiitis obliterans, 36
Vascular headache, and pheochromocytoma, 409
Vascular infections, and Takayasu arteritis, 35
Vascular lesions, and encephalitides, 284
Vascular stenoses, and Williams syndrome, 270
Vasculitic neuropathy, and Guillain-Barré syndrome, 535
Vasculitis, and alpha 1-antitrypsin deficiency, 671
  and Eales disease, 646
  and eosinophilic gastroenteritis, 342
  and microscopic polyangiitis, 27–27
  and mixed cryoglobulin syndrome, 5

  and Parsonage-Turner syndrome, 577
  and polyarteritis nodosa, 28–29
  and thromboangiitis obliterans, 36
  and thrombotic thrombocytopenic purpura, 416
Vasculopathy, and scleroderma, 33–34
Vasoactive intestinal peptide, and acute respiratory distress syndrome, 670
Vasoconstrictors, and hepatorenal syndrome, 344
Vasodilators, and scleroderma, 33
Vasopressin deficiency, and diabetes insipidus, 313–314
Vasulitis, and Kawasaki disease, 15
VATER, and caudal regression syndrome, 166
VATER association, and Townes-Brocks syndrome, 262
Vein of Galen malformation, and hydrocephalus, 539
Velocardiofacial syndrome, 70–71
  and CHARGE syndrome, 167
  and floating harbor syndrome, 195
  and Pierre Robin sequence, 235–236
  and Smith-Magenis syndrome, 254
  and Williams syndrome, 270
Venezuelan hemorrhagic fever, 282
Venooclusive disease, and Banti syndrome, 377
Venous angioma, 117–118
Venous congestion, and endomyocardial fibrosis, 48
Venous disease, and erythromelalgia, 113
Venous insufficiency, and hereditary lymphedema, 396
Venous malformations, 117–118
  and blue rubber bleb nevus syndrome, 160
Venous thrombosis, and antiphospholipid syndrome, 2
  and factor XII deficiency, 382
  and MELAS, 469
Venous varicosities, and Klippel-Trenaunay syndrome, 212
Ventricular enlargement, and Dandy-Walker syndrome, 526–527
Ventricular septal defect, and atrial septal defects, 43
  and chromosome 7, monosomy 7p2, 80
Ventricular tachyarrhythmias, and Jervell and Lange-Nielsen syndrome, 51–52
  and Romano-Ward long QT syndrome, 54

Ventricular volume overload, and persistent truncus arteriosus, 56

Ventriculo-cystoperitoneal shunt, and Dandy-Walker syndrome, 526

Ventriculoatrial shunt, and hydrocephalus, 539

Ventriculocisternal shunt, and hydrocephalus, 539

Ventriculoperitoneal shunt, and hydrocephalus, 539

Ventriculopleural shunt, and hydrocephalus, 539

Ventriculostomy, and hydrocephalus, 539

Vermian aplasia, and Dandy-Walker syndrome, 526–527

Verneuil disease, 118–119

Verruca vulgaris, and Bowen disease, 97

Vertebral anomalies, and caudal regression syndrome, 166
    and Dubowitz syndrome, 179–180
    and Goldenhar syndrome, 716
    and Jarcho-Levin syndrome, 207–208
    and multiple pterygium syndrome, 241
    and spondyloepiphyseal dysplasia tarda, 729–730
    and 3-M syndrome, 259

Vertebral fusion, and Klippel-Feil syndrome, 720

Vertigo, and Arnold-Chiari syndrome, 516
    and Camurati-Engelmann disease, 707–708
    and episodic ataxia type II, 601–602
    and Ménière disease, 558
    and syringobulbia, 589

Very-long-chain acyl-CoA dehydrogenase deficiency, 439–440

Vestibular schwannomas, and neurofibromatosis type 2, 564–565

Vigabatrin, and hyperekplexia, 540
    and Lennox-Gastaut syndrome, 550
    and succinic semialdehyde dehydrogenase deficiency, 499

Vinblastine sulfate, and Langerhans cell histiocytosis, 393

Vincent infection, and Sutton disease, 138

Vincristine, and idiopathic thrombocytopenic purpura, 416

Viral exanthem, and erythema multiforme, 110

Viral hemorrhagic fevers, 282

Viral hepatitis, and liver fluke disease, 286
    and Q fever, 293

Viral infections, and dengue fever, 281
    and ebola, 282
    and encephalitides, 284
    and giant hypertrophic gastritis, 341
    and large granular lymphocyte leukemia, 394
    and West Nile fever, 296

Viral myocarditis, and hypersensitivity myocarditis, 53

Viral warts, and bowenoid papulosis, 98

Virilizing adrenal hyperplasia, 304

Visceral abnormalities, and Wyburn-Mason syndrome, 667

Visceral defects, and Simpson dysmorphia syndrome, 251

Visceral heterotaxy, 54–55

Visceral pain-associated disability syndrome, and intestinal pseudoobstruction, 348

Visceroatrial heterotaxia, 205–206

Vision anomalies, and deletion of the short arm of chromosome 1, 58

Vision blurring, and hydrocephalus, 539
    and keratoconus, 650–651
    and pars planitis, 656–657
    and posterior uveitis, 666

Vision loss, and acute posterior multifocal placoid pigment epitheliopathy, 642
    and Camurati-Engelmann disease, 707–708
    and carotid artery insufficiency, 659
    and Coats disease, 643
    and infantile neuroaxonal dystrophy, 634
    and Leber hereditary optic neuropathy, 653
    and pseudotumor cerebri, 582
    and Refsum disease, 604–605
    and retinal arterial occlusion, 658
    and retinitis pigmentosa, 660
    and Rosenbert-Chutorian syndrome, 585
    and Santavuori disease, 585–586
    and Wyburn-Mason syndrome, 667
    and X-linked juvenile retinoschisis, 662

Vision problems, and peroxisomal biogenesis disorders, 487

Visual agnosia, and Kluver-Bucy syndrome, 545

Visual deficits, and sialidosis, 498

Visual disturbances, and primary empty sella syndrome, 530

Visual impairment, and Loken-Senior syndrome, 692

Visual inattentiveness, and Sandhoff disease, 497

Vitamin A, and epidermolytic hyperkeratosis, 110
    and retinitis pigmentosa, 660
    and transient acantholytic dermatosis, 104

Vitamin A deficiency, and chylomicron retention disease, 380
    and Stargardt disease, 663

Vitamin B_6, and type V glycogen storage disease, 455

Vitamin B_{12}, and methylmalonic acidemias, 429

Vitamin B_{12} deficiency, and giant axonal neuropathy, 569
    and hereditary spastic paraplegia, 575
    and primary lateral sclerosis, 548

Vitamin C, and alkaptonuria, 431
    and glutathione synthetase deficiency, 449
    and human cytochrome oxidase deficiency, 436

Vitamin D intoxication, and Singleton-Merten syndrome, 252

Vitamin D–dependent rickets, and hypophosphatasia, 317–318

Vitamin D–resistant rickets, 326–327
    and Lowe syndrome, 466–467

Vitamin E, and Friedreich ataxia, 602
    and glucose-6-phosphate dehydrogenase deficiency, 385
    and glutathione synthetase deficiency, 449
    and human cytochrome oxidase deficiency, 436
    and Peyronie disease, 26
    and retinitis pigmentosa, 660
    and tardive dyskinesia, 591

Vitamin E deficiency, and ataxia, 606–607
    and ataxia-telangiectasia, 605–606
    and chylomicron retention disease, 380

Vitamin K, and human cytochrome oxidase deficiency, 436

Vitiligo, and Cronkhite-Canada syndrome, 338
    and lichen sclerosis, 126

Vitrectomy, and pars planitis, 657
    and X-linked juvenile retinoschisis, 662

Vitreoretinal hemorrhage, and Norrie disease, 656

Vitreous hemorrhage, and X-linked juvenile retinoschisis, 662

Vitreous veils, and X-linked juvenile retinoschisis, 662

Vocal cord spasms, and laryngeal dystonia, 613–614
Vocal tics, and Tourette syndrome, 594
Vogt-Koyanagi-Harada syndrome, 36–37
Voice strain, and laryngeal dystonia, 613–614
Vomiting, rapid-fire, and cyclic vomiting syndrome, 525–526
Von Gierke disease, 451
von Hippel-Lindau disease, 265–266
von Hippel-Lindau syndrome, and Wyburn-Mason syndrome, 667
Von Recklinghausen disease, 563–564
von Willebrand disease, and Glanzmann thrombasthenia, 383
and hereditary hemorrhagic telangiectasia, 418
Vrolik disease, 227–228

W
Waardenburg anophthalmia, and Norrie disease, 656
Waardenburg syndromes, 732–733
Waddling gait, and Camurati-Engelmann disease, 707–708
and Duchenne muscular dystrophy, 623
and multiple epiphyseal dysplasia, 187–188
and Schmid metaphyseal chondrodysplasia, 248
WAGR syndrome, 699
Wakefulness, and locked-in syndrome, 554
Waldenström disease, 37–38
Waldenström hypergammaglobulinemic purpura, and Sjögren syndrome, 34
Waldenström macroglobulinemia, 37–38
and mixed cryoglobulin syndrome, 5
Waldmann syndrome, 346
Walker-Warburg syndrome, 597–598
and megalocornea, 556
Warburg syndrome, 597–598
Warfarin, and carotid artery insufficiency, 659
and primary pulmonary hypertension, 678
Warfarin exposure, and Conradi-Hünermann syndrome, 173
Warm antibody hemolytic anemia, 371–372
Warm autoimmune hemolytic anemias, and cold hemolytic anemia syndromes, 368
Watson-Alagille syndrome, 332

Watson syndrome, and Noonan syndrome, 722
Weaver syndrome, 266–267
and Beckwith-Wiedemann syndrome, 518
and Marshall-Smith syndrome, 219
and Simpson dysmorphia syndrome, 251
and Sotos syndrome, 255
Webbed neck, and chromosome 9, trisomy 9p, 84
and chromosome 22, trisomy mosaic, 72
and Noonan syndrome, 722–723
Weber-Christian disease, and mesenteric panniculitis, 350
Wegener disease, 422–423
Wegener granulomatosis, 422–423
and chronic granulomatous disease, 386
and Churg-Strauss syndrome, 674
and lymphomatoid granulomatosis, 48
and microscopic polyangiitis, 27
and polyarteritis nodosa, 28
and relapsing polychondritis, 29
and Sutton disease, 138
Weight gain, and chronic lymphocytic thyroiditis, 329
Weight loss, and acquired generalized lipodystrophy, 320–321
and acquired partial lipodystrophy, 321
and angioimmunoblastic lymphadenopathy-type T-cell lymphoma, 398
and Churg-Strauss syndrome, 674
and giant hypertrophic gastritis, 341
and Lambert-Eaton myasthenic syndrome, 621
and mantle cell lymphoma, 399
and pulmonary alveolar proteinosis, 677
and Wegener granulomatosis, 422
Weill disease, 289
Weill-Marchesani syndrome, *fig. 40*, 267–268
and Leri pleonosteosis, 217
and megalocornea, 556
Weismann-Netter-Stuhl syndrome, 268
Wells syndrome, 99
Werdnig-Hoffman disease, 637
Werner syndrome, *fig. 41*, 269
and congenital generalized lipodystrophy, 322
and Rothmund-Thomson syndrome, 135

Wernicke encephalopathy, and Korsakoff syndrome, 546
Wernicke-Korsakoff syndrome, 546
Wernicke syndrome, and Korsakoff syndrome, 546
West Nile encephalitis, 296
West Nile fever, 296
West syndrome, 541
Whipple disease, 297–298
Whistling face syndrome, 714
White fibrous papulosis, and pseudoxanthoma elasticum, 133–134
Wickham striae, and lichen planus, 125
Wieacker-Wolff syndrome, 638
Wiedemann-Beckwith syndrome, 518
Wiedemann-Rautenstrauch syndrome, 238
and acquired generalized lipodystrophy, 320–321
and congenital generalized lipodystrophy, 322
and De Barsy syndrome, 6
and Hallermann-Streiff syndrome, 202
Wildervanck syndrome, and Klippel-Feil syndrome, 720
Williams-Beuren syndrome, 270
Williams syndrome, 270
and Coffin-Lowry syndrome, 171–172
and Noonan syndrome, 722
and Smith-Magenis syndrome, 254
Wilms tumor, and Denys-Drash syndrome, 686
and trisomy 18 syndrome, 88
and WAGR syndrome, 699
Wilms tumor aniridia syndrome, and Russel-Silver syndrome, 245–246
Wilson disease, 506
and alpha 1-antitrypsin deficiency, 671
and Hallervorden-Spatz syndrome, 620
and Huntington disease, 537
and Niemann-Pick disease, 485
and tardive dyskinesia, 591
and Tourette syndrome, 594
and warm antibody hemolytic anemia, 371–372
Winchester syndrome, 271
Wiskott-Aldrich syndrome, 38–39
and Glanzmann thrombasthenia, 383
and severe combined immunodeficiency, 14
Wolf-Hirschhorn syndrome, 272
and chromosome 4, monosomy 4q, 74
and chromosome 4 ring, 76
and Pallister-Killian syndrome, 231
Wolfram syndrome, 273